D1223768

Handbook of
Oxidants and Antioxidants
in Exercise

Handbook of Oxidants and Antioxidants in Exercise

Editors:

Chandan K. Sen, Ph.D., FACSM
Lawrence Berkeley National Laboratory
University of California, Berkeley, USA
and
Department of Physiology
University of Kuopio, Finland

Lester Packer, Ph.D., FOS
Department of Molecular and Cell Biology
University of California, Berkeley, USA

Osmo O.P. Hänninen, M.D., Ph.D.
Department of Physiology
University of Kuopio, Finland

2000

ELSEVIER

Amsterdam – Lausanne – New York – Oxford – Shannon – Singapore – Tokyo

ELSEVIER SCIENCE B.V.
Sara Burgerhartstraat 25
P.O. Box 211, 1000 AE Amsterdam, The Netherlands

© 2000 Elsevier Science B.V. All rights reserved.

This work is protected under copyright by Elsevier Science, and the following terms and conditions apply to its use:

Photocopying
Single photocopies of single chapters may be made for personal use as allowed by national copyright laws. Permission of the Publisher and payment of a fee is required for all other photocopying, including multiple or systematic copying, copying for advertising or promotional purposes, resale, and all forms of document delivery. Special rates are available for educational institutions that wish to make photocopies for nonprofit educational classroom use.

Permissions may be sought directly from Elsevier Science Rights & Permissions Department, PO Box 800, Oxford OX5 1DX, UK; phone: (+44) 1865 843830, fax: (+44) 1865 853333, e-mail: permissions@elsevier.co.uk. You may also contact Rights & Permissions directly through Elsevier's home page (http://www.elsevier.nl), selecting first 'Customer Support', then 'General Information', then 'Permissions Query Form'.

In the USA, users may clear permissions and make payments through the Copyright Clearance Center, Inc., 222 Rosewood Drive, Danvers, MA 01923, USA; phone: (978) 7508400, fax: (978) 7504744, and in the UK through the Copyright Licensing Agency Rapid Clearance Service (CLARCS), 90 Tottenham Court Road, London W1P 0LP, UK; phone: (+44) 171 631 5555; fax: (+44) 171 631 5500. Other countries may have a local reprographic rights agency for payments.

Derivative Works
Tables of contents may be reproduced for internal circulation, but permission of Elsevier Science is required for external resale or distribution of such material.
Permission of the Publisher is required for all other derivative works, including compilations and translations.

Electronic Storage or Usage
Permission of the Publisher is required to store or use electronically any material contained in this work, including any chapter or part of a chapter.

Except as outlined above, no part of this work may be reproduced, stored in a retrieval system or transmitted in any form or by any means, electronic, mechanical, photocopying, recording or otherwise, without prior written permission of the Publisher.
Address permissions requests to: Elsevier Science Rights & Permissions Department, at the mail, fax and e-mail addresses noted above.

Notice
No responsibility is assumed by the Publisher for any injury and/or damage to persons or property as a matter of products liability, negligence or otherwise, or from any use or operation of any methods, products, instructions or ideas contained in the material herein. Because of rapid advances in the medical sciences, in particular, independent verification of diagnoses and drug dosages should be made.

First edition 2000

Library of Congress Cataloging in Publication Data
A catalog record from the Library of Congress has been applied for.

ISBN: 0-444-82650-5

⊗ The paper used in this publication meets the requirements of ANSI/NISO Z39.48-1992 (Permanence of Paper).

Printed in the Netherlands

Preface

Through the ages man has sought to harness the knowledge of exercise; interest in exercise science dates back at least to ancient Greece. Today, exercise is seen as not merely a leisure activity, but as an effective preventive and therapeutic tool in medicine. The study of exercise physiology and biochemistry has had a revolutionary overall impact on biomedical research, and exercise has been used as a model for studying the response of physiological regulatory mechanisms to stress. At the same time, advances in oxygen free radical biochemistry have lured exercise biochemists to study the effects of the increased oxygen consumption that accompanies exercise. The first reports in this field, published in the early 1970s, indicated that strenuous physical exercise might cause oxidative lipid damage in various tissues. Since then, a considerable body of research has accumulated concerning the effects of exercise, nutrition and training on indices of oxidative stress and antioxidant responses in various tissues. Most studies support the contention that during strenuous exercise, generation of reactive oxygen species (highly reactive, partially reduced metabolites of oxygen) is elevated to a level that overwhelms tissue antioxidant defence systems. The result is oxidative stress. The magnitude of the stress depends on the ability of the tissues to detoxify reactive oxygen species; i.e., antioxidant defences. Endurance training enhances such defence in various tissues, especially in skeletal muscle and heart. Antioxidants produced by the body act in concert with their exogenous (mainly dietary) counterparts to provide protection against the ravages of reactive oxygen as well as nitrogen species.

Exercise and Oxygen Toxicity was first published in 1994. The purpose of this multiauthor volume — the first of its kind — was to examine different aspects of exercise-induced oxidative stress, its management, and how reactive oxygen may affect the functional capacity of various vital organs and tissues. Remarkable interest of the readers and favourable critical reviews published in leading journals provided the impetus to put together an enlarged second edition. We started to accomplish that goal. After two years of tireless effort of many, the current volume was ready to go the press. This volume was over double in size of the original edition. Key related issues such as analytical methods, environmental factors, nutrition, aging, organ function and several pathophysiological processes were thoroughly addressed. Leading experts provided unprecedented insight into the understanding of the role of reactive species and antioxidants. The combination of these properties makes this volume an authoritative treatise.

During the course of review of the finalized manuscripts at the publishing house it was brought to our attention that the structure and contents of this volume more closely resembled a *Handbook* than just a second edition of *Exer-*

cise and Oxygen Toxicity. This view was shared by many of our colleagues and peers, and thus we decided to name this volume as the *Handbook of Oxidants and Antioxidants in Exercise.*

Since *Exercise and Oxygen Toxicity* was published, interest in exercise, reactive species and the possible role of endogenous and supplemented antioxidants has soared. Search of the PubMed database of the National Library of Medicine using a combination of the keywords "exercise" and "antioxidant" show that the number of research reports in 1997 is more than double of that in 1994. This handbook is therefore a timely publication. It is relevant to all those who have interest in biomedical sciences and is designed to be intelligible to a general scientific audience.

We are delighted to be involved in this project. The excellent editorial assistance of Dr. Savita Khanna and the outstanding contribution of authors are gratefully acknowledged. We hope that this volume will contribute to the further development of this important late-breaking field of research.

Chandan K. Sen
Lester Packer
Osmo Hänninen

Contents

Preface   v

Part I: Introduction to free radicals

1. Free radical chemistry
    K.-D. Asmus and M. Bonifačić   3

Part II: Reactive species in tissues

2. Exercise and oxygen radical production by muscle
    M.J. Jackson 57

3. Exercise and xanthine oxidase in the vasculature:
    superoxide and nitric oxide interactions
    *C.R. White, J.E. Shelton, D. Moellering, H. Jo, R.P. Patel and
    V. Darley-Usmar* 69

Part III: Oxidative stress: Mechanisms and manifestations

4. Chemical bases and biological relevance of protein oxidation
    O. Tirosh and A.Z. Reznick 89

5. Lipid peroxidation in healthy and diseased models:
    influence of different types of exercise
    H.M. Alessio 115

6. Metal binding agents: possible role in exercise
    R.R. Jenkins and J. Beard 129

7. The role of xanthine oxidase in exercise
    Y. Hellsten 153

8. Acute phase immune responses in exercise
    J.G. Cannon and J.B. Blumberg 177

9. Oxidative DNA damage in exercise
    A. Hartmann and A.M. Niess 195

Part IV: Antioxidant defenses

10. Physiological antioxidants and exercise training
     S.K. Powers and C.K. Sen   221

11. Superoxide dismutases in exercise and disease
     K. Suzuki, H. Ohno, S. Oh-ishi, T. Kizaki, T. Ookawara, J. Fujii,
     Z. Radák and N. Taniguchi   243

12. Antioxidants and physical exercise
     C.K. Sen and A.H. Goldfarb   297

Part V: Nutrition

13. Dietary sources and bioavailability of essential and nonessential
     antioxidants
     E.A. Decker and P.M. Clarkson   323

14. Vitamin E
     M.G. Traber   359

Part VI: Cellular and molecular mechanisms

15. Biological thiols and redox regulation of cellular signal transduction
     pathways
     C.K. Sen   375

16. Regulation and deregulation of vascular smooth muscle cells by
     reactive oxygen species and by α-tocopherol
     A. Azzi, D. Boscoboinik, N.K. Özer, R. Ricciarelli and E. Aratri   403

Part VII: Analytical methods

17. Oxidative stress indices: analytical aspects and significance
     D. Han, S. Loukianoff, and L. McLaughlin   433

18. Noninvasive measures of muscle metabolism
     T. Hamaoka, K.K. McCully, T. Katsumura, T. Shimomitsu and
     B. Chance   485

Part VIII: Environmental factors

19. Air pollution and oxidative stress
     D.M. Meacher and D.B. Menzel   513

20. Risk of oxidative stress at high altitude and possible benefit of
    antioxidant supplementation
    I.M. Simon-Schnass 555

21. Oxidants in skin pathophysiology
    S. Weber 579

Part IX: Organ functions

22. Muscle fatigue: mechanisms and regulation
    M.B. Reid 599

23. Oxidative stress in muscular atrophy
    H. Kondo 631

24. Protection against free radical injury in the heart and cardiac
    performance
    D.K. Das and N. Maulik 655

25. Exercise-induced oxidative stress in the heart
    L.L. Ji 689

26. Influence of exercise-induced oxidative stress on the
    central nervous system
    S.M. Somani and K. Husain 713

Part X: Aging

27. Oxidants and aging
    K.B. Beckman and B.N. Ames 755

28. Caloric restriction, exercise and aging
    R.J.M. McCarter 797

29. Oxidative stress and the pathogenesis of sarcopenia
    M.E. Lopez, T.A. Zainal, S.S. Chung, J.M. Aiken and
    R. Weindruch 831

30. Molecular mechanisms of oxidative stress in aging: free radicals,
    aging, antioxidants and disease
    M. Pollack and C. Leeuwenburgh 881

Part XI: **Disease processes**

31. Oxidative stress, antioxidants and cancer
    M. Gerber 927

32. Alcohol and oxidative stress
     C.S. Lieber   951

33. Cigarette smoking as an inducer of oxidative stress in relation to
     disease pathogenesis
     G.G. Duthie, J.R. Arthur and S.J. Duthie   977

34. Regulation of inflammation and wound healing
     J.J. Maguire   995

35. Oxidative stress induced by the metabolism of medical and
     nonmedical drugs
     M. Paolini and G. Cantelli-Forti   1021

36. The paradoxical relationship of aerobic exercise and the oxidative
     theory of atherosclerosis
     R. Shern-Brewer, N. Santanam, C. Wetzstein, J.E. White-Welkley,
     L. Price and S. Parthasarathy   1053

37. Claudication, exercise and antioxidants
     P.V. Tisi and C.P. Shearman   1069

38. Exercise and oxidative stress in diabetes mellitus
     D.E. Laaksonen and C.K. Sen   1105

39. Exercise induces oxidative stress in healthy subjects and in chronic
     obstructive pulmonary disease patients
     J. Viña, E. Servera, M. Asensi, J. Sastre, F.V. Pallardó, A. Gimeno,
     L. Heunks, P.N.R. Dekhuijzen and J.A. Ferrero   1137

40. Hypoxia, oxidative stress and exercise in rheumatoid arthritis
     S. Jawed, S.E. Edmonds, V. Gilston and D.R. Blake   1147

Index of authors   1189

Subject index   1191

Part I

Introduction to free radicals

©2000 Elsevier Science B.V. All rights reserved.
Handbook of Oxidants and Antioxidants in Exercise.
C.K. Sen, L. Packer and O. Hänninen, editors.

3

Part I • Chapter 1

Free radical chemistry

Klaus-Dieter Asmus[1] and Marija Bonifačić[2]

[1]*Radiation Laboratory, University of Notre Dame, Notre Dame, IN 46556, USA*
[b]*Ruđer Bočković Institute, Department of Physical Chemistry, P.O. Box 1016, 10001 Zagreb, Croatia*

1 INTRODUCTION
2 PROPERTIES AND DETECTION OF FREE RADICALS
     2.1 What is a free radical?
     2.2 How fast are free radical reactions?
     2.3 Detection of free radicals by time-resolved optical spectroscopy
     2.4 Detection of free radicals by electron spin resonance
     2.5 Spin trapping
     2.6 Product analysis
     2.7 Reduction potentials
     2.8 Where to find rate constants, ESR splittings, reduction potentials, etc.
3 OXYGEN RADICALS
     3.1 The hydroxyl radical
     3.2 Peroxyl radicals
     3.3 Reversible oxygen addition
     3.4 Alkoxyl radicals
     3.5 Phenoxyl radicals
     3.6 Semiquinone radicals
     3.7 Superoxide ($O_2^{\bullet -}$ / $HO_2^{\bullet}$)
4 SULFUR-CENTERED FREE RADICALS
5 CONCLUSION
6 SUMMARY
7 ACKNOWLEDGEMENTS
8 ABBREVIATIONS
9 NOTES
10 REFERENCES

1   INTRODUCTION

It is well accepted these days in the scientific community that free radicals participate in many biological processes, often in a quite decisive manner [1—8]. This clearly emerges from the still rapidly increasing number of studies on this subject and the very important fact that such investigations are not restricted to the views of just one particular group of researchers. Free radical studies in biological systems embrace practically all fields from fundamental chemistry to applied clinical studies these days and have proved to be particularly successful when scientists of the various fields engage in collaborative work and extensive interdisciplinary discussions.

In living systems, including humans, the presence of free radicals is something very natural. The decision of nature to provide the enzyme superoxide dismutase

(SOD), for example, clearly hints on the existence of the superoxide radical, $O_2^{\bullet-}$, – considered to be one of the most prominent radical species in oxygenated biological systems – and it also shows the obvious need of cellular systems to regulate its concentration [9–15]. While this serves as an example that a "too much" of a particular radical species is not in the interest of a biological system there are, on the other hand, also observations where a "too little" of radicals seems equally unwanted. For example, healthy cervix tissue has been reported to contain quite a measurable radical concentration whereas a cancerous tissue is almost completely devoid of radical species [16]. In general, however, it seems that the majority of malignant disturbances is associated with an increase in free radical concentration [17]. Free radicals are undoubtedly involved in many degenerative processes including aspects of aging, cancer, cardiovascular diseases, arteriosclerosis, neural disorders, skin irritations and inflammations. Reperfusion injuries, e.g., in the aftermath of surgery, are also typically characterized by an enhanced formation of free radicals [18]. Actually, any metabolism involving redox active centers is, per se, a possible source of continuous free radical production. This certainly allows the extrapolative conclusion that any stress situation, including exercise, carries the potential of excess free radical production associated with all the chemical consequences arising thereof.

Most of the radicals relevant in biological systems are either derived from or associated with the presence of molecular oxygen, in particular, the already mentioned superoxide anion ($O_2^{\bullet-}$) and peroxyl radicals ($ROO^{\bullet}$). Other oxygen-centered and highly reactive radical species are hydroxyl ($^{\bullet}OH$) and oxyl radicals ($RO^{\bullet}$). Their biological significance is not in doubt but somewhat more in the debate than that of $O_2^{\bullet-}$ and $ROO^{\bullet}$. Of course, it is not only oxygen-centered free radicals which are of importance and interest. Many others, generated both from endogenous as well as exogenous substrates are also of significance. A particularly relevant example is the thiyl radical, $RS^{\bullet}$, which is the one-electron redox intermediate between thiols and disulfides, two vital classes among the biologically abundant substrates [19,20].

The action of free radicals is generally determined by their chemical reactivity and the availability of a suitable reaction partner in the vicinity of their production site. In some cases such a radical-molecule interaction may directly lead to a biological damage in a few or even just one reaction step [7]. Thus, an $^{\bullet}OH$ reaction with the sugar moiety of DNA can result in a strand break due to a radical specific phosphate cleavage reaction. Such a singular event does, however, not necessarily imply cell death as there are enzymatic and chemical, possibly even radical associated repair mechanisms. Accumulation of hazardous compounds as a result of free radical reactions is often the reason for long-term effects. In this case it may even be difficult to prove the free radical's responsibility. It should also be pointed out that the appearance of free radicals does not automatically imply their direct participation in the disturbance of vital biological functions. In other words, free radical reactions are not necessarily the cause of disorders but may equally well just be a consequence thereof. In this case free radicals and their reactions may, however, serve as useful markers.

Nature and modern medicine related science have provided us with mechanisms and substrates to cope with free radicals by "deactivation". Enzymes such as the above already mentioned SOD serve this function. Another important group of compounds in this respect are the so-called antioxidants [22,23]. Most prominent representatives in this respect are vitamin E (α-tocopherol) and vitamin C (ascorbate) which are most effective free radical scavengers in the lipid cell membrane and adjacent, more aqueous compartments, respectively. The same function is assigned to many other redox-active compounds such as, for example, thiols, carotenoids, quinones, etc.

Whenever a free radical reacts with a molecular compound it loses its identity but at the same time it proliferates its general radical properties to a new radical formed in this reaction. In order to assess the action of free radicals it is, therefore, necessary to know not only the properties of the initiating but also of all subsequently generated species. The aim of the present article is, therefore, to elucidate on all these aspects and to provide an understanding for the chemical basis of free radical processes. In the first part of our essay we shall focus on the general properties of free radicals, their generation in chemical model systems, and provide some basic information on the most common methods of their detection. Later we shall focus on the identification and chemical properties of specific groups or individual free radical species which are considered to be of potential significance in biological processes. To find out whether the latter actually applies is then a challenge for the biochemist, biologist and medical researcher. It must, of course, always be remembered that a chemical "test tube" or *in vitro* experiment can only provide the basic information what a free radical can and will do chemically when meeting a suitable reaction partner. Such knowledge is an absolute prerequisite to understand a free radical's potential action. By no means can an *in vitro* experiment, however, substitute for the *in vivo* situation where many more parameters need to be taken into the consideration.

2 PROPERTIES AND DETECTION OF FREE RADICALS

2.1 What is a free radical?

A free radical is, per definition, a molecule or just a single atom with an unpaired electron, conventionally symbolized by a radical dot "$^\bullet$". Examples, extremes from the molecular size point of view, would be a DNA radical (4′ in sugar moiety) and a bromine atom.

Both are species of interest in certain biological processes. The DNA radical is generated, for example, by reaction of an •OH radical with this vital macro-molecule in any cellular system exposed to ionizing radiation and is a direct pre-cursor for a potential strand lesion [7]. The bromine atom, on the other hand, is formed *en route* of reductive degradation of 1,2-dibromoethane, a well-known toxin [24−30].

What means "unpaired" electron? Typically, any electron seeks the association with another of its kind, so that they can pair up their spins in a system of lower energy. A spin is the rotational motion of an electron which can attain two direc-tions and, viewed in a simplified picture, sort of represent a right handed (or "up") and a left handed (or "down") version. Two radicals "shaking hands", i.e., teaming up two individually provided unpaired electrons of opposite spin, form a new bond with this process:

$$\uparrow \quad + \quad \downarrow \quad \rightarrow \quad \uparrow\downarrow \tag{1}$$

A chemical example would be the combination of two bromine atoms which results in the formation of the Br−Br σ-bond:

$$\text{Br}^{•\uparrow} \quad + \quad \text{Br}^{•\downarrow} \quad \rightarrow \quad \text{Br} - \text{Br (with the spins } \uparrow\downarrow \text{ in the bond)} \tag{2}$$

Generally, any even number of electrons in a molecule arranges in "up"-"down" spin coupled pairs, both in bonds or as nonbonding electron pairs. Usually this is an energetically quite favorable process. Sometimes, however, it may be more economic from the energy point of view that two electrons remain uncoupled, even within the same molecule. In this case the two unpaired electrons attain the same spin direction and the chemist talks about a "triplet state" or, if they are located at different atoms, a biradical. A most important example for this situation is the molecular oxygen which we generally view as a molecule with a double bond (a). The two electrons of its p-bond seem, however, to some extent separated and may thus act as if there were two centers providing one unpaired electron each (b):

$$\text{O} = \text{O} \quad \text{(a)} \qquad\qquad {}^{\uparrow}{}^{•}\text{O} - \text{O}{}^{•}{}^{\uparrow} \quad \text{(b)}$$

The presence of unpaired electrons or unpaired spins has a most important con-sequence, namely the generally very high reactivity of such species.[1] This, of course, reflects the genuine desire of the radical species to attain the most favor-able energetic state by coupling its unpaired spin with that of an opposing sign in a new bond between two spin carrying atoms. Accordingly, most radical-radical and also many radical-molecule reactions occur as soon as the two react-ing species meet each other. Such a reaction is, as we say, a diffusion controlled process. The time it actually takes for completion of any chemical reaction depends on two parameters, a reaction specific rate constant (which attains its highest value for a diffusion controlled reaction) and the concentration of the reacting species. In biological systems the free radical concentration is usually very low and rarely acquires values high enough so that a radical-radical reaction could beat a reaction of a radical with a suitable molecular partner. The latter are typically present at much higher concentration in the near-by vicinity.

In order to illustrate this, let us discuss a simple example. Carbontretrachloride, CCl_4, known as a potent liver toxin, is readily reduced by the enzymatic P-450 system of the endoplasmic reticulum [31]. In the presence of oxygen this results in the formation of $CCl_3OO^\bullet$, i.e., trichloromethylperoxyl radicals as an important intermediate in the CCl_4 degradation process (further mechanistic details on peroxyl radical decay will be presented later in this article). Its steady state concentration is, however, extremely small and only few research groups with highly sensitive equipment and great experience have been able to actually detect this radical *in vivo* [32]. It is probably even lower or, at most, comparable to the steady state radical concentration of $\leqslant 1$ pM ($\leqslant 10^{-12}$ M) prevailing in systems which are subjected to γ-irradiation in an average research ^{60}Co-source. In the absence of any suitable reaction partner the above peroxyl radicals have, indeed, no other chance than to react with each other:

$$CCl_3OO^\bullet + CCl_3OO^\bullet \quad \rightarrow \quad \text{products} \quad (2k = 2 \times 10^8 \text{ M}^{-1} \text{ s}^{-1}) \text{ [33] (3)}$$

The half-life for such a so-called second order process is mathematically given by an equation which includes the rate constant (for this kind of second order process defined as "2k") and the radical concentration (in molar units) [34]:

$$t_{1/2} = 1 \: / \: \{(2k) \times [CCl_3OO^\bullet] \} = 1 \: / \: \{2 \times 10^8 \times 10^{-12}\} = 5\ 000 \text{ s} \qquad \text{(I)}$$

On the other hand, if a scavenger such as vitamin E (α-tocopherol) was around in just nanomolar (10^{-9} M) concentration the following reaction would successfully take over:

$$CCl_3OO^\bullet + \text{Vit E} \quad \rightarrow \quad \text{products} \quad (k = 5 \times 10^8 \text{ M}^{-1} \text{ s}^{-1}) \text{ [35]} \qquad \text{(4)}$$

When the concentration of the molecular reaction partner (Vit E) significantly exceeds that of the radical ($CCl_3OO^\bullet$) the reaction becomes of pseudo-first order (reflecting the fact, that the concentration of the excess component hardly changes during the course of the reaction). For such a condition, the mathematical equation attains a slightly different form, the most important difference being that it contains the concentration of the molecular reaction partner and not that of the radical:

$$t_{1/2} \quad = \quad \ln 2/ \: \{k \times [\text{Vit E}] \} \quad = \quad 1 \: / \: \{5 \times 10^8 \times 10^{-9}\} \quad = \quad 1.4 \text{ s} \qquad \text{(II)}$$

By comparison, these two half-lives show that the scavenging of the $CCl_3OO^\bullet$

radical by Vit E is several orders of magnitude faster, i.e., more probable to occur than the mutual radical-radical deactivation.

While this example, from the biological point of view, pertains more to the lipid phase (where Vit E is preferentially located) a similar system may be considered for the aqueous compartments. Thiyl radicals, RS$^\bullet$, although not oxygen-centered but nonetheless equally frequent and important as any oxygen-centered free radical in cellular systems, readily react with the water-soluble ascorbate (Vit C), as formulated in the following equation for the thiyl radical, GS$^\bullet$, from the probably most abundant thiol, glutathione (GSH):

$$GS^\bullet + ascorbate\ (AH^-) \rightarrow GS^- + A^{\bullet-} \tag{5}$$

With a rate constant of k = 6 x 10^8 M^{-1} s^{-1} [36] and an estimated Vit C concentration (e.g., in liver tissue) in the low millimolar range (10^{-3} M) the half-life of this process, calculated according to eq.(II), assumes a value of about 1 ms. For a second order thiyl radical recombination process (2k$_6$ $\approx$ 10^9 M^{-1} s^{-1}) [37] to compete, i.e., to occur with a comparable half-life, a GS$^\bullet$ concentration of about 1 mM would be necessary (calculated with eq. (I)). Such a high steady-state radical concentration is, however, pretty unrealistic in any biological system.

$$GS^\bullet + GS^\bullet \rightarrow GSSG \tag{6}$$

Therefore, any radical-radical reaction is extremely unlikely to occur and the discussion of radical reactions in biological systems should accordingly always be checked first with respect to possible radical-molecule processes. Even if the latter are slow they may still benefit from the usually considerably higher concentration of the molecular reaction partner as compared to the free radical concentration.

2.2 How fast are free radical reactions?

As mentioned above most radical reactions are essentially controlled just by the diffusion of the reacting species. In liquid environment this typically results in rate constants within the order of 10^9 M^{-1} s^{-1} with the individual value depending on the size and structure of the respective species, on solvation effects, and also on the viscosity of the environment. One intrinsic parameter lowering this value could be an internal stabilization of the free radical, meaning delocalization of spin and electron density into the existing regular bonds or to atoms of particularly high electron affinity. Often it is feasible to characterize such radicals by resonance structures, especially when aromatic π-systems are involved. For example, phenoxyl type radicals (structurally similar to the chromanoxyl radical obtained upon oxidation of Vit E) mostly behave as oxygen-centered radicals (a) but certain reactions such as di- and oligomerizations can only be understood in terms of their carbon-centered resonance forms (b) and (c) [38]:

(a)   (b)   (c)

Sometimes such resonance structures are so stable that the radical becomes more and more persistent and may, in extreme cases, even be bottled. At the same time the reactivity towards other radicals and molecular substrates becomes lower and lower, and rate constants accordingly diminish, possibly by many orders of magnitude.

A second parameter which influences the rate of a radical reaction pertains to radical-molecule reactions:

$$R^{\bullet} \quad + \quad A-B \quad \rightarrow \quad R-B \quad + \quad A^{\bullet} \tag{7}$$

In this case, the initial radical $R^{\bullet}$ succeeds in pairing up its lonesome electron, a process certainly beneficial for a high rate constant. At the same time, however, it is necessary to break the molecular $A-B$ bond, and this is a process which requires energy and is, therefore, of adverse influence on the overall rate of reaction. In fact, the complete assessment of the kinetics of such processes must also take into account the energy contents of the product species and, in particular, of the transition state in going from the educt to the product system. This transition state, in which (with reference to the above example) $R^{\bullet}$ has associated already with $A-B$ but $A^{\bullet}$ has not left yet (i.e., $[R...B...A]^{\bullet}$, has, per definition, always the highest energy content along the reaction trajectory. The energy difference between the educts and the transition state is the so-called activation energy, and this is essentially the parameter which decides on the overall rate constant of a reaction. For a typical diffusion controlled process the activation energy is so small that it is essentially provided by the Brownian motion of the reacting partners. However, if this activation energy becomes higher statistically fewer and fewer of the reacting species provide the necessary internal energy to, literally spoken, push the reaction over the transition state mountain. Such reactions are not any more *diffusion* but *activation energy controlled*. An example, quite relevant and important from the biological point of view, would be an oxidative cleavage of a $C-H$ bond by, e.g., a trichloromethyl peroxyl radical:

$$-\overset{|}{\underset{|}{C}}-H \quad + \quad CCl_3OO^{\bullet} \quad \longrightarrow \quad -\overset{|}{\underset{|}{C}}{}^{\bullet} \quad + \quad CCl_3OOH \tag{8}$$

Abstraction of a bisallylic hydrogen atom from linoleic acid, for example, has been reported to occur with a rate constant on the order of 10^6 M^{-1} s^{-1} [39], i.e., three orders of magnitude below the diffusion limit. This means that, despite the strong activation these hydrogen atoms receive from the allylic double bonds of this PUFA, statistically only one in about a thousand encounters actually leads to completion of the above reaction.

An important consequence of these rate constant considerations is the following: radicals which are generated in the vicinity of substrates will definitely undergo fast and quantitative reaction with the latter whenever this reaction is a diffusion or near-diffusion controlled process. Such a situation does not allow any migration of the radicals over larger distances and must, therefore, not be considered for any direct action at distant sites or longer times after their generation.

In this respect it may, in fact, be interesting to know how far a species can actually move until it reacts. Let us consider, for example, a hydroxyl radical $^{\bullet}OH$ generated e.g., in a radiation exposed biological sample. These radicals are known to react with almost any available C–H bond with rate constants $> 10^7$ M^{-1} s^{-1} [40,41]. Assuming potential targets of this kind in a cellular fluid of at least millimolar concentration this translates into a half-life of the $^{\bullet}OH$ radical of $\leqslant 70$ µs and after ten half-lives, i.e., 700 µs, the reaction can, by all practical means, considered to be completed. The simplest mathematical equation relating time (t) with the mean displacement of a diffusing species (Δx) and the diffusion coefficient (D) is:

$$(Dx)^2 = 2\,D\,t \qquad \text{or} \qquad Dx = (2\,D\,t)^{1/2} \qquad \text{(III)}$$

With a typical diffusion coefficient of about 10^{-5} cm^2 s^{-1} the linear free pathway would thus calculate to $\Delta x \leqslant (2 \times 10^{-5} \times 7 \times 10^{-4})^{1/2} \approx 10^{-4}$ cm. For diffusion controlled processes ($k \geqslant 10^9$ M^{-1} s^{-1}) the distance shrinks for another order of magnitude (because of the square root dependence) to $\approx 10^{-5}$ cm. These are clearly no macroscopically interesting distances.

Larger pathways can only be envisaged for lower concentrations of the target molecules, or for lower than the above applied rate constants. An extreme case is given when the radical cannot find a suitable molecular partner and lives until it meets another radical of its kind. As calculated for the particular example of the trichloromethyl peroxyl radical (see Eqs. 3 and I) with an estimated steady state radical concentration of 1 pM the half-life extends to about 5,000 seconds, or more than one hour. In this case, the Δx calculation becomes, however, rather meaningless since convectional motion of the cellular fluid is likely to take over with respect to mass transport.

In conclusion, all the previous discussion has hopefully shown how important it is to know the exact rate constants for the all possible radical reactions as well as the local concentrations of both the radicals and their potential molecular reaction partners. Both parameters are an essential prerequisite for any mechanistic assessment in a free radical containing biological system.

2.3 Detection of free radicals by time-resolved optical spectroscopy

As the reader may have realized from the previous chapter, free radical reactions are usually very fast and thus clearly escape any direct detection in an *in vivo* real-time experiment. Fortunately, absolute rate constants are an inherent property of any particular reactive system and may, therefore, be determined, without introducing any error, outside the biological compartment in suitable and often even much better defined *in vitro* model studies.

The basic problem one has to deal with in case of free radical reactions is the usually high rate at which most of these processes occur. The typical time window for the lifespan of a free radical, reacting in solution via a diffusion controlled process with molecular substrates which are present at µM to mM concentrations, lies in the millisecond time scale. Any technique for direct study of such fast reactions must, therefore, comprise of a correspondingly fast detection system. For quantitative kinetic analysis it is highly desirable, in fact almost mandatory, that the formation of the radical of interest is completed within a time period that is short compared to the lifetime of the radical. Only then becomes it possible to directly "see" such a species. A further prerequisite is, of course, that the radical exhibits a detectable property. A very suitable parameter, in this respect, is the optical absorption. In fact, most radicals are colored, not necessarily in the visible part of the spectrum, but IR and UV regions are equally accessible by modern time-resolving optical spectroscopy. In principle, also any other property detectable with appropriate time resolution is equally suitable [42]. The most frequently used is conductivity which helps, in particular, to study charged species, i.e., radical ions [43,44].

Two techniques have been especially successful to study fast processes and to determine absolute rate constants for free radical reactions, namely, the radiation chemical method of pulse radiolysis [42,45,46] and laser flash photolysis [6,47]. The principle idea is the same for both methods and shall briefly be introduced in the following simplified scheme. It depicts the formation and decay of a transient which is generated in the "cell", typically an all-quartz vessel of $0.5-10$ cm^3 volume containing the chemical solution to be investigated. For convenience and rapid sample exchange the cell is often attached to a flow system. Irradiation is achieved by admitting short pulses of either high energy electrons (MeV range), generated in a Van de Graaff or Linear Accelerator (pulse radiolysis), or photons from a laser (laser flash photolysis). For kinetic studies the duration of these pulses is typically in the pico- to microsecond time range. The result of such a pulse is an energy deposit in the solution contained in the "cell". This, in turn, is responsible for the free radical production.

Despite the principle similarities of these two techniques the actual detailed picture includes some differing aspects. The somewhat easier to understand system is the photolytic one. Here, the incoming photons from the laser pulse interact directly with a target molecule in the "cell" compartment in a process which may lead to its excitation and ionization. A prerequisite is, however, that this target molecule absorbs light at the wavelength of the incoming photons with a sufficiently high extinction coefficient and the energy of the photon is sufficient to initiate the desired process.

In case of pulse radiolysis the energy of the incoming electrons is significantly

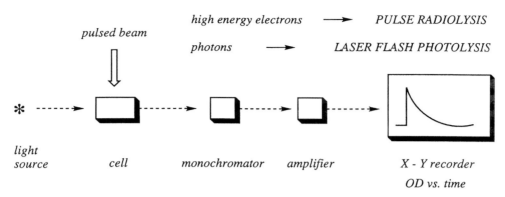

Scheme 1. Time-resolved optical spectroscopy.

higher compared to that of a laser photon. Considering that ionization of a molecule typically requires energies in the 5—20 eV range one might, in fact, get quite scared about such a "bombardment" with MeV electrons. Fortunately, those high energy particles lose their energy in small packages via many consecutive steps rather than at once. In simple terms, while flying through the atomic world of matter a high energy electron very rarely hits any of the atomic electrons or positively charged nuclei directly. Typically, it just passes those charged centers at more or less larger distance. Since charges can "see" each other over quite a distance (coulombic interaction) the "flying" electron becomes deflected from its original path at each of these encounters. Physics tells us that any such event is accompanied by an exchange of energy. As a consequence, all the kinetic energy is deposited in small portions which, on average, are of 50—100 eV magnitude. These energy islands (also called spurs) are more or less homogeneously distributed in the irradiated sample. This amount of energy is just sufficient for molecular excitations and one or two ionizations, i.e., events which lead directly to free radicals. There are, of course, some more particulars to it which do not, however, need to be elaborated further in this context. Certainly they do not involve any unresolved magic with respect to the chemistry initiated by radiation. Basically, everything is described in common radiation chemistry [45,48–50] or radiation biology [6,7] textbooks, for example.

When comparing the two time-resolved methods one more important feature must be pointed out. In pulse radiolysis the high energy electron, while flying through matter, does not distinguish between the various molecules since it interacts with the coulombic field of any atomic electron or nucleus it passes by. Statistically, the respective energy deposits are, therefore, preferentially located in the solvent rather than near any low concentration solute. This results, in the first instance, in solvent-derived radicals, and the free radicals of interest would then be formed in a subsequent reaction of these primary radicals with the solute. We call this an "indirect" formation of free radicals.

In principle, however, both the photolysis as well as the pulse radiolysis method are equally suited to generate and study free radicals and their reactions. In fact, they are in many ways complementary.

Let us now return to the time-resolved experiment outlined in the above schematic drawing. Perhaps we would like to study the free radical induced oxidation of ascorbate (Vitamin C). In a pulse radiolysis experiment our irradiation cell would then probably contain an aqueous solution of typically about 100 µM ascorbate and the sample would have been saturated with nitrous oxide (N_2O). The latter serves two functions. Firstly, by purging the solution with this gas oxygen will be removed (O_2 usually disturbs because it scavenges many free radicals before they can undergo the reaction of interest). The second function of the N_2O is to establish defined chemical conditions as will become apparent in the following discussion of the general reaction scheme in irradiated aqueous solutions.

Irradiation of this ascorbate solution leads, in accordance with our above considerations, primarily to reactive species from the solvent water (Eq. 9):

$$H_2O \quad \rightarrow \quad e_{aq}^-, \ ^\bullet OH, \ H^\bullet, \ H_{aq}^+, \ H_2O_2, \ H_2 \qquad (9)$$

The two most important ones are the hydrated electrons (e_{aq}^-) and hydroxyl radicals ($^\bullet OH$) which together account for 90% of the initial free radicals. They are typically formed at about µM-concentrations per pulse.[2] However, while the hydrated electron is a strong reductant the hydroxyl radicals is a powerful oxidant.[3] This potentially disturbing problem can be overcome by the presence of nitrous oxide which converts hydrated electrons into hydroxyl radicals:

$$N_2O \quad + \quad e_{aq}^- \quad + \quad H_2O \quad \rightarrow \quad ^\bullet OH \quad + \quad OH^- + N_2 \qquad (10)$$

At N_2O saturation this process is completed within a few nanoseconds and consequently the only reactive species available for further reaction is the hydroxyl radical. In our model experiment this would then react with the ascorbate (denoted as AH^-) to generate the ascorbyl radical, $A^{\bullet-}$:

$$^\bullet OH \quad + \quad AH^- \quad \rightarrow \quad A^{\bullet-} \quad + \quad H_2O \qquad (11)$$

At millimolar ascorbate concentration this reaction is completed within less than a few ms. The ascorbyl radical, now, has an important property: it absorbs light and the maximum of its absorption lies at about 360 nm [51]. Accordingly, if we shine light through the irradiation cell while the system is exposed to the pulse of high energy electrons the intensity of this light will be diminished as soon as the absorbing ascorbyl radical is generated. In order to scan this event the analyzing light beam, after having penetrated the irradiated solution, enters a monochromator which allows to select a suitable wavelength. After conversion of the optical signal into an electrical signal and amplification it is finally displayed on an X–Y-recorder in terms of a time-dependent voltage which actually represents the change in optical density at a selected wavelength as a function of time. The signal shown on our scheme is thus a true fingerprint of a transient which is formed in a fast process and then eventually decays away again. Exactly this is the type of signal we observe in our above example on the oxidation of the ascorbate under the discussed conditions and which is attributable to the ascorbyl radical.

The intensity of such signals recorded at varying wavelengths provides the complete absorption spectrum. Kinetic analysis of both the formation and decay of the absorption yields the respective rate constants of the underlying processes, here the reaction of $^\bullet OH$ with ascorbate and the subsequent disproportionation of the ascorbyl radical.

Generally, such studies conveniently allow to investigate the reactivity of just any absorbing transient with other substrates. In this case we just need to add the suspected reaction partner in small quantities (small enough so that it does not react directly with one of the primary radicals) prior to irradiation. If it does indeed react with our transient this will show up as an accelerated decay of the transient signal which, furthermore, depends on the concentration of the added substrate. Such experiments are actually the general basis for the evaluation of absolute rate constants.[4]

2.4 Detection of free radicals by electron spin resonance

As mentioned already, the time-resolved detection techniques discussed above, as excellent as they are for relatively simple model studies, they do usually not permit investigations with more complex biological material. Whenever a direct proof of free radicals in tissue is at stake another technique, namely, electron spin resonance (ESR) is probably the better method of choice [52—54].

The principle idea behind this method is to take advantage of the spin of the radical's unpaired electron. As a "moving" charge an electron has an associated magnetic moment which can be aligned either in (parallel to) or against (antiparallel to) the direction of an external magnetic field. Now, it is important to realize that the energy level of the magnetic moment of the unpaired electron is higher for the antiparallel than for the parallel alignment and, furthermore, that the resulting energy difference, or split in energy levels, depends linearly on the external magnetic field as shown in the simple pictorial. All this is basically controlled by quantum mechanics.

The energy separation, expressed in terms of $h\nu$, increases with increasing magnetic field, here depicted for a deliberately chosen experimental field strength H_e. The energy difference between the two levels is given by

$$h\nu = g\beta H$$

where g denotes a spectroscopic splitting factor and β the Bohr magneton. While β is a constant, g varies with the nature of the free radicals. For a single free electron, which is solely characterized by the angular momentum of the spin, it

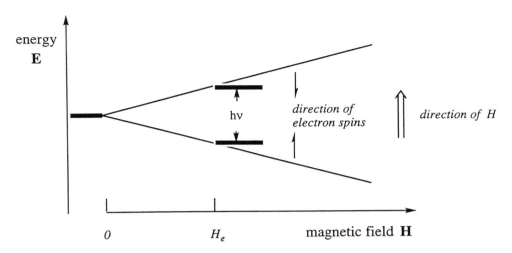

energy
E

hν

*direction of
electron spins*

direction of H

0   H_e magnetic field **H**

Scheme 2. Splitting of energy levels in magnetic field.

assumes a value of 2.0023. However, if this electron interacts with its surroundings this number may deviate, usually within $\leqslant \pm0.01$. The g-factor thus provides the information on the molecular orbital of the unpaired electron and in that respect is a property of the radical as a whole [55].

How is it possible to verify this concept experimentally? We need to measure the energy level difference $h\nu$ at a given magnetic field H_e. One possibility to do this would be to offer a varying spectrum of electromagnetic energies $h\nu$ (in ESR typically within the microwave range) at constant magnetic field and see which of the frequencies is absorbed in order to promote the electron from the low (parallel) to the high (antiparallel) energy alignment. Experimentally this procedure is, however, more difficult to realize than the second possibility where the microwave frequency is kept constant (e.g., $\approx$ 9 GHz X-band or $\approx$ 36 GHz Q-band microwaves) and the probe is exposed to a varying external magnetic field. Wherever in such a scan the separation of the two energy levels matches the offered microwave energy $h\nu$ there will be a resonance absorption, i.e., energy will be transferred from the microwave field into the molecule. Generally, the absorption signal is not recorded as such but as its first derivative. Both are depicted in the following scheme.

With H_r, $h\nu$ and the natural constant β we now have all parameters to evaluate g. (For most known free radicals g values have explicitly been measured and many of them are tabulated in data collections) [56].

Some of the radical assignments rely pretty much on such g factor determinations, a prominent example being the superoxide anion, $O_2^{\bullet-}$. There are, however, further effects which give even more insight into the molecular structure of a free radical. Just as all the other electrons contribute to the position of the two spin energy levels with their orbital magnetism, a corresponding effect is caused

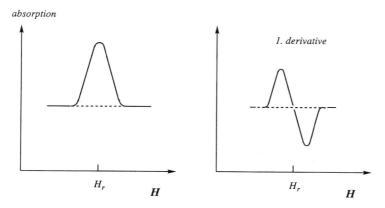

Scheme 3. Microwave absorption in magnetic field.

by the magnetic fields of nuclear spins. This influence is not very big and thus usually restricted to the atoms in the immediate vicinity of the unpaired radical electron, but this makes it actually a very specific probe for a partial structure of the free radical. One prerequisite must be met though, and that is the presence of a nuclear spin in the atom of interest. Typically, atoms with all even numbers of protons and neutrons do not have any nuclear spin. Therefore, the most abundant carbon isotope, ^{12}C, is of no use in this respect; ^{13}C, on the other hand, would be a most suitable atom since it has an unpaired neutron (nuclear spin of $1/2$). Because of its low abundance this isotope is, nevertheless, only of lesser importance in ESR, but it serves a very significant role in the related field of NMR (nuclear magnetic resonance). Two other atoms with nuclear spin play, however, an important, almost decisive role in ESR, namely, nitrogen and hydrogen with nuclear spins of 1 and $1/2$, respectively.

Let us briefly discuss just one simple example, a methyl radical, $^{\bullet}CH_3$. Here, the unpaired electron "sees" the magnetic fields exerted by the three protons (spin $1/2$). Following quantum mechanical rules these nuclear magnetic moments will couple with that of the electron spin in either parallel or antiparallel fashion. Since there are three protons a total of four possibilities arises: all three parallel (total spin $+3/2$), two parallel and one antiparallel (total spin $+1/2$), one parallel and two antiparallel (total spin $-1/2$), all three antiparallel (total spin $-3/2$), and the statistical probability that they do so is 1:3:3:1. What is the consequence? Each of the two original spin energy levels of the free, unpaired electron will be further split into four new levels as shown in the following scheme:

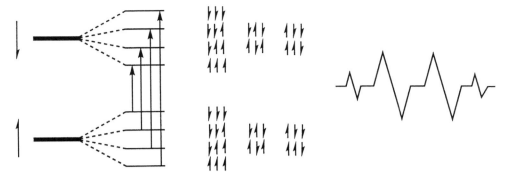

Scheme 4. ESR spectrum of methyl radical.

Considering the selectivity rules, four transitions become possible and thus the ESR signal of the $^\bullet CH_3$ radical will consist of four lines the intensities of which reflect the above mentioned statistics.

Had there been only one proton the two possible nuclear spin directions, $+1/2$ and $-1/2$, would have caused a split into two levels and the resulting absorption spectrum would have been a doublet of equal (1:1) intensity. In case of two interacting protons nuclear spin combinations assume values of $+1$, 0, and -1 yielding a triplet with a 1:2:1 intensity ratio.

For larger radicals influences from even further distant groups may become visible. For example, in an ethyl radical, $^\bullet CH_2-CH_3$, the two energy levels of the "free" electron will be split into three levels due to the nuclear spin interaction of the two α-protons (CH_2-group), and then each of these resulting levels will be further split into four levels due to the interaction of the three β-positioned protons in the CH_3-group. This provides the possibility of a total of twelve transitions and accordingly the microwave absorption spectrum consists of twelve lines. Such secondary effects, generally referred to a hyperfine interaction, become smaller and smaller the further distant the interacting nuclei are positioned.

Of course, there is much more about ESR, impossible to cope with in detail in this short and anyway diversifying introductory article. This pertains, in particular, to the vast amount of structural information which may also be extracted from these hyperfine splittings, from anisotropy effects, and special techniques such as ENDOR [52,57]. However, it can hopefully be appreciated how potent, in principle, ESR is to identify free radicals and to determine their structure. It is generally less suited for kinetic studies as compared to the optical measurements although several time-resolved ESR studies have provided very useful specific kinetic data as well. Innovative research will certainly depend on both of these, in the best sense, complementary approaches.

2.5 Spin trapping

One of the problems, particularly with respect to biological samples, is the generally extremely small steady-state concentration of the free radicals, either because only few radicals are produced, or their lifetimes are too short for accumulation. It often helps to freeze the sample in order to slow down the kinetics. Furthermore, certain radicals exhibit rather unspecific spectral characteristics with perhaps just one broad line and lack of any fine structure information. In fact, four biologically quite relevant radicals belong to this group, superoxide ($O_2^{\bullet-}$), thiyl radicals ($RS^{\bullet}$), peroxyl ($ROO^{\bullet}$), and alkoxyl radicals ($RO^{\bullet}$) [52,58].

One possibility to overcome many of these problems is to trap the free radical of interest by a suitable scavenger and thus convert it into a better detectable and usually longer-lived secondary radical. This procedure is generally known as "spin trapping" [48,59].

What is a good spin trapping agent? Probably the best studied and one of the most efficient class of compounds in this respect are nitrones. They usually incorporate free radicals in fast addition processes and the resulting nitroxyl radicals are generally highly persistent and thus subject of convenient ESR investigations. The underlying chemical reaction is formulated in its general form in Eq. 12. A specific example, namely, the trapping of a glutathiyl radical which was generated as metabolite in a horseradish peroxidase induced oxidation process [60] is given in Eq. 13:

$$R'' - CH = \overset{\overset{\displaystyle O^-}{|}}{\underset{+}{N}} - R' \quad + \quad R^{\bullet} \quad \longrightarrow \quad R'' - \overset{\overset{\displaystyle O^{\bullet}}{|}}{\underset{\underset{\displaystyle R}{|}}{CH}} - N - R' \qquad (12)$$

$$(13)$$

The radical of interest, $R^{\bullet}$, adds to the carbon in the C=N double bond of the nitrone, and the unpaired electron becomes located at the oxygen with some spin delocalization also to the nitrogen. An ESR investigation of such nitroxyl radicals usually allows to reveal the identity of R through the hyperfine splitting.

Spin trapping has become one of the most sensitive in situ methods for the detection of free radicals in tissue. Despite its unquestionable success a word of caution should be issued though. Whenever free radicals are suspected and spin trapping agents are introduced it is certainly necessary to confirm by independent measurements that the ultimately trapped radicals are not themselves a metabolic product of the spin trap compound, or generated because of an interference of the spin trap with a mechanism which, in the absence of the spin trap, would not produce these radicals.

2.6 Product analysis

Besides these two powerful tools for the direct study of free radicals, time-resolved spectroscopy and ESR, there is, of course, still the most classical method to prove free radicals and that is stable product analysis. Many free radical reaction routes have been revealed in thorough and often sophisticated chemical studies. For example, the formation of phosgene ($COCl_2$) as a transient, and CO_2 and HCl as stable end products upon reductive degradation of the liver toxin carbon tetrachloride can quantitatively be described by a free radical mechanism [61,62]. A corresponding statement holds for the products from one of the frequently used anaesthetics, halothane (CF_3-CHClBr), namely, CF_3-COOH, CF_2-CHCl, CF_2-CHO, CO_2, F^-, Cl^-, Br^-, and some others [63—65]. All these result from free radical reactions under particular conditions, such as oxidative or reductive initiation, and the presence or absence of oxygen. The identity of the products found both *in vitro* (radiation chemical and photocatalytic free radical studies) and as a result of metabolism suggests, in fact, that the biological degradation of halothane involves most likely free radicals.

While these examples leave little doubt how the final molecular products are generated and which kind of free radicals participate *en route*, again a word of caution must be given. Not always is it possible to extrapolate straight back from a final molecular product to an initiating or transient free radical generated in the course of a reaction sequence. Quite a number of highly speculative and strange mechanisms are offered once in a while, much to the amusement of a free radical chemist. Clearly, in order to unravel an unknown mechanism a certain degree of imagination is necessary. Final products should, however, better be viewed as just the ultimate proof of a proposed mechanism which ought to be sustained by a separate study of as many as possible intermediate steps. Again, it hopefully becomes apparent that the most beneficial approach is the cooperative one.

2.7 Reduction potentials

As stated in our introductory chapter the main driving force for a reaction of a free radical is its desire to retain an even number of electrons. Whenever this is achieved by either donating the unpaired or accepting an additional electron (without incorporation of any further atomic or molecular constituents) such a reaction qualifies as a classical one-electron transfer or redox process.[5]

How potent a free radical species is with respect to any oxidative or reductive electron transfer is usually quantified by the standard redox or better, by IUPAC recommendation, *reduction* potential $E°$. The actual figures for $E°$ refer to reactions of the general form

$$\text{oxidant} \quad + \quad \text{n e}^- \quad \rightarrow \quad \text{reductant} \tag{14}$$

and are denoted as standard reduction potentials $E°(Ox/Red)$. (The term "standard" refers to unit activity, i.e., ca 1 M in concentration for liquids and solids, and unit fugacity, i.e., 1 atm at 298 K for gases). For one-electron processes either the oxidant or the reductant is a radical.

Let us now consider a chemical redox reaction which involves two pairs of redox couples, namely, $A^•/A^-$ and $B^•/B^-$ with the respective standard reduction potentials $E°(A^•/A^-)$ and $E°(B^•/B^-)$. ($A^•$, $B^•$ and A^-, B^- refer to the oxidized and reduced forms, respectively, irrespective of the actual state of charge). The deciding factor into which direction the equilibrium reaction

$$A^• \quad + \quad B^- \quad \rightleftharpoons \quad A^- \quad + \quad B^• \tag{15}$$

actually proceeds depends on the relative desire of $A^•$ and $B^•$ to accept an electron, in other words, on the difference in the respective reduction potentials:

$$\Delta E° \quad = \quad E°(B^•/B^-) \quad - \quad E°(A^•/A^-)$$

If this figure is negative the reaction proceeds from left to right, and vice versa. (Please note: The couple with the reduced form on the left hand side of the equation appears first, here the $B^•/B^-$ couple).

The difference in reduction potentials is related to the equilibrium constant, K, for reaction 15 via the standard free enthalpy $G°$:

$$\Delta G° \quad = \quad -nF\Delta E° \quad = \quad -RT \ln K$$

For a one-electron reaction (n=1) $\Delta E°$ calculates to

$$\Delta E° \, [mV] \quad = \quad 59.1 \log K$$

If K is not known it may be determined through measurement of equilibrium concentrations or the ratio of rate constants for the forward and back reactions. In the above example $K_{15} = [A^-][B^•] / [A^•][B^-] = k_{15}/k_{-15}$. In order to achieve this experimentally within appropriate accuracy the $E°$ values for the individual couples should not differ too much. Finally, the reduction potentials $E°$ can be calculated from $\Delta E°$ by knowing the other $E°$ involved, or by measurement of $\Delta E°$ against the standard (normal) hydrogen electrode (NHE) whose $E°(H^+ / \frac{1}{2} H_2) = 0$ per definition.

For practical assessments just this reminder: any deviations from standard conditions affects, of course, the actual potential (E) through the influence of the concentrations ($E = E° + RT/nF \ln [Ox]/[Red]$). This is particularly relevant for all redox processes involving protons (e.g., $RS^\bullet + e^- + H^+ \rightleftharpoons RSH$) where the reduction potential becomes pH dependent. When looking up potential values attention should also be turned to the reference potential. This is not always that of the normal hydrogen electrode (NHE) but often refers to other standards. Many systems have been measured against the saturated calomel (SCE) or a Ag/AgCl electrode. These values can be converted to NHE values by adding 244 mV and 222 mV, respectively (both correction terms referring to 298 K).

Another important source of confusion is particularly relevant for one of the biologically most interesting redox couples, namely that of $O_2/O_2^{\bullet-}$. Thus, the potential amounts to $E° = -325$ mV if standardized according to the gas phase rules, namely, to one atmosphere of partial oxygen pressure. In aqueous solution this refers accordingly to saturation concentration, namely, $[O_2]_{sat} \approx 1.3$ mM. Applying, however, the liquid phase standardization rules the reference concentration is 1 M and, extrapolated to this figure, the liquid phase "standard" potential assumes quite a different value, namely, $E_{liq}° = -155$ mV.

2.8 Where to find rate constants, ESR splittings, reduction potentials, etc.

Fortunately, it is not necessary anymore to determine all the rate constants, spectroscopic data, redox properties and many other physico-chemical parameters which one may need to know for a complete understanding of a free radical mechanism. In fact, a huge amount of such data have been gathered already and are now compiled in special reference books. For convenience we shall mention just a few of the most comprehensive editions.

The probably largest collection of rate constants for free radical reactions in solution is to be found in a five volume issue of the "Landolt-Börnstein" (Springer Verlag) [66], including an extensive recent supplement. A most valuable source of information is also several issues of the *Journal of Physical and Chemical Reference Data* (former NSRDS-Series) [40,68,69]. ESR data have also be compiled in a "Landolt-Börnstein" series (including recent supplements) [56]. For reduction potentials, finally, an excellent and well commented survey is given by P. Wardman in an issue of the *Journal of Physical and Chemical Reference Data Series* [70]. We like to add though that this is, nevertheless, only a very personal selection and shall not discredit other textbooks or compilations not mentioned nor any singular result in the regular scientific literature.

3   OXYGEN FREE RADICALS

In the following we shall now present and discuss the most abundant and important oxygen centered free radicals as there are:

the hydroxyl radical	$^\bullet OH$
the peroxyl radical	$ROO^\bullet$
the alkoxyl radical	$RO^\bullet$

the phenoxyl and semiquinone radicals $ArO^{\bullet}$, $HO{-}Ar{-}O^{\bullet}$
the superoxide $O_2^{\bullet-}$

In doing this, we will restrict ourselves, however, to the fundamental physico-chemical and chemical properties in order to provide just the basis for an understanding of their reactivity. For illustration some specifically selected examples will be included.

3.1 The hydroxyl radical

By far the most reactive oxygen containing species is the hydroxyl radical, $^{\bullet}OH$. Whenever discussed in biological context it must, therefore, be recognized that its direct chemical action is strictly confined to the close vicinity of the site of its generation. There may, of course, be an indirect effect through an $^{\bullet}OH$-induced process at further distance but the actually active species would then always be a secondary radical or molecular product.

What makes the hydroxyl radical such a reactive species, and what means "high reactivity"? The answer to the first question lies in the versatility of this radical which can undergo three types of reactions. Thus it is a potentially powerful oxidant from the thermodynamic point of view with a reduction potential of 1.9 V for the $^{\bullet}OH/OH^-$ couple (2.7 V for $^{\bullet}OH,H^+/H_2O$). In other words, the hydroxyl radical is, in principle, very eager to accept an electron and convert to the hydroxide ion (or water). Most interestingly, this is, however, a rather rare process although, from the mere redox point of view, a large amount of molecules should be prone for such an electron transfer mechanism. One of the few reactions of this kind is the oxidation of hexacyano ferrate (II):

$$^{\bullet}OH \quad + \quad Fe(CN)_6^{4-} \quad \rightarrow \quad OH^- \quad + \quad Fe(CN)_6^{3-} \tag{16}$$

It should perhaps be noted that this inorganic complex is electronically unique in the sense that the central Fe^{2+} ion, through interaction with the six cyano ligands, has attained completely filled s-, p-, and d-orbitals in its M shell (n = 3) and completely filled s- and p-orbitals in its outer-most N shell (n = 4). This leaves practically no chance anymore for the hydroxyl radical to enter the ligand sphere as a molecular entity or, in other words, to add on to a molecule.

Addition of $^{\bullet}OH$ to atoms and molecules is, in fact, the most preferred process this radical species undergoes. This reflects two important parameters. Firstly, the hydroxyl group is an excellent ligand and, therefore, any OH^- formed in an electron transfer process with, e.g., a metal ion, may stick to the oxidized form of the latter. An example is the $^{\bullet}OH$-induced oxidation of Tl^+ to Tl^{2+} which proceeds via a short-lived but unambiguously identifiable intermediate adduct:

$$Tl^+ \quad + \quad ^{\bullet}OH \quad \rightarrow \quad Tl(OH)^+ \tag{17}$$

This is then involved in acid/base equilibria

$$Tl(OH)_2 \;\rightleftharpoons\; Tl(OH)^+ \;+\; OH^- \;\rightleftharpoons\; Tl_{aq}^{2+} \;+\; 2\,OH^- \quad (18)$$

with pKs of 7.7 and 4.6, respectively [71,72]. Biologically perhaps more relevant examples refer to the corresponding oxidations of copper or iron in many vital complexes of these metals. Just recently, such a transient hydroxyl adduct has been identified in the •OH-induced oxidation of a copper-(I)-thia-crown-ether [73], a model for certain copper proteins.

A further important property of the hydroxyl radical is its pronounced electrophilic character. Thus it likes to add to centers of high electron density as they are provided by aromatic π-systems, olefinic double bonds or free (lone) electron pairs. In each case the hydroxyl clearly draws on the offered electron density but remains in close contact with the potential donor at least for some limited time. An intensively studied example is the oxidation of organic sulfides where the hydroxyl radical adds to the lone p-electron pair of sulfur [74—76]:

$$-\overset{..}{\underset{..}{S}}- \quad + \quad {}^{\bullet}OH \quad \longrightarrow \quad >\overset{\overset{\displaystyle OH}{\displaystyle |}}{\underset{..}{S}}{}^{\bullet} \qquad (19)$$

The resulting sulfuranyl radical typically decays within less than a microsecond but in some cases it may be stabilized through hydrogen bridging and then assume considerably longer lifetimes [76]. Such an adduct constitutes, for example, an important intermediate *en route* to an oxidative decarboxylation of the essential amino acid methionine [77—79] where it is a direct precursor of a sulfur-nitrogen linked (three-electron-bonded) species which, in turn, is the key transient which transfers the reactive site from sulfur to the amino acid moiety. (For further information on three-electron bonds see chapter on "Sulfur-centered Free Radicals").

$$CH_3\text{-}S\text{-}CH_2\text{-}CH_2\text{-}CH \overset{\displaystyle NH_3^+}{\underset{\displaystyle COO^-}{}} \quad + \quad {}^{\bullet}OH \quad \longrightarrow \qquad (20)$$

$$\xrightarrow{\;-H_2O\;} \qquad (21)$$

$$CH_3\text{-}S\text{-}CH_2\text{-}CH_2\text{-}CH \overset{\displaystyle \overset{\bullet}{N}H_2^+}{\underset{\displaystyle COO^-}{}} \quad \longrightarrow \quad CH_3\text{-}S\text{-}CH_2\text{-}CH_2\text{-}\overset{\bullet}{C}H\text{-}NH_2 \quad + \quad CO_2 \qquad (22)$$

By the way, the α-amino radical, $CH_3SCH_2CH_2C^{\bullet}HNH_2$, formed in this reaction sequence is a highly reductive species and readily transfers an electron to oxygen and NAD^+, for example [80]. Considering that the initiating species was the oxidizing hydroxyl radical this constitutes a complete turnover of the redox properties along the reaction coordinate. Many more corresponding examples with other sulfur containing amino acids and peptides have been described recently [81−83].

Similar redox considerations apply to many $^{\bullet}$OH-adducts to double bonds. Biologically striking examples are the pyrimidine bases which are vital constituents of the DNA. Uracil, with its C-5/C-6 double bond, provides such a target for an electrophilic $^{\bullet}$OH-addition. Two possible radicals may be generated: a 6-yl radical, when $^{\bullet}$OH adds to C-5, and a 5-yl radical, when it adds to C-6. Both are indeed formed, with an 82:18 relative ratio [84]. Most important, the 6-yl radical has reducing properties while the 5-yl radical, on the other hand, is an oxidant. For rationalization, please note the α-positioned amino group relative to the radical site in the 6-yl species. This, therefore, resembles the α-amino radical from methionine mentioned above. In the oxidizing 5-yl radical the unpaired spin can probably be delocalized to some extent into the carbonyl group to yield an oxyl radical resonance form.

Other pyrimidine bases show different 5-yl/6-yl ratios since other substituents affect the electron density at C-5 and C-6 differently, and may exert also some steric constraints [7,21,84]. In general, the 6-yl radical prevails.

The third type of reaction a hydroxyl radical frequently undergoes is abstraction or displacement. If, for example, an $^{\bullet}$OH radical was formed in the vicinity of a thiol, such as cysteine or glutathione, it would most likely abstract (or displace) a hydrogen atom:

$$RS–H \quad + \quad ^{\bullet}OH \quad \rightarrow \quad RS^{\bullet} \quad + \quad H_2O \tag{24}$$

This reaction is fast, i.e., almost diffusion controlled [40] since the S–H bond energy is considerably smaller than that of the O–H bond energy in water.

A prime target are also C–H bonds, and in this context it must be recognized that practically all biologically relevant material contains plenty of them. The general reaction

$$-\overset{|}{\underset{|}{C}}-H \quad + \quad {}^{\bullet}OH \qquad \rightarrow \qquad -\overset{|}{\underset{|}{C}}{}^{\bullet} \quad + \quad H_2O \tag{25}$$

usually requires some more activation energy than the ${}^{\bullet}OH$ reaction with thiols since C–H bonds are, on average, stronger than S–H bonds [85]. Of course, not all C–H bonds are of equal strength and, therefore, there will be preferred and less probable reaction sites in a molecule which contains various kinds of C–H bonds. Some general rules can be applied. Thus, the most difficult C–H bond to break is that in CH_3-groups (primary H-atom), while it becomes increasingly easier to displace a secondary (CH_2-group) or tertiary (CH-group) hydrogen. Particularly labile are the bisallylic hydrogens in polyunsaturated fatty acids; they can even be abstracted by thiyl radicals [86]. However, in the case of PUFAs it must be recognized that the double bonds do not only serve the function of activating the bisallylic hydrogens but are themselves a sink for ${}^{\bullet}OH$ via electrophilic addition [87].

Although there are differences in C–H bond energies and, as a result of that, different reaction rates with respect to hydrogen abstraction, a selective process in a larger target molecule is highly improbable. The reason is that the associated activation energies for an ${}^{\bullet}OH$-induced abstraction process are generally low and do not allow complete discrimination. Take the simple alcohol ethanol where three types of hydrogens (primary and secondary C–H, and O–H bonds) may be cleaved [88]:

$$
{}^{\bullet}OH + CH_3\text{–}CH_2\text{–}OH \rightarrow
\begin{array}{lll}
{}^{\bullet}CH_2\text{–}CH_2\text{–}OH & (13.2\%) & (26a) \\
CH_3\text{–}C^{\bullet}H\text{–}OH & (84.3\%) & (26b) \\
CH_3\text{–}CH_2\text{–}O^{\bullet} & (2.5\%) & (26c)
\end{array}
$$

Such relative abstraction yields vary, of course, with the individual compound and will have to be determined experimentally for any quantitative assessment. However, quite many of them have been documented in the meantime, particularly for the sugar moiety of DNA [7].

A question arises, of course, on how to distinguish between the various possible abstraction routes. One possibility is product analysis and knowledge of the mechanism by which the initially formed radicals convert to the analyzable stable substrates. Another successful approach is time-resolved direct observation of the intermediates, e.g., through their optical absorptions. Considering the above alcohol example, a discrimination is possible on the basis of the redox properties of the three radicals formed in reaction 26. Thus, the α-hydroxyl radical (formed at the highest, i.e., 84.3% yield) exhibits reasonably strong reducing properties; the oxyl radical (formed with 2.5% yield), on the other hand, is a strong oxidant; and the remaining β-hydroxyl radical (13.2% yield) is practically redox inert [88]. Similar considerations have been applied for the above mentioned $^\bullet$OH/pyrimidine adducts and show the value of free radical redox studies [7,84].

The variety of possible $^\bullet$OH reactions can still be enlarged since several of the three mechanisms discussed (electron transfer, addition, abstraction) may occur simultaneously. Just one example shall briefly be mentioned, namely, the oxidation of disulfides. The reaction with simple aliphatic disulfides thus proceeds with about equal probability via a one-electron oxidation to yield the disulfide radical cation and a, pH dependent, displacement process [89]:

$$
\text{RSSR} + {}^\bullet\text{OH} \quad \rightarrow \quad
\begin{array}{ll}
(\text{RSSR})^{\bullet+} + \text{OH}^- & \quad(27a)\\
\text{RS}^\bullet + \text{RSOH} \ (\text{neutral pH}) & \quad(27b)\\
\text{RSH} + \text{RSO}^\bullet \ (\text{low and high pH}) & \quad(27c)
\end{array}
$$

The high reactivity of the hydroxyl radicals is, as mentioned already at the beginning of this chapter, the reason why its reactions are usually confined to the immediate vicinity of their generation. Within this reaction sphere a great variety of final products may, nevertheless, be formed. The latter is a direct reflection of the "reactivity-selectivity" principle which, incidentally, applies for all free radical reactions: The more reactive a radical species (i.e., the lower the activation energies for potentially competing reaction routes) the less selective it becomes.

One further property of the hydroxyl radicals needs to be mentioned although this is not of any direct relevance to real biological systems. It is the acid/base equilibrium

$$
{}^\bullet\text{OH} \quad + \quad \text{OH}^- \quad \rightleftharpoons \quad \text{O}^{\bullet-} \quad + \quad \text{H}_2\text{O} \tag{28}
$$

which the $^\bullet$OH is involved in. As can be appreciated from the high pK of 11.9 the conjugate base, O$^{\bullet-}$, may at best serve a function in principle mechanistic *in vitro* studies. But it points out a general and important property of many α-functionalized free radicals, namely, the existence of acid/base equilibria. Two examples mentioned already in this article belong to this group, namely, the α-hydroxyl radical from alcohols and the α-amino radical from amines. The pKs of the particular equilibria

$$
\text{CH}_3-\text{C}^\bullet\text{H}-\text{OH} \quad \rightleftharpoons \quad \text{CH}_3-\text{C}^\bullet\text{H}-\text{O}^- \quad + \quad \text{H}^+ \tag{29}
$$

$$
\text{CH}_3\text{S}(\text{CH}_2)_2\text{C}^\bullet\text{H}-\text{NH}_3^+ \quad \rightleftharpoons \quad \text{CH}_3\text{S}(\text{CH}_2)_2\text{C}^\bullet\text{H}-\text{NH}_2 \quad + \quad \text{H}^+ \tag{30}
$$

are 11.6 [90] and 3.85 [80], respectively, i.e., by orders of magnitude lower than for their molecular parents, ethanol and (3-methylthio)propyl amine. Could this have any general implication? Yes, because acidic and basic form often exhibit different properties. Generally, the basic form is a stronger reductant (or weaker oxidant) than the acidic form, and these radical equilibria thus constitute a redox regulating parameter. Another possible change becomes apparent in the hydroxyl radical system where the $O^{\bullet-}$, because of its negative charge, has completely lost the electrophilicity of its conjugate $^{\bullet}OH$ partner.

3.2 Peroxyl radicals

While the hydroxyl radical clearly is the most reactive among the oxygen radicals, peroxyl radicals are probably the most abundant radicals in biological systems. This conclusion emerges merely from the fact, that they are readily formed in any oxygen containing environment and generally are not as reactive as other free radical species. In principle, this group of transients would include both organic peroxyl radicals as well as superoxide. Considering their different modes of formation and chemical properties it is certainly justified, however, to deal with them in separate chapters.

Organic peroxyl radicals, generally denoted as $ROO^{\bullet}$, result from oxygen addition to practically any carbon-centered free radical ($R^{\bullet}$).

$$R^{\bullet} \quad + \quad O_2 \quad \rightarrow \quad ROO^{\bullet} \tag{31}$$

This is typically a fast, i.e., diffusion or close-to-diffusion controlled process with rate constants close or within the 10^9 M^{-1} s^{-1} range [66,69]. Variations are explained to some extent by differences in electron density at the radical site exerted by near substituents in connection with the electrophilic character of the oxygen molecule. However, this is not the only parameter. Addition of oxygen to trichloromethyl radicals, for example, – a process of great significance in the toxicology of carbontetrachloride –

$$^{\bullet}CCl_3 \quad + \quad O_2 \quad \rightarrow \quad CCl_3OO^{\bullet} \tag{32}$$

proceeds with a rate constant of 3.3×10^9 M^{-1} s^{-1}, i.e., practically as fast as that of the O_2-addition to the $^{\bullet}CH_3$ radical, despite the strong electron density withdrawing chlorine substituents [62]. A plausible explanation is provided by steric arguments. While $^{\bullet}CH_3$ is planar, $^{\bullet}CCl_3$ is pyramidal. The chlorinated radical thus offers a much more exposed site for the oxygen addition which obviously compensates for the reduced electron density.

A direct observation of organic peroxyl radicals is, in the majority of cases, difficult or impossible. ESR spectra are generally characterized by rather unspecific broad single lines, and the optical absorptions reported are usually weak and confined to the $UV < 300$ nm where they can easily be missed because of other radicals absorbing in this wavelength range. An interesting example with a VIS absorption near 500 nm has, however, been reported [91], namely, vinylperoxyl radicals of the general structure:

$$\begin{array}{c}\diagdown\\ \diagup\end{array}C=C\begin{array}{c}\diagup^{O-O^{\bullet}}\\ \diagdown\end{array}$$

The possibility of electronic resonance with the π-systems of the vinyl double bond is undoubtedly the advantageous parameter for a shift of the optical transition energy to lower values and thus higher wavelengths.

However, for the study of most peroxyl radicals and their reactions one has to rely on indirect measurements. The rate constant for the oxygen addition to the trichloromethyl radical, for example, was derived from a reaction sequence where reaction 32 was followed by reaction 33 [62,92]:

$$CCl_3OO^{\bullet} \quad + \quad phenothiazine\ (PZ) \quad \rightarrow \quad PZ^{\bullet+} \quad + \quad CCl_3OO^- \quad (33)$$

The phenothiazine radical cations (PZ = promethazine, chlorpromazine, metiazinic acid, etc.), in contrast to $CCl_3OO^{\bullet}$, show very strong and thus easily detectable absorptions [93,94]. Therefore, in order to measure the rate constant for reaction 32, it was only necessary to look at the rate of $PZ^{\bullet+}$ formation at high phenothiazine concentrations, i.e., under conditions were reaction 33 became faster than reaction 32 and consequently the oxygen addition to $^{\bullet}CCl_3$ became the rate determining step.

Reaction 33 indicates already one of the chemical properties of peroxyl radicals, particularly if they are substituted with electron withdrawing atoms like halogens: they are oxidants. Reduction potentials for $ROO^{\bullet}/ROO^-$ couples are almost unknown and only two estimates have been reported, ca 0.6 V and >1 V for the $CH_3OO^{\bullet}$ and $CCl_3OO^{\bullet}$ systems, respectively [95]. One difficulty for an unambiguous determination of such potentials arises from the fact that peroxyl radicals may not only get involved in true electron transfer processes but often oxidize their reaction partners via an addition-elimination mechanism. This seems to apply, for example, for the peroxyl radical induced oxidation of organic sulfides (R_2S, e.g., methionine) where the first step *en route* to a sulfide radical cation is an addition, followed by a substitution and equilibration of the transient three-electron bonded dimer radical cation to the molecular radical cation $R_2S^{\bullet+}$ [96].

$$R_2S \quad + \quad CCl_3OO^{\bullet} \quad \rightarrow \quad CCl_3OO-^{\bullet}SR_2 \tag{34}$$

$$CCl_3OO-^{\bullet}SR_2 \quad + \quad R_2S \quad \rightarrow \quad CCl_3OO^- \quad + \quad (R_2S \therefore SR_2)^+ \tag{35}$$

$$(R_2S \therefore SR_2)^+ \quad \rightleftharpoons \quad R_2S^{\bullet+} \quad + \quad R_2S \tag{36}$$

It will not be difficult to appreciate that such a complex mechanism cannot be linearly related to any redox potentials. Even more so, because the adduct radical, in competition with reaction 35, enters yet another pathway in which the sulfuranyl radical electron is transferred intramolecularly to the hydroperoxide moiety (under participation of water) to yield sulfoxide and a reduced hydroperoxide (which decays into the oxyl radical):

$$CCl_3-O-O-SR_2 \xrightarrow{\ H_2O\ } (CCl_3OOH)^{\bullet -} + R_2S(OH)^+$$

$$CCl_3O^\bullet + OH^- \quad H^+ + R_2SO \tag{37}$$

This latter process constitutes a most interesting mechanism in the sense that it actually describes the second step of an overall two-electron transfer initiated by a peroxyl radical. The two-electron oxidation product is the sulfoxide and the corresponding two-electron reduction counter part is the oxyl radical. Formally, this peroxyl-radical-induced sulfoxide formation via Eqs. 34 and 37, may also be viewed as oxygen atom transfer, however, studies with labeled oxygen indicate that the sulfoxide oxygen is coming from the solvent water [96]. (This does not mean that the possibility of oxygen transfer has to be dismissed in all cases; it seems to be a real possibility in the peroxyl induced oxidation of certain organic tellurides, for example) [97].

The capability of peroxyl radicals to undergo both, one-electron and two-electron processes pertains particularly for the sulfide-to-sulfoxide oxidation and would, therefore, be of special biological relevance for methionine and methionine-containing peptides and proteins. Generally, the sulfoxide yields, produced via the 2-e-mechanism, are higher than via the 1-e-mechanism [96,98] where, e.g., competing radical cation deprotonation may come into play.

Absolute rate constants for addition reactions of peroxyl radicals have hardly been measured so far but can reasonably be anticipated, at least for the above addition to sulfides, to be in the range of diffusion controlled values. Electron transfer reactions from a donor to the peroxyl show a distinct dependence on the electron density at the peroxyl radical site. The lower the latter the faster, in general, the reaction. This is nicely exemplified by a series of chloromethylperoxyl radical induced oxidations of ascorbate where the rate constant increases from 2.2×10^6 to 2.0×10^8 M^{-1} s^{-1} from $CH_3OO^\bullet$ to $CCl_3OO^\bullet$, respectively [99]. These early figures have, in the meantime, been corroborated by many more examples for 1-e-oxidation reactions of peroxyl radicals with different degrees of halogenation [69,92,95,99−102].

Besides electron transfer and addition reactions peroxyl radicals also undergo hydrogen atom abstraction reactions, and thus resemble quite similar reactivity features as $^\bullet OH$. The most important abstraction process is probably the chain carrying reaction in lipid peroxidation (with $R-H =$ PUFA) and other autoxidation processes [1,7,13,15,17,103−106]. In principle, any carbon-centered radical, $R^\bullet$, may get involved in the following reaction sequence:

$$R^\bullet \quad + \quad O_2 \quad \rightarrow \quad ROO^\bullet \tag{38}$$

$$ROO^\bullet \quad + \quad R-H \quad \rightarrow \quad ROOH \quad + \quad R^\bullet \tag{39}$$

Reaction 39 is the slower of the two processes and thus rate controlling. Not too many rate constants are known. Published values range from the $10^{-4} - 10^4$ M^{-1} s^{-1} order of magnitude [66,69] and, to mention a biologically relevant example, $k_{39} = 36$ M^{-1} s^{-1} has been reported for the peroxyl radical reaction in the autoxidation of linoleic acid [106]. It should further be mentioned that the chain length involving the above two processes significantly increases when going from homogeneous solutions to micellar aggregates [107,108] and, by extrapolation, lipids. A plausible explanation for this is the restricted diffusion of the radicals and, as a result thereof, a much lower probability for radical-radical termination processes.

In all the discussion of peroxyl radical reaction kinetics, including those for the abstraction processes, it must be recognized that peroxyl radicals are highly polarizable [109] and its electron density distribution depends to a significant extent on the polarity of the solution. Therefore, absolute rate constants will vary with the nature of the environment [110,111] in which these reactions occur and caution is advised when trying to extrapolate aqueous or specific organic solvent *in vitro* figures to, for example, cellular conditions. In first approximation, it is probably safe though to operate within the given order of magnitude.

In the absence of suitable molecular reaction partners, or if the corresponding reactions are too slow, peroxyl radicals may decay via unimolecular processes [7,21,112]. The most prominent and, from the biological point of view, most significant mechanism is a superoxide elimination. Prerequisite for this process is a sufficiently large electron delocalization into the peroxyl group. This may be achieved by simultaneous stabilization of a positive, i.e., electron deficient entity as it would be the case upon liberation of a proton. Since the latter is easily cleaved from hydroxyl groups, for example, any α-hydroxyl peroxyl radical is prone for such a process [113−117].

$$\underset{OH}{\overset{OO^\bullet}{\underset{\diagup}{\searjoin}}C} \quad \longrightarrow \quad {\overset{\diagdown}{\underset{\diagup}{}}}C{=}O \quad + \quad H^+ \quad + \quad O_2^{\bullet-} \tag{40}$$

This elimination is considered to be assisted by a transient cyclic five-membered ring structure in which the hydroxyl proton interacts with the terminal peroxyl oxygen. Typical rate constants for this first-order decay are on the order of $10^5 - 10^6$ s^{-1}, corresponding to half-lives in the lower microsecond region. The superoxide elimination becomes even faster in basic solutions [114,117] where the α-hydroxyl group increasingly equilibrates to its conjugate anion ($-OH \rightleftharpoons -O^-$).

The positive charge may also be stabilized within the remaining molecule. With a dialkylamine substituent, for example, the peroxyl radical becomes even so unstable that it actually escapes detection [118]:

$$\text{(structure)} \longrightarrow \text{(structure)} \quad C = \overset{+}{N}R_2 \quad + \quad O_2^{\bullet-} \qquad (41)$$

Steric arguments can also be forwarded to rationalize intramolecular hydrogen abstraction or addition reactions by peroxyl groups. Five- and six-membered ring structures would thus facilitate hydroperoxide and epoxide formations (the latter via an endoperoxide radical) [21,119]. Respective examples are given in the following:

$$\qquad (42)$$

$$\qquad (43)$$

The actual rates of these processes depend very much on the electronic influence exerted by the substituents near the reactive sites.

Finally, if there are neither suitable reaction partners nor the possibility for intramolecular conversion, the peroxyl radicals will suffer the ultimate free radical fate, namely, a bimolecular radical-radical deactivation. The actual mechanism of the generalized process

$$\text{ROO}^\bullet \quad + \quad \text{ROO}^\bullet \quad \rightarrow \quad [\text{ROO}-\text{OOR}] \quad \rightarrow \quad \text{products} \quad (44)$$

may be quite manifold but is considered, in any case, to proceed via an intermediate tetroxide. At room temperature these tetroxides are usually not stable enough for analytical detection. Their transitory existence seems beyond doubt though as emerges from low temperature studies [120,122] as well as from the following mechanistic considerations.

Generally, the bimolecular termination reactions (Eq. 44) are quite fast in terms of rate constants, and long lifetimes result mostly only because of the low steady-state concentrations of these radicals. This pertains, in particular for primary and secondary peroxyl radicals, i.e., those which still carry at least one hydrogen atom at the peroxyl carbon. Many measured bimolecular rate constants on the order of 10^9 M^{-1} s^{-1} ($2k_{40}$) indicate diffusion controlled processes

[66,69]. Deviations to lower values can mostly be rationalized in terms of steric hindrance. Tertiary peroxyl radicals, on the other hand, terminate with significantly lower rate constants, e.g., $2k = 2 \times 10^4 \text{ M}^{-1} \text{ s}^{-1}$ for *tert*-butylperoxyl [123]. This probably does not only reflect steric constraints but also the smaller number of possible reaction channels available, as compared with primary and secondary peroxyl radicals.

Tertiary peroxyl radicals, $R_3COO^\bullet$, practically all decay via the tetroxide and by subsequent oxygen elimination to the respective oxyl radicals (the three substituents R do not need to be identical):

$$2 \, R_3COO^\bullet \quad \rightarrow \quad [R_3COOOOCR_3] \quad \rightarrow \quad 2 \, R_3CO^\bullet \; + \; O_2 \qquad (45)$$

The further chemistry is then that of the oxyl radical which will be discussed in detail in a later chapter.

This type of reaction may also apply to primary and secondary peroxyl radicals where at least one R=H. However, for these species additional routes become possible. The most preferred pathway is, in fact, a cyclic mechanism known as "Russell mechanism", the key element of which is considered to be a cyclic six-membered transition structure of the tetroxide [124]. Three bond ruptures and a hydrogen transfer directly yields one molecule of oxygen, an alcohol and an aldehyde or ketone. From the redox point of view this constitutes a disproportionation.

$$\text{(46)}$$

An interesting aspect in this mechanism is the possible generation of single oxygen, $^1O_2$, which has been claimed to be formed in organic solutions [125,126]. In aqueous solutions, on the other hand, the natural triplet oxygen, $^3O_2$, seems to be cleaved which is then, however, accompanied by a triplet excited carbonyl compound [127].

Another decay mode of the tetroxide leads to two carbonyl molecules and, instead of oxygen, to hydrogenperoxide (R = H and $\neq$ H):

$$[R_2HCOOOOCHR_2] \quad \rightarrow \quad 2 \, R_2C{=}0 \; + \; H_2O_2 \qquad (47)$$

This alternative pathway is also considered to involve cyclic transition structures which, in aqueous solution, probably include water molecules [21,112,128].

In addition to these general features there are further specific characteristics to certain peroxides which are mainly attributable to individual structural and electronic parameters. This is not the place to present and discuss any of them in greater detail (for more information see [21,112]), and just one group-specific example shall be mentioned here. Thus, all peroxyl radicals generated as a result of oxidative or reductive radical attack at aromatics show a high tendency to embark on reaction routes which re-establish the aromaticity. This clearly reflects thermodynamic stability criteria. A specific example is the ·OH-induced oxidation of benzene in oxygenated solution for which phenol is formed as final product with about 60% efficiency via the following route [21]:

(48)

Some further words also about halogenated peroxyl radicals: As mentioned above most bimolecular peroxyl termination processes lead to alcohols and aldehydes as stable molecular products. If any of the hydrogen substituents at the hydroxyl-carrying or carbonyl carbon is a halogen atom then these compounds (α-halo-alcohols, "α-haloaldehydes" = acyl halides) assume, in fact, a higher oxidation state and, upon hydrolysis, directly convert into aldehydes/ketones and acids, respectively [65,129,130]:

$$> CH-OH \qquad > CX-OH \xrightarrow{\quad (H_2O) \quad} \quad > C=O \qquad (49)$$
alcohol   *α-haloalcohol*   *aldehyde/ketone*

$$-CH=O \qquad -CX=O \xrightarrow{\quad (H_2O) \quad} \quad -COOH \qquad (50)$$
aldehyde   *acyl halide*   *acid*

Any metabolic degradation of halogenated organic material, proceeding via peroxyl radicals as intermediates, would thus yield aldehydes and acids. The bad reputation of aldehydes as toxins is well known [131], and the organic acid (in combination of the inorganic acid H^+/X^- released in the hydrolysis processes) may exert a harmful influence due to pH changes.

3.3 Reversible oxygen addition

Addition reactions, as organic chemistry has shown in many examples, inherently seem to include the possibility to be reversed. Free radical addition to a double bond and subsequent β-scission, in principle, also fall into this category although the cleaved radical may not be identical with the incoming one:

$$R^· \; + \; -C(Y) = C< \; \rightleftharpoons \; -C(R)(Y) - C^·< \; \rightleftharpoons \; -C(R) = C< \; + \; Y^· \qquad (51)$$

The question whether a reaction is reversible or not is of principle significance.

Any irreversible process is a once-and-forever event. A reversible reaction, however, always means an equilibrium which may have a preferred side but has not closed the door yet for the back reaction. And most important, any substrate which engages a "minority" component in an irreversible reaction pulls eventually the entire equilibrium back to the "wrong side". An instructive example is a thiyl radical mediated degradation of carbontetrachloride in the presence of *iso*-propanol [132—135] where the equilibrium

$$\text{RS}^{\bullet} \quad + \quad (\text{CH}_3)_2\text{CHOH} \quad \rightleftharpoons \quad \text{RSH} \quad + \quad (\text{CH}_3)_2\text{C}^{\bullet}\text{OH} \tag{52}$$

lies far on the left hand side. It may, nevertheless, completely be shifted to the right in the presence of CCl_4 which engages the iso-propanol radical in a dissociative, i.e., irreversible electron transfer reaction:

$$(\text{CH}_3)_2\text{C}^{\bullet}\text{OH} + \text{CCl}_4 \quad \rightleftharpoons \quad (\text{CH}_3)_2\text{CO} + \text{H}^+ + \text{Cl}^- + {}^{\bullet}\text{CCl}_3 \tag{53}$$

What about a possible reversibility of oxygen addition to free radicals? The answer is: Yes, it may well occur but it depends on the nature of the addition center and seems connected with the electrophilicity of the molecular oxygen [21]. Practically no addition has ever been observed, at least at room temperature, to organic oxygen-centered radicals, i.e., the possible reaction if occurring at all, must be reversible with the equilibrium way on the left hand side.

$$-\text{O}^{\bullet-} \quad + \quad \text{O}_2 \quad \rightleftharpoons \quad -\text{O}-\text{OO}^{\bullet} \tag{54}$$

This pertains to all oxyl and peroxyl radicals. An interesting exception is the basic form of the hydroxyl radical, $\text{O}^{\bullet-}$, which in the presence of oxygen has been reported to form the ozonide radical anion, $\text{O}_3^{\bullet-}$ [136].

Carbon-centered free radicals are generally prone for irreversible oxygen addition. However, there are some examples also for a reversible process. One of them is the addition of O_2 to the hydroxyhexadienyl radical formulated in Eq. 48. Here, the peroxyl radical is formed with a rate constant of $3.1 \times 10^8 \text{ M}^{-1} \text{ s}^{-1}$ ($t_{1/2} \approx 8$ ms in air saturated solution) and the back reaction, i.e., the re-elimination of oxygen occurs with $1.2 \times 10^4 \text{ s}^{-1}$ ($t_{1/2} \approx 57$ ms [137].

A biologically most relevant example is the oxygen addition to those pentadienyl-type PUFA radicals [138,139] which result from abstraction of the particularly labile bisallyllic hydrogens by practically any kind of reactive free radical, even $\text{RS}^{\bullet}$ [86] and $\text{ROO}^{\bullet}$ [69]. An interesting feature in this context is also that oxygen preferentially does not add to the bisallylic site but to a resonance form thereof with the result of a thermodynamically favorable conjugate double bond structure [139—141]:

$$\tag{55}$$

The peroxyl radical, incidentally, exhibits the same UV absorption (234 nm) which is characteristic for conjugated dienes, in general.

Another example for reversible oxygen addition, and also of particular biological relevance, is provided by thiyl free radicals. For quite some time and various reasons in dispute, there seems to be convincing evidence now for an equilibrium between thiyl and thioperoxyl radicals [142−145]:

$$RS^{\bullet} \quad + \quad O_2 \quad \rightleftharpoons \quad RSOO^{\bullet} \tag{56}$$

Rate constants for the forward reaction and back reactions of about 2×10^9 M^{-1} s^{-1} and 6×10^5 s^{-1}, respectively, have been measured and they appear to be independent on the nature of R. Accordingly, an equilibrium constant of about 3×10^3 M^{-1} applies. (Measured values refer to cysteine, glutathione and 2-mercaptoethanol).

Does such a reversible oxygen addition to a sulfur-centered free radical make sense? From the electronic point of view certainly yes. The electronegativity of sulfur lies in between that of oxygen and carbon, and, as we have seen before, oxygen does not add to oxygen-centered free radicals (i.e., an "addition" is highly reversible) while most of the respective processes with carbon-centered free radicals seem irreversible.

The chemistry of thioperoxyl radicals has not yet completely been revealed and still leaves open questions particularly with respect to the redox properties of RSOO$^{\bullet}$. In part, this is probably due to the above equilibrium (Eq. 56). Further complicating factors with respect to establishing a reliable and quantitative picture arise from side reactions [145−150]. A most interesting one is a rearrangement by which the oxygen-centered is converted to a sulfur-centered sulfonyl free radical [146]. This process, depicted in Eq. 57, is of considerable significance because the sulfonyl radical can add another molecule of oxygen to yield a sulfonyl peroxyl radical [146,151] which itself is considered to be a precursor of sulfonic acids.

$$R-S-O-O^{\bullet} \quad \xrightarrow{\quad O \quad} \quad R-\overset{\overset{\displaystyle O}{\|}}{\underset{\underset{\displaystyle O}{\|}}{S}}^{\bullet} \quad \left(RSO_2^{\bullet}\right) \tag{57}$$

$$RSO_2^{\bullet} \quad + \quad O_2 \quad \rightarrow \quad RSO_2OO^{\bullet} \quad \rightarrow \rightarrow \rightarrow \quad RSO_3H \tag{58}$$

3.4 Alkoxyl radicals

We have learned already that oxyl radicals may be formed *en route* of the peroxyl radical decay. One direct possibility to generate them is by hydrogen atom abstraction from a hydroxyl group, e.g., in the $^{\bullet}$OH reaction with an alcohol:

$$R-OH \quad + \quad {}^{\bullet}OH \quad \rightarrow \quad R-O^{\bullet} \quad + \quad H_2O \qquad\qquad (59)$$

This reaction competes, of course, with the C–H cleavage in other parts of the molecule, particularly in α-position to the hydroxyl group, as discussed already in the chapter on ${}^{\bullet}OH$ reactions. The yield of O–H cleavage in aliphatic compounds or, better, detectable alkoxyl radicals appears pretty small and attains, at most, ca 7% relative to the reacting ${}^{\bullet}OH$ in the case of methanol [88]. This figure might, however, only represent a lower limit. As we shall see later there is a fast intramolecular rearrangement (1,2-hydrogen shift) which may take place with certain oxyl radicals and thus obscure part of the initial yield.

Oxyl radicals are also generated upon reductive degradation of peroxides and hydroperoxides. The key feature of the underlying reaction is that the incoming electron is accommodated in an antibonding σ* orbital which causes an O–O bond lengthening and thus prepares it for easier rupture.

$$R-O-O-R(H) \; + \; e^- \; \rightarrow \; [R-O\therefore O-R(H)]^- \; \rightarrow \; RO^{\bullet} \; + \; {}^-OR(H) \quad (60)$$

This mechanism is, incidentally the same, as for the reduction of H_2O_2 (resulting in ${}^{\bullet}OH + OH^-$ formation) and disulfides [75,149–153] (resulting in $RS^{\bullet} + RS^-$ formation) (for further details on this latter process and the three-electron bond "$\therefore$" notation, see section on sulfur-centered free radicals below). The intermediate $(R-O \therefore O-R)^-$ radical anion is generally much too short-lived as to become of direct chemical significance or to establish a measurable equilibrium with the oxyl radical.

Reaction 60 reminds us of the well-documented Fenton-Haber-Weiss process. Whenever the reductive power of enzymatic systems may not be sufficient for an electron transfer to peroxides and hydroperoxides this function can be served by low oxidation state metal ions, particularly iron-(II) or copper-(I). The biologically most relevant reaction

$$ROOH \quad + \quad Fe\text{-}(II) \quad \rightarrow \quad RO^{\bullet} \quad + \quad OH^- \quad + \quad Fe\text{-}(III) \quad (61)$$

thus becomes understandable in view of the same electronic concept as outlined above for the general peroxide reduction mechanism.

The most basic chemical property of alkoxyl radicals is that they are oxidizing species and may be detected through their reaction with an electron donor, e.g., iodide [88,154]:

$$RO^{\bullet} \quad + \quad 2\,I^- \quad \rightarrow \quad I_2^{\bullet -} \quad + \quad RO^- \qquad\qquad (62)$$

Alkoxyl radicals also engage in hydrogen atom abstraction reactions, a process which usually requires, however, considerable activation energy:

$$RO^\bullet \quad + \quad R'–H \quad \rightarrow \quad ROH \quad + \quad R'^\bullet \tag{63}$$

Although these oxidizing reactions are quite significant they probably do not constitute the most important characteristic of the alkoxyl radicals. Two features need particular attention, a 1,2-hydrogen shift and a β-scission process. Both occur at very short time scales and result in completely different chemical systems.

The 1,2-hydrogen shift may be formulated as an intramolecular process but, at least in aqueous or protic environment, it has probably to be viewed as solvent assisted [155–157]:

$$
\begin{array}{ccc}
\overset{\displaystyle H}{\underset{\displaystyle |}{|}} & & \\
-\overset{|}{\underset{|}{C}}-O^\bullet & \xrightarrow{\quad O \quad} & -\overset{\bullet}{\underset{|}{C}}-OH \\
\end{array}
\tag{64}
$$

For our further discussion two aspects are important. First, the half-life of this rearrangement is typically on the order of a microsecond. In order to compete, even a diffusion controlled bimolecular reaction of the oxyl radical requires as much as 100 μM or more of oxidizable substrate. As pointed out above, this fast rearrangement may be a likely cause for α-hydrogen substituted oxyl radicals to escape direct detection. The second important consequence of the 1,2-hydrogen shift is that it converts the oxidizing oxyl radical into a, usually strongly, reducing α-hydroxyl radical. In other words, it dramatically changes the redox properties of the radical species.

Whenever the oxyl carrying carbon is not substituted with hydrogen, as in the case of a tertiary oxyl radical, a β-scission process becomes a dominant pathway:

$$
\begin{array}{ccc}
\overset{\displaystyle R}{\underset{\displaystyle |}{|}} & & \\
R-\overset{|}{\underset{|}{C}}-O^\bullet & \xrightarrow{\hspace{2cm}} & R^\bullet \quad + \quad R_2CO \\
\overset{\displaystyle |}{\underset{\displaystyle R}{}} & & \\
\end{array}
\tag{65}
$$

This elimination process constitutes practically the reverse of a radical addition to a C=O double bond and, therefore, reaction 65 should, in principle, be formulated as an equilibrium. Efficient back reaction would require $R^\bullet$, however, to be a good nucleophile since the site of addition is the carbon atom, i.e., the more positive of the two atoms in the carbonyl bond. But as the majority of radicals seem electrophilic in nature most β-scissions appear, indeed, fast and irreversible. The actual rates involved, both for the cleavage and possible readdition, depend, of course, on the identity of $R^\bullet$, possible resonance stabilizations, and steric parameters.

Some biologically relevant consequences of this β-scission are probably be worth pointing out. Firstly, there is no reason to restrict this process only to tertiary oxyl radicals. The same may happen with hydrogen substituted species as well, e.g.,

$$
\begin{array}{ccc}
\text{H} & & \text{HCHO} \\
| & & \\
\text{R} - \text{C} - \text{O}^{\bullet} & \longrightarrow & \text{R}^{\bullet} \quad + \\
| & & \\
\text{H(R)} & & \text{RCHO}
\end{array}
\tag{66}
$$

It must only be recognized, however, that β-cleavage of a hydrogen atom itself, i.e., $R_2CHO^{\bullet} \rightarrow H^{\bullet} + R_2CO$ does not take place. Whether or not reaction 66 occurs effectively is mainly a question of competition with the 1,2-hydrogen shift (Eq. 64). If it has a chance against the latter then it opens a route to aldehyde formation.

Another potentially interesting aspect is associated with halogenated oxyl radicals. The radical cleaved by β-scission may, in this case, be a halogen atom. For example, the carbon tetrachloride derived $CCl_3O^{\bullet}$ would liberate $Cl^{\bullet}$ atoms, leaving behind a molecule of phosgene, CCl_2O:

$$
CCl_3O^{\bullet} \quad \rightarrow \quad Cl^{\bullet} \quad + \quad CCl_2O
\tag{67}
$$

What about other halogen atoms? The following observation [158], made with oxyl radicals from halogenated acetic acids, reveals not only some significant (although, in view of bond strength considerations, probably not unexpected) difference between fluorine and the other halogens but it also stresses the need for individual product analysis before final conclusions on mechanisms and potential toxicity should be made. For example, in the following fluorinated model oxyl radical, $^{\bullet}OCF_2-CO_2^-$, in principle two β-cleavage processes may be envisaged, one involving C–F bond breakage with $F^{\bullet}$ elimination (Eq. 68a) and the other involving C–C breakage with $CO_2^{\bullet-}$ as remaining radical (Eq. 68b).

$$
\begin{array}{l}
\text{F} \\
| \\
^{\bullet}\text{O} - \text{C} - \text{CO}_2^- \\
| \\
\text{F}
\end{array}
\qquad
\begin{cases}
\longrightarrow\!\!\!/\!\!/ & F^{\bullet} \quad + \quad CF(O){-}CO_2^- \tag{68a} \\
\\
\longrightarrow & CO_2^{\bullet-} \quad + \quad CF_2O \tag{68b}
\end{cases}
$$

The actual mechanism proceeds exclusively via C–C cleavage, as proven by the ultimate products CO_2 and fluoride (involving Eqs. 69 and 70 in oxygenated solution).

$$
CO_2^{\bullet-} \quad + \quad O_2 \quad \rightarrow \quad CO_2 \quad + \quad O_2^{\bullet-}
\tag{69}
$$

$$
CF_2O \quad + \quad H_2O \quad \rightarrow \quad CO_2 \quad + \quad 2\,F^- \,/\, 2\,H^+
\tag{70}
$$

Corroborating support is provided by the complete lack of oxalate which has been shown to result upon hydrolysis of $CF(O)-CO_2^-$ [159].

The bromine and chlorine analogues, on the other hand, decay quantitatively via carbon-halogen bond cleavage, i.e., under formation of bromine and chlorine atoms. In this case all the halogens also end up as halide ions, Br^- and Cl^-, eventually.

$$
\begin{array}{c}
Br^\bullet \;+\; CBr(O)\text{--}CO_2^- \\
Cl^\bullet \;+\; CCl(O)\text{--}CO_2^-
\end{array} \qquad (71a)
$$

$$
\underset{\overset{|}{Br\,(Cl)}}{\overset{\overset{|}{Br\,(Cl)}}{^\bullet O - C - CO_2^-}}
$$

$$
CO_2^{\bullet-} \;+\; \begin{array}{c} CBr_2O \\ CCl_2O \end{array} \qquad (71b)
$$

With respect to the fate of the carbon skeleton, however, yet another interesting and perhaps surprising aspect emerged. Both, the oxaloyl bromide and chloride do not hydrolyse to oxalic acid as the oxaloyl fluoride but suffer $C\text{--}C$ cleavage to generate CO and CO_2 at a 1:1 molecular ratio [159].

$$
CBr(O)\text{--}CO_2^- \,/\, CCl(O)\text{--}CO_2^- \;\underline{\quad\quad}\; (H_2O) \;\rightarrow\; CO \;+\; CO_2 \;+\; Br^- \,/\, Cl^- \quad (72)
$$

The formation of carbon monoxide as well as of the halogen atoms is, of course, a most significant outcome from a toxicological point of view.

Finally, a general consequence of any $C\text{--}C$ cleavage in the β-scission process in an oxyl radical should be recognized, namely, the shortening of the carbon chain by one carbon unit. The eliminated radical $R^\bullet$ is, of course, again a potential target for oxygen addition, and after going through another possible peroxyl and oxyl radical chemistry cycle, it may be prone for a further β-scission. This may carry on and on until eventually a long aliphatic chain has been completely broken down into C_1-units.

3.5 Phenoxyl radicals

Most features displayed and discussed for the formation and properties of alkoxyl radicals in the previous chapter also apply for phenoxyl-type free radicals, i.e., for species where the aliphatic (R) has been replaced by an aromatic substituent (Ar). Thus formation of $ArO^\bullet$ is easily achieved by oxidation of the phenolic group, either by hydrogen abstraction or one-electron oxidation of the phenolate. The latter is a much more feasible process than for the aliphatic substrates, particularly in view of its biological relevance, since the pK of phenols is much closer to physiological pH than that of alcohols.

Mechanistically the free radical induced oxidation of a phenolic hydroxyl group is, however, often not a simple one-step process. Hydroxyl radicals, for example, typically add to the aromatic π-system in the first instance and subsequently eliminate H_2O in an acid-catalyzed second step:

$$(73)$$

This is important, for example, in view of the radical's reactivity towards molecular oxygen. Whilst the phenoxyl, being an oxygen-centered radical, is practically unreactive in this respect, the carbon-centered $^\bullet$OH-adduct radical is prone for peroxyl radical formation. And furthermore, as we have seen before, hydroxylated peroxyl radicals may cleave superoxide. In other words, any $^\bullet$OH-induced oxidation of a phenol in oxygenated environment bears the potential of superoxide formation [21,112].

Phenoxyl radicals are moderately good oxidants with reported reduction potentials for the ArO$^\bullet$/ArO$^-$ couples in the 400—1,000 mV range for phenol derivatives at pH 7 [70]. The actual values differ considerably and depend strongly on the other substituents. Naturally, the possibility to delocalize electron density within aromatic structures affects the actual oxidative power of the radical oxygen site.

An important reaction phenoxyl-type free radicals readily undergo is the oxidation of ascorbate (AH$^-$, Vit C). This pertains, in particular, to the most prominent of them, the chromanoxyl radical derived from α-tocopherol (Vit E) [160]. The reaction

$$\text{VitE } (-O^\bullet) \quad + \quad AH^- \quad \rightarrow \quad \text{VitE } (-OH) \quad + \quad A^{\bullet-} \qquad (74)$$

presumably constitutes the most important repair mechanism of this vital antioxidant. Although the stoichiometry looks like a hydrogen transfer reaction 74 appears, nevertheless, to be based on an electron transfer.

Finally, let us consider a very special problem which, however, touches on a general aspect of phenoxyl radicals, particularly those derived from Vit E and related substrates. Some recent studies with the water soluble Vit E analogue Trolox C (I) [161,162] have revealed (and in part substantiate earlier findings) [163] that certain quinoid and prequinoid products arise from the chromanoxyl radical which cannot be explained exclusively on the basis of an oxygen-centered radical (II) alone. Assuming, however, participation of carbon-centered resonance forms such as (III), a disproportionation process via a carbocation (IV) intermediate can be envisaged which leads directly to a lactone (V) and, after hydrolysis of the latter, to an open-chain substituted quinone (VI), both of which have been identified as products in the $^\bullet$OH-induced oxidation of Trolox C.

$$(75)$$

(III) $\xrightarrow{\text{disproportionation}}$ (structure) (IV)

(75a)

(IV) $\longrightarrow$ (structure V) $\xrightarrow{\text{hydrolysis}}$ (structure VI)

(V)   (VI)

(75b)

The general message is, not to neglect possible electronic resonance structures, particularly when the predominant form of the radical is relatively unreactive.

3.6 Semiquinone radicals

Semiquinones may be viewed as just a special kind of phenoxyl radicals. They typically involve resonance structures under participation of another oxygen function at the aromatic ring. To some extent even the chromanoxyl radicals fall into this category. The classical semiquinone is a one-electron intermediate between two relatively stable compounds, hydroquinones and quinones.

(structure) $\underset{}{\overset{-e^-/-H^+}{\rightleftharpoons}}$ (structure) $\underset{}{\overset{-e^-/-H^+}{\rightleftharpoons}}$ (structure)

(76)

As many free radicals do, also the semiquinone establishes an acid-base equilibrium in which the remaining hydroxyl group deprotonates. The respective pK_a values of

$$Q(H)^\bullet \;\; \rightleftharpoons \;\; Q^{\bullet -} \;\; + \;\; H^+ \tag{77}$$

are typically in the range around 4, i.e., the prevailing form under physiological conditions is the anionic species, $Q^{\bullet -}$.

A characteristic feature of the semiquinone radicals is that they are not as good oxidants as simple phenoxyl radicals, with pH 7 reduction potentials of the semiquinone/ hydroquinone couples being around 400 mV for various 1,4-dihydroxybenzenes [66e,70]. In fact, semiquinones are generally more of a reductant. This is reflected, for example, in their role of biological electron shuttle agents in the photosystem, and also in an electron transfer equilibrium with molecular oxygen and quinone (Q) [164]:

$$Q^{\bullet-} \;+\; O_2 \;\rightleftharpoons\; Q \;+\; O_2^{\bullet-} \tag{78}$$

Semiquinones may thus effectively contribute to the superoxide formation in biological systems. The actual reduction potentials of the $Q/Q^{\bullet-}$ couples depend, of course, on the structure of the individual quinone involved but they are generally close to that of the $O_2/O_2^{\bullet-}$ couple (see chapter 2.7 on reduction potentials, pp. 19–21).

3.7 Superoxide ($O_2^{\bullet-}$, $HO_2^{\bullet}$)

Superoxide is probably the most discussed and investigated among the biologically relevant oxygen radicals. Chemically, it is, however, a rather simple species and, in addition what has been said already in previous chapters, there is little more to add (see also two informative review articles [165,166]). As mentioned, superoxide is formed either by direct electron attachment to molecular oxygen, through some electron transfer reactions from other free radicals (e.g., disulfide radical anions or $CO_2^{\bullet-}$), or via elimination reactions from certain peroxyl radicals. It exists in an acid-base equilibrium with a pK_a of 4.8 [67], i.e., under physiological conditions the anionic form clearly prevails:

$$HO_2^{\bullet} \;\rightleftharpoons\; O_2^{\bullet-} \;+\; H^+ \tag{79}$$

It must be recognized though that any $O_2^{\bullet-}$ which might find access to a less polar environment may protonate due to a shift in pK_a, and thus assume the properties of the undissociated $HO_2^{\bullet}$.

$O_2^{\bullet-}$ itself is a moderate reductant and transfers an electron to, for example, cytochrome-c-(III) [167], and is involved in electron exchange equilibria with quinones, as mentioned above. $HO_2^{\bullet}$, on the other hand, is not as good a reductant but rather engages in oxidation reactions [67] and it would not be surprising if some of the reported oxidations by $O_2^{\bullet-}$ of, e.g., hydroquinones were, in fact, due to the conjugate acid radical.

The decay of superoxide, unless enzymatically assisted by SOD [9], proceeds fastest via the mutual $HO_2^{\bullet}/O_2^{\bullet-}$ reaction (with a rate constant of 10^8 M^{-1} s^{-1} [67])

$$HO_2^{\bullet} \;+\; O_2^{\bullet-} \;\rightarrow\; HO_2^- \;(H_2O_2) \;+\; O_2 \tag{80}$$

while both the $HO_2^{\bullet} + HO_2^{\bullet}$ and $O_2^{\bullet-} + O_2^{\bullet-}$ reactions occur much more slowly [168]. This is particularly true for the superoxide anion decay. The $O_2^{\bullet-}$ is, in fact, a very stable species in the absence of a suitable reaction partner, a property which translates, of course, into relatively long pathways over which it may be transported.

One other reaction of superoxide must, however, also be mentioned in this context and that is its possible cross-termination with peroxyl radicals. Although only few data exist so far [169−171], it appears that this process, namely,

$$ROO^\bullet \quad + \quad O_2^{\bullet-} \quad \rightarrow \rightarrow \rightarrow \quad \text{products} \tag{81}$$

kinetically dominates over the competing mutual self-terminations (described in Eqs. 44–47, and 80). In a recent extensive study involving a halogenated model peroxyl radical, $^\bullet CF_2CO_2^-$, it was, in fact, quantitatively demonstrated that cross-termination under any circumstances accounted for at least 80%, often 100% of the peroxyl or superoxide decay [171]. The difficulty of these studies is that the products from reaction 81 and the peroxyl self-termination are often identical, thus preventing a distinction. Unambiguous quantification may, however, become possible through the hydrogen peroxide yields since cross-termination typically does not result in H_2O_2 formation and thus significantly lowers the yield of this product otherwise derived from the superoxide self-termination.

4 SULFUR-CENTERED FREE RADICALS

In several chapters we have come across free radicals with the unpaired electron located at the higher homologue atom to oxygen, namely, sulfur. In view of the very interesting redox chemistry of sulfur-centered free radicals and the recently increased focus on redox regulation of molecular processes in the bio sciences it is probably quite appropriate not only to summarize once more these various aspects under this separate headline but also to elaborate a little further on the role such radicals play in the context of thiol and disulfide chemistry.

The most important of the sulfur-centered intermediates is probably the thiyl radical, $RS^\bullet$ [172,173]. It may be generated via oxidation of thiols as well as by reduction of the corresponding disulfides. The former typically occurs as hydrogen atom abstraction by, in principle, almost any radical whenever the thiol prevails in its neutral form. Examples have been formulated in reaction 24 and in the back reaction of Eq. 52. Oxidation of thiolate, the conjugate base of the thiol, is likely to occur via an electron transfer, as formulated in the following equation with a general oxidizing radical $X^\bullet$:

$$RS^- \quad + \quad X^\bullet \quad \rightarrow \quad RS^\bullet \quad + \quad X^- \tag{82}$$

The possibility of this reaction is basically controlled by the respective redox potentials which for the $RS^\bullet/RS^-$ couple typically are of the order of 0.7–0.8 V (vs. NHE) [70,173a]. Accordingly, any oxidant more potent than $RS^\bullet$ may, in principle, engage in this process. This has been verified, for example, for the $Br_2^{\bullet-}$ reactions with $CysS^-$ [174] and $PenS^-$ [175], respectively, the $(CH_3SSCH_3)^{\bullet+}$-induced oxidation of $CysS^-$, $CyaS^-$ and $PenS^-$ [175] and, possibly even more relevant from the biological point of view, for the reaction of the lipoate radical cation Lip(SS)$^{\bullet+}$ (E° = 1.10 V) with these conjugate bases of cysteine, cysteamine and penicillamine [175]. Rate constants, ranging from $(1.1–3.7) \times 10^9$ M^{-1} s^{-1} for the above-mentioned reactions, indicate that the electron transfer occurs almost diffusion controlled.

With respect to the oxidation of thiolate (e.g., RS$^-$ of cysteine, cysteamine, *N*-acetyl-L-cysteine) it is noted that the rate constants for the reaction of $^{\bullet}$OH + RS$^-$ are practically the same as for the reaction of $^{\bullet}$OH with RSH [176,177] ($\approx 3 \times 10^9$ M^{-1} s^{-1}) although the respective mechanisms are presumably quite different. While the reaction with the thiols clearly has to be viewed as a hydrogen atom abstraction, the corresponding reaction with the thiolate is likely to be an electron transfer. The positive redox potential of the hydroxyl radical, E°[$^{\bullet}$OH/OH$^-$] = 1.9 V [70], provides the necessary driving force.

The other mechanism by which thiyl radicals are readily formed is by reduction of disulfides as formulated in the following general reaction:

$$RSSR \quad + \quad e^- \quad \rightarrow \quad RS^{\bullet} \quad + \quad RS^- \tag{83}$$

This process is generally very fast and efficient, i.e., controlled only by the diffusion of the reaction partners. The electron itself may be, for example, a hydrated (solvated) electron, an electron transferred from a reducing radical, electrode, semiconductor, or an enzymatically provided one.

For a full understanding of the disulfide reduction it must be recognized that Eq. 83 gives only a very simplified overall summary of this process [153,172]. The detailed mechanism is much more complex and interesting. Please note that the incoming electron finds two electronically already rather satisfied sulfur atoms (total of eight electrons around each sulfur with four in bonding and four in nonbonding mode). So, where does it go? Sulfur-d-orbitals may be one consideration but this is energetically not feasible, nor are the alkyl groups suitable sites for electron attachment. The answer is an antibonding σ*-orbital of the existing S–S bond, so that this bond after the reduction contains two bonding σ-electrons and one bond-weakening σ*-electron. This 2-center-3-electron bond is generally denoted with a "∴" symbol. The effect of the antibonding σ*-electron, in fact, drives the two sulfur atoms apart and provides the basis for the establishment of a reversible dissociation equilibrium, i.e.:

$$RS-SR \quad + \quad e^- \quad \rightarrow \quad [RS \therefore SR]^- \quad \rightleftharpoons \quad RS^{\bullet} \quad + \quad RS^- \tag{84}$$

One immediately emerging consequence is that the transient disulfide radical cation is not only formed via disulfide reduction but also by association of thiyl radicals with thiolate. Furthermore, the lifetime of [RS∴SR]$^-$ is practically controlled by the thiolate concentration which, in turn, in thiol containing systems is a function of both, the total thiol concentration and the pH. In thiol-free solutions, half-lives of as short as a few hundred nanoseconds have been measured for the above equilibrium (K $\approx 10^{-3}$ M), involving the reduction of simple aliphatic disulfides. Here, the RS$^\bullet$ and RS$^-$ components may freely diffuse apart once the sulfur-sulfur bond has been broken. Much longer lifetimes (up to milliseconds) are, however, obtained with increasing thiolate concentration or, and this is particularly interesting, if RS$^\bullet$ and RS$^-$ are prevented from diffusing apart through backbone linkage. The latter is the case in, for example, lipoic acid but may also be anticipated in proteins and many other macromolecular structures with either disulfide linkage or closely positioned thiol groups.

The [RS$\therefore$SR]$^-$/RS$^\bullet$ equilibrium is of utmost importance because it strongly affects the overall redox behavior of the environment in which these two species coexist. While the thiyl radical is a moderately good oxidant [178], as outlined above in connection with Eq. 82, the disulfide radical anion is a reductant (E$^\circ$ $\approx$ −1.6 V) [154], capable of reducing, for example, molecular oxygen [179−181].

$$[RS\therefore SR]^- \quad + \quad O_2 \quad \rightarrow \quad RSSR \quad + \quad O_2^{\bullet-} \tag{85}$$

Reaction 85 leads us directly into the chemistry (and potential problems) of superoxide.

The variety of other reactions the thiyl radical RS$^\bullet$ may undergo need not be repeated here since they have been mentioned and discussed already in connection with Eqs. 52, 55 and 56. In summary, it is, however, noteworthy that thiyl radicals may engage in quite a number of equilibria and reactions involving molecular oxygen and oxygen-centered free radicals.

5 CONCLUSION

In this survey we have discussed the majority of the oxygen-centered and some sulfur-centered radicals with particular emphasis on general features of free radical chemistry. Nevertheless, this article can still not claim to provide a comprehensive coverage of all detailed information available up to now, nor was it intended to do. The exciting chemistry of singlet oxygen [1,6,182−185] or ozone [13,184], and species derived therefrom certainly warrants equal attention. Or, to go beyond the oxygen-centered species, many more sulfur-centered radicals [19], or the nitrogen-centered NOX (particularly NO [186−188]) free radicals are undoubtedly of similar interest and biological significance. Much has been documented in books, reviews and summarizing conference reports, and more information will unquestionably emerge from present days and future research. All of this will reflect, however, the fundamental chemical characteristics of radicals, and it is hoped that this article has provided some useful basis for the chemical understanding of those biological phenomena which can be related to these highly reactive species.

6 SUMMARY

This chapter on *Free Radical Chemistry* comprises of two main sections. In the first part some important general properties of free radicals are discussed. (i) A free radical is introduced as a species with an unpaired electron. (ii) As a consequence thereof, free radicals are usually highly reactive species. (iii) The knowledge of their chemical properties and absolute rate constants for their reactions is an indispensable requirement to assess any possible activity of free radicals. (iv) This information is best obtained by application of time-resolved detection techniques such as the radiation chemical method of pulse radiolysis and, complementary to this, laser flash photolysis. (v) Structural information on free radicals is mainly achieved by application of electron spin resonance (ESR); in biological systems spin trapping techniques are of particular value. (vi) Further useful information on the reactivity of free radicals may be obtained from redox potential measurements, and can also be deduced from stable products of free radical reactions.

In the second part of this article the most important oxygen-centered and thiyl free radicals are discussed in some detail as there are: (1) the hydroxyl radical $^\bullet OH$, (2) peroxyl radicals $ROO^\bullet$, (3) alkoxyl radicals $RO^\bullet$, (4) phenoxyl radicals $ArO^\bullet$, (5) semiquinone radicals $^-O-Ar-O^\bullet$, (6) superoxide $O_2^{\bullet-}$, and (7) for comparison the redox-active species in disulfide/thiol systems. The examples chosen try to illustrate characteristic features of general interest such as: (a) acid-base equilibria of certain groups of free radicals, (b) the change of redox properties within a free radical reaction mechanism, (c) the possible involvement of electronic resonance forms of free radicals, and (d) the consideration of free radical lifetimes with respect to possible reactions and migration of these reactive species in solution or biological systems.

In conclusion, it is hoped that the biologically or medically oriented reader appreciates the wealth of fundamental information free radical chemistry can provide for the understanding of probably many biochemical mechanisms.

7 ACKNOWLEDGEMENTS

Some of our own work referred to in this article has been supported by the International Association for Cancer Research (AICR) and the Office of Basic Energy Sciences of the U.S. Department of Energy. This is gratefully acknowledged (this is publication No NDRL-4045 of the Notre Dame Radiation Laboratory).

8 ABBREVIATIONS

b:	Bohr magneton
γ-rays:	gamma-rays (> 0.1 MeV electromagnetic radiation)
Δx:	mean diffusion distance
ν:	frequency

π:	molecular pi orbital
σ:	molecular sigma orbital
σ^*:	molecular antibonding sigma*orbital
Φ:	quantum yield
$AH^-/A^{\bullet-}$:	ascorbate anion / ascorbate radical anion
Ar:	aromatic substituent (aryl)
$CyaS^-$:	cysteamine thiolate
$CysS^-$:	cysteine thiolate
D:	diffusion coefficient
DNA:	deoxyribonucleic acid
E:	reduction potential
E°:	standard reduction potential
ENDOR:	electron nuclear double resonance
ESR:	electron spin resonance
e:	electron
e_{aq}^-:	hydrated electron
eV:	electron-volt
F:	Faraday constant
G:	radiation chemical yield (species per 100 eV absorbed energy)
G°:	standard free enthalpy
GSH:	glutathione
Gy:	Gray
g:	gyromagnetic factor
H:	magnetic field intensity
h:	Planck's constant
$h\nu$:	photon, quantum of electromagnetic radiation
IR:	infrared light range
IUPAC:	International Union of Pure and Applied Chemistry
J:	Joule
K:	equilibrium constant
K:	(as temperature unit) Kelvin
k:	rate constant
2k:	radical-radical termination rate constant
Lip(SS):	lipoic acid, thioctic acid
MeV:	mega electron-volt
NAD:	nicotinamide adenine dinucleotide
NHE:	standard (normal) hydrogen electrode
NMR:	nuclear magnetic resonance
NOX:	nitric oxide-derived reactive oxygen species
n:	number of electrons transferred in a redox process
OD:	optical density
$PenS^-$:	penicillamine thiolate
PUFA:	polyunsaturated fatty acid
PZ:	phenothiazine

pH: negative decadic logarithm of proton concentration
pK: negative decadic logarithm of acid dissociation constant
Q: quinone
R: (in $\Delta G°$ equation) gas constant
R: aliphatic substituent
SCE: saturated calomel electrode
SOD: superoxide dismutase
T: absolute temperature (in K)
$t_{1/2}$:   half-life
UV: ultraviolet light range
VIS: visible light range
Vit C: vitamin C, ascorbic acid
Vit E: vitamin E, α-tocopherol
●   unpaired electron
∴   three-electron-bond

9   NOTES

1. There are exceptions, however, molecular oxygen, for example, is in fact relatively unreactive towards nonradical molecules.
2. In radiation chemistry the yield of chemically changed species is usually expressed in terms of G which denotes the number of species per 100 eV absorbed energy. This is approximately equivalent to μmoles per 10 J, or μM concentration per 10 J/kg (1 J/kg = 1 Gy); (Gy = Gray). In N_2O saturated aqueous solution $G(^•OH) \approx 6$.
    In photochemistry the efficiency of a photo-induced process is generally expressed in terms of the quantum yield Φ, i.e., the number of product species formed per quantum of absorbed light.
3. If necessary the effect of $H^•$ atom reactions can be studied separately, and H_2O_2 and H_2 do usually not interfere at the early pulse radiolysis time scale. Any effect by protons is usually controlled by the solution pH rather than the small amount generated as the result of the irradiation.
4. Free radical studies may also be conducted by γ-radiolysis. They can equally be trusted as the pulse radiolysis studies since it involves the same chemistry. In γ-radiolysis the initial energy carrier is a high energy photon (γ-ray) which on interaction with matter generates high energy electrons (up to MeV) in a Compton process. From any chemical point of view the situation is, therefore, the same as in the pulse radiolysis.
5. Formally, a reduction process is not restricted to a full and isolated electron transfer. Thus, the oxidation state of a particular atom is also changed if a free radical adds to it. For example, the oxidation number of sulfur in an organic sulfide like methionine, CH_3-S-CH_2CH_2–$CH(NH_2)COOH$ is –2. Addition of a hydroxyl radical to the sulfur, CH_3–$S^•(OH)$–CH_2...., changes it to –1 and thus constitutes an oxidation.

10   REFERENCES

1. Halliwell B, Gutteridge MC. Free Radicals in Biology and Medicine, 2nd edn. Oxford: Clarendon Press, 1989; Methods Enzymol 1990;186:1—85.
2. Witmer CM, Snyder RR, Jollow DJ, Kalf OF, Kocsis JJ, Sipes IG (eds). Biological Reactive Intermediates IV. New York: Plenum Press, 1991.

3. Cheeseman KH, Slater TF (eds). Free radicals in medicine. Br Med Bul. Edinburgh: Churchill Livingstone, 1993;49:479—723.
4. Slater TF. Biochem J 1985;222: 1—15.
5. Rice-Evans C (ed). Free Radicals, Disease States and Anti-Radical Interventions. London: Richelieu Press, 1989.
6. Bensasson RV, Land EJ, Truscott TO. Excited States and Free Radicals in Biology and Medicine: Contributions from Flash Photolysis and Pulse Radiolysis. Oxford: Oxford University Press, 1993.
7. von Sonntag C. The Chemical Basis of Radiation Biology. London: Taylor and Francis, 1987.
8. Quintanilha A (ed). Reactive Oxygen Species in Chemistry, Biology, and Medicine. NATO ASI Series A, vol 146. New York: Plenum Press, 1988.
9. Oberley LW (ed). Superoxide Dismutase. Boca Raton, FL: CRS Press, 1982.
10. Rotiglio G (ed). Superoxide and Superoxide Dismutase in Chemistry, Biology and Medicine. Amsterdam: Elsevier, 1986.
11. Sies H (ed). Oxidative Stress, Oxidants and Antioxidants. London: Academic Press, 1991.
12. Sies H. Angew Chem Int Ed Engl 1986;25:1058—1071.
13. Elstner EF. Der Sauerstoff, Biochemie, Biologie, Medizin. Mannheim: Wissenschaftsverlag, 1990.
14. Greenwald RA (ed). CRC Handbook of Methods for Oxygen Radical Research. Boca Raton, FL: CRC Press, 1985.
15. Yagi K (ed). Active Oxygens, Lipid Peroxides and Antioxidants. Tokyo: Jap. Sci Soc Press/Boca Raton: CRC Press, 1993;39—56.
16. Slater TF, Cook JWR. In: Evans DMD (ed) Cytology Automation. Edinburgh: E. and S. Livingstone, 1970;108—120.
17. McBrien DCH, Slater TF (eds). Free Radicals, Lipid Peroxidation and Cancer. London: Academic Press, 1982.
18. Bulkley GB. Br J Cancer 1987;55(Suppl 8):66—73.
19. Chatgilialoglu C, Asmus K-D (eds). Sulfur-Centered Reactive Intermediates in Chemistry and Biology. NATO ASI Series, A: Life Sciences, vol 197. New York: Plenum Press, 1990.
20. Sies H, Ketterer B (eds). Glutathione Conjugation: Mechanisms and Biological Significance. London: Academic Press, 1988.
21. von Sonntag C. Basic Life Science 1991;58:287—321.
22. Packer L, Glazer AN (eds). Methods Enzymol, vol 186. San Diego: Academic Press, 1990.
23. Emerit I, Packer L, Auclair C (eds). Antioxidants in Therapy and Preventive Medicine. New York: Plenum Press, 1990.
24. Lal M, Mönig J, Asmus K-D. Free Rad Res Comms 1986;1:235—241.
25. Guha SN, Schöneich C, Asmus K-D. Arch Biochem Biophys 1993;305:132—140.
26. Rannug U. Mutat Res 1980;76:269—295.
27. van Bladeren PJ, Hoogeterp JJ, Breimer DD, van der Gen A. Biochem Pharmacol 1981;30: 2983—2987.
28. Kluwe WM, McNish R, Smithson K, Hook JB. Biochem Pharmacol 1981;30:2265—2271.
29. Nachtomi E. Biochem Pharmacol 1970;19:2853—2860.
30. Albano E, Poli G, Tomasi A, Bini A, Vannini V, Dianzani MU. Chem Biol Interact 1984;50: 255—265.
31. Slater TF. Free Radical Mechanisms in Tissue Injury. London: Pion, 1972.
32. Albano E, Lott KAK, Slater F, Stier A, Symons MCR, Tomasi A. Biochem J 1982;204: 593—603.
33. Shen X, Lind J, Eriksen TE, Merenyi G. J Phys Chem 1989;93:553—557.
34. For comprehensive kinetics analysis the reader is refered to:.
    a) Frost AA, Pearson RG. Kinetics and Mechanism. New York: Wiley, 1961; b) Capellos C, Bielski BHJ. Kinetic Systems: Mathematical Description of Chemical Kinetics in Solution. New York: Wiley-Interscience, 1972; c) Hammes GG. Investigations of Rates and Mechanisms

of Reactions: Elementary Reaction Steps in Solution and Very Fast Reactions. vol VI, part II of the series: Techniques of Chemistry. New York: Wiley Interscience, 1974 d) Espenson JH. Chemical Kinetics and Reaction Mechanisms. New York: McGraw-Hill, Inc., 1981.

35. Packer JE, Slater TF, Willson RL. Nature (London) 1979;278:737—738.
36. Forni LG, Mönig J, Mora-Arellano VO, Willson RL. J Chem Soc Perkin Trans 2 1983;961—965.
37. Quintiliani M, Badiello R, Tamba M, Esfandi A, Gorin G. Int J Radiat Biol 1977;32:195—202.
38. Butler J, Land EJ, Swallow AJ, Prütz W. Radiat Phys Chem 1984;23:265—270.
39. Brault D, Neta P, Patterson LK. Chem-Biol Interact 1985;54:289—297.
40. Buxton GV, Greenstock CL, Helman PW, Ross AB. J Phys Chem Ref Data 1988;17:513—886.
41. Asmus K-D. In: Quntanilha A (ed) Reactive Oxygen Species in Chemistry, Biology, and Medicine. NATO ASI Series A, vol 146. New York: Plenum Press, 1988;37—54.
42. Baxendale JH, Busi F (eds). The Study of Fast Processes and Transient Species by Electron Pulse Radiolysis. NATO ASI Series. Dordrecht: Reidel, 1982.
43. Asmus K-D, Janata E. In: Baxendale JH, Busi F (eds) The Study of Fast Processes and Transient Species by Electron Pulse Radiolysis. NATO ASI Series. Dordrecht: Reidel, 1982;115—128.
44. Beck G. Rev Sci Instr 1979;50:1147—1150.
45. Farhataziz, Rodgers MA (eds). Radiation Chemistry, Principles and Applications. Weinheim: VCH, 1987.
46. Asmus K-D. Methods Enzymol 1984;105:167—178.
47. Fleming GR, Siegman AK (eds). Ultrafast Phenomena V. Springer Series in Chem Phys, vol 46. Berlin: Springer Verlag, 1986.
48. Henglein A, Schnabel W, Wendenburg J. Einführung in die Strahlenchemie. Weinheim: Verlag Chemie, 1969.
49. Draganic IG, Draganic ZD. The Radiation Chemistry of Water. New York: Academic Press, 1971.
50. Spinks JWT, Woods RJ. An Introduction to Radiation Chemistry, 3rd edn. New York: Wiley, 1990.
51. Bielski BHJ. In: Seib TA, Tolbert BM (eds) Ascorbic Acid: Chemistry, Metabolism, and Uses. Washington DC: Am Chem Soc, 1982;81—100.
52. Symons MCR. Chemical and Biochemical Aspects of Electron-Spin Resonance Spectroscopy. New York: Van Nostrand Reinhold, 1978.
53. Trifunac AD. In: Baxendale JH, Busi F (eds) The Study of Fast Processes and Transient Species by Electron Pulse Radiolysis. NATO ASI Series. Dordrecht: Reidel, 1982;163—178.
54. Fessenden RW, Schuler RH. Adv Radiat Chem 1970;2:1—176.
55. Grody W. In: West W, Weissberger A (eds) Techniques of Chemistry, vol 15. New York: Wiley, 1980.
56. Landolt-Börnstein. Numerical Data and Functional Relationships in Science and Technology, New Series, Hellwege K-H (ed) Group II: Atomic and Molecular Physics, vol 9: Magnetic Properties of Free Radicals. Fisher H. Hellwege K-H (eds) Berlin: Springer Verlag, 1977—1980. Supplement and Extension: vol 17, 1987—1990.
57. Kurreck H, Kirste B, Lubitz W. Electron Nuclear Double Resonance Spectroscopy. Weinheim: VCH, 1988.
58. Janzen KG. Meth Enzymol 1984;105:188—198.
59. Mason RP, Ramakrishna Rao DN. In: Chatgilialoglu C, Asmus K-D (eds) Sulfur-Centered Reactive Intermediates in Chemistry and Biology. NATO ASI Series, A: Life Sciences, vol 197. New York: Plenum Press, 1990;401—408.
60. Ross D, Norbeck K, Moldeus P. J Biol Chem 1985;260:15028—15032.
61. Slater TF. In: McBrien DCH, Slater TF (eds) Free Radicals, Lipid Peroxidation and Cancer. London: Academic Press, 1982;243—270.
62. Mönig J, Bahnemann D, Asmus K-D. Chem-Biol Interact 1983;47:15—27.
63. Mönig J, Asmus K-D. J Chem Soc Perkin Trans 2 1984;2057—2063.
64. Mönig J, Krischer K, Asmus K-D. Chem-Biol Interact 1983;45:43—52.

65. Asmus K-D, Bahnemann D, Krischer K, Lal M, Mönig J. Life Chem Rep 1985;3:1—15.
66. Landolt-Börnstein. Numerical Data and Functional Relationships in Science and Technology, New Series, Hellwege K-H, Madelung O (eds) Group II: Atomic and Molecular Physics, vol 13.: Radical Reaction Rates in Liquids. Fischer H. ed. Berlin: Springer: Part a: Beckwith ALJ, Griller D, Lorand JP. Carbon-Centered Radicals I, 1984. Part b: Asmus K-D, Bonifacic M. Carbon-Centered Radicals II, 1984. Part c: Ingold KU, Roberts BP. Radicals Centered on N, S, P and other Heteroatoms. Nitroxyls, 1983. Part d: Howard JA, Scaiano JC. Oxyl, Peroxyl and Related Radicals, 1984. Part e: Dohrmann JK, Scaiano JC, Steenken S. Proton and Electron Transfer. Biradicals, 1985 and Supplement additions, 1995/96.
67. Bielski BHJ, Cabelli DE, Arudi RL. Reactivity of $HO_2^\bullet/O_2^{\bullet-}$ radicals in aqueous solution. J. Phys Chem Ref Data 1985;14:1041—1100.
68. Neta P, Huie RE, Ross AB. Rate constants for reactions of inorganic radicals in aqueous solution. J Phys Chem Ref Data 1988;17:1027—1284.
69. Neta P, Huie RE, Ross AB. Rate constants for reactions of peroxyl radicals in fluid solutions. J Phys Chem Ref Data 1990;19:413—513.
70. Wardman P. Reduction potentials of one-electron couples involving free radicals in aqueous solution. J Phys Chem Ref Data 1989;18:1637—1723.
71. O'Neill P, Steenken S, Schulte-Frohlinde D. Angew Chem 1975;87:417—418.
72. Bonifačić M, Asmus K-D. J Chem Soc Dalton 1976;2074—2076.
73. Sanaullah, Hungerbühler H, Schöneich Ch, Morton M, Vander Velde DG, Wilson GS, Asmus K-D, Glass RS. J Am Chem Soc 1997;119:2134—2145.
74. Bonifačić M, Möckel H, Bahnemann D, Asmus K-D. J Chem Soc Perkin Trans 2 1975; 675—685.
75. Asmus K-D. Acc Chem Res 1979;12:436—442.
76. Bobrowski K, Schöneich Ch. J Chem Soc Chem Commun 1993;795—797.
77. Hiller K-O, Masloch B, Göbl M, Asmus K-D. J Am Chem Soc 1981;103:2734—2743.
78. Mönig J, Göbl M, Asmus K-D. J Chem Soc Perkin Trans 2 1985;647—651.
79. Asmus K-D, Göbl M, Hiller K-O, Mahling S, Mönig J. J Chem Soc Perkin Trans 2 1985; 641—646.
80. Hiller K-O, Asmus K-D. J Phys Chem 1983;87:3682—3688.
81. Bobrowski K, Holcman J. Int J Radiat Biol 1987;52:139—144.
82. Bobrowski K, Schöneich Ch, Holcman J, Asmus K-D. J Chem Soc Perkin Trans 2 1991; 353—362.
83. Bobrowski K, Pogocki D, Schöneich Ch. J Phys Chem 1993;97:13677—13684.
84. Fujita S, Steenken S. J Am Chem Soc 1981;103:2540—2545.
85. McMillen DF, Golden DM. Ann Rev Phys Chem 1982;33:493—532.
86. Schöneich Ch, Asmus K-D, Dillinger U, Bruchhausen F. Biochem Biophys Res Commun 1989; 161:113—120.
87. Schöneich Ch, Dillinger U, Bruchhausen F, Asmus K-D. Arch Biochem Biophys 1992;292: 456—467.
88. Asmus K-D, Möckel H, Henglein A. J Phys Chem 1973;77:1218—1221.
89. Bonifačić M, Schäfer K, Asmus K-D. J Phys Chem 1975;79:1496—1502.
90. Asmus K-D, Henglein A, Wigger A, Beck G. Ber Bunsenges Phys Chem 1966;70:756—758.
91. Mertens R, von Sonntag C. Angew Chem Int Ed Engl 1994;33:1262—1264.
92. Lal M, Schöneich Ch, Mönig J, Asmus K-D. Int J Radiat Biol 1988;54:773—785.
93. Bahnemann D, Asmus K-D, Willson RL. J Chem Soc Perkin Trans 2 1983;1661—1668.
94. Bahnemann D, Asmus K-D, Willson RL. J Chem Soc Perkin Trans 2 1981;890—895.
95. Huie RE, Neta P. Int J Chem Kinet 1986;18:1185—1191.
96. Schöneich Ch, Aced A, Asmus K-D. J Am Chem Soc 1991;113:375—376.
97. Engman L, Persson J, Merenyi, Lind J. Organometallics 1995;14:3641—3648.
98. Aced A. PhD Thesis, Technical University Berlin, Germany, D 83, 1991.
99. Packer JE, Willson RL, Bahnemann D, Asmus K-D. J Chem Soc Perkin Trans 2 1980:296—299.

100. Huie RE, Brault D, Neta P. Chem Biol Interact 1987;62:227–235.
101. Neta P, Huie RE, Mosseri S, Shastri LV, Mittal JP, Maruthamuthu P, Steenken S. J Phys Chem 1989;93:4099–4104.
102. Mönig J, Asmus K-D. In: Bors W, Saran M, Tait D (eds) Oxygen Radicals in Chemistry and Biology. Berlin: Walter de Gruyter, 1984;57–63.
103. Martin RA, Richard C, Rousseau-Richard C. In: Vigo-Pelfrey C (ed) Membrane Lipid Oxidation. Boca Raton, FL: CRC Press, 1989;63–100.
104. Vigo-Pelfrey C (ed). Membrane Lipid Oxidation. Boca Raton, FL: CRC Press, 1989.
105. Korcek S, Chenier JHB, Howard JA, Ingold KU. Can J Chem 1972;50:2285–2297.
106. Gebicki JM, Bielski BHJ. J Am Chem Soc 1981;103:7020–7022.
107. Gebicki JM, Allen AO. J Phys Chem 1969;73 2443–2445.
108. Patterson LK, Redpath JL. In: Mittal KL (ed) Micellization, Solubilization, and Micro-emulsions, vol 2. New York: Plenum Press, 1977;589–601.
109. Fessenden RW, Carton PM, Shimamori H, Scaiano JC. J Phys Chem 1982;86:3803–3811.
110. Neta P, Huie RE, Maruthamuthu P, Steenken S. J Phys Chem 1989;93:7654–7659.
111. Alfassi ZB, Huie RE, Neta P. J Phys Chem 1993;97:7253–7257.
112. von Sonntag C, Schuchmann H-P. Angew Chem 1991;103:1255–1279.
113. Rabani J, Klug-Roth D, Henglein A. J Phys Chem 1974;78:2089–2093.
114. Ilan Y, Rabani J, Henglein A. J Phys Chem 1976;80:1558–1565.
115. Bothe E, Behrens G, Schulte-Frohlinde D. Z Naturforsch 1977;32b:886–889.
116. Bothe E, Schulte-Frohlinde D, von Sonntag C. J Chem Soc Perkin Trans 2 1978;416–420.
117. Bothe E, Schuchmann MN, Schulte-Frohlinde D, von Sonntag C. Photochem Photobiol 1978; 28:639–644.
118. Das S, Schuchmann MN, Schuchmann H-P, von Sonntag C. Chem Ber 1987;120:319–323.
119. Bloodworth AJ, Courtneidge JL, Davies AG. J Chem Soc Perkin Trans 2 1984;523–527.
120. Adamic K, Howard JA, Ingold KU. Can J Chem 1969;47:3803–3808.
121. Howard JA. ACS Symposium Ser 1978;69:413–432.
122. Furimsky E, Howard JA, Selwyn J. Can J Chem 1980;58:677–680.
123. Bennett JE. J Chem Soc Faraday Trans 1990;86:3247–3252.
124. Russell GA. J Am Chem Soc 1957;79:3871–3877.
125. Nakano M, Takayama K, Shimizu Y, Tsuji Y, Inaba H, Migita T. J Am Chem Soc 1976;98: 1974–1975.
126. Niu Q, Mendenhall GD. J Am Chem Soc 1990;112:1656–1657.
127. Lee S-H, Mendenhall GD. J Am Chem Soc 1988;110:4318–4323.
128. Bothe E, Schulte-Frohlinde D. Z Naturforsch 1978;33b:786–788.
129. Asmus K-D. In: Fielden EM, Fowler JF, Hendry JH, Scott D (eds) Radiation Research, Proceeding 8th International Congress of Radiation Research, vol 2. London: Taylor and Francis, 1987;48–53.
130. Lal M, Mönig J, Asmus K-D. J. Chem Soc Perkin Trans 2 1987;1639–1644.
131. Esterbauer H, Zollner H, Schaur RJ. In: Vigo-Pelfrey C (ed) Membrane Lipid Oxidation. Boca Raton, FL: CRC Press, 1989;239–268.
132. Schöneich Ch, Bonifačić M, Asmus K-D. Free Radical Res Communs 1989;6:393–405.
133. Schöneich Ch, Asmus K-D. Radiat Environ Biophys 1990;29:263–271.
134. Schöneich Ch, Bonifačić M, Asmus K-D. J Chem Soc Faraday Trans 1995;91:1923–1930.
135. Schöneich Ch, Bonifačić M, Dillinger U, Asmus K-D. In: Chatgilialoglu C, Asmus K-D (eds) Sulfur-Centered Reactive Intermediates in Chemistry and Biology. NATO ASI Series, A: Life Sciences, vol 197. New York: Plenum Press, 1990;367–376.
136. Czapski G, Dorfman LM. J Phys Chem 1964;68:1169–1177.
137. Pan X-M, von Sonntag C. Z Naturforsch 1990;45b:1337–1340.
138. Porter NA, Lehman LS, Weber BA, Smith KJ. J Am Chem Soc 1981;103:6447–6455.
139. Porter NA, Wujek DG. In: Quintanilha A (ed) Reactive Oxygen Species in Chemistry, Biology, and Medicine. NATO ASI Series A, vol 146. New York: Plenum Press, 1988;55–79.

140. Frankel EN. In: Simic MG, Taylor KA, Ward JF, von Sonntag C (eds) Oxygen Radicals in Biology and Medicine. New York: Plenum Press, 1988;265—282.
141. Barclay LRC. In: Minisci F (ed) Free Radicals in Synthesis and Biology. Dordrecht: Kluwer, 1989;391—406.
142. Mönig J, Asmus K-D, Forni LG, Willson RL. Int J Radiat Biol 1987;52:589—602.
143. Tamba M, Simone G, Quintiliani M. Int J Radiat Biol 1986;50:595—600.
144. Wardman P. In: Chatgilialoglu C, Asmus K-D (eds) Sulfur-Centered Reactive Intermediates in Chemistry and Biology. NATO ASI Series, A: Life Sciences, vol 197. New York: Plenum Press, 1990;415—427.
145. Zhang X, Zhang N. Schuchmann H-P, von Sonntag C. J Phys Chem 1994;98:6541—6547.
146. Swarts SG, Becker D, DeBold S, Sevilla MD. J Phys Chem 1989;93:155—161.
147. Chatgilialoglu C, Guerra M. In: Chatgilialoglu C, Asmus K-D (eds) Sulfur-Centered Reactive Intermediates in Chemistry and Biology. NATO ASI Series, A: Life Sciences, vol 197. New York: Plenum Press, 1990;31—36.
148. Chatgilialoglu C. In: Patai S (ed) The Chemistry of Sulfenic Acids and Their Derivatives. New York: Wiley, 1990;549—569.
149. Asmus K-D, Schöneich Ch. Oxidative Damage & Repair. In: Davies KEJ (ed) Chemical, Biological and Medical Aspects. New York: Pergamon Press, 1991;226—233.
150. Asmus K-D. In: Yagi K (ed) Active Oxygen, Lipid Peroxides, and Antioxidants. Tokyo: Japan Sci Press; Boca Raton: CRC Press, 1993;57—67.
151. Chatgilialoglu C, Schöneich Ch, Asmus K-D. Unpublished results.
152. Asmus K-D. In: Nygaard OF, Simic MG (eds) Radioprotectors and Anticarcinogens. New York: Academic Press, 1983;23—42.
153. Asmus K-D. In: Chatgilialoglu C, Asmus K-D (eds) Sulfur-Centered Reactive Intermediates in Chemistry and Biology. NATO ASI Series, A: Life Sciences, vol 197. New York: Plenum Press, 1990;155—172.
154. Dainton FS, Janovsky IV, Salmon GA. Proc Roy Soc Ser A 1972;327:305—316.
155. Berdnikov VM, Bazhin NM, Fedorov VK, Polyakov OV. Kinet Catal 1972;13:986—987.
156. Gilbert BC, Holmes RGG, Laue HAH, Norman ROC. J Chem Soc Perkin Trans 2 1976; 1047—1052.
157. Schuchmann H-P, von Sonntag C. J Photochem 1981;16:289—295.
158. Makogon O, Fliount R, Asmus K-D. J Adv Oxid Techn 1998;3:11—21.
159. Fliount R, Makogon O, Asmus K-D. To be published.
160. Packer JE, Slater TF, Willson RL. Nature 1979;278:737—738.
161. Willnow A. PhD Thesis, Technical University Berlin, D83, 1994.
162. Willnow A, Liebler DC, Asmus K-D. To be published.
163. Thomas MJ, Bielski BHJ. J Am Chem Soc 1989;111:3315—3319.
164. Patel KB, Willson RL. J Chem Soc Faraday Trans I 1973;69:814—825.
165. von Sonntag C, Schuchmann H-P. Angew Chem Int Ed Engl 1991;30:1229—1253.
166. Bielski BHJ, Cabelli DE. Int J Radiat Biol 1991;59:291—319.
167. Bielski BHJ, Richter HW. J Am Chem Soc 1977;99:3019—3023.
168. Bielski BHJ. Photochem Photobiol 1978;28:645—649.
169. Shastri LV, Shrinavasan K, Rama Rao KVS Proc Nucl & Radiat Chem Symp, University of Pune. Poona, India 1967;49 ff.
170. Schuchmann MN, von Sonntag C. J Am Chem Soc 1988;110:5698—5701.
171. Fliount R, Magogon O, Asmus K-D. J Phys Chem 1997;101:3547—3553.
172. Asmus K-D. In: Packer L, Glazer AN (eds) Methods of Enzymology, vol 186. San Diego: Academic Press 1990;168—180.
173. see following articles in ref 19: a) Armstrong DA: 121—134 and 341—352; b) von Sonntag C: 359—366; c) Dunster C, Willson RL: 377—388; d) Mason RP, Rao DNR: 401—408; e) von Sonntag C, Schuchmann HP: 409—414;f) Wardman P: 415—428;Quintiliani M: 435—443.
174. Adams GE, Aldrich JE, Bisby RH, Cundall RB, Redpath JL, Willson RL. Radiat Res 1972;49:

278—289.

175. Bonifačić M, Asmus K-D. Int J Radiat Biol 1984;46:35—45.
176. Mezyk SP. Radiat Res 1996;145:102—106.
177. Mezyk SP. J Phys Chem 1996;100:8295—8301.
178. Surdhar PS, Armstrong DA. J Phys Chem 1987;91:6532—6537.
179. Chan PC, Bielski BHJ. J Am Chem Soc 1973;95:5504—5508.
180. Willson RL. Chem Commun 1970;1425—1426.
181. Micic OI, Nenadovic MT, Carapellucci PA. J Am Chem Soc 1978;100:2209—2212.
182. Frimer AA (ed). Singlet O_2. Boca Raton, FL: CRC Press, 1985.
183. Wilkinson F, Brummer JG. Rate constants for the decay and reactions of the lowest electronically excited singlet state of molecular oxygen in solution. J Phys Chem Ref Data 1981;10: 809—1000.
184. Hippeli S, Elstner EF. In: Sies H (ed) Oxidative Stress, Oxidants and Antioxidants. London: Academic Press, 1991;3—55.
185. Foote CS. In: Quintanilha A (ed) Reactive Oxygen Species in Chemistry, Biology, and Medicine. NATO ASI Series A, vol 146. New York: Plenum Press, 1988;107—116.
186. Saran M, Michel C, Bors W. Free Rad Res Commun 1990;10:221—226.
187. Noack E, Murphy M. In: Sies H (ed) Oxidative Stress, Oxidants and Antioxidants. London: Academic Press, 1991;445—489.
188. Snyder SH, Bredt DS. Sci Am 1992;May:28—35.

Part II

Reactive species in tissues

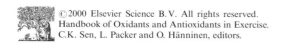
©2000 Elsevier Science B.V. All rights reserved.
Handbook of Oxidants and Antioxidants in Exercise.
C.K. Sen, L. Packer and O. Hänninen, editors.

Part II • Chapter 2

Exercise and oxygen radical production by muscle

Malcolm J. Jackson

Muscle Research Centre, Department of Medicine, University of Liverpool, P.O. Box 147, Liverpool, L69 3GA, UK

1   INTRODUCTION
2   EXERCISE
3   POTENTIAL SOURCES OF FREE RADICAL GENERATION IN EXERCISING MUSCLE
    3.1   Primary sources of free radicals
          3.1.1   Mitochondrial generation of free radical species
          3.1.2   Xanthine oxidase
          3.1.3   Prostanoid metabolism
          3.1.4   Catecholamines
          3.1.5   NAD(P)H oxidase
    3.2   Secondary sources of free radicals
          3.2.1   Radical generation by phagocytic white cells
          3.2.2   Generation of radicals secondary to muscle calcium accumulation
          3.2.3   Free radical formation due to disruption of iron-containing proteins
4   CONSEQUENCES OF EXERCISE-INDUCED FREE RADICAL PRODUCTION
5   CONCLUSIONS
6   ABBREVIATIONS
7   REFERENCES

1   INTRODUCTION

The idea that oxygen radicals might be produced in excess during physical exercise and that these substances are responsible for some of the deleterious effects of excessive or unaccustomed exercise has been widely discussed for about 20 years [1]. In the initial stages it became clear that oxygen radicals could be produced in excess under certain exercise regimens [2], but this was not an inevitable consequence of all forms of exercise and did not always initiate cellular damage or degeneration (see Jackson et al. [3] for a review). Much of the confusion in this area can probably be attributed to the different types of exercise examined in various studies and the predominant manner in which muscle is used in different protocols. Prior to a discussion of the potential sites, and effects, of oxygen radical generation during exercise this review will therefore briefly consider these different forms of exercise with a view to a clearer recognition of the implications for oxygen radical production.

2   EXERCISE

The "umbrella" title of exercise is used to describe a wide range of physical activity ranging from a small number of repeat contractions of single or small groups of muscles (e.g., "hand exercises") to extensive, rapid and exhaustive contractions of many of the major muscle groups of the body (such as occurs in many competitive sports events). It would therefore be reasonable in discussion of free radical generation during exercise to refine the question from "is exercise associated with increased free radical generation?" to more specific ones such as "are free radicals generated during muscle contractions?" or "are free radicals generated by increased oxygen consumption by muscle?" However, it is clear that this logical approach has not been widely followed and most studies have examined whole body exercise in man or animals. Such exercise is very complex and any observed changes in indicators of increased free radical activity may be theoretically derived from many tissues (e.g., lungs, heart, liver) in addition to skeletal muscle or may be associated with a variety of factors such as mechanical stresses, increased mitochondrial activity or increased supply of blood borne substrates in addition to muscular contraction.

   A number of such compounding factors therefore potentially influence free radical generation during exercise and it is also clear that the intensity and duration of the exercise will play a major role in the process. Thus high intensity, short term exercise is essentially anaerobic while longer term and endurance exercise is aerobic and dependant on substantial increases in mitochondrial oxygen consumption. Various theories for the production of free radicals in these two extreme areas have been proposed (e.g., see Sjodin et al. [4] for a review), but clear comparisons of the production of free radicals in these two extreme areas do not appear to have been undertaken.

   A further complication concerning the study of potential damaging processes during exercise is the predominant manner in which the muscle is used. Muscle may contract in three ways: where the active muscle is allowed to shorten (concentric contractions), remains at fixed length (isometric contractions) or is lengthened (eccentric contractions). A number of comparisons between experimental concentric and eccentric contractions have demonstrated that repetitive eccentric contractions are much more damaging that concentric contractions [5—9], although the time course of onset of the pain and damage is much slower than seen following excessive concentric contractions. Most standard exercise protocols (e.g., running, cycling, etc.) involve a combination of concentric and eccentric contractions with some muscles being used primarily in a concentric and some in an eccentric manner. Occasional forms of exercise, such as predominantly downhill running involve extensive use of a number of muscles in an eccentric manner and, are therefore very damaging to muscle tissue. Further characteristics of these different forms of muscle activity are presented in Table 1.

   It is therefore clear that any consideration of the potential role of free radicals in exercise-induced muscle injury should carefully control the nature of the con-

Table 1. Characteristics of different types of contractile activity.

	Eccentric	Isometric	Concentric
Movement of muscle	Lengthening	Static	Shortening
Mechanical forces	High	Low	Low
Electrical activity	Low	High	High
Metabolic cost	Low	High	High
Oxygen consumption	Low	High	High
Tendency to induce:			
Damage	High	Low	Low
Fatigue	High	Low	Low
Pain	High	Low	Low

tractile activity undertaken and the intensity and duration of that activity. The different types of exercise discussed have such different energy requirements, oxygen consumption, and mechanical stresses on the tissue that it is unlikely that similar mechanisms for generation of damaging free radicals are active in each situation. It is entirely feasible that different mechanisms in each model predispose to the excessive generation of free radicals, since many potential mechanisms for generation of free radical species in exercising tissue exist. These are discussed in the next section.

3   POTENTIAL SOURCES OF FREE RADICAL GENERATION IN EXERCISING MUSCLE

There are a number of potential sites for the generation of free radical species within exercising muscle tissue and further possible mechanisms by which free radical species may be increased secondary to damage induced by other mechanisms. One of the major problems with assessment of the role of free radicals in any situation where tissue damage occurs is to differentiate between free radicals mediating the cell damage and occurring secondarily to it. Halliwell and Gutteridge [10] have pointed out that free radicals are produced by degenerating tissue in a number of situations and this possibility must always be considered.

3.1 Primary sources of free radicals

3.1.1 *Mitochondrial generation of free radical species*

Oxidative metabolism in mammals involves the reduction of molecular oxygen in mitochondria. Where oxygen is not limiting, this highly regulated system provides a means for the continuous generation of "high energy" phosphates (ATP) for muscular contraction. The ability of muscle to undertake co-ordinated increases in mitochondrial oxygen consumption is substantial. As part of the process for delivery of energy supplies molecular oxygen generally undergoes four electron reduction catalysed by cytochrome oxidise. This process has been claimed to account for 95—98% of the total oxygen consumption of tissues, but the remainder (i.e., 2—5% of the total) may undergo one electron reduction with the production of the superoxide radical $[O_2^-]$. Further one electron reduction of superoxide produces hydrogen peroxide which has been shown to be released by isolated mitochondria [11,12].

The site of this apparent "loss" of electrons to oxygen has been proposed to be coenzyme Q [4]. Thus it is envisaged that the quinones which constitute coenzyme Q are reduced to semiquinones by electrons from NADH and that these lipophilic compounds are able to readily diffuse to come into contact with oxygen with the generation of superoxide radial [11]. this hypothesis agrees well with what is known about the radical species which are visible by electron spin resonance studies of exercising muscle [2,13]. The only free radical signal observed in intact normal muscle has a g-value of approximately 2.004 and has been claimed to derive mainly from the mitochondria of cells [14]. The actual nature of the radical species has been disputed [15] although it is likely that it primarily derives from semiquinones [16]. It is therefore apparent that substantial aerobic exercise could theoretically lead to an increased production of superoxide radicals because of the vastly increased electron flux through the mitochondrial electron transport chain. However, it should also be noted that the mitochondrion has well-developed systems for protection against oxygen radical mediated damage with the presence of a specific mitochondrial superoxide dismutase to prevent local superoxide-mediated degeneration. There is increasing evidence that aerobic exercise leads to release of mitochondria-derived superoxide radicals from the muscle cell. Reid and co-workers [17,18] found that superoxide produced in contracting myocytes was released into the interstitial fluid and O'Neill and co-workers have recently reported clear evidence of increased hydroxyl radical production by contracting skeletal muscle [19]. In this elegant study the authors used L-phenylalanine as a probe for hydroxyl radicals and examined stimulated intermittent static contractions of the triceps surae muscle in anaesthetised cats. Contractile activity induced a rapid and substantial rise in the content of *m*-, and *o*-tyrosines (formed by reaction of phenylalanine with hydroxyl radicals) indicating production of hydroxyl radicals during intermittent contractions (Table 2).

This production appeared to be related to the tension developed by the muscle. Furthermore these authors pretreated animals with desferrioxamine and were able to show a reduction in hydroxyl radical production (Table 2).

The overall conclusion of these disparate studies appears to be that superoxide is generated within mitochondria during contractile activity. Superoxide (and probably hydrogen peroxide) are subsequently lost from the muscle cell into the interstitial fluid. Hydroxyl radicals are then generated from the released superoxide/hydrogen peroxide by an iron-catalysed system (the lack of cell penetration of desferrioxamine indicate that this latter process must occur extracellularly).

Table 2. Hydroxyl radical production during intermittent static contractions of triceps surae muscles in cats.

	Hydroxyl radical production	Hydroxyl radical production with desferrioxamine treatment
1 min precontractions	0.30 ± 0.08	0.26 ± 0.15
After 1 min contractions	7.98 ± 2.30	4.10 ± 1.80
After 3 min contractions	10.70 ± 3.50	5.16 ± 1.56[a]
After 4.5 min contractions	11.65 ± 2.03	6.71 ± 1.37[a]
1 min postcontractions	5.09 ± 1.90	1.65 ± 0.78[a]

Hydroxyl radical production will calculated from the increase in isomeric tyrosines formed from L-phenylalanine. Blood was sampled from the venous output (popliteal vein) of triceps surae muscles stimulated to contract via the sciatic nerve. Muscle received 15 s of stimulation followed by 15 s recovery for the period shown. An alternative group of animals received desferrioxamine (10 mg/kg iv) 15 min prior to commencement of stimulation. [a]$p < 0.05$ compared to control untreated animals. Data derived from O'Neill et al. [19].

One implication of the above process is that radical species are present at increased concentrations in the extracellular fluid following contractile activity and may therefore be detectable in exercising humans or animals. Recent electron spin resonance studies by Ashton and co-workers [20] appear to support this possibility.

It is also worthy of comment that all of these studies have examined relatively nondamaging forms of aerobic exercise, although the exercise was primarily exhaustive.

3.1.2 Xanthine oxidase

The possible role of xanthine oxidase in the generation of free radical species has been promoted by McCord and co-workers [21]. These workers have proposed that the process of ischaemia may lead to formation of xanthine oxidase from xanthine dehydrogenase (via activation of a calcium-dependant protease) and also to a breakdown of ATP with the formation of AMP via the adenylate kinase reaction. This substance is then further metabolised to hypoxanthine which is a substrate for both xanthine dehydrogenase and xanthine oxidase. Xanthine oxidase utilises molecular oxygen as an electron acceptor with the formation of xanthine (eventually uric acid) and the superoxide radical (Fig. 1).

In order for such a process to provide an important source of free radial species in exercising muscle a number of criteria must be achieved. Firstly the enzyme (xanthine dehydrogenase/oxidase) must be present in skeletal muscle; secondly a failure of calcium homeostasis must occur (to stimulate the calcium-activated protease) in exercising muscle and finally the substrate hypoxanthine must be produced in substantial amounts by exercising muscle.

Most human tissues have only very low activities of xanthine dehydrogenase/

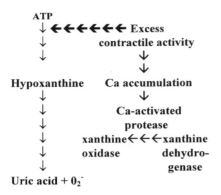

Fig. 1. Scheme for production of superoxide radicals by increased xanthine oxidase activity dependent upon production of hypoxanthine and stimulation of calcium-activated protease (Adapted from McCord [21]).

oxidase in comparison to other species [22–24], but this enzyme has been local-ised to the capillary epithelium of human muscle providing a potential source for superoxide production adjacent to skeletal muscle tissue. The second pre-requisite, that exercising muscle show a failure of calcium homeostasis, also appears to be true. A number of studies have demonstrated that calcium metabo-lism is deranged during excessive contractile activity of skeletal muscles [25,26] and that contractile activity-induced damage to skeletal muscle can be reduced or prevented by modification of muscle calcium levels [27] or inhibition of calcium-mediated pathological processes [28]. Evidence that calcium-activated proteases are activated in skeletal muscle postexercise is indirect, but may be inferred from the characteristic z-line "streaming" which is observed on ultra-structural examination [29].

The production of hypoxanthine by muscle during exercise has received con-siderable attention. Most forms of exercise have been associated with some changes in purine metabolism [30,31] although changes in hypoxanthine are par-ticularly evident in subjects undertaking ischaemic exercise [32,35]. Furthermore hypoxanthine is rapidly released from exercising muscle to the serum [32,33] and hence could also provide a substrate for xanthine oxidase within the capil-lary endothelium.

It is therefore clear that xanthine oxidase within muscle, or the closely asso-ciated capillary endothelium, could play a role in superoxide radical generation during or after exercise. The requirement for both hypoxanthine (as a substrate) and calcium-activation of a protease to allow the reaction to occur, suggests that this is most likely to occur in metabolically compromised muscle where the rate of ATP breakdown is greater than its generation and cellular ion homeostasis is lost. Such a situation is more likely to occur in very high intensity short duration exercise than in a chronic form of exercise at a moderate or low intensity. Finally it should be noted that if the site of generation of the xanthine oxidase-derived radicals is within the endothelium then the protease-mediated conversion of the enzyme and activation of other calcium-mediated degenerative processes should occur in that tissue. To the author's knowledge this has not been demonstrated.

3.1.3 Prostanoid metabolism

Prostaglandins are released from various cell types in response to stimuli and appear to be released from skeletal muscle subjected to various stresses, including excessive contractile activity [34—36]. Many of the intermediates in prostaglandin metabolism are free radical species and the active oxygen metabolites are produced during prostanoid biosynthesis [37]. Arachidonic acid (the precursor of prostaglandins) can also be converted to active metabolites by lipoxygenase enzymes. This process also involves the production of free radical intermediates, but such enzymes do not appear to have been demonstrated in skeletal muscle. However, products of lipoxygenase metabolism have been suggested to be mediators of some forms of damage to skeletal muscle [38].

The potential role of prostanoids as a source of oxidative stress in exercise is therefore not yet clear. At the present time the increase in prostaglandin production during muscle contractile activity does not have any known physiological role although it is unlikely to be surreptitious. Further examination of this area is necessary to evaluate whether this represents a beneficial or deleterious effect of excessive muscular contraction.

3.1.4 Catecholamines

Catecholamine release is increased during exercise and has a number of metabolic effects on substrate availability and blood flow [39]. It has been reported that catecholamines can autoxidise leading to free radical production [40] or undergo metal ion-catalysed oxidation to free radical products [41] and hence provide another potential source of free radical production during exercise.

3.1.5 NAD(P)H oxidase

A further site of free radical production is the NAD(P)H oxidase which is known to occur in neutrophils and various other cell types [42,43]. However, it is unclear whether this enzyme system is present in skeletal muscle and whether it would be influenced by contractile activity [44]. Hence, in the absence of this crucial information, this potential source remains speculative.

3.2 Secondary sources of free radicals

A number of other sources of radicals within muscle are likely to be important following the onset of damage initiated by other sources. These secondary sources of radicals may be important in propagation or exacerbation of damaging processes or may merely be a part of the body's adaptive responses ensuing efficient preparation of the damaged tissue to allow regeneration to occur.

3.2.1 Radical generation by phagocytic white cells

It is clear that substantial injury to muscle fibres is followed by invasion of the area by macrophages and other phagocytic cells from the blood and interstitium [8]. These infiltrating cells appear to be essential to prepare the tissue to allow fast, effective regeneration to occur. As part of the phagocytic process they release substantial amounts of oxygen radicals [45,46] to aid in the degeneration of necrotic areas, but which may also contribute to damage to surrounding viable tissue. It is relevant to note that this increase in free radical generation is non-specific and will occur in all tissue damaged "in vivo" regardless of the mechanism by which the cellular damage occurs. Thus direct trauma to muscle during exercise can cause damage which will eventually lead to a secondary increase in intramuscular free radical generation from phagocytic cells, but this does not equate to an "exercise-induced" increase in free radical generation although measurements of indicators of free radical activity may be abnormal.

Similarly, supplementation with antioxidants could not influence the extent of the initial muscle damage although they might theoretically modify the "scavenging" role of the phagocytic cells. Such changes can be inferred from the work of Cannon and co-workers [47].

3.2.2 Generation of radicals secondary to muscle calcium accumulation

It was previously mentioned that activation of a calcium-dependant protease appeared necessary to form xanthine oxidase in ischaemic tissue [21]. Many workers have suggested that a failure of muscle calcium homeostasis is a key step in the degenerative process in exercise-induced muscle damage [9,26,27,48]. It is possible that this failure of calcium in homeostasis occurs secondarily to an increase in free radical activity as has been proposed for other tissues [49–52] but a number of studies argue against this for skeletal muscle [53–56].

If it is assumed that a failure of muscle calcium homeostasis is a primary event in exercise-induced muscle damage this could lead to increased free radical activity in a number of ways. A rise in intramuscular calcium will activate endogenous phospholipase and proteolytic enzymes leading to release of free fatty acids and disruption of intracellular membrane structures. Furthermore in an attempt to "buffer" the rise in intracellular calcium, mitochondria will become overloaded with calcium leading to an eventual failure of ATP production with an increase in superoxide production, for recent reviews see Gower et al. [57] and McArdle and Jackson [56].

Increased oxidative stress induced by intracellular calcium overload is therefore a potential secondary form of oxidative stress indirectly caused by exercise. Again, simple measurements of indicators of free radical activity will only indicate a rise in oxidative reaction products without any evidence for whether they are primary or secondary and should therefore be evaluated with caution.

3.2.3 *Free radical formation due to disruption of iron-containing proteins*

The potential of "delocalised", "loosely-bound" or "free" iron to catalyse free radical reactions is well known [37]. Endurance running and other sports with a high mechanical impact may theoretically cause destruction of erythrocytes with a release of iron and hence a potential source of "catalytic" iron. Damage to muscle tissue is also known to release relatively large amounts of the iron-containing protein, myoglobin, into the circulation. Rice-Evans and co-workers [58] have demonstrated the potential of this and other haem proteins to catalyse the production of oxygen radical species and hence this is an alternative mechanism for possible secondary production of further oxidants following the initiation of cellular damage.

4 CONSEQUENCES OF EXERCISE-INDUCED FREE RADICAL PRODUCTION

A number of other chapters in this book will discuss the potential deleterious effects of an increase in free radical activity. However, it can be argued that the apparent contradiction between the clear increase in free radical production reported in muscle undergoing repeated fatiguing aerobic concentric contractions and the relative lack of subsequent tissue damage indicates that the muscle cell has evolved appropriate defences to deal with the increased oxidative stress. Furthermore, there is also increasing evidence that such a stress may be used by cells to signal an adaptive response.

Cells exposed to a nonlethal increase in free radical activity have been shown to respond by the induction of a number of genes. These can be thought of as two types: the cellular adaptation to free radical insult, and the use of free radicals as intracellular messengers. The mechanism of induction of gene expression and the absolute number of genes involved remains to be clarified. Generally an increase in free radical activity triggers a signal transduction pathway which terminates in the production of active transcription factors which are then able to bind to the promoter region of their target genes and activate transcription. Currently there is much interest in three transcription factors, nuclear factor kappa b (NF-κB), activator protein -1 (AP-1) and heat shock factor (HSF), all of which have been shown to be modulated by oxidative stress (for review see [60]).

In muscle it is now clear that there is an adaptive response of the protective enzymes (SOD etc.) to repeated bouts of exercise (see other chapters in this volume) which is prompted by oxidative stress. Recent data also indicates that exhaustive exercise leads to an increase in the synthesis of muscle stress (or heat shock) proteins. This has been reported to be triggered by the increased oxidative stress associated with exercise [61]. In tissues such as the heart, stimulation of increased expression of stress proteins results in protection against a subsequent bout of (normally lethal) oxidative stress [62—65] and preliminary data supports a similar action in skeletal muscle [66,67]. Sublethal oxidative stress may therefore play a crucial initiating role in several aspects of the adaptive response of skeletal muscle to exercise.

5   CONCLUSIONS

It is therefore clear that there are a number of potential sites for the generation of oxygen radicals in muscle during exercise and that the form of exercise which is studied may influence both the site of formation and the relative quantity of radical species produced. Much more difficult to assess is the possible production of oxygen radicals secondarily to damage caused by other mechanisms. This complicates interpretation of quantitative data on production of radical products following exercise and in combination with the known multiplicity of action of pharmacological agents and antioxidants [54,59] may cause misinterpretation of the mechanisms involved.

6   ABBREVIATIONS

AMP: adenosine monophosphate
AP-1:   activator protein-1
ATP: adenosine triphosphate
HSF: heat shock factor
NF-κB: nuclear factor kappa B
SOD: superoxide dismutase

7   REFERENCES

 1. Dillard CJ, Litov RE, Savin WM, Dumelin EE, Tappel AL. J Appl Physiol 1978;45:927—932.
 2. Davies KJA, Packer L, Brooks GA. Biochem Biophys Res Comm 1982;107:1199—1205.
 3. Jackson MJ. Proc Nutr Soc 1987;46:77—80.
 4. Sjodin B, Westing YM, Apple FS. Sports Med 1990;10:236—254.
 5. Newham DJ, Mills KR, Quigley BM, Edwards RHT. Clin Sci 1983;64:55—62.
 6. Newham DJ, Jones DA, Edwards RHT. Muscle Nerve 1986;9;54-63.
 7. Newham DJ, Jones DA, Tolfree SEJ, Edwards RHT. Eur J Appl Physiol 1986;55:106—112.
 8. Armstrong RB. Sports Med 1986;3:370-381.
 9. Armstrong RB. Med Sci Sports Exercise 1990;22:429-435.
10. Halliwell B, Gutteridge JMC. Lancet 1984;ii:1396-1397.
11. Loschen G, Azzi A, Richter C, Flohe L. FEBS Lett 1974;42:68-72.
12. Boveris A, Chance BC. Biochem J 1973;134:707-716.
13. Jackson MJ, Edwards RHT, Symons MCR. Biochim Biophys Acta 1985;847:185-190.
14. Borg DC. In: Swatz HM, Bolton JR, Borg DC (eds) Biological Applications of Electron Spin Resonance. New York: John Wiley and Sons, 1972;265-280.
15. Swartz HM. In: Swatz HM, Bolton Jr, Borg DC (eds) Biological Applications of Electron Spin Resonance. New York: John Wiley and Sons, 1972;155—165.

16. Chetverikov A, Kalmanson A, Kharitonenkor I, Blumenfield L. Biofizika 1964;9:18—23.
17. Reid MB, Hoack KE, Franchek KM, Valberg PA, Kobzik L, Wert MS. J Appl Physiol 1992;73: 1797—1804.
18. Reid MB, Shoji T, Moody MR, Fentman MC. J Appl Physiol 1992;73:1805—1809.
19. O'Neill CA, Stebbins CL, Bonigiet S, Halliwell B, Longhurst JC. J Appl Physiol 1996;81: 1197—1206.
20. Ashton A, Rowlands CC, Jones E, Young IS, Jackson SK, Davies B, Peters JR. Eur J Appl Physiol 1998;77:498—502.
21. McCord JM. N Eng J Med 1985;312:159—163.
22. Al-Khalidi UAS, Chaglasscain TH. Biochem J 1965;97:318—320.
23. Wajner M, Harkness RA. Biochim Biophys Acta 1989;991:79—84.
24. Jarasch E-D, Grund C, Bruder G, Heid HW et al. Cell 1981;25:67—82.
25. Claremont D, Jackson MJ, Jones DA. J Physiol 1984;353:57P.
26. McArdle A, Edwards RHT, Jackson MJ. Clin Sci 1992;82:455—459.
27. Jones DA, Jackson MJ, McPhail G, Edwards RHT. Clin Sci 1984;66:317—322.
28. Jackson MJ, Jones DA, Edwards RHT. Eur J Clin Invest 1984;14:369—374.
29. Friden J, Sjöström M, Ekblom B. Int J Sports Med 1983;4:170—176.
30. Sutton JR, Toews CJ, Ward GR, Fox IH. Metabolism 1980;29:254—260.
31. Helstron-Westling Y, Sollevi A, Sjödin B. Eur J Appl Physiol 1991;62:380—384.
32. Patterson VH, Kaiser KK, Brooke MH. J Neurol Neurosurg Psychiat 1982;45:552—553.
33. Bothuis PA, Zwart R, Bär PR, de Vissor M, van der Helm HJ. Clin Chem 1988;34:1607—1610.
34. Rodemann HP, Goldberg AL. J Biol Chem 1982;257:1632—1638.
35. Smith R, Palmer RM, Reeds PJ. Biochem J 1982;214:142—161.
36. McArdle A, Edwards RHT, Jackson MJ. Clin Sci 1991;80:367—371.
37. Halliwell B, Gutteridge JMC. Free Radicals in Biology and Medicine. Oxford: Clarendon Press, 1985.
38. Jackson MJ, Wagenmakers AJM, Edwards RHT. Biochem J 1987;241:403—407
39. Terjuing RL. In: Strauss RH (ed) Sports Medicine and Physiology. Philadelphia: Sauders 1979: 147—165.
40. Jewett SL, Eddy LJ, Hockstein P. Free Radical Biol Med 1989;6:185—188.
41. Singal PK, Kapur N, Dhillon KS, Beamish RE, Dhalla NS. Can J Physiol Pharmacol 1982;60: 1390—1397.
42. Babior BM. Blood 1984;64:956—966.
43. Rossi F. Biochim Biophys Acta 1986;853:65—89.
44. Duncan CJ. In: Duncan CJ (ed) Calcium, Oxygen Radicals and Cellular Damage. Cambridge: Cambridge University Press, 1991;97—113.
45. Malech HL, Gallin JI. N Engl J Med 1987;317:687—694.
46. Kleban SJ. In: Gallin JI, Fauci AS (eds) Advances in Host Defense Mechanisms, vol 1. New York: Raven Press, 1982;111—162.
47. Cannon JG, Orencole SF, Fielding RA, Meydani M, Meydani SN, Fiatrone MA, Blumberg JB, Evans WJ. Am J Physiol 1990;259:R214—R219.
48. Gollnick PD, Hodgson DR, Byrd SK. In: Benzi G (ed) Advances in Myochemistry: 2. London: John Libbey Eurotext, 1989;339—350.
49. Burton KP, Morris AC Massey KD, Buja LM, Hagler HK. J Mol Cell Cardiol 1988;20(Suppl V):59.
50. Vandeplassche G, Bernier M, Thone F, Borges M, Kusama Y, Hearse DJ. J Mol Cell Cardiol 1990;22:287—301.
51. Shattock MJ, Matsuura H, Hearse DJ. In: Duncan CJ (ed) Calcium, Oxygen Radicals and Cellular Damage. Cambridge: Cambridge University Press, 1991;77—95.
52. Nicotera P, Kass GEN, Duddy SK, Orrenius S. In: Duncan CJ (ed) Calcium, Oxygen Radicals and Cellular Damage. Cambridge: Cambridge University Press, 1991;17—33.
53. Phoenix J, Edwards RHT, Jackson MJ. Biochem J 1989;287:207—213.

54. Phoenix J, Edwards RHT, Jackson MJ. Biohim Biophys Acta 1991;1097:212—218.
55. Jackson MJ, McArdle A, Edwards RHT. In: Duncan CJ (ed) Calcium, Oxygen Radicals and Cellular Damage. Cambridge University Press, 1991;139—148.
56. McArdle A, Jackson MJ. Basic Appl Myol 1994;4:43—50.
57. Gower, JD, Cotterill LA, Green CJ. In: Duncan CJ (ed) Calcium, Oxygen Radicals and Cellular Damage. Cambridge: Cambridge University Press 1991;165—188.
58. Rice-Evans C. In: Dass DK (ed) Oxygen Radicals: Systemic Events and Disease Processes. Basel: Karger, 1990;1—30.
59. Jackson MJ, Jones DA, Harris EJ. Biosci Rep 1984;4:581—587.
60. Jackson MJ, McArdle, McArdle F. Proc Nutr Soc 1998;57:301—305.
61. Salo DC, Donovan CM, Davies KJA. Free Rad Biol Med 1991;11:239—246.
62. Currie RW, Karmazyn M, Kloz M, Mailes K. Circ Res 1988;63:543—549.
63. Donnelly TJ, Sieves RE, Vissen FLJ, Welch WJ, Wolfe CC. Circulation: 1992;85:7709—778.
64. Yellon DM, Pasinc E, Corgoni A, Marber MS, Latchman DS, Ferrari R. J Mol Cell Cardiol 1992;24:895—907.
65. Marber MS, Mestrill R, Chi SH, Sayen MR, Yellon DM, Dillman WH. J Clin Invest 1995;95:1446—1456.
66. McArdle A, McArdle C, Jackson MJ. J Physiol 1997;499:9P.
67. McArdle A, Beaver A, Edwards RHT, Jackson MJ. J Physiol 1995;483:84P.

©2000 Elsevier Science B.V. All rights reserved.
Handbook of Oxidants and Antioxidants in Exercise.
C.K. Sen, L. Packer and O. Hänninen, editors.

Part II • Chapter 3

Exercise and xanthine oxidase in the vasculature: superoxide and nitric oxide interactions

C. Roger White[1,3], Jonathan E. Shelton[1], Douglas Moellering[2], Hanjoong Jo[2], Rakesh P. Patel[2,3] and Victor Darley-Usmar[2,3]

[1]*Departments of Medicine, Vascular Biology and Hypertension Program,*
[2]*Departments of Pathology, Division of Molecular and Cellular Pathology, and*
[3]*Center for Free Radical Biology, University of Alabama at Birmingham, Birmingham, Alabama, USA.*
E-mail: darley@path.uab.edu

1 INTRODUCTION
   1.1 Oxidant stress
   1.2 Oxidants, exercise and vascular injury
2 NITRIC OXIDE AND SUPEROXIDE INTERACTIONS
   2.1 Nitric oxide production by endothelial cells
   2.2 Reactive oxygen species and atherosclerosis
   2.3 Endothelium-dependent relaxation is impaired in atherosclerosis
   2.4 Vascular responses to peroxynitrite
3 XANTHINE OXIDASE AS A SOURCE OF SUPEROXIDE
   3.1 Xanthine oxidase and cardiovascular injury
   3.2 Glycosaminoglycans interact with both oxidants and antioxidants
4 EXERCISE AND OXIDANT STRESS
   4.1 Exercise and purine degradation
   4.2 Exercise and oxidant formation
   4.3 Adaptations to exercise training
   4.4 Exercise and antioxidant defense mechanisms
   4.5 Exercise and nitric oxide production
5 SUMMARY
6 PERSPECTIVES
7 ACKNOWLEDGEMENTS
8 ABBREVIATIONS
9 REFERENCES

1   INTRODUCTION

1.1 Oxidant stress

Reactive oxygen species (ROS) are generated during the molecular reduction of O_2 to H_2O and in response to the activation of a variety of cellular enzyme systems including cyclooxygenase, lipoxygenase, NAD(P)H oxidase and xanthine oxidase (XO) [1]. Cells possess antioxidant defense mechanisms which normally metabolize ROS before they reach the critical concentrations at which they may produce vascular injury [2,3]. Among these antioxidants are the enzymes superoxide dismutase (SOD), catalase and glutathione peroxidase. Superoxide dismutase catalyzes the dismutation of superoxide (O_2^-) to hydrogen peroxide (H_2O_2) while catalase reduces H_2O_2 to H_2O. Glutathione peroxidase also serves an important role as a scavenger of H_2O_2 with the concomitant oxidation of glutathione [1].

1.2 Oxidants, exercise and vascular injury

In recent years, numerous studies have shown that vascular function is compromised in a number of cardiovascular conditions including stroke, hypertension, and atherosclerosis. In atherosclerosis, blood vessels undergo marked changes in both structure and function which may predispose for angina and myocardial infarction. Defects in lipoprotein metabolism and vascular reactivity are fundamental pathological responses to hypercholesterolemia, with extensive evidence suggesting that reactive oxygen species play an important role in the initiation and progression of these lesions. Recent studies have shown that nitric oxide (NO) interactions with ROS are an important route to the biochemical changes which occur in the compromised vasculature. Some of these critical pathways and their interactions are summarized in Fig. 1.

Physical exercise also induces oxidative stress. On initial inspection, this would appear to be a paradoxical response, since it is generally agreed that long-term

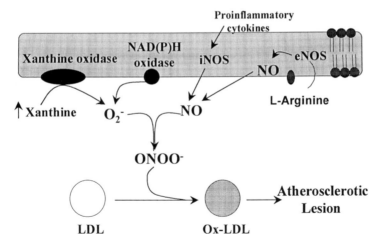

Fig. 1. Generation of reactive oxygen and nitrogen species in the vasculature. The oxidant peroxynitrite (ONOO$^-$) is formed from the reaction between superoxide (O_2^-), and nitric oxide (NO). Superoxide is generated from metabolism of purines such as xanthine and/or oxygen reduction mediated by membrane localized NAD(P)H oxidases. Nitric oxide is synthesized by NO synthases which can be stimulated by calcium-calmodulin dependent processes (NOS III) or by pro-inflammatory cytokines (NOS II). Peroxynitrite causes oxidative modification of low-density lipoprotein (LDL) leading to atherogenic lesion development. This process can occur in the vessel wall and is associated with an increased cellular production of O_2^- and hence ONOO$^-$, which is thought to be a critical event in atheroma formation.

compliance with an exercise program decreases the risk for development of cardiovascular disease. In this review, we shall explore cellular pathways involved in the formation of reactive species in the vessel wall under normal and pathophysiological conditions. As will be discussed, the induction of oxidant stress under exercise conditions occurs through similar mechanisms to those identified in disease processes.

2 NITRIC OXIDE AND SUPEROXIDE INTERACTIONS

2.1 Nitric oxide production by endothelial cells

The dynamic role of the endothelium in the regulation of vascular tone has become well established since Furchgott and Zawadsky [4] reported that the relaxation of isolated blood vessels to vasoactive agents such as acetylcholine and the calcium (Ca^{2+}) ionophore, A23187, was dependent on the presence of an intact endothelium. They postulated that endothelial cells produced a diffusible "endothelium-derived relaxing factor" (EDRF) which stimulated cGMP-dependent mechanisms of relaxation in vascular smooth muscle cells (VSMC). It has subsequently been shown that EDRF and NO share similar chemical and pharmacological properties [5], are derived from the oxidation of a terminal guanidino-group of L-arginine [6,7] and are believed by many to be the same compound. Three distinct enzymes are involved in NO formation in different cell types, each of them utilizing NADPH as a cofactor [5]. In the central nervous system, a neuronal isoform of NO synthase is expressed constitutively and has been designated NOS I [8]. In the vascular endothelium, a Ca^{2+}-calmodulin-dependent NO synthase (NOS III) is also expressed constitutively, and increases in intracellular calcium ($[Ca^{2+}]_i$), following agonist stimulation increase NO formation and thereby induce vascular relaxation [9]. In contrast, an inducible isoform of NO synthase (NOS II) may be produced in macrophages, hepatocytes, VSMCs and the endothelium in response to endotoxin, cytokines and other pro-inflammatory factors [5,10,11].

2.2 Reactive oxygen species and atherosclerosis

Reactive oxygen species have been implicated in both the pathogenic mechanisms and altered physiologic responses characteristic of atherosclerosis. Oxidation of low-density lipoprotein (LDL), thought to be a critical event in the initiation of atheroma formation [12,13], is associated with enhanced cellular production of O_2^- [14,15]. Low-density lipoprotein is normally incorporated in cells via a high affinity, ligand-receptor binding interaction [16,17]. Modification of LDL (acetylation, oxidation) reduces the affinity of the lipoprotein for this uptake mechanism. Macrophages and other cell types are able to incorporate modified LDLs, however, via an acetylated-LDL (Ac-LDL) or "scavenger" receptor, leading to the formation of lipid-enriched foam cells [16]. Evidence suggests that multiple "scavenger" receptor types exist which bind modified LDLs with high affinity but have overlapping ligand specificity [18—23].

Oxidized lipoproteins may promote further injury by initiating chain-propagating oxidation reactions within the cell, thus it is no surprise that the efficacy of the antioxidant probucol in preventing the development of intimal lesions in Watanabe hyperlipidemic rabbits is due to its radical scavenging properties [24]. In addition, the presence of oxidized-LDL in atheromatous plaque correlates with the progression of atherosclerotic carotid disease [25]. Oxidized LDL has also been shown to directly inhibit endothelium-dependent vasorelaxation [26,27]. Currently, the precise role of oxidants (including O_2^-) in the initiation of lipoprotein oxidation and impairment of vascular function in hypercholesterolemia remains unclear.

2.3 Endothelium-dependent relaxation is impaired in atherosclerosis

In recent years, it has been suggested that alterations in vascular reactivity associated with atherosclerosis are related to changes in endothelium-dependent mechanisms of relaxation. Isolated blood vessels from both atherosclerotic patients [28,29] and hypercholesterolemic animal models [30—34] exhibit this defect. Numerous mechanisms have been proposed to explain the impaired vascular relaxation associated with atherosclerosis and hypercholesterolemic animal models. These include an increased diffusional barrier for NO due to intimal cell proliferation and lipid deposition [35], L-arginine substrate depletion [30,36,37], changes in endothelial cell receptor-coupling mechanisms [38], as well as modification of NO via its reaction with oxygen-derived free radical species such as O_2^- [34]. Intimal thickening as a barrier to NO does not appear to be a critical factor since cessation of a high cholesterol diet restores normal endothelium-dependent relaxation in *cynomolgus* monkey arteries despite the continued presence of an enlarged intima [39]. There appears to be little evidence supporting the hypothesis that defects in receptor-mediated calcium mobilization in endothelial cells result in impaired relaxation, since dietary restriction and antioxidant therapy improve the agonist-mediated release of NO.

Other reports suggest that impaired endothelium-dependent relaxation is due a depletion of L-arginine substrate, the precursor for NO synthesis [30,36,37], with a reduction of L-arginine in hypercholesterolemic rabbits possibly accounting for the diminished response of isolated vascular preparations to calcium-mobilizing agonists such as acetylcholine. These studies [30,36,37] showed that prolonged incubation of vessels with L-arginine restores endothelium-dependent relaxation. Other reports, however, suggest that NO production is actually enhanced in vessels of hypercholesterolemic rabbits [40]. Using chemiluminescence techniques, it was shown that the basal release of NO and its metabolites was increased in the aorta of hypercholesterolemic rabbits [40]. This suggests that NO synthesis is actually enhanced, and again supports the view that the impaired relaxation response is due to the rapid reaction of NO with other molecules such as O_2^-, leading to a reduction in its vasoactive properties. Superoxide anion is generated in both intracellular and extracellular compartments and reacts with the more membrane-permeable and diffusible NO, yielding peroxynitrite (ONOO$^-$) [34]. Peroxynitrite may promote atherogenesis by reducing the normal physiological actions of NO and by acting as a potent oxidant capable of oxidizing lipoproteins (Fig. 1). Liposome-entrapped SOD and polyethylene glycol-derivatized SOD have been used to enhance vascular endothelial anti-oxidant enzyme levels in vessels of hypercholesterolemic rabbits [34,41]. These treatments effectively restored endothelium-dependent relaxation, suggesting that O_2^--mediated injury resulted in a functional modification of NO. Similar protective effects are observed when ring segments are treated with allopurinol or oxypurinol, inhibitors of the free radical generating enzyme XO [42,43]. Thus, O_2^- derived from XO may react with NO produced in the vessel wall and play an important role in the modification of vascular function.

2.4 Vascular responses to peroxynitrite

Peroxynitrite has been targeted as a potential mediator of endothelial cell injury in cardiovascular disease [44]. The reaction of O_2^- with NO is kinetically favored over the spontaneous and even the enzymatically catalyzed dismutation of O_2^- [45], with several reports suggesting ONOO$^-$ plays an important role in athero-genesis [34,46]. First, impaired vascular reactivity may result from the production of ONOO$^-$ which acts as only a relatively weak stimulus for guanylate cyclase activity in VSMCs [47,48]. Second, due to its potent oxidizing properties, ONOO$^-$ will participate in the oxidation of lipoproteins whose modification is involved in the production of the fatty streak and subsequent plaque formation characteristic of the atherosclerotic lesion [34]. Finally, downregulation of cell growth kinetics and other beneficial actions of NO will be lost upon its reaction with O_2^- to yield ONOO$^-$ (Fig. 1).

Relatively few studies have examined the direct effect of ONOO$^-$ on vascular relaxation. One problem associated with in vitro studies of ONOO$^-$ function is its relatively short half-life at physiological pH ($t_{1/2} = 1-2$ s). Still, it has been observed that ONOO$^-$ produces a rapid relaxation of bovine pulmonary artery ring segments [49]. This response was blunted by inhibitors of guanylate cyclase but was insensitive to dimethyl sulfoxide, a $^\bullet$OH radical scavenger. Treatment of ring segments with diethyl maleate, an agent which depletes tissue glutathione and therefore thiol groups, reduced the thiol-dependent conversion of ONOO$^-$ to a vasorelaxant metabolite. It was suggested that ONOO$^-$ exerts its relaxant actions by nitrosating tissue sulfhydryl groups, yielding nitrosothiol derivatives, which then slowly release NO [49]. Peroxynitrite may also react with glucose, gly-cerol and other molecules containing multiple hydroxy groups, resulting in the formation of NO donors [50,51]. These reaction products share similar biochem-ical properties with organic nitrates and nitrites and are also dependent on thiols for the liberation of free NO [50,51].

Peroxynitrite has also been implicated in the enhanced contractility of canine coronary arteries from hearts subjected to ischemia-reperfusion [52]. Contractions in hypoxic perfusate were blocked by the NO synthase inhibitor L-NMMA, suggesting that reperfusion following ischemia stimulates the production of $ONOO^-$ which is itself metabolized to form an endothelium-dependent contracting factor or stimulates the release of such a factor. In contrast, $ONOO^-$ is reported to produce a dose-dependent relaxation of canine coronary artery rings [53]. The relaxant effect of $ONOO^-$ was similar in intact and endothelium-denuded vessels and was potentiated by the addition of SOD to the tissue bath.

The diversity of these responses to $ONOO^-$ underscores the gaps which exist in our understanding of this reactive species and the role it plays in vascular reactivity. While sites of NO formation in the vessel wall have been well characterized in recent years, sources of O_2^-, with which NO reacts to form $ONOO^-$, remain to be clearly defined. Potential sources of O_2^- which have been recently identified include a plasma membrane NAD(P)H oxidase [54,55], the enzyme NO synthase when deprived of its substrate L-arginine [56] and the oxidative enzyme XO [57].

3   XANTHINE OXIDASE AS A SOURCE OF SUPEROXIDE

3.1 Xanthine oxidase and cardiovascular injury

Xanthine oxidase is produced via sulfhydryl oxidation or limited proteolysis of xanthine dehydrogenase (XDH) [57]. In the presence of purine substrate and molecular O_2, XO catalyzes the formation of uric acid and the oxidants O_2^- and H_2O_2 [58]. Increases in circulating plasma XO are associated with numerous pathological conditions including ischemia-reperfusion injury [59,60], hepatotoxicity [61], respiratory distress syndrome [62], thermal stress [63], viral infections [64] and ethanol intake [65]. The vascular endothelium is a common site of injury associated with these conditions, and the oxidative damage at this locus has been linked to the enhanced production of O_2^- by XO [59—64]. The importance of XO in cardiovascular injury has been the subject of debate since several reports suggest that human tissues exhibit low or undetectable levels of XO [66—68]. Other investigators, however, have detected XO in a variety of human tissues including cardiac and skeletal muscle [69], liver, intestine, lung and kidney [70]. At the cellular level, XO expression was localized in hepatocytes [70], endothelial cells, VSMCs, macrophages and mast cells [71]. Recently, XO has also been found associated with human atherosclerotic tissues including vessels surgically removed in the repair of aneurysm and endarterectomy [72]. It is suggested that in atherosclerosis, a localized hypoxia in the vessel wall may favor the conversion of XDH to XO, thus promoting oxidative injury to the vessel wall [73].

Regional ischemia in organs such as the liver and intestine results in a significant release of XO into the circulation after aortic cross-clamping procedures [74]. Remote cardiac and pulmonary injury are characteristic responses to ischemia-reperfusion and the elevation of plasma XO [74,75]. Increases in myocardial lipid peroxidation [76] and purine efflux [77] are correlated with increased XO activity following human coronary bypass grafting. Plasma XO concentration is also elevated in patients with inflammatory and autoimmune rheumatic diseases [78]. In these patients, plasma XO activity increased up to 50-fold, concomitant with a 45–74% reduction in serum sulfhydryls, a marker of oxidative injury. Allopurinol, an inhibitor of XO, is effective in preventing remote tissue injury following ischemia-reperfusion. In a porcine model of reperfusion injury, pretreatment with allopurinol prevented the occurrence of focal arrhythmias [66]. Similarly, preoperative treatment of patients undergoing cardiac bypass surgery with allopurinol results in an accelerated recovery of myocardial performance with cardiac output and left ventricular function returning to normal more rapidly than in untreated control patients [79]. Additionally, plasma XO and uric acid levels were significantly reduced in these patients. Protective effects of allopurinol and its metabolites are also reported in the treatment of pulmonary inflammation [75] and intestinal [80] and renal [81] reperfusion injury. Increases in circulating XO have also been reported in atherosclerotic humans [82]. A recent report also shows that infusion of oxypurinol, an active metabolite of allopurinol, in hypercholesterolemic humans increases forearm blood flow and decreases vascular resistance, suggesting that XO modulates vascular tone in these patients [83]. The beneficial effects of allopurinol in these diverse pathological conditions are consistent with an inhibition of XO-mediated free radical formation.

3.2 Glycosaminoglycans interact with both oxidants and antioxidants

Vascular endothelial cells possess glycosaminoglycan (GAG)-rich proteoglycan receptors which serve to both concentrate molecules at the cell surface and participate in signal transduction processes [84–86]. With regard to free radical events, GAGs reversibly bind both prooxidant (XO) and antioxidant (extracellular SOD type C) molecules via saturable, high affinity receptors [87,88]. Oxidative injury occurs to both vascular functional and structural elements as the concentration of reactive species exceeds the capacity for removal by endogenous antioxidant enzyme systems [34]. Glycosaminoglycan association can also promote the endocytic incorporation of bound molecules [89,90]. Thus, XO may be internalized by endothelial cells to react with intracellular purines and produce reactive oxygen species in the intracellular compartment.

Heparin and heparan sulfate GAGs are prominently expressed in endothelial cells and in the interstitial matrix where they bind substances including fibroblast growth factor [92] and lipoprotein-associated coagulation inhibitor [86,91,92]. Association of LDL with human macrophage and smooth muscle cell GAGs increases the susceptibility of the lipoprotein to oxidation as compared to native LDL [93]. The increased oxidative capacity was associated with a modification of apolipoprotein A and a reorganization of lipids within the lipoprotein.

Extracellular SOD type C (EC-SOD) is an SOD isozyme exhibiting high affinity, saturable binding to heparin sulfate proteoglycans [87,94]. Incubation of arterial ring segments with EC-SOD results in a substantial increase in enzyme bound to the vessel wall [87]. Washout of the incubation media results in minimal recovery of the enzyme. EC-SOD treatment protected against the inhibition of NO bioactivity induced by treatment of ring segments with pyrogallol, an O_2^- generating system. Treatment with heparin, which competitively binds and displaces GAG-associated molecules, eliminated the protective effect of EC-SOD, suggesting that heparin had displaced the enzyme from binding sites on sulfated proteoglycans. Native Cu-Zn SOD, which lacks affinity to heparin sulfate proteoglycans and is electrostatically repelled from cell surfaces, failed to provide protection against pyrogallol-mediated injury in these studies [87]. In studies of EC-SOD transgenic mice, a 5-fold increase in brain activity was shown to protect against edema resulting from cold-stress [94]. The edema was mediated by $ONOO^-$, since inhibitors of NO synthase also protected against injury [94]. Other studies have shown that heparin treatment increases plasma EC-SOD activity due to the ability of heparin to compete with heparin-sulfated GAGs for binding with and thus displacement of EC-SOD [95,96].

The pro-oxidant enzyme XO readily interacts with GAGs on the endothelial cell surface. Adachi and coworkers have shown that XO binds electrostatically to GAGs on the surface of cultured endothelial cells, and that this binding phenomenon can be reversed by treatment of cells with heparin or by enzymatically cleaving GAGs with heparinase and heparitinase [97]. Recent evidence suggests that numerous oxidizing agents, including xanthine/XO, stimulate the synthesis of GAGs [98] and reduce the expression of EC-SOD and antioxidant activity [99]. Oxidative injury due to O_2^- production has been linked to increases in circulating XO in ischemia-reperfusion models [66]. A protective effect of heparin, which displaces XO from GAG binding sites, has been described under these conditions [96]. Acetylcholine-mediated relaxation of isolated rat hindlimbs was severely compromised when the vascular bed was reperfused after an ischemic period. Heparin treatment, however, permitted a dose-dependent recovery of endothelium-dependent relaxation under the same experimental conditions [100]. In a hemorrhagic shock model of ischemia-reperfusion, XO activity is concentrated in the rat vasculature after reperfusion [88]. Perfusion with heparin generated a substantial increase in plasma XO activity. These investigators also demonstrated that XO binds in a heparin-reversible fashion to endothelial cells, suggesting that in ischemia-reperfusion injury, XO can gain access to the circulation after release from injured tissues and become concentrated on the vessel wall at sites remote from the primary location of injury [88].

A protective effect of heparin on vasomotor function has also been described in the aorta of rabbits after balloon catheter injury [101]. Balloon injury results in a diminished relaxant response of blood vessels to NO. Chronic heparin treatment, however, significantly restored endothelium-dependent relaxation compared to untreated, experimental groups. The mechanism for this protective effect of heparin is unknown and does not appear to be related to antiproliferative effects of the free GAG [101]. The generation of O_2^- by XO requires purine substrates such as hypoxanthine (HX) and xanthine. Under atherosclerotic conditions, adequate amounts of xanthine and XO are present in blood vessels to support O_2^- production. It has been suggested that a localized hypoxia develops in the vessel wall under hypercholesterolemic conditions, stimulating both the intracellular degradation of ATP to HX and xanthine [102] and the release of purines from the cell [103]. Exercise-induced oxidative injury may occur through similar mechanisms. As will be discussed in the next section, a component of the hypoxic response to exercise is the enhanced formation of HX and xanthine via purine degradation pathways.

4   Exercise and oxidant stress

4.1 Exercise and purine degradation

In conditioned athletes undergoing normal exercise regimens, energy consumption occurs primarily by aerobic mechanisms [104]. Oxygen uptake can be used as an index for the resynthesis of high-energy phosphate compounds such as adenosine triphosphate (ATP) under these conditions of aerobic metabolism [105]. With intensive exercise, however, a reduction in the generation of ATP leads to the accumulation of adenosine 5'-diphosphate (ADP), lactic acid, and purine nucleotide metabolites such as HX in the plasma [105]. The generation of these metabolites reflects the activation of anaerobic respiratory mechanisms with exercise [104].

Phosphocreatine (PCr) and stored ATP are additional sources of high energy phosphate compounds which may be tapped under conditions of intensive exercise [104]. The enzyme creatine kinase catalyzes the transfer of the phosphate group from PCr to ADP, resulting in the formation of ATP and creatine. Under conditions of intensive exercise, ATP formation from PCr may be diminished due to a significant reduction in muscle PCr content [106]. As a result, cellular ADP concentration increases. During exhaustive exercise, the enzyme adenylate kinase is activated in muscle cells resulting in the degradation of ADP to AMP. AMP may be further metabolized to form adenosine and inosine 5'-monophosphate (IMP). After high-speed treadmill running, there is a prominent accumulation of IMP in skeletal muscle, and metabolism of IMP results in an increase in plasma concentrations of inosine and HX [107]. Studies using venous and arterial erythrocytes also show a reduction in ADP and AMP and an increase in IMP with intensive exercise [108]. This initiates a cascade of purine catabolism, which has important implications for exercise-induced oxidant formation (Fig. 2).

Muscle fatigue, which occurs after exhaustive exercise, is due to a reduced capacity to generate ATP and is correlated with an increased muscle content of IMP and HX [109,110]. Following exercise and metabolic stress, HX and uric acid release from skeletal muscle have been noted both in vivo and in vitro

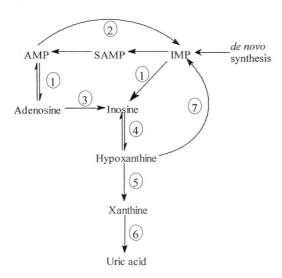

Fig. 2. Catabolism and salvage synthesis of purine nucleotides. Adenosine monophosphate (AMP), formed during normal metabolism, can be either dephosphorylated to adenosine by a specific cytosolic 5'-nucleotidase (reaction 1) or deaminated to the purine nucleotide, inosine 5'monophosphate (IMP) (reaction 2). Adenosine is further metabolized to inosine by adenosine deaminase (reaction 3). IMP can also be dephosphorylated to inosine (reaction 1). Inosine undergoes phosphorolysis to hypoxanthine (reaction 4) and hypoxanthine is oxidized to xanthine and ultimately to uric acid. These latter two reactions are catalyzed by xanthine oxidase (reactions 5 and 6) and are irreversible. Hypoxanthine can be salvaged through phosphorylation in a reaction catalysed by hypoxanthine phosphoribosyltransferase (reaction 7).

[108,111]. Hypoxanthine, xanthine, and uric acid are thus significantly elevated in plasma under conditions of muscle fatigue and during the recovery period after exercise [111]. While muscle appears to be a major source of HX during exercise, its conversion to xanthine and uric acid may occur in distal tissues [112,113].

Dietary ingestion of creatine effectively increases muscle content of both creatine and PCr [106]. A major benefit of this oral supplement may be to facilitate PCr formation during and after exercise. Further, ATP degradation and the accumulation of HX and other respiratory metabolites in plasma are minimized during exercise. Creatine loading may thus improve performance and reduce oxidative muscle injury after exercise [106].

4.2 Exercise and oxidant formation

Increases in oxygen demand and energy utilization during exercise result in the formation of oxidants [114]. From the previous section, it is evident that the substrates for XO are elevated under conditions of even mild hypoxia. Drawing from our understanding of oxidant formation in atherosclerosis, it is likely that

XO is an important source of O_2^-, H_2O_2 and other oxidative metabolites during acute exercise and may thus contribute to exercise-induced muscle injury [115]. Both human and animal studies show that tissue XO activity is significantly increased during acute exercise [111,116]. Exhaustive exercise in humans results in increases in plasma concentrations of HX and uric acid [117]. Using immuno-histological techniques, Hellesten and co-workers reported that XO content of muscle after strenuous exercise was up to 8-fold higher (measured $1-4$ days after exercise) compared to control muscle biopsies [117]. The increase was ascribed to an increased production of XO by endothelial cells and to the infiltration of XO-containing leukocytes [117]. The action of XO in the presence of HX substrate is to generate O_2^-, H_2O_2 and secondary reactive nitrogen species with potential damaging effects on muscle membranes. Increases in plasma XO activity are correlated with the formation of lipid peroxides and oxidized glutathione, markers of oxidative injury. Administration of the XO inhibitor, allopurinol, or the O_2^- scavenger, SOD, prior to exercise markedly reduces the modification of lipids and thiols [113,118]. Furthermore, allopurinol treatment increases plasma concentrations of xanthine and HX, substrates for XO, while plasma urate, a product of XO-mediated purine oxidation, is significantly reduced [113].

Exhaustive treadmill running in rats increases XO and glutathione peroxidase activities and the formation of thiobarbituric acid-reactive substances (TBARS), a nonspecific marker of lipid oxidation, in the liver and kidney. Administration of SOD to these animals, prior to the exercise regimen, reduced both XO activity and TBARS formation [118]. The effect of SOD on the reduction in XO activity may reflect an inhibition of the oxidative conversion of xanthine dehydrogenase to XO [118]. In support of this idea, treadmill running in mice also enhances the oxidation of glutathione in skeletal muscle. Administration of allopurinol to mice after exercise, however, results in a rapid restoration of the reduced form of glutathione in these tissues [115]. These are the results of acute training episodes. In the next section, we will discuss long-term effects.

4.3 Adaptations to exercise training

Plasma concentrations of HX and lactic acid may remain within the normal range under conditions of nonstrenuous exercise, however, when anaerobic respiration is evoked, the metabolism of purine nucleotides is accelerated [119]. Muscle injury due to oxidant stress may be minimized by limiting exercise to aerobic conditions [119]. There are differences in human skeletal muscle purine nucleotide metabolism before and after a chronic training regimen. Stathis and co-workers reported that exercise training reduces the depletion of ATP after exercise compared to pre-training levels [120]. During the recovery period after a short, strenuous exercise bout, there was a similar reduction in the accumulation of IMP, inosine, and ammonia after training. Plasma HX levels were similarly reduced. The reduced loss of ATP after training was ascribed to an improved balance between ATP metabolism and resynthesis [120].

A report by Hellsten-Westing and co-workers suggests that exercise training alters the activities of enzymes involved in purine metabolism [121]. They found that the activity of AMP deaminase was reduced, while HX phosphoribosyl transferase (HPRT) and phosphofructokinase activities were increased after a 6-week training period compared with pretraining levels. Increased HPRT activity is associated with an increase in the phosphorylation of intracellular HX to IMP. This effectively reduces the available substrate for oxidative enzymes in the trained muscle. Accumulation of plasma HX and uric acid was also significantly lower following training compared with pretraining values. It was suggested that a major beneficial response to exercise training is a reduction in the release of purines from muscle [121].

4.4 Exercise and antioxidant defense mechanisms

Increased antioxidant enzyme production may play an important role in the prevention of oxidative tissue injury under acute exercise conditions [122]. Antioxidants may also contribute significantly to the long-term beneficial effects of exercise on cardiovascular function. Exercise-trained rats show a marked increase in the expression of mRNA for manganese SOD (MnSOD), a mitochondrial isoform of SOD [123,124]. Both basal and postexercise MnSOD activity and content in skeletal muscle are also elevated in exercise-trained rats compared to untrained controls [123]. Results of human studies also show an increase in the activity of Cu-Zn SOD, MnSOD and glutathione peroxidase in skeletal muscle of trained versus untrained subjects [125]. No differences in plasma antioxidant activity were noted between trained and sedentary individuals however. Platelets from exercised-trained human subjects and isolated rat hearts have an increased activity of antioxidant enzymes such as catalase, glutathione peroxidase, as well as SOD [122,126]. Other reports suggest that acute exhaustive exercise promotes a greater increase in MnSOD, catalase and glutathione peroxidase in untrained humans compared to trained individuals [122].

4.5 Exercise and nitric oxide production

Recent studies show that exercise training leads to an increase in NO production, which in turn, may have long-term protective effects on the cardiovascular system in humans [127–129]. Increased blood flow to muscles is an important response to exercise, allowing the replenishment of nutrients and oxygen in tissues. The increased flow may be due to an elevation of shear stress forces on the vascular endothelium, resulting in the stimulation of NO production [130]. Enhanced NO production and release during acute exercise plays a crucial role in modulation of vascular tone [131–134]. The vascular sensitivity to exogenous endothelium-dependent vasodilators and to endogenous NO produced in response to activation of parasympathetic, cholinergic neural pathways is enhanced in exercise-trained animals [135,136]. These treatments enhance coronary artery blood flow during periods of exercise to a greater extent in trained compared to untrained animals [136].

Beneficial effects of exercise on cardiovascular function in humans may thus be due, in part, to the increased production of NO, resulting in enhanced tissue perfusion. Nitric oxide release in response to shear forces on the vascular endothelium may inhibit processes associated with the development and progression of atherosclerosis, including platelet adhesion and the proliferation of cells within the lesioned vessel [130]. Other studies, however, suggest that NO does not play a major role in the adaptive vascular response to exercise [137—138]. Thus, controversy exists regarding the efficacy of long-term exercise and its correlation with NO production [139,140].

5   SUMMARY

1. A prominent response to acute exercise may be to stimulate the production of oxidants such as O_2^- and $ONOO^-$. A comparison of atherosclerosis, as a model system for oxidative injury in the vasculature, indicates that tissue damage in response to exercise occurs through similar mechanisms.
2. Hypoxia appears to play a major role in tissue injury, and facilitates the formation of both XO and its substrates HX and xanthine after acute bouts of

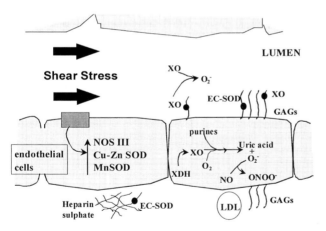

Fig. 3. Exercise and antioxidant defense mechanisms. Increased blood flow to muscles in response to exercise increases shear stress forces on the vascular endothelium. This enhanced shear stress increases endothelial NOS III activity and hence NO production. There is also a concomitant increase in native copper-zinc (Cu-Zn SOD) and manganese superoxide dismutase (MnSOD) activities after *sustained* exercise. During *acute* exercise, xanthine oxidase (XO) bound by glycosaminoglycans (GAGs) may be an important source of superoxide (O_2^-), which can react to form other oxidative metabolites such as peroxynitrite ($ONOO^-$) and thus may contribute to exercise-induced injury. Extracellular SOD (EC-SOD) exhibits high affinity and saturable binding to heparin sulfate proteoglycans which are upregulated after sustained exercise and may protect against free radical-induced vascular injury.

exercise in untrained individuals.
3. Chronic training, on the other hand, is associated with an enhanced perfusion of tissues such as skeletal muscle and a reduction in the hypoxic response. These adaptations may contribute significantly to the reduced cardiovascular risk in individuals who adhere to chronic exercise programs.
4. Nitric oxide may be a critical mediator of these beneficial effects by facilitating tissue perfusion under exercise conditions. The concurrent upregulation of anti-oxidant defense mechanisms may minimize oxidative injury in response to exercise. These putative cellular reaction mechanisms are summarized in Fig. 3.

6   PERSPECTIVES

The importance of exercise is underlined by its emphasis in trend setting documents such as "Healthy People 2000" and the prominent discussion of cardio-vascular disease in the popular literature. We are now extending the insights from basic research into this arena, and these studies will provide an interesting perspective on how and when we should exercise to gain maximum beneficial effects. The focus of this article has been on the effects of acute and chronic exercise on free radical production in the vasculature. Since exercise can increase oxidative damage, it again emphasizes a holistic approach to our health which must also encompass diet and mental aspects. This will no doubt lead to considerable reflection and pause for thought, preferably while partaking of a full bodied glass of red wine, in planning future research endeavors in this interesting and topical area.

7   ACKNOWLEDGEMENTS

The authors are grateful for support from the National Institutes of Health HL 53601 (HJ), HL 54815 (CRW), HL 58031 (VDMU) and the American Heart Association - South East Affiliate (HJ and VMDU) and the American Diabetes Association (VMDU). R.P.P is Parker B. Francis Fellow in Pulmonary Research.

8   ABBREVIATIONS

EDRF: endothelium-derived relaxing factor
GAG: glycosaminoglycan
HX: hypoxanthine
LDL: low-density lipoprotein
NO: nitric oxide
NOS: nitric oxide synthase
$ONOO^-$: peroxynitrite
O_2^-:   superoxide
ROS: reactive oxygen species
SOD: superoxide dismutase
VSMC: vascular smooth muscle cell

XDH: xanthine dehydrogenase
XO: xanthine oxide

9   REFERENCES

1. Rubanyi GM. Free Rad Biol Med 1988;4:107—120.
2. Lindsay SL, Freeman BA. In: Fishman AP (ed) Pulmonary Circulation: Normal and Abnormal. Univ Penn Press, 1990;217—229.
3. Hiraishi H, Terano A, Razandi M, Sugimoto T, Harada T, Ivey KJ. J Biol Chem 1992;267(21): 14812—14817.
4. Furchgott F, Zawadski JV. Nature 1980;288:373—376.
5. Moncada S, Palmer RMJ, Higgs EA. Pharmacol Rev 1991;43:109—142.
6. Palmer RMJ, Ferrige AG, Moncada S. Nature 1987;327:524—526.
7. Ignarro LJ, Buga GM, Wood KS, Byrns RE, Chaudhuri G. Proc Natl Acad Sci USA 1987;84: 9265—9269.
8. Pollack JS, Forstermann U, Tracey WR, Nakane M. Histochem J 1995;27(10):738—744.
9. Lopez-Jaramillo P, Gonzalez MC, Palmer RMJ, Moncada S. Br J Pharmacol 1990;101: 489—493.
10. Radomski MW, Palmer RMJ, Moncada S. Proc Natl Acad Sci USA 1990;87:10043—10047.
11. Beasley D, Schwartz JH, Brenner BM. J Clin Invest 1991;87:602—608.
12. Panasenko OM, Vol'nova TV, Azizova OA, Vladimirov YA. Free Rad Biol Med 1991;10: 137—148.
13. Berliner JA, Navab M, Fogelman AM, Frank JS, Demer LL, Edwards PA, Watson AD, Lusis AJ. Circulation 1995;91:2488—2496.
14. Steinbrecher UP. Biochim Biophys Acta 1988;959(1):20—30.
15. Witzum JL, Steinberg D. J Clin Invest 1991;88:1785—1792.
16. Schwartz CJ, Valente AJ, Sprague EA, Kelley JL, Nerem RM. Clin Cardiol 1991;14:I1—I16.
17. Krieger M. Trends in Biol Sci 1992;17:141—146.
18. Steinbrecher UP, Zhang H, Lougheed M. Free Rad Biol Med 1990;9:155—168.
19. Arai H, Kita T, Yokode M, Narumiya S, Kawai C. Biochem Biophys Res Comm 1989;159: 1375—1382.
20. Sparrow CP, Parathasarathy S, Steinberg D. J Biol Chem 1989;264(5):2599—2604.
21. Ottnad E, Parathasarathy S, Sambrano GR, Ramprasad MP, Quehenberger O, Kondratenko N, Green S, Steinberg D. Proc Natl Acad Sci USA 1995;92(5):1391—1395.
22. Acton SL, Scherer PE, Lodish HF, Kreiger M. J Biol Chem 1994;269(33):21003—21009.
23. Stanton LW, White RT, Bryant CM, Protter AA, Endemann G. J Biol Chem 1992;267(31): 22446—22451.
24. Carew TE, Schwenke DC, Steinberg D. Proc Natl Acad Sci (USA) 1987;84(21):7725—7729.
25. Salonen JT, Yla-Herttuala S, Yamamoto R, Butler S, Korpela H, Salonen R, Nyyssonen L, Palinski W, Witztum JL. Lancet 1992;339:883—887.
26. Jacobs M, Plane F, Bruckdorfer KR. Br J Pharmacol 1990;100(1):21—26.
27. Plane F, Kerr P, Bruckdorfer KR, Jacobs M. Biochem Soc Transact 1990;18(6):1177—1178.
28. Bossaler C, Habib GB, Yamamoto H, Williams C, Wells S, Henry PD. J Clin Invest 1987;79: 170—174.
29. Forstermann U, Mugge A, Alheid U, Haverich A, Frolich JC. Circ Res 1988;62:185—190.
30. Shimokawa H, Kim P, VanHoutte PM. Circ Res 1988;63:604—612.
31. Harrison DG, Freiman PC, Armstrong ML, Marcus ML, Heistad DD. Circ Res 1987;61(II): 74—80.
32. Jayakody L, Senaratne M, Thomson A, Kappagoda T. Circ Res 1987;60:251—264.
33. Chappell SP, Lewis MJ, Henderson AH. Cardiovasc Res 1987;21:34—38.
34. White CR, Brock TA, Chang LY, Crapo J, Briscoe P, Ku D, Bradley WA, Gianturco SA, Gore J,

Freeman BA, Tarpey MM. Proc Natl Acad Sci USA 1994;91:1044—1048.

35. Lopez JAG, Armstrong ML, Harrison DG, Piegors DJ, Heistad DD. Circ Res 1989;65: 1078—1086.
36. Cooke JP, Andon NA, Girerd XJ, Hirsch AT, Creager MA. Circulation 1991;83:1057—1062.
37. Schini VB, Vanhoutte PM. Circ Res 1991;68:209—216.
38. Cohen RA, Zitnay KM, Haudenschild CC, Cunningham LD. Circ Res 1988;63:903—910.
39. Harrison DG, Armstrong ML, Freiman PC, Heistad DD. J Clin Invest 1987;80:1808—1811.
40. Minor RL, Myers PR, Guerra R, Bates JN, Harrison DG. J Clin Invest 1990;86:2109—2116.
41. Mugge A, Elwell JH, Peterson TE, Hofmeyer TG, Heistad DD, Harrison DG. Circ Res 1991;69: 1293—1300.
42. Ohara Y, Peterson TE, Harrison DG. J Clin Invest 1991;91:2546—2551.
43. White CR, Darley-Usmar V, McAdams M, Berrington WR, Gore J, Thompson JA, Parks DA, Tarpey MM, Freeman BA. Proc Natl Acad Sci USA 1996;93:8745—8749.
44. Beckman JS, Beckman TW, Chen J, Marshall PA, Freeman BA. Proc Natl Acad Sci USA 1990; 87:1620—1624.
45. Darley-Usmar VM, Hogg N, O'Leary VJ, Wilson MT, Moncada S. Free Rad Res Commun 1992; 17(1):9—20.
46. Hogg N, Darley-Usmar VM, Graham A, Moncada S. Biochem Soc Trans 1993;21:358—362.
47. Tarpey MM, Beckman JS, Ishiropolous H, Gore JZ, Brock TA. FEBS Lett 1995;364:314—318.
48. Mayer B, Schrammel A, Klatt P, Koesling D, Schmidt K. J Biol Chem 1995;270(29): 17355—17360.
49. Wu M, Pritchard KA, Kaminski PM, Fayngersh RP, Hintze TH, Wolin MS. Am J Physiol 1994; 266:H2108—2113.
50. Moro MA, Darley-Usmar VM, Lizasoain I, Su Y, Knowles RG, Radomski MW, Moncada SM. Br J Pharmacol 1995;116: 1999—2004.
51. White CR, Moellering D, Kirk M, Barnes S, Darley-Usmar VM. Biochem J 1997;328: 517—524.
52. Pearson PJ, Lin PJ, Schaff HV. Annals Thor Surg 1991;51(5):788—793.
53. Liu S, Beckman JS, Ku DD. J Pharm Exp Ther 1994;268(3):1114—1121.
54. Mohazzab KM, Wolin MS. Am J Physiol 1994;267(1):L823—L831.
55. Munzel T, Sayegh H, Freeman BA, Tarpey MM, Harrison DG. J Clin Invest 1995;95(1): 187—194.
56. Pritchard KA, Grosneck L, Smalley DM, Sessa WC, Wu M, Villalon P, Wolin MS, Stemerman MB. Circ Res 1995;77(3):510—518.
57. Amaya Y, Yamazaki K, Sato M, Noda K, Nishino T, Nishino T. J Biol Chem 1990;265(24): 14170—14175.
58. Dupont GP, Huecksteadt TP, Marshall BC, Ryan US, Michael JR, Hoidal JR. J Clin Invest 1992;89:197—202.
59. Linas SL, Whittenburg D, Repine JE. Am J Physiol 1990;258:F711—716.
60. Terada LS, Dormish JJ, Shanley PF, Leff JA, Anderson BO, Repine JE. Am J Physiol 1992;263 (3):L394—401.
61. Ramboer C, Piessens F, de Groote J. Digestion 1972;7:183—195.
62. Grum CM, Ragsdale RA, Ketai LH, Simon RH. J Crit Care 1987;2:22—26.
63. Friedl HP, Till GO, Trents O, Ward PA. Am J Pathol 1989;135:203—217.
64. Oda T, Akaike T, Homamoto T, Suzuki F, Hirano T, Maeda H. Science 1989;244:974—976.
65. Zima T, Novak L, Stipek S. Alcohol Alcoholism 1993;28(6):693—694.
66. Hopson SB, Lust RM, Sun YS, Zeri RS, Morrison RF, Otaki M, Chitwood WR. J Natl Med Assoc 1995;87(7):480—484.
67. Toivonen HJ, Ahotupa M. J Thor Cardio Surg 1994;108(1):140—147.
68. Dorion D, Zhong A, Chiu C, Forrest CR, Boyd B, Pang CY. J Appl Physiol 1993;75(1): 246—255.
69. Wright RM, Vaitaitis GM, Wilson CM, Repine TB, Terada LS, Repine JE. Proc Natl Acad Sci

USA 1993;90(22):10690—10694.
70. Moriwaki Y, Yamamoto T, Suda M, Nasako Y, Takahashi S, Agbedana OE, Hada T, Higashino K. Biochem Biophys Acta 1993;1164(3):327—330.
71. Hellsten-Westing Y. Histochemistry 1993;100(3):215—222.
72. Swain J, Gutteridge JM. FEBS Lett 1995;368(3):513—515.
73. Crawford DW, Blankenhorn DH. Atherosclerosis 1991;89(2—3):97—108.
74. Tan S, Gelman S, Wheat JK, Parks DA. Southern Med J 1995;88(4):479—482.
75. Till GO, Friedl HP, Ward PA. Free Rad Biol Med 1991;10(6):379—386.
76. Lazzarino G, Raatikainen P, Nuutinen M, Nissinen J, Tavazzi B, Di Pierro D, Giardina B, Peuh-kurinen K. Circulation 1994;90(1):291—297.
77. Vlessis AA, Ott G, Cobanoglu A. J Thor Cardio Surg 1994;107(2):482—486.
78. Miesel R, Zuber M. Inflammation 1993;17(5):551—561.
79. Castelli P, Condemi AM, Brambillasca C, Fundaro P, Botta M, Lemma M, Vanelli P, Santoli C, Gatti S, Riva E. J Cardio Pharmaco 1995;25(1):119—125.
80. Vaughn WG, Horton JW, Walker PB. J Pediatric Surg 1992;27(8):968—972.
81. Dillon JJ, Grossman SH, Finn WF. Renal Failure 1993;15(1):37—45.
82. Mohacsi A, Kozlovsky B, Kiss I, Seres I, Fulon T. Biochim Biophys Acta 1996;1316:210—216.
83. Cardillo C, Kilcoyne CM, Cannon RO, Quyyumi AA, Panza JA. Hypertension 1997;30(1): 57—63.
84. D'Amore PA. Haemostasis 1990;20(1):159—165.
85. Frebilius S, Nydahl S, Swendenborg J. Blood Coag Fibrinol 1990;1(3):285—292.
86. Novotny WF, Palmier M, Wun TC, Broze GJ, Miletich JP. Blood 1991;78(2):394—400.
87. Abrahamsson T, Brandt U, Marklund SL, Sjoqvist PO. Circ Res 1992;70:264—271.
88. Tan S, Yokoyama Y, Dickens E, Cash TG, Freeman BA, Parks DA. Free Rad Biol Med 1993;15 (4):407—414.
89. Lindstedt KA, Kokkonen JO, Kovanen PT. J Lipid Res 1992;33:65—75.
90. Srinivasan SR, Vijayagopal P, Eberle K, Radhakrishnamurthy B, Berenson GS. Biochem Bio-phys Acta 1991;1081:188—196.
91. Bourin MC, Lindahl U. Biochem J 1993;289:313—330.
92. D'Amore PA. Haemostasis 1990;20(1):159—165.
93. Hurt-Camejo E, Camejo G, Rosengren B, Lopez F, Ahlstrom C, Faber G, Bondjers G. Arterio-scler Thromb 1992;12(5):569—583.
94. Oury TD, Piantadosi CA, Crapo JD. J Biol Chem 1993;268(21):15394—15398.
95. Karlsson K, Marklund SL. Biochem J 1988;255:223—228.
96. Karlsson K, Marklund SL. J Clin Invest 1988;82:762—766.
97. Adachi T, Fukushima T, Usami Y, Hirano K. Biochem J 1993;289(2):523—527.
98. Tanaka H, Okada T, Konishi H, Tsuji T. Archiv Dermatol Res 1993;285(6):352—355.
99. Stralin P, Marklund SL. Biochem J 1994;298(2):347—352.
100. Sternbergh WC, Makhoul RG, Adelman B. J Vasc Surg 1993;17(2):318—327.
101. Light JT, Bellan JA, Roberts MP, Force SD, Chen IL, Kerstein MD, Kadowitz PJ, McNamara DB. Circulation 1993;88(2):413—419.
102. Swain J, Gutteridge JM. FEBS Lett 1995;368(3):513—515.
103. Vlessis AA, Ott G., Cobanoglu A. J Thor Cardio Surg 1994;107(2):482—486.
104. Bangsbo J. J Sports Sciences 1994;12:S5—12.
105. Zhang YY, Wasserman K, Sietsema KE, Ben-Dov I, Barstow TJ, Mizumoto G. Chest 1993;103 (3):735—741.
106. Greenhaff PL. Intl J Sport Nutr 1995;5:S100—S110.
107. Tullson PC, Arabadejis PG, Rundell KW, Terjung RL. Am J Physiol 1996;270(4, Pt 1): C1067—C1074.
108. Yamamoto T, Moriwaki Y, Takahashi S, Ishizashi H, Higashino K. Horm Metabol Res 1994;26 (11):504—508.
109. Waern MJ, Fossum C. Am J Veterinary Res 1993;54(4):596—601.

110. Norman B, Sollevi A, Kaijser L, Jansson E. Clin Physiol 1987;7(6):503—510.
111. Hellsten-Westing Y, Kaijser L, Ekblom B, Sjodin B. Am J Physiol 1994;266(1 Pt 2):R81—R86.
112. Sahlin K, Ekberg K, Cizinsky S. Acta Physiol Scand 1991;142(2):275—281.
113. Mills PC, Smith NC, Harris RC, Harris P. Res Veterin Sci 1997;62(1):11—16.
114. Ji LL. Med Sci Sports Exer 1993;25(2): 225—231.
115. Duarte JA, Appell HJ, Carvalho F, Bastos ML, Soares JM. Intl J Sports Med 1993;14(8): 440—443.
116. Radak Z, Asano K, Inoue M, Kizaki T, Oh-Ishi S, Suzuki K, Taniguchi N, Ohno H. J Appl Physiol 1995;79(1):129—135.
117. Hellsten Y, Frandsen U, Orthenblad N, Sjodin B, Richter EA. J Physiol 1997;498(Pt 1): 239—248.
118. Radak Z, Asano K, Inoue M, Kizaki T, Oh-Ishi S, Suzuki K, Taniguchi N, Ohno H. Eur J Appl Physiol Occ Physiol 1996;72(3):189—194.
119. Yamanaka H, Kawagoe Y, Taniguchi A, Kaneko N, Kimata S, Hosoda S, Kamatani N, Kashiwazaki S. Metabolism: Clinical and Experimental 1992;41(4):364—369.
120. Stathis CG, Febbraio MA, Carey MF, Snow RJ. J Appl Physiol 1994;76(4):1802—1809.
121. Hellsten-Westing Y, Balsom PD, Norman B, Sjodin B. Acta Physiol Scand 1993;149(4): 405—412.
122. Somani SM, Frank S, Rybak LP. Pharmacol Biochem Behav 1995;51(4):627—634.
123. Oh-Ishi S, Kizaki T, Nagasawa J, Izawa T, Kamabayashi Y, Nagata N, Suzuki K, Taniguchi N, Ohno H. Clin Exp Pharmacol Physiol 1997;24(5):326—332.
124. Powers SK, Criswell D, Lawler J, Martin D, Lieu FK, Ji LL, Herb RA. Am J Physiol 1993;265 (6, Pt 2):H2094—H2098.
125. Ortebland N, Madsen K, Djurhuus MS. Am J Physiol 1997;272(4 Pt 2):R1258—R1263.
126. Kedziora J, Buczynski A, Kedziora-Kornatowska K. Intl J Occ Med Envir Health 1995;8(1): 33—39.
127. Wang J, Wolin MS, Hintze TH. Circ Res 1993;73(5):829—838.
128. Koller A, Huang A, Sun D, Kaley G. Circ Res 1995;76(4)544—550.
129. Shen W, Zhang X, Zhao G, Wolin MS, Sessa W, Hintze TH. Med Sci Sports Exer 1995;27(8): 1125—1134.
130. Niebauer J, Cooke JP. J Am Coll Cardiol 1996;28(7):1652—1660.
131. Dietz NM, Engelke KA, Samuel TT, Fix RT, Joyner MJ. J Physiol 1997;498(Pt 2):531—540.
132. Gilligan DM, Panza JA, Kilcoyne CM, Waclawiw MA, Casino PR, Quyyumi AA. Circulation 1994;90(6):2853—2858.
133. Node K, Kitakaze M, Sato H, Koretsune Y, Katsube Y, Karita M, Kosaka H, Hori M. Am J Cardiol 1997;79(4):256—258.
134. Green DJ, O'Driscoll G, Blanksby BA, Taylor RR. Sports Med 1996;21(2):119—146.
135. Delp MD. Med Sci Sports Exer 1995;27(8):1152—1157.
136. Zhao G, Zhang X, Xu X, Pchoa M, Hintze TH. Circ Res 1997;80(6):868—876.
137. Endo T, Imaizumi T, Tagawa T, Shiramoto M, Ando S, Takesita A. Circulation 1994;90(6): 2886—2890.
138. Altman JD, Kinn J, Duncker DJ, Bache RJ. Cardiovasc Res 1994;28(1):119—124.
139. Parker JL, Mattox ML, Laughlin MH. J Appl Physiol 1997;83(2):434—443.
140. McAllister RM, Laughlin M. J Appl Physiol 1997;82(5):1438—1444.

Part III

Oxidative stress:
Mechanisms and manifestations

©2000 Elsevier Science B.V. All rights reserved.
Handbook of Oxidants and Antioxidants in Exercise.
C.K. Sen, L. Packer and O. Hänninen, editors.

Part III • Chapter 4

Chemical bases and biological relevance of protein oxidation

Oren Tirosh[1] and Abraham Z. Reznick[2]

[1] *Department of Molecular and Cell Biology, University of California, Berkeley, California, USA*
[2] *Department of Anatomy and Cell Biology, The Bruce Rappaport Faculty of Medicine, Technion-Israel Institute of Technology, P.O. Box 9649, 31096 Haifa, Israel. E-mail: reznick@tx.technion.ac.il*

1   CHEMICAL BASES FOR PROTEINS OXIDATION
    1.1 Introduction to the chemistry of protein oxidation
    1.2 Tryptophan oxidation
    1.3 Tyrosine oxidation
        1.3.1 Tyrosine nitration
        1.3.2 Tyrosine chlorination
    1.4 Oxidation of aliphatic amino acids and the peptide bond
        1.4.1 Oxygen mediated cleavage of proteins
    1.5 Protein oxidation chain reaction
    1.6 Hypochlorous acid mediated oxidation of dipeptides
    1.7 Oxidation of other amino acids
    1.8 Lipid peroxidation derived aldehydes and protein damage
2   BIOLOGICAL RELEVANCE OF PROTEIN OXIDATION
    2.1 Introduction
    2.2 Oxidative stress, protein oxidation, and aging
    2.3 Protein oxidation in pathologic conditions and various diseases
        2.3.1 Diabetes and the modification and oxidation of proteins
        2.3.2 Protein oxidation in atherosclerosis
        2.3.3 Protein oxidation in cancer
        2.3.4 Protein oxidation and neurological diseases
        2.3.5 Protein oxidation in other pathologies
    2.4 The role of protein oxidation in the process of protein inactivation and degradation
    2.5 Exercise, immobilization, and protein oxidation
    2.6 Plasma protein oxidation and cigarette smoke
3   SUMMARY
4   ACKNOWLEDGEMENT
5   ABBREVIATIONS
6   REFERENCES

1   CHEMICAL BASES FOR PROTEINS OXIDATION

1.1 Introduction to the chemistry of protein oxidation

The complex structure of proteins and the numerous different oxidizable functional groups of the amino acids make them a prime target for interaction with oxidants.

The constant flux of reactive oxygen species (ROS) in living cells can cause damage to acyl chain in membranes, to phospholipid polar head groups of phosphatidylethanolamine and phosphatidylserine, and to DNA and proteins. Oxidation of proteins can lead to the formation of reversible disulfide bridges, or to chemical modified derivatives that are nonbiologically reducible e.g., schiff's base [1,2]. Proteins can be attacked by membrane originated ROS or by ROS generated in the aqueous phase such as nitric oxide, hydroxyl radical, and hydrogen peroxides. Alkoxy or peroxy radicals and also carbon-centered radicals may also cause oxidative protein damage. For example, alkoxy radicals can attack tryptophan and cysteine residues. Aldehydes can react with sulfhydryl (SH) and amine (NH_2) groups on proteins to form both intramolecular cross-links and also cross-links between different proteins, or between proteins and the amino group of lipids such as phosphatidylethanolamine (PE) and phosphatidylserine (PS).

Oxidative modification of proteins may occur by two different mechanisms. (I) a site-specific formation of ROS via redox-active transition metals which are loosely bound to protein binding site. This might promote damage via metal-catalyzed oxidation (MCO). MCO leads to the formation of keto groups on the proteins (carbonyl derivatives) [3,4]. Examples of amino acids which are sensitive to MCO are PRO, ARG, LYS, and HIS. (II) Non-metal-dependent ROS-induced oxidation of amino acids such as MET, HIS, TRP, and CYS which are sensitive to peroxyl and alkoxyl radicals. In these processes there is direct damage to the amino acid or oxidative degradation of the protein by cleavage of the peptide bond [3,4]. The principles and mechanisms involved in the oxidation of ROS sensitive amino acids is discussed in the following sections.

1.2 Tryptophan oxidation

Tryptophan has a unique chemical structure, the tryptophenyl residue has no similarity to any other amino acid and therefore its function cannot be replaced by any other amino acid by site-directed mutagenesis [5]. However, tryptophan residues can be easily altered by oxidation. The indole residue in tryptophan can undergo oxidation by several pathways. The end result as well as the oxidative products distribution, depends on the oxidizing species and the conditions under which the reaction was performed.

Oxidation of proteins by ozone is one way to achieve high yield of tryptophan oxidation without damaging other amino acids [5—7]. The main oxidation product of tryptophan by ozone is cleavage of the pyrrole ring which results in formation of. N'-formylkynurenine (NFK) which is also a metabolite of tryptophan, Freezing and thawing of NFK in acidified solution converts it to kynurenine (Fig. 1). Circular dichroic and fluorescence spectra of γ-immunoglobulin light chains, ribonuclease, and hen egg-white lysozyme treated by ozone for tryptophan oxidation, demonstrated that the tertiary structure of protein is maintained. However, the slight modification of even a single tryptophan residue produced a large decrease in the stability of these proteins when treated with guanidine

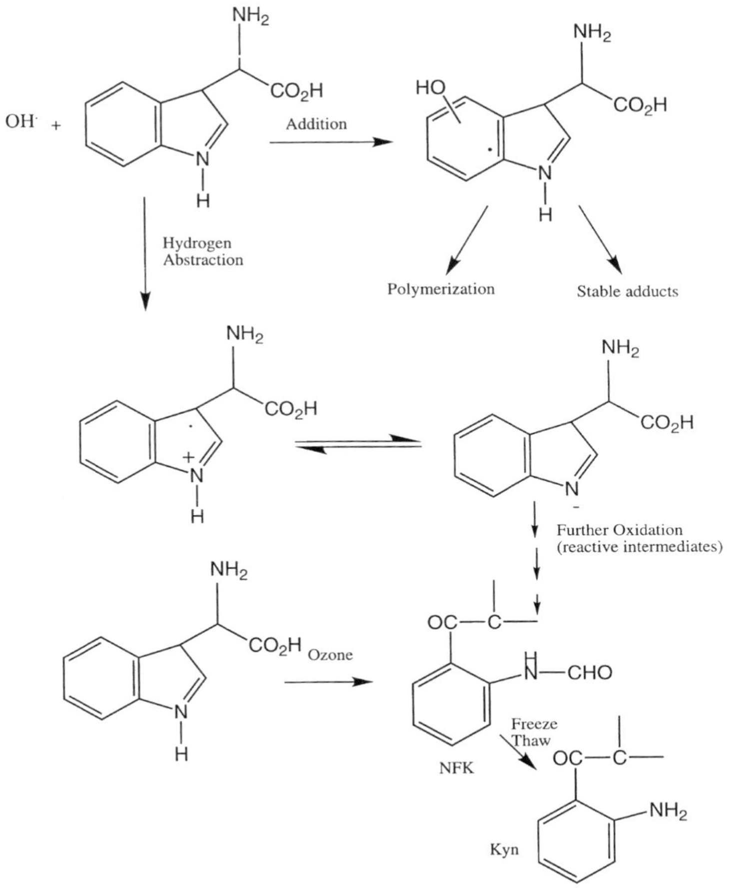

Fig. 1. Oxidation pathways of tryptophan, N'-formylkynurenine (NFK), kynurenine (kyn).

hydrochloride and heat [5]. Stability studies have shown that the lower the mobility or solvent accessibility of tryptophan residue, the greater is the extent of the decrease in the stability upon modification [8]. Studies of the changes in stability of *Staphylococcus* nuclease with amino acid substitutions of a buried hydrophobic residue with a bulkier and more polar residue showed that the enthalpy and the entropy changes for thermal unfolding of the protein are both larger, and that the free energy change is smaller for the mutant protein compared with values for the wild protein. These findings may be explained by a greater disruption of interchain interactions in the unfolded state of the mutant protein. The same explanation can be valid for the oxidative modification of tryptophans [9].

   Hydroxyl radical, which is the most potent oxidant in biology, can trigger two types of reaction: hydroxylation (especially on aromatic rings), and hydrogen abstraction (especially with electron donors) [1]. The complex chemical integrity of tryptophan makes it subject to both type of reaction cited above [10,11]. Pulse radiolysis experiments have shown that hydroxyl radicals react with tryptophan to form two kinds of species [11]: a hydroxycyclohexadienyl radical or hydroxyl radical adduct, and a tryptophenyl radical in equilibrium with its cation radicals (Fig. 1). Radiolysis of a nitrous oxide-saturated, unbuffered tryptophan solution at neutral pH produces six primary products: 4-OHtrp, 5-OHtrp, 6-OHtrp, 7-OHtrp, NFK, and oxindole-3-alanine. Also a yellow polymeric product is formed, as result of radical-radical interactions. The main product during γ-radiation of tryptophan solutions saturated with nitrous oxide is a yellow product with a maximum absorbance at 425 nm. This is a product of dimerization and polymerization of the hydroxyl-radical-tryptophan-adduct intermediate which is also a radical [11]. In this situation, the yield of stable hydroxylation products is very low (4%) [11]. However, in the presence of iron the radical intermediate can undergo a disproportional reaction that generate back the tryptophan molecule and a stable hydroxylation adduct. The maximum yield achieved at high concentrations of Fe(III)-ethylenediaminetetraacetic acid (EDTA) (0.5 mM) is 27 hydroxylation products for every 100 hydroxyl radicals [11].

The second type of products that originate as a result of hydrogen abstraction, specially from the pyrrole ring, provide the tryptophenyl radical itself as an intermediate. Further oxidation, spontaneous or enhanced, in the presence of dioxan facilitates the transformation of ring cleavage rearrangement and the formation of NFK.

Treatment of peptides containing tryptophans as well as N-*tert*-butyloxycarbonyl (BOC)-L-tryptophan with superoxide in the presence of iron-EDTA or H_2O_2/horseradish peroxidase selectively transform tryptophan into NFK, and oxygenation of the pyrrole ring of the indole nucleus (3-(3-oxindolyl) propionic acid) without any formation of hydroxylation products [12]. This suggests that in these systems hydroxyl radical was not involved and that higher valent iron oxygen complexes served as the oxidizing species. Thus, iron oxygen species may play a central role in tryptophan oxidation. When tryptophan reacts with oxidants generated by Fenton reaction (reduce iron and hydrogen peroxide) or Udenfriend reaction (vitamin C, oxidized metal, and oxygen), NFK is predominantly produced and the yield of hydroxylation product is low. This product distribution may also indicate a lower involvement of hydroxyl radicals or higher scavenging of hydroxyl radicals by the vitamin C which is used in the Udenfriend reaction [11].

An interesting aspect of tryptophan oxidation by metal ions such as Cu^{+2} is the possible ability of intermediate tryptophan radicals to initiate lipid peroxidation. This type of chemistry (Fig. 1) which include, tryptophan oxidation in the formation of a tryptophan radical, and in the presence of oxygen, formation of tryptophanperoxy radical can initiate lipid peroxidation chain reaction [13,14]. In low density lipoprotein (LDL) five tryptophan residues are lost within few minutes of exposure to copper. This implies that LDL oxidation is initiated through oxidative modification of proteins rather than that of lipids [13,14].

Another powerful oxidant that possesses a significant biological relevancy is peroxynitrite. This oxidizing species can be formed by the combination of super-oxide and NO• radical in biological systems. Alternatively peroxynitrite can be prepared synthetically by reaction between hydrogen peroxide and nitrite. Hydrogen peroxide by itself cannot induce tryptophan oxidation. The mechanism by which peroxynitrite degrades tryptophan residues remain obscure. Using (Boc)-tryptophan (trp) as a model for tryptophan oxidation in proteins and by reverse phase-HPLC, NMR and FAB/MS analysis it has been identified that peroxynitrite does not cause nitration of tryptophan residues. Another explanation for the lack of nitration is that the nitration products were not identified by HPLC [15]. The oxidized product that were identified were Boc-NFK, Boc-oxindole, and Boc-hydropyrroloindole (Fig. 1). Using different techniques such as liquid chromatography-MS other groups have reported that peroxynitrite can induce tryptophan nitration [16,17].

1.3 Tyrosine oxidation

1.3.1 Tyrosine nitration

A major mechanism of injury associated with the production of nitric oxide and its reaction with superoxide radical to generate peroxynitrite. The reaction rate constant of these two radicals is 6.7×10^9 $M^{-1}s^{-1}$. At physiological concentrations, nitric oxide can compete with superoxide dismutase (SOD) to produce peroxynitrite [18]. Peroxynitrite is a remarkably stable compound in alkaline pH [19]. The stability of peroxynitrite allows it to diffuse through cells and hit a distant target. At pH 7.4, 80% of peroxynitrite is ionized and 20% of it forms peroxynitrous acid a strong oxidant that can oxidize iron/sulfur centers [20,21], zinc finger protein [22] and proteins thiols [23]. Peroxynitrite lead to the formation of end products that are similar to hydroxyl radical caused damage [24,25]. However, the direct reaction of peroxynitrite accounts for most of its toxic effect [26]. One important reaction of peroxynitrite is catalyzed by transition metals, including the metal centers of SOD and myeloperoxidase (MPO). Transition metals catalyze a heterolytic cleavage to produce hydroxyl anion and nitronium ion (NO_2^+). Nitronium ion is well known to react with phenols and produce nitrophenols. The nitration of protein tyrosine to 3-nitrotyrosine is a finger-print left by peroxynitrite in vivo [18]. This reaction also produces nitrosotyrosine. The nitroso group can apparently interchange between the carbon and oxygen. Nitrosotyrosine is unstable in water, because water can interact with the NO group to form nitrite and tyrosine [1,2].

Auto-oxidation of NO· in aqueous solution lead to the formation of nitrite via a mechanism that may involve intermediate formation of NO_2· radical. Decomposition of peroxynitrous acid results in intermediates possessing the reactivity of hydroxyl radical and NO_2·. These intermediates may induce hydroxylation and nitration of aromatic amino acid residues [27]. Spontaneous nitration and aromatic hydroxylation of tyrosine in the absence of transition metals also results in the formation of dimers suggesting the involvement of a radical mechanism. In this reaction a phenoxyl radical is formed together with $NO_2\cdot$, which combines to form nitrated phenol or the dimers. In pH-dependent experiments of tyrosine oxidation it has been shown that the production of 3-nitrotyrosine is maximal at physiological pH [27]. The formation of 3-nitrotyrosine declined rapidly at pH values higher than 8. The maximum formation of dityrosine was at pH 8.5. The formation of both dityrosine and 3-nitrotyrosine is linearly increased with the concentration of reacting peroxynitrite. The formation of dityrosine is significantly increased at concentration above 0.1 mM of tyrosine. These results imply that tyrosine radical is intermediate in the nitration as well as dimerization of tyrosine residue caused by peroxynitrite or any other $NO_2\cdot$ generating systems (Fig. 2). However, the formation of 3-nitrotyrosine via the tyrosyl radical intermediate is currently only a hypothesis that requires better consideration. One way to address such an issue and to elucidate the actual mechanism of tyrosine

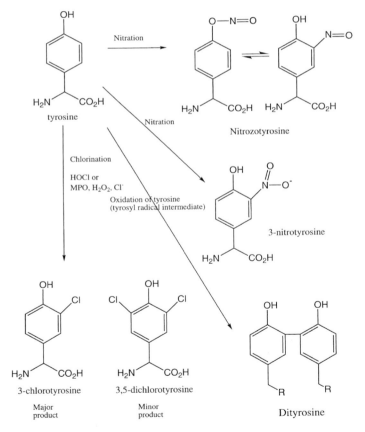

Fig. 2. Oxidation pathways of tyrosine.

nitration in metal free solutions is to use esters or ethers of tyrosine where the radical cannot be formed but the reactivity of the aromatic ring towards electrophilic addition remains unchanged.

Reaction of peroxynitrite with phenylalanine results in formation of *para, meta* and *ortho*-tyrosine residues [28]. Other products of the reaction are 3-nitrotyrosine and 4-nitrophenylalanine. Thus, the formation of hydroxylated products of phenylalanine may serve as a mark of peroxynitrite induce damage in vivo. Peroxynitrite is most stable when folded into a *cis*-conformation when it is protonated it isomerizes to trans-peroxynitrous acid and form an exited state that can react like hydroxyl radical. The distal peroxy oxygen in trans-peroxynitrite can also swing around to attack by the nitrogen to form nitrate [18]. The question whether peroxynitrite decomposes to release free hydroxyl radicals into the solution to damage biological protein targets, or peroxynitrite reacts by itself can be considered from a simple aromatic chemistry point of view. Through resonance, the π electrons of the benzene ring are loosely held and are available to reagents that are seeking electrons. The aromatic ring can be looked upon as a source of electrons, e.g., a base. So the typical reactions of the ring are electrophilic substitution reactions which include nitration, halogenation, and sulfonation. Any kind of substituent on the aromatic ring can be classified into one of two categories, ring activator or ring deactivator. Hydroxylation of the aromatic ring will result in strong activation and will direct the nitration on the ring to the *ortho* position, while ring nitration by nitro group will strongly deactivate the ring towards any further aromatic substitution that will occur only as minor products. Based on this understanding it may be thought that the reaction of peroxynitrite with phenylalanine to form tyrosine by decomposition of peroxynitrite into hydroxyl radical and $NO_2\cdot$ radicals is highly improbable. This is because the tyrosine formed by phenylalanine hydroxylation is more reactive than the phenylalanine itself, and the tyrosine should continue to react to become *ortho* nitrated or dihydroxy phenylalanine. The isolation of tyrosine residues indicate a direct interaction between peroxynitrite and phenylalanine and implies that the hydroxylation mechanism is not accompanied by further nitration suggesting that their are no nitrogen radicals or nitronium ions in a close proximity.

Formation of nitrogen dioxide ($NO_2\cdot$) from NO_2^- by oxidation catalyzed enzymatically was recently suggested as an alternative mechanism for protein nitration and halogenation [29]. Nitrite, the primary metabolic end of nitric oxide, can be oxidized by the heme peroxidases, horseradish peroxidase, MPO, and lactoperoxidase in the presence of hydrogen peroxide to the $NO_2\cdot$ which can contribute to tyrosine nitration. The phenolic nitration by MPO-catalyzed NO_2^- oxidation is only partially inhibited by chloride. At low concentrations nitrite catalyzed MPO mediated oxidation of chloride, that can be monitored by increased chlorination of 4-hydroxyphenylacetic acid. Based on this observation it has been proposed that MPO compound 1 can oxidize chloride and nitrite by a two-electron oxidation mechanism with regeneration of ferric MPO. Alternatively, nitrite can be oxidized by one electron oxidation to form compound 2 and $NO_2\cdot$. Compound 2 was suggested to regenerate the ferric MPO by oxidation of another molecule of nitrite [29].

Nitration of a single amino acid or a short peptide does not necessarily resemble the case of nitration inside a protein. The state of tyrosyl residues in the enzyme thermolysin was examined by nitration and pH-dependent ionization [30]. The state of 28 tyrosyl residues of thermolysin have been characterized by means of a pH jump procedure. The ionization of 16 tyrosyl residues was completed within 15 min suggesting the occurrence of conformational changes that leads to the exposure of the buried tyrosyl residues to the solvent. Sixteen tyrosyl residues were nitrated by tetranitromethane. The second-order rate constants of the respective classes of tyrosyl residues, for nitration were evaluated as $3.32 \ M^{-1}min^{-1}$ of the first class of six tyrosyl residues and $0.52 \ M^{-1}min^{-1}$ and $0.18 \ M^{-1}min^{-1}$ for the second (seven tyrosyl residues) and third class (three tyrosyl residues), respectively. The pK_a values suggested that the tyrosyl residues in the first class are not entirely free on the surface, but are slightly constrained. However, the second and third group pK_a that were 11.4 and 11.8, respectively, reflect a biological micro-environment unfavorable to pH ionization. This results demonstrate that nitration of tyrosine is highly dependent on the location of the residue in the protein and its exposure to the surface solvent.

1.3.2 Tyrosine chlorination

Gas chromatography mass spectroscopy analysis of the reaction of L-tyrosine with HOCl indicates that five components are present in the reaction product. These products included ring chlorination [31]. Eighty six% of the product was identified as 3-chlorotyrosine, and 7% was found to be 3,5-dichlorotyrosine (Fig. 2).

Chlorotyrosine, as a product of the reaction between the oxidant HOCl and tyrosine, is formed in a mixture containing MPO, hydrogen peroxide, chloride and protein. This reaction may occur in activated neutrophils [32,33]. Thus, chlorotyrosine may served as a useful marker to establish the role of hypochlorous acid in host defence and inflammation.

Tyrosyl residues of peptides and bovine serum albumin (BSA) are found to be substrates for halogenation by HOCl at neutral pH [33,34]. Chlorination has been proposed to take place via intramolecular attack by chloramine intermediate [34]. It recently has been demonstrated that phagocytes use molecular chlorine (Cl_2), that is in equilibrium with MPO-generated HOCl, to chlorinate the aromatic ring of free or protein-bound L-tyrosine [35—37] and that this reaction is optimal at slightly acidic pH (the pH of the phagolysosomal compartment). HOCl can oxidize the amine moiety of tyrosine to an aldehyde (*p*-hydroxyphenyl-acetaldehyde).

Another mechanism for the in vivo chlorination as well as nitration of tyrosine residues involves hypochlorous acid and nitrite (the oxidation product of nitric oxide). The intermediate that is possibly formed in the reaction is $Cl-NO_2$

(nitrylchloride) [38]. The reaction between nitrylchloride and tyrosine results in the formation of 3-chlorotyrosine and 3-nitrotyrosine in a ratio of 4:1, respectively.

1.4 Oxidation of aliphatic amino acids and the peptide bond

The oxidation products and pathway of aliphatic amino acids by ionizing irradiation is strongly affected by the reaction conditions. In the presence of oxygen, hydroxyl radical attacks the α-carbon of the amino acid possessing a relatively high partial positive charge in a hydrogen abstraction reaction. The free radical amino acid thus formed continues to react with molecular oxygen to form a amino acid peroxy radical. The amino acid peroxy radical interacts with superoxide radical to form the unstable amino acid hydroperoxide and molecular oxygen. Spontaneous decomposition of the alkylperoxide yields hydrogen peroxide and an imino derivative of the amino acid that undergoes hydrolysis to form either ammonium CO_2 and an aldehyde or ammonium and an α-keto acid which could then be transformed by oxidative decarboxylation to a one-carbon shorter amino acid [39] (Fig. 3). The yield of expected oxidation products is dependent on the complexity of the amino acid and it decreases linearly as a function of the number of carbon atoms in the aliphatic side chain [40,41]. Alternatively, an α-amino acid can react with hypochlorous acid to form an imine intermediate which subsequently results in the formation of the corresponding aldehydes and carboxylic acid [42,43] (Fig. 3).

In the absence of oxygen, the oxidative pathway of irradiated proteins is quite

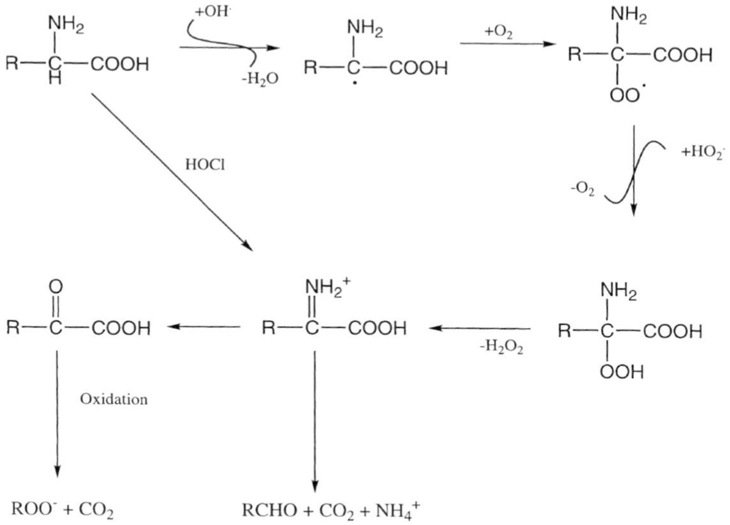

Fig. 3. Reaction mechanism for aliphatic amino acid oxidation (oxidative deamination).

different. Lack of oxygen suppressor the formation of the amino acid peroxy radical and favors reductive deamination by the hydrated electrons generated by decomposition of water. Reductive deamination may result in the formation of mono carboxylic acid, dicarboxylic acid or amino acids-carboxylic acid adducts from the precursor amino acid. Another type of adduct is simply the di-amino acid connected at the two α-amino acid carbons, i.e., di-amino-dicarboxylic acid derivative [39].

Metal catalyzed oxidation of free amino acid include the production of hydroxyl radicals by Fenton reaction. The oxidation leads to the formation of ammonium ions, α-ketoacids, carbon dioxide, oximes and aldehydes or carboxylic acid containing one less carbon atom. The Fenton chemistry of iron which leads to proteins oxidation depends on the presence of bicarbonate ions and its is stimulated by iron chelators such as ethelendiaminetetraacetic acid, desferrioxamine and nitrilotriacetic acid [39,44]. The importance of bicarbonate ions in Fenton chemistry is highlighted by the fact that Mn (II) is able to catalyze oxidation of amino acids and the disproportionation of hydrogen peroxide to oxygen and hydrogen only in the presence of bicarbonate ions [45,46]. When an amino acid such as leucine is added to the above reaction mixture a hetero-complex of amino acid with the metal and two equivalents of bicarbonate ions {M-$(HCO_3)_2{}^-$ AA} with greatly enhanced catalytic potential is formed. As a result of the aforesaid reaction a 16 fold increase in oxidative deamination of amino acid may occur [39]. The metal ion catalyzed oxidation of amino acids may be viewed as on a caged process since the oxidation is not inhibited by hydroxyl radical scavengers [44,47].

1.4.1 Oxygen mediated cleavage of proteins

The effects of radiolysis on proteins under aerobic conditions differ from those observed under anaerobic conditions. In the absence of oxygen there is almost no fragmentation of protein and aggregation of the macromolecules is the major pathway in response to oxidation. However, under aerobic conditions there is little or no protein aggregation and considerable fragmentation is visible [48,49]. Oxygen mediated cleavage of proteins is assumed to occur by the α-amidation pathway [39] (Fig. 4). The first step for the cleavage of the peptide bond involves hydrogen abstraction from an α-carbon from the peptide or protein backbone, and formation of a protein peroxy radical. The protein peroxy radical is then converted by radical-radical interaction with superoxide to the corresponding protein hydroperoxide. Protein hydroperoxide thus generate imine intermediate on the protein backbone by releasing hydrogen peroxide. The imine intermediate is then hydrolysed to protein fragments. Deamination of the N-terminal amino acid residue and the protein fragmentation both leads to the formation of α-ketoacyl derivatives, which are reactive to dinitrophenylhydrazine [39]. Nevertheless, the formation of carbonyl groups in protein upon exposure to hydroxyl radical generating systems cannot be taken as an evidence for protein fragmentation.

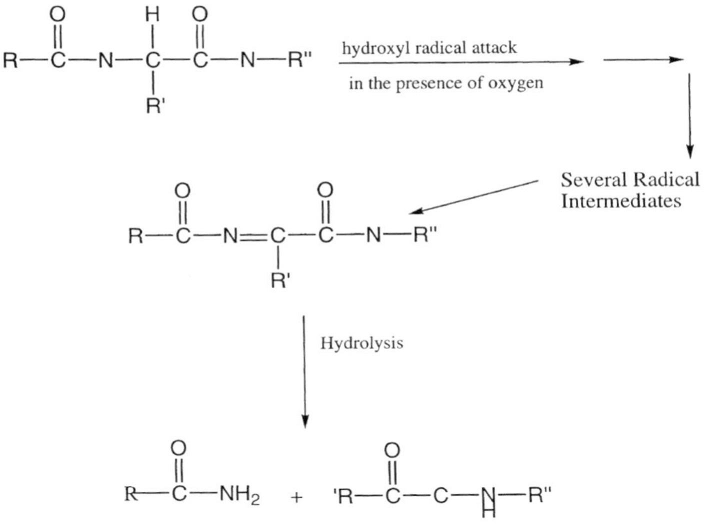

Fig. 4. Reaction mechanism for peptide bond cleavage by hydroxyl radical attack.

This is because oxidation of side chains of some amino acids residues (lys, Arg) may also lead to the formation of carbonyl groups [50—54].

Under anaerobic conditions of radiolysis, the protein is converted to higher molecular weight aggregates because of covalent cross-linking [48,49,55] as well as noncovalent interactions such as hydrophobic and electrostatic interactions [55,56].

1.5 Protein oxidation chain reaction

Under aerobic conditions a remarkable loss of amino acid occurs in proteins exposed to ionizing radiation. Calculation of the amount of radicals produced with the oxidative damage show that for each radical generated approximately 15 amino acid groups of BSA were consumed [57]. Such a massive oxidation of amino acid does not occur when radiation is carried under anaerobic conditions. The mechanism of protein oxidation chain reaction and the nature of the propagation radicals are not known at present.

1.6 Hypochlorous acid mediated oxidation of dipeptides

Dipeptides are a good model for the study of oxidation reaction of the protein backbone. This is because dipeptides have a simple chemical structure that allows to distinguish between susceptibility of the peptide bond toward oxidation and other functional groups on the amino acid residues. Reaction of four different dipeptides with two equivalents of hypochlorous acid demonstrate that the main product formed is dichloramine (Fig. 5) [31]. Dichloramine can undergo further

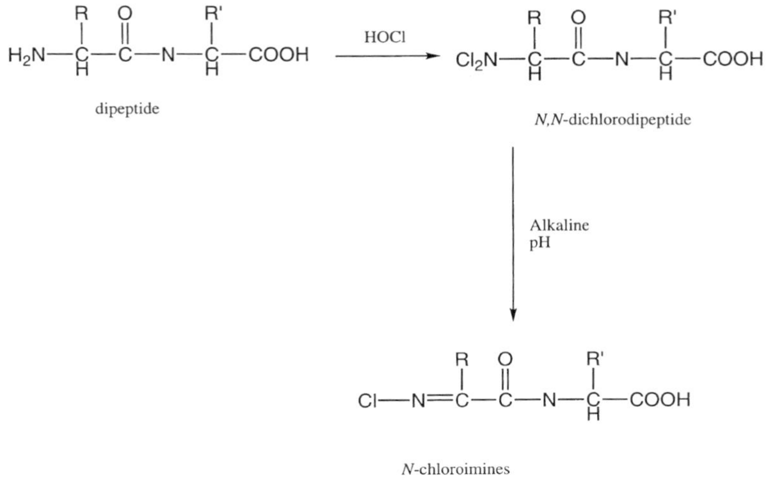

Fig. 5. Hypochlorous acid as an oxidant and its interaction with dipeptides to form chloroamines and chloroimines.

hydrolysis to form *N*-chlorimines and eventually may undergo deamination to form carbonyls. The peptide bond has been formed to be extremely stable in response to hypochlorous treatment. Exposure to hypochlorous acid even for several days did not result in no chlorination of the peptide bond [31].

1.7 Oxidation of other amino acids

Metal catalyzed oxidation (MCO) systems such as NADPH oxidase/NADPH/ oxygen/Fe(III), xanthine/xanthine oxidase/Fe(III), ascorbate/ transition metals, thiols/Fe(III), and reduced metal/hydrogen peroxide can inflict oxidative damage to proteins. Studies of amino acid homopolymers [52] peptides [39] and several enzymes [39,47,50—54,58—62] have established that His, Arg, Lys, Pro Met and Cys are among the most common sites of oxidation by MCO systems. Histidine is oxidized to aspartate, asparagine, and 2-oxo-imidazoline; arginine residues are converted to glutamic semialdehydes; proline residues are converted to glutamate, pyroglutamate, cis/trans-4-hydroxyproline, 2-pyrrolidone, glutamic semialdehyde, and γ-aminobutiric acid; and arginine is converted to glutamic semialdehyde [39]. The conversion of some amino acid residues (e.g., arginine, proline, lysine) to carbonyl derivatives provide a mechanism other than peptide bond cleavage for incorporation of carbonyls into proteins.

Proteins which are exposed to oxidation by ozone, a non-metal-dependent oxidation system, show loss of amino acids in the following order: Met > Trp > His=Tyr > Phe [63]. The loss of Histidine matched to the formation of aspartate or of a derivative that is a precursor of aspartic acid. Ozone induced loss of His residues in BSA is 1.5—2 times faster than in glutamine synthetase indicating that the susceptibility to oxidation is dependent on the primary, secondary, tertiary, and quaternary structure of proteins.

Oxidative modification of residues may be mediated by physiologic and non-physiologic systems including oxidases, ozone, hydrogen peroxide, superoxide, and ionizing irradiation. Methionine residues are remarkable for their high susceptibility toward oxidation by most of these systems [64] with the product generally being methionine sulfoxide.

Cysteine, when oxidized at room temperature by 1 or 2 equivalents of hypochlorous acid produced cysteic acid as the only product [31].

1.8 Lipid peroxidation derived aldehydes and protein damage

Lipid peroxidation processes that occurs in biological membranes results in membrane instability. Peroxidation processes has been connected to changes in both chemical and physical properties of the biological membrane, and to impairment of activity of enzymes located in the membrane environment [65]. Aldehydes are stable end products of lipid peroxidation. Unlike reactive free radicals, aldehydes are rather long lived and can therefore diffused from the site of their origin to reach distant targets. Aldehydes are formed during the peroxidation process mainly in the presence of transition metals which catalyzed the breakdown of the acyl chains and the release of reactive aldehydes [1]. Aldehydes can react with –SH and –NH_2 groups on proteins to form both intramolecular cross-links, and also cross-links between different proteins or between proteins and lipids such as in phosphatidylethanolamine (PE) and phosphatidylserine (PS). Among the aldehydes that originate from the peroxidation of cellular membrane lipids, 4-hydroxy-2-nonenal (HNE) is believed to be a product which responsible for pathological effects observed during oxidative stress [2,66]. HNE reacts with sulfhydryl groups leading to the formation of thioether adducts that further undergo cyclization to form hemiacetales. HNE also reacts with histidine and lysine residue of proteins to form stable Michael addition type adducts [67,68].

Reaction of SH containing amino acids, peptides or proteins with HNE involves a classical Michael addition and the formation of a stable adduct [2]. This 1,4 addition as described in Fig. 6 requires the formation of a sulfhydryl ion by dissociation of the thiol. The ionized thiol can then attack the aldehydes on the fourth carbon which possesses a relatively high partial positive charge due to delocalization of the double bond electrons of the aldehydes. The enol which is then formed is rearranged in keto-enol tautomerism to the corresponding saturated aldehyde. In reactions with 2-alkenals without the hydroxy group this is the final adducts. Cyclization occurs in alkenals containing hydroxy residue at a carbon-4 position. Since all the individual steps in this pathway are reversible, the overall reaction is also reversible.

4-Hydroxyalkenals may react with various amino acid residues of a protein. For example, the binding to lysine is reversible and in order to stabilize the bond the

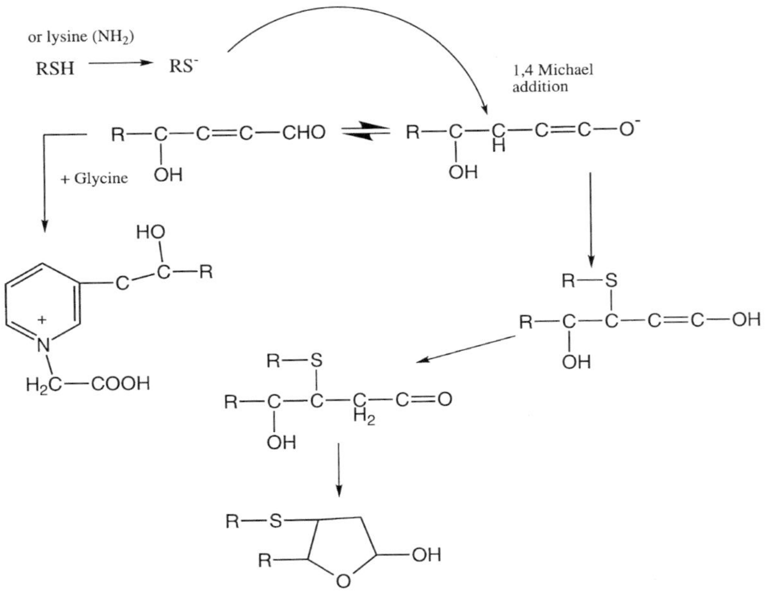

Fig. 6. Reaction mechanism for the formation of protein-aldehyde conjugates.

formed Schiff base has to be reduced to an secondary amine. HNE is highly reactive against amino acids such as Pro, Gly, His, Lys, and Ser; and the lowest reactivity is seen with Ala, Phe, Ile, Arg, Asp, Leu, Asn, Val, Gln and Glu [2]. HNE was found to react with the simplest amino acid glycine to form a pyridinium, derivative, 1-(1-carboxymethyl)-3-(2-hydroxypropyl)-pyridinium betaine [69] (Fig. 6). Uchida and Stadtman proposed [67] that HNE reacts with lysine also by a Michael addition mechanism as showed in Fig. 6.

2.   BIOLOGICAL RELEVANCE OF PROTEIN OXIDATION

2.1 Introduction

There are several major areas which are the subject of this review concerning protein oxidation and its biological relevance:
— Oxidative stress, protein oxidation, and aging.
— Protein oxidation in pathological conditions and various diseases.
— The role of protein oxidation in the process of protein inactivation and degradation.
— Exercise, immobilization, and protein oxidation.
— Plasma protein oxidation and modification due to exposure to cigarette smoke.

2.2 Oxidative stress, protein oxidation and aging

The aging phenomenon is a gradual, multifactorial process that has been an enigma for humanity since time immemorial. Many theories have been put forward in this century in order to attempt to explain the causes and processes of aging. However, one can divide the important theories into two main categories, as seen in Fig. 7: the molecular and cellular theories and the systemic and physiological theories. The molecular and cellular theories can be further subdivided into genetic and nongenetic theories (see Fig. 7). Among this multitude number of theories, the free radical theory of aging has gained tremendous support and become the most popular hypothesis to explain the ubiquitous process of aging. The reason for this stems from the fact that this is the only theory for which extensive experimental evidence today supports the involvement of free radical damage in aging and age-related diseases.

It was Harman [70] who first suggested, in 1956, that free radicals produced during respiration and cellular metabolism might cause oxidative damage to biological macromolecules. In addition, external factors such as toxic agents, irradiation, and excessive exercise may also raise the level of oxidative stress, and its cumulative effects over the years will lead to cellular damage, tissue and organ malfunctioning, and subsequently aging and death. This can be seen in Fig. 8. Several interesting findings in the last few decades have provided support and credibility to the free radical theory of aging. It was the discovery of the enzyme superoxide dismutase (SOD) [71] that showed that evolution has provided the living organism with antioxidant capacity to neutralize oxygen free radicals such as superoxide. Later, Cutler [72] observed that the metabolic rate of organisms is inversely related to the life span and aging rate in many animals. The higher the metabolic rate and, thus, the greater the increase in mitochondrial respiration and production of oxygen free radicals, the shorter the life span observed in aging

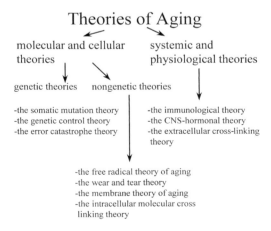

Fig. 7. Theories of aging.

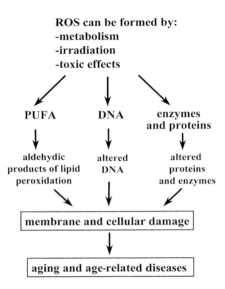

Fig. 8. Effects of reactive oxygen species on biological systems.

mammals with some number of exceptions. Finally, very compelling evidence was presented several years ago which demonstrated that the increase of expression of the two antioxidant enzymes catalase and SOD retarded the age-related oxidative damage of *Drosophila melanogaster* [73] and increased the life span of these flies [74].

As seen in Fig. 8, the free radical theory of aging predicts that one should be able to observe elevated oxidative damage to proteins and enzymes with advanced age. Using the carbonyl assay for protein oxidation [75], the content of protein carbonyls has been found to increase considerably in several aging systems [3,73,75–81]. Protein carbonyls refer to aldehydes or ketone groups which maybe introduced into proteins by either metal-catalyzed oxidation reactions, the reaction of proteins with carbohydrates or lipids, or by Michael addition of aldehydes to proteins. Accordingly, it has been found that protein carbonyls increase by almost 50% in muscles of old versus young rats [75]. Similarly, protein oxidative damage estimated by the carbonyl assay was associated with the life expectancy of houseflies [73]. The use of estimation of carbonyl content as a measure for protein oxidation in biological tissues and in aging was questioned by Cao and Cutler [76,77] when they encountered some technical difficulties in measuring protein carbonyls. Thus, they could not detect any changes in the level of protein carbonyls in gerbil liver and brain with age or with α-phenyl-*N*-tert-butyl nitrone (PBN)-treated animals. This is in contrast to the work of Carney et al. [78] who could detect such changes in protein oxidation in aging gerbils and with PBN treatment. However, Dubey et al. [79] later repeated the work of Carney et al. [78] and confirmed the original finding that PBN treatment causes a decrease of age-related elevation of protein carbonyls in gerbil brain cortex.

In other studies it was observed that the carbonyl content of proteins dramatically increased in oxidized proteins during the final third of the life span of several species such as human, rat, and the housefly *D. melanogaster* [82]. Stadtman [3] estimated that oxidized protein content of old tissues represents at least 30—50% of the total protein content. This observation was compared to the finding that many enzymes such as aldolase, superoxide dismutase and inolase have lower catalytic activity in aging animals in the range of 25—50% [82]. A very interesting work was reported that showed that accumulation of protein carbonyls in mitochondrial proteins increased considerably with age [81]. This study showed that protein oxidation during aging was not a random process, it was show that high molecular weight mitochondrial proteins were relatively more oxidatively damaged than small molecular weight proteins during aging [81].

In addition to carbonyl accumulation of protein oxidation were measured by the loss of the membrane protein-sulfhydryl (–SH) group, Agarwal and Sohal [80] could show a decrease of membrane protein-SH content in old male houseflies with a concomitant decrease in the activity of alcohol dehydrogenase and glucose-6-phosphate dehydrogenase using the quantitation of O,O'-dityrosine and O-tyrosine in proteins as a measure of protein oxidation. Recent work showed a marked increase of dityrosine with age in cardiac and skeletal muscles, but not in liver and brain, of aging mice [83]. O-tyrosine did not change with age in any of the above-mentioned tissues studied. However, caloric restriction to 60% of an ad libitum diet was capable of attenuating the dityrosine increase in cardiac and skeletal muscle [83]. It is interesting to note that elevation of protein oxidation with age is a relatively new area of research in the biology of aging compared to the previous observation of increased lipid peroxidation in aging tissues. Nonetheless, oxidative damage to biological molecules and their role in the aging process are not clear at this time, and more research is needed to elucidate this point.

2.3 Protein oxidation in pathological conditions and various diseases

2.3.1 Diabetes and the modification and oxidation of proteins

In diabetes, long-term elevation of glucose has been shown to cause the phenomenon of non-enzymatic glycosylation or "glycation" of proteins. Indeed, an increased level of glycosylated hemoglobin has been observed in vivo in diabetic patients [84], and the extent of hemoglobin glycation has been used in the clinic as an index of progression of glycemia [85]. The molecular mechanism of protein modification due to reaction of glucose with proteins leads to the formation of Schiff base reaction between the protein amines and the aldehydic moiety of sugars (see Fig. 9). Upon rearrangement, these Schiff base compounds formed what has been called Amadori adducts containing a single group of ketosugars that can be further degraded into deoxyglucosomes containing dicarbonyl deriva-

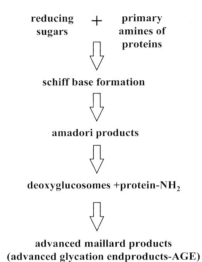

Fig. 9. Nonenzymatic glycation and formation of AGE.

tives. These latter compounds are very reactive and cross-react with proteins to form adducts known as Maillard reaction products or advanced glycation end products [86]. The physiological consequences of this phenomenon has been the modification and alteration of many proteins like collagen [87] and serum albumin [88] and the aggregation of lens proteins in glycosilation associated cataracts [89]. Indeed, the stiffness of joints and arteries of diabetic patients has been attributed to increased cross-linking of collagen, possibly due to non-enzymatic glycosylation of collagen [87].

2.3.2 Protein oxidation in atherosclerosis

In the process of formation of atherosclerotic plaques, oxidized low-density lipoprotein (LDL) plays a major role. In a review article, the major oxidative changes to the protein component of LDL were summarized [90]. These include the appearance of tyrosyl radical reactive nitrogen intermediates and the formation of hypochlorous acid. In contrast, protein oxidation products that are characteristics of metal-catalyzed oxidation like carbonyls were not elevated in vitro models of LDL oxidation [90]. More specifically, 3-chlorotyrosine, which is a specific marker for myeloperoxidase-catalyzed oxidation, was found to be markedly elevated in LDL isolated from human atherosclerotic plaques [37]. Moreover, careful work has validated that hypochlorite-oxidized proteins including oxidized apolipoprotein B, are present in atherosclerotic plaques [91]. Nitrotyrosine, which is used as a marker for peroxynitrite formation in diseased tissues, could not be detected in atherosclerotic lesions [92]. However, 3-nitrotyrosine was elevated [93]. In a recent publication, a significant increase of dityrosine and not *O*-tyrosine was observed in fatty streaks of atherosclerotic plaques [94]. This finding supported the notion that tyrosyl radical is involved in the oxidative damage occurring in human atherosclerosis [94] and also suggest that MCO plays a minor role in this process.

2.3.3 *Protein oxidation in cancer*

The involvement of free radicals and oxidative stress has been documented in a number of malignancies. The proposed mechanisms have been postulated to range from free radicals causing DNA double-strand breaks to the possibility of free-radical activation of oncogenes [95]. However, evidence for direct changes in the level of protein oxidation in cancer cells has been quite meager. In vitro studies of red blood cells from cancer patients compared to controls that were exposed to lipid or protein oxidation showed that methemoglobin formation was significantly higher in cancer patients [96]. Free radicals can cause oxyhemoglobin oxidative stress, which will result in an increase of methemoglobin [96]. The conclusion of the above authors was that free radicals in cancer alter erythrocyte permeability, which results in higher susceptibility to oxidative stress. A recent report on the capacity of benzo[a]pyrine of carcinogenesis initiation relates this chemical to the formation of a so-called micronucleus [97]. Evidence was presented that micronucleus formation in rat skin fibroblasts is connected to the elevation of oxidation of protein (carbonyl formation) and oxidation of DNA. The main conclusion of the above work was that carcinogenic initiation requires enzymatic bioactivation and it is peroxidase dependence and probably mediated by oxidation of proteins and DNA [97].

2.3.4 *Protein oxidation and neurological diseases*

Up to the present day, the etiology of many neurological and neurodegenerative diseases remains unclear. An interesting hypothesis was put forward by Beal [98] in which a defect in energy metabolism will lead to neuronal depolarization and an increase in intracellular calcium, which will, in turn, result in increased free radical generation [98]. A similar hypothesis was recently advanced by Markesbery [99] in which the etiology of Alzheimer disease (AD) was attributed to increased oxidative stress observed in the brain of AD patients.

A corollary of the above hypothesis is that one should be able to detect increased oxidation to protein and lipids in neurodegenerative diseases. Indeed, studies in human have demonstrated an increase in oxidized proteins in the brains of patients with different neurological diseases (Alzheimer, Parkinson, and Huntington disease) [100]. A more detailed study of the level of oxidative damage to proteins, lipids, and DNA in seven different brain areas of AD patients was reported [101]. Overall, only a slight increase of protein carbonyls was found in areas such as frontal, occipital, and temporal lobes. In the parietal lobes the increase was quite significant. In addition, measuring some oxidized

DNA bases showed that there was a significant elevation of DNA oxidation in a number of brain regions [101]. These findings partially support the notion that oxidative damage may play a role in the pathogenesis of AD, at least in some brain regions. On the other hand measuring protein carbonyls in motor cortex of sporadic motor neurons disease could not detect a significant elevation of protein oxidation compare to control patients [102].

2.3.5 *Protein oxidation in other pathologies*

Protein oxidation as measured by protein thiol loss and protein carbonyls has been detected in chronic ethanol-induced liver pathology [103], in inflammation [104], and in synovial fluid of patients with rheumatoid arthritis [105]. Elevated protein carbonyls and oxidation of protein thiols has also been observed in muscles of chickens with inherited muscular dystrophy [106]. A more recent report of measuring protein carbonyls in six human patients afflicted with Duchenne muscular dystrophy indicated that in quadriceps femoris there was an increase of 211% in protein oxidation compared to normal control subjects [107]. The latter finding was related to the fact that in Duchenne muscular dystrophy the protein dystrophin was missing, along with neuronal-type nitric oxide synthase. This was postulated to alter calcium homeostasis and to increase intracellular calcium levels, resulting in activation of the xanthine dehydrogenase/xanthine oxidase system, which causes elevation of superoxide radicals [107].

2.4 The role of protein oxidation in the process of protein inactivation and degradation

Early studies on glutamine synthetase from *E. coli* showed that oxidative damage renders the enzyme inactive. Oxidation of the enzyme could be generated by the cytochrome P-450 system or by ascorbic acid and oxygen [51]. After the enzyme was oxidized and inactivated, it was susceptible to proteolytic degradation systems of bacterial extracts [51]. In later studies in the mid-1980s, Davis and co-workers [55,108–110] showed that oxidation of proteins by hydroxyl radicals caused rapid protein denaturation and increased hydrophobicity, which was followed by protein degradation. The above process was dependent on the extent of denaturation and hydrophobicity, which seem to be the main signals for initiation of the proteolytic process [111]. Mild oxidative modification of protein caused a linear increase of denaturation and hydrophobicity. However, more severe protein oxidation (usually in the absence of oxygen) resulted in stabilization of the proteins, due to both intra- and intermolecular cross-links. This process prevented further denaturation, which caused the proteins to become less susceptible to proteolytic degradation [111]. The latter finding may explain the phenomenon observed in aging when a number of proteins and enzymes are found to have longer half-lives and degrade more slowly [112,113]. This seemingly contradicts the observation that mildly oxidized proteins are degraded more rapidly.

There have been at least two explanations for the above finding. One is that oxidized proteins in aging may result in cross-linked in some proteins that render them more resistant to proteolytic degradation [114]. Indeed, cross-linked extracellular proteins like collagen and elastin are known to accumulate in aging tissues. The second explanation is that with aging there is a gradual reduction and loss of activity in the proteolytic system responsible for the removal of faulty proteins in aging [115]. In a later work, the increase in activity of neutral proteases was suggested to be responsible for the accumulation of oxidized proteins in aging [116]. Support for the above contention was found when an increased relationship was observed between the amount of abnormal protein accumulated in aging hepatocytes and the level of activity of neutral proteases found in these cells [47].

In the last decade there have been several attempts to identify the specific proteolytic system responsible for the degradation of oxidized proteins. Several works have suggested that it is the 19s multicatalytic cytosolic protease, part of the intracellular proteolytic system, known as proteosome, that is mainly responsible for degradation of oxidized proteins [117,118].

2.5 Exercise, immobilization, and protein oxidation

It is suggested that with strenuous exercise there is a marked elevation of oxidative stress to muscles. The first report to demonstrate that rats subjected to exhaustive exercise accumulate higher level of protein carbonyls was published in 1992 [119]. However, several weeks of pre-exercise feeding with high levels of vitamin E could ameliorate the accumulation of protein carbonyls [120]. Rats exercised for long-term training of 12 weeks also exhibited an increase in the level of protein carbonyls from 2.6 to 5.4 nmol/mg protein. However, after 2 weeks of cessation from exercise this value of protein oxidation was reduced to 3.6 nmol/mg protein [120]. More recent reports have also demonstrated an increase of protein carbonyls in muscle of rats subjected to high-altitude training [121]. In that study, however, a concomitant increase of lipid peroxidation products was not observed. In another recent study, long-term exercise for 8 weeks increased protein carbonyls and lipid peroxidation measured by thiobarbituric acid-reactive substances. Moreover, 8 weeks of vitamin E supplementation to animals supplemented with fish and soy oils markedly reduced the level of protein oxidation and lipid peroxidation [122]. Table 1 summarizes reports in which an increase protein oxidation was observed in exercised animals.

Immobilization of hind-limb muscles of rats was shown to be associated with an increase of lipid peroxidation that could be reduced to some extent when immobilized animals were administered vitamin E [123]. A xanthine oxidase dependent molecular mechanism for this oxidative stress observed in immobilization has been proposed [124]. More recently, the increase of protein carbonyls in immobilized muscles of aging rats was also reported [125,126]. Administration of rat growth hormone to the immobilized animals could retard some of the protein oxidation and lipid peroxidation as well as other parameters of immobilization-

Table 1. Summary of protein carbonyl levels in exercise and immobilization.

Type of tissue	Experimental conditions	Results	Reference
Red and white muscle, quadriceps muscle	Running until exhaustion	↑	Reznick et al., 1992 [119]
Total hind-limb muscle	8 weeks of running	↑	Witt et al., 1992 [120]
Quadriceps femoris muscle	4 weeks of high-altitude running	↑	Radak et al., 1997 [121]
	4 weeks of running at sea level	↔	
Muscles and liver	8 weeks of running	↑	Sen et al., 1997 [122]
Gastrocnemius muscles	4 weeks of immobilization	↑	Carmeli et al., 1993 [125]
Plantaris muscle	4 weeks of immobilization	↑	Fares et al., 1996 [126]
Various brain areas	Immobilization	↑	Liu et al., 1996 [127]

associated damage [125,126]. Another paper [127] reported that immobilization causes increased levels of protein oxidation as well as lipid and DNA oxidative damage in several areas of the brain, supporting the notion that general stress such as immobilization may cause oxidative damage to brain and contribute to degenerative diseases observed in aging [127].

It is noteworthy that both severe modes of exercise and immobilization result in elevated lipid and protein oxidation. Nevertheless, the mechanism of these two phenomena may not be the same.

2.6 Plasma protein oxidation and cigarette smoke

In early studies it was shown that exposure of human plasma, in vitro, to gas-phase CS resulted in oxidative damage to lipids. Concomitant with the increase of lipid hydroperoxide due to CS exposure, there was a marked depletion of plasma and antioxidants such as rapid decrease of ascorbic and uric acids and slower disappearance of plasma α-tocopherol [128].

In subsequent studies, the effect of exposure of plasma to CS on protein carbonyl levels was investigated. Interestingly, exposure of humane plasma to nine puffs of CS over a period of 3 hours produced a 500% increase in plasma protein carbonyls that could not be inhibited by the addition of glucose, ascorbate, or desferrioxamine. Only small thiols containing molecules like glutathione or dihydrolipoic acid could ameliorate the time-dependent accumulation of protein carbonyls [129].

In a later study, an attempt was made to elucidate the mechanism of these protein modifications. It was found that with the increase of protein carbonyl accumulation due to CS exposure, there was a concomitant decrease in protein-SH groups. Using purified unsaturated volatile aldehydes, such as acrolein and crotonaldehyde, known to be present in CS, it was possible to show that increase of protein carbonyl due to exposure to aldehydes was accompanied by a 1:1 molar ratio decrease of protein-SH groups. This explained quite clearly that aldehydes in CS interact with the SH group of proteins in a Michael addition reaction, leading to accumulation of carbonyls contributed by the aldehydic groups acrolein and crotonaldehyde [130].

3   SUMMARY

A wide variety of chemical protein modifications do occur during protein oxidation. The modification of a protein by either a direct oxidation of a specific amino acid or cleavage of the protein backbone might results in impaired biological activity and changes in the secondary and tertiary structure of the protein. In this chapter we reviewed the chemistry and the patho-physiological relevancy of biologically irreversible protein oxidation. The physiological relevancy of the fine tuning of redox regulation on proteins activity was not included. Indeed oxidative stress in proteins results in faulty proteins accumulation in the organism's cells, tissues and body fluid. The numerous publications that describes the accumulation of oxidized proteins in the aging process and in various pathological disorders including diabetes, atherosclerosis, and brain disorders clearly demonstrate the relevancy of oxidative stress in these pathologies.

4   ACKNOWLEDGEMENT

Many thanks to Dr. Christiaan Leeuwenburgh for critically reading this work and providing comments. Part of this work was supported by the Krol Foundation, Lakewood, N.J., USA, to AZR

5   ABBREVIATIONS

ROS: reactive oxygen species
MCO: metal-catalyzed oxidation
NFK: N'-formylkynurenine
LDL: Low-density lipoprotein
SOD: superoxide dismutase
EDTA: ethylenediaminetetraacetic acid
BOC: *tert*-butyloxycarbonyl
BSA: bovine serum albumin
MPO: myeloperoxidase
HNE: 4-hydroxy-2-nonenal
AD: Alzheimer disease

PBN: α-phenyl-*N-tert*-butyl nitrone
CS: cigarette smoke

6   REFERENCES

1. Halliwell B, Gutridge J (eds). Free Radicals in Biology and Medicine, 2 edn. Oxford Press, 1989.
2. Esterbauer H, Schaur RJ, Zollner H. Free Radic Biol Med 1991;11(1):81–128.
3. Stadtman ER. Science 1992;257(5074):1220–1224.
4. Stadtman ER, Oliver CN, Starke-Reed PE, Rhee SG. Toxicol Ind Health 1993;9(1–2): 187–196.
5. Okajima T, Kawata Y, Hamaguchi K. Biochemistry 1990;29(39):9168–9175.
6. Bobrowski K, Holcman J, Poznanski J, Wierzchowski KL. Biophys Chem 1997;63(2–3): 153–166.
7. Mudd JB, Dawson PJ, Tseng S, Liu FP. Arch Biochem Biophys 1997;338(2):143–149.
8. Fukunaga Y, Katsuragi Y, Izumi T, Sakiyama F. J Biochem (Tokyo) 1982;92(1):129–141.
9. Shortle D, Meeker AK. Biochemistry 1989;28(3):936–944.
10. Maskos Z, Rush JD, Koppenol WH. Arch Biochem Biophys 1992;296(2):521–529.
11. Maskos Z, Rush JD, Koppenol WH. Arch Biochem Biophys 1992;296(2):514–520.
12. Itakura K, Uchida K, Kawakishi S. Chem Res Toxicol 1994;7(2):185–190.
13. Giessauf A, van Wickern B, Simat T, Steinhart H et al. FEBS Lett 1996;389(2):136–140.
14. Giessauf A, Steiner E, Esterbauer H. Biochim Biophys Acta 1995;1256(2):221–232.
15. Kato Y, Kawakishi S, Aoki T, Itakura K et al. Biochem Biophys Res Commun 1997;234(1): 82–84.
16. Alvarez B, Rubbo H, Kirk M, Barnes S et al. Chem Res Toxicol 1996;9(2):390–396.
17. Pietraforte D, Minetti M. Biochem J 1997;321(Pt 3)):743–750.
18. Beckman JS, Koppenol WH. Am J Physiol 1996;271(5, Pt 1):C1424–C1437.
19. Bohle DS, Glassbrenner PA, Hansert B. Meth Enzymol 1996;269:302–311.
20. Castro L, Rodriguez M, Radi R. J Biol Chem 1994;269(47):29409–29415.
21. Hausladen A, Fridovich I. J Biol Chem 1994;269(47):29405–29408.
22. Crow JP, Beckman JS, McCord JM. Biochemistry 1995;34(11):3544–3552.
23. Radi R, Rodriguez M, Castro L, Telleri R. Arch Biochem Biophys 1994;308(1):89–95.
24. Crow JP, Spruell C, Chen J, Gunn C et al. Free Radic Biol Med 1994;16(3):331–338.
25. Beckman JS, Beckman TW, Chen J, Marshall PA et al. Proc Natl Acad Sci USA 1990;87(4): 1620–1624.
26. Zhu L, Gunn C, Beckman JS. Arch Biochem Biophys 1992;298(2):452–457.
27. van der Vliet A, Eiserich JP, O'Neill CA, Halliwell B, Cross CE et al. Arch Biochem Biophys 1995;319(2):341–349.
28. van der Vliet A, O'Neill CA, Halliwell B, Kaur H, Cross CE et al. FEBS Lett 1994;339(1–2) :89–92.
29. van der Vliet A, Eiserich JP, Halliwell B, Cross CE. J Biol Chem 1997;272(12):7617–7625.
30. Lee SB, Inouye K, Tonomura B. J Biochem (Tokyo) 1997;121(2):231–237.
31. Pereira WE, Hoyano Y, Summons RE, Bacon VA et al. Biochim Biophys Acta 1973;313(1): 170–180.
32. Kettle AJ, Winterbourn CC. Meth Enzymol 1994;233:502–512.
33. Kettle AJ. FEBS Lett 1996;379(1):103–106.
34. Domigan NM, Charlton TS, Duncan MW, Winterbourn CC et al. J Biol Chem 1995;270(28): 16542–16548.
35. Hazen SL, Hsu FF, Duffin K, Heinecke JW. J Biol Chem 1996;271(38):23080–23088.
36. Hazen SL, Hsu FF, Mueller DM, Crowley JR et al. J Clin Invest 1996;98(6):1283–1289.
37. Hazen SL, Heinecke JW. J Clin Invest 1997;99(9):2075–2081.
38. Eiserich JP, Cross CE, Jones AD, Halliwell B et al. J Biol Chem 1996;271(32):19199–19208.

39. Stadtman ER. Annu Rev Biochem 1993;62:797–821.
40. Holian J, Garrison WM. J Phys Chem 1968;72(13):4721–4723.
41. Holian J, Garrison WM. Nature 1969;221(175):57.
42. Yan LJ, Traber MG, Kobuchi H, Matsugo S et al. Arch Biochem Biophys 1996;327(2):330–334.
43. Yan LJ, Lodge JK, Traber MG, Matsugo S et al. J Lipid Res 1997;38(5):992–1001.
44. Stadtman ER, Berlett BS. J Biol Chem 1991;266(26):17201–17211.
45. Berlett BS, Chock PB, Yim MB, Stadtman ER. Proc Natl Acad Sci USA 1990;87(1):389–393.
46. Stadtman ER, Berlett BS, Chock PB. Proc Natl Acad Sci USA 1990;87(1):384–388.
47. Stadtman ER, Oliver CN. J Biol Chem 1991;266(4):2005–2008.
48. Schuessler H, Herget A. Int J Radiat Biol Relat Stud Phys Chem Med 1980;37(1):71–80.
49. Schuessler H, Schilling K. Int J Radiat Biol Relat Stud Phys Chem Med 1984;45(3):267–281.
50. Stadtman ER, Wittenberger ME. Arch Biochem Biophys 1985;239(2):379–387.
51. Levine RL, Oliver CN, Fulks RM, Stadtman ER. Proc Natl Acad Sci USA 1981;78(4): 2120–2124.
52. Amici A, Levine RL, Tsai L, Stadtman ER. J Biol Chem 1989;264(6):3341–3346.
53. Climent I, Tsai L, Levine RL. Anal Biochem 1989;182(2):226–232.
54. Szweda LI, Stadtman ER. J Biol Chem 1992;267(5):3096–3100.
55. Davies KJ, Delsignore ME, Lin SW. J Biol Chem 1987;262(20):9902–9907.
56. Yim MB, Berlett BS, Chock PB, Stadtman ER. Proc Natl Acad Sci USA 1990;87(1):394–398.
57. Neuzil J, Gebicki JM, Stocker R. Biochem J 1993;293(Pt 3)):601–606.
58. Fucci L, Oliver CN, Coon MJ, Stadtman ER. Proc Natl Acad Sci USA 1983;80(6):1521–1525.
59. Stadtman ER. Free Radic Biol Med 1990;9(4):315–325.
60. Kim K, Rhee SG, Stadtman ER. J Biol Chem 1985;260(29):15394–15397.
61. Cooper B, Creeth JM, Donald AS. Biochem J 1985;228(3):615–626.
62. Farber JM, Levine RL. J Biol Chem 1986;261(10):4574–4578.
63. Berlett BS, Levine RL, Stadtman ER. J Biol Chem 1996;271(8):4177–4182.
64. Levine RL, Mosoni L, Berlett BS, Stadtman ER. Proc Natl Acad Sci USA 1996;93(26): 15036–15040.
65. Uchida K, Itakura K, Kawakishi S, Hiai H et al. Arch Biochem Biophys 1995;324(2):241–248.
66. Yoritaka A, Hattori N, Uchida K, Tanaka M et al. Proc Natl Acad Sci USA 1996;93(7): 2696–2701.
67. Uchida K, Stadtman ER. Proc Natl Acad Sci USA 1992;89(10):4544–4548.
68. Uchida K, Szweda LI, Chae HZ, Stadtman ER. Proc Natl Acad Sci USA 1993;90(18): 8742–8746.
69. Napetschnig S, Schauenstein E, Esterbauer H. Chem Biol Interact 1988;68(3–4):165–177.
70. Harman DJ. J Gerontol 1956;11:298–300.
71. McCord JM, Fridovich I. J Biol Chem 1969;244(22):6049–6055.
72. Cutler RG. In: Smith KC (ed) Aging, Carcinogenesis, and Radiation Biology. New York: Plenum Press, 1976. QU 58 A267 1975.
73. Sohal RS, Agarwal S, Dubey A, Orr WC. Proc Natl Acad Sci USA 1993;90(15):7255–7259.
74. Orr WC, Sohal RS. Science 1994;263(5150):1128–1130.
75. Reznick AZ, Packer L. Meth Enzymol 1994;233:357–363.
76. Cao G, Cutler RG. Arch Biochem Biophys 1995;320(1):106–114.
77. Cao G, Cutler RG. Arch Biochem Biophys 1995;320(1):195–201.
78. Carney JM, Starke-Reed PE, Oliver CN, Landum RW et al. Proc Natl Acad Sci USA 1991;88 (9):3633–3636.
79. Dubey A, Forster MJ, Sohal RS. Arch Biochem Biophys 1995;324(2):249–254.
80. Agarwal S, Sohal RS. Mech Ageing Dev 1994;75(1):11–19.
81. Agarwal S, Sohal RS. Mech Ageing Dev 1995;85(1):55–63.
82. Levine RC, Stadtman ER. In: Schneider EL, Rowe JW (eds) Handbook of the Biology of Aging, 4th edn. New York: Academic Press, 1997.
83. Leeuwenburgh C, Wagner P, Holloszy JO, Sohal RS et al. Arch Biochem Biophys 1997;346(1):

74—80.
84. Trivelli LA, Ranney HM, Lai HT. N Engl J Med 1971;284(7):353—357.
85. Kennedy L, Baynes JW. Diabetologia 1984;26(2):93—98.
86. Wolff SP, Jiang ZY, Hunt JV. Free Radic Biol Med 1991;10(5):339—352.
87. Bailey AJ, Kent KJC. In: Baynes JW, Monnier VM (eds) The Maillard Reaction in Aging, Diabetes and Nutrition. New York: Alan R. Liss, 1989.
88. Shaklai N, Garlick RL, Bunn HF. J Biol Chem 1984;259(6):3812—3817.
89. Monnier VM, Stevens VJ, Cerami A. J Exp Med 1979;150(5):1098—1107.
90. Heinecke JW. Curr Opin Lipidol 1997;8(5):268—274.
91. Hazell LJ, Arnold L, Flowers D, Waeg G et al. J Clin Invest 1996;97(6):1535—1544.
92. Evans P, Kaur H, Mitchinson MJ, Halliwell B. Biochem Biophys Res Commun 1996;226(2): 346—351.
93. Leeuwenburgh C, Hardy MM, Hazen SL, Wagner P et al. J Biol Chem 1997;272(3):1433—1436.
94. Leeuwenburgh C, Rasmussen JE, Hsu FF, Mueller DM et al. J Biol Chem 1997;272(6): 3520—3526.
95. Reizenstein P. Med Oncol Tumor Pharmacother 1991;8:229—233.
96. Della Rovere F, Granata A, Broccio M, Zirilli A et al. Anticancer Res 1995;15(5B):2089—2095.
97. Kim PM, DeBoni U, Wells PG. Free Radic Biol Med 1997;23(4):579—596.
98. Beal MF. Ann Neurol 1995;38(3):357—366.
99. Markesbery WR. Free Rad Biol Med 1997;23(1):134—147.
100. Carney JM, Carney AM. Life Sci 1994;55(25—26):2097—2103.
101. Lyras L, Cairns NJ, Jenner A, Jenner P et al. J Neurochem 1997;68(5):2061—2069.
102. Lyras L, Evans PJ, Shaw PJ, Ince PG et al. Free Rad Res 1996;24(5):397—406.
103. Rouach H, Fataccioli V, Gentil M, French SW et al. Hepatology 1997;25(2):351—355.
104. Krsek-Staples JA, Webster RO. Free Radic Biol Med 1993;14(2):115—125.
105. Chapman ML, Rubin BR, Gracy RW. J Rheumatol 1989;16(1):15—18.
106. Murphy ME, Kehrer JP. Biochem J 1989;260(2):359—364.
107. Haycock JW, MacNeil S, Jones P, Harris JB et al. Neuroreport 1996;8(1):357—361.
108. Davies KJ, Delsignore ME. J Biol Chem 1987;262(20):9908—9913.
109. Davies KJ. J Biol Chem 1987;262(20):9895—9901.
110. Davies KJ, Lin SW, Pacifici RE. J Biol Chem 1987;262(20):9914—9920.
111. Davis KJA. Biochem Soc Trans 1993;21:346—352.
112. Reznick AZ, Gershon D. Mech Ageing Dev 1979;11(5—6):403—415.
113. Reznick AZ, Lavie L, Gershon HE, Gershon D. FEBS Lett 1981;128(2):221—224.
114. Grant AJ, Jessup W, Dean RT. Biochim Biophys Acta 1992;1134(3):203—209.
115. Lavie L, Reznick AZ, Gershon D. Biochem J 1982;202(1):47—51.
116. Starke-Reed PE, Oliver CN. Arch Biochem Biophys 1989;275:559—567.
117. Rivett AJ. Curr Top Cell Regul 1986;28:291—337.
118. Pacifici RE, Salo DC, Davies KJ. Free Rad Biol Med 1989;7(5):521—536.
119. Reznick AZ, Witt E, Matsumoto M, Packer L. Biochem Biophys Res Commun 1992;189: 801—806.
120. Witt EH, Reznick AZ, Viguie CA, Starke-Reed P et al. J Nutr 1992;122(3 Suppl):766—773.
121. Radak Z, Asano K, Lee KC, Ohno H et al. Free Radic Biol Med 1997;22(6):1109—1114.
122. Sen CK, Atalay M, Agren J, Laaksonen DE et al. J Appl Physiol 1997;83(1):189—195.
123. Kondo H, Miura M, Itokawa Y. Acta Physiol Scand 1991;142(4):527—528.
124. Kondo H, Nakagaki I, Sasaki S, Hori S et al. Am J Physiol 1993;265(6, Pt 1):E839—E844.
125. Carmeli E, Hochberg Z, Livne E, Lichtenstein I et al. J Appl Physiol 1993;75(4):1529—1535.
126. Fares FA, Gruener N, Carmeli E, Reznick AZ. Ann N Y Acad Sci 1996;786:430—443.
127. Liu J, Wang X, Shigenaga MK, Yeo HC et al. Faseb J 1996;10(13):1532—1538.
128. Frei B, Forte TM, Ames BN, Cross CE. Biochem J 1991;277(Pt 1)):133—138.
129. Reznick AJ, Cross CE, Hu M-L, Suzuki YJ. Biochem J 1982;286:607—611.
130. O'Neill CA, Halliwell B, van der Vliet A, Davis PA et al. J Lab Clin Med 1994;124(3):359—370.

©2000 Elsevier Science B.V. All rights reserved.
Handbook of Oxidants and Antioxidants in Exercise.
C.K. Sen, L. Packer and O. Hänninen, editors.

Part III • Chapter 5

Lipid peroxidation in healthy and diseased models: influence of different types of exercise

Helaine M. Alessio

Miami University, Oxford, Ohio 45056, USA. Tel.: +1-513-529-2707. E-mail: alessih@muohio.edu

1   INTRODUCTION
    1.1   Lipid peroxidation: What is it and why is it important?
    1.2   How is lipid peroxidation measured?
2   LIPID PEROXIDATION AND EXERCISE
    2.1   Healthy models
        2.1.1   Acute exercise
        2.1.2   Regular exercise
        2.1.3   Aerobic and nonaerobic exercise
        2.1.4   Antioxidant supplementation
    2.2   Diseased models
        2.2.1   Cardiovascular disease
        2.2.2   Diabetes
3   SUMMARY
4   PERSPECTIVES
5   ACKNOWLEDGEMENTS
6   ABBREVIATIONS
7   REFERENCES

1   INTRODUCTION

Free radicals and lipid peroxides play an important role in the oxidative stress balance between prooxidant and antioxidant activities. If the balance tilts towards prooxidants, the functional health of an organism is jeopardized. The major site for oxidative metabolism is the mitochondria. Energy-releasing reactions of oxidation-reduction for transporting electrons cause a proton (H^+) gradient across the inner mitochondrial membrane. Energy stored in the proton gradient combined with the inner mitochondrial membrane potential, provide the electrochemical basis for coupling electron transport with ADP phosphorylation. This is how large amounts of ATP are produced. Uncoupling may occur if an electron escapes the inner mitochondrial membrane, leaving the final electron receiver, oxygen, with one less electron in its possession. Uncoupling of oxidative phosphorylation results in the generation of oxygen radicals and lipid peroxides. Many of these radicals are derived from normal mitochondrial oxygen consumption and electron transport flux or movement across the inner mitochondrial membrane. Examples of free radicals formed in part by oxygen consumption and electron transport flux include superoxide radical ($O_2^{\bullet-}$), hydroxyl radical

(•OH), perhydroxyl radical (HO$_2$•), and conjugated peroxyl radical (LOO•), all of which may induce lipid peroxidation reactions [1–3].

1.1 Lipid peroxidation: what is it and why is it important?

Lipid peroxidation reactions involve free radical attack on polyunsaturated fatty acids. The availability of polyunsaturated fatty acid substrates and the antioxidant protection in lipid-rich cell membranes, control the pathophysiology of lipid per-oxidation chain reactions that can produce free radicals and lipid peroxides. The way in which lipid peroxides may ultimately harm an organism is when the fatty acid under radical attack becomes a lipid radical with allylic double bonds. These double bonds are relatively weak and can combine with oxygen to produce lipid peroxy radicals and ultimately lipid peroxides. Lipid peroxides usually decom-pose to form aldehydes (e.g., malonaldehyde) which can cross-link or change the structures of proteins, lipids, carbohydrates, and DNA.

Lipids are generally hydrophobic, and act as fuel for metabolism, support for membrane structure, and selective cell membrane transport. Unsaturated fatty acids are vulnerable to free radical attack, especially by the hydroxyl radical. When a hydrogen is removed from a hydrocarbon chain and a lipid peroxide is formed, the unsaturated fatty acid becomes more hydrophilic than usual. This new characteristic of fatty acids being attracted to water, alters the ability of lipids to selectively transfer metabolites through the cell membrane. As a result, excess water may enter the cell and inflammation may occur. Inflammation may trigger more O$_2$•$^-$ release, thus contributing to a positive feedback system that facilitates or propagates lipid peroxidation reactions, and produces more aldehydes, moving the cell towards destruction.

Active oxygen species, including O$_2$•$^-$, •OH, HO$_2$•, and LOO• can initiate and propagate lipid peroxidation reactions (Fig. 1). Free radical mediated lipid per-oxidation generally requires radicals and weakly bonded polyunsaturated fatty acids for the initial steps. Oxygen and a lipid radical are necessary for the inter-mediate or propagation steps which ultimately produce lipid peroxidation by-products.

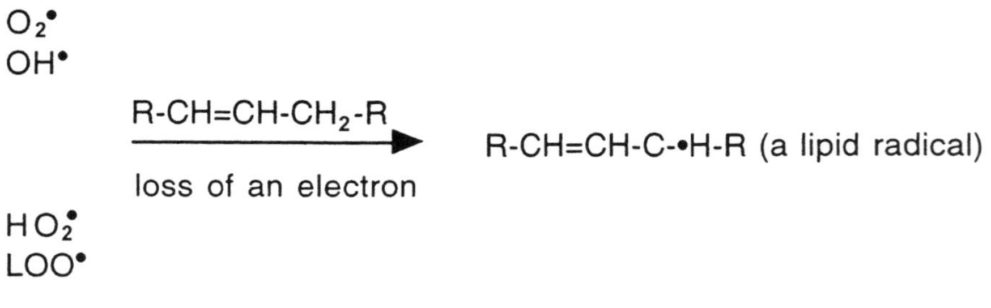

O$_2$•
OH•

$$\xrightarrow[\text{loss of an electron}]{\text{R-CH=CH-CH}_2\text{-R}}$$ R-CH=CH-C-•H-R (a lipid radical)

HO$_2$•
LOO•

Fig. 1. Summary of initial step for free radical initiation of lipid peroxidation reactions. O$_2$•: super-oxide radical; OH•: hydroxyl radical; HO$_2$•: perhydroxyl radical; LOO•: conjugated peroxyl radical; R: alkyl group; R-CH=CH-CH$_2$-R: unsaturated lipid; –: single bond; =: double bond; R-CH=CH-C-•H-R: lipid radical.

1.2 How is lipid peroxidation measured?

Malonaldehyde (MDA), thiobarbituric acid reactive substances (TBARS), lipid hydroperoxides (LH), and 4-hydroxyalkenals (4-HNE) are examples of lipid peroxidation by-products that have been used as barometers of lipid peroxidation reaction rates. By-products of lipid peroxidation reactions have been investigated in many studies that have focused on exercise using both healthy and diseased models. Increases in MDA, TBARS, LH, or 4-HNE are directly linked to increased lipid peroxidation rates, and indirectly related to electron transport disturbances, uncoupling of oxidative phosphorylation, increased mitochondrial respiration, and/or elevated oxygen uptake (VO_2). These lipid peroxidation by-products are, themselves, toxic.

Aldehydes such as MDA may be harmful because of their carcinogenic [4,5], mutagenic [6], and protein cross-linking [7] properties. The basis of the TBARS method is the measurement of MDA, which is one of the secondary products formed during the oxidation of polyunsaturated fatty acids. There are, however, other endogenous sources of MDA in tissues, which come from a variety of reactions such as side products of prostaglandin and thromboxane synthesis [8,9]. LH are the first separate products of oxidation, and interaction between LH and proteins or any other compounds, can damage membranes and enzymes [10]. 4-HNE is a well characterized oxidation product of polyunsaturated fatty acids and increases in direct proportion to both LDL oxidation and lipid peroxidation reactions [11].

Steady-state MDA, TBARS, LH, and 4-HNE content of a tissue is the net result of the endogenous rate of lipid peroxidation chain reactions, the metabolic removal of lipid peroxidation by-products, and the antioxidant status of the tissue. It is generally agreed that oxygen toxicity is often accompanied by lipid peroxidation by-products However, it is not clear whether lipid peroxidation by-products themselves are directly harmful to cells or if lipid peroxidation reaction rates coincidentally increase when oxygen radicals overwhelm antioxidants. An interesting side to the incubus perception of lipid peroxidation is that lipid peroxidation has been shown to be essential for normal cell development. Sevanian and Hochstein [12] suggested that only when lipid peroxidation takes place in uncontrolled free radical chain reactions that overwhelm antioxidant cell protection does lipid peroxidation cause cell damage. The implication that lipid peroxidation is necessary for normal growth and development is intriguing. Nevertheless, much evidence has accumulated implicating lipid peroxidation to a number of diseases including diabetes mellitus, atherosclerosis, rheumatoid arthritis, ischemia-reperfusion [11], hemolytic anemias, and pulmonary dysfunction [12]. Thus, an elevated lipid peroxidation rate as indicated by elevated MDA, TBARS, LH, or 4-HNE levels, implies that those cells that accumulate lipid peroxidation by-products, are less apt to function properly.

Lipid peroxidation can also be driven by agents other than oxygen or oxygen derived radicals, such as chelated iron, redux metal irons, ascorbate, enzymes such as cyclooxygenase-dependent peroxidation of arachidonate to prostaglandin and thromboxane precursors or the NADPH-cytochrome P450 reductase dependent reactions in microsomes. The rate of lipid peroxidation can also be moderated by the amount and/or activity of certain antioxidants. That lipid peroxidation by-products can increase without evidence of higher oxygen consumption or oxygen derived radical activity, is of interest in studies on lipid peroxidation, disease, and research using different modes of exercise.

2   LIPID PEROXIDATION AND EXERCISE

Many studies have hypothesized that physical exercise can induce oxidative stress and accelerate lipid peroxidation reactions in humans [13−17]. Virtually all of these studies implicate aerobic exercise in producing either increased active oxygen species (e.g., $O_2^{\bullet-}$, $^{\bullet}OH$, $HO_2^{\bullet}$, and $LOO^{\bullet}$) that overwhelm antioxidant defenses to the point where free radicals and lipid peroxidation reactions run amuck. Most of the protocols used to study exercise-induced lipid peroxidation have used healthy models that participate in aerobic exercise such as running or swimming with durations of at least 20 min to exhaustion.

2.1 Healthy models

Most studies on exercise and lipid peroxidation have used healthy subjects. Exercise-induced oxidative stress in healthy subjects has been shown to increase above baseline levels, but has not been blamed for serious health problems or compromised performance. Virtually all studies on aerobic exercise report that healthy and fit persons generally have a higher capacity to consume oxygen compared to age-matched unhealthy or unfit persons, and have less oxidative stress associated with aerobic exercise.

2.1.1 Acute exercise

How dangerous can oxygen be if it is such a key component in aerobic exercise? Figure 2 gives a theoretical estimate of superoxide radicals produced by oxygen consumption at rest and during exercise. In this example, a 150 pound person is estimated to have a resting VO_2 equivalent to about 1 MET or 3.5 ml· kg^{-1}· min^{-1}. This basal metabolic rate translates to about 353 l of oxygen consumed in a day or 14.7 moles oxygen consumed in a day. Halliwell [18] has speculated that 1% of VO_2 escapes univalent reduction in the electron transport system and 0.146 moles of superoxide radicals are formed. Over a year time, 0.146 moles of $O_2^{\bullet-}$ would be equivalent to 1.72 kg of $O_2^{\bullet-}$.

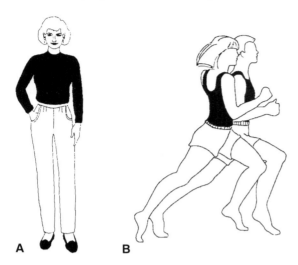

Fig. 2. Estimation of VO_2 and $O_2^{\bullet-}$ production per year if a person does not exercise and if a person engages in daily moderate exercise. **A:** A 150 lb adult consumes 3.5 ml/kg/min, 352.8 l O_2/day or 14.7 moles O_2/day. Assuming 1% of VO_2 becomes $O_2^{\bullet-}$, then 0.146 moles $O_2^{\bullet-}$/day is produced adding 1.72 kg $O_2^{\bullet-}$ each year. **B:** If a 150 lb adult consumes the same amount of oxygen at rest but exercises for 40 min each day at approximately 35 ml/kg/min, then this person consumes 441 l O_2/day or 18.4 moles O_2/day. Assuming 1% of VO_2 becomes $O_2^{\bullet-}$, then 0.184 moles $O_2^{\bullet-}$/day is produced adding 0.43 more $O_2^{\bullet-}$ for a total of 2.15 kg $O_2^{\bullet-}$ each year.

2.1.2 Regular exercise

The second scenario has this same 150 pound person raising their basal metabolic rate 10-fold (with a $VO_2 = 35$ ml$\cdot$kg$^{-1}\cdot$min^{-1}), by exercising regularly for 40 min each day. Under the same assumption that 1% of the oxygen consumed will become $O_2^{\bullet-}$, this person, by adding a regular exercise regime, will produce 2.15 kg of $O_2^{\bullet-}$ in a year. One can hypothesize that the effect on oxidative stress balance will vary quantitatively, with exercise time and intensity. It is likely that with no further antioxidant protection arising from either endogenous or exogenous sources, 2.15 kg of $O_2^{\bullet-}$ compared to 1.72 kg of $O_2^{\bullet-}$ would result in greater production of $O_2^{\bullet-}$, lipid peroxidation by-products, oxidative stress, and cell damage.

2.1.3 Aerobic and nonaerobic exercise

Exhaustive exercise has been shown to incur the most signs and symptoms of oxidative stress. Radak et al. [19] reported that exhaustive running induced xanthine oxidase-derived oxidative damage in liver. Kidney tissue showed an increased lipid peroxidation after the run, which the authors suggested was due to a washout-dependent accumulation of peroxidized metabolites. When treated with antioxidants, a superoxide dismutase derivative, before exercising to exhaustion, rats showed lower levels of TBARS and xanthine oxidase activity after the exercise [19]. Based on these results, oxidative stress associated with exhaustive exercise resulted in higher levels of lipid peroxidation by-products, namely MDA, and anti-oxidant supplement attenuated lipid peroxidation activity and MDA production.

Swimming to exhaustion caused some forms of chemical change and oxidative damage to the membranes of erythrocytes, cardiac and skeletal muscle tissue of rats [20]. Following exhaustive exercise MDA increased, phospholipids decreased, protein oxidation increased and total cellular sulfyhdryls in blood plasma and skeletal muscle, increased. Sulfhydryl group oxidation was reported in another exercise study where seven moderately trained males completed a marathon race [13]. It is important to protect sulfhydryl groups, because a decrease in sulfhydryls resulting from their oxidation or a change in the di-sulfide/sulfhydryl ratio can inactivate certain enzymes and damage cells [21]. Although plasma TBARS did not change significantly, plasma protein-bound sulfhydryl group levels were 22, 12, and 13% lower than baseline immediately, 1 day, and 2 days, respectively, following the race [13]. These sulfhydryl levels may have been lower following exercise due to oxidization, and may tilt the di-sulfide/sulfhydryl ratio in a way that inactivates enzymes and causes cell damage.

Few studies have focused on nonaerobic types of exercise that last only a minute or two. Radicals that initiate lipid peroxidation reactions are not always generated aerobically. Superoxides have been observed during the autooxidation of catechol-amines, hemoglobin, and thiols [22,23]. By-products of lipid peroxidation accumulate under conditions of both and low and high oxygen consumption. Alessio, Goldfarb and Cutler [24] reported increased lipid peroxidation following both aerobic and nonaerobic exercise in rats. One minute of high-intensity running (45 m·min^{-1}) resulted in 167 and 157% elevated TBARS in red slow-twitch and white fast-twitch muscle, respectively and in 34 and 31% elevated LH in red slow-twitch and white fast-twitch muscle, respectively. Since the high-intensity running only lasted for 1 min, it is likely that increased oxygen consumption may not be the exclusive rate limiting factor for lipid peroxidation. A pilot study by Alessio, Fulkerson and Wiley, [25] lends support to this suggestion. In this study, blood levels of prooxidant and antioxidant biomarkers were compared in six volunteers who exercised to exhaustion on a treadmill and a week later, exercised to exhaustion by squeezing a hand grip dynamometer at 50% of 1 repetition max (RM) at 45 s on/off intervals for the same amount of treadmill exercise time. Results showed that aerobic exercise resulted in a 14-fold increase in VO_2 compared to a 2-fold increase in VO_2 with isometric exercise (Fig. 3). MDA increased 5.6% above rest following aerobic exercise compared to 25.4% ($p < 0.05$) for isometric. An antioxidant biomarker, oxygen radical absorbance capacity (ORAC), increased 52.6% ($p < 0.05$) pre- to postaerobic exercise compared to 23.3% pre- to post-isometric (Fig. 4). Antioxidant activation indirectly suggests that pro-oxidant forces are increased. So, biomarkers of oxidative stress were observed following exhaustive bouts of both aerobic and nonaerobic exercise, and isometric exercise showed more oxidative stress than aerobic exercise.

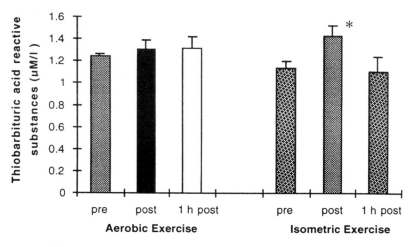

Fig. 3. Thiobarbituric acid reactive substances before and after aerobic and isometric exercise.

A study by Ortenblad, Madsen and Djurhuus [26] supported some but not all of the results from Alessio, Fulkerson and Wiley [25]. In their study, subjects performed six bouts of 30 s strenuous jumping with 2-min rest in between bouts. Lipid peroxidation did not increase significantly, however, the increase of several key antioxidants (e.g., superoxide dismutase, glutathione peroxidase, and glutathione reductase) did reach significance. Higher antioxidant activity may have been partly responsible for attenuating lipid peroxidation by-products.

Mechanical stress has been proposed to explain why exercise can damage muscle fibers. In particular, eccentric exercise, where the muscle generates high levels of force while lengthening, has been shown to initiate cytokine activity which regulates inflammation. Lipid peroxidation by-products, including cyclo-oxygenase- and lipid peroxidation-derived products, are potent vasoactive and chemoattractant factors [27]. It is likely that lipid peroxidation reactions may play a mediating role in inflammation. Yet, not all studies have reported that lipid

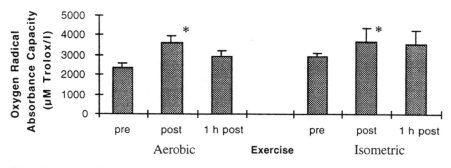

Fig. 4. Oxygen radical absorbance capacity for peroxyl radicals before and after aerobic and isometric exercise.

peroxidation indices increase following either eccentric or concentric strength exercise. In a study by Saxton, Donnelly and Roper [28], both eccentric and concentric arm and leg exercise were performed and muscle soreness peaked 2 days after eccentric exercise. Protein carbonyl derivatives and serum creatine kinase activity, but not TBARS, increased immediately following concentric leg exercise in this study. Creatine kinase is a marker for tissue damage. So, in this case, protein but not lipid oxidation was associated with muscle damage following intense mechanical exercise stress.

2.1.4 Antioxidant supplementation

When challenged with the extreme aerobic and mechanical stress of a marathon or other long-distance race, some studies have reported increased oxidative stress biomarkers and others have not. Hartman et al. [29] reported that urinary excretion of the oxidized base, 8-hydroxy-2′deoxyguanosine did not change during 5 consecutive days following a short distance (average time 2.5 h) triathlon. All six subjects had trained between 1 and 7 years and took antioxidants except for 1 week before and after the test. Rokitzki et al. [3] suggested that part of the explanation for the discrepancy of previous results may be that some athletes supplemented with antioxidants and some did not. They controlled for supplementation by dividing 24 long-distance runners into a placebo group and a group that supplemented with α-tocopherol (400 IU·day^{-1}) and ascorbic acid (200 mg·day^{-1}) for 4.5 weeks prior to a marathon race. Following the marathon race, MDA increased in both groups, but the antioxidant supplement group showed higher levels of select antioxidants as well as a much smaller change in serum creatine kinase compared to the placebo group. It appeared that antioxidant supplementation protected body tissues from oxidative and mechanical stress during the marathon race. So, exhaustive aerobic exercise, in this case, resulted in oxidative stress, but both regular exercise training and antioxidant supplementation combined to reduce the extent of the oxidative stress.

Kosugi et al. [30] measured TBARS in urinary samples following different types of stresses. Daily levels of TBARS varied over a 1.53 fold range under normal lifestyle conditions, with higher levels reported in the afternoon and evening compared to the morning. The daily level of TBARS was increased 3-fold by remaining awake all night compared to 7-fold following exhaustive exercise.

One explanation for the regulation of oxidative stress by factors other than VO$_2$ alteration is the spontaneous oxidation of epinephrine when exposed to oxygen (Fig. 5). When this happens, epinephrine may lose a hydrogen atom as well as an electron, leaving the phenolic as a radical. The electrons involved are the ones in the phenolic OH groups. The hydrogen and its associated electron is easily lost and the compound which picks up the hydrogen and electron is reduced. When the second H (and electron) is removed, a quinone is produced. Another possibility is for only loss of just one hydrogen (and one electron), forming a ROO• radical and leaving the phenolic as a radical cation, which then

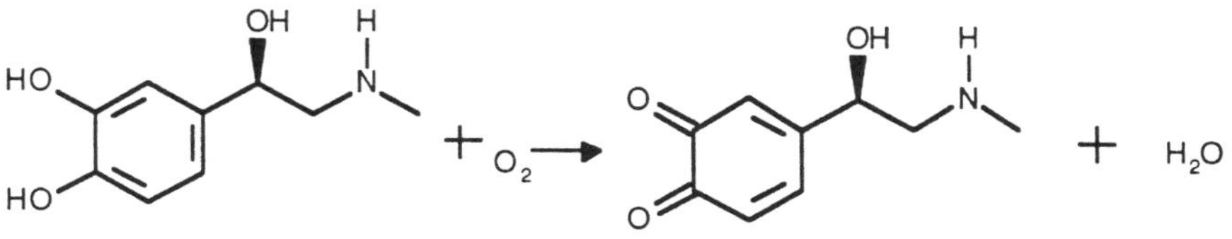

Fig. 5. Oxygen is reduced by gaining electrons from oxidized epinephrine.

may then give up H^+ to become a phenolic radical. It is agreeable but not essential for the phenolic radical to lose another H and electron and become the quinone. Regardless of the way that electrons from epinephrine are released, once the oxidized epinephrine forms, it would be able to oxidize other substrates, including lipids, and be reduced back to epinephrine. This scenario and some evidence suggest that influences other than large metabolic shifts can contribute to lipid peroxidation and oxidative stress (e.g., provocations that trigger catecholamine response). Training tends to lower circulating levels of epinephrine at rest and submaximal exercise [31,32]. It is possible that lower blood levels of epinephrine reduce the chances of epinephrine becoming oxidized, so that autooxidation reactions, including lipid peroxidation, are reduced. In contrast, higher levels of circulating epinephrine, whether due to increased adrenal secretion or the pooling of epinephrine as a result of pharmaceutical blockade (e.g., β-blockers) at the cell membrane, are simply more vulnerable to oxidation. Superoxides produced from oxidized epinephrine can initiate and facilitate lipid peroxidation reactions. This idea has yet to be studied in a systematic way, but has many ramifications for the prophylactic recommendations of exercise in disease prevention, especially cardiovascular disease.

2.2 Diseased models

Despite the observations that exercise increases oxidative stress, voluntary physical exercise, performed on a regular basis, has the potential to positively influence the oxidative stress balance toward antioxidant protection rather than prooxidant assault. Table 1 summarizes some of the mechanisms by which regular exercise may reduce prooxidant activity or increase antioxidant defense. If research continues to support these effects, then exercise may be useful in reducing risk for and the treatment of certain diseases.

Table 1. Summary of regular aerobic exercise-induced effects on oxidative stress.

Effect	Significance
Oxidative capacity increases	Enhanced coupling in oxidative phosphorylation
Muscle mass increases	Muscle proteins increase cell membrane integrity
Immune function is enhanced	Increases efficiency of respiratory bursts, so less cell damage occurs
Antioxidants increase	Protects against production of free radicals; supplements

2.2.1 Cardiovascular disease

Cardiovascular disease (CVD) has been related to oxidative stress and, particularly, lipid peroxidation. A common index for risk of CVD is an above average level of low density lipoproteins (LDL). LDLs are more likely to be oxidized than high density lipoproteins (HDL) because of their size, large surface area, and high concentration of polyunsaturated fatty acids [33]. High-fat diets are often blamed for contributing to CVD. The reasons behind this connection may be due to either what fat does or does not do-in relation to oxidative stress. High fat diets do increase the amount of LDLs available and vulnerable to oxidation. High fat diets do not usually contain a significant amount of antioxidants to deter oxidation, and attenuate lipid peroxidation reactions.

Kujala et al. [34] compared LDL oxidation between endurance athletes and sedentary persons during a rested state. Athletes had lower plasma LDL cholesterol diene conjugation (an indicator of LDL oxidation) compared to the sedentary group. The authors reported a significant inverse relation between intensive physical exercise energy expenditure and LDL diene conjugation ($r = -0.41$, $p=0.021$), supporting their contention that regular exercise is associated with reduced oxidative stress. Sanchez-Quesada et al. [35] recently supported Kujala's observations reporting that LDL in aerobically trained persons were more resistant to oxidative modification compared to sedentary subjects. In this study, they measured conjugated diene formation as an index of LDL oxidation and reported a 12% lower susceptibility of LDL to oxidation in athletes compared to sedentary persons of similar age and body composition.

Lipid peroxidation depends in large part on the levels of lipid substrate. Chen, Hsu, and Lee [36] studied the effect of 10 mg·day^{-1} Pravastatin, a lipid lowering medication, on lipid, platelet activation, and lipid peroxidation markers in a group of hypercholesterolemic and a control group consisting of persons with average cholesterol levels. Persons with total cholesterol > 240 mg·dl^{-1} were considered to be hypercholesterolemic. They had higher levels of MDA, thromboxane $\beta2$ and β-thromboglobulin compared to the control group. Following approximately 10 min of graded treadmill exercise, platelet activation and lipid peroxidation increased in both groups, but returned to baseline more quickly in the control group. Exercise-induced changes in MDA, thromboxane $\beta2$ and β-thromboglobulin were more pronounced in the hypercholesterolemic group. Pravastatin attenuated the increase in MDA, β-thromboglobulin and prostanoids, but their platelet activation and lipid peroxidation markers were still higher than the control group.

2.2.2 Diabetes

In addition to CVD, LDLs appear to contribute, in part, to diabetes. Lipid peroxidation processes may be involved in adult-onset diabetes, where the *B*-cells are still viable, but blood glucose transport and regulation is compromised. Laaksonen et al. [37] compared lipid peroxidation in men with and without insulin dependent diabetes mellitus (IDDM). Resting plasma TBARS was more than twice as high in IDDM men compared to a matched control group of men without diabetes. In diabetic patients only, resting plasma TBARS was inversely correlated with VO_2max ($r = -0.82$, $p = 0.006$). Diabetic men with low cardiovascular capacity tended to have faster resting lipid peroxidation rates as indicated by higher TBARS. A 40-min submaximal exercise session where the men cycled at 60% of VO_2max resulted in a 50% increase in TBARS for both IDDM and non-IDDM men. Although TBARS increased at the same relative level, the non-IDDM men had an absolute TBARS level that was lower than the IDDM both at rest and after submaximal exercise. Possible explanations include: a) less superoxide radicals were produced in the non-IDDM group (despite exercise-induced VO_2 increases), b) less propagation of lipid peroxidation reactions (possibly due to activation of antioxidants which interfered with lipid peroxidation chain reactions), and c) less vulnerable fatty acids were available. Another possibility involves the type of LDLs, since small, dense LDL particles rather than large, buoyant LDLs, accumulate more often in diabetes, arthritis, and perhaps other types of coronary heart diseases [38].

3   SUMMARY

1. Free radicals and lipid peroxides play an important role in oxidative stress balance. Lipid peroxidation reactions involve free radical attack on polyunsaturated fatty acids and form lipid peroxides. Lipid peroxides usually decompose to form aldehydes (e.g., malonaldehyde) which can cross-link or change the structures of proteins, lipids, carbohydrates, and DNA.
2. Just as oxygen is both necessary and harmful to life, lipid peroxidation has been shown to be essential for normal cell development.
3. Most studies that have reported exercise-induced lipid peroxidation used healthy models who participated in aerobic exercise. Few studies have focused on nonaerobic types of exercise-and those that did also reported increased lipid peroxidation.
4. Studies that have investigated lipid peroxidation in diseased models (e.g., cardiovascular disease and diabetes), generally agree that healthy controls have lower lipid peroxidation levels compared to persons with disease.
5. Lipid peroxidation not driven by high levels of oxygen consumption may be driven by high levels of circulating epinephrine. Lower circulating epinephrine levels is associated with regular exercise training. Higher levels of epinephrine may contribute to lipid peroxidation and diseases, including cardiovascular disease and diabetes.

4   PERSPECTIVES

Research on lipid peroxidation in both healthy and diseased models will continue to shed light on several distinctive processes, namely aging versus disease, and favorable versus adverse responses to stress. Exercise is a good stress model because, in most cases, it can be performed by persons of all ages with different health status. Exercise-induced oxidative stress is often accompanied by lipid peroxidation, with more lipid peroxidation by-products accumulating in unhealthy compared to healthy models. The challenge for scientists and practitioners is to continue to understand the implications of lipid peroxidation for health and develop ways to interrupt or slow down lipid peroxidation. Implications of such developments may include remission or postponement of some diseases.

5   ACKNOWLEDGEMENTS

The author is grateful to Dr. Ron Cox and Dr. Ann Hagerman for their helpful comments and assistance.

6   ABBREVIATIONS

4-HNE:	4-hydroxyalkenals
CVD:	cardiovascular disease
HDL:	high density lipoproteins
$HO_2^\bullet$:	perhydroxyl radical
IDDM:	insulin dependent diabetes mellitus
LDL:	low density lipoproteins
LH:	lipid hydroperoxides
$LOO^\bullet$:	conjugated peroxyl radical
MDA:	malonaldeyhyde
$O_2^{\bullet-}$:	superoxide radical
$^\bullet OH$:	hydroxyl radical
TBARS:	thiobarbituric acid reactive substances
VO_2:	oxygen consumption

7   REFERENCES

1. Dekkers JC, van Doornen LJ, Kemper HC. Sports Med 1996;21:213—238.
2. Pyne DB. Austral J Sci Med Sport 1994;26:49—58.
3. Rokitzki L, Logemann E, Sagredos AN, Murphy M, Wetzel-Roth W, Keul J. Acta Physiol Scand 1994;151:149—158.
4. Trush MA, Kensler TW. Free Rad Biol Med 1991;10:201—209.
5. Shamburger RJ, Andreone TL, Willis CE. J Natl Cancer Inst 1974;53:1771—1773.
6. Basu AK, Marnett LJ. Carcinogenesis 1984;4:331—333.
7. Kikugawa, K. Adv Free Rad Biol Med 1986;2:389—417.
8. Esterbauer H. In: McBrien T, Slater D (eds) Free Radicals, Lipid Peroxidation, and Cancer.

London: Academic Press, 1982:101—128.
9. Viinikka L, Vuori L, Ylikorkala O. Med Sci Sports Exer 1984;16:275—277.
10. Frankel E. Chem Physics Lipids 1987;44:73—85.
11. Requena JR, FuMX, Ahmed MU, Jenkins AJ, Lyons TJ, Thorpe SR. Nephrology 1996;11(Suppl 5):48—53.
12. Sevanian A, Hochstein P. Ann Rev Nutr 1985;1985:365—390.
13. Inayama T, Kumagai, Y, Sakane M, Saito M, Matsuda M. Life Sci 1996;59:573—578.
14. Leeuwenburgh C, Ji LL. J Nutr 1996;126:1833—1843.
15. Davies KJA, Quintanilha AT, Brooks GA, Packer L. Biochem Biophysics Res Comm 1982,107: 1198—1205.
16. Alessio H, Goldfarb AH. J Appl Physiol 1988;64:1333—1336.
17. Jenkins RR, Frieland R, Howard H. Int J Sports Med 1984;5:11—14.
18. Halliwell B. Lancet 1994;344:721—724.
19. Radak Z, Asano K, Inoue M, Kizaki T, Oh-Ishi S, Suzuki K, Taniguchi N, Ohno O. Eur J Appl Physiol Occup Physiol 1996;72:189—194.
20. Raiguru SU, Yeargans GS, Seidler NW. Life Sci 1994;54:149—157.
21. Leibovitz BE, Siegal BV. J Gerontol 1980;35:45—56.
22. Fridovich I. Science 1978;201:875—880.
23. Cohen G and Heikkila RE. J Biol Chem 1974;249:2447—2452.
24. Alessio H, Goldfarb AH, Cutler RG. Am J Physiol 1988;255:C874—C877.
25. Alessio HM, Fulkerson BK, Wiley R. Med Sci Sport Exer 1998;30:(Under review).
26. Ortenblad N, Madsen K, Djurhuus MS. Am J Physiol 1997;272:R1258—1263.
27. Samuelsson B. Harvey Lect Series 1980;75:1—40.
28. Saxton JM, Donnelly AE, and Roper HP. Eur J Appl Physiol Occup Physiol 1994;68:189—193.
29. Hartmann A, Pfuhler S, Dennog C, Germadnik D, Pilger A, Speit G. Free Rad Biol Med 1998; 24:245—251.
30. Kosugi H, Enomoto H, Ishizuka Y, Kikugawa K. Biol Pharmac Bull 1994;17:1645—1650.
31. Cox RH, Hubbard JW, Lawler JE, Sanders BS, Mitchell VP. J Appl Physiol 1985;58: 1207—1214.
32. Greenen D, Buttrick P, Scheuer J. J Appl Physiol 1988;65:116—123.
33. Jacob RA, Burri BJ. Am J Clin Nutr 1996;63:985S—990S.
34. Kujala UM, Ahotupa M, Vasankari T, Kaprio J, Tikkanen MJ. Scand J Med Sci Sports 1996;6: 303—308.
35. Sanchez-Quesada JL, Ortega H, Payes-Romero A, Serrat-Serrat J, Gonzalez-Sastre F, Lasuncion MA, Ordonez-Llanos J. Atheroscl 1997;132:207—213.
36. Chen MF, Hsu HC, Lee YT. Prostaglandin 1994;48:157—174.
37. Laaksonen DE, Atalay M, Niskanen L, Uusitupa M, Hanninen O, Sen CK. Diab Care 1996;9: 569—574.
38. Slyper AH. JAMA 1994;272:305—308.

©2000 Elsevier Science B.V. All rights reserved.
Handbook of Oxidants and Antioxidants in Exercise.
C.K. Sen, L. Packer and O. Hänninen, editors.

Part III • Chapter 6

Metal binding agents: possible role in exercise

Robert R. Jenkins[1] and John Beard[2]

[1]*Biology Department, Ithaca College, 953 Danby Road, Ithaca, New York, NY 14850, USA*
[2]*Nutrition Department, The Pennsylvania State University, 125 S Henderson Bldg., University Park, PA 16802, USA*

1   INTRODUCTION
2   BASIC IRON CHEMISTRY
3   IRON TRANSPORT
    3.1   Nutritional influences
    3.2   Iron cycle
4   IRON TRANSPORT AND STORAGE
    4.1   Transferrin
    4.2   Ferritin
    4.3   Hemosiderin
    4.4   Regulation and uptake
5   LOW-MOLECULAR MASS IRON
    5.1   Utilization pool
6   IRON OVERLOAD
    6.1   Incidence of overload
    6.2   Ferritin as an indicator
    6.3   Iron and disease
    6.4   Epidemiological evidence
7   IRON LOADING MODELS
    7.1   Mongolian gerbil
    7.2   Carbonyl iron
    7.3   Transfusions
    7.4   Chelators
8   IRON AND RADICAL CHEMISTRY
    8.1   Fenton reaction
    8.2   Haber-Weiss reaction
9   IRON AND PHYSICAL ACTIVITY
    9.1   Nutrition, activity and anemia
    9.2   Iron deficiency and aerobic performance
    9.3   Exercise and iron mobilization
10   MUSCLE INTEGRITY
11   INFLUENCE OF pH
12   BLOOD IRON AND EXERCISE
13   HEMOGLOBIN AND MYOGLOBIN
14   SUMMARY
15   PERSPECTIVE
16   ABBREVIATIONS
17   REFERENCES

1   INTRODUCTION

The transition elements zinc (Zn), manganese (Mn), copper (Cu), and iron (Fe) are essential for the normal biochemistry of virtually all cells. This chapter will focus on the potential harmful consequences of transition elements. Iron will be singled out for attention since there is an abundant literature concerning that element's relationship to physical activity and to radical chemistry.

Transition elements must be very closely regulated. In general, they are not believed to exist in a free form in human plasma but may exist in low molecular weight complexes. Although such complexes are near or below detection limits May and Williams [1] used computer simulation modeling and estimated their approximate concentrations to be: 10^{-9} M for Zn, 10^{-12} M for Mn, 10^{-18} M for Cu, 10^{-23} M for Fe $^{3+}$ and 10^{-11} M for Fe $^{2+}$. Iron which is the second most abundant element in the earth's crust exhibits certain undesirable properties that impose rigid biochemical constraints. For instance, the tendency of Fe ions to hydrolyze, oxidize and polymerize into iron hydroxide reduces its bioavailability. The poor solubility of iron makes its transport outside of cells, through cells, and even within cells a considerable challenge. In addition, iron is potentially toxic if its redox activity is not strictly regulated. It is not surprising then that an elaborate biochemistry has evolved to regulate the availability of iron and to protect against its untoward effects. Iron and its potential for interaction with oxygen have imposed a considerable challenge to our most basic understanding of life function. The import of Fe-oxygen chemistry touches virtually every area of life science. For instance, evidence suggesting an early presence of an oxidizing atmosphere and the rich abundance of iron has resulted in the need to reassess standard models of molecular evolution that assumed the existence of a reducing atmosphere [2,3]. Iron has had a long history in medicinal biochemistry. It was used in China as a cure for anemia as long ago as 2735 B.C. [4]. The importance of iron as a prosthetic group for many enzymes and other proteins such as hemoglobin, myoglobin, hydroxylases, dioxygenases, reductases, and lyases is well known [5]. Most reviews related to trace elements and sports science or medicine have centered on nutritional adequacy and its influence on performance [6,7].

2   BASIC IRON CHEMISTRY

This section is meant to acquaint or reacquaint the reader with the rudiments of inorganic iron chemistry pertinent to physiological environments. Those requiring additional information should find the reviews by Spiro and Saltman [8] or by Hawker [9] helpful. Iron is a transition metal of the 3d series. It has an electron configuration 3d64s2 in the uncharged state. Although iron can occur in oxidation states ranging from II to VI its common oxidation states in biochemical systems are the ferrous [Fe(II)] and ferric [Fe(III)] forms [7]. The ferric form is the most stable oxidation state of iron but the Fe $^{2+}$ form oxidizes under aerobic conditions to Fe $^{3+}$ at a rate that depends on the pH, O_2 tension and ligands present. That reaction proceeds as in reaction [1] and results in the formation of the superoxide free radical.

$$Fe^{2+} \quad + \quad O_2 \quad \rightarrow \quad Fe^{3+} \quad + O_2^- \qquad (1)$$

Additionally, Fe (IV) occurs at active sites of peroxidases and many other heme proteins after reaction with H_2O_2 [10]. Iron has six orbitals which can form bonds along three axes. An octahedral geometry commonly results as bonds are formed along those axes. In aqueous solutions iron exists as the aquated ions Fe $(H_2O)_6^{2+}$ and Fe (H2O) $_6^{3+}$. The ferric cations abstract OH^-, forming H^+ as in reaction [2]. The reaction continues until the iron is converted to hydrated Fe $(OH)_3$ and the solution becomes quite acidic.

$$Fe (H_2O)_6^{3+} \quad \rightarrow \quad Fe (OH) (H_2O)_5^{2+} \quad + \quad H^+ \qquad (2)$$

The ionic states of transition metals are influenced by ligands and chelates. A ligand is a neutral molecule or ion having a lone electron pair that can be used to form a bond to a metal ion. Some ligands have more than one atom with a lone electron pair that can be used to bond a metal ion. Such ligands are said to be chelating ligands or chelates (from the Greek word chele for "claw"). Schubert [11] has provided an excellent outline of the chemistry of chelation as it applies to biochemical events and Halliwell [10] has recently reviewed the development and use of chelators in clinical chemistry.

The typical geometry of iron complexes will vary according to the oxidation states of iron. For instance Fe^{3+} bonds to reacting molecules with shorter bond distances than Fe^{2+}. The geometry will also be altered by the characteristics of any ligands present.

3 IRON TRANSPORT

3.1 Nutritional influences

Figure 1 illustrates the events related to absorption and metabolism of iron that have been quite well understood since the early work of Crosby [12]. Kushner [13] and Haymes and Lamanca [7] have provided reviews of factors influencing iron uptake. For instance, the average diet rich in animal protein will also be rich in heme and will provide about 17 mg of iron per day. The bioavailability of heme iron is greater than that of inorganic iron which is absorbed by a different pathway [14]. In addition, something in meat itself serves as a promoter of non-heme iron absorption thus increasing overall absorption more than expected. Diets abundant in plant protein will also be phytate and polyphenol rich. These chelators are potent inhibitors of iron absorption. By contrast, vitamin C increases absorption by converting the poorly absorbable Fe^{3+} to absorbable Fe^{2+} and also increasing solubility [15]. Iron absorption by the gastrointestinal

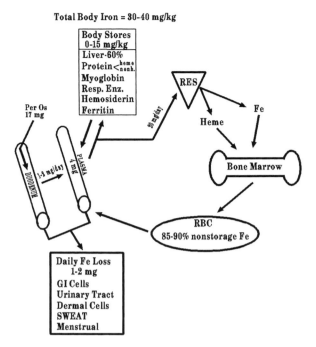

Fig. 1. Normal iron distribution and exchange pools. Fe, Iron; RBC, red blood cell, RES, reticulo-endothelial system; Resp. Enz., respiratory enzymes.

tract is not complete, and the amount absorbed depends not only on the constituents of the diet and the type of iron absorbed but also on the iron storage status of the body as well. The absolute mass of iron is important as well. An increased load of iron as in a supplement, may have limited bioavailability, but the total amount absorbed may be increased because of mass action. On average, about 10% of the nonheme iron consumed is transported out of the intestine to the blood where it is found attached to transferrin protein. Transferrin transports iron to cells for incorporation into various stores, enzymes etc. Approximately 80% of absorbed iron is directed to the bone marrow for new red cell production. Senescent erythrocytes are degraded by the reticuloendothelial system after about 120 days and the constituent heme iron is recycled to the erythropoietic tissue to be reincorporated into hemoglobin. The overall regulation normally balances a 1−2 mg/day iron loss with an equal intestinal uptake.

Supplement use provides the additional needed iron to some people who cannot derive appropriate amounts of iron from their diets. Pregnancy and early childhood are two such cases. In addition, strict vegetarians and certain individuals with compromised G.I. function may require supplements. Since these supplements usually enter the nonheme iron pool their absorption is regulated much the same as iron from grains, cereals, or nonmeat products.

3.2 Iron cycle

Although the exact mechanisms of iron uptake are still not well understood, several reviews have provided helpful insights to recent advances in iron metabolism [16—20]. As we trace the flow of iron through the iron cycle we will note how carefully it is maintained in proteins. In Fig. 2 we notice that at the acidic pH of the stomach iron combines with a variety of compounds including mucins and perhaps integrins. It now seems that iron crosses an intestinal membrane channel bound to mucin where at the neutral or slightly alkaline intracellular pH the iron is released to a protein known as mobilferrin [17]. It is then either temporarily stored in the protein ferritin or moved on to the blood. The amount of ferritin within the cell is proportional to the amount of iron previously in the cell. This proportionality is obtained by the regulation of the stability of the ferritin mRNA by an iron response element (IRE). The blood contains an iron binding protein known as apotransferrin which is called transferrin as iron accumulates within it. Virtually all plasma iron is bound to this glycoprotein with a $K_d = 10^{-22}$ M. Under normal conditions it is believed that transferrin is in excess relative to

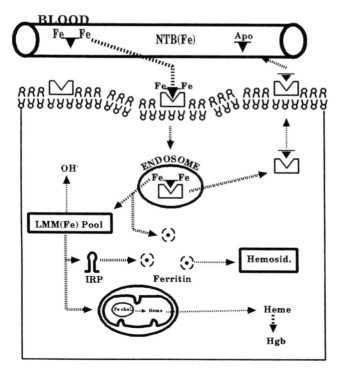

Fig. 2. Iron transport and cellular uptake. (▼), apotransferrin; NTB, nontransferrin bound iron; LMM (Fe), low-molecular mass iron; Fe ch., iron chelates; IRP, iron responsive protein; Hemosid., hemosiderin; Hgb, hemoglobin.

iron and this binding capacity is referred to as the UIBC (unbound iron binding capacity). For that reason there appears to be no significant amount of iron complexed to low molecular mass molecules in blood plasma [21–23].

Winzerling and Law [24] have recently pointed out the importance of copper in the mechanisms related to iron absorption. As early as 1927 Waddell and colleagues [25] showed that the administration of iron salts alone failed to reduce anemia in pigs. However, if iron salts were combined with ashed food low hemoglobin levels were corrected. The active ingredient of the ashed food turned out to be a copper ion [26] which is now generally considered to be provided by ceruloplasmin [27]. It has also been shown that iron is taken up into mucosal cells but is not cleared to the blood in copper-deficient animals [28]. This suggested that copper-mediated reduction of iron was necessary for the binding of iron to transferrin.

4   TRANSPORT AND STORAGE

4.1 Transferrin

The iron uptake of most mammalian cells occurs by way of a transferrin receptor in most cells. The importance of this receptor in the regulation of the flow of iron into cells has been the subject of several recent reviews [16,29]. Since it has been shown that iron is rapidly removed from the circulation while the transferrin protein recycles, the concept of a transferrin-cell cycle has been suggested. According to this notion the protein apotransferrin travels in search of iron, binds the iron, transports iron in the plasma pool, and then attaches it to the transferrin receptor. The receptor-Fe complexes are then believed to move into the cell by endocytosis where iron is released to a poorly defined LMW (low molecular weight) iron pool. The LMW iron can go to ferritin for storage, to the mitochondrion for heme synthesis or to other Fe-requiring subcellular compartments. Ferritin is found in all tissues but primarily in liver, spleen and bone marrow, and about 25% of the total body iron is contained in this protein. Apotransferrin is then released to the plasma for another cycle. This is illustrated in Fig. 3.

4.2 Ferritin

On the average tissue ferritin is normally only about 20% saturated with iron. The iron within ferritin exists as a hydrous ferric oxide core which is capable of containing as many as 4,500 atoms Fe/molecule [30]. Each ferritin molecule is composed of 24 subunits designated as either H or L depending on their molecular weight. The distribution of H or L predominant subunits varies by tissue and stage of development and possible also by iron status. Mobilization of iron from ferritin for intracellular transport requires conversion from the ferric to ferrous form [31]. A membrane ferrireductase performs that reduction [32]. Once inside the cell, a multi copper oxidase is believed to be responsible for the reoxidation

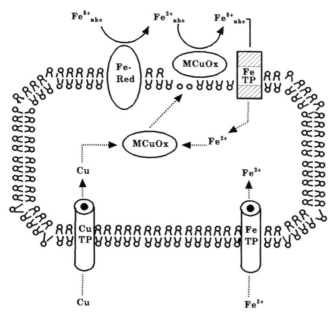

Fig. 3. Putative linkage between copper and iron uptake. Fe-Red, ferrireductase; McuOxy multi-copper oxidase; nhe; nonheme iron; FeTP, iron transport protein; Cu TP, copper transport protein.

of Fe(II) back to Fe(III) which is then stored [33]. This explains, at least in part, the obligatory role of copper in iron metabolism. The amount of ferritin detected in the plasma is proportional to the amount of storage iron in ferritin.

4.3 Hemosiderin

Hemosiderin is a water-insoluble iron storage protein believed to be formed by lysosomal attack and/or free radical damage to ferritin. It is the predominant Fe-storage protein in Fe-overloaded patients and tissue damage is correlated with increased deposition of this protein [34]. O'Connell et al. [35] have suggested that it is a safer form of iron than ferritin because iron is less easily mobilisable from it.

4.4 Regulation of uptake

Klausner et al. [18] reviewed the recent work related to the control of cellular iron metabolism. They point out that iron taken up by cells can be divided into three pools including what they call the utilization pool, the sequestration/ storage pool and the regulatory pool. The amount of iron flowing to the various pools seems to related to the overall metabolic requirements and the amount of iron available. The regulatory pool involves compounds that have been called the Fe-responsive element-binding proteins (IRE-BP$_1$ + IRE-BP$_2$). According to Cook et al. [16] iron homeostasis can be envisaged as a posttranscriptional regulatory circuit that controls the level of expression of the transferrin receptor and ferritin. The IRE-BPs bind to IREs on the 3' or 5' ends of the mRNAs for the TFR and ferritin. Thus the amount of iron received by the cell is controlled by the number of receptors available and the potential for iron sequestration is determined by ferritin availability. When cellular iron levels are decreased the IRE-BPs bind to the IREs which results in decreased ferritin mRNA translation and increased stability of the transferrin receptor mRNA. The result is increased capacity for acquisition of iron. Klausner et al. [18] emphasized the importance of a new view of the Fe-sulfur clusters. They have reviewed the evidence indicating that the Fe-sulphur clusters of aconitase and similar enzymes are able to switch between the enzymatic form and an RNA-binding form. That ability to switch seems to be related to the presence or absence of the fourth iron. In an iron replete state the protein is cytoplasmic aconitase; while in the cellular iron depletion state the 3-Fe-4S complex is an IRE-BP$_1$. The authors point out that the 100 plus proteins containing Fe-sulfur clusters must now be considered to function as potentially important gene regulatory systems in addition to their well-defined role in enzymes.

5   LOW MOLECULAR MASS IRON

A variety of terms such as "free", "labile", "low molecular weight" and "chelated" have been applied to what Klausner [18] called the utilization pool. There are conceptual problems associated with each of those terms. For instance Halliwell and Gutteridge [36] have pointed out that 'iron salts will never exist "free" in biological systems'. Iron will be bound to something such as inorganic phosphate, phosphate esters, proteins, membrane lipids or organic acids such as citrate. We will refer to this pool as the low molecular mass iron pool (LM-Fe). The binding of iron by various ligands may alter its ability to participate in radical chemistry by keeping iron in solution, altering its redox chemistry to favor or disfavor reduction by superoxide or reaction with H_2O_2, and/or by directing any reactive radicals produced onto the ligand itself, thus protecting other potential targets of damage [10].

5.1 Utilization pool

The proposition that a utilization pool exists has emerged from a variety of lines of reasoning. Various investigators point out that determination of tissue iron by analysis of hemoproteins, ferritin, hemosiderin, Fe-sulfur proteins etc. fails to account for all iron. Jacobs [37] was among the first to show that there appears to be an intracellular transit pool of iron. By the 1970s he and his colleagues provided evidence for LM-Fe in a variety of cells including reticuloendothelial, polymorphonuclear leukocytes, small intestinal epithelial cells and cultured liver cells.

White et al. [38] estimated the cytosol iron in liver cells by atomic absorption spectrometry to be in the order of 20 fg/cell. Other workers such as Mulligan et al. [39] reported that liver, kidney, heart and spleen contain LM-Fe ranging from 3–8 mg/g, whereas brain tissue contains about 20 µg/g LM-Fe. Additionally, many investigators employ in their studies an exogenous iron chelator known as deferoxamine. Iron chelation by deferoxamine has been shown to influence such diverse biochemical processes as DNA synthesis [40], activity of various hydroxylase enzymes [41], 6-phosphogluconate dehydrogenase [42], and skeletal muscle α-glycerophosphate dehydrogenase [43]. It has been argued that LM-Fe may result as an artifact of tissue homogenization. However, Kozlov et al. [44] recently provided direct electron paramagnetic resonance spectroscopy evidence for LM-Fe in liver tissue. Furthermore, they demonstrated that this iron would complex with nitric oxide. This is of interest since it is now known that nitric oxide is synthesized by a variety of tissues and appears to influence iron in a variety of ways that might relate to free radical events. This topic has recently been reviewed by Reif [45]. A variety of sources of LM-Fe exist. O'Connell [46] showed that iron capable of stimulating lipid peroxidation was released from ferritin at physiological pH when ascorbate was added. Iron overloaded hemochromatosis subjects have an appreciable amount of plasma iron bound to citrate [22] in a form capable of inducing both single and double strand breaks in DNA [47]. Reif [45] pointed out that the rapid release of iron from ferritin requires reduction of the iron core. He recently reviewed the evidence demonstrating that the superoxide anion (O_2^{-}) is capable of mobilizing ferritin iron in a form capable of initiating oxidative damage. The superoxide could be formed enzymatically, radiolytically or by metal-catalyzed oxidation. The importance of this source of iron is unsettled. For instance, the amount of O_2^{-} mobilisable iron in ferritin is very small, amounting to less than 1% of the total iron present [48]. Superoxide cannot mobilize iron from hemosiderin [49]. While Flint et al. [50] showed that O_2^{-} can release iron from Fe-S clusters in *Escherichia coli*, it is not yet clear whether this happens in mammalian cells. In in vitro experiments, iron can be mobilized from ferritin either by direct chelation of Fe^{3+} or by reduction of Fe^{3+} to Fe^{2+}. Direct chelation by biological chelators is slow in comparison with release by reducing agents. Ferritin iron release is facilitated most efficiently by reductive processes. Various agents have been shown to be effective in reducing ferritin. These include adrenaline [51], thiols [52], ascorbate [53], xanthine [55], xanthine oxidase [54], NADH and NADPH [55].

6 IRON OVERLOAD

6.1 Incidence of overload

During negative iron balance, storage iron is gradually depleted and ferritin and hemosiderin iron deposits disappear. Once these stores are close to zero, iron balance is directly dependent on absorbed dietary or supplemental iron. Iron depletion up to the end stage, anemia, is without severe consequences. The incidence of iron deficiency anemia in countries that have eliminated parasitic infestations is very low in most parts of the population. For instance, in the USA the rates of iron deficiency anemia range from 1—3% for men, premenopausal women, and postmenopausal women [56]. Approximately 2 or 3 times that number may be considered iron depleted. Despite this fact, there has been a general tendency for the medical community to focus on iron status solely as a deficiency disorder.

6.2 Ferritin as an indicator

Herbert [57] recently reviewed the topic of iron disorders. He points out the usefulness of following serum ferritin as an indicator of iron balance. Normal serum ferritin values range from 12 to 325 ng/ml with a mean of about 125 ng for adult men and 55 ng for women [58]. Ferritin values less than 10 ng/ml are considered Fe-deficient. Iron deficiency anemia is usually designated by low serum ferritin and hemoglobin less than 13 g/dl. A new perspective relative to iron is beginning to emerge. For instance Edwards and colleagues [59] reported that it is likely that twice as many American men have hemochromatosis, an inherited tendency for iron loading (1 in 250) as have clinically significant iron deficiency (1 in 500). There have been many excellent reviews in recent years related to iron loading disorders [60—62]. Warnings that nonjudicious use of iron supplements may do more harm than good are beginning to appear.

6.3 Iron and disease

Iron is implicated in a variety of problems. Salonen et al. [63] found that men with serum ferritin concentrations of 200 µg/l or more had a 2.2 fold increased risk for myocardial infarction than did men with lower serum ferritin levels. High serum ferritin was second only to cigarette smoking as a predictor of heart disease. For every 1% increase in serum ferritin the incidence of heart attack rose 4%. This epidemiologic evidence has not been easily reproduced in the United States. Investigations utilizing data from the Framingham, NHANGS I, and NHANGS II studies have found little correlation between iron status, iron intake, or heme iron intake and CVD. However, Fe-overloaded patients often suffer cardiac malfunction, and this is a common cause of death in thalassemics [61,62]. Although gender difference is a major risk factor for heart disease it is usually ignored since it is assumed to be unmodifiable. Cook et al. [56] reported that in the USA, tissue iron increases throughout life in males. In females there is a gradual increase in iron stores to the time of menopause and then a substantial increase occurs as iron balance becomes much more positive. For instance, if we use the standard conversion factor of 1 µg ferritin/l = 8 mg of storage iron than males mean storage iron would range from about 350 mg at age 20 to about 1.2 g at age 80. Females mean storage iron on the other hand rises from 170 mg at 20 years to only about 320 mg by age 50. However, by age 60, females mean storage values rise to over 600 mg and to between 700—800 mg at age 80. At the time of the postmenopausal rise in iron the females susceptibility to heart disease also increases. There is a significant rise in other risk factors associated with heart disease (body weight, hyperlipidemia, diabetes, etc.) At this time as well suggesting a synergistic relationship. However, if tissue stores of iron are implicated in heart disease, blood donation 3 times a year could lower the serum ferritin of a male to that of a young woman and perhaps reduce the risk of heart disease [15]. Dietary changes in males to decrease iron intake would also reduce this accumulation.

Epidemiological studies by Selby and Friedman [64] and Stevens et al. [65] provide data consistent with the hypothesis that large tissue iron stores may be a risk factor for cancer. The levels of LM-Fe in synovial fluid was shown to correlate with disease severity in rheumatoid arthritis patients [66]. The severity of ocular inflammation and tissue damage was shown to be reduced by the iron chelator desferoxamine mesylate suggesting the inflammatory reaction was Fe-catalyzed [67]. We found there was an increased level of LM-Fe in neonatal hearts, associated with a reduced ability of the tissues to defend against hydroperoxide induced oxidative stress [68]. Sullivan [69] suggested that what are now considered "normal" levels for serum ferritin actually may be a strong risk factor for certain diseases. Desirable iron status may need to be redefined if these hypothesis are proven correct. Decreased iron stores without anemia may eventually become regarded as optimal for long-term health. How we achieve this without significant risk to the vulnerable parts of the population is a tremendous public health question.

7 IRON LOADING MODELS

7.1 Mongolian gerbil

Although iron uptake is normally tightly coupled to its removal from the body, the growing awareness of iron loading disorders and the relative refractoriness of such conditions to treatment has stimulated interest in understanding animal models that exhibit loading. Attempts for many years using iron doses orders-of-magnitude beyond that consumed by humans fail to replicate the pathology of human hereditary hemochromatosis. The Mongolian gerbil appears to be the only animal that responds to prolonged iron overload in a manner common to that of iron overloaded humans [70]. For instance, overloaded gerbils typically develop both hepatic and cardiac fibrosis.

7.2 Carbonyl iron

The inclusion of dietary carbonyl iron results in hepatic but not cardiofibrosis in rats [71]. Recent studies employing various iron compounds to induce loading in rats reveal a broader panorama of involvement including alteration of intestinal growth and morphology [72], pancreatic mitochondria damage [73] and skeletal muscle protein degradation [74].

7.3 Transfusions

A number of hemolytic anemias result in the accumulation of iron in the Fe-recycling system involving RE cells of the spleen and liver. Periodic transfusions are employed in animals to study the deranged iron metabolism that commonly results from thalassemia [75]. Erythrocytes are catabolized by reticuloendothelial cells and a significant proportion of the iron released is found within those cells in low molecular weight complexes [76]. Increased transfusions only worsen the situation as these RBCs also have a decreased lifespan and thus contribute to the RE cell accumulation of iron. A nonprotein bound iron detectable in thalassemia has been implicated in the organ toxicity related to this disorder [77].

7.4 Chelators

A third alternative to the study of iron involves the addition of a variety of chelators. The preponderance of work with these compounds was motivated by the desire to provide an clinical alternative to desferrioxamine. Zanninelli et al. [78] recently reviewed the chemical characteristics of the commonly employed chelators. They vary greatly in their hydrophobicity and lipid solubility. Chelators could be applied to exercise related studies to determine whether an experimental condition might increase the availability of loosely bound iron. However, the interpretation of results from chelator studies must be approached with caution since under certain circumstances chelators actually serve as a source of iron capable of inducing radical reactions [79,80].

Unfortunately, to date, there has been little interest in employing these various models in the study of the impact of exercise upon iron metabolism.

8   IRON AND RADICAL CHEMISTRY

8.1 Fenton reaction

Although a minute amount of iron must be kept available in the intracellular pool as a source for obligatory cell requirements, excessive amounts must be avoided. Excess iron triggers deleterious reactions such as protein and nucleic acid degradation, and peroxidative decomposition of polyunsaturated fatty acids. A growing number of workers in the field of free radical chemistry consider that transition metals play a major role in generating deleterious free radicals [81–85]. But what is the mechanism of such potentially harmful chemistry? Fenton [86] was the first to provide evidence that a transition metal in combination with H_2O_2 could serve as an effective oxidant of organic substances. Koppenol [87] provided an extensive review of Fenton's work [87]. The mixture of hydrogen peroxide and ferrous salts is known as the "Fenton reagent". The reaction is usually characterized as in reaction [3] shown below, where -L represents ligand(s) and the highly reactive hydroxyl radical results.

$$H_2O_2 \quad + \quad Fe_2{+}\text{-}L \quad \rightarrow \quad HO\bullet \quad + \quad OH^- \quad + \quad Fe^{3+}\text{-}L \qquad (3)$$

8.2 Haber-Weiss reaction

Although the term "Fenton reagent" is generally used to apply to a mixture of H_2O_2 and ferrous salts, other metal ions in their lower oxidation states react in a similar manner and are referred to as "Fenton-like" reagents [88]. In 1934 Haber and Weiss [89] proposed reaction [4]. What is generally known as the Haber-Weiss reaction may also be considered a superoxide driven Fenton reaction.

$$H_2O_2 \quad + \quad O_2^- \quad \rightarrow \quad O_2 \quad + \quad OH\bullet \quad + \quad OH^- \qquad (4)$$

It was subsequently shown that the original Haber-Weiss reaction was not likely to occur in vivo. However, if transition metals such as iron or copper are available then the hydroxyl radical may be formed. This has become known as the Fe-catalyzed Haber-Weiss reaction which is shown in reaction [5,36].

$$O_2^- \quad + \quad H_2O_2 - Fe \text{ catalyst} \quad \rightarrow \quad O_2 + OH\bullet + OH^- + Fe^{3+} \quad (5)$$

Ryan and Aust [82] recently reviewed published work and discuss the important role of iron in determining rates of lipid peroxidation. They argue that the simultaneous presence of Fe^{2+} and Fe^{3+} in a ratio of approximately 1 is the essential factor rather than the rate of formation of oxygen radicals. While in general, data seem to support that notion, it has not held for all experimental situations [90]. A number of workers in this area [36,82] point out that reactive species in addition to $OH\bullet$ may be generated from the interaction of iron chelates with H_2O_2. However, there is no clear evidence for the importance of these other species at physiological pH [91]. Tissue damage and destruction appear to lead to the release of iron ions and haem proteins in forms that can catalyze free radical damage [92].

It should be pointed out that transition metals are especially toxic to the nervous system, liver and kidney [93]. While the reason for the difference in susceptibility to oxidative stress is unclear, the mechanism involving transition metal induction seems consistent.

The influence of iron and copper in the involvement of DNA damage has received considerable attention recently [94,95]. Iron [96], ferritin [97], and iron-sulfur clusters [98] are present in the nucleus in certain circumstances. There is evidence that a metallothionein may serve to protect the nuclear environment against iron driven radical chemistry [99].

Cabanatchik and colleagues [100] recently developed a fluorescence assay which should provide an important tool for measuring chelated intracellular iron. The technique has been applied successfully to the study of the labile (low molecular) iron pool of the cell [101].

9   IRON AND PHYSICAL ACTIVITY

9.1 Nutrition, sport and anemia

It is not difficult to understand the preoccupation of sports medicine investigators with iron deficiency since it is the most common single nutrient deficiency for about 15% of the world's population [102]. In developing countries, successful pregnancy outcomes and infant growth are highly dependent on nutrition interventions. In more developed countries, people make food choices for other reasons. The decision by many athletes to reduce food quantity and to reduce meat consumption might reasonably be expected to result in a marginal provision of iron. [103,104]. However, there is now an increasing amount of evidence indicating that the typical emphasis on correcting any appearance of low iron levels in athletes may be misdirected. For instance the body exerts a homeostatic adaptation to the stimulus of low iron stores by increasing iron absorption [105]. While habitual runners may be at an increased risk for iron deficiency, full-blown anemia is rare [106] and should be diagnosed carefully by assessing serum ferritin and hemoglobin markers. The relationship between these two markers in the clinical stages of iron-deficiency states are illustrated in Table 1. Although serum

Table 1. States iron-deficiency

Stage	Indicator = Low serum ferritin and:	Cutoff values
I. Storage Fe depletion	Normal total Fe binding capacity	$250-500$ µg/dl
	Normal percent transferrin saturation	$> 15\%$
	Normal serum iron concentration	> 80 µg/dl
	Normal hemoglobin	> 12 g/dl
II. Fe deficient erythropoiesis	Increased total Fe binding capacity	$350-650$ µg/dl
	Decreased percent transferrin saturation	$< 15\%$
	Normal hemoglobin	> 12 g/dl
	Or Decreased serum Fe concentration	$< 60-80$ µg/dl
	Normal hemoglobin	> 12 g/dl
III. Iron deficiency anemia	Increased total Fe binding capacity	$350-650$ µg/dl
	Decreased percent transferrin saturation	$< 15\%$
	Decreased serum iron concentration	< 60 µg/dl
	Low hemoglobin	< 12 g/dl

Adapted from [111].

ferritin alone is generally considered the most sensitive and specific marker of iron deficiency [107] it must be kept in mind that serum ferritin values ranging from 12 to 135 ng/ml are considered normal [108]). While athletes and investigators studying athletes generally resort to iron tablets it should be pointed out that simple dietary changes are typically sufficient to maintain ferritin levels during moderate exercise [109] and as little as 39 mg of elemental iron or 125 mg of ferrous sulfate sufficed to maintain ferritin in competitive swimmers [110].

9.2 Iron deficiency and aerobic performance

It is possible to increase VO_2 max and treadmill running endurance in Fe-deficient rats through a mild running protocol [112]. Those beneficial effects occurred despite the fact that iron dependent enzyme pathways were unchanged in skeletal muscle. Celsing and co-workers [113] arrived at a similar conclusion in a study involving humans. They artificially induced iron deficiency by a combination of repeated venesections and a low iron content diet. After 9 weeks the subjects were clinically iron deficient with serum-iron of 4.3 $\mu mol.l^{-1}$, serum-ferritin of 7.3 $\mu g.l^{-1}$, per cent saturation of 7.1, and hemoglobin of 11 g/dl. The subject's hemoglobin values were restored to control level by transfusion and aerobic endurance capacity was tested within 24 h. Neither the iron dependent enzyme cytochrome c oxidase nor the activities of marker enzymes for the glycolytic and citric acid routes, nor endurance capacity were reduced by this procedure. Rector et al. [114] studied polycythemia vera subjects who had been rendered iron deficient by venesection therapy. They found no deficit in work performance. LaManca and Haymes [115] supplemented anemic female subjects (plasma ferritin < 20 μg l^{-1}) and significantly increased plasma ferritin and hemoglobin. The endurance times of the subjects were not improved. Garza et al. [111] recently reviewed 33 studies involving subjects described as iron deficient. They noted that while iron supplementation increased serum ferritin levels, there was no improvement in performance unless the ferritin increase was accompanied by increased hemoglobin concentration. Such observations support the contentions of Gutteridge et al. [116] and Evans and Cannon [117] that physical training associated reductions in hematocrit, hemoglobin concentration, and plasma iron that have been labeled "runners anemia" may actually be an adaptive mechanism to reduce "oxidative stress". Alternatively, the reduction in plasma iron and subsequent reductions in hemoglobin and hematocrit could result from the immune systems response to exercise [117].

9.3 Exercise and iron mobilization

It appears that exercise does influence tissue chemistry in such a way as to increase the availability of Fe for participation in peroxidative damage. For instance, Serbinova et al. [118] compared the effects of iron loading and loading combined with additional oxidative stressors. They found that loading signifi-

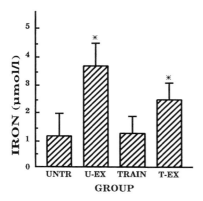

Fig. 4. Influence of exercise on iron tissue iron. Data are means ± SD of low-molecular mass iron in gastrocnemius muscle of UNTR, untrained and TRAIN, trained rats prior to and subsequent to a 2-h exhaustive treadmill run. U-EX, untrained exhausted; T-EX trained exhausted. *p < 0.05 (from [80]).

cantly increased liver lipid peroxidation products, and decreased liver vitamin E and cytochrome P-450 (a family of liver enzymes involved in the detoxification of xenobiotics). Furthermore, they found that these changes were potentiated by exposure to hyperoxia or exercise. Recently we have shown that exhaustive exercise resulted in a significant increase of LM-Fe in the gastrocnemius of rats. The rise in this form of tissue iron occurred both in trained and untrained animals and was associated with significantly elevated peroxidation products as measured by the thiobarbituric acid method [119]. These data are shown in Figs. 4 and 5. This supports the contention of Halliwell [120] that iron mobilization can occur as result of tissue injury and then create oxidative stress.

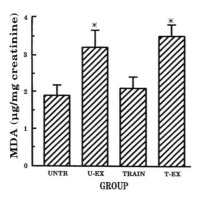

Fig. 5. Influence of exercise on urinary malondialdehyde. Data are means ± SD of UNTR, untrained and TRAIN, trained rats prior to and subsequent to a 2-h exhaustive treadmill run. U-EX, untrained exhausted; T-EX trained exhausted. *p < 0.05 (from [80]).

10 MUSCLE INTEGRITY

The integrity of muscle may be compromised both by activity and inactivity. Factors related to disruption of muscle integrity may induce oxidative stress. For instance Kondo and co-workers [121] studied the influence of disuse atrophy on trace elements in rat soleus muscles. They found that whole muscle iron was increased. The subcellular distribution was also altered with the microsomal fraction showing the largest change. The appearance of increased lipid peroxidation and glutathione disulfide provided evidence that oxidative stress may play a role in the events leading to atrophy. That conclusion was strengthened by their finding that vitamin E decreased the rate of atrophy. They also noted an increased tissue calcium level which may have initiated the atrophy process. Recently, Byrd [122] reviewed the role of calcium overload in exercise-induced muscle injury. In that review changes in muscle pH, high energy phosphates, ionic balance and temperature were all offered as possible exercise related factors that might hinder sarcoplasmic reticular regulation of calcium. This might activate proteases and phospholipases that degrade membranes and proteins. It is possible that such degradation could, in turn, result in an increased presence of LW-Fe. Furthermore, a clear link between cell injury by oxidative stress and by excess Ca^{2+} was demonstrated by Orrenius and coworkers [123,124] demonstrated that iron loading altered membrane integrity of heart cell cultures. They noted changes in the cell's electrophysiological behavior and contractility as well as a significant release of lactate dehydrogenase. Kanner et al. [125] studied oxidative stress in muscle stimulated by a redox cycle system. They concluded that iron-ascorbate initiated peroxidation in muscle membranes resulted from a site-specific attack by OH• on unsaturated fatty acid double bonds. They contend that OH• formed exogenous to membranes is not able to initiate peroxidation. Instead they suggest that normally stable, nontoxic compounds such as ascorbic acid, thiols or what they called "free iron" are more likely to be involved in the initiation. They reasoned that such stable compounds could diffuse in to the membrane and be converted to highly active compounds in site-specific reactions near unsaturated fatty acids. The lysosomal enzyme marker N-acetyl-b-glucosaminidase and the urinary marker of protein degradation, 3-methylhistidine both were shown to increase after rats were run downhill for 200 min [126]. It is possible that proteins other than structural proteins such as the iron containing proteins are also attacked and may provide a source of LM-Fe.

11 INFLUENCE OF pH

Although pH is one of the most closely regulated parameters in the body, cell pH is altered by intense exercise. For instance Pan et al. [127], using ^{1}H-NMR recorded a resting intramuscular pH of 7.01 which fell to 6.1 after exhausting exercise. Similarly Hood et al. [128], using nuclear magnetic resonance, reported that intracellular muscle pH fell from 7.06 to 6. 29 postexercise. Lactic acid accelerates lipid peroxidation in kidney homogenates [129]. That observation may be explained by the fact that a low pH helps to keep Fe ions in solution. For instance, Bralet et al. [130] showed that LM-Fe in tissue was significantly increased as the buffer pH was made more acidic. They also found that anoxia increased the availability of this LM-Fe and that the iron was in a form that could stimulate lipid peroxidation.

12 BLOOD IRON AND EXERCISE

Exercise may induce a variety of mechanisms that provide potential sources of LM-Fe. For instance it appears that erythrocyte fragility is increased at the outset of training [131,132] and there is evidence of hemolysis induced by intense endurance exercise [133,134]. Gastrointestinal bleeding is another common finding in distance runners. Some studies found evidence of bleeding in 70 to 80% of the runners [135,136]. Hemolysis associated with uphill and downhill running is presumably related to the direct physical trauma to the blood cells from foot strikes [135]. Gimenez et al. [137] studied 14 physically trained males as they performed an exhaustive, 45 min, interval training program. That protocol resulted in increases of 32% in serum iron, and a 13% increase in serum transferrin which was estimated by an antibody method. Although the transferrin change could be explained by the observed change in hemoconcentration the serum iron change could not. The authors commented that the readily available iron might be used in myoglobin synthesis or lost in sweat or urine. Several authors have shown that transition metals appear in sweat subsequent to exercise [116,138] though the quantity was quite varied between subjects and no obvious relationship to whole body metal metabolism was detected. According to Jacob et al. [139] loss of iron through sweat is insignificant while Cu loss by that route may account for 25–30% of the dietary requirement for that transition metal. Exercise often induces a physiological reaction similar to a mild acute phase response [15,138,140,141]. Lauffer [15] theorized that the acute phase response may, at least in part, be responsible for inducing an increase in ferritin synthesis and reducing iron availability. A generalization such as Lauffer's overlooks the tremendous variability of response to exercise intensity. For instance, though exercise has been shown to increase serum ferritin after moderate exercise, more intense exercise resulted in a significant decrease [142] and, in general, plasma levels of transition metals have not been shown to be decreased in exercising populations.

13 HEMOGLOBIN AND MYOGLOBIN

In a review on work-related muscle injury Armstrong [143] pointed out the evidence for muscle cell necrosis caused by invading macrophages. Tissue injury was evidenced by increased plasma levels of myoglobin and intramuscular enzymes. It is quite possible that LM-Fe might become available from either hemoglobin or myoglobin in the face of unaccustomed or severe exercise stress. The concentration of free plasma haemoglobin is normally kept very low. It normally ranges from 3 to 5 mg/dl and is bound to haptoglobin [12]. However, plasma hemoglobin was found to be elevated both after a marathon [144] and even shorter 4-km runs [145]. According to Roxin et al. [146] older skiers and less experienced skiers had higher plasma myoglobin levels after a ski race. After cycle exercise myoglobin began to rise 1.2 h after the exercise. That rise was not related to fitness and there was considerable differences in protein leakage. Seven days of prolonged jogging by moderately fit men resulted in elevated serum myoglobin, and intracellular enzymes and a decrease in haptoglobin [147]. Unaccustomed weight lifting also may increase plasma myoglobin [148]. Uberoi et al. [149] reported that seven healthy individuals were hospitalized with acute renal failure subsequent to cross country runs or an extended military march. Four of the subjects required dialysis. They exhibited myoglobinuria which was attributed to exertional rhabdomyolosis. Halliwell [10] has pointed out that hemoglobin and myoglobin are potentially dangerous proteins when released from cells since the proteins can be degraded by H_2O_2 to release Fe ions and heme, both of which can stimulate lipid peroxidation.

14 SUMMARY

The purpose of this chapter has been to show that:
1. Iron and other transition metals are very closely regulated by biochemical systems.
2. Iron plays a pivotal role in free radical chemistry.
3. There is now evidence that LM- Fe may be increased by tissue injury and exercise and can participate in free-radical chemistry.
4. The current trend to supplement the general public and especially athletes with iron may in fact be ill advised.

A more targeted approach is needed. The advice of Sullivan [150] that we 'consider "iron depletion" the physiologically normal state until proven otherwise' is premature and may be too extreme. However, we may have ignored an important clue to general health by failing to notice that, in general, women have a derived longevity benefit even though they live in a state of iron depletion relative to men during their reproductive years. In fact, the female's protection against cardiovascular disease seems to diminish after menopause when they tend to become iron sufficient and CVD risk factors tend to rise dramatically in developed western countries.

15 PERSPECTIVE

As we attempt to understand the complex relationship of physical activity and free radical chemistry upon the human body we would do well to attend to the advice of Aruoma et al. [138]. They pointed out the great variability between subjects in parameters relating to exercise and metal content of sweat and plasma. They cautioned that, 'statistical analysis of "pooled" data from large numbers of subjects is unlikely to lead to identification of generalized deficiencies in body metal content'. It is unlikely that we shall uncover a deficiency in the human organism's vast antioxidant defense that will apply to the general population. It is much more likely that as we gain additional information we shall be able to pick out individuals that may require special supplementation of either trace metals or compounds to protect against transition metals. Iron chemistry and its relationship to oxidative stress especially in physically active populations has been largely ignored. At the moment there is no reason to expect that exercising populations are protected from iron driven oxidative stress reactions. There is a need for studies of the susceptibility to oxidative stress in relation to iron status.

16 ABBREVIATIONS

Cu TP:	copper transport protein
Cu:	copper
DNA:	deoxyribonucleic acid
Fe:	iron
Fe ch.:	iron chelates
Fe(II):	ferrous
Fe(III):	ferric
Fe-Red	ferrireductase
FeTP:	iron transport protein
^{1}H-NMR:	nuclear magnetic resonance
H_2O:	water
Hemosid:	hemosiderin
Hgb:	hemoglobin
IRE:	iron response element
IRE-BP$_1$ + IRE-BP$_2$:	Fe-responsive element-binding proteins
IRP:	iron responsive protein
-L:	ligand(s)
LM-Fe:	low molecular mass iron pool
LMW:	low molecular weight
MCu:	Ox multicopper oxidase
MDA:	malondialdehyde
Mn:	manganese
mRNA:	messenger ribonucleic acid
NADH:	reduced nicotinamide adenine dinucleotide
NADPH:	reduced nicotinamide adenine dinucleotide phosphate
nhe:	nonheme iron
$O_2^{.-}$:	oxygen
OH$^.$:	hydroxyl radical

OH⁻:   hydroxyl ion

OH⁻:	hydroxyl ion
RES:	reticuloendothelial system
Resp. Enz.:	respiratory enzymes
T-EX:	trained exhausted
TRAIN:	trained
U-EX:	untrained exhausted
UIBC:	unbound iron binding capacity
UNTR:	untrained
Zn:	zinc

17 REFERENCES

1. May PM, Williams DR. FEBS Lett 1977;78:134—138.
2. Awaramik S et al. In: Holland H, Schidlowski M (eds) Mineral Deposits and the Evolution of the Biosphere. New York: Springer-Verlag, 1982;314.
3. Bilinski T. BioSystems 1991;24:305—312.
4. Mettler CC. History of Medicine. New York: McGraw-Hill, Inc, Blakiston Division, 1947;177.
5. Wrigglesworth JM, Baum H. In: Jacobs A, Worwood M (eds) Iron in Biochemistry and Medicine II. London: Academic Press, 1980;29—86.
6. McDonald R, Keen CL. Sports Med 1988;5:171—184.
7. Haymes EM, Lamanca JJ. Sports Med 1989;7: 277—285.
8. Spiro TG, Saltman P. In: Jacobs A, Worwood M (eds) Iron in Biochemistry and Medicine. London: Academic Press, 1974;1—28.
9. Hawker PN. In: Wilkinson G, Gillard RD, McCleverty JA (eds) Comprehensive Coordination Chemistry, Vol 4. New York: Pergamon Press, 1987;1179—1187.
10. Halliwell B. In: Bergeron RJ, Brittenham GM (eds) The Development of Iron Chelators for Clinical Use. Boca Raton: CRC Press, 1994;33—56.
11. Schubert J. In: Gross F (ed) Iron Metabolism. Berlin: Springer-Verlag, 1964;466—493.
12. Crosby WH. Am J Med 1955;18: 112—122.
13. Kushner JP. In: Wyngaarden JB, Smith LH, Bennett JC (eds) Cecil Textbook of Medicine, 19th edn. Philadelphia: WB Saunders, 1992;839—846.
14. Bezkorovainy A. Biochemistry of Nonheme Iron. New York: Plenum Press, 1980;47—51.
15. Lauffer RB. In: Lauffer RB, ed. Iron and Human Disease. Boca Raton, FL: CRC Press, 1992; 459—476.
16. Cook JD, Skikne BS, Baynes RD. Annu Rev Med 1993;44:63—74.
17. Conrad ME, Umbreit JN. Am J Hematol 1993;42:67—73.
18. Klausner RD, Rouault TA, Harford JB. Cell 1993;72:19—28.
19. Mascotti DP, Rup D. Thach RE. Annu Rev Nutr 1995;15:239—261.
20. Beard Jl, Dawson H, Pinero DJ. Nutr Rev 1996;54:295—317.
21. Gutteridge JMC, Rowley DA, Halliwell B. Biochem J 1981;199:263—265.
22. Grootveld M, Bell JD, Halliwell B, Aruoma OI, Bomford A, Sadler PJ. J Biol Chem 1989;264: 4417—4422.
23. Evans PJ, Evans RW, Bomford A, Williams R, Halliwell B. Free Rad Res Comms 1994;20: 139—144.
24. Winzerling JJ, Law JH. Annu Rev Nutr 1997;17:501—526.
25. Waddell J, Steenbock H, Elvenhjem CA, Hart EB. J Biol Chem 1927;77:777—795.
26. Hart EB, Steenbock H, Waddell J, Elvehjem CA. J Biol Chem 1927;77:797—812.
27. Osaki S, Johnson DA, Frieden E. J Biol Chem 1966;241:2746—2751.
28. Lee GR, Nacht S, Lukens JN, Cartwright GE. J Clin Invest 1968;47:2058—2069.
29. Crichton RR, Ward RJ. In: Lauffer RB (ed) Iron and Human Disease. Boca Raton, FL: CRC

Press, 1992;33−68.
30. Theil EC. In: Theil EC, Eichhorn GL, Marzil LG (eds) Iron Binding Proteins Without Cofactors or Sulfur Clusters. New York: Elsevier, 1983;1−38.
31. Sirivech S, Frieden E, Osaki S. Biochem J 1974;143:311−315.
32. Eide D, Davis-Kaplan S, Jordan I, Sipe D, Kaplan J. J Biol Chem 1992;267:20774−20781.
33. Askwith C, Eide D, Van Ho A, Bernard PS, Li L, Davis-Kaplin JJ, Sipe DM, Kaplan J. Cell 1994;76:403−410.
34. Richter GW. Am J Pathol 1978;91:363−397.
35. O'Connell MJ, Halliwell B, Moorhouse CP, Aruoma OI, Baum H, Peters TJ. Biochem J 1986; 234:727−731.
36. Halliwell B, Gutteridge JMC. Arch Biochem Biophys 1986;246:501−514.
37. Jacobs A. Blood 1977;50:433−439.
38. White GP, Jacobs A, Grady RW, Cerami A. Blood 1976;48:923−929.
39. Mulligan M, Althaus B, Linder MC. Int J Biochem 1986;18:791−798.
40. Hoffbrand AV, Ganeshaguru K, Tattersall MHN, Tripp E. Br J Haematol 1976;33:517−526.
41. Prockop DJ. Fed Proc 1971;30:984−990.
42. Bailey-Wood R, Blayney LM, Muir JR, Jacobs A. Br J Exp Pathol 1975;56:193−198.
43. Finch CA, Miller LR, Inandar AR, Person R, Seiler K, Mackler B. J Clin Invest 1976;58: 447−453.
44. Kozlov AV, Yegorov DY, Vladimirov YA, Azizova OA. Free Rad Biol Med 1992;13:9−16.
45. Reif DW. Free Rad Biol Med 1992;12:417−427.
46. O'Connell MJ, Ward RJ, Baum H, Peters TJ. Biochem J 1985;229:135−139.
47. Toyokuni S, Sagripanti J-L. Free Rad Biol Med 1993;15:117−123.
48. Bolann BJ, Ulvik RJ. Eur J Biochem 1990;193:899.
49. Evans PJ, Halliwell B. Unpublished data. 1994.
50. Flint DH, Tuminello JF, Emptage MH. J Biol Chem 1993;268:22369−22376.
51. Watt GD, Frankel PB, Papaefthymiou GC. Proc Natl Acad Sci USA 1985;82:3640−3643.
52. Green S, Mazur A, Shorr E. J Biol Chem 1956;220:237−255.
53. Boyer RF, McCleary CJ. Free Rad Biol Med 1987;3:389−395.
54. Topham R, Goger M, Pearce, Schultz P. Biochem J 1989;261:137−143.
55. Thomas CE, Morehouse LA, Aust SD. J Biol Chem 1985;260:3275−3280.
56. Looker AC, Dallmen PR, Canal MD, Ganter EW, Johnson A. JAMA 1997;277:973−976.
57. Herbert V. Blood Rev 1992;6:125−132.
58. Lushner K. In: Wyngaarden JB, Smith LH, Bennett JC (eds) Cecil Textbook of Medicine, 19th edn. Philadelphia: W.B. Saunders Co, 1992;840−843.
59. Edwards CQ, Griffen LM, Goldgar D, Drummond C, Skolnick MH, Kushner JP. N Engl J Med 1988;318:1355−1362.
60. Weintraub LR, Edwards CQ, Krikker M. Ann NY Acad Sci 1988;526:370.
61. Bank A. Ann NY Acad Sci 1990;612:590.
62. Iancu TC. Pediatr Pathol 1990;10:281−296.
63. Salonen JT, Nyyssonen K, Korpela H, Tuomilehto J, Seppanen R, Salonen R. Circulation 1992;86:803−811.
64. Selby JV, Friedman GD. Int J Cancer 1988;41:677−682.
65. Stevens RG, Jones YD, Micozzi MS. N Engl J Med 1988;319:1047−1052.
66. Rowley DA, Gutteridge JMC, Blake DR, Farr M, Halliwell B. Clin Sci 1984;66:691−695.
67. Rao NA, Romero JL, Fernandez MAS, Sevanian A, Marak GE. Arch Opthalmol 1986;104: 1369−1371.
68. Jenkins RR, Kohman LJ, Veit LJ. Free Rad Biol Med 1994;16:627−631.
69. Sullivan JL. Circulation 1992;86:1036−1037.
70. Carthew P, Smith AG, Hider RC, Dorman B, Edwards RE, Francis JE. Biometals 1994;7: 267−271.
71. Park CH, Bacon BR, Brittenham EM, Tavil AS. Lab Invest 1987;57:555−563.

72. Oates PS, Morgan EH. Anat Rec 1996;246:364—371.
73. Tandler B, Horne WI, Brittenham GM, Tsukamoto. Anat Rec 1996;245:65—75.
74. Nagasawa T, Hatayama T, Watanabe Y, Tanaka M, Niisato Y, Kitts DD. Biochem Biophys Res Com 1997;231:37—41.
75. Porter JB, Morgan J, Hoyes KP, Burke LC, Huehns ER, Hider RC. Blood 1990;11:2389—2396.
76. Siegenberg D, Baynes RD, Bothwell TH, Macfarlane BJ, Lamparelli RD. Proc Soc Exp. Biol Med 1990;193:65—72.
77. Burkitt MJ, Mason RP. Proc Natl Acad Sci USA 1991;88:8440—8444.
78. Zanninelli G, Glickstein H, Breuer W, Milgram P, Brissot P, Hider RC, Konijn AM, Libman J, Shanzer A, Ioav Cabantchik Z. Molec Pharmacol 1997;51:842—852.
79. Roginsky VA, Barsukova TK, Bruchelt G, Stegmann HB. Biochim Biophys Acta 1997;1335:33—39.
80. Young IS, Tate S, Lightbody JH, McMaster D, Trimble ER. Free Radic Biol Med 1995;18:833—840.
81. Halliwell B, Gutteridge JMC. Biochem J 1984;219:1—14.
82. Ryan TP, Aust SD. Crit Rev Toxicol 1992;22:119—141.
83. McCord JM. Circulation 1991;83:1112—1114.
84. Sutton HC, Winterbourn CC. Free Rad Biol Med 1989;6:53—60.
85. Minotti G. Arch Biochem Biophys 1992;287:189—198.
86. Fenton HJH. J Chem Soc 1894;65:899—910.
87. Koppenol WH. Free Rad Biol Med 1993;15:645—651.
88. Goldstein S, Meyerstein D, Czapski G. Free Rad Biol Med 1993;15:435—445.
89. Haber F, Weiss J. Proc Roy Soc 1934;147:332—351.
90. Aruoma OI, Halliwell B, Laughton MJ, Quinlan GJ, Gutteridge JM. Biochem J 1989;258:617—620.
91. Halliwell B, Gutteridge JMC. FEBS Lett 1992;307:108—112.
92. Halliwell B, Cross CE, Gutteridge JMC. J Lab Clin Med 1992;119:598—620.
93. Stohs SJ, Bagchi D. Free Radic Biol Med 1995;18:321—336.
94. Tokoyokuni S, Sagripanti J-L. Free Radic Biol Med 1996;20:859—864.
95. Meneghini R. Free Radic Biol Med 1997;23:783—792.
96. Csermely P, Fodor P, Somogyi J. Carcinogenesis 1987;8:1663—1666.
97. Smith AG, Carthew P, Francis JE, Edwards RE, Dinsdale D. Hepatology 1990;12:1399—1405.
98. Prince RC, Grossman MJ. Trends Biochem Sci 1993;18:153—154.
99. Thornalley PJ, Vasak M. Biochim Biophys Acta 1985;827:36—44.
100. Cabantchik AI, Glickstein H, Milgram P, Breuner W. Anal Biochem 1966;233:221—227.
101. Epsztejn S, Kakhlon O, Glickstein H, Breur W, Cabantchik ZI. Anal Biochem 1997;248:31—40.
102. Demaeyer E, Adiels-Tegman M. World Health Stat Quart 1985;38:302.
103. Weaver CM, Rarjaram S. J Nutr 1994;122:782.
104. Cook JD. Sem Hematol 1994;31:146—154.
105. Cook JD, Dassenko SA, Lynch SR. Am J Clin Nutr 1991;54:717.
106. Pate RR, Miller BJ, Davis M, Slentz CA, Klingshirn LA. Int J Sport Nutr 1993;3:222—231.
107. Guyatt GH, Oxman AD, Ali M. Gen Intern Med 1992;7:145—153.
108. Cook JD. Baillieres Clin Haematol 1994;7:787—804.
109. Lyle RM, Weaver CM, Sedlock DA et al. Am J Clin. Nutr 1992;56:1049—1055.
110. Brigham DE, Beard JL, Krimmel R, Kenney WL. Nutrition 1993;9:418—422.
111. Garza D, Shrier I, Kohl HW, Ford P, Brown M, Matheson GO. Clin J Sports Med 1997;7:46—53.
112. Willis WT, Dallman PR, Brooks GA. J Appl Physiol 1988;1:256—263.
113. Celsing F, Blomstrand E, Werner W, Pihlstedt P, Ekblom B. Med Sci Sports Exerc 1986;18:156—161.
114. Rector WG, Fortuin NJ, Conley CL. Medicine 1982;61:382—389.
115. Lamanca JJ, Haymes EM. Med Sci Sports Exerc 1993;25:1386—1392.

116. Gutteridge JMC, Rowley DA, Halliwell B, Cooper DF, Heeley DM. Clin Chim Acta 1985;145: 267—273.
117. Evans WJ, Cannon JG. In: Holloszy JO (ed) Exercise and Sports Sciences Reviews. Baltimore: Williams & Wilkins, 1991;19:99—125.
118. Serbinova EA, Kadiiska MB, Bakalova RA, Koynova GM, Stoyanovsky, DA, Karakashev PC, Stoytchev TsS, Wolinsky I, Kagan VE. Toxicol Lett 1989;47:119—123.
119. Jenkins RR, Krause K, Schofield LS. Med Sci Sports Exerc 1993;25:213—217.
120. Halliwell B. FASEB J 1987;1:358—364.
121. Kondo H, Miura M, Nakagaki I, Sasaki S, Itokawa Y. Am J Physiol 1992;262:583—590.
122. Byrd SK. Med Sci Sports Exerc 1992;24:531—536.
123. Orrenius S, McConkey DJ, Bellomo G, Nicotera P. Trends Pharm Sci 1989;10:281—285.
124. Link G, Athias P, Grynberg A, Pinson A, Hershko C. J Lab Clin Med 1989;113:103—111.
125. Kanner J, Harel S, Hazan B. J Agric Food Chem 1986;34:506—510.
126. Kasperek GJ, Snider RD. Eur J Appl Physiol 1985;54:30—34.
127. Pan JW, Hamm JR, Rothman DL, Shulman RG. Proc Natl Acad Sci USA 1988;85:7836—7839.
128. Hood VL, Schubert C, Keller U, Muller S. Am J Physiol 1988;255:F479—F485.
129. Fauconneau B, Tallineau C, Huguet F, Pontcharraud R, Piriou A. Toxicology 1993;77:249—258.
130. Bralet J, Schreiber L, Bouvier C. Biochem Pharmacol 1992;43:979—983.
131. Puhl JL, Runyan WS, Kruse SJ. Res Quart Exer Sport 1981;52:484—494.
132. Shiraki K, Yoshimura J, Yamada T. 20th World Congress in Sports Medicine Proceedings. Melbourne: 1974;405—415.
133. Falsetti JL, Klee G, Huss C, Hamilton H. Physiologist 1979;22:36.
134. Miller B. Sports Med 1990;9:1—6.
135. Robertson JD, Maughan RJ, Davidson RJL. Br Med J 1987;295:303—305.
136. Stewart JG, Ahlquist DA, McGill DB, Ilstrup DM, Schwartz S, Owen RA. Ann Int Med 1984; 100:843—845.
137. Gimenez M, Uffoltz H, Paysant P, Bellville F, Nabet P. Eur J Appl Physiol 1988;57:154—158.
138. Aruoma OI, Reilly T, MacLaren D, Halliwell B. Clin Chim Acta 1988;177:81—88.
139. Jacob RA, Sandstead HH, Munoz JM, Kleavay LM, Milne DB. Am J Clin Nutr 1981;34: 1379—1383.
140. Weight LM, Alexander D, Jacobs P. Clin Sci (Colch) (Diz) 1991;81:677—683.
141. Fielding RA, Manfredi TJ, Ding W, Fiatarone MA, Evans WJ, Cannon JG. Am J Physiol 1993; 265:R166—R172.
142. Pattini A, Schena F, Guidi GC. Eur J Appl Physiol 1990;61:55—60.
143. Armstrong RB. Sports Med 1986;3:370—381
144. Dickson DN, Wilkinson RL, Noakes TD. J Sports Med 1982;3:111—117.
145. Fredrickson LA, Puhl JL, Runyan WS. Med Sci Sports Ex 1983;15:271—276.
146. Roxin LE, Hedin G, Venge P. Int J Sports Med 1986;7:259—263.
147. Dressendorfer RH, Wade CE, Claybaugh J, Cucinell SA, Timmis GC. Int J Sports Med 1991;12: 55—61.
148. Paul GL, DeLany JP, Snook JT, Seifert JG, Kirby TE. Eur J Appl Physiol 1989;58:786—790.
149. Uberoi HS, Dugal JS, Kasthuri AS, Kolhe VS, Kumar AK, Cruz SA. J Assoc Physicians India 1991;39:677—679.
150. Sullivan JL. Free Rad Biol Med 1992;13:703.

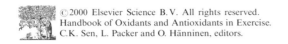
©2000 Elsevier Science B.V. All rights reserved.
Handbook of Oxidants and Antioxidants in Exercise.
C.K. Sen, L. Packer and O. Hänninen, editors.

Part III • Chapter 7

The role of xanthine oxidase in exercise

Y. Hellsten

Copenhagen Muscle Research Centre, August-Krogh Institute, University of Copenhagen, 13 Univer-sitetsparken, DK-2100 Copenhagen Ø, Denmark. Tel.: +45-35-321550. Fax: +45-35-321600.

1 INTRODUCTION
2 XANTHINE DEHYDROGENASE/OXIDASE
   2.1 Structure and function
   2.2 Distribution
3 PURINE METABOLISM
   3.1 Degradation of adenine nucleotides in muscle with exercise
   3.2 Formation of purines during exercise
   3.3 Salvage of purines
   3.4 Urate as a scavenger
4 XO AND TISSUE INJURY
   4.1 Conversion of XDH to XO
   4.2 XO in ischemia/reperfusion-induced injury
5 THE ROLE OF XO IN EXERCISE-INDUCED MUSCLE DAMAGE
   5.1 Evidence for oxygen radical generation via XO in skeletal muscle
   5.2 Generation of oxygen radicals via XO in muscle during exercise
6 XO IN INFLAMMATORY PROCESSES
7 SUMMARY
8 PERSPECTIVES
9 ACKNOWLEDGEMENTS
10 ABBREVIATIONS
11 REFERENCES

1   INTRODUCTION

The enzyme xanthine dehydrogenase (XDH) participates in the purine degradation pathway in which it oxidizes hypoxanthine to xanthine and xanthine to urate. The main localization of XDH is in the vessel walls of most tissues including cardiac and skeletal muscle but the enzyme is also present in e.g. mammary gland epithelial cells and in large amounts in milk [1—3]. XDH can exist both in a dehydrogenase form, which utilizes nicotinamide adenine dinucleotide (NAD^+) as electron acceptor, and in an oxidase form (xanthine oxidase; XO) which utilizes molecular oxygen as electron acceptor. The univalent reduction of oxygen in the XO catalyzed reaction leads to the formation of reactive superoxide radicals [4] which are proposed to contribute to free radical-induced injury to cells [5]. Although the main proportion of the enzyme exists in the harmless dehydrogenase form in normal tissue, the enzyme can be converted to the oxidase form during conditions of metabolic stress, such as ischemia [5,6]. The possible involvement of XO in tissue damage has lead to a growing clinical interest in the enzyme where the main research focus has been in reperfusion of ischemic tissue [7—9] and there is good evidence from animal models that XO in part may be the cause of the cellular damage that occurs during this form of metabolic stress [10—12]. XO has also been suggested to participate in immunological events, such as activation of neutrophils, that may occur subsequent to cellular damage and that can escalate the extent of tissue injury [13].

The role of XO in exercise-induced muscle damage has not been extensively investigated and only a limited amount of information is presently available on this topic. The metabolic conditions of skeletal muscle during strenuous exercise do, however, appear to resemble those of ischemic tissue in several aspects. Similar to during ischemia intense exercise causes the degradation of nucleotides in the muscle, which leads to the formation of hypoxanthine and xanthine, both of which are substrates for XDH/XO. Exercise may also indirectly lead to a conversion of XDH to XO.

The present review describes some of the properties of XDH/XO and brings up adenine nucleotide catabolism and purine formation in the muscle during exercise as these events may be prerequisites for generation of radicals from XO. Evidence for conversion of XDH to XO and for oxygen radical generation via XO in tissues during ischemia/reperfusion are briefly presented. Finally, the possible implications of XDH/XO in exercise-induced muscle damage and inflammatory events are discussed.

2   XANTHINE DEHYDROGENASE/OXIDASE

2.1 Structure and function

XDH (E.C. 1.1.1.204; XD) is a dimer consisting of two similar 150-kDa monomers. Each monomer contains a molybdenum atom, four non-heme iron-sulfur groups and one flavine adenine nucleotide molecule [14,15]. XDH can exist in two forms, a dehydrogenase and an oxidase form. Both forms of the enzyme catalyze two reactions in which hypoxanthine is oxidized to xanthine and xanthine is oxidized to urate. However, the electron acceptor specificity is different for the two forms. In the XDH catalyzed reaction, NAD^+ is utilized as the sole electron acceptor (1) whereas XO utilizes molecular oxygen. The univalent reduction of oxygen leads to the formation of superoxide radicals (2).

$$Hx \; + \; NAD^+ \; + \; H_2O \quad \rightarrow \quad X \; + \; NADH \; + \; H^+ \qquad (1)$$

$$Hx \; + \; O_2 \; + \; H_2O \quad \rightarrow \quad X \; + \; O_2^- \; + \; H^+ \qquad (2)$$

In normal tissue, between 10—30% of the total enzyme activity exists in the oxidase form [9,16,17] but during certain conditions a conversion from the dehydrogenase to the oxidase form can occur. It was Della Corte and Stirpe [18,19] who discovered that XDH could undergo either a reversible or an irreversible conversion to XO in vitro in rat liver. The reversible transformation of XDH to XO was found to occur with various treatments, such as sulphydryl agents, storage at $-20°C$, and in the presence of sulphydryl oxidase [18—21]. The conversion was reversed in the presence of thiol groups and Waud and Rajagopalan [22] hypothesized that the reversible alteration of the enzyme occurred through reduction of disulfide bonds to sulfhydryl groups resulting in a change in conformation. The irreversible transformation of XDH was found to take place in the presence of proteases [19,23] and the proteolytic action was later observed to cause the removal of a 20 kDa peptide [22]. Roy and McCord [5] showed the protease to be calcium-dependent and proposed that calpain was responsible for the conversion. Subsequent findings indicated, however, that calpain is not a likely candidate for the conversion of the enzyme [24].

2.2 Distribution

There are some discrepancies between reports on the distribution of XDH/XO in human and animal tissues. Early studies, utilizing histochemical techniques for the localization of XDH/XO activity reported the enzyme to be present in hepatocytes [25,26] and duodenal epithelial cells [27]. A recent study applied more specific histochemical methods and demonstrated enzyme activity in hepatocytes but also in endothelial cells of hepatic micro vessels [28]. Immuno-histochemical examinations utilizing polyclonal antibody have described the enzyme to be present solely in endothelial cells of micro-vessels and epithelial cells of mammary glands [2]. The use of monoclonal antibody to XDH/XO has, furthermore, revealed XO immunoreactivity in smooth muscle cells of vessel walls, as well as capillary endothelial cells [3]. The two latter studies have both reported absence of XO in skeletal muscle cells and in endothelial cells of larger vessels [2,3]. The presence of the enzyme in capillary endothelial cells of skeletal muscle has been confirmed by the demonstration of XDH mRNA in this cell-type [29].

It has been reported that XDH/XO in human muscle is irregularly distributed among microvessels with some vessels showing prominent immunoreactivity and others showing weak or no staining [3]. As the mRNA of XDH, at least in horse, appears to be expressed in most microvessels in muscle [29], the finding of an irregular presence of the enzyme could imply that XDH protein may be induced in cells. The hypothesis is supported by the observation of a higher level of XDH/XO in damaged than in normal skeletal muscle [30]. This topic is discussed in detail below.

The activity of XDH differs between animal species, as well as between tissues but there is also a large discrepancy between reports on the level of XDH/XO activities [31]. The latter variation is maybe due to sample collection, sample treatment or differences in assay conditions, such as the substrate concentration. Wajner and Harkness [32] proposed that some of the deviation between reports could be due to the presence of an unknown inhibitor which could be overcome by the use of a high concentration of substrate in the assay. In general, it appears safe to conclude that the enzyme activity is low in skeletal and cardiac muscle and relatively high in liver (Table 1). The two forms of the enzyme also differ slightly in their activity levels. For example, XDH derived from rat liver has an activity of approximately 810 mol min^{-1} mol flavin adenine dinucleotide (FAD^{-1}) for xanthine-NAD$^+$, whereas XO from the same tissue holds an activity of 1,030 mol min^{-1} mol FAD^{-1} for xanthine/O$_2$ [33].

3   PURINE METABOLISM

3.1 Degradation of adenine nucleotides in muscle with exercise

The presence of the substrates of XDH/XO, hypoxanthine (HX) and xanthine (X), is clearly a requirement for flux through the reaction and, thus, for the formation of oxygen radicals via the enzyme. Hypoxanthine and xanthine are products in the degradation pathway of nucleotides. In the muscle, nucleotides can be degraded during intensive exercise when the rate of adenosine 5′-triphosphate (ATP) utilization exceeds the rate of ATP regeneration. In humans, reductions in muscle nucleotides of up to 40% of resting levels have been found following short term sprint exercise [38], and in rats reductions of approximately 50% of the total nucleotide pool have been observed in fast-twitch white fibers subjected to intense electrical stimulation [39]. During these conditions a drastic accumulation of adenosine 5′-diphosphate (ADP) and adenosine 5′-monophosphate (AMP) is prevented through two enzymatic reactions, the adenylate kinase reaction and the AMP deaminase reaction. In the adenylate kinase reaction two ADP form one ATP and one AMP molecule and in the AMP deaminase reaction AMP is deaminated to inosine 5′-monophosphate (IMP) (Fig. 1). Thus, during intensive exercise, ADP is degraded first to AMP and then further to IMP [40].

Table 1. Xanthine dehydrogenase/oxidase activities in human tissues.

Tissue	XDH/XO activity (nmol· min^{-1}· g^{-1} protein)		Number of observations	References
Skeletal muscle	420	(200—660)	10	[32]
	35.5	(0—320)	7	[31]
	0.12	(0.04—0.19)	2	[34]
Cardiac muscle	1200	(750—1980)	9	[32]
	0.27	(0.16—0.38)	2	[34]
	0.0018			[35]
	0.0000			[36]
Liver	900		2	[37]
	710	(360—-980)	8	[32]
	580	(60—1050)	4	[31]
	90	(40—250)	6	[34]

Data presented as means. Numbers in brackets indicate range.

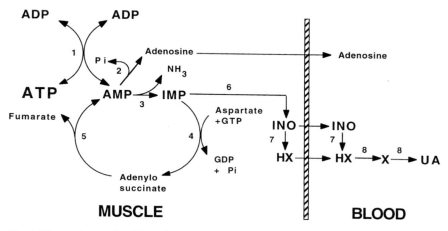

Fig. 1. The purine nucleotide cycle and the purine degradation pathway. Numbers indicate enzymes. 1. Adenylate kinase, 2. AMP 5'nucleotidase, 3. AMP deaminase, 4. adenylosuccinate synthetase, 5. adenylosuccinate lyase, 6. IMP 5'nucleotidase, 7. purine nucleoside phosphorylase, 8. xanthine dehydrogenase/oxidase (XDH/XO). ATP: Adenosine triphosphate; ADP: Adenosine diphosphate; AMP: Adenosine monophosphate, IMP: Inosine monophosphate; INO: Inosine; HX: Hypoxanthine; X: Xanthine; UA: Urate; GTP: Guanosine triphopshate, GDP: Guanosine diphosphate.

The physiological role of nucleotide degradation has been debated and propositions such as regulation of phosphofructokinase and phosphorylase b activity have been made [see 41]. As the catabolism of ATP to IMP prevents large increases in ADP and AMP concentrations [38,42,43] one of the more certain outcomes of this degradation is an upkeep of the energy charge in the muscle, allowing for continued contraction [44].

3.2 Formation of purines during exercise

The cell membrane is impermeable to IMP and, thus, during intensive exercise the majority of catabolized nucleotides remain as IMP within the muscle [40,43,45]. In recovery from exercise the accumulated IMP is reaminated to AMP via adenylosuccinate synthetase and adenylosuccinate lyase in the purine nucleotide cycle (Fig. 1). A fraction of the IMP formed in the muscle is, however, dephosphorylated to inosine in a reaction catalyzed by 5' nucleotidase which is localized intracellularly in the muscle cells, as well as in the membrane of both muscle and capillary endothelial cells [46,47]. Inosine (INO) can also be formed from adenosine which is generated through dephosphorylation of AMP via 5' nucleotidase. Although important in cardiac muscle, the flux through this pathway appears to be minor in skeletal muscle [48,49]. INO can be further degraded to hypoxanthine via purine nucleoside phosphorylase which, in cardiac muscle, has been reported to be present mainly in the cytosol of endothelial cells [50]. The concentration of hypoxanthine in muscle at rest is low relative to the adenine nucleotide levels and following short-term intense exercise the increase in muscle hypoxanthine only amounts to less than one percent of the increase in IMP [49]. In human muscle, hypoxanthine levels have even been found unaltered, despite large elevations in muscle IMP following a few minutes of all-out cycling [51]. It is, however, clear that hypoxanthine is formed in the muscle during intense exercise as there is a marked release of this purine from muscle into the blood [52—54]. Thus, it is likely that the majority of purine bases leave the muscle cells in the form of inosine and are subsequently degraded to hypoxanthine, possibly in the vascular walls.

The extent to which hypoxanthine accumulates in the blood is mainly dependent on the intensity of exercise and, the highest plasma levels have been found following exhaustive exercise performed during only a few minutes [55] (Fig. 2A). During short term intense exercise the magnitude of hypoxanthine formation appears to be associated with the accumulation of IMP in muscle which is also related to the intensity of exercise [56]. It remains unclear what determines the degree of nucleotide degradation and formation of purines [57]. It has been proposed that the degradation of nucleotides in the muscle is coupled to the level of creatine phosphate. In a study by Katz et al. [58] it was found that the rate of in vivo AMP deamination, as calculated from the rate of IMP formation, was

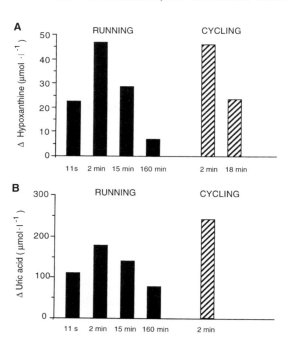

Fig. 2. Peak accumulation of plasma A) hypoxanthine and B) urate following exhaustive running and cycling of various durations. Accumulation is calculated as the difference between peak plasma concentration and pre-exercise values. Running data from Hellsten-Westing et al. [65], cycling data from Hellsten-Westing et al. [73] 2 min and Sahlin et al. [52] 18 min.

related to the degree of ATP turnover and to low creatine phosphate levels. In accordance, Balsom et al. [59] showed that the accumulation of hypoxanthine in plasma during repeated intermittent 6 s sprints was lower in subjects that had ingested creatine during the days prior to the exercise. Although muscle creatine phosphate levels were not determined, it is reasonable to believe that the concentration of creatine phosphate was higher after the supplementation, as previously observed [60], and that this was the factor affecting the lower degree of IMP dephosphorylation. The extent of AMP deamination could, moreover, be regulated by binding of AMP deaminase to myosin. AMP deaminase binds to myosin in rat skeletal muscle during intense contraction and the enzyme kinetics are thereby altered so that the Km for AMP deaminase is markedly lower [61,62]. Recent findings indicate, however, that the binding of AMP deaminase to myosin may not occur in human skeletal muscle during high intensity exercise [51].

IMP and purines are also formed during long term exercise performed to exhaustion. It has been demonstrated that IMP and hypoxanthine formation occurs first towards the end of prolonged exhaustive exercise, suggesting that nucleotides are degraded when the resynthesis of ATP is limited due to low glycogen levels [63,64]. The accumulation of hypoxanthine in plasma is, however, markedly lower after endurance exercise than after short-term exercise [65] (Fig. 2A).

The two final reactions in the degradation of nucleotides where hypoxanthine is oxidized to xanthine and xanthine to urate are both catalyzed by XDH/XO (Fig. 1). Urate (UA) is an end-product in man and is renally cleared whereas most other mammals can oxidize urate further to allantoin via the enzyme uricase. INO and hypoxanthine are membrane permeable and plasma hypoxanthine is, thus, a source of substrate for XDH/XO in the vessels walls of all organs. Considering the localization of XDH/XO, the formation of xanthine and urate must occur after hypoxanthine has left the muscle cell and reached the blood vessel wall of the muscle or of any other tissue. In humans, the formation of urate in the bloodvessels of skeletal muscle tissue appears to be small as there is no detectable release of urate from the muscle during or after intense exercise [52—54]. In a study examining the exchange of purines in human skeletal muscle and liver with intense exercise, it was found that the liver was a major source of urate after exercise, which agrees well with the much higher activity of XDH/XO in liver than in muscle (Table 1) [54]. The exercised muscle released hypoxanthine into the blood stream in recovery and a proportion of the hypoxanthine was extracted by the liver. There was a marked release of urate from the liver, indicating that the extracted hypoxanthine had been oxidized to urate.

The observation of a lack of significant release of urate from muscle may, however, not necessarily mean that there is no formation of urate in muscle in man. The method of subtracting the arterial from the venous plasma concentration of a metabolite it is not very sensitive for a substance such as urate which has a resting concentration of about 250—350 $\mu mol \cdot l^{-1}$ in plasma. Thus, it cannot be excluded that small amounts of urate are formed in the vascular walls in skeletal muscle. In rat skeletal muscle, an accumulation of urate has been found following intense electrical stimulation [66] and ischemia [67] suggesting that urate may be formed in muscle tissue, at least in some species. The discrepancy between man and animals may be explained by a higher activity of XDH in muscle tissues of some species compared to that of humans [31]. This difference is important to take into consideration when findings regarding the role of XO in animals are translated to man.

There is a relationship between the peak concentration of hypoxanthine and that of urate in plasma following high intensity exercise [31,54] (Fig. 3). This observation indicates that the plasma hypoxanthine concentration is important for the flux through the XDH/XO pathway where a high level of plasma hypoxanthine may enhance the magnitude of superoxide radical formation in a situation where a conversion to the oxidase form has occurred. For exercise of long duration the ratio of peak plasma hypoxanthine to plasma urate concentration is much lower than for intense exercise (Fig. 2). A possible explanation for this finding is the difference in metabolic fate for the two purines. Hypoxanthine may be taken up by tissues where it can be converted to urate or to IMP, or it can be renally cleared. This means that during exercise of moderate intensity when the release rate of hypoxanthine from muscle is low [52] the accumulation of hypoxanthine in plasma is minor. In comparison, the relatively slow clearance rate of plasma urate allows urate to accumulate and to remain elevated for many hours after exercise [55].

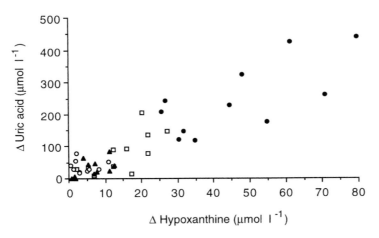

Fig. 3. The relation between the peak concentration change of hypoxanthine and urate in plasma after 2 min of cycling performed at a mean estimated oxygen demand of 106 (filled triangle), 113 (open circle), 123 (open square) and 135, all out (filled circle)% of maximal oxygen uptake (n = 11).

3.3 Salvage of purines

There appears to be negligible uptake of purines from plasma by the exercised muscle as indicated by a net release of hypoxanthine from activated muscle still at 75 min after exercise [54]. The lack of uptake of hypoxanthine by the muscle suggests that purines released to plasma represent a loss of nucleotides from the muscle. Hypoxanthine within the muscle may, however, be rephosphorylated to IMP via the enzyme hypoxanthine phosphoribosyl transferase (HPRT). The importance of HPRT for salvage of hypoxanthine has been demonstrated in a study on HPRT deficient patients who were found to excrete markedly larger amounts of urate than healthy individuals [68]. It has also been shown that lymphoblasts deficient in HPRT successively deplete their adenine nucleotide pool during active growth suggesting that HPRT is necessary for salvage of purine bases [69].

Nucleotides lost through the release of purines from the muscle into the blood are replenished by de novo biosynthesis. This pathway originates in ribose-5-phosphate which is formed in the pentose phosphate pathway (Fig. 4). Ribose-5-phosphate is converted to phosphoribosyl pyrophosphate (PRPP) which is used both in the de novo synthesis of nucleotides and in the HPRT pathway. The accumulation of hypoxanthine within the muscle during and after intense exercise is minor which suggests that the rate of hypoxanthine formation in the muscle is similar to the rate of flux of hypoxanthine through the HPRT pathway and the rate of hypoxanthine release from the muscle. Several studies have shown that a

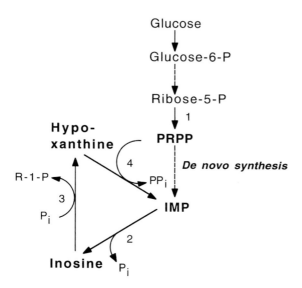

Fig. 4. Pathways for purine salvage and de novo synthesis of IMP. Numbers indicate enzymes. 1. PRPP synthetase, 2. 5'nucleotidase, 3. purine nucleoside phosphorylase, 4. hypoxanthine phosphoribosyl transferase (HPRT). PRPP: phosphoribosylpyrophosphate.

single bout of exhaustive short-term exercise does not lead to a detectable loss of adenine nucleotides [36,70] and it has been proposed that the loss of nucleotides via the formation of purines is negligible. However, two recent studies have shown that repeated high intensity intermittent exercise can lead to a lowered resting level of adenine nucleotides in muscle [71,72]. In one of the studies [71] subjects performed intermittent cycle sprints three times per week for 6 weeks directly followed by 1 week of the same training performed twice per day, everyday. The resting muscle adenine nucleotide levels were significantly lower after the 6-week period but remained at the post 6-week level during the one additional week of training. The study provided no mechanistic explanation for the decrease in nucleotide levels, however, as there was no indication of protein leakage with the exercise regime it can be postulated that the decrease was, at least in part, due to a repeated loss of nucleotides from the muscle through a release of purines. This hypothesis is supported by the finding of a lower accumulation of hypoxanthine in plasma following a given intense exercise bout performed after compared to before a period of intermittent sprint training [73]. The period of sprint training also induced an increase in the activity of HPRT which could allow for a greater flux of hypoxanthine through this salvage pathway in trained muscle, with a consequent reduction in the release of purines into the blood [73].

Another plausible explanation for a reduced formation of muscle hypoxanthine during intensive exercise in the trained subjects could be an improved capacity for anaerobic energy regeneration which is known to occur with sprint training [31,74]. These observations may provide an explanation as to why, in the study by Hellsten-Westing et al. [71], an additional week of more frequent training, performed after a 6-week training period, did not cause a further reduction in muscle nucleotides.

A lowered level of muscle nucleotides would probably only have a minor effect on exercise performance. However, it is possible that there may be local decreases in nucleotides which may cause the muscle cell to more easily become injured. For example, a loss of muscle nucleotides may impair the activity of the calcium pumps, resulting in a greater intracellular calcium concentration and an activation of calcium-dependent proteases. Activated proteases could per se cause damage or act on XDH and convert the enzyme to the potentially damaging oxidase form.

3.4 Urate as a scavenger

An interesting aspect of the XO reaction is that, simultaneous to an oxygen free radical formation, the reaction also provides radical protection as urate is a potent scavenger of radicals [75]. Although there is little evidence for a scavenger function of urate in vivo, several in vitro studies have shown that urate attenuates damage to cells subjected to free radical formation [76,77]. It has, moreover, been shown that addition of urate to the perfusion medium lowers the reperfusion associated damage in ischemic rat liver and the level of lipid peroxidation products in the perfusate [78]. Becker et al. [79] found that ischemic rat hearts perfused with urate had a lowered reduction in functional capacity and stability than ischemic controls. Other investigators have suggested that urate is the main antioxidant in human plasma [80] and that a rise in plasma urate following eccentric exercise improves the plasma radical scavenging capacity [81]. More direct evidence for whether urate may function as a scavenger in muscle may be obtained by assessing the formation of the oxidation product of urate, allantoin. Since the enzyme responsible for the enzymatic conversion of urate to allantoin, uricase, is absent in human tissues, an increase in the allantoin concentration is likely to indicate formation of free radicals. The concentration of allantoin in plasma in rheumatoid patients has been found to be significantly higher than that of healthy subjects [82]. Plasma allantoin exchange has also been determined in the pulmonary bed where a low level of allantoin release could be detected [75]. Moreover, in a recent study the concentration of urate in human muscle was observed to decrease markedly during exhaustive cycling exercise of a few minutes duration after which it rapidly increased to pre-exercise levels [83]. In parallel with the decrease in muscle urate, the concentration of muscle allantoin was increased, indicating an oxidation of urate to allantoin. The rapid recovery of urate after exercise may appear puzzling considering the low activity of XDH/XO in human muscle. However, in a subsequent study, in which subjects perfomed one legged knee-extensor exercise, it was demonstrated that the intensely exercised leg extracted urate from plasma, during the first few minutes of recovery [84]. The uptake did not appear to simply be due to an elevated plasma urate concentration as the resting leg did not extract urate. Thus, hypoxanthine released from the muscle may enter the muscle again as urate to replenish intracellular urate stores, oxidized by reactive oxygen species (Fig. 5). It may be speculated that the reason for urate formation occurring in the liver as opposed to the muscle is because a high activity of XDH/XO may be harmful to a tissue such as muscle, which is subjected to large alterations in metabolic demand.

4   XO AND TISSUE INJURY

4.1 Conversion of XDH to XO

In 1981 Granger and co-workers [6] demonstrated that treatment of feline intestine with superoxide dismutase prior to ischemia attenuated the extent of membrane leakage during the subsequent reperfusion phase, suggesting a role of the superoxide ion in causing tissue damage. These authors proposed that the ischemic phase caused a conversion of XDH to XO and a degradation of adenine nucleotides to hypoxanthine, hence, with the re-introduction of molecular oxygen during reperfusion, a burst of superoxide radicals would be formed in the XO catalyzed reaction [5,6] (Fig. 6). After these observations, an array of studies followed concerning conversion of XDH to XO in a variety of tissues such as lung tissue of rats [85] and rabbits [10], rat liver and kidney [86], canine heart [87],

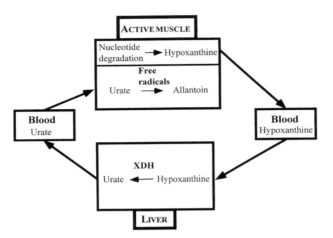

Fig. 5. Schematic representation of the metabolic circuit of hypoxanthine and urate during and after exercise. Strenuous exercise causes a release of hypoxanthine from the active muscle into the blood stream. Blood hypoxanthine is taken up by the liver where it is oxidized to urate via XDH. Urate is released from the liver into the blood stream and may be taken up by the previously active muscle for replenishment of muscle urate stores which have been depleted during exercise due to a free radical induced oxidation of urate to allantoin.

and skeletal muscle of dog [8,12], rat [88] and man [89]. Studies on the in vivo conversion of the dehydrogenase to the oxidase form show conflicting results. Several investigations have shown none or only a minor change in the proportion of XO to XDH during ischemia [17,90]. The magnitude of conversion appears to vary depending on the tissue investigated [5] and there may also be a species difference [35].

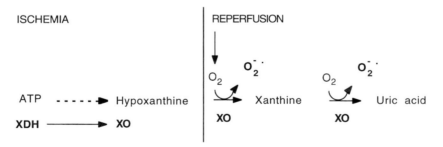

Fig. 6. Schematic representation of the theory proposed by Granger and co-workers [6] and Roy and McCord [5] on the mechanisms underlying XO induced radical formation during ischemia followed by reperfusion. Scheme modified from that of Granger et al. [6].

4.2 XO in ischemia/reperfusion-induced injury

The most abundant evidence for the role of XO in tissue injury stems from studies involving treatment of animals with XDH/XO inhibitors and free radical scavengers prior to ischemia. A frequently used inhibitor of XDH/XO is allopurinol, which is a purine analog that, after being metabolized to oxypurinol, forms a tight binding complex with the enzyme [14,91]. Pretreatment of animals with allopurinol has been shown to attenuate ischemia/reperfusion-induced damage in a variety of animal tissues [7,10,92—94] suggesting that XO may contribute to reoxygenation injury of tissue. Evidence for that radical formation is the mechanism by which XO causes damage during reperfusion has furthermore, been provided in studies which show both an attenuated free radical signal and reduced tissue injury in animals treated with XO inhibitors [11,95]. Generation of oxygen radicals by XO is also supported by findings of a similar effect of allopurinol and oxygen radical scavengers in reducing reperfusion injury [8,10,94].

Although most reports demonstrate a significant contribution by XO to re-oxygenation induced-damage, some investigators have suggested that XO is not involved in tissue damage, based on findings of no effect of allopurinol in preventing reperfusion injury. Kehrer et al. [96] found that rat hearts pretreated with allopurinol for 48 h and then perfused with the inhibitor after a 30 min period of hypoxia, did not prevent protein release from the tissue despite an almost complete inactivation of XDH. These authors also found infusion of the radical scavengers superoxide dismutase and catalase ineffective in protecting against tissue injury. Downey et al. [35] induced infarct in rabbit hearts and found that the infarct injured area was similar in allopurinol treated rabbits and in controls. However, treatment with superoxide dismutase significantly reduced the infarct area suggesting a source of superoxide radicals other than XO. In support of this observation, the authors were unable to detect any XDH activity in rabbit cardiac muscle [35]. The effect of allopurinol in reducing radical induced tissue injury could in part be due to the scavenging property of the inhibitor. It has been observed that allopurinol is only effective in reducing reperfusion damage at doses previously reported to be well over those required to inhibit XDH/XO [17,97]. Nevertheless, it does not appear as if the scavenging effect of allopurinol can fully explain the observations of attenuated damage and superoxide formation in ischemic tissue. Studies involving the use of the XDH/XO inhibitor oxypurinol, which only holds a weak scavenging property, have shown attenuation of tissue damage [98], as well as free radical generation [11] during ischemia and reperfusion. In addition, the extent of tissue injury after ischemia/reperfusion has been demonstrated to be markedly lower in animals fed tungsten than in control animals [85,86,99]. The tungsten molecule replaces molybdenum in the active site of XO and animals fed a diet supplemented with tungsten consequently get a pronounced reduction in XO activity [99,100].

5   THE ROLE OF XO IN EXERCISE ICNDUCED MUSCLE DAMAGE

There are two ways by which XO potentially could be involved in muscle damage induced by exercise. XO could initiate damage by causing lipid peroxidation of the cell membranes, with consequent cytosolic leakage, loss in cell viability and possibly tissue necrosis. This hypothesis would require that exercise induced a conversion of XDH to XO in the muscle and that a sufficient amount of hypoxanthine was available. Alternatively, XO may play a role first after damage to the muscle has occurred via other mechanisms such as mechanical disruption of the muscle fibres or radical attack through generation of reactive oxygen species from other sources. In the latter scenario, radical formation via XO may serve to mediate inflammatory processes. The below sections bring up some of the support for a role of XO as a generator of oxygen radicals in muscle during exercise.

5.1 Evidence for oxygen radical generation via XO in skeletal muscle

As mentioned earlier, the activity of XDH/XO in skeletal muscle is relatively low and the contribution of XO to free radical generation during metabolic stress has thus, been debated. In addition, Roy and McCord [5] reported that although the conversion of XDH to XO occurred during ischemia in most rat tissues tested they were unable to detect a change in the proportion of XO in ischemic skeletal muscle. Later investigations have, nevertheless, provided some evidence for that the conversion to XO can occur also in ischemic skeletal muscle and that the enzyme may participate in tissue damage. Lindsay et al. [101] showed that the proportion of XO in canine skeletal muscle increased from 10% to 35% with 5 hrs of ischemia. Similarly, Smith and co-workers [12] demonstrated that ischemic rat skeletal muscle had a significantly higher proportion of XO than non-ischemic muscle, 59% vs. 30%. XDH has been shown to be converted to XO also in human skeletal muscle. In human skeletal muscle subjected to ischemia at room temperature the activity of XO was found to increase, whereas keeping the tissue at low temperatures during the ischemic phase prevented the conversion [89].

Several studies have shown that inactivation of XDH/XO leads to a reduction in ischemia/reperfusion induced-muscle damage. Pretreatment of animals with either tungsten or oxypurinol has been found to result in a marked attenuation of the reperfusion induced increase in vascular permeability in the muscle [8,12,88]. Xanthine oxidase has also been found to contribute to lipid peroxidation [102,103], impaired contractile function [104], oxidative stress and edema [105] of rat skeletal muscle subjected to ischemia/reperfusion.

5.2 Generation of oxygen radicals via XO in muscle during exercise

Based on the numerous reports in the area of ischemia/reperfusion, it is reasonably clear that radical generation via XO may be a cause of tissue damage, including damage to skeletal muscle, during these conditions. It is also rather clear that exercise can induce generation of free radicals in skeletal muscle. The question may now be raised as to whether XO may be one of the sources of radical generation in muscle during exercise. High intensity exercise and, potentially, prolonged exhaustive exercise, subjects the active muscle to a marked level of metabolic stress and may lead to the two main conditions required for a major formation of radicals to occur via XO: a significant conversion of XDH to the oxidase form, and a greatly enhanced presence of hypoxanthine as substrate for the enzyme. However, to date little direct documentation exists for the role of XO in exercise induced-muscle damage. A limited number of studies have shown that free radical generation occurs in muscle of rodents during exercise [106,107]. XO has, furthermore, been demonstrated to be involved in exercise-induced oxidative stress, as assessed by a decrease in muscle glutathione levels, and morphological changes of exercised muscle in mice [108,109].

Although a proportion of XDH exists in the oxidase form in skeletal muscle it would appear that a conversion of XDH to XO would have to occur in the muscle during exercise to enable a large burst of superoxide radicals via XO. A transformation of the enzyme via activated calcium-dependent proteases would require a change in the intracellular calcium homeostasis. Studies on sprint running horses have shown disturbances of the sarcoplasmatic reticulum with consequent abnormal increases in intracellular calcium in the muscle [110]. Highly intensive exercise may also lead to local reductions in adenine nucleotides that possibly could lower the activity of the calcium pumps. However, in order for activated proteases in the muscle cells to act on XDH/XO localized in the vessel walls, the cell membrane would already have to be disrupted. Alternatively, a transformation to the oxidase form could arise via calcium-activated proteases within the vascular cells or through other mechanisms such as oxidation of free sulphydryl groups [20]. The latter mechanism could occur via oxygen radicals.

The other requirement for a marked generation of oxygen radicals via XO is a high concentration of the substrate hypoxanthine. The extent of hypoxanthine formation is related to the level of adenine nucleotide degradation and several studies have shown that intensive short-term exercise leads to a pronounced release of hypoxanthine into plasma [54]. Hypoxanthine does not accumulate to any great extent in human muscle during intense exercise but as the purine can diffuse through membranes, plasma also serves as a source of substrate for XO. This is especially true in light of the findings that exercise can induce an increase in the plasma XDH/XO level in horses [111] and rats [112].

In support of a role for XO in exercise-induced muscle damage are findings of morphological disturbances of capillary endothelium, one of the primary sites of XO, in muscle after long term endurance exercise [108,113]. Duarte and co-workers [100] found mitochondrial swelling in endothelial cells of muscle of control animals after 1 h of exhaustive running whereas animals treated with allopurinol showed no endothelial alterations. Moreover, human muscle that has been subjected to prolonged strenuous exercise [114] and rat muscle subjected to ischemia [115] show major increases of insulin like growth factor-I in the capillary endothelium implying regeneration of previously injured cells.

6   XO IN INFLAMMATORY PROCESSES

As stated in the beginning of this chapter, the only known physiological role of XDH is in the catabolism of purines. However, investigators have attempted to find a possible additional role of XDH that fits with the property of the enzyme to convert to an oxidase form. Several hypotheses have been suggested and among them is an involvement of XO in iron mobilization [116], and in regulation of vaso-tone [117]. A third possibility is that XO may function as a mediator in immunological events [13]. There are many reports in the literature that point at the latter function. It has been proposed that XO is involved in immunological processes through an influence of the enzyme on neutrophil attraction [13,118]. The authors of these studies suggested that superoxide radicals generated by XO activated a chemotactic factor that in turn attracted neutrophils. Later it was also found that neutrophils added to a culture of endothelial cells could cause the conversion of XDH to XO, possibly via cell to cell contact [119]. In a rat ischemia-reperfusion model of skeletal muscle it was observed that pretreatment with a xanthine oxidase inhibitor attenuated both muscle injury and vascular leukocyte adherence [120].

Treatment of mice with interferon and interferon precursors has been shown to elevate the activity of XO without an effect on the XDH/XO ratio, possibly suggesting an increase in protein [121]. In subsequent studies it was found that interferon induced an increase in the level of XDH mRNA in a variety of tissues [122]. An additional interesting observation was that, in contrast to most tissues, an interferon induced XDH mRNA expression in cultured fibroblastic cells was not accompanied by an elevation in enzyme activity [123]. This could indicate that the enzyme lies inactive in certain cell-types as suggested by Nishino [124]. The ratio of XO to XDH has also been found to increase in plasma of rats subjected to burn injury [125]. A similar effect on the XO activity in rat pulmonary artery endothelial cells was obtained by treatment with histamine, where it was observed that the activity of XO had increased 2- to 3-fold after 5 min of histamine exposure [125].

The level of XDH/XO protein has been examined in human skeletal muscle before and after prolonged strenuous exercise and it was found that the presence of XDH/XO, as assessed immunohistochemically, was higher in muscle microvasculature after the exercise [30]. The exercise appeared to have caused some damage to the muscle as the level of creatine kinase in plasma was markedly increased after the exercise. The study also showed an increase in the muscle content of hydroxyproline, a major protein of collagen, and of insulin like growth factor-(16F-1), suggesting that the tissue had gone through regeneration [115, 126−128]. In this context it is also of interest to note that reactive oxygen species have been found to stimulate the synthesis of IGF-1 [129]. To examine whether the increase in XDH/XO had occurred specifically due to muscle damage a follow-up study was conducted in which the subjects performed strictly eccentric exercise. Damage was evident by muscle soreness and markedly elevated plasma creatine kinase levels ($\approx$ 13,000 U/l). Forty-eight hours after exercise the number of xanthine oxidase positive cells, identified as capillary endothelial cells and infiltrating leukocytes, was 8-fold higher than before exercise [30]. Thus, it seems that exercise-induced muscle damage is associated with an increased amount of XDH/XO in the muscle.

The above findings do not reveal whether the increased presence of XDH/XO reflected an elevated expression of the enzyme in the muscle. Alternatively, the elevated enzyme level could be due to an attachment of XDH/XO to the surface of endothelial cells [130]. Studies have shown an increased activity of XO in plasma with a variety of clinical conditions such as adult respiratory distress syndrome [131], myocardial infarction [132,133], rheumatic diseases [134] and influenza [135], as well as with exercise [111,112] which suggests that there is a release or leakage of XO out into the blood stream. Thus, as shown by Adachi et al. [130], XO in plasma could bind to membranes of endothelial cells via a proteoglycan. A heparin reversible binding of XO to glycosaminoglycans on the surface of endothelial cells has also been demonstrated by Tan and co-workers [136].

There is good support in the literature for an inflammatory response subsequent to severe exercise [137]. Figure 7 shows a theoretical representation of the

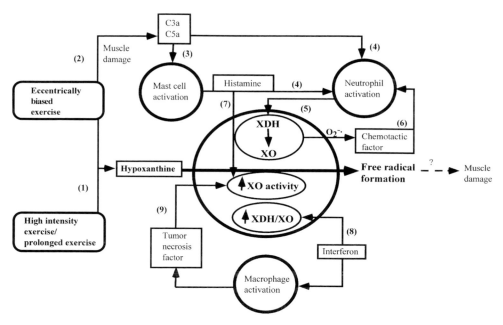

Fig. 7. A hypothetical schematic representation of an exercise initiated interaction between xanthine dehydrogenase/oxidase and various components of inflammation. The large circle represents an endothelial cell or a smooth muscle cell. For detailed description of Fig. 7, see text.

interaction between XO and inflammatory mediators and cells and how they may relate to exercise-induced muscle damage. The figure provides two possible initial causes of damage: metabolic stress with a decline in adenine nucleotide levels, an increase in hypoxanthine formation, and the possible conversion to XO through an increased level of intracellular calcium (1). This scheme of events would occur during exercise of very high intensity or towards the end of prolonged exercise where energy regeneration is limited due to low levels of glycogen. The second possible initiation of immunological events could be through rupture of the muscle fibers due to mechanical stress, which mainly occurs with eccentric exercise [138]. Eccentric exercise also leads to an increase in plasma hypoxanthine [30]. Tissue debris from disruption of the muscle fibers could activate the complement system through the alternative pathway with a consequent formation of the complement fragments C3a and C5a (2). The complement fragments can cause the release of histamine from mast cells (3), which together with the fragments cause the attraction of neutrophils (4). The neutrophils may then, as suggested by Phan et al. [119], cause the conversion of XDH to XO (5). In the scenario in which exercise-induced metabolic stress is theorized to initiate the conversion of XDH to XO, neutrophils may consequently be activated via a chemoattractant which has been activated by XO generated superoxide radicals (6) [13]. Histamine can directly affect the catalytic activity of XO (7) [125], which consequently would lead to an enhanced formation of harmful radicals, but histamine can also cause an increase in the permeability of the capillaries. These two effects could in part explain the observed protein release following some forms of strenuous exercise [see 139].

Macrophages are attracted to the site of injury by a macrophage chemotactic factor and activation can occur through γ-interferon. Interferon is, furthermore, an inducer of XO (8) [121]. The activated macrophages release interleukin-1 that activates neutrophils, with a subsequent potential escalation of radical damage but interleukin-1 can also induce an increase in the protective radical scavenger enzymes superoxide dismutase and catalase [140], thereby regulating the hazardous effect of a substantial generation of oxygen radicals. Tumor necrosis factor, released by macrophages, can cause an increase in circulating neutrophils and an enhanced catalytic activity of XO (9) [125]. Combined, the interaction between XO and the various immunological components could lead to a cascade of free radicals, which, potentially could overpower the well structured radical defense systems and thus, lead to tissue damage.

7 SUMMARY

1. Although studies on the distribution and activity of XDH/XO in tissues show inconsistent results, it is reasonable to conclude that the main localization of the enzyme is in the vascular cells of most tissues, including skeletal muscle, and that the activity of XDH/XO is low in skeletal muscle relative to several other tissues such as the liver.

2. During intensive exercise, and towards the end of long-term exercise to exhaustion, adenine nucleotides in the muscle are degraded to IMP of which a small proportion is further catabolized to hypoxanthine. Hypoxanthine formed in the muscle is in part released into the blood from where it may be taken up and oxidized to urate via XDH/XO in cells of the blood vessel walls of any tissue. The liver is a major site for urate formation after intense exercise in man, whereas the active muscle does not appear to release any measurable amounts of urate.

3. Muscle shows only a negligible uptake of hypoxanthine from plasma in recovery after exercise and, thus, a release of hypoxanthine from the muscle during exercise represents a loss of nucleotides. Lost nucleotides have to be replenished via de novo synthesis. If intense exercise is repeated frequently resting levels of adenine nucleotides in the exercised muscle decrease, which may render the muscle more susceptible to damage.

4. High intensity training reduces the loss of nucleotides from the muscle by an improved capacity to rephosphorylate hypoxanthine to IMP via the enzyme HPRT within the muscle and through an enhanced capacity for anaerobic energy generation.

5. During intensive exercise the concentration of urate decreases in the muscle and, in parallel, the oxidation product of urate, allantoin, increases. The muscle urate levels are probably replenished after exercise via an uptake of urate from plasma. These findings suggest that urate is utilized as a scavenger of radicals in the muscle.

6. A multitude of studies performed on different tissues and animals have shown that XDH is converted to XO during ischemia and that the enzyme is a significant contributor to reperfusion-induced tissue injury.

7. To date there is not much direct evidence for a role of XO in exercise-induced muscle damage. Nevertheless, exhaustive exercise leads to metabolic stress to the muscle and an extensive adenine nucleotide degradation. This metabolic state could lead to a conversion of XDH to XO in the blood vessel walls of the muscle, possibly through the action of proteases or through oxidation of free sulfhydryl groups. The catabolism of nucleotides in the active muscle also provides XO with a substantial amount of the substrate hypoxanthine.

8. Based on the many observations of an interaction of XO with several immunological factors and cells it is proposed that XO may be involved in inflammatory processes that occur subsequent to muscle damage and that may escalate the extent of injury.

8   PERSPECTIVES

Studies on the involvement of XO in free radical damage during ischemia/reperfusion show rather clear evidence that XO contributes to reperfusion injury in a variety of animal tissues including skeletal muscle. However, as there are some discrepancies between the metabolic conditions in the muscle during ischemia compared to during exercise, results from the ischemia/reperfusion model are not directly transferable to the exercise situation. Thus, in order to truly evaluate the role of xanthine oxidase as a source of reactive oxygen species in exercising skeletal muscle more evidence is needed from studies using exercise as a model, including studies on human subjects. Here, key questions that remain to be answered are, for example, whether and by what mechanisms a conversion of XDH to XO occurs in muscle during exercise and whether radical formation via XO is an important step in inflammatory processes in skeletal muscle.

9   ACKNOWLEDGEMENTS

Work cited by the author was supported by The Swedish Work Environment Fund, The Swedish Sports Research Council, Karolinska Institute and the Swedish Medical Research Council and the Danish Natural Research Foundation (Jnr 504–14).

10   ABBREVIATIONS

XDH: xanthine dehydrogenase
XO: xanthine oxidase
NAD^+:   nicotinamide adenine dinucleotide
FAD: flavin adenine dinucleotide
ATP: adenosine triphosphate
ADP: adenosine diphosphate
AMP: adenosine monophosphate
IMP: inosine monophosphate
INO: inosine
HX: hypoxanthine
X: xanthine
UA: urate
GTP: guanosine triphopshate
GDP: guanosine diphosphate
HPRT: hypoxanthine phosphorybosyl transferase
PRPP: phosphoribosyl pyrophosphate
R-1-P: ribose-1-Phosphate
P_i: inorganic phosphate

11   REFERENCES

1. Nathans GR, Hade EPK. Biochim Biophys Acta 1978;526:328–344.
2. Jarasch ED, Grund C, Bruder G, Heid HW, Keenan TW, Franke WW. Cell 1981;25:67–82.
3. Hellsten-Westing Y. Histochemistry 1993;100:215–222.
4. McCord JM, Fridovich I. J Biol Chem 1969;244:6049–6055.
5. Roy RS, McCord JM. In: RA Greenwald, G Cohen, (eds) Oxy Radicals and their Scavenger Systems, Cellular and Medical aspects, vol. 2, Elsevier New York 1983;145–153.

6. Granger DN, Rutili G, McCord JM. Gastroenterology 1981;81:22−29.
7. Parks DA, Granger DN. Am J Physiol 1983;245:G285−G289.
8. Korthuis RJ, Granger DN, Townsley MI, Taylor AE. Circ Res 1985;57:599−609.
9. Chambers DE, Parks DA, Patterson G, Roy R, McCord JM, Yoshida S, Parmley LF, Downey JM. J Molec Cell Cardiol 1985;17:15−152.
10. Kennedy TP, Rao NV, Hopkins C, Pennington L, Tolley E, Hoidal JR. J Clin Invest 1989;83: 1326−1335.
11. Thompson-Gorman SL, Zweier JL. J Biol Chem 1990;265:6656−6663.
12. Smith JK, Carden DL, Korthuis RJ. J Appl Physiol 1991;70:2003−2009.
13. McCord JM. Adv Free Radical Biol and Med 1986;2:325−345.
14. Hille R, Massey V. Pharmac Ther 1981;14:249−263.
15. Waud WR, Brady FO, Wiley RD, Rajagopalan KV. Arch Biochem Biophys 1975;169:695−701.
16. Parks DA, Williams TK, Beckman JS. Am J Physiol 1988;254:G768−G774.
17. Lindsay S, Liu T-H, Xu J, Marshall PA, Thompson JK, Parks DA, Freeman BA, Hsu CY, Beckman JS. Am J Physiol 1991;261:H2051−H2057.
18. Della Corte E, Stirpe F. Biochem J 1968;108:349−351.
19. Della Corte E, Stirpe F. FEBS letters 1968;2:83−84.
20. Della Corte E, Stirpe F. Biochem J 1972;126:739−745.
21. Clare DA, Blakestone BA, Swaisgood HE, Horton HR. Arch Biochem Biophys 1981;211: 44−47.
22. Waud WR, Rajagopalan KV. Arch Biochem Biophys 1976;172:354−364.
23. Batelli MG, Della Corte E, Stirpe E. Biochem J 1972;126:747−749.
24. Stark K, Seubert P, Lynch G, Baudry M. Biochem Biophys Res Comm 1989;165:858-864.
25. McIndoe WM, Wight PAL, MacKenzie GM. Histochem J 1974;6:339−345.
26. Auscher C, Amory N, Pasquier C, Delbarre F. Int Adv Exp Med Biol 1977;76A:605−609.
27. Sackler ML. J Histochem Cytochem 1966;14:326−333.
28. Kooij A, Frederiks WM, Gossrau R, Van Noorden CJF. J Histochem Cytochem 1991;39:87−93.
29. Räsänen LA, Karvonen U, Pösö AR. Biochem J 1993;292:639−641.
30. Hellsten Y, Frandsen U, Ørthenblad N, Sjödin B, Richter EA. J. Physiol. 1997;498.1:239−248.
31. Hellsten Y. Doctoral Thesis, Karolinska Institute, Stockholm, Sweden 1993.
32. Wajner M, RA Harkness. Biochim Biophys Acta 1989;991:79−84.
33. Nishino T. In: Curti D, Ronchi S, Zanetti S (eds) Flavins and flavoproteins. Proceeding X int symposium, Como Italy, G Walter de Gruyter Co Berlin 1990;885−894.
34. Watts RWE, Watts JEM, Seegmiller JE. J Lab Clin Med 1965;66:688−697.
35. Downey JM, Hearse DJ, Yellon DM. J Mol Cell Cardiol 1988;Suppl II 20:55−63.
36. Eddy LJ, Stewart JR, Jones HP, Engerson TD, McCord JM, Downey JM. Am J Physiol 1987; 253:H709−H711.
37. Krenitsky TA, Spector T, Hall WW. Arch Biochem Biophys 1986;247:108−119.
38. Cheetham M E, Boobis LH, Brooks S, Williams C. J Appl Physiol 1986;61:54−60.
39. Dudley GA, Terjung RL. Am J Physiol 1985;48:C37−C42.
40. Sahlin K, Palmskog G, Hultman E. Pflügers Arch 1978;374:193−198.
41. Tullson PC, Terjung RL. In: Holloszy JO (ed) Ex Sci Sports Rev, vol 19. Baltimore: Williams and Wilkins, 1991;507−537.
42. Jansson E, Dudley GA, Norman B, Tesch PA. Acta Physiol Scand 1990;139:147−152.
43. Bangsbo J, Graham T, Johansen L, Strange S, Christensen C, Saltin B. Am J Physiol 1992;263: R891−899.
44. Löwenstein JM. Physiol Rev 1972;52:382−414.
45. Jansson E, Dudley GA, Norman B, Tesch PA. Clin Physiol 1987;7:337−345.
46. Rubio R, Berne RM, Dobson JG. 1973. Am J Physiol 1973;225:938−953.
47. Hellsten Y, Frandsen U. J Physiol 1997;504,695−704.
48. Meyer RA, Terjung RL. Am J Physiol 1980;239:C32−C38.
49. Sabina RL, Swain JL, Olanow CW, Bradley WG, Fishbein WN, Dimauro S, Holmes EW. J Clin

Invest 1984;73:720—730.

50. Rubio R, Berne RM. Am J Physiol 1980;239:H721—H30.
51. Tullson PC, Bangsbo J, Hellsten Y, Richter EA. J Appl Physiol 1995;78:146—152.
52. Sahlin K, Ekberg K, Cizinsky S. Acta Physiol Scand 1991;142:275—281.
53. Bangsbo J, Hellsten-Westing Y, Sjödin B. Acta Physiol Scand 1992;146:549-550.
54. Hellsten-Westing Y, Ekblom B., Kaijser L, Sjödin B. Am J Physiol 1994;266:R81—R86.
55. Hellsten-Westing Y, Ekblom B, Sjödin B. Acta Physiol Scand 1989;137:341—345.
56. Sahlin K, Broberg S, Ren JM. Acta Physiol Scand 1989;136:193—198.
57. Löwenstein JM. Int J Sports Med 1990;11:S37—S46.
58. Katz A, Sahlin K, Henriksson J. Am J Physiol 1986;250:C834—C840.
59. Balsom PD, Ekblom B, Söderlund K, Sjödin B, Hultman E. Scand J Med Sci Sports 1993;3:
     143—149.
60. Harris RC, Söderlund K, Hultman E. Clin Sci 1992;83:367—374.
61. Rundell KW, Tullson PC, Terjung RL. Am J Physiol 1992;263:C294—299.
62. Rundell KE, Tullson PC, Terjung RL. Am J Physiol 1992;263:C287—C293.
63. Norman B, Sollevi A, Kaijser L, Jansson E. Clin Physiol 1987;7:503—510.
64. Spencer MK, Yan Z, Katz A. Am J Physiol 1992;262:C975—C979.
65. Hellsten-Westing Y, Sollevi A, Sjödin B. Eur J Appl Physiol 1991;62:380—384.
66. Arabadjis PG, Tullson P, Terjung RL. Am J Physiol 1993;254:C1246—C1251.
67. Idström JP, Soussi B, Elander A, Bylund-Fellenius AC. Am J Physiol 1990;258:H1668—H1673.
68. Edwards NL, Recker D, Fox IH. J Clin Invest 1979;63:922—930.
69. McCreanor GM, Harkness RA. Biochem Soc Trans 1987;15:1060.
70. Hultman E, Bergström J, McLennan Anderson N. Scand J Clin Lab Invest 1967;19:56—66.
71. Hellsten-Westing Y, Norman B, Balsom PD, Sjödin B. J Appl Physiol 1993;74:2523—2528.
72. Stathis CG, Febbraio MA, Carey MF, Snow RJ. J Appl Physiol 1994;76:1802—1809.
73. Hellsten-Westing Y, Balsom PD, Norman B, Sjödin B. Acta Physiol Scand 1993;149:405—412.
74. Simoneau J-A, Lortie G, Boulay MR, Marcotte M, Thibault MC, Bouchard C. J Appl Physiol
     1987;56:516—521.
75. Becker BF. Free Rad Biol Med 1993;14:615—631.
76. Ames BN, Cathcart R, Schwiers E, Hochstein P. Proc Nat Acad Sci USA 1981;78:6858—6862.
77. Smith RC, Lawing L. Arch Biochem Biophys 1983;223:166—172
78. Zhong Z, Lemasters JJ, Thurman RG. J Pharmacol Exp Therap 1989;250:470—475.
79. Becker BF, Reinholz N, Özçelic T, Leipert B, Gerlach E. Pflügers Arch 1989;415:127—135.
80. Wayner DDM, Burton GW, Ingold KU, Barclay LRC, Locke SJ. Biochim Biophys Acta 1987;
     924:408—419.
81. Maxwell SRJ, Jakeman P, Thomason H, Leguen C, Thorpe GHG. Free Rad Res Comms 1993;
     19:191—202.
82. Grootveld M, Halliwell B. Biochem J 1987;243:803—808.
83. Hellsten Y, Tullson PC, Richter EA, Bangsbo J. Free Rad Biol Med 1997;22:169—173.
84. Hellsten Y, Richter EA, Sjödin B, Bangsbo J. Am J Physiol 1998 (In press).
85. Waintrub ML, Terada LS, Beehler CJ, Anderson BO, Leff JA, Repine JE. J Appl Physiol 1990;
     68:1755—1757.
86. McKelvey TG, Höllwarth ME, Granger DN, Engerson TD, Landler U, Jones HP. Am J Physiol
     1988;254:G753—G760
87. Charlat ML, O'Neill PG, Egan JM, Abernethy DR, Michael LH, Myers ML, Roberts R, Bolli
     R. Am J Physiol 1987;252:H566—H577.
88. Sexton WL, Korthuis RJ, Laughlin MH. J Appl Physiol 1990;68:2329—2336.
89. Wilkins EG, Rees RS, Smith D, Cashmer B, Punch J, Till GO, Smith DJ. Annals Plastic Surg
     1993;31:60—65.
90. Bindoli A, Cavallini L, Rigobello MP, Coassin M, Di Lisa F. Free Rad Biol Chem 1988;4:
     163—167.
91. Elion GB, Kovensky A, Hitchings GH, Metz E, Rundles RW. Biochem Pharmacol 1966;15:

863—880.
92. Hansson R, Gustafsson B, Jonsson O, Lundstam S, Pettersson S, Scherstén T, Waldenström J. Transpl Proc 1982;14:51-58.
93. Stewart JR, Crute SL, Loughlin V, Hess ML, Greenfield LJ. J Thor Cardiovasc Surg 1985;90: 68—72.
94. Chambers DJ, Braimbridge MV, Hearse DJ. Ann Thorac Surg 1987;44:291—297.
95. Zweier JL, Flaherty JT, Weisfeldt ML. In: Gerutti et al. (eds) Oxy Radicals in Molecular Biology and Pathology, Liss Ar Inc, New York, 1988;365—383.
96. Kehrer JP, Piper HM, Sies H. Free Rad Res Commun 1987;3:69—78.
97. Betz AL, Randall J, Martz D. Am J Physiol 1991;260:H563—H568.
98. Zager RA, Gmur DJ. Am J Physiol 1989;257:F953—F958.
99. Linas SL, Whittenburg D, Repine JE. Am J Physiol 1990;258:F711—F716.
100. Smith JK, Grisham MB, Granger DN, Korthuis RJ. Am J Physiol 1989;256:H789—H793.
101. Lindsay TF, Liauw S, Romaschin AD, Walker PM. J Vasc Surg 1990;12:8—15.
102. Kawasaki S, Sugiyama S, Ishiguro N, Ozawa T, Miura T. Eur Surg Res 1993;25:129—136.
103. Asami A, Orii M, Shirasugi N, Yamazaki M, akiyama Y, Kitajima M. J Cardiovasc Surg 1996; 37:209—216.
104. McCutchan HJ, Schwappach JR, Enquist EG, Walden DL, Terada LS, Reiss OK, Leff JA, Repine JE. Am J Physiol 1990;258:H1415—H1419.
105. Appell HJ, Duarte JA, Gloeser S, Remiao F, Carvalho F, Basytos ML, Soares JMC. Arch Orth Trauma Surg 1997;116:101—105.
106. Davies KJA, Quintanilha AT, Brooks GA, Packer L. Biochem Biophys Res Commun 1982;107: 1198—1205.
107. Jackson MJ, Edwards RHT, Symons MCR. Biochem Biophys Acta 1985;847:185—190.
108. Duarte JAR, Appell HJ, Carvalho F, Bastos ML, Soares JMC. Int J Sports Med 1994;14: 440—443.
109. Duarte JA, Carvalho F, Bastos ML, Soares JMC, Appell HJ. Eur J Appl Physiol 1994;68: 48—53.
110. Byrd SK. Med Sci Sports Ex 1992;24:531—536.
111. Räsänen LA, Wiitanen PAS, Lilius EML, Hyyppä S, Pösö AR. Comp Biochem Physiol 1996; 114B:139—144
112 Radak Z, Asano K, Inoue M, Kizaki T, Oh-Ishi S, Suzuki K, Taniguchi N, Ohno H. J Appl Physiol 1995;79:129—135.
113. Crenshaw AG, Fridén J, Hargens AR, Lang GH, Thornell L-E. Acta Physiol Scand 1993;148: 187—198.
114. Hellsten Y, Hansson HA, Johanson L, Frandsen U, Sjödin B. Acta Physiol Scand 1996;157: 191—197
115. Jennische E, Skottner A, Hansson H-A. Acta Physiol Scand 1987;129:9—15.
116. Biemond P, Swaak AJG, Beindorff CM, Koster JF. Biochem J 1986;239:169—173.
117. Hong KW, Rhim BY, Lee WS, Jeong BR, Kim CD, Shin YW. Am J Physiol 1989;257: H1340—H1346.
118. Petrone WF, English DK, Wong K, McCord JM. Proc Natl Acad Sci 1980;77:1159—1163.
119. Phan SH, Gannon DE, Varani J, Ryan US, Ward PA. Am J Pathol 1989;134:1201—1211.
120. Suematsu M, Delano FA, Poole D, Engler RL., Miyasaka M, Zweifach BW, Scmid-Scoenbein GW. Lab Invest 1994;70:684—695.
121. Ghezzi P, Bianchi M, Mantovani A, Spreafico F, Salmona M. Biochem Biophys Res Commun 1984;119:44—149.
122. Terao M, Cazzaniga G, Ghezzi P, Bianchi M, Falciani F, Perani P, Garattini E. Biochem J 1992; 283:863—870
123. Falciani F, Ghezzi P, Terao M, Cazzanigi G, Garattini E. Biochem J 1992;285:1001—1008.
124. Nishino T, Usami C, Tsushima K. Proc Natl Acad Sci USA 1983;80:1826—1829.
125. Friedl HP, Till GO, Trentz O, Ward PA. Am J Pathol 1989;135:203—217.

126. Myllylä R, Salminen A, Peltonen L, Takala TES, Vihko V. Pflügers Arch 1986;427:78—90.
127. Edwall D, Schalling M, Jennische E, Norstedt G. Endocrinology 1989;124:820—825.
128. Jennische E. Acta Endocrinol 1989;121:733—738.
129 Delafontaine P, Ku L. Cardiovasc Res 1997;33:216—222
130. Adachi T, Fukushima T, Usami Y, Hirano K, Biochem J. 1993;289:523—527.
131. Grum CM, Ragsdale RA, Ketai LH, Simon RH. J Crit Care 1987;2:22—26.
132. Friedl HP, Smith DJ, Till GO, Thompson PD, Louia DS, Ward PA. Am J Pathol 1990;136: 491—495.
133. Yokoyama Y, Beckman JS, Beckman TK, Wheat JK, Cash TG, Freeman BA, Parks DA. Am J Physiol 1990;258:G564—G570.
134. Miesel R, Zuber M. Inflammation 1993;17:551—561.
135. Akaike T, Ando M, Oda T, Doi T, Ijiri S, Araki S, Maeda H. J Clin Invest 1990;85:739—745.
136. Tan S, Yokoyama Y, Dickens E, Cash TG, Freeman BA, Parks DA. Free Rad Biol Med 1993;15: 407—414.
137. Smith L. Med Sci Sports Ex 1991;23:542—551.
138. Fridén J, Lieber RL. Med Sci Sports Ex 1991;24:521—530.
139. Ebbeling CB, Clarkson PM. Sports Med 1989;7;207—234.
140. White CW, Ghezzi P, McMahon S, Dinarello CA, Repine JE. J Appl Physiol 1989;66: 1003—1007.

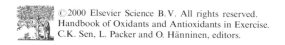

©2000 Elsevier Science B.V. All rights reserved.
Handbook of Oxidants and Antioxidants in Exercise.
C.K. Sen, L. Packer and O. Hänninen, editors.

Part III • Chapter 8

Acute phase immune responses in exercise

Joseph G. Cannon[1] and Jeffrey B. Blumberg[2]

[1] *Noll Physiological Research Center, Pennsylvania State University, Pennsylvania, USA*
[2] *Antioxidants Research Laboratory, USDA Human Nutrition Research Center on Aging, Tufts University, 711 Washington Street, Boston, Massachusetts 02111, USA. E-mail: blumberg@hnrc.tufts.edu*

1 INTRODUCTION
2 THE ACUTE PHASE RESPONSE
3 GENESIS OF THE ACUTE PHASE RESPONSE
4 OXYGEN RADICAL PRODUCTION BY LEUKOCYTES
5 ANTIOXIDANT MECHANISMS OF THE ACUTE PHASE RESPONSE
6 REACTIVE OXYGEN SPECIES IN THE ACUTE PHASE RESPONSE
7 EXERCISE-INDUCED ACUTE PHASE RESPONSE
8 EXERCISE-INDUCED CTOKINE PRODUCTION
9 THE ACUTE RESPONSE IN TRAINING ADAPTATIONS
10 THE ROLE OF ANTIOXIDANT VITAMINS IN LEUKOCYTE FUNCTION
11 POLYUNSATURATED FATTY ACIDS, ANTIOXIDANTS, AND IMMUNE RESPONSES
12 ECCENTRIC EXERCISE AS A TOOL FOR STUDYING AGE- AND NUTRITION-INDUCED CHANGES IN ACUTE PHASE RESPONSES
13 SUMMARY
14 PERSPECTIVES
15 ABBREVIATIONS
16 REFERENCES

1 INTRODUCTION

Oxygen consumption may rise several fold during physical exercise. Muscle damage is found after intense and/or exhaustive exercise even in highly trained athletes as assessed by a decrease in mitochondrial respiratory control, loss of structural integrity of sarcoplasmic reticulum, increased lipid peroxidation, and/or release of myoglobin and muscle enzymes into the circulation. The increase in oxidant stress following exercise is usually associated with a decline in antioxidant status, although careful training regimens can increase the activity of superoxide dismutase, catalase, and glutathione peroxidase. Long-duration or damaging exercise often initiates reactions that resemble the acute phase response to infection. Neutrophils are mobilized and activated within the first few hours of the response. These cells phagocytize pathogenic organisms and destroy them with oxygen free radicals and nonspecific proteases. However, inappropriate release of these agents can damage host tissues and may be the basis of noninfectious inflammatory diseases. Understanding the nature and role of the acute phase immune response during exercise may provide a rationale for optimal physical training regimens, dietary requirements of antioxidants for physically active people, and the prevention and treatment of noninfectious inflammatory diseases.

2   THE ACUTE PHASE RESPONSE

Infection and trauma induce a coordinated, invariant sequence of host responses that do not rely upon recognition of particular antigens, and involve a wide variety of tissues. In addition to the lymphoid/reticuloendothelial cells normally associated with host defense, cells of the central nervous system, liver, pancreas, kidney, and skeletal muscle are involved in bringing about major metabolic adjustments. Collectively, these nonspecific host defense responses are referred to as "the acute phase response".

The acute phase response includes fever, leukocytosis, redistribution of iron from extracellular to intracellular compartments, and accelerated hepatic production of certain plasma proteins. These are beneficial adaptations for the host: bacteria cannot grow well at elevated body temperatures, especially when the essential nutrient iron is not readily available [1]. Activated leukocytes phagocytize infectious microorganisms and acute phase plasma proteins such as C reactive protein opsonize (coat) bacteria and cellular debris in a manner that enhances phagocytosis [2]. Moreover, elaboration of reactive oxygen species by neutrophils and monocytes is a primary mechanism involved in destruction of invading pathogens [3].

The acute phase response is modulated and sustained through the action of protein mediators known as cytokines, notably interleukin (IL)-1, IL-6, and tumor necrosis factor (TNF) [4]. Infectious microorganisms and cellular fragments from damaged tissue directly stimulate blood monocytes or resident tissue macrophages to produce these cytokines. In addition, other host defense effectors such as the complement system and reactive oxygen species can modulate cytokine production.

The acute phase response can contribute to the production of reactive oxygen species during exercise, as well as during infection. This chapter presents the ways in which an acute phase response is generated and controlled during these events and how they can be modulated by nutrients. Furthermore, the acute phase response involves up-regulation of several processes that provide protection of host tissues from reactive oxygen species. These processes may be valuable adaptations of exercise training.

3   GENESIS OF THE ACUTE PHASE RESPONSE

Foreign pathogens or damaged cells trigger the proteolytic cleavage of circulating inactive precursors of the complement system [5]. When cleaved, these precursors become active proteolytic enzymes themselves that subsequently cleave other components of the complement system, resulting in a self-amplifying cascade [6]. Certain activated complement components have direct antibacterial activities, while others promote phagocytosis or draw leukocytes to the site of infection or injury (chemotaxis). The complement system is activated within minutes of an injury or infection.

The number of circulating neutrophils increases several-fold within a few hours of infection. This mobilization of neutrophils can be induced by certain microbial products, such as endotoxin, as well as endogenous factors such as cortisol [7] and activated complement [8]. These cells rapidly accumulate at the site of injury, drawn by bacterial toxins, complement components and cytokines. Neutrophils kill pathogens and clear cellular fragments through phago-cytosis and subsequent release of proteolytic enzymes and reactive oxygen species into the phagosome. Over a slightly longer time frame (days as opposed to hours) monocytes localize at the site of injury. These cells are also capable of phagocytosis, secretion of catabolic enzymes, and reactive oxygen species, as well as delivery of factors that promote repair and regeneration [9]. Of the three phagocytic cell types, neutrophils produce the greatest quantities of reactive oxygen species, monocytes produce intermediate amounts, and macrophages secrete the least [3].

The secretion of cytokines within the first few hours after injury or infection trigger increased hepatic synthesis of acute phase plasma proteins including α_1-antitrypsin, ceruloplasmin and C reactive protein. Due to the time necessary for de novo protein synthesis to occur, significantly higher concentrations of these proteins in the plasma may not be evident until 12 to 24 h later. Likewise, the sequestration of iron from extracellular fluids to intracellular stores depends in part upon de novo synthesis of binding proteins. Therefore, the fall of plasma iron follows a time course similar to the rise in acute phase plasma proteins. IL-1 or TNF will induce the full spectrum of the acute phase response when injected into laboratory animals or humans, through direct action on target cells or by inducing other cytokines such as IL-6 [10].

4   OXYGEN RADICAL PRODUCTION BY LEUKOCYTES

Neutrophils and monocytes generate an "oxidative burst" in response to receptor-mediated binding to various particulate or soluble factors (Table 1). The first step in this oxidative burst involves the assembly of protein subunits into the NADPH oxidase, a membrane-associated enzyme complex of the lysosome that

Table 1. Relative activity of reactive oxygen species in phagocytic cells.

Species	Catalyst	Compartment	Reduction potential (V)	2nd Order rate constant (m^{-1}s^{-1})
O^{2-}	NADPH oxidase	Membrane	−0.33 (at pH7)	$10^{-1}-10^2$
H^2O^2	—	—	1.776	—
HOCl	Myelo-peroxidase	Cytosolic granules	1.63 (at low pH)	—
·OH	Iron	Extracellular	2.7 (at low pH)	10^9-10^{10}

Reduction potential data obtained from [13–16].

catalyzes the transfer of electrons from NADPH to molecular oxygen, yielding superoxide anions [11]. Although superoxide has some cytotoxic activity of its own, it serves primarily as the precursor to other reactive oxygen species with far greater activity. Dismutation of superoxide yields antimicrobial hydrogen peroxide. Furthermore, in the presence of myelo-peroxidase, an enzyme stored in the azurophilic granules of neutrophils and cytoplasmic granules in monocytes, cytotoxic agents such as hypochlorous acid (bleach) are produced [12]. The relative differences in the oxidative activity of neutrophils, monocytes and macrophages mentioned earlier is paralleled by relative differences in cellular concentrations of myeloperoxidase [3].

Most of these cytotoxic reactive oxygen species are secreted into phagosomes, but some leakage occurs that can cause unwanted damage to "innocent bystander" host tissue in site of inflammation. Any reactive oxygen leakage into a tissue containing iron may be particularly damaging since iron catalyzes production of the highly active hydroxyl radical from superoxide and hydrogen peroxide [17]. Iron is rarely free in solution, but instead bound to various proteins (see below). The potential for iron to catalyze the formation of hydroxyl radicals depends upon the degree of saturation of these binding proteins [18].

Furthermore, reactive oxygen species can partially denature these binding proteins, thus, making the bound iron accessible to act as a catalyst [17].

5   ANTIOXIDANT MECHANISMS OF THE ACUTE PHASE RESPONSE

An integral part of the acute phase response involves production of antioxidant proteins that help limit the destruction of host tissue by reactive oxygen species (Table 2). For example systemic concentrations of ceruloplasmin, an oxygen radical scavenger, increase via IL-6-induced hepatic protein synthesis [10]. Intracellular concentrations of Mn-superoxide dismutase (SOD), metallothionein and catalase increase in response to IL-1 and TNF [19—21]. Furthermore, iron is redistributed, with a net increase in intracellular iron and net decrease in extracellular iron, thus, limiting the potential for hydroxyl radical formation.

The mechanism for iron redistribution involves changes in the expression of iron binding proteins [22]. Normally, macrophages (primarily in the liver) phagocytize senescent red blood cells and the iron contained in these cells is recycled

Table 2. Cytokine-mediated regulation of reactive oxygen species.

Cytokine	Action
IFN, TNF	Increases oxygen radical production
IL-1, TNF	Increases intracellular Mn-SOD, metallothionein, catalase
IL-6	Increases hepatic ceruloplasmin synthesis
IL-1	Promotes iron sequestration
IL-1	Induces nitric oxide synthase

to the major extracellular transport protein transferrin. However, during infection or inflammation, there is a rapid up-regulation of ferritin, the intracellular storage iron in hepatocytes and other cells, with a concurrent downregulation of hepatic production of transferrin [22]. The reciprocal changes in these iron-binding proteins appear to be regulated, at least in part by IL-1 [23,24]. In addition, neutrophils release lactoferrin which binds extracellular iron. The iron-lactoferrin complex is subsequently cleared from the extracellular space by macrophages. Iron-free lactoferrin, or lactoferrin at physiological levels of saturation ($\sim 20\%$), inhibit lipid peroxidation in an in vitro liposome preparation, whereas fully saturated lactoferrin has no inhibitory effect [18].

6   REACTIVE OXYGEN SPECIES IN THE ACUTE PHASE RESPONSE

In addition to their roles as effectors of pathogen killing, reactive oxygen species also modulate other effector mechanisms during an acute phase response (Table 3). Several proteolytic enzymes are stored in latent forms that are activated by reactive oxygen species [12]. Likewise, reactive oxygen species promote complement activation [25], as well as facilitate vascular translocation of leukocytes by inducing expression of adhesion molecules [26]. Superoxide anions have been shown to induce IL-1 bioactivity from isolated human mononuclear cells in vitro [27] and hydrogen peroxide enhanced lipopolysaccharide (LPS)-induced TNF production by murine peritoneal macrophages in vitro [28]. Furthermore, IL-1 upregulates inducible nitric oxide synthase in target cells [29] and the nitric oxide produced has been implicated in signal transduction pathways [30].

7   EXERCISE-INDUCED ACUTE PHASE RESPONSE

A sequence of events similar to an infection-induced acute phase response, but of smaller magnitude, occurs after various forms of exercise. A 2-fold increase in activated complement components has been observed in the circulation immediately after a 2.5-h run [31]. In another study, significant increases in activated complement components were observed in plasma following 45 mins of downhill running, an activity that involves damaging (eccentric) muscle actions [32]. It seems likely that activation of the complement system by exercise occurs via the so-called "alternative pathway" which can be stimulated by fragments of damaged tissue [5].

Table 3. Modulatory actions of reactive oxygen species.

Upregulation	Downregulation
Complement activation	Antiproteases
Proteolytic enzymes	
Leukocyte vascular translocation	
Cytokine production	

An increase in circulating leukocytes, primarily neutrophils, was documented as early as 1903 in a study of men completing the Boston marathon [33]. Leukocytosis was also observed after much shorter duration exercise, such as 5 mins of gymnastics [34] and 10 mins of running upstairs [35]. Transient increases after short-duration exercise may stem from epinephrine or hemodynamic shear forces that release neutrophils from their usual (marginated) location on blood vessel walls (especially lung vasculature). However, conflicting reports have been published regarding the influence of β-blockers on the increases observed immediately after exercise [36,37]. A study of supine vs. upright exercise showed that posture can influence the magnitude of leukocytosis, consistent with the hemodynamic shear hypothesis [38]. Longer-duration exercise causes more prolonged increases in circulating neutrophils that are more consistent with increases in cortisol or IL-1, both of which cause neutrophilia [4,7]. In recent cycle ergometry experiments, subjects were thermally clamped by immersion in water at specified temperatures [39]. Blocking the rise in core temperature in this way inhibited the increase in circulating neutrophils and eliminated the association with cortisol.

In addition, activated complement components promote neutrophilia [8]. Recent reports support the hypothesis that muscle damage and complement activation contribute to exercise-induced neutrophilia. Downhill running (involving damaging eccentric muscle actions) has been found to cause a greater increase in circulating neutrophils than uphill exercise at the same intensity [40]. Further, individuals exhibiting the greatest increases in complement activation have been noted to have the greatest increases in circulating neutrophils [32].

There is considerable evidence that neutrophils become activated during exercise (Table 4). Activation in vivo can be inferred through observations of elevated plasma concentrations of enzymes stored in neutrophil granules. In vitro, increased release of reactive oxygen species has been detected in cells isolated after exercise.

Based on muscle biopsies taken immediately after eccentric exercise, it is evident that neutrophils rapidly infiltrate damaged muscle tissue. Furthermore, the magnitude of infiltration is proportional to the extent of z-band damage [45]. Infusing technicium-labeled leukocytes into humans performing eccentric exercise indicated that the cells localized in the affected muscle, with significant accumulation at 24 h postexercise which was coincident with delayed onset muscle soreness [46]. Monocytes also accumulate in muscle tissue by 24 h following a marathon [47], and in other studies of damaging exercise in humans, several days elapse

Table 4. Evidence of exercise-induced neutrophil activation.

Increased superoxide production in vitro after downhill running [41]
Increased plasma elastase after a 10-km run [42]
Increased plasma lactoferrin after a triathlon [43]
Increased plasma myeloperoxidase after graded ergometer exercise [44]

Table 5. Repair factors from macrophages.

Factor	Function
PDGF, TFGß, bFGF	Modulate satellite cell proliferation, chemotaxis [51]
Fibronectin	Cell adhesion, extracellular matrix stabilization [52]
Proteoglycans	Cell adhesion, extracellular matrix stabilization [52]
IL-1	Fibroblast proliferation [53], collagen synthesis [54]

before significant numbers of monocytes are observed in muscle [48,49]. It is important to recognize that these cells appear after the damage has occurred. Rather than cause damage, the phagocytic actions of neutrophils, monocytes and macrophages appear to help promote clearance of damaged tissue. In rodent models of muscle damage [50], different subpopulations of macrophages have been identified during the early phagocytic stage compared to the later regenerative phase of muscle recovery. These observations suggest that specialized macrophage phenotypes carry out phagocytosis and others deliver growth regulatory factors. Robertson et al. [51] have shown that macrophages produce platelet-derived growth factor (PDGF), transforming growth factor β (TGFβ), and basic fibroblast growth factor (bFGF), all of which are chemotactic for muscle precursor cells, as well as stimuli for myogenic cell proliferation (Table 5).

8   EXERCISE-INDUCED CYTOKINE PRODUCTION

Since the first report noting circulating IL-1 activity after exercise in 1983 [55], additional studies have demonstrated increased IL-1 production in vitro by cells isolated after exercise [56], increased IL-1 localization in skeletal muscle [57], and increased IL-1 concentrations in urine [58]. These studies have been carried out with in vivo and in vitro bioassays, as well as immunoreactive detection systems. There is also evidence of increased IL-6 secretion [56] and elevated concentrations of IL-6 in plasma and urine after exercise [58]. The data indicating changes in TNF are more equivocal [56], in contrast to the dramatic changes in this cytokine observed after an infectious challenge [59]. Modest increases in plasma interferon activity have been reported as well [60].

Several mechanisms have been proposed for the cytokine appearance following exercise (Table 6). Increased IL-1 secretion and plasma concentrations have been detected after moderate cycling exercise involving little tissue damage [55],

Table 6. Potential factors influencing cytokine synthesis during exercise.

Inducers	Modulators
LPS from gastrointestinal tract	Epinephrine
Tissue fragments inducing phagocytosis	Cortisol
Lipid peroxides	Reactive oxygen species complement

as well as after eccentric exercise that causes extensive damage to muscle sarcomeres [61]. Therefore, tissue damage does not appear to be a requisite. Viti et al. [60] have suggested that skeletal muscle compression of lymphatic vessels increases drainage of cytokine-rich lymph into the vena cava. Humoral mechanisms have been studied in vitro to a limited extent. Both epinephrine and cortisol in physiological concentrations will augment basal IL-1 secretion, but in combination, these hormones have no net effect [62]. In a dynamic system in vivo, it is possible that rapid increases in plasma epinephrine up-regulate cytokine secretion and that more slowly increasing concentrations of cortisol eventually downregulate the response. Increased intestinal permeability during exercise [63] can allow entry of LPS from gut flora which is a direct stimulus for cytokine production. As discussed above, mononuclear cells can become primed for cytokine release by reactive oxygen species, and cytokine production is induced by lipid peroxidation products [64]. Recent findings indicate that post-exercise increases in IL-1 secretion are proportional to lipid peroxide levels and the time course of cytokine release may be further influenced by arachidonic acid levels [65]. Exercise-induced increases in oxidant stress arise from numerous sources, including mitochondrial superoxide production, ischaemia-reperfusion events, and auto-oxidation of catecholamines [66,67]. While most studies report an association between intense exercise and measures of oxidative stress, the literature is not entirely consistent in this regard [68,69].

9   THE ACUTE PHASE RESPONSE IN TRAINING ADAPTATIONS

Elevated IL-1 bioactivity (but not immunoactivity) in plasma [62] and elevated IL-1 immunoactivity in urine [58] have been reported in resting samples taken from highly trained individuals. Likewise, plasma iron levels are chronically lower [70] and acute phase plasma protein levels are chronically higher [71] in trained individuals. These changes may indicate the cumulative effects of repeated exercise-induced acute phase responses. Such cumulative effects would tend to enhance antioxidant capabilities and thus, training should tend to reduce susceptibility to reactive oxygen species produced via mitochondrial leakage.

10   THE ROLE OF ANTIOXIDANT VITAMINS IN LEUKOCYTE
FUNCTION

The antioxidant vitamins ascorbic acid and α-tocopherol have been found to play an important role in the ability of leukocytes to function normally. Vitamin C is found in large (millimolar) amounts in the cytosol of human neutrophils where it serves to preserve the cell's integrity and protect host tissues by acting as a reducing agent to neutralize the bactericidal products produced during the respiratory burst [72]. It is also possible that some cytosolic ascorbic acid may be secreted into the extracellular environment to reduce oxidants near the neutrophil surface. In experimental animals, vitamin C deficiency is associated with altered leukocyte morphology, diminished bactericidal activity of neutrophils and macrophages, and loss of chemotactic responses in vitro, even though phagocytic activity remains unchanged; addition of ascorbate to scorbutic animals reverses these indices [73]. It is relevant to note that degranulated leukocytes release ascorbate (and lactoferrin) that can chelate iron, an essential mineral for microorganisms. Neutrophils are responsive to intracellular vitamin deficiency and can make rapid adjustments via absorption of plasma ascorbate by both low- and high-affinity membrane transporters to correct it [74].

The vitamin E content of lymphocytes and mononuclear cells is approximately 10 times greater than that found in platelets and red blood cells [75]. When macrophages are exposed to oxidative stress, the vitamin E content of these cells is significantly reduced [76]. Vitamin E deficiency compromises neutrophil functions including directed cell movement and ingestion of C3b and IgG opsonized particles [77]. Boxer [78] has suggested that the membrane-associated NADPH-oxidase responsible for the generation of oxyradicals in vitamin E deficient neutrophils is situated in an abnormal lipid milieu which facilitates greater activation of the enzyme and generation of auto-toxic concentrations of hydrogen peroxide. This hypothesis is consistent with increases in metabolic activity and malonyl-dialdehyde formation in neutrophils with low concentration of α-tocopherol. On the other hand, large increases in vitamin E content of neutrophils achieved by high dose supplementation in healthy adults significantly enhance the phagocytic uptake of opsonized particles, although it may mildly reduce their bactericidal activity [79]. This observation may be due to a decreased release of hydrogen peroxide by vitamin E supplemented neutrophils which protects their membranes from oxidative damage and increases the efficiency of phagocytosis but reduces the peroxide-mediated attack on ingested microorganisms. However, this phenomenon does not appear to translate to impaired cellular immune responsiveness in vivo.

Several studies have confirmed that vitamin E is also a potent inhibitor of superoxide generation by activated neutrophils in vitro [80,81] and, when administered to healthy human volunteers, is associated with decreased generation of reactive oxidants by neutrophils ex vivo [82]. However, in these situations vitamin E may not act to scavenge either superoxide or hydrogen peroxide, but rather interferes with the activation of NADPH-oxidase in the neutrophil plasma membrane, indicating that this property of vitamin E may be unrelated to its classical antioxidant properties. Vitamin E-mediated inhibition of superoxide generation by activated phagocytes may be related to interference with transductional mechanisms involved in activation of NADPH-oxidase, perhaps via inhibiting the activation and translocation of cytosolic protein kinase C [83].

Various mechanisms have been proposed for the involvement of vitamins C and E in the maintenance of optimum immune responsiveness (Table 7). While each of these elements have been demonstrated to be relevant, they may be directly or indirectly modulated by an antioxidant-mediated neutralization of phagocyte-derived autoreactive, immuno-suppressive oxidants. As noted, these reactive oxi-

Table 7. Potential mechanisms of antioxidant vitamins in immune responsiveness.

Inhibition of protein kinase C and NADPH-oxidase activation [81]
Neutralization of immunosuppressive reactive oxidants [85]
Modulation of intracellular cyclic nucleotides [86]
Synthesis of immunoregulatory prostaglandins [87]
Protection of 5'lipoxygenase [88]
Enhancement of cytokine production [89]
Antagonism of immunosuppression by histamine [90]

dant species, particularly hydrogen peroxide and hypochlorous acid, inhibit chemotaxis, phagocytosis, and antimicrobial activity. Further, these compounds also inhibit the proliferation of bystander T- and B-lymphocytes, as well as natural killer cell activity [84]. Anderson et al. [85] have demonstrated that vitamin C can protect against the immunosuppressive effects of hypochlorous acid (but not hydrogen peroxide) in human neutrophils by preventing the inactivation of glyceraldehyde-3-phosphate dehydrogenase and ATP generation.

It is important to appreciate the apparent paradox in this relationship, i.e., the capacity of phagocytes to generate reactive oxidants is increased by challenges like bacterial infections and trauma but this increased oxidative activity can compromise host defenses through auto-oxidative inhibition of neutrophil functions and inhibition of the proliferation of lymphocytes and natural killer cells. Increased numbers and metabolic activity of neutrophils in individuals with infections or trauma are often accompanied by anergy and decreased levels of plasma and leukocyte ascorbate [91]. Consumption of vitamins C and E during neutrophil activation is due in part to their scavenging of reactive oxidants. Thus, the availability of these antioxidants at sites of vigorous phagocyte activity may be a determinant of local cellular immunocompetence. More globally, pre-race training status and racing intensity have been related to immunosuppression in athletes after competitive marathon events. Vitamin C supplementation has been shown to reduce the incidence of upper respiratory tract infection symptoms following competitive distance events, a benefit attributed to its inhibition of the auto-oxidative activity of phagocytes [92].

The role of other antioxidant compounds such as the bioflavonoids and carotenoids in acute phase immune responses are much less well characterized than vitamins C and E. However, Mobarhan et al. [93] have reported that supplementing healthy young men with β-carotene significantly lowered serum lipid peroxide levels but had no effect on neutrophil superoxide production stimulated by phorobol myristate acetate, formyl-methionyl-leucyl phenyl-alanine or opsonized zymosan.

11 POLYUNSATURATED FATTY ACIDS, ANTIOXIDANTS, AND IMMUNE RESPONSES

It is worth noting that changes in the intake and utilization of polyunsaturated fatty acids (PUFA) can affect immune responses in a fashion interdependent with antioxidant status [94]. For example, increased intakes of fish oil and other fats rich in eicosapentaenoic (EPA) and docosahexaenoic n-3 fatty acids have been demonstrated to decrease neutrophil chemotaxis and leukotriene (LT) B4 production in healthy volunteers [95] and in patients with asthma [96]. Increasing n-3 PUFA intake via diet or supplements is associated with a suppressed synthesis of IL-1α, IL-1β, IL-6 and TNF, possibly via decreased production of LTB4 and generation of the biologically less active metabolite LTB5 from EPA [97,98]. This effect is consistent with the decreased inflammatory responses reported in patients receiving n-3 PUFA supplementation and the lower incidence of inflammatory diseases such as asthma and type I diabetes mellitus in populations with high intakes of n-3 PUFA.

It is well established that the dietary requirement for α-tocopherol is dependent on the level of PUFA in the diet. More recently recognized is an appreciation of a delicate balance existing among the immunostimulatory, antiinflammatory, and immunosuppressive actions of n-3 fatty acids and vitamin E. For example, Virella et al. [99] observed a depression of neutrophil function and B cell responses following fish oil supplementation. On the other hand, Kremer et al. [100] reported that increasing vitamin E intakes restored fish oil-induced suppression of blastogenesis in mitogen-stimulated T lymphocytes. As noted above, Cannon et al. [65] found that alterations in elastase (reflecting in vivo neutrophil degranulation) and IL-1β secretion induced by eccentric exercise correlated with plasma fatty acids and lipid peroxidation following fish oil supplementation. Specifically, elastase responses correlated with plasma arachidonic acid/EPA ratios and exercise-induced changes in IL-1β correlated with urinary lipid peroxides and plasma arachidonic acid.

The potential mechanisms underlying this dynamic interrelationship between n-3 PUFA and vitamin E are unknown. However, the n-3 PUFA-induced suppression of immune responsiveness could potentially involve:
1) an elevated α-tocopherol requirement due to the peroxidative stress associated with increased PUFA intake;
2) an increased formation of EPA-derived eicosanoids such as prostaglandin (PG) E3 and LTB5 which are potentially more immunosuppressive than PGE2 and LTB4; and/or
3) changes in membrane composition which affect signal transduction pathways, e.g., in protein kinase C activation.

12 ECCENTRIC EXERCISE AS A TOOL FOR STUDYING AGE- AND NUTRITION- INDUCED CHANGES IN ACUTE PHASE RESPONSES

Eccentric exercise serves as a model which allows measurements before and after an endogenous in vivo inflammatory stress in humans. The relatively benign nature of the eccentric stress allows studies to be carried out in older people, thus, we are able to compare responses in older vs. younger subjects, as well as the influence of dietary factors [101]. Apparent aging effects on certain acute phase responses have been observed although many of these parameters can be modulated by dietary factors (Table 8).

Zerba et al. [102] have observed that muscle from senescent mice is more susceptible to injury and is damaged more severely by lengthening contractions than muscle from young and adult mice. Pre-treatment of old mice with polyethylene glycol-SOD provided immediate protection against injury. Thus, although the activity of antioxidant enzymes in muscle may increase with age, the ability of these enzymes to protect against oxidative injury may be inadequate to meet demands under conditions of oxidative stress [103].

Rates of lipid peroxidation, as well as antioxidant enzyme activities in skeletal muscle increase with advancing age [103]. However, the age-related accumulation of oxidized proteins in muscle suggests there is a relatively greater increase in pro-oxidant reactions than in antioxidant defenses. This imbalance may contribute to the reduced ability of the elderly to mount an acute phase response to muscle damage. As noted above, Cannon et al. [41,61] observed a greatly attenuated neutrophil and plasma creatine kinase (CK) responses in untrained older men (> 55 years) when compared to young men (< 30 years) during the 24-h period following 45 mins of downhill running; vitamin E supplementation significantly increased the postexercise rise in circulating neutrophils and CK activity in the older subjects to levels similar to those of the younger men. At the time of peak concentrations in the plasma, CK was significantly correlated with superoxide release from neutrophils. Urinary 3-methylhistidine excretion after the exercise

Table 8. Aging, nutrition and the acute phase response.

Acute phase reactant	Apparent aging effect	Nutritional effect
Complement	No change	Not affected [33]
Neutrophilia	Decreased	Vitamin E supplementation had no effect on the stress-induced neutrophilia of young subjects, but "restored" responses of older subjects [41]
Elastase	Decreased	Neutrophil degranulation, measured by plasma elastase levels, is related to plasma arachidonic acid/eicosapentaenoic acid (AA/EPA) ratios changed by fish oil supplementation [31]
Cytokine	No change	Lipid peroxide and AA levels are production correlated with cytokine production; dietary factors that change lipid peroxide and AA levels change cytokine production [61,65]

was correlated with mononuclear cell secretion of both IL-1β and PGE2. Moreover, increases in superoxide production by circulating neutrophils and in vitro endotoxin-induced IL-1 and TNF production by neutrophils were attenuated when subjects were supplemented with vitamin E. These data indicate that enhancing antioxidant status via vitamin E supplementation may affect the rate of repair of skeletal muscle following muscle damage and that these effects may be more pronounced in older subjects. The alterations observed in fatty acid composition, vitamin E, and lipid conjugated dienes in muscle and in urinary lipid peroxides after the eccentric exercise were consistent with the concept that vitamin E provides protection against exercise-induced oxidative injury [104].

The disruption of the contractile properties of human skeletal muscle following eccentric exercise-induced muscle damage also results in a substantial loss in maximal voluntary contraction and a selective loss of contractile force at low compared to high stimulation frequencies [105,106]. This selective low-frequency fatigue has been attributed to oxidative stress and free radical injury to the sarcoplasmic reticulum [107]. Thus, Jakeman and Maxwell [108] tested the effects of vitamins C and E supplementation on muscle function prior to an eccentric box-stepping exercise in physically active young people. They found a reduction in the loss of contractile function after the eccentric exercise and in the first 24 h of recovery in the group supplemented with vitamin C but not vitamin E; this protective effect was most evident with the low-frequency fatigue component (20/50 Hz tetanic tension).

Interestingly, recent studies of a more severe form of tissue injury, blunt trauma, suggest that the major mechanism involved in neutrophil dysfunction in these patients is the triggering of the complement cascade and release of complement-derived chemotactic factors, followed by inappropriate activation and subsequent deactivation of these cells [109]. These changes are associated with increased rates of auto-oxidation, declines in serum and neutrophil concentrations of vitamins C and E (but not glutathione), and loss of reducing capacity [110]. Employing a randomized clinical trial, Maderazo et al. [111] found that intravenous infusion of vitamins C and E to victims of serious blunt trauma (from motor vehicle accidents) significantly reverses neutrophil locomotory dysfunction.

13 SUMMARY

Heavy exercise, especially when muscle injury occurs, initiates an acute phase response that contributes to the breakdown and clearance of overloaded tissue. Following the exercise, the mobilization and activation of neutrophils appear to contribute to increased myocellular enzyme efflux. The acute phase reactions are unified by a common set of cytokine mediators including IL-1β, IL-6, and TNF which in turn influence some of their target tissues via induction of eicosanoids like PGE2. Importantly, these events are all modulated by peroxide tone and antioxidant defense status. The antioxidant vitamins C and E are consumed during acute phase immune reactions. A limited numuber of studies employing interventions with these vitamins have shown a beneficial impact on some aspects of the acute phase immune response, including improvements in neutrophil function.

14 PERSPECTIVES

The ability to modulate acute phase immune responses through nutritional means suggests new approaches to determining the fundamental role of the acute phase response in exercise. Despite several unsuccessful attempts to demonstrate a direct ergogenic effect of antioxidant nutrients, these compounds appear very important to the process of repair and recovery following intensive exercise. Thus, there may be a potential for increasing the intensity and/or frequency of physical training to improve performance following appropriate increases in antioxidant defenses as optimal physical performance capacity cannot be achieved without optimum cellular function. Further, as some data already suggests, information about the relationship between nutrition, exercise, and acute phase immune reactions may be directly applicable to the prevention and/or treatment of noninfectious inflammatory diseases such as rheumatoid arthritis and ankylosing spondylitis.

15 ABBREVIATIONS

AA: arachidonic acid
bFGF: basic fibroplast growth factor
CL: creatine kinase
EPA: eicosapentaenoic acid
IFN: interferon
IL-1:   interleukin-1
LPS: lipopolysaccharide
LT: leukotriene
PDGF: platelet-derived growth factor
PG: prostaglandin
PUFA: polyunsaturated fatty acids
SOD: superoxide dimutase
TGFβ: transforming growth factor β
TNF: tumor necrosis factor

16 REFERENCES

1. Kluger MJ, Rothenburg BA. Science 1979;203: 374–376.
2. Rees RF, Gewurz H, Siegel JN, Coon J et al. Clin Immunol Immunopath 1988;48:95–107.
3. Klebanoff SJ. In: Gallin JI, Goldstein IM, Snyderman R (eds) Inflammation: Basic Principles and Clinical Correlates. New York: Raven Press, 1992;541–588.
4. Dinarello CA, Cannon JG, Wolff SM. Rev Infect Dis 1988;10:168–189.
5. Gelfand JA, Donelan MB, Burke JF. Ann Surg 1983;198:58–62.

6. Muller-Eberhard HJ. In: Gallin JI, Goldstein IM, Snyderman R (eds) Inflammation: Basic Principles and Clinical Correlates. New York: Raven Press, 1992;33—61.
7. Dale DC, Fauci AS, Wolff SM. N Engl J Med 1974;291:1154—1158.
8. Rother K. Eur J Immunol 1972;2:550—558.
9. Massimino ML, Rapizzi E, Cantini M, Dalla Libera L et al. Biochem Biophys Res Comm 1997; 235:754—759.
10. Gauldie J, Baumann H. In: Kimball ES (ed) Cytokines and Inflammation. Boca Raton: CRC Press, 1991;275—305.
11. Roos D, Bolscher BGJM, Boer MD. In: van Furth R (ed) Mononuclear Phagocytes. Dordrecht: Kluwer Academic Publ, 1992;243—253.
12. Weiss SJ, Peppin G, Ortiz X, Ragsdale C, Test ST. Science 1985;227:747—749.
13. Bielski BHJ, Cabelli DE, Aurndi RV, Ross AB. J Phys Chem Ref Data 1985;14:1041—1092.
14. Buxton GV, Greenstock CL, Helman WP, Ross AB. J Phys Chem Ref Data 1988;17:513—531.
15. Drago RS. Principles of Chemistry. Boston: Allyn and Bacon, 1975.
16. Slater TF. In: Lachmann PJ, Peters DK, Rosen FS, Walport MJ (eds) Clinical Aspects of Immunology. Cambridge, Massachusetts: Blackwell Scientific Publications, 1993;377—393.
17. Halliwell B, Gutteridge JMC. Meth Enzymol 1990;186:1—85.
18. Gutteridge JMC, Paterson SK, Segal AW, Halliwell B. Biochem J 1981;199:259—261.
19. Karin M, Imbra RJ, Heguy A, Wong G. Molec Cell Biol 1985;5:2866—2869.
20. White CW, Ghezzi P, McMahon S, Dinarello CA, Repine JE. J Appl Physiol 1989;66: 1003—1007.
21. Wong GHW, Goeddel DV. Science 1988;242:941—944.
22. Weinberg ED. Phys Rev 1984;64:65—75.
23. Perlmutter DH, Dinarello CA, Punsal PI, Colten HR. J Clin Invest 1986;78:1334—1338.
24. Rogers JT, Bridges KR, Durmowicz, GP, Glass J et al. J Biol Chem 1990;265:14572—14578.
25. Shingu M, Nobunaga M. Am J Pathol 1984;117:35—40.
26. Patel KD, Zimmerman GA, Prescott SM, McEver RP et al. Cell Biol 1991;112:749—759.
27. Kasama T, Kobahashi K, Fukushima T, Tabata M et al. Clin Immunol Immunopathol 1989;53: 439—448.
28. Chaudhri G, Clark IA. J Immunol 1989;143:1290—1294.
29. Oddis CV, Simmons RL, Hattler BG, Finkel MS. Am J Physiol 1996;271:C429—C434.
30. Anggard E. Lancet 1994;343:1199—1206.
31. Dufaux B, Order U. Clin Chim Acta 1989;179:45—50.
32. Cannon JG, Fiatarone MA, Fielding RA, Evans WJ. J Appl Physiol 1994;76:2626—20.
33. Blake JB, Larrabee RC. Boston Med Surg J 1903;148:195—205.
34. Martin HE. J Physiol (London) 1932;75:113—129.
35. Steel CM, Evans J, Smith MA. Nature 1974;247:387—388.
36. Ahlborg B, Ahlborg G, Acta Med Scand 1970;187:241—246.
37. Foster NK, Martyn JB, Rangno RE, Hogg JC et al. J Appl Physiol 1986;61:2218—2223.
38. Muir AL, Cruz M, Martin BA, Thommasen H et al. J Appl Physiol 1984;57:711—719.
39. Cross MC, Radomski MW, VanHelder WP, Rhind SG et al. J Appl Physiol 1996;81:822—829.
40. Smith LL, McCammon M, Smith S, Chamness M et al. Eur J Appl Physiol 1989;58:833—837.
41. Cannon JG, Orencole SF, Fielding RA, Meydani M et al. Am J Physiol 1990;259: R1214—R1219.
42. Kokot K, Schaefer RM, Teschner M, Gilge U et al. Adv Exp Med Biol 1988;240:57—63.
43. Taylor C, Rogers G, Goodman C, Baynes RD et al. J Appl Physiol 1987;62:464—469.
44. Pincemail J, Camus G, Roesgen A, Dreezen E et al. Eur J Appl Physiol 1990;61:319—322.
45. Fielding RA, Manfredi TJ, Ding W, Fiatarone MA et al. Am J Physiol 1993;265:R166—R172.
46. MacIntyre DL, Reid WD, Lyster DM, Szasz IJ et al. J Appl Physiol 1996;80:1006—1013.
47. Hikida RS, Staron RS, Hagerman FC, Sherman WM et al. J Neuro Sci 1983;59:185—203.
48. Jones DA, Newham DJ, Round JM, Tolfree SEJ. J Physiol (London) 1986;75:435—448.
49. Round JM, Jones DA, Cambridge G. J Neurol Sci 1987;82:1—11.

50. St Pierre BA, Tidball JG. J Appl Physiol 1994;77:290—297.
51. Robertson TA, Maley AL, Grounds MD, Papadimitriou JM. Exper Cell Res 1993;207: 321—331.
52. Nathan CF. J Clin Invest 1987;79:319—326.
53. Schmidt JA, Mizel SB, Cohen D, Green I. J Immunol 1982;28:2177—2182.
54. Krane SM, Dayer JM, Simon LS, Byrne S. Collagen Res 1985;5:99—117.
55. Cannon JG, Kluger MJ, Science 1983;220:617—619.
56. Haahr PM, Pedersen BK, Fomsgaard A, Tvede N et al. Int J Sports Med 1991;12:223—227.
57. Cannon JG, Fielding RA, Fiatarone MA, Orencole SF et al. Am J Physiol 1989;257:R451—455.
58. Sprenger H, Jacobs C, Nain M, Gressner AM et al. Clin Immunol Immunopathol 1992;63: 188—195.
59. Cannon JG, Tompkins RG, Gelfand JA, Michie HR et al. J Infect Dis 1990;161:79—84.
60. Viti A, Muscettola M, Paulesa L, Bocci V et al. J Appl Physiol 1985;59:426—428.
61. Cannon JG, Meydani SN, Fielding RA, Fiatarone MA et al. Am J Physiol 1991;260: R1235—R1240.
62. Cannon JG, Evans WJ, Hughes VA, Meredith CN et al. J Appl Physiol 1986;61:1869—1874.
63. Pals KL, Change RT, Ryan AJ, Gisolfi CV. J Appl Physiol 1997;82:571—576.
64. Ku G, Thomas CE, Akeson AL, Jackson RL. J Biol Chem 1992;267:14183—14188.
65. Cannon JG, Fiatarone MA, Meydani M, Gong J-X et al. Am J Physiol (In press).
66. Packer L. J Sports Sci 1997;15:353—363.
67. Karlsson J. World Rev Nutr Diet 1997;82:81—100.
68. Leaf DA, Kleinman MT, Hamilton M, Barstow TJ. Med Sci Sports Exercise 1997;29:1036—1039.
69. Margaritis I, Tessier F, Richard MJ, Marconnet P. Int J Sports Med 1997;18:186—190.
70. Magnusson B, Hallberg L, Rossander L, Swolin B. Acta Med Scand 1984;216:157—164.
71. Liesen H, Dufaux B, Hollmann W. Eur J Appl Physiol 1977;37:243—254.
72. Anderson R, Theron AJ, Ras GJ. Am Rev Resp Dis 1987;135:1027—1032.
73. Goldschmidt MC. Am J Clin Nutr 1991;54:1214S—1220S.
74. Bergsten P, Amitai G, Kehrl J, Dhariwal RK et al. J Biol Chem 1990;265:2584—2587.
75. Bendich A. Adv Exp Med Biol 1990;262:35—55.
76. Coquette A, Vray B, Vanderpas J. Arch Int Physiol Biochem 1986;94:S29—S34.
77. Harris RE, Boxer LA, Baehner RL. Blood 1980;55:338—341.
78. Boxer LA. Adv Exp Med Biol 1990;262:19—33.
79. Baehner RL, Boxer LA, Allen JM, Davis J. Blood 1977;50:327—331.
80. Engle WA, Yoder MC, Baurley JL, Yu PL. Pediatr Res 1988;23:245—248.
81. Anderson R, Theron AJ, Myer MS, Richards GA et al. J Nutr Immunol 1992;1:43—63.
82. Baehner RL, Boxer LA, Ingraham LM, Butterick et al. Ann NY Acad Sci 1982;293:237—250.
83. Azzi A, Boscoboinik, Szewczwyk A. Arch Biochem Biophys 1991;286:264—269.
84. El-Hag A, Clark RA. J Immunol 1987;139:2406—2413.
85. Anderson R, Smit MJ, Joone GK, Van Staden AM. Ann NY Acad Sci 1990;587:3448.
86. Esposito AL. Am Rev Resp Dis 1986;133:643—647.
87. Meydani SN, Barklund PM, Liu S, Meydani M et al. Am J Clin Nutr 1990;52:557—563.
88. Steinhilber D, Moser U, Roth HJ, Schmidt KH. Ann NY Acad Sci 1987;498:522—524.
89. Siegel BV, Leibovitz B. Int J Vit Nutr Res 1982;23(Suppl):9—22.
90. Johnston CS, Martin LJ, Cai X. Am Coll Nutr 1992;11:172—176.
91. Maderazo EG, Woronick CL, Albano SD, Breaux SP et al. J Infect Dis 1986;154:471—477.
92. Peters EM. Internatl J Sports Med 1997;18:S69—S77.
93. Mobarhan S, Bowen P, Andersen, Evans M et al. Nutr Cancer 1990;14:195—206.
94. Blumberg JB. Clin Appl Nutr 1991;1:53—61.
95. Lee TH, Hoover RI, Williams JD, Ravalese J et al. N Engl J Med 1985;312:1217—1224.
96. Payan DG, Wong MY, Chernov—Rogan T, Valone FH et al. J Clin Immunol 1986;6:402—410.
97. Endres S, Ghorbani BS, Kelley VE, Georgilis K et al. N Engl J Med 1989;320:265—271.

98. Meydani SN, Endres S, Woods MN, Goldin RD et al. J Nutr 1991;121:546—555.
99. Virella G, Kilpatrick JM, Rugeles MT, Hyman B et al. Clin Immun Immunopathol 1989;52: 257—270.
100. Kremer JR, Schoene N, Dougless LW, Judd JT et al. Am J Clin Nutr 1991;54:896—902.
101. Fielding RA, Meydani M. Aging 1997;9:12—18.
102. Zerba E, Komorowski TE, Faulkner JA. Am J Physiol 1990;258:C429—C435.
103. Oliver CN, Ahn B, Moerman EJ, Goldstein S et al. J Biol. Chem 1987;262:5488—5491.
104. Meydani M, Evans WJ, Handleman G, Biddle L et al. Am J Physiol 1993;264:R992—R998.
105. Newham DJ, Jones DA, Clarkson PM. J Appl Physiol 1987;63:1381—1386.
106. Evans WJ, Cannon JG. Exerc Sport Sci Rev 1991;19:99—125.
107. Byrd SK. Med Sci Sports Exerc 1992;24:531—536.
108. Jakeman P, Maxwell S. Eur J Appl Physiol 1993;67:426—430.
109. Maderazo EG, Woronick CL, Albano SD, Breaux SP et al. J Infect Dis 1986;154:471—477.
110. Maderazo EF, Woronick CL, Hickingbotham N, Mercier E et al. Crit Care Med 1990;18: 141—147.
111. Maderazo EG, Woronick CL, Hickingbotham N, Jacobs L et al. J Trauma 1991;31:1142.

©2000 Elsevier Science B.V. All rights reserved.
Handbook of Oxidants and Antioxidants in Exercise.
C.K. Sen, L. Packer and O. Hänninen, editors.

Part III • Chapter 9

Oxidative DNA damage in exercise

Andreas Hartmann[1] and Andreas M. Niess[2]

[1] *Andreas Hartmann, Novartis Pharma AG, Genetic Toxicology, WS2881.5.14 CH-4002 Basel, Switzerland*

[2] *Andreas M. Niess, Medical Clinic and Polyclinic, Department of Sports Medicine, University of Tuebingen, Hoelderlinstr. 11, D-72074 Tuebingen, Germany. E-mail: andreas.niess@uni-tuebingen.de*

1 INTRODUCTION
2 DNA: CARRIER OF GENETIC INFORMATION
3 OXIDATIVE DNA DAMAGE
4 DNA DAMAGE AFTER EXERCISE
    4.1 Exercise-induced damage in cellular DNA
    4.2 Analysis of oxidized bases in cellular DNA
    4.3 Urinary excretion of oxidized DNA bases and nucleosides
    4.4 Cytogenetic methods
    4.5 Exercise-induced apoptosis: Secondary induction of DNA fragmentation
5 FREE RADICAL GENERATION IN EXERCISE: POTENTIAL MECHANISMS FOR DNA DAMAGE INDUCTION
    5.1 Generation of radicals during exercise
    5.2 Generation of radicals after exercise: inflammatory processes
6 BIOLOGICAL SIGNIFICANCE OF EXERCISE-INDUCED DNA DAMAGE: EPIDEMIOLOGICAL EVALUATION
7 SUMMARY
8 PERSPECTIVES
9 ACKNOWLEDGEMENTS
10 ABBREVIATIONS
11 REFERENCES

1   INTRODUCTION

Oxidative stress due to vigorous exercise is a well-described phenomenon. In living cells, reactive oxygen species are formed continuously and physical exercise leads to an increased generation of radicals. Free radicals are also generated as part of the reparative process following muscular injury. If not adequately removed by antioxidant defenses, free radicals react with membranes, proteins, nucleic acids, and other cellular components to initiate cellular damage or degeneration. Indicators of free radical damage, such as oxidized proteins and products of lipid peroxidation have been widely described. Recent reports provide evidence that certain regimens of physical exercise are also capable of inducing DNA modifications. Induction of DNA damage after excessive exercise was described, whereas moderate exercise was shown to have no effects on cellular DNA. Antioxidants, as well as regular training seem to have a protective effect against the occurrence of DNA damage after exercise and the involvement of oxidative stress as one underlying mechanism was proposed. Further evidence for oxidative stress as one underlying mechanism was provided by demonstrating a concomitant increase of heat shock proteins in leukocytes. The induction of structural DNA alterations by exposure to reactive oxygen species is of great interest since such modifications seem to play a key role in human cancer development. However, the relationship between oxidative stress due to vigorous exercise and induction of DNA modifications is unknown and their long-term effects on health have yet to be elucidated. The aim of this chapter is to provide insight into the relatively new field of exercise-induced DNA damage, the techniques used to detect this specific damage, and the biological significance of these findings.

2   DNA: CARRIER OF GENETIC INFORMATION

All living organisms, prokaryotes and eukaryotes, are composed of cells. The genetic information of cells is encoded in their deoxyribonucleic acid (DNA). Nucleic acids are macromolecules assembled from nucleotides. The sequence in which the individual blocks are joined together is the critical factor that determines the property of the resulting macromolecule. The maintenance of the exact structure is important for both, cellular metabolism and passing the correct information from one generation to the next. The unit of inheritance is called a gene and each gene constitutes a specific sequence of DNA that carries the information representing a particular protein. Genes are carried on chromosomes and the set of genes of a particular organism is called a genome.

   Genetic material is subjected to a number of stresses including oxidative damage and damage due to environmental mutagens/carcinogens. These agents induce structural alterations in DNA such as modified bases or chromosome breaks. The alterations induced have a certain probability of remaining damaged or being misrepaired. When a cell divides, such damage may manifest in changes in the DNA sequence, a mutation. The sequence of bases in the polynucleotide chain is important not in a sense of structure per se, but because it codes for the sequence of amino acids that constitutes the corresponding protein. Therefore, mutations may result in dysfunctional proteins but may not affect the maintenance of DNA itself. Certain proteins are important for the regulation and control of the cell cycle and before a cell can become malignant, disturbance of homeostasis in a number of cellular systems is necessary. Neoplastic expansion of a mutated cell may result from activation of stimulatory mechanisms or the inactivation of inhibitory mechanisms. It is assumed that dynamic processes and several genetic changes are required before a normal cell can become tumorigenic [1]. However, DNA is continuously damaged by oxidative reactions and DNA damage induced by endogenous mechanisms is high [2,3].

   Cells are able to respond to DNA damage with a variety of repair mechanisms to restore DNA structure and sequence. Oxidative DNA damage can be repaired by excising damage bases or nucleotides. Deficiencies in DNA repair systems may lead to the accumulation of genetic changes and can have deleterious effects on organisms. Several human hereditary diseases are known which are caused by mutations in DNA repair genes or genes involved in eliminating reactive oxygen species [4]. The rare human disease Xeroderma Pigmentosum is caused by a defect in nucleotide excision repair and is characterized by photodermatoses including skin cancer at an early age [5]. The importance of an intact defense system against reactive oxygen species is further underscored by another rare genetic disease, Amyotrophic Lateral Sclerosis. Some of the familial forms are associated with mutations in Cu/Zn-superoxide dismutase which are accounted for the accumulation of reactive oxygen species with catastrophic effects on motor neurons [6].

3   OXIDATIVE DNA DAMAGE

Oxygen is the terminal oxidant for respiration and other oxidative reactions in aerobic organisms. Some reactive oxygen species have important physiological functions, but also represent a source of endogenous damage to the genome. It is generally accepted that a certain amount of oxidative DNA damage occurs in animals and humans. Ames and colleagues [7] estimated that each liver cell from adult rats contain 10^6 oxidative lesions and that 10^5 new lesions are added daily. Cells possess mechanisms to minimize, but not necessarily eliminate, the effects of normal levels of oxidative damage. Oxidized DNA is abundant in human tissues and it is suggested that damaged DNA bases accumulate with age [7,8]. A relationship between oxidative modification of mitochondrial DNA and the process of aging has emerged [9]. Subjecting tissue to oxidative stress, and thereby overwhelming the antioxidative capacity of a cell can result in severe metabolic dysfunctions [2,10], including un- or misrepaired DNA lesions as demonstrated in Fig. 1. Different types of oxidative DNA damage are known

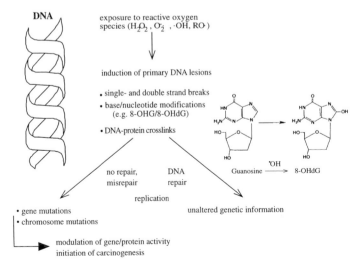

Fig. 1. DNA damage induced by reactive oxygen species and their biological consequences.

such as base lesions, sugar lesions, single- and double-strand breaks, abasic sites, and DNA-protein crosslinks. The oxidized desoxynucleoside 8-hydroxy-7,8-dihydro2'-deoxyguanosine (8-OHdG) is of special interest. Due to its mispairing properties it has been suggested that it is directly involved in the process of carcinogenesis [11,12]. The cell is able to rapidly remove this DNA lesion from nuclear DNA and from the nucleotide pool by different repair mechanisms. This might explain, why elevated levels of activated endogenous oxygen species are rather inefficient at inducing gene mutations, but tend to generate gross chromosomal rearrangements [13]. The carcinogenic impact of oxygen radicals may be based on oncogene activation or suppressorgene inactivation through chromosomal rearrangements. Furthermore, oxygen radicals may induce genotoxic effects by indirect mechanisms leading to the formation of chromosome breaking agents (clastogenic factors) [14].

Besides its key role in human cancer development, oxidative DNA damage also seems to be of causal importance in various other disease processes. It has been suggested that damage to mitochondrial DNA is related to age-associated degenerative diseases. Mitochondrial DNA (mtDNA) is a major source and target site of reactive oxygen species. An accumulating rate of mtDNA mutations as a result of oxidative DNA damage will result in deficient mitochondrial respiratory function which, in turn, leads to cellular energy deficit [9,15]. Mounting evidence suggests that mitochondrial dysfunction and oxidative stress contribute to the pathogenesis in several neuro-degenerative diseases such as Parkinson disease, Amyotrophic Lateral Sclerosis, Alzheimer disease and Huntington disease [16]. An elevated content of 8-OHdG in mtDNA extracted from cerebrums and cerebellums [17], as well as increased levels of other oxidized DNA bases in different brain areas [18] have been shown in patients with Alzheimer disease. However, it remains unclear whether oxidative DNA damage is a primary or secondary event in this disease. Furthermore, other energy-requiring postmitotic tissues such as skeletal and heart muscle also seem to be sites in which mutations of mtDNA are associated with chronic degenerative diseases [15]. Measurements of an accumulated content of 8-OHdG in human heart mitochondria with age confirms the assumption that oxidative damage to mitochondrial DNA may be involved in failure of the aging heart [19,20].

Induction of DNA damage is measured using a variety of techniques. Primary DNA lesions induced by free radicals such as strand breaks, abasic sites, and DNA-protein crosslinks are determined with biochemical methods. These methods allow the detection of DNA strand breaks and DNA adducts with high sensitivity. However, primary DNA lesions are usually repaired by repair enzymes with high efficiency and for the assessment of the biological significance of DNA damage, cytogenetic techniques and mutation assays are employed. These methods allow the detection of DNA lesions which remained unrepaired or misrepaired and were transformed into chromosome modifications or mutations during cell proliferation [21].

4   DNA DAMAGE AFTER EXERCISE

Only recently, an increasing number of studies demonstrated the induction of DNA modifications in human subjects as a consequence of exhaustive exercise. Oxidative stress has been discussed as a mechanism causing these effects. In principle, three different endpoints were used to investigate exercise-induced DNA damage:

1. Analysis of the steady-state level of DNA alterations as an indicator of the balance between damage (analysis of primary DNA lesions) and repair. This analysis was performed in DNA from peripheral leukocytes or lymphocytes which are well-established indicators of exposure to DNA damaging agents in human biomonitoring studies [21].
2. An index of the total oxidative DNA damage which has been repaired. This is provided by analysis of DNA base damage products excreted in the urine.
3. Analysis of exercise-induced chromosome alterations.

The following overview provides an insight into the techniques and endpoints used to assess exercise-induced DNA damage and discusses differences in the findings. Figure 2 summarizes the techniques used to measure DNA damage after exercise.

4.1 Exercise-induced damage of cellular DNA

DNA lesions such as strand breaks, abasic sites, and DNA-protein crosslinks are measured with biochemical methods. In the majority of the studies reported so far, the comet assay (single-cell gel test) was used to demonstrate elevated DNA breaks in leukocytes of human subjects after exercise. The comet assay is a microgel electrophoresis technique which enables the detection of DNA damage and

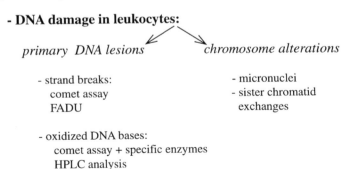

- DNA damage in leukocytes:

primary DNA lesions   *chromosome alterations*

- strand breaks: - micronuclei
  comet assay   - sister chromatid
  FADU   exchanges

- oxidized DNA bases:
  comet assay + specific enzymes
  HPLC analysis

- oxidized DNA bases
HPLC-analysis of urinary excretion of 8-OHdG and 8-OHG

Fig. 2. Techniques used to demonstrate exercise-induced DNA damage. FADU, fluorescence analysis of DNA unwinding; 8-HdG, 8-hydroxy guanosine; 8-OHG, 8-hydroxy guanine.

DNA repair in individual cells with high sensitivity [22]. This technique has wide-spread potential applications and is becoming an established tool in biomonitor-ing studies, as well as in genotoxicity testing [23]. Detailed protocols for the assay have been described [24]. In brief, a single-cell suspension (e.g., whole blood or isolated lymphocytes) is dispersed in agarose and spread on a microscope slide. Then, the cells are lysed with high salt and detergents, alkali-denatured and elec-trophoresed. After staining, the microscopic image of cells with increased DNA damage displays increased migration of chromosomal DNA out of the nucleus, resembling the shape of a comet. The amount of DNA migration indicates the amount of DNA breakage in the cell. Unlike other methods, results of the comet assay are believed not to be confounded by dead cells, which might have under-gone programmed cell death (apoptosis, see below) or necrosis [25]. Using the comet assay, various exercise protocols have been studied, such as incremental runs to exhaustion on a treadmill [26–28], half marathons [29,30], triathlon competitions [31] or repeated bouts of anaerobic runs (Zankl, personal com-munication). The results with the comet assay unequivocally show the induction of DNA damage in human leukocytes independent of the exercise protocols used. In all studies, DNA damage was detected with a delay of several hours after the exercise. Interestingly, the exercise protocol used seems to have an influence on the induction of DNA damage. Figure 3 compares the effects of an single bout of exhaustive exercise on the treadmill with the occurrence of DNA damage after a triathlon competition. After a run on a treadmill, the highest increase in DNA damage was found 24 h postexercise, whereas after the triathlon, an addi-tional and very strong increase in DNA damage was found 72 h after the race. The results indicate that the exercise protocol used has an important influence

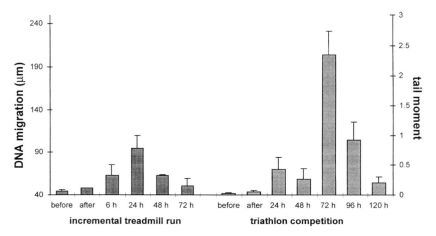

Fig.3. DNA damage in leukocytes of humans measured as increased DNA migration, (mean and SEM of 50 cells per data point), in the comet assay. a: DNA damage after a run on a treadmill (n = 3); b: DNA damage after a triathlon competition (n = 6). Reprinted with the permission of Oxford University Press 26] and also with permission from Elsevier Sciences Inc [31].

on occurrence and persistence of DNA damage. It should be stressed that the treadmill run was performed by untrained individuals, whereas the triathlon was done by well-trained athletes. Another study described a difference in the extent of DNA damage induced in trained vs. untrained individuals. The results of a comparative study on trained and untrained individuals after a treadmill run are shown in Fig. 4.

In most of the studies discussed above, either whole leukocytes or isolated lymphocytes were analyzed. One investigation studied DNA damage in ten trained individuals after a half marathon and a differential analysis was performed with leukocytes and separated mononuclear cells [30]. It was shown that the percentage of damaged cells 24 h after the race was higher in total leukocytes than in mononuclear cells (Fig. 5). The authors concluded that the exercise protocol used induces DNA damage primarily in granulocytes. This might also explain negative or equivocal findings using techniques with which only proliferating cells (lymphocytes) could be used for an analysis (see section 4.4, Cytogenetic methods).

Using a fluorometric analysis of DNA unwinding (FADU), Sen and colleagues [32] detected an association between a single bout of exercise and the induction of DNA strand breaks in leukocytes. In this study, two submaximal exercises were carried out 7 days apart, each lasting 30 min. Blood samples were taken before and 2 min after each exercise. This study found an induction of DNA damage in 13 out of 18 samples. In contrast to the studies described above, DNA damage was detected directly after the runs suggesting that the technique used might be more sensitive. Unfortunately, no blood samples were analyzed at later time points after the runs.

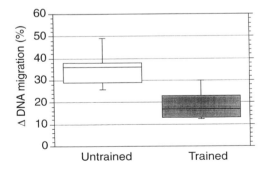

Fig. 4. Effects of a run on a treadmill on DNA damage in leukocytes of trained (n = 6) and untrained (n = 5) individuals. The results are presented as percent changes of DNA migration in the comet assay from resting to 24 h postexercise values (Δ DNA migration) and displayed as boxplots, in which the horizontal line represents the median, the edges of the box the 25% and 75% quantiles and the end of the bars the extremes. Data modified from [28] with kind permission.

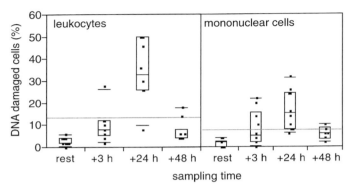

Fig.5. Effects of a half marathon on the induction of DNA damage in total leukocytes (left panel) and separated mononuclear cells (right panel) of human subjects. The results are displayed as quantile boxplots, which visualize the median (horizontal line within the box) 25% and 75% quantiles (edges of the box), 10% and 90% quantiles (lower and upper lines), mean of the total sample (horizontal line) and the single values (points). Data modified from [30] with permission.

4.2 Analysis of oxidized bases in cellular DNA

Besides measuring DNA strand breaks and lesions converted to strand breaks, DNA can also be assayed for oxidized bases. This specific class of DNA damage is detected with the comet assay in conjunction with lesion-specific endo-nucleases. The enzymes, applied to the microscope slides for a short time after lysis, nick DNA at sites of base alterations and the resulting single-strand breaks can be quantified. Using this modification of the comet assay, free radical induced oxidative DNA base modifications have been detected with high sensitiv-ity in vitro [33,34] and in vivo with human subjects undergoing hyperbaric oxygen treatment [35]. However, only one study has been published so far using this assay to investigate the effects of a strenuous exercise on the induction of oxida-tively modified DNA bases in leukocytes and found no increased base damage directly after the exercise [31]. In contrast, unpublished data suggests that the amount of oxidatively modified DNA bases clearly increased 72 h after a medium distance triathlon (Pfuhler and Dennog, personal communication). This prelimi-nary data suggests that leukocyte DNA may not be oxidatively damaged during exhaustive exercise, however, the exercise may result in the initiation of second-ary mechanisms leading to oxidative damage.

The specific base modification 8-hydroxy-2′-deoxyguanosine (8-OHdG) can be detected by high-performance liquid chromatography (HPLC) analysis of iso-lated nuclear DNA. To our knowledge, so far only two reports assessing this end-point in human lymphocytes have been published and the results are conflicting. While no alterations were found in 10 well-trained long-distance runners after an 8-day training camp [36], an unexpected statistically significant decrease in the 8-OHdG-content of lymphocyte-DNA was reported [37]. Similarly, an endur-ance test with dogs running on a treadmill for 7 h found a significant decrease in lymphocyte 8-OHdG [38]. The latter two studies discuss that the decreased 8-OHdG level may be caused by an exercise-induced elevated efficiency of DNA repair systems to remove oxidative DNA damage. The studies, however, did not take into account that strenuous exercise induces sudden temporary changes in the immune system called acute responses [reviewed in 39]. A dramatic change in both, total leukocyte count and subpopulations of lymphocytes is detected and results from a redistribution of cells from the spleen, bone marrow or the endothelia [40]. Certain exercise protocols result in a transient increased lymphocyte count. Within 30 min of recovery from exercise, lymphocyte count decreases from 30 to 50% below pre-exercise levels [39]. Therefore, data on nuclear content of 8-OHdG in lymphocytes before and after exercise should be interpreted with great caution because the leukocytes analyzed before vs. after exercise might consist of different subpopulations with different degrees of endogenous damage.

4.3 Urinary excretion of oxidized DNA bases and nucleosides

A widely used indicator for oxidative DNA damage is the HPLC analysis of oxidized nucleosides or DNA bases excreted in the urine. These lesions are rapidly removed from nuclear DNA by various repair mechanisms. The repair of 8-OHdG in DNA involves the pathways of base excision repair yielding 8-hydroxy-guanine (8-OHG) and nucleotide excision repair, yielding 8-OHdG which are excreted in urine [8,41—43]. The use of 8-OHdG and/or 8-OHG as markers for oxidative DNA damage in humans is well-established [2,44] and some studies have investigated the influence of exercise on the induction of 8-OHdG. Since a relationship between oxygen consumption and urinary excretion of this base modification was suggested [45,46] a concomitantly elevated level of 8-OHdG in the urine of athletes after strenuous exercise should be expected. However, this suggestion is not completely supported by data published so far. While no alterations were found directly after distance running [38], consecutive days of cycling [47], long-distance training of athletes [43], or in triathletes 0—96 h after a competitive race [31], elevated levels were, however, found in samples from marathon runners 10 h after a run [48], in soldiers participating in 30 days of exercise [49] and in endurance athletes during a training camp [36]. It appears that several variables have to be considered, including the extent of exercise, urinary collection periods, and creatine concentrations used for correction of 8-OHdG data. Furthermore, although the majority of urinary 8-OHdG is believed to originate from nuclear DNA, it should be stressed that this base modification is also derived from oxidation of mitochondrial DNA and the nucleotide pool, as well as from cell turnover [10]. Since cell disruption (which is commonly observed after strenuous exercise) can increase free radical reactions [50], one must be cautious in using the amounts of 8-OHdG excreted from the body as a marker of the extent of repair for cellular oxidative damage.

4.4 Cytogenetic methods

Primary DNA lesions detected after exercise may be repaired error-free and may not result in chromosome damage or mutation induction. To gain more insight into the biological significance, and to assess a potential mutagenic risk of DNA strand breaks and base oxidation after exercise, it is necessary to compare these effects with other markers of genotoxicity. Cytogenetic methods give a specific indication of mutagenic effects. Various methods have been used routinely for many years and are established as sensitive markers in human biomonitoring studies [21]. The classical method is the measurement of chromosomal aberrations which demonstrate structural alterations of single chromosomes or exchanges between different chromosomes. Sister chromatid exchanges (SCE) are a reciprocal exchange between DNA molecules of a replicating chromosome. Micronuclei (MN) are small chromosome fragments or whole chromosomes which were not integrated into the daughter cell during cell division. The use of cytogenetic techniques is restricted to proliferating cells.

So far, only three studies measured DNA damage with the comet assay and also analyzed cytogenetic endpoints. One study reports no influence of an exhaustive run on a treadmill on the frequency of SCE in lymphocytes of humans [26]. However, an unaltered SCE frequency is not unexpected because direct strand-breaking agents like oxygen radicals are weak inducers of SCE [51]. Two studies assessing MN in lymphocytes show conflicting results. A strong increase of MN was found 24 and 48 h after repeated anaerobic runs [52] with a concomitant increase of DNA damage in the comet assay (Zankl, personal communication). In contrast, a triathlon competition had no effect on MN frequency 0–96 h after the race despite very strong effects in the comet assay [31]. Although data on chromosome alterations after exercise are still very limited, these results suggest that DNA effects found in the comet assay after exercise represent DNA lesions which may be repaired error-free and may not necessarily result in chromosome alterations. In vitro studies underscore the hypothesis that effects seen in the comet assay are not closely related to mutagenic effects but rather relate to other biomarkers of primary DNA damage [53–55]. Further studies on chromosome alterations and mutation induction are necessary to assess the biological significance of DNA damage after exercise. Table 1 summarizes the results of studies published so far on exercise-induced DNA damage.

4.5 Exercise–induced apoptosis: secondary induction of DNA fragmentation

Apoptosis is a term for a specific form of cell death. Oxidative stress can induce apoptosis [56] or be a result of cells undergoing apoptosis. It has recently been suggested that cellular free radical damage can result from cells dying by apoptotic and/or necrotic processes [57]. This underscores the proposal of Halliwell and Gutteridge that oxidative stress in tissue causing cell death, can also cause secondary tissue injury due to oxidative reactions [58]. Recent reports describe

Table 1. Techniques used to demonstrate exercise-induced DNA damage.

Assay/endpoint	Tissue/specimen investigated	Exercise protocol	Results	Ref.
Comet assay/DNA breaks	Leukocytes	Incremental treadmill runs	DNA damage 6–48 h after exercise	26
			Preventive effect of vitamin E on DNA damage	27
			DNA damage in trained volunteers	28
		Triathlon competition	DNA damage 24–120 h postrace	31
		Half marathon	Increased DNA damage 24 h postexercise	29
	Lymphocytes	Repeated sprints	Increased DNA damage 24 h after sprints	*
	Leukocytes and mononuclear cells	Half marathon	Higher DNA damage in whole leukocytes vs. Mononuclear cells	30
FADU / DNA breaks	Leukocytes	30 min run	Increased DNA damage Directly after a run	32
Oxidized DNA bases	Leukocytes	Triathlon competition	No effects before vs. directly after the race	31
HPLC / 8-OHdG	Lymphocytes	Intermittent swim	Lower amount of 8-OHdG after swim	37
		Distance run	No effect	37
		8-days training	No effect	36
		Endurance training	No effect	43
HPLC / 8-OHdG	Urine	Distance run	No effect	37
		9-days cycling	No effect	47
		6 min all-out rowing	No effect	122
		Triathlon competition	No effects 0–96 h after race	31
		8-days training	Increase during training; no effect post-training	36
		marathon	Increase 10 h after race	48
		30-days training	Increase before vs. end of exercise period	49
Micronuclei (MN)	Lymphocytes	2 subsequent sprints	Increased MN frequency 24 and 48 h postexercise	52
		Triathlon competition	No altered MN frequency 0–120 h postexercise	31
Sister chromatid exchanges (SCEc)	Lymphocytes	Incremental treadmill run	No altered SCE frequency 048 h postexercise	26

* Zankl, personal communication

the induction of apoptosis in muscle cells after eccentric exercise. Apoptosis occurred due to mechanical damage of myofibers and resulting inflammatory and necrotic processes [59—61]. Furthermore, apoptosis was also detected in thymocytes of rats undergoing two separated runs to exhaustion [62]. In cells undergoing apoptosis, fragmentation of DNA due to endonuclease-induced cleavage is commonly observed [63]. There are important differences in terms of the biological significance of apoptosis-induced DNA fragmentation and DNA damage detected in leukocytes after exercise. Apoptosis-induced DNA fragmentation only occurs in dying cells, whereas DNA damage detected in leukocytes occurs in living/viable cells in which misrepair of the damage may lead to mutations.

In conclusion, using tests to detect DNA strand breaks, several studies have shown the induction of DNA damage in leukocytes of humans by various exercise protocols. Damage was observed with a delay of several hours after exercise and was persistent. Comparative investigations with cytogenetic assays show that exercise-induced DNA strand breaks do not necessarily lead to chromosome alterations. Studies quantifying the oxidatively modified DNA nucleoside 8-OHdG did not yield clear results; therefore, it can be assumed that this modification may not be the only cause of the DNA strand breaks detected. The differences in results of the various test systems used may reflect differences in the sensitivity of assays, and the fundamental differences between assaying for primary DNA lesions or chromosome alterations.

5 FREE RADICAL GENERATION IN EXERCISE: POTENTIAL MECHANISMS FOR DNA DAMAGE INDUCTION

Numerous studies have shown that excessive exercise can result in oxygen radical-mediated injury, and various biochemical mechanisms of free radical generation after strenuous exercise have been identified [64—67]. During and after exercise, radicals are generated at different potential sites and by mechanisms which may cause DNA damage. Indirect evidence for oxidative stress as one underlying mechanisms to induce DNA damage after exercise is provided from a study in which volunteers supplemented with antioxidants before a run showed a significantly reduced amount of DNA damage [27]. The results of this study are shown in Fig. 6. It was also shown that the expression of the antioxidative stress proteins HSP70 (heat shock protein 70) and HO-1 (heme oxygenase 1) were enhanced in leukocytes concomitant to increased DNA damage after exercise [30]. Potential mechanisms of exercise-induced generation of oxygen radicals are summarized in Fig. 7 and their possible role in inducing DNA damage are discussed below.

5.1 Generation of radicals during exercise

In the exercising muscle, chemically bound energy is converted to mechanical energy. Energy is provided from adenosine triphosphate (ATP) which is limited

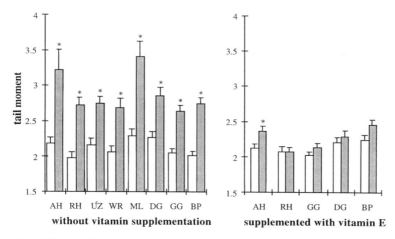

Fig.6. Effect of vitamin E on DNA damage in leukocytes of humans measured as increased DNA migration in the comet assay. Open bars, before exercise; filled bars, 24 hours after exercise. Mean and SEM of 50 cells per data point. *Significantly different from preexercise values. Reprinted from [27] with kind permission from Elsevier Science NL, Sara Burgerhaartstraat 25, 1055 KV Amsterdam.

in cells and must continuously be regenerated. The most efficient pathway of ATP regeneration is through oxidation of glycogen and fat stored in the musculature. Molecular oxygen is the final acceptor of electrons in the respiratory chain located in the mitochondria. This reduction process is very accurate, however, a small fraction of the oxygen consumed in cells may lead to the formation of highly reactive intermediate oxygen species due to monovalent reduction of oxygen [68]. Therefore, mitochondria represent a potential site for elevated oxygen free radical formation during oxidative stress. Another well-described source of

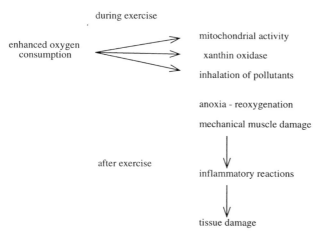

Fig.7. Potential mechanisms by which exhaustive exercise could induce DNA damage.

oxygen radicals is xanthine dehydogenase/xanthine oxidase (XDH/XO). The role of XDH/XO as an inducer of oxidative stress in exercise has been described extensively in the first vol. of this book [69]. It is also possible that the increased inhalation caused by higher oxygen utilization may increase the uptake of environmental pollutants containing free radicals and/or initiators of free radical generating reactions in the body (e.g., ozone, $NO_2^\bullet$) [70]. Inhaled ozone can cause oxidative reactions, including lipid peroxidation, which generates free radicals [58]. However, oxygen radicals generated by mitochondria, xanthine oxidase or from the uptake of pollutants would more likely lead to DNA damage during or directly after exercise. This does not provide an explanation for delayed effects, as observed in the majority of the studies. Therefore, the involvement of secondary mechanisms causing DNA damage after exercise are more likely.

5.2 Generation of radicals after exercise: inflammatory mechanisms

Endogenous sites are an important source of radicals. Oxygen radicals are produced in inflammatory processes as a result of tissue injury or due to infections. Neutrophils and phagocytic cells are able to fight pathogenic organisms by generating nitric oxide and superoxide (which react to form peroxynitrite, a powerful oxidizing agent), hypochloride and hydrogen peroxide. Release of these agents protects humans from immediate death by pathogens, but also causes oxidative DNA damage. Host tissue can be damaged by inappropriate release of reactive oxygen species which is thought to be a basis of noninfectious inflammatory diseases [71]. Infection and injury initiate a similar series of host defense reactions known as the acute phase response [72]. Release of reactive oxygen species following disruption of muscle tissue, especially after eccentric exercise, was described [73] and marked similarities exist between effects seen after exercise and events typically seen in acute inflammation [72]. A single bout of exercise induced an increased production of reactive oxygen species by neutrophils [74] and biomarkers of oxidative stress were found secondary to muscle tissue damage by infiltrating phagocytic cells as part of the reparative process [75,76]. The sequence of events involved in muscle tissue injury is not well-defined but common mechanisms include initial induction of muscle damage and a secondary or delayed onset injury of muscle tissue [73]. The initial injury is thought to be of mechanical, as well as chemical origin and can result in activation of polymorphonuclear neutrophils. Physiological changes detected after muscle injury resemble those seen in acute inflammation, like increased body temperature, concentration of cytokines and acute phase proteins [77], and increased numbers of circulating granulocytes [72–74,78] and rise of plasma myeloperoxidase [79].

The infiltration of damaged muscle by immunocompetent cells and subsequent macrophage infiltration may be maintained through several days postexercise. Therefore, a relationship might also exist between the induction of DNA damage detected with delay after exercise and temporary immunomodulations such as changes in activities of immunocompetent cells. These mechanisms include a rise in cytokines like IL-6 and TNF α [80], which are known to augment the expression of the inducible NO• (nitric oxide) synthase [81]. As shown in in vitro studies, stimulation of macrophages is capable of inducing the production of NO•, which peaks after 12 h and results in DNA damage in these cells another 12 h [82]. Physiological levels of NO• are able to induce DNA damage, as demonstrated with the comet assay [83]. In this context it is also likely that DNA effects in leukocytes after exercise may result from a secondary release of reactive products by activated inflammatory cells. This would be an explanation for the persistent DNA damage seen in leukocytes. Interestingly, an unpublished investigation of athletes after strenuous endurance exercise revealed that leukocytes maintained for several hours in vitro, after blood sampling showed a reduced amount of DNA damage compared to cells analyzed immediately (Pfuhler and Dennog, personal communication). This strongly suggests that DNA damage is repaired in vitro in contrast to in vivo, where cells persistently show a high amount of DNA damage. The persistent damage seen in vivo probably results from a continuous exposure to reactive oxygen species. Activated neutrophils were shown to induce prolonged DNA damage in co-cultivated cells [84]. Furthermore, it has been suggested that these cells play a causative role in inducing DNA damage in the comet assay with leukocytes of children suffering from infections [85]. The induction of DNA damage due to inflammatory reactions is of increasing interest, because in various inflammatory diseases an elevated risk of cancer development has been suggested [2]. Furthermore, heavy exertion, in contrast to moderate exercise, has adverse effects on the immune system, however, underlying mechanisms are not fully understood. It would be of interest whether DNA damage in leukocytes is a cause of increased susceptibility to infection, as observed in the postexercise recovery period [86].

6 BIOLOGICAL SIGNIFICANCE OF EXERCISE-INDUCED DNA DAMAGE: EPIDEMIOLOGICAL EVALUATION

Since DNA damage may result in mutations and subsequently initiate carcinogenesis, indices of exercise-induced DNA damage promote the question, whether physical activity is associated with a higher risk of cancer. Various epidemiological studies were performed to investigate the influence of regular physical activity on the incidence of cancer, especially of the most common sites such as lung, prostate, colon and breast. Most of the studies investigating the influence of regular physical exercise on the risk of lung cancer found a trend towards a preventive effect of regular exercise in men [87,88]. In contrast, one report suggested a higher incidence in physically active individuals [89]. A more recent prospective study of 81,516 men and women demonstrated a protective effect of leisure physical activity on lung cancer risk in male individuals after adjustment for other confounding factors such as smoking habits [90]. In the same study, no association between physical activity and lung cancer in women was seen, probably due to the small number of cases in the female participants. A protective effect of aerobic exercise against the development of breast cancer and an inverse relation between the amount of training and cancer risk became apparent, when the amount of regular physical conditioning was at least 3.8 h a week [91]. An overall reduced risk of breast cancer among active women was confirmed by other studies [92–94]. A reduced risk of breast cancer was reported more recently in a study of 25,624 women performing a higher level of physical activity at work, as well as in their leisure time [95]. This effect was even more pronounced in premenopausal women. In contrast, findings by Chen et al. [96] could not confirm these results. They reported no influence of regular exercise on the incidence of breast cancer in the adolescent years or in adulthood of young women. Furthermore, no protective effect of physical activity on the occurrence of breast cancer in postmenopausal women was seen, suggesting a statistically not significant trend towards a higher incidence [97]. The most likely mechanism accounting in large part for a lower risk of breast cancer in active women seems to be a reduced lifetime exposure to estrogens as a result of exercise-induced reduction of follicle stimulation hormone levels. Lower estrogen levels may also account for a lower incidence of other estrogen-dependent tumors [98] such as endometrial cancer [99,100]. Studies concerning the influence of regular physical conditioning on the incidence of prostate cancer show conflicting results. Most of these studies report a protective or no effect of sports [87,101–103]. Recent investigations, including 12,975 men, found a protective role of cardiorespiratory fitness towards the development of prostate cancer [104]. However, there are also some reports suggesting a greater prevalence of prostate cancer in physically active men [105,106]. Therefore, it remains unclear whether physical activity affects the risk of prostate cancer. Also, no evidence could be found for an association between physical activity and testicular cancer [107]. Most of the studies found that regular physical activity decreased the incidence of colon cancer [108]. In contrast to studies investigating other types of cancer, data of these studies are in fair agreement. Furthermore, physical inactivity appears to increase the prevalence of colon cancer [109] and some authors reported a greater protective effect of intense exercise [110,111]. The protective effect, however, seems to be lower in women compared to men [112]. A shorter colon transit time [113] and probably a lower concentration of fecal bile acid concentration as shown in endurance athletes [114] are believed to diminish the lifetime exposure of the colon mucosa to potential carcinogens and, therefore, may explain in part a reduced risk for colon cancer in active individuals.

Exercise-induced DNA damage has predominantly been detected after long-term [31,48,49] or intensive exercise [26,28]. Keeping this in mind, considerations have to be focused on epidemiological data concerning the risk of cancer in highly trained athletes, performing a long-standing training of a high quantity and intensity over many years. In contrast to the studies discussed above, only a few reliably controlled epidemiological studies are available which focused on the incidence of cancer in highly trained or former athletes. Moreover, most of these studies investigated the all-cause mortality and do not separately evaluate the prevalence of cancer. A study of 8,393 athletes participating in competitive sports reported a higher incidence of cancer in active individuals [115]. Other authors did not confirm this finding, and reported a lower risk of reproductive system cancers in 2,622 former collegiate athletes [116]. Karvonen and co-workers reported a 2.8- to 4.3-year longer life expectancy in male champion skiers compared to a control group [117]. More recently, a study including 2,259 male long-distance skaters detected a lower all cause mortality in the athlete group [118]. Nevertheless, a statistically non significant trend towards a higher mortality of competitive participants compared to the noncompetitive athletes could be observed in the same study. No relationship between long-term athletic training and life expectancy was apparent in another study comparing former male college athletes and nonathletes [119]. An enhanced life expectancy in world class athletes (n = 2613) compared to healthy non active controls was reported [120], and the cause was explained by a decreased cardiovascular and cancer mortality. It is noteworthy that, life expectancy was highest in endurance athletes in this investigation. The results of a lower all cause mortality in athletes as shown in a few studies must be assessed carefully because they may be influenced by regular training and also by confounding variables. These factors include better health habits, better living conditions and also the influence of selection in terms of the genotype. The genotype may influence both, propensity for physical conditioning leading to regular training for competitive sports, and predisposition to cancer or cardiovascular disease.

In conclusion, epidemiological data suggest that moderate physical activity does not increase the incidence of cancer. Moreover, several lines of evidence exist that there is a negative correlation between regular physical exercise and the risk of certain types of cancer [121]. At present, no clear evidence has been provided suggesting an increased risk of cancer in athletes performing long-term athletic training and participating in competitive sports. However, recent epidemiological data also show that, compared to moderate physical exercise, competitive sports do not provide an additional protective effect against the occurrence of cancer. A summary of representative studies and the results are given in Table 2.

7 SUMMARY

Firstly, a great body of evidence shows that strenuous physical exercise can result in the induction of DNA damage in humans, as demonstrated by elevated DNA strand breaks in leukocytes. DNA strand breaks are detectable after various exercise protocols in untrained and well-trained individuals.

Secondly, oxidative stress may present one underlying mechanism for the induction of DNA damage after exercise. However, analysis of oxidized DNA nucleosides excreted in the urine as a biomarker of oxidative DNA damage showed conflicting results. This might reflect a difference in the sensitivity of this biomarker compared to strand break analysis and/or suggests that oxidative

Table 2. Influence of physical activity on the incidence of cancer: comparison of epidemiological data.

Physical activity	Subjects	Results	Ref.
Self-reported physical activity	7080 women and 25.341 men	lower risk for death from cancer in physical active men, no association in women	121
Physical activity in leisure time	81.516 men and women	protective effect on the risk of lung cancer in men, no association in women	90
Recreational physical activity	1090 pre-menopausal women	reduction of breast cancer risk by 50% (at least 4 h exercise per week)	91
Everyday exercise in leisure time and at work	25.624 women	lower risk of breast cancer, more pronounced effect among pre-menopausal women	95
Occupational and recreational	2321 women	no protective effect on breast cancer risk, increased risk in more active women (marginally significant)	97
Assessment of the cardio respiratory fitness by treadmill testing	12.975 men	protective effect of cardiorespiratory fitness against prostate cancer	104
Occupational and recreational	204 women, 180 men	greater protective effect of intense exercise against colon cancer	110
Walking or cycling > 4 h/ week	53.242 men, 28.274 women	Inverse dose-response effect on colon cancer risk	111
Competitive	8393 athletes	higher incidence of cancer in active individuals	115
long-term athletic training	2622 former college athletes	lower risk of reproductive system cancer	116
Champion skiers	396 athletes	longer life expectancy (2.8-4.3 years) compared to inactive controls	117
regular endurance training, competitive and non-competitive athletes	2259 male long-distance skaters	statistically non-significant trend towards higher all-cause mortality in competitors compared to non-competitors	118
endurance sports; power athletes; team sports	2613 athletes	life expectancy was highest in endurance athletes	120

base modifications may not be the predominant DNA lesion. Because DNA damage occurs with delay after exercise, it is likely that secondary mechanisms, possibly inflammatory-like reactions, are involved.

Thirdly, it is not clear whether DNA lesions found after exercise are repaired error free or may result in chromosome alterations. Very few studies, so far, assessed the induction of chromosome alterations after exercise, and results are conflicting.

Finally, the biological significance of exercise-induced DNA damage has yet to be determined. It is generally accepted that DNA damage has a certain potential to result in the initiation of processes leading to carcinogenesis. However, epidemiological data on athletes suggest that the overall cancer incidence in physically active individuals is lower compared with non active individuals, and that even strenuous endurance exercise does not seem to have adverse effects. Therefore, although the rate of DNA damage may be enhanced by physical exercise, beneficial mechanisms induced by regular physical conditioning seem to prevail and counterbalance exercise-induced DNA damage.

8   PERSPECTIVES

Most of the studies discussed in this chapter used peripheral leukocytes as an indicator of the DNA-damaging effect of exercise. Since muscle tissue is likely to be directly damaged by exercise-induced oxidative stress, it would be of interest whether DNA damage can also be detected in muscle cells or other cell types. Furthermore, mitochondria are one major site of free radical generation, and research should also be encouraged on exercise-induced DNA damage in mitochondria. Damaged mitochondria possibly lead to deterioration of respiratory enzyme activities and modulate muscular energy metabolism. Regarding the consequences of exercise-related DNA damage it would also be reasonable to conduct epidemiological studies investigating whether there is an upper threshold for an additional cancer risk in athletes performing vigorous and high-volume training.

9   ACKNOWLEDGMENTS

Andreas Hartmann is supported by a postdoctoral fellowship from the "Deutsche Forschungsgemeinschaft" Germany. Support for the work of Andreas Niess is received in part from the "Bundesinstitut fuer Sportwissenschaft" Germany. We are grateful to Maike Sander and Robert Gonzales for critically reading the manuscript.

10 ABBREVIATIONS

ATP: adenosine triphosphate
8-OHdG: 8-hydroxy-7,8-dihydro2′-deoxyguanosine
8-OHG: 8-hydroxyguanine
DNA: deoxyribonucleic acid
FADU: fluorometric analysis of DNA unwinding
HPLC: high-performance liquid chromatography
H_2O_2:   hydrogen peroxide
IL-6:   interleukine 6
MN: micronuclei
mtDNA: mitochondrial DNA
$NO^{\bullet}$: nitric oxide
$NO_2^{\bullet}$: nitrogen dioxide
$O^{2-\bullet}$: superoxide anion
SCE: sister chromatid exchanges
TNFα: tumor necrosis factor α
XDH: xanthine dehydrogenase
XO: xanthine oxidase

11 REFERENCES

1. Tlsty TD, Briot A, Gualberto A, Hall I, Hess S, Hixon M, Kuppuswamy D, Romanov S, Sage M, White A. Mutat Res 1995;337:1−7.
2. Wiseman H, Halliwell B. Biochem J 1996;313:17−29.
3. Ames BN, Shigenega MK, Hagen TM. Proc Natl Acad Sci USA 1993;90:7915−7922.
4. Sancar A. Ann Rev Genet 1995;29:69−105.
5. Cleaver JE, Kraemer KH. In: Scriver CR, Beaudet AL, Sly WS, Valle D (eds) The Metabolic Basis of Inherited Disiease. New York: McGraw-Hill, 1989;2949−2971.
6. Rosen DR, Siddique T, Patterson D, Figlewicz DA, Sapp P. Nature 1993;362:59−62.
7. Ames BN, Gold LS, Willett WC. Proc Natl Acad Sci USA 1995;92:5258−5265.
8. Shigenaga MK, Ames BN. Free Radic Biol Med 1991;10:221−225.
9. Lee HC, Wei YH. J Biomed Sci 1997;4:319−326.
10. Halliwell B, Aruoma OI. FEBS Lett 1994;281;9−19.
11. Floyd RA. Carcinogenesis 1990;11:1447−1450.
12. Grollman AP, Moriya M. Trends Genet 1993;9:246−249.
13. Gille JJP, van Berkel CGM, Joenje H. Carcinogenesis 1994;15:2695−2699.
14. Emerit I. Free Radic Biol Med 1994;16:99−109.
15. DeFlora S, Izzotti A, Randerath K, Randerath E, Bartsch H, Nair J, Balansky R, vanSchooten F, Degan P, Fronza G, Walsh D, Lewtas J. Mutat Res Rev 1996;366:197−238.
16. Bowling AC, Beal MF. Life Sci 1995;56:1151−1171.
17. Mecocci P, Beal MF, Cecchetti R, Polidori MC, Cherubini A, Chionne F, Avellini L, Romano G, Senin U. Molec Chem Neuropathol 1997;31:53−64.
18. Lyras L, Cairns NJ, Jenner A, Jenner P, Halliwell B. J Neurochem 1997;68:2061−2066.
19. Tanaka M, Kovalenko SA, Gong JS, Borgeld HJ, Katsumata K, Hayakawa M, Yoneda M, Ozawa T. Ann NY Acad Sci 1996;786:102−111.
20. Hayakawa M, Sugiyama S, Hattori K, Takasawa M, Ozawa T. Molec Cell Biol 1993;119: 95−103.

21. Carrano AV, Natarajan AT. Mutat Res 1988;204:379—406.
22. Singh NP, McCoy MT, Tice RR, Schneider EL. Exp Cell Res 1988;175:184—191.
23. Tice RR. In: Butterworth FM (ed) Biomonitors and Biomarkers as Indicators of Environmental Change. New York: Plenum Press, 1995;314—327.
24. Speit G, Hartmann A. In: Henderson D, (ed) Methods in Molecular Biology: DNA Repair Protocols. New York: Humana Press, (In press).
25. Hartmann A, Haupter S, Speit G. Toxicol Lett 1997;90:183—188.
26. Hartmann A, Plappert U, Raddatz K, Grünert-Fuchs M, Speit G. Mutagenesis 1994;9: 269—272.
27. Hartmann A, Niess AM, Grünert-Fuchs M, Poch B, Speit. Mutat Res 1995;346:195—202.
28. Niess AM, Hartmann A, Grünert-Fuchs M, Poch B, Speit G. Int J Sports Med 1996;17: 397—403.
29. Niess AM, Hartmann, A, Baumann M, Roecker K, Mayer F, Dickhuth HH. Med Sci Sport Exerc 1997;29:S297.
30. Niess AM, Veihelmann S, Passek F, Roecker K, Dickhuth HH, Northoff H, Fehrenbach E, Dtsch Z Sportmed 1997;48:330—341.
31. Hartmann A, Pfuhler S, Dennog C, Germadnik D, Pilger, A, Speit G. Free Radic Biol Med 1998;24:245—251.
32. Sen CK, Rankinen T, Väisänen S, Rauramaa R. J Appl Physiol 1994;76:2570—2577.
33. Collins AR, Duthie SJ, Dobson VL. Carcinogenesis 1993;14:1733—1735.
34. Collins AR, Ai-guo A, Duthie SJ. Mutat Res 1995;336:69—77.
35. Dennog C, Hartmann A, Frey G, Speit. Mutagenesis 1996;11:605—609.
36. Okamura K, Doi T, Hamada K, Sakurai M, Yoshioka Y, Mitsuzono R, Migita T, Sumida S, Sugawa-Katayama Y. Free Radic Res Commun 1997;26:507—14.
37. Inoue T, Mu Z, Sumikawa K, Adachi K, Okochi T. Jpn J Cancer Res 1993;84:720—725.
38. Okamura K, Doi T, Sakurai M, Hamada K, Yoshioka Y, Sumida S, Sugawa-Katayama Y. Free Radic Res 1997;26:523—528.
39. Nieman DC, Nehlsen—Cannarella SL. Sem Hematol 1994;31:166—179.
40. Shek PN, Sabiston BH, Buguet A, Radomski MW. Int J Sports Med 1995;16:466—474.
41. Germadnik D, Pilger A, Rüdiger HW. J Chromatogr B 1997;689:399—403.
42. Suzuki J, Inoue Y, Suzuki S. Free Radic Biol Med 1995;18:431—436.
43. Pilger A, Germadnik D, Formanek D, Zwick H, Winkler N, Rüdiger HW. Eur J Appl Physiol Occ Physiol 1997;75:467—469.
44. Loft S, Poulsen HE. Molec Med 1996;74:297—312.
45. Loft S, Astru A, Buemann B, Poulsen HE. FASEB J 1994;8:534—537.
46. Loft S, Wierik EJMV, van der Berg H, Poulsen HE. Cancer Epiderm Biomark Prev 1995;4: 515—519.
47. Vigui CA, Frei B, Shigenega MK, Ames BN, Packer L, Brooks GA. Med Sci Sports Exerc 1984; 22:514—521.
48. Alessio HM. Med Sci Sports Exerc 1993;25:218—224.
49. Poulsen, HE, Loft S, Vistisen K. J Sports Sci 1996;14:343—346.
50. Gutteridge JMC, Halliwell B. Trends Biochem Sci 1990; 15:129—135.
51. Speit G, Hochsattel R, Vogel W. In: Tice RR, Hollaender A (eds) Sister Chromatid Exchanges. New York: Plenum Press, 1984;229—243.
52. Schiffl C, Zieres C, Zankel H. Mutat Res 1997;389:243—246.
53. Bastlová T, Vodicka P, Peterková K, Hemminki K, Lambert B. Carcinogenesis 1995;16: 2357—2362.
54. Speit G, Hanelt S, Helbig R, Seidel A, Hartmann A. Toxicol Lett 1996;88:91—98.
55. Hanelt S, Helbig R, Hartmann A, Lang M, Seidel A, Speit G. Mutat Res 1997;390:179—188.
56. Polyak K, Xia Y, Zweier JL, Kinzler KW, Vogelstein B. Nature 1997:389:300—305.
57. Limoli CL, Hartmann A, Shephard L, Yang C, Boothman DA, Bartholomew J, Morgan WF. Cancer Press 1998;58:3712—3718.

58. Halliwell B. Lancet 1994;244:721−724.
59. Sandri M, Podhorska-Okolow M, Geromel V, Rizzi C, Arslan P, Francheschi C, Carrano U. J Neuropathol Exp Neurol 1997;56:145−57.
60. Carrano U, Franceschi C. Aging Clin Exp Res 1997;9:19−34
61. Carrano U. Basic Appl Myol 1995;5:371−374.
62. Concordet JP, Ferry A. Am J Physiol 1993;265:C626−C629.
63. Brown DG, Sun XM, Cohen GM. J Biol Chem 1993;268:3037−3039.
64. Aruoma OI. J Nutr Biochem 1994;5:370−381.
65. Cannon JG, Blumberg JH. In: Sen CK, Packer L, Häninnen O (eds) Exercise And Oxygen Toxicity. Amsterdam: Elsevier, 1994;447−462.
66. Ji LL. Free Radic Biol Med 1995;18:1079−1086.
67. Sjödin B, Hellsten-Westing Y, Apple FS. Sports Med 1990;10:236−254.
68. Boveris A, Chance B. Biochem J 1973;134:707−716.
69. Hellsten Y. In: Sen CK, Packer L, Häninnen O (eds) Exercise And Oxygen Toxicity, Amsterdam: Elsevier, 1994;211−234.
70. Singh VN: A current perspective of nutritition and exercise. J Nutr 1992;122:760−765.
71. Malech HL, Gallin JI. N Engl J Med 317:687−694.
72. Smith LL. Med Sci Sports Exerc 1991;23:542−551.
73. Zerba E, Komorowski T, Faulkner JA. Am J Physiol 1990;258:C429−C435.
74. Smith JA, Telford RD, Mason IB, Weidemann MJ. Int J Sports Med 1990;11:179−187.
75. Ebbeling C B, Clarkson P M. Sports Med 1989;7:207−234.
76. Salminen A. Acta Physiol Scand 1986;124(Suppl 539):5−31.
77. Nieman DC. J Appl Physiol 1997;82:1385−1394.
78. Benoni G, Bellavite P, Adami A, Chirumbolo S, Lippi G, Brocco L, Cuzzolin L. Eur J Appl Physiol 1995;70:187−191.
79. Camus G, Pincemail J, Ledent M, Juchmès-Ferir A, Lamy M, Deby-Dupont G, Deby C. Int J Sports Med 1992;13:443−446.
80. Northoff H, Weinstock C, Berg A. Int J Sports Med 1994;15:S167−S171.
81. Stuehr DJ, Cho HJ, Kwon NS, Weise MF, Nathan CF. Proc Natl Acad Sci USA 1991;88:7773.
82. deRojas-Walker T, Tamir S, Ji H, Wishnok JS, Tannenbaum, SR. Chem Res Toxicol 1995;8: 473−477.
83. Delaney CA, Green MH, Lowe JE, Green IC. FEBS Lett 1993;333:291−295.
84. Shacter E, Beecham EJ, Covey JM, Kohn KW, Potter M. Carcinogenesis 1988;9:2297−2304.
85. Betancourt M, Ortiz R, Gonzales C, Perez P, Cortes L, Rodriguez L, Villasenor. Mutat Res 1995;331:65−77.
86. Fitzgerald R. Int J Sports Med 1991;11:5−8.
87. Severson RK, Nomura AMY, Grove JS, Stemmermann GN. Am J Epidemiol 1989;130: 522−529.
88. Lee IM, Paffenberger Jr RS. Med Sci Sports Exerc 1994;26:831−837.
89. Brownson RC, Chang JC, Davis JR, Smith CA. Am J Pub Health 1991;81:639−642.
90. Thune I, Lund E. Int J Cancer 1997;70:57−62.
91. Bernstein L, Henderson BE, Hansich R, Sullivan-Halley J, Ross RK. J Natl Cancer Inst 1994; 86:1403−1408.
92. Friedenreich CM, Rohan TE. Eur J Cancer Prevent 1995;4:145−151.
93. Mittendorf R, Longnecker MP, Newcomb PA et al. Cancer Cause Control 1995;6:347−353.
94. DeAvanzo B, Nanni O, La Vecchia C et al. Cancer Epiderm Biomark Prev 1996;5:155−160.
95. Thune I, Brenn T, Lund E, Gaard M. N Engl J Med 1997;336:1269−1275.
96. Chen CL, White E, Malone KE, Daling JR. Cancer Cause Control 1997;8:77−84.
97. Dorgan JF, Brown C, Barrett M, Splansky GL, Kreger BE, DeAgostino RB, Albanes D. Am J Epidemiol 1994;139:662−669.
98. Kramer MM, Wells CL. Med Sci Sports Exerc 1996;28:322−334.
99. Hirose K, Tajima K, Hamajima N, Takezaki T, Inoue M, Kuroishi T, Kuzuya K, Nakamura S,

Tokudome S. Jpn J Cancer Res 1996;87:1001—1009.

100. Olson SH, Vena JE, Dorn JP, Marshall JR, Zielezny M, Laughlin R, Graham S. Ann Epidemiol 1997;7:46—53.
101. Vena JE, Graham S, Zielezny M, Brasure J, Swanson MK. Am J Clin Nutr 1987;45:318—327.
102. Yu H, Harris RE, Wynder EL. Prostate 1988;13:17—25.
103. Lee IM, Paffenberger Jr RS, Hsieh CC. Am J Epidemiol 1992;135:169—179.
104. Oliviera SA, Kohl HW III, Trichopoulos D, Blaier. Med Sci Sports Exerc 1996;28:97—104.
105. Whittemore AS, Paffenberger RS, Anderson K, Lee JE. J Natl Cancer Inst 1985;74:43—51.
106. LeMarchand L, Kolonel LN, Yoshizawa CN. Am J Epidemiol 1991;133:103—111.
107. Thune I, Lund E. Cancer Cause Control 1994;5:549—556.
108. HoffmannGoetz L, Husted J. In: Shepard RJ (ed) Exercise Immunology Review. Human Kinetics Publishers Inc, 1995;1:81—96.
109. Slattery ML, Potter J, Caan B, Edwards S, Coates A, Ma KN, Berry. Cancer Res 1997;57:75—80.
110. Slattery ML, Schumacher MC, Smith KR, West DW, AbdElghany. Am J Epidemiol 1988;128:989—999.
111. Thune I, Lund E. Br J Cancer 1996;73:1134—1140.
112. Thun MJ, Calle EE, Namboodiri MM, Flanders WD, Coates RJ, Boffetta P, Garfinkel L, Heath CW. J Natl Cancer Inst 1992;84:1491—1500.
113. Gerhardson M, Floderus B, Norell SE. Int J Epidemiol 1988;17:743—746.
114. Sutherland WHF, Nye ER, MacFarlane DJ, Robertson MC, Williamson SA. Int J Sports Med 1991;12:533—536.
115. Polednak AP. Cancer 1976;38:382—387.
116. Frisch RE, Wyshak C, Albright NL et al. Am J Clin Nutr 1987;45:328—335.
117. Karvonen MJ, Klemola H, Virkajdrvi I, Kekkonen A. Med Sci Sports Exerc 1984;6:49—51.
118. van Saase JLCM, Noteboom WMP, Vandenbrouke JP. Br Med J 1990;301:1409—1411.
119. Quinn TJ, Spraque HA, van Huss WD, Olson HW. Med Sci Sports Exerc 1990;22:742—750.
120. Sarna S, Sahi T, Koskenvuo M, Kaprio J. Med Sci Sports Exerc 1993;25:237—244.
121. Kampert JB, Blair SN, Barlow CE, Kohl HW III. Ann Epidemiol 1996;6:452—457.
122. Nielsen HB, Hanel B, Loft S, Poulsen HE, Pedersen BK, Diamant M, Vistisen K, Secher NH. J Sport Sci 1995;84:720—725.

Part IV

Antioxidant defenses

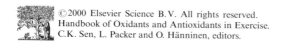 ©2000 Elsevier Science B.V. All rights reserved.
Handbook of Oxidants and Antioxidants in Exercise.
C.K. Sen, L. Packer and O. Hänninen, editors.

Part IV • Chapter 10

Physiological antioxidants and exercise training

Scott K. Powers[1] and Chandan K. Sen[2]

[1]*Department of Exercise and Sport Sciences, University of Florida, Gainesville, FL 32611 USA. Tel.: +1-352-392-9575. Fax: +1-352-392-0316. E-mail: spowers@hhp.ufl.edu*
[2]*Lawrence Berkeley National Laboratory, University of California, One Cyclotron Road, Building 90, Room 3031, Berkeley, CA 94720-3200, USA. Fax: +1-510-644-2341.*
E-mail: cksen@socrates.berkeley.edu

1 INTRODUCTION
2 CELLULAR STRATEGIES TO DETOXIFY REACTIVE OXYGEN SPECIES
   2.1 Overview of antioxidant enzymes
      2.1.1 Superoxide dismutase
      2.1.2 Glutathione peroxidase
      2.1.3 Catalase
      2.1.4 Thioredoxin antioxidant enzyme system
      2.1.5 Glutaredoxin antioxidant enzyme system
   2.2 Nonenzymatic antioxidants
      2.2.1 Glutathione
      2.2.2 Vitamin E
      2.2.3 Vitamin C
      2.2.4 α-Lipoic acid
      2.2.5 Carotenoids
      2.2.6 Uric acid
      2.2.7 Bilirubin
      2.2.8 Ubiquinone
3 EXERCISE TRAINING AND SKELETAL MUSCLE ANTIOXIDANT CAPACITY
   3.1 Superoxide dismutase
   3.2 Glutathione peroxidase
   3.3 Catalase
   3.4 Glutathione
   3.5 Vitamin E and other nonenzymatic antioxidants
4 SUMMARY
5 PERSPECTIVES
6 ACKNOWLEDGEMENTS
7 ABBREVIATIONS
8 REFERENCES

1   INTRODUCTION

Muscular exercise results in an increased production of radicals and other forms of reactive oxygen species (ROS) [1–6]. Further, evidence exists to implicate cytotoxic ROS as an underlying etiology in exercise-induced disturbances in muscle which could result in muscle fatigue and/or injury [4,5,7–10]. Given the potential role of ROS in contributing to a disturbance in muscle redox status, it is not surprising that myocytes contain defense mechanisms to reduce the risk of oxidative injury. Two major classes of endogenous protective mechanisms (i.e., enzymatic and nonenzymatic antioxidants) work together to ameliorate the harmful effects of oxidants in the cell. The purpose of this chapter is to provide a brief overview of cellular antioxidants and summarize the current understanding of how endurance exercise training modifies the antioxidant capacity of skeletal muscle. We begin with a discussion of the major components that comprise the endogenous antioxidant-defense system in cells.

2   CELLULAR STRATEGIES TO DETOXIFY REACTIVE OXYGEN SPECIES

Both enzymatic and nonenzymatic antioxidants detoxify ROS in the intracellular and extracellular environments; these antioxidants work as a complex unit to remove different ROS. To provide maximum intracellular protection, these scavengers are strategically compartmentalized throughout the cell. Illustrated in Fig. 1 are the cellular locations of important antioxidants and Table 1a,b provides a brief overview of the antioxidant function of these molecules.

Several strategies are applied by antioxidants to protect against ROS toxicity. These include conversion of ROS into less active molecules (i.e., scavenging) and prevention of the transformation of less reactive ROS into more deleterious forms (i.e., H_2O_2 into $^\bullet OH$). In the following sections we discuss important antioxidant enzymes and key nonenzymatic antioxidants in the skeletal muscle myocyte.

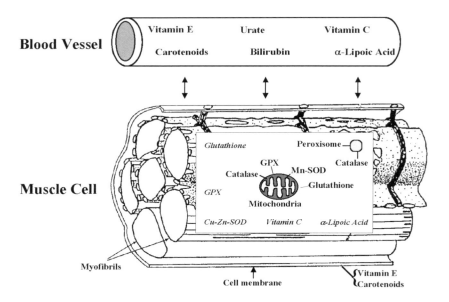

Fig. 1. Localization of major intracellular and extracellular antioxidants within the skeletal muscle myocyte. See text and Table 1 for details on antioxidant function.

Table 1A. Major enzymatic physiological antioxidants.

Enzymatic antioxidants	Properties
Superoxide dismutase	•located in both mitochondria and cytosol •dismutates superoxide radicals
Glutathione peroxidase	•located in mitochondria, cytosol and cell membrane •removes hydrogen peroxide and organic hydroperoxides
Catalase	•located primarily in peroxisomes •removes hydrogen peroxide
Thioredoxin	•12 kDa oxidoreductase found in both eukaryotes and prokaryotes •repairs oxidized sulfhydryl proteins •antioxidant properties include removal of hydrogen peroxide and radical scavenging
Glutaredoxin	•(also called thioltransferase); a thiol-disulfide oxidoreductase enzyme involved in the protection and repair of protein and nonprotein thiols under oxidative stress

Table 1B. Major nonenzymatic physiological antioxidants.

Nonenzymatic antioxidants	Properties
Vitamin E	•lipid soluble phenolic compound; major chain breaking antioxidant found in cell membranes, •major classes: tocopherols and tocotrienols
Vitamin C	•located in aqueous phase of cell; acts of radical scavenger and recycles vitamin E
Vitamin A	•derived from cleavage of carotene in intestine •has biological activity of retinol •unsaturated lipid •inhibits lipid peroxidation
Uric acid	•by-product of purine metabolism in humans and higher apes; may be an important physiological antioxidant; scavenges hydroxyl radicals
Glutathione	•nonprotein thiol in cells; serves multiple roles in the cellular antioxidant defense
α-Lipoic acid	•effective as an antioxidant and in recycling vitamin C •potent pro-glutathione agent
Carotenoids	•lipid soluble antioxidants located primarily in membranes of tissues
Flavonoids and polyphenols	•major component of "phytochemicals" •lipid soluble radical savenger and metal chelators
Bilirubin	•by-product of heme metabolism; may serve as an extracellular antioxidant
Ubiquinones	•lipid soluble quinone derivatives; reduced forms are efficient antioxidants
Melatonin	•pineal hormone •thought to be localized in nucleus of cell •lipid soluble radical scavenger

2.1 Overview of antioxidant enzymes

Primary antioxidant enzymes in cells include superoxide dismutase (SOD), glutathione peroxidase (GPX) and catalase (CAT). Each of these antioxidant enzymes performs detoxification of a particular ROS. Growing evidence also suggests that the thiol-disulfide oxidoreductase enzymes, thioredoxin and glutaredoxin may also be important in prevention of oxidative stress in cells. A brief discussion of each of these enzymes follows.

2.1.1 Superoxide dismutase

The primary cellular defense against superoxide radicals is provided by SOD. SOD dismutates superoxide radicals to form hydrogen peroxide and O_2:

$$2O_2^{\bullet -} \quad + \quad 2H^+ \quad \rightarrow \quad H_2O_2 \quad + \quad O_2 \tag{1}$$

In humans and other mammals, two isozymes of SOD exist in skeletal muscle that vary in both cellular location, as well as the metal ion bound to its active site. The CuZn SOD is primarily located in the cytosol whereas the MnSOD is principally found in the mitochondrial matrix [12–14]. Both enzymes catalyze the dismutation of superoxide anions with similar efficiency [13]. In humans, the CuZnSOD is a dimer with a molecular weight of $\sim 32,000$ kDa whereas the MnSOD is a tetramer (MW = $\sim 88,000$ kDa) [13].

The distribution of the SOD isoforms varies from tissue to tissue. In skeletal muscle, 15 to 35% of the total SOD activity is in the mitochondria with the remaining 65 to 85% being in the cytosol [10]. SOD activity is highest in highly oxidative muscles (i.e., high percentage of type I and IIa fibers) compared to muscles with low oxidative capacity (i.e., high percentage of type IIb fibers) [15,16].

2.1.2 Glutathione peroxidase

GPX catalyzes the reduction of H_2O_2 or organic hydroperoxide to H_2O and alcohol, respectively, using reduced glutathione (GSH) as the electron donor (12):

$$2GSH \quad + \quad H_2O_2 \quad \rightarrow \quad GSSG \quad + \quad 2H_2O \tag{2}$$

or

$$2GSH \quad + \quad ROOH \quad \rightarrow \quad GSSG \quad + \quad ROH \tag{3}$$

GPX is a selenium-dependent enzyme that exists in one isoform. Although GPX is highly specific for its electron donor (GSH), this enzyme has a low specificity for hydroperoxides. Indeed, GPX will reduce a wide range of hydroperoxides ranging from H_2O_2 to a wide range of complex organic hydroperoxides [12]. This characteristic makes GPX an important cellular protectant against ROS-mediated damage to membrane lipids, as well as proteins and nucleic acids.

GPX activity varies across muscle fiber types with type I fibers containing the highest activity and type IIb fibers possessing the lowest activity [10,16]. Similar to SOD, GPX is located in, cytosol, and the mitochondria. In skeletal muscle, approximately 45% of the GPX activity is found in the cytosol whereas the remaining 55% is found in the mitochondria [10]. The fact that GPX is located in mitochondria, cytosol, as well as plasma membrane allows it to remove hydrogen peroxide and hydroperoxides from a variety of sources [11].

To function, GPX requires a supply of GSH. Since GSH is oxidized by GPX to form GSSG, cells must possess a pathway capable of regenerating GSH. This is accomplished by the enzyme GSSG reductase (GR) which uses NADPH as the reducing power for the reaction:

$$GSSG \quad + \quad NADPH \quad \rightarrow \quad 2GSH \quad + \quad NADP \tag{4}$$

In many tissues, NADPH is largely produced by glucose-6-phosphate dehydrogenase via the pentose pathway [17]. However, in skeletal muscle, NADPH is primarily produced by isocitrate dehydrogenase [18–20].

GR has a cellular distribution similar to GPX and its activity is greater in highly oxidative muscles compared to muscles with low oxidative capacity. Although GR is not considered to be a primary antioxidant enzyme, it is essential for the normal antioxidant function of GPX.

2.1.3 Catalase

The primary function of CAT is to catalyze the decomposition of H_2O_2:

$$2H_2O_2 \quad \rightarrow \quad 2H_2O \quad + \quad O_2 \tag{5}$$

CAT is a tetramer with a molecular weight of $\sim 240,000$ kDa. Fe^{3+} is a required cofactor that must be bound to the enzyme's active site [12].

Although there is some overlap between the function of CAT and GPX, the two enzymes differ in their affinity for H_2O_2 as a substrate. Mammalian GPX has a much greater affinity for H_2O_2 at low concentrations compared to CAT (e.g., GPX $K_m = 1 \ \mu M$ vs. CAT $K_m = 1$ mM). This means that at low concentrations, GPX plays a more active role in removing H_2O_2 from the muscle cell.

CAT is widely distributed in the cell; however, high concentrations are found in both peroxisomes and mitochondria [12]. Similar to SOD and GPX, CAT activity is highest in highly oxidative muscles and lowest in muscle with a large percentage of fast (type II) fibers [16].

2.1.4 Thioredoxin antioxidant enzyme system

The thioredoxin antioxidant system is composed of three proteins with enzymatic properties: thioredoxin (Trx), thioredoxin reductase, and thioredoxin peroxidase. Thioredoxin is a highly conserved 12 kDa protein expressed in both eukaryotes and prokaryotes [21]. Functionally it is an oxidoreductase that catalyzes the reduction of protein S-S bridges; this reduction activity plays an important role in the redox regulation of the redox status of protein thiols [22–37]. A key feature of thioredoxins is the presence of a catalytic site containing the conserved amino acid sequence of Trp-Cys-Gly-Pro-Cys-Lys in a protrusion of the three-dimensional structure of the protein. The two cysteine residues of this site can be reversibly oxidized to form a disulfide bridge; this disulfide bridge can be reduced via the selenoenzyme thioredoxin reductase in the presence of NADPH [20a].

The antioxidant properties of Trx include the removal of both hydrogen peroxide (35) and radicals [36]. Collectively these properties have been shown to provide protection against oxidative stress in cells [30,34].

Cellular sulfhydryl proteins are targets for oxidation during periods of oxidative stress [23,24]. Since Trx catalyzes the reduction of protein disulfides, this enzyme system has been implicated in the repair of sulfhydryl proteins [23,28]. In particular, the thioredoxin system has been shown to repair and/or prevent oxidative damage to key sulfhydryl enzymes that participate in steps in intermediary metabolism; these include glucose-6 phosphate dehydrogenase, phosphofructokinase, phosphoglycerate kinase, and pyruvate kinase [23].

Thioredoxin reductase has been shown to participate as part of the antioxidant team by regenerating ascorbate. Indeed, it has been shown that purified liver thioredoxin reductase functions as a NADPH-dependent dehydroascorbate reductase [37]. Details of the importance of recycling ascorbate (vitamin C) will be discussed in detail later.

Further, there is growing evidence that thioredoxin peroxidase is an important cellular antioxidant. Thioredoxin peroxidase is a cytosolic protein that catalyzes the conversion of hydroperoxide and alkyl hydroperoxides to water and alcohols [33]. It may also be important in removing thiyl radicals from cells [32]. During oxidative stress, thiols react with radical species to neutralize the radical; as a result of this reaction, thiyl radicals are formed [21]. These radicals are capable of triggering oxidative damage to a variety of biological macromolecules (e.g., lipids, proteins). Hence, removal of thiyl radicals by thioredoxin peroxidase maybe an important means of reducing cellular oxidative stress.

2.1.4 Glutaredoxin antioxidant enzyme system

Like thioredoxin, glutaredoxin (also called thioltransferase) is a thioldisulfide oxidoreductase enzyme involved in the protection and repair of protein and non-protein thiols under oxidative stress [23,28]. This is achieved by the transfer of electrons from NADPH to disulfide substrates; this glutaredoxin (Grx) catalytic cycle is coupled with glutathione and glutathione reductase.

Although Trx and Grx both repair molecules with sulfhydryl groups, their simultaneous presence in many cells suggests different functions for each protein [27]. In this regard, Grx displays a high degree of selectivity for glutathionyl disulfides and catalyzes their reduction efficiently whereas Trx does not a high affinity for these substrates [24,25]. Since glutathione is the major nonprotein thiol in cells, it forms the majority of mixed sulfides exposed to oxidative stress [23]. Hence, it follows that Grx would be expected to play a key role in reducing oxidized glutathione [23]. By comparison, Trx is more efficient in catalyzing the reduction of protein disulfides [26]. Therefore, it seems likely that the Grx and Trx systems cooperate in a synergistic manner to repair oxidatively damaged protein and nonprotein thiols [23].

Finally, although both Trx and Grx repair oxidatively damaged thiols, recent evidence suggests that each of these enzymes are subject to oxidative damage and that damage to each of these sulfhydryl proteins results in a loss of enzymatic activity [23]. Additional research that improves our understanding of the relative sensitivities of Grx and Trx to deactivation by oxidative stress is warranted.

2.2 Nonenzymatic antioxidants

Many nonenzymatic antioxidants exist in cells. Important nonenzymatic defenses include glutathione, vitamin E, vitamin C, lipoic acid, carotenoids, uric acid, bilirubin, and ubiquinone.

2.2.1 Glutathione

GSH is the most abundant nonprotein thiol source in cells [38]. GSH is primarily synthesized in the liver and transported to tissues via the circulation. Because of the peptide structure of GSH, it is degraded in the small intestine when ingested; therefore, cellular levels of GSH are not directly influenced by diet.

GSH concentration in the cell is in the millimolar range for most tissues, but there is wide variability in GSH content across organs depending on their function. For example, the two highest GSH levels in the body are found in the lens of the eye (10 mM) and the liver (5—7 mM) [12]. Other key organs such as the lung, kidney, and heart contain $\sim 2-3$ mM of GSH [11]. Skeletal muscle GSH concentration varies depending on muscle fiber type and animal species [11,39]. In rats, (slow) type I fibers contain 600% higher GSH content (~ 3 mM) compared to (fast) type IIb fibers (0.5 mM) [11].

GSH serves multiple roles in the cellular antioxidant defense. First, GSH readily interacts with a variety of radicals including hydroxyl and carbon radicals, by donating a hydrogen atom [40]. Secondly, one of the most important antioxidant functions of GSH is to remove both hydrogen and organic peroxides (e.g., lipid peroxide) during a reaction catalyzed by GPX, forming water and alcohol, respectively. By donating a pair of hydrogen atoms, two GSH are oxidized to glutathione disulfide (GSSG). As mentioned earlier, reduction of GSSG is catalyzed by glutathione reductase (GR), a flavin-containing enzyme, wherein nicotinamide-adenine dinucleotide phosphate (NADPH) is used as the reducing power. This reaction takes place in conjunction with GPX, thus, providing a redox cycle for the regeneration of GSH [11]. GSSG levels in most tissues are kept very low, and the intracellular ratio of GSH:GSSG has recently been shown to be much higher than previously reported in the literature [41,42].

Also, GSH has been shown to be involved in reducing a variety of antioxidants in the cell. For example, GSH has been postulated to reduce vitamin E (tocopheroxyl) radicals which are formed in the chain-breaking reactions with alkoxyl or lipid peroxyl radicals [43]. GSH may also be used to reduce semidehydroascorbate radical (vitamin C radical) derived in the recycling of vitamin E. This reaction has recently been hypothesized to play an important role in the recycling of ascorbic acid [44].

2.2.2 Vitamin E

Vitamin E is the most widely distributed antioxidant in nature and is the primary chain breaking antioxidant in cell membranes [45–47]. The generic term vitamin E refers to at least eight structural isomers of tocopherols or tocotrienols. Among these, α-tocopherol is the best known and possesses the most potent antioxidant activity [45,46].

Because of it's high lipid solubility, vitamin E is associated with lipid-rich membranes such as mitochondria, sarcoplasmic reticulum, and the plasma membrane. Under most dietary conditions the concentration of vitamin E in tissues is relatively low. For example, the ratio of vitamin E to lipids in the membrane may range from 1:1000 in red blood cells to 1:3000 in other tissues and organelles [45,48]. However, vitamin levels in tissues and organelles can be elevated with dietary supplementation [46].

As an antioxidant, vitamin E is particularly important because of its ability to convert superoxide, hydroxyl, and lipid peroxyl radicals to less reactive forms. Vitamin E can also break lipid peroxidation chain reactions that occurs during free radical damage to membranes [45].

While vitamin E is an efficient radical scavenger, the interaction of vitamin E with a radical results in a reduction of functional vitamin E and the formation of a vitamin E radical. Oxidative stress has been shown to significantly reduce tissue vitamin E levels [45,46,49]. However, the vitamin E radical can be "recycled" back to its native state by a variety of other antioxidants [45,49]. Therefore, it is postulated that the ability of vitamin E to serve as an antioxidant is synergistically connected to other antioxidants that are capable of recycling vitamin E during periods of oxidative stress. This point is discussed in more detail in the sections on vitamin C and α-lipoic acid.

2.2.3 Vitamin C

In contrast to vitamin E, vitamin C (ascorbic acid) is hydrophilic and functions better in aqueous environments than vitamin E. Because the pKa of ascorbic acid is 4.25, the ascorbate anion is the predominant form existing at physiological pH [40]. Ascorbate is widely distributed in mammalian tissues, but is present in relatively high amounts in the adrenal and pituitary glands [40].

Vitamin C's role as an antioxidant is twofold. First, vitamin C can directly scavenge superoxide, hydroxyl, and lipid hydroperoxide radicals. Secondly, vitamin C plays an important role in recycling vitamin E [49]. However, in the process of recycling vitamin E, native vitamin C is consumed which results in the formation of a vitamin C (semiascorbyl) radical [49]. This radical can be reduced back to native vitamin C by NADH semiascorbyl reductase, or cellular thiols such as glutathione and dihydrolipoic acid [59].

Increasing cellular levels of vitamin C should provide protection against radical-mediated injury [40]. However, in high concentrations (i.e., ~ 1 mM) vitamin C is a pro-oxidant in the presence of transition metals such as Fe^{3+} or Cu^{2+}. Ascorbate's pro-oxidant action comes from its ability to reduce Fe^{+3} to the Fe^{+2} state. This is significant because Fe^{+2} is known to be a potent radical inducer. Therefore, the wisdom of mega-dose supplementation of vitamin C has been questioned by some investigators [40].

2.2.4 α-Lipoic acid

α-Lipoic acid (LA) is a naturally occuring compound that serves as a cofactor for α-dehydrogenase complexes and participates in S-O transfer reaction [48]. Normally, LA is present in very small quantities (5—25 nmol/g) in animal tissues and is generally bound to an enzyme complex and is, therefore, unavailable as an antioxidant. [48]. However, exogenous free unbound LA may be effective as an antioxidant and in recycling vitamin C [48,50]. LA can be consumed in the diet and has no known toxic side effects [48]. After dietary supplementation, LA is reduced to dihydrolipoic acid (DHLA) which is a potent antioxidant against all major ROS [48]. Further, DHLA has been shown to be an important agent in recycling vitamin C during periods of oxidative stress [48,50].

Figure 2 illustrates the role of vitamin C and DHLA in the recycling of vitamin E during periods of oxidative stress. Again, the interaction of vitamin E with a radical results in the formation of a vitamin E radical. The vitamin E radical can be recycled by vitamin C at the cost of forming a vitamin C (semiascorbyl) radical. This radical can be reduced back to vitamin C by DHLA; DHLA is then converted to LA in this process and can be reconverted to DHLA by cellular enzymatic mechanisms [48].

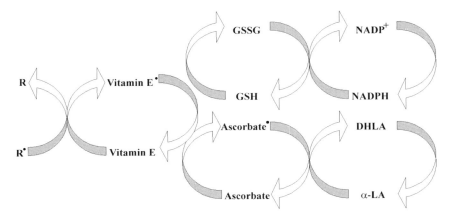

Fig. 2. Illustration of the interaction between α-lipoic acid (α-LA), glutathione (GSH), vitamin C (ascorbate) in the recycling of vitamin E. Ascorbate˙ = ascorbate radical; vitamin E˙ = vitamin E radical; DHLA = dihydrolipoic acid; GSSG = oxidized glutathione. Figure is modified from reference [11].

2.2.5 Carotenoids

Carotenoids (e.g., β-carotene) are lipid soluble antioxidants located primarily in membranes of tissues. The antioxidant properties of carotenoids comes from their structural arrangement consisting of long chains of conjugated double bonds; this arrangement permits the scavenging several ROS including superoxide radicals and peroxyl radicals [40,51,52,68]. Indeed, carotenoids display a efficient biological antioxidant activity as evidenced by their ability to reduce the rate of lipid peroxidation induced by radical generating systems [51].

Similar to vitamin C, β-carotene can function both as an antioxidant and a pro-oxidant. Under physiological oxygen partial pressures (i.e., < 100 Torr), β-carotene exhibits radical scavenging activity. However, exposure to hyperoxic partial pressures (i.e., > 150 Torr) results in β-carotene exerting pro-oxidant properties with a concomitant loss of its antioxidant capacity [53,54].

2.2.6 Uric acid

Uric acid, a by-product of purine metabolism in humans and other primates, has been argued to be an important physiological antioxidant. The role of urate as a scavenger of hydroxyl radicals was first reported in 1960 [55]. Since this first report, numerous investigators have provided additional evidence that urate is a significant intracellular and extracellular physiological antioxidant [56—58]. Although the precise mechanism of how urate provides antioxidant protection is unknown, evidence exists that uric acid may preserve ascorbate by chelating transition metals such as iron and copper [57,59].

2.2.7 Bilirubin

Bilirubin is a product of hemoprotein catabolism and can be found in both intercellular and extracellular environment (e.g., plasma). Bilirubin is only partially soluble in water and is typically found bound to albumin in concentrations of 5 to 17 µM in human plasma [60,61]. At high plasma concentrations bilirubin is considered to be toxic. Indeed, plasma concentrations greater than 300 µM are associated with the risk of development of neurologic dysfunction because of the deposition of bilirubin in the brain [62,63].

Stocker et al. [60,61] proposed that bilirubin may serve as an antioxidant. However, at present, the importance of bilirubin as a physiological antioxidant is not well-described [64]. Nonetheless, it appears that bilirubin is capable of protecting albumin-bound fatty acids from lipid peroxidation under conditions of low oxygen tension [60,61]. Further, recent evidence suggests that both synthetic and natural bilirubin can be a potent circulating antioxidant in some conditions [65–67]. Additional research is required to determine if circulating bilirubin is an important antioxidant for skeletal muscle myocytes during exercise-induced oxidative stress.

2.2.8 Ubiquinone

Ubiquinones are lipid-soluble quinone derivatives that contain an isoprene or farnesyl tail. Ubiquinone homologues containing 1 to 12 isoprene units occur in nature. Reduced forms of ubiquinones, ubiquinols, are efficient antioxidants. Indeed, when compared to ubiquinones, ubiquinols are better antioxidants by several orders of magnitude [69].

The predominant form of ubiquinone in humans and many mammals is ubiquinone-10 (often called coenzyme Q) [70]. The major sources of ubiquinone-10 (UQ-10) in the diet are soybean oil, meats, fish, nuts, wheat germ, and vegetables (beans, garlic, spinach, cabbage) [71]. The concentration of UQ-10 in human plasma varies between 0.4 and 1.0 µmol/liter; approximately 80% is present in the reduced (ubiquinol) state [72,73]. In human tissue, UQ-10 is found in relative high levels (60–110 µg/g) in heart, liver, and kidney; 70–100% of which is in the reduced state [73]. With regard to the intracellular location, approximately 40–50% of the total cellular ubiquinone is located within the mitochondria, 25–30% in the nucleus, 15–20% in the endoplasmic reticulum, and the remaining 5–10% in the cytosol [74].

The antioxidant effect of ubiquinone was reported by in 1966 by Mellors and Tappel [69]. In recent years numerous reports have described the antioxidant role of ubiquinones and the consensus is that the antioxidant properties of ubiquinones are due to its phenol ring structure [70,75]. Ubiquinones react with oxygen radicals and singlet oxygen to prevent lipid peroxidation in membranes and other lipid structures in the cell 70). Also, some ubiquinones play an important role in the recycling of vitamin E during periods of oxidative stress via an NADPH-dependent system [75,76].

3. EXERCISE TRAINING AND SKELETAL MUSCLE ANTIOXIDANT CAPACITY

The antioxidant capacity of mammalian organ systems is well-matched to the rates of oxygen consumption and radical production. Indeed, body tissues with the highest oxygen consumption (e.g., liver, brain, kidney), have the greatest antioxidant enzyme activity. Further, skeletal muscles with high oxidative capacities possess higher antioxidant capacities compared to those muscles with lower oxidative potential.

It is well-established that the antioxidant defense systems of many mammalian tissues are capable of adaptation in response to chronic exposure to ROS. For example, it has been shown that irradiation of the mouse heart results in an increased expression of MnSOD [77]. Since prolonged exercise results in an increased production of ROS in skeletal muscle, it seems logical that regular exercise training would upregulate muscle antioxidant enzyme activities. Although there is growing evidence that endurance exercise training results in an increase in skeletal muscle antioxidant enzyme activity, several studies have failed to find a link between exercise training effects and muscle antioxidant enzyme activity. In this section we critically summarize the major findings regarding the effects of regular endurance training on the enzymatic and nonenzymatic antioxidants in skeletal muscle [11,78,79].

3.1 Superoxide dismutase

Although some investigators have reported that endurance training does not promote an increase in SOD activity in skeletal muscles [80,81], many studies have reported a training-induced increase in total SOD activity [15,16,84,85,94,97]. Differences in the experimental techniques used to assay SOD activity, variances in the type of exercise training protocol employed, and fiber composition of the muscles investigated may explain the variation in the literature. For example, the relative sensitivity to detect SOD activity differs widely between assays. Indeed, when comparing seven common assays to estimate SOD activity, Oyanagui [86] reported that 10-fold differences in the relative SOD sensitivity exist between methods. Therefore, investigations using SOD procedures with low sensitivity, might fail to observe small to moderate changes in tissue SOD activity due to the lack of analytical resolution.

Another potential explanation for the variable SOD findings is the differences in the type of exercise training protocols employed by investigators. For example, studies that have reported training-induced increases in muscle antioxidant enzymes have generally employed rigorous exercise training programs (i.e., high intensity and duration of exercise). This observation suggests that rigorous exercise training programs may be required to promote antioxidant enzyme activity in skeletal muscle. To test the postulate that high intensity and long duration exercise training is required to increase SOD activity in skeletal muscle, Powers et al.

[16] experimentally analyzed the relationship between the training stimulus (i.e., exercise intensity and daily duration) and the activity of skeletal muscle SOD. Nine groups of rats ran at three different daily durations (i.e., 30, 60, 90 min/day) and three different exercise intensities (i.e., 55, 65, 75% of VO_2 max). The results are illustrated in Fig. 3. These data clearly show that high intensity exercise training is generally superior to low intensity exercise in the upregulation of skeletal muscle SOD activity.

Also, close examination of training studies reveals that exercise induction of SOD may be fiber type specific with highly oxidative muscles being most responsive [10,15,16,81,82] (see Fig. 4). It seems likely that differences in fiber recruitment patterns (i.e., size principle) may account for these differences. However, the direct influence of exercise intensity and fiber recruitment on the upregulation of SOD activity in individual muscle fibers is difficult to evaluate. The influence of exercise on a muscle fiber is determined by the force of contraction, the frequency of fiber contraction, and trophic neuroendocrine influences [87,88]. Hence, it remains unknown as to whether the selective upregulation of antioxidant enzyme activity in highly oxidative muscles is due to ordered fiber type recruitment alone or due to fiber type regulated differences in antioxidant enzyme activities.

At present, only a few studies have examined which SOD isoforms in skeletal muscle are upregulated in skeletal muscle following endurance exercise training and the findings are inconsistent. For example, work by Higuchi et al. [84] and Pereira et al. [89] have shown that exercise training results in an increase in the activity of MnSOD only. In contrast, Leeuwenburgh et al. [97] reported that

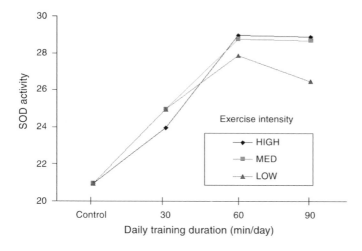

Fig. 3. The influence of endurance training daily duration and exercise intensity on total SOD activity in the rat soleus muscle. Note that training-induced increases in SOD activity are influenced by both the daily training duration and the exercise intensity. SOD activity is expressed as units per mg protein. Data are from reference [16].

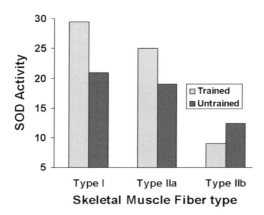

Fig. 4. The influence of skeletal muscle fiber type on endurance training induced changes in total SOD activity in rat skeletal muscle. Note that training-induced increases in SOD activity appears to be limited to highly oxidative muscle. SOD activity is expressed as units per mg protein. Data are from reference [16].

endurance training promotes an increase in the CuZn isoform of SOD in locomotor muscle. Two recent studies have provided new evidence that intense exercise training results in an upregulation of both MnSOD and CuZnSOD in rat skeletal muscle. First, Oh-Ishi et al. [90] reported that endurance exercise training results in an increased expression of both MnSOD and CuZnSOD in the rat diaphragm. Further, the effects of endurance training on the activity of SOD isoforms in skeletal muscles of rats have been recently examined [82]. Adult female Sprague-Dawley rats ran on a motorized treadmill for 10 weeks (60 min/day; 4 days/week at $\sim 70\%$ VO$_2$ max). At the completion of the training program, hindlimb skeletal muscles were isolated and homogenized to determine the activities of MnSOD and CuZnSOD using the technique described by Oyanagui [86]. Similar to the findings of Oh-Ishi et al. [90], these experiments support the notion that regular endurance training increases the activity of both MnSOD and CuZnSOD in the rat locomotor muscles (Fig. 5). In summary, there is growing evidence that endurance exercise training results in an increase in the activity of both MnSOD and CuZnSOD in rodent skeletal muscle.

Although endurance training promotes an increase in the activity of both oxidative enzymes and SOD, the increase in oxidative capacity is not matched by a proportional increase in SOD activity. Several studies have shown that endurance training does not result in parallel increases in both oxidative and antioxidant enzymes [15,16,91]. Indeed, the correlation between oxidative enzyme activity (e.g., Krebs cycle enzyme) and SOD activity is relatively low (r = 0.17) when compared in several rodent hindlimb muscles following exercise training [91]. The physiological significance of this observation is worthy of further investigation.

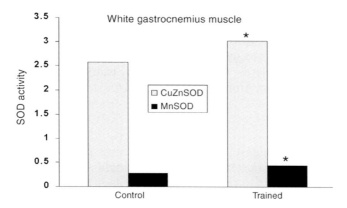

Fig. 5. Effects of endurance training on SOD isoforms in locomotor skeletal muscle. These results indicate that training promotes an increase in both MnSOD and CuZnSOD activity in muscle. Data are from reference [82]. Activity is expressed as units per mg of protein.

3.2 Glutathione peroxidase

The literature concerning the effects of endurance training on skeletal muscle GPX activity is reasonably consistent. It is generally agreed that endurance exercise training results in an increase GPX activity in active skeletal muscles [15,16,81,83,91—93]. A review of the literature indicates that long duration exercise training is superior to short duration exercise training in the upregulation of muscle GPX activity. This point is illustrated in Fig. 6.

Also, training-induced upregulation of GPX activity is generally limited to oxidative skeletal muscles (i.e., type I and IIa fibers). Further, endurance training promotes an increase in both cytosolic and mitochondrial GPX activity with the greater increase occurring in the mitochondrial fraction [10].

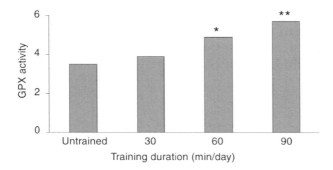

Fig. 6. Influence of daily training duration on glutathione peroxidase (GPX) activity in the rat plantaris muscle. GPX activity is expressed as μM substrate converted per min per 100 mg protein. Data are from reference [16].

Finally, similar to SOD activity, endurance training does not result in parallel and predictable increases in oxidative enzyme activity and GPX activity. Specifically, training-induced increases in Krebs cycle enzyme activities may increase by 40–100% in rat locomotor skeletal muscles whereas training-induced increases in GPX activity generally range from 10 to 30% [15,16,91].

3.3 Catalase

To date, there is little evidence to suggest that exercise training promotes an increase in catalase activity in skeletal muscle [16,84]. Interestingly, several studies have shown that exercise training may result in reduced catalase activity in some locomotor muscles [80,81]. The explanation for why endurance training may result in lowered catalase activity in muscle remains unclear.

3.4 Glutathione

There is growing evidence that skeletal muscle adapts to exercise-induced oxidative stress by increasing the GSH content. However, the effect of training on GSH content seems to vary greatly between animal species and tissues [11]. High intensity and long duration endurance training has been shown to increase GSH content in the hindlimb muscles of dogs [95,96,98] and rats [94,97]. This increased GSH content in trained muscles may be explained by an enhanced ability to take up GSH from the blood which may be due, at least in part, to increased activities of γ-glutamyl cycle enzymes (i.e., γ-glutamyltranspeptidase, γ-glutamylcysteine synthase, and GSH synthase) [11].

Careful examination of the literature reveals that training adaptation of GSH in muscle is fiber type specific. The explanation for this muscle fiber type variation in adaptation may be related to the rate of GSH utilization vs. the capacity of GSH uptake within each fiber type. In this regard, activities of the γ-glutamyl cycle enzymes may play an important role. For example, endurance training results in significant increases in GSH within the deep vastus lateralis muscle rats. In contrast, the GSH levels in the soleus and superficial vastus lateralis muscles were not elevated in response to training [97]. A potential explanation for this findings is that compared to the soleus and superficial vastus lateralis muscles, the deep vastus lateralis muscle has a higher γ-glutamyltranspeptidase activity [97]. Interestingly, no significant differences existed in γ-glutamylcysteine synthase activity between these skeletal muscles; this suggests that the translocation of amino acids across the muscle sarcolemma may be the limiting factor in the intracellular assembly of GSH [11].

While it appears clear that endurance training promotes an increase skeletal muscle GSH content, results on the effects of training on GR (required to recycle GSSG back to GSH) are less clear. Although some investigators report that endurance training results in little or no change in GR activity in locomotor muscles [94,97,98], others report that training promotes in increases in GR activity in skeletal muscle of trained rats [83]. The explanations for these divergent findings are unclear and warrant further study.

3.5 Vitamin E and other nonenzymatic antioxidants

To date, studies on the effects of endurance training on tissue levels of nonenzymatic antioxidants are limited. Of the nonenzymatic antioxidants, vitamin E and coenzyme Q are the only nonenzymatic antioxidants that have received experimental attention. In this regard, several studies have examined the effects of both chronic exercise (i.e., endurance training) and acute exercise on tissue levels of vitamin E in rodents. Unfortunately, the results are not consistent. Indeed, some investigations have reported that acute or chronic exercise in young adult rodents is associated with a significant reduction in skeletal muscle vitamin E levels [99,100] whereas others have reported no change [101–103]. The explanation for the divergent findings is not clear and additional experiments are required to provide a clear picture of the effects of exercise on vitamin E concentrations in rodent skeletal muscles.

To date, only published report exists regarding the effects of acute exercise on vitamin E levels in human skeletal muscle. Meydani et al. [104] reported that a bout of eccentric exercise resulted in a small but significant decrease in skeletal muscle vitamin E concentrations when expressed per gram wet weight. However, if muscle vitamin E levels were expressed per milligram of arachidonic acid (a membrane specific measure), exercise did not alter muscle vitamin E levels.

On a related issue, Packer et al. [105] have postulated that acute exercise results in an interorgan transport of vitamin E. Support for this notion comes from studies which indicate that plasma levels of vitamin E increase following exercise [104]. This could occur due to a release of vitamin E from adipose tissue, liver, and other tissues [105]. This type of interorgan transport may play an important role in maintain skeletal muscle vitamin E concentrations during acute exercise and/or chronic exercise training.

In summary, more research is required to clarify the effects of acute and chronic exercise training on vitamin E levels in skeletal muscle. Furthermore, the possibility that exercise results in interorgan transport of vitamin E is interesting and should receive additional research attention.

Studies investigating the effects of endurance exercise training the ubiquinone content of rat skeletal muscle are in agreement that training results in a significant increase in oxidative muscles [106–108]. Further, ubiquinone content in human skeletal muscle is higher in physically active subjects [106]. This training-induced increase in skeletal muscle ubiquinone content may be important in reducing exercise-induced lipid peroxidation.

4 SUMMARY

1. Muscular exercise results in an increased production of radicals and other

forms of reactive oxygen species. Further, growing evidence implicates cytotoxic as an underlying etiology in exercise-induced disturbances in muscle
redox status which could result in muscle fatigue and/or injury.

2. Muscle cells contain complex cellular defense mechanisms to reduce the risk
    of oxidative injury. Two major classes of endogenous protective mechanisms
    work together to reduce the harmful effects of oxidants in the cell: a) enzy-
    matic; and b) nonenzymatic antioxidants.

3. Key antioxidant enzymes include superoxide dismutase, glutathione peroxi-
    dase, and catalase; these enzymes are responsible for removing superoxide
    radicals, hydrogen peroxide/organic hydroperoxides, and hydrogen peroxide,
    respectively. Also, the thioredoxin and glutaredoxin enzyme systems play an
    important role in regulating cellular redox status by repairing oxidatively
    damaged thiols.

4. Important nonenzymatic antioxidants include vitamins E and C, β-carotene,
    GSH, uric acid, ubiquinone, and bilirubin. Vitamin E, β-carotene, and ubi-
    quinone are located in lipid regions of the cell whereas uric acid, GSH, and
    bilirubin are in aqueous compartments of the cell.

5. Regular endurance training promotes an increase in both total SOD and GPX
    activity in active skeletal muscles. In this regard, high intensity exercise train-
    ing is superior to low intensity exercise in the upregulation of muscle SOD
    and GPX activities. Also, training-induced upregulation of antioxidant
    enzymes is limited to highly oxidative skeletal muscles. In contrast to the
    observation that SOD and GPX are upregulated, training does not result in
    an increase in muscle catalase activity.

6. Regular endurance training improves GSH antioxidant reserve in skeletal
    muscle by increasing GSH levels in selected fibers, thus, attenuating exercise-
    induced oxidative stress.

7. To date, there is limited information on the effects of endurance training on
    nonenzymatic antioxidants. Of the nonenzymatic antioxidants, vitamin E
    and coenzyme Q have received the most attention. Several studies have exam-
    ined the effects of both chronic exercise (i.e., endurance training) and acute
    exercise on tissue levels of vitamin E in rodents. Unfortunately, the results are
    not consistent. Indeed, some investigations have reported that acute or
    chronic exercise in young adult rodents is associated with a significant reduc-
    tion in skeletal muscle vitamin E levels [61,62] whereas others have reported
    no change [63–65]. The explanation for the divergent findings is not clear
    and additional experiments are required to provide a clear picture of the
    effects of exercise on vitamin E concentrations in rodent skeletal muscles.

5   PERSPECTIVES

Although progress has been made toward identifying key physiological antioxidants, additional research is needed in this area. Indeed, improving our understanding of how individual antioxidants work in as a unit in both the intracellular

and extracellular environment is of paramount importance. Thus, work should focus on developing models to enhance our understanding of the cooperative action of both enzymatic and nonenzymatic antioxidants. Further, more research is required to fully understand individual antioxidant systems such as the thioredoxin and glutaredoxin antioxidant systems.

While previous studies have clearly demonstrated that regular endurance exercise promotes an increase in certain antioxidant defenses in the skeletal muscle myocyte, many additional questions remain. For example, it is unclear if exercise training alters the thioredoxin or glutaredoxin antioxidant systems in skeletal muscles. Further, there is a paucity of data regarding the effects of endurance training on nonenzymatic antioxidants.

While it is clear that endurance training promotes changes in skeletal muscle antioxidant capacity, an important mechanistic question is, "how does exercise-induced production of ROS promote the expression of antioxidant defense proteins"? Specifically, a key area for future research is to elucidate how exercise-induced changes in cellular redox status influences the cellular signal transduction processes that trigger antioxidant defense protein expression (see chapter 12 by Sen and Goldfarb in this volume, pp. 297–320).

There are a growing number of investigations regarding the influence of dietary antioxidants on the prevention of oxidative stress in a variety of experimental conditions. However, most of this work has not focused on the area of exercise and nutritional antioxidants. Hence, there is a need for well-designed experiments to explore the many unanswered questions regarding the potential effects of nutritional antioxidants on exercise metabolism and performance. For example, does regular endurance exercise increase the need for dietary antioxidants? Further, what is the optimal combination of dietary antioxidants to reduce exercise-induced oxidative stress? A pragmatic but answered question is, "will the consumption of optimal levels of nutritional antioxidants improve athletic performance in endurance events"?

6   ACKNOWLEDGEMENTS

This work was supported by grants from the American Heart Association, Florida (SKP), American Lung Association, Florida (SKP), National Institute of Aging (SKP) and by grants from the Ministry of Education, Finland and Juho Vainio Foundation, Helsinki (CKS).

7   ABBREVIATIONS

CAT: catalase
DHLA: dihydrolipoic acid
GPX: glutathione peroxidase
GR: GSSG reductase
Grx: glutaredoxin

GSH: reduced glutathione
GSSG: glutathione disulfide or oxidized GSH
LA: α-lipoic acid
ROS: reactive oxygen species
SOD: superoxide dismutase
Trx: thioredoxin
UQ: ubiquinone
VO$_2$ max: maximal aerobic capacity

8   REFERENCES

1. Davies KJ, Quintanilha AT, Brooks GA, Packer L. Biochem Biophys Res Commun 1982;107:1198—1205.
2. Jackson M, Edwards R, Symons M. Biochem Biophys Acta 1985;847:185—190.
3. O'Neill C, Stebbins C, Bonigut S, Halliwell B, Longhurst J. J Appl Physiol 1996;81: 1197—1206.
4. Reid M, Haack K, Franchek K, Valberg P, Kobzik L, West S. J Appl Physiol 1992a;73: 1797—1804.
5. Reid M, Shoji T, Moody M, Entman M. J Appl Physiol 1992b;73:1805—1809.
6. Borzone G, Zhao B, Merola A, Berliner L, Clanton T. J Appl Physiol 1994;77:812—818.
7. Nashawati E, DiMarco A, Supinski G. Am Rev Respir Dis 1993;147:60—65.
8. Shindoh C, DiMarco A, Thomas A, Manubay P, Supinski G. J Appl Physiol 1990;68: 2107—2113.
9. Barclay J, Hansel M. Can J Physiol Pharmacol 1991;69:279—284.
10. Ji L, Stratman F, Lardy H. Arch Biochem Biophys 1988;263:150—160.
11. Ji L. Exercise and Sport Science Reviews. Baltimore: Williams and Wilkins, 1995.
12. Halliwell B, Gutteridge JM. Free radicals in biology and medicine. Oxford: Clarendon Press, 1989.
13. Ohno H, Suzuki K, Ffujii J, Yamashita H, Kizaki T, Oh-ishi S, Taniguchi N. Exercise and Oxygen Toxicity. Amsterdam: Elsevier Publishers, 1994.
14. Grisham M, McCord J. Physiology of oxygen radicals. Baltimore: Williams and Wilkins, 1986.
15. Criswell D, Powers S, Dodd S, Lawler J, Edwards W, Renshler K, Grinton S. Medicine and Science in Sports and Exercise, 1993.
16. Powers S, Criswell D, Lawler J, Ji L, Martin D, Herb R, Dudley G. Am J. Physiol;1994;266: R375—R380.
17. Mathews C, van Holde K. Biochemistry. Redwood City: Benjamin Cummings, Publishing, 1990.
18. Lawler J, Powers S, Criswell D. Acta Physiol Scand 1993;149:177—181.
19. Smith CM, Plautt GW. Eur J Biochem 1977;97:283—295.
20. Pfeifer R, Karl G, Scholz R. Biol Chem Hoppe-Seyler 1986;367:1061—1068.
21. Sen C. Biochem Pharmacol 1998;55:1747—1758.
22. Goldman R, Stoyanovsky D, Day B, Kagan V. Biochemistry 1995;11:4765—4772.
23. Starke D, Chen Y, Bapna C, Lesnefsky EJ et al. Free Rad Biol Med 1997;23:373—384.
24. Mieyal J, Gravina S, Mieyal P. In: Packer L, Cadenas E (eds) Biothiols in Health and Disease. New York: Marcel Dekker Inc, 1995:305—372.
25. Gravina S, Mieyal J Biochem 1993;32: 3368—3376.
26. Yoskitake S, Nanri H, Fernando M, Minakami. J Biochemistry 1994;116:42—46.
27. Martinez-Galisteo E, Padilla C, Holmgren A, Barcena JA. Comp Biochem Physiol 1995;111B: 17—25.
28. Holmgren A. J Biol Chem 1989;264:13963—13966.
29. Fernando M, Nanri H, Yoshitake S Nagata-Kuno K et al. Eur J Biochem 1992;209:917—922.

30. Nakamura H, Nakamura K, Yodoi J. Annu Rev Immunol 1997;15:351—369.
31. Chae H, Rhee S. Biofactors 1994;4:177—180.
32. Yim M, Chae H, Rhee S. J Biol Chem 1994;269:1621—1626.
33. Netto L, Chae H, Kang S, Rhee SG et al. J Biol Chem 1996;271:15315—15321.
34. Tanaka T, Nishiyama Y, Okada K, Hirota K et al. Lab Invest 1997;77:145—155.
35. Spector A, Yan G, Huang R, McDermontt MJ et al. J Biol Chem 1988;263:4984—4990.
36. Schallreuter K, Wood J. Biochem Biophys Res Commun 1986;136:630—637.
37. May J, Mendiratta S, Hill K, Burk RF. J Biol Chem 1997;272:22607—22610.
38. Meister A, Anderson ME. Ann Rev Biochem 1983;52:711.
39. Ji L, Stratman FW, Lardy HA. J Am Coll Nutr 1992;11:79—86.
40. Yu B. Physiol Rev 1994;74:139—162.
41. Asuncion JG, Millan A, Pla R, Bruseghini L et al. FASEB J, 1996;10:333.
42. Vina,J, Sastre J, Asensi M, Packer L. Meth Enzymol 1995;251:237.
43. Packer L. Am J Clin Nutr 1991; 53:1050S.
44. Niki E, Noguchi N, Tsuchihashi H, Gotoh N. Am J Clin Nutr 1995;62(Suppl):1322S.
45. Burton G, Traber M. Annu Rev Nutr 1990;10:357—382.
46. Janero D. Free Rad Biol Med 1991;10:315—324.
47. Burton G, Ingold K. Ann N Y Acad Sci 1989;570;7—22.
48. Packer L. Ann N Y Acad Sci 1994;257—264.
49. Packer J, Slater T, Wilson R. Nature 1979;278:737—738.
50. Kagan V, Shvedova A, Serbinova E, Khan S, Swanson C, R Powell, Packer L. Biochem Pharmocol 1992;44:1637—1649.
51. Krinsky N, Deneke S. J Natl Cancer Inst 1982;69:205—209.
52. Krinsky N. In: Frei B (ed) Natural antioxidants in human health and disease. San Diego: Academic Press, 1994:239—262.
53. Burton G, Ingold K. Science 1984;224: 569—573.
54. Palozza P, Luberto C, Calviello G. Free Rad Biol Med 1997;22:1065—1073.
55. Howell RR, Wyngarden JB. J Biol Chem 1960;235:3544—3550.
56. Cutler R. In: Armstrong D, Sohal R, Cutler R, Slater T (eds) Free radicals in molecular biology, aging, and disease. New York: Raven Press, 1984:235—266.
57. Davies K. Free Radical Biol Med 1986;2:155—173.
58. Ames B, Cathcart E, Schwiers E, Hochstein P. Proc Natl Acad Sci USA 1981;78:6858—6862.
59. Sevanian A, Davies K, Hochstein P. Free Rad Biol Med 1985;1:117—124.
60. Stocker R, Glazer A, Ames B Proc Natl Acad Sci 1987;84:5918—5922.
61. Stocker R, Yamamoto Y, McDonach A, Glazer AN et al. Science 1987;235;1043—1046.
62. Meuwissen J, Heirwegh K. In: Heirwegh K, Brown S (eds) Bilirubin, vol 2. Boca Raton: CRC Press, 1982:39—83.
63. Schenker S, Hoyumpa A, McCandless D. In: Ostrow J (ed) Bile pigments and jaundice. New York: Marcel Dekker, 1986:395—419.
64. Belanger S, Lavoie JC, Chessex P. Biol Neonate 1997;71:233—238.
65. Yamaguchi T, Terakado M, Horio F, Aoki K et al. Biochem Biophys Res Comm 1996;223: 129—135.
66. Yamaguchi T, Horio F, Hashizume T, Tanaka M et al. Biochem Biophys Res Comm 1995;214: 11—19.
67. Wu T, Wu J, Li RK, Mickle D et al. Biochem Cell Biol 1991;69:683—688.
68. Briviba K, Sies H. In: Frei B (ed) Natural antioxidants in health and disease. San Diego: Academic Press, 1994:107—128.
69. Mellors A, Tappel A. J Biol Chem 1966;241:4353—4356.
70. Karlsson J. Antioxidants and exercise. Champaign: Human Kinetics Publishers, 1997.
71. Kamei M, Fujita T, Kanbe T, Sasaki K et al. Int J Vitam nutr Res 1986;56:57—63
72. Stocker R, Frei B. In: Sies H (ed) Oxidative stress: oxidants and antioxidants. San Diego: Academic Press, 1991:213—243.

73. Abert F, Appenlkwist E, Dallner G et al. Arch Biochem Biophys 1992;295:230—234.
74. Sustry P, Jayaraman J, Ramasarma T. Nature 1961:189;577—580.
75. Kagan V, Bakalova R, Serbinova E, Staychev TS. In: Packer L, Glazer A (eds) Methods in Enzymology, vol 186. San Diego: Academic Press, 1990:355—367.
76. Maquire J, Kagan V, Ackrel B Arch Biochem Biophys 1992;292:47—53.
77. Oberley L, St Clair D, Autor A, Oberley T. Arc Biochem Biophys 1987;254:69—80.
78. Sen CK. J Appl Physiol 1995;79:675—686.
79. Dekkers JC, van Doornen L, Kemper CG. Sports Med 1996;213—238.
80. Alessio H, Goldfarb A. J Appl Physiol 1988;64:1333—1336.
81. Laughlin MH, Simpson T, Sexton WL, Brown OR, Smith JK, Korthuis RJ. J Appl Physiol 1990;68:2337—2343.
82. Winters M. Unpublished masters thesis. University of Florida. 1998.
83. Venditti P, Di Meo S. Int J Sports Med 1997;18:497—502.
84. Higuchi M, Cartier LJ, Chen M, Holloszy JO. J Gerontol 1985;40(3):281—286.
85. Jenkins R. In: H Knuttgen (ed) Biochemistry of Exercise. Vol 13. Champaign: Human Kinetics Publishers, 1983:467—471.
86. Oyanagui Y. Anal Biochem 1984;142:290—296.
87. Pette D, Dusterhoft S. Am J Physiol 1992;262:R333—R338.
88. Vandenburgh H. Am J Physiol 1992;262:R350—R355.
89. Pereira B, Costa Rosa L, Safi D, Medeiros M, Curi R, Bechara E. Physiol Behav 1994;56:1095—1099.
90. Oh-Ishi S, Kizaki T, Ookawara Sakurai T, Izawa T, Nagata N, Ohno H. Am J Respir Crit Care Med 1997;156:1579—1585.
91. Hammeren J, Powers S, Lawler J, Criswell D, Martin D, Lowenthal D, Pollock M. Int J Sports Med 1992;13:412—416.
92. Hellsten Y, Apple F, Sjodin B. J Appl Physiol 1996;81:1484—1487.
93. Ji L, Wu E, Thomas D. Gerontology 1991;37:317—325.
94. Leeuwenburg C, Fiebig R, Chandwaney R, Ji L. Am J Physiol 1994;267:R439—R445.
95. Kretzschmar M, Muller D. Sports Med 1993;15:196.
96. Marin E, Kretzschmar M, Arokoski J, Hanninen O, Klinger W. Acta Physiol Scand 1993;147:369.
97. Leeuwenburgh C, Hollander J, Leichtweis S, Griffiths M et al. Am J Physiol 1997:272;R363—R369.
98. Sen CK, Marin E, Kretzschmar M, Hanninen O. J Appl Physiol 1992;73:1265—1272.
99. Bowles D, Torgan C, Ebner S, Kehrer JP et al. Free Rad Res Commun 1991;14:139—143.
100. Gohil K, Packer L, deLumen B, Terblanche SE. J Appl Physiol 1986;60:1986—1991.
101. Tiidus P, Houston M. J Nutr 1993;123: 834—840.
102. Salminen A, Vihko V. Acta Physiol Scand 1983;117:109—113.
103. Starnes J, Cantu G, Farrar R, Kehrer JP. J Appl Physiol 1989;67:69—75.
104. Meydani M, Evans W, Handelman G, Biddle L et al. Am J Physiol 1993;264:R992—R998.
105. Packer L, Almada A, Rothfuss L. Ann N Y Acad Sci 1989;570:311—321.
106. Karlsson J, Lin L, Sylven C. Mol Cell Biochem 1996;156:169—172.
107. Beyer RE, Morales-Corral P, Ramp B, Kreitman KR et al. Arch Biochem Biophys 1984;234:323—329.
108. Gohil K, Rothfuss L, Lang J, Packer L. J Appl Physiol 1987;63:1638—1641.

©2000 Elsevier Science B.V. All rights reserved.
Handbook of Oxidants and Antioxidants in Exercise.
C.K. Sen, L. Packer and O. Hänninen, editors.

Part IV • Chapter 11

Superoxide dismutases in exercise and disease

K. Suzuki[1]*, H. Ohno[2]*, S. Oh-ishi[2], T. Kizaki[2], T. Ookawara[2], J. Fujii[1],
Z. Radák[3] and N. Taniguchi[1]

[1]*Department of Biochemistry, Osaka University Medical School, 2-2, Yamadaoka Suita 565-0871, Osaka, Japan. Tel.: +81-6-6879-3421. Fax: +81-6-6879-3429. E-mail: seika@biochem.med.osaka-u.ac.jp*
[2]*Department of Hygiene, National Defence Medical College, 3-2 Namiki, Tokorozawa 359-8513, Saitama, Japan. Tel.: +81-429-95-1563. Fax: +81-429-96-5195. E-mail: eisei@ndmc.ac.jp and*
[3]*Laboratory of Exercise Physiology, Hungarian University of Physical Education, H-1123 Budapest, Alkotás u. 44, Hungary. Tel.: +36-1-156-4180. Fax: +36-1-156-6337. E-mail: radak@mail.hupe.hu*

1   INTRODUCTION
2   GENERAL PROPERTIES AND ASSAYS OF SOD
    2.1   General properties of SOD
    2.2   Assays of SOD
3   SOD IN EXERCISE
    3.1   Effect of exercise on SOD activity in humans
        3.1.1   Acute exercise
        3.1.2   Chronic exercise
    3.2   Effect of exercise on SOD activity in animals
        3.2.1   Acute exercise
        3.2.2   Chronic exercise
    3.3   Effect of exercise on SOD level in humans
        3.3.1   Acute exercise
        3.3.2   Chronic exercise
    3.4   Effect of exercise on SOD level in animals
        3.4.1   Acute exercise
        3.4.2   Chronic exercise
    3.5   Combined effects of dietary calcium restriction and acute exercise on SOD in animals
    3.6   Combined effects of hypoxia and chronic exercise on SOD in animals
    3.7   Combined effects of SOD treatment and acute exercise on oxidative stress in animals
4   SOD IN DISEASES
    4.1   Knockout mice of SODs
        4.1.1   Cu,Zn-SOD-deficient mice
        4.1.2   Mn-SOD-deficient mice
        4.1.3   EC-SOD-deficient mice
    4.2   Cu,Zn-SOD
        4.2.1   Clinical significance of Cu,Zn-SOD
        4.2.2   ALS
        4.2.3   Diabetes mellitus
        4.2.4   Werner's syndrome
    4.3   Mn-SOD
        4.3.1   Clinical significance of Mn-SOD
        4.3.2   Expression of Mn-SOD in vitro
        4.3.3   Mn-SOD in diseases
5   SUMMARY
6   PERSPECTIVES
7   ABBREVIATIONS
8   REFERENCES

*K.S. and *H.O. contributed equally to the work and should both be equal as first authors.

1   INTRODUCTION

Spitzer [1] has summarized that the formation of highly reactive oxygen-containing molecular species is a normal consequence of a variety of essential biochemical reactions. Oxygen free radicals can injure lipids, proteins, and DNA, and thus, may contribute to the development or exacerbation of many human diseases, including ischemia-reperfusion injury in heart attacks, organ transplantation, stroke, cancer, and emphysema, various inflammatory-immune injuries and the disorders of aging, as well as in several neurodegenerative disorders [1—9]. Moreover, there is growing evidence that strenuous physical exercise imposes oxidative stress on the body due to oxygen free radical generation, including an increase of lipid peroxidation in various tissues [3,4,8,10—20]. As a result of the potential for free radicals to damage cells and tissues, an intricate system consisting of both enzymes and small molecular weight molecules with antioxidant capabilities has evolved to protect against the adverse effects of free radical reactions. There exists ultimately a critical balance between free radical generation and antioxidant defenses.

Superoxide dismutase (SOD) is one of the most important enzymes in the antioxidant defense system. The enzyme scavenges superoxide anion (O_2^-),which is the first product of O_2 radicals, and thus, leads others in the antioxidant system [21]. An increasing number of papers have also been published concerning the effect of physical exercise on SOD in humans and animals (for reviews see Clark et al. [3], Jenkins [4], Sjödin et al. [10], Ji [17], and Ohno et al. [20]). With the exception of our works, almost all the experiments on physical exercise and SOD have been conducted to determine the enzymatic activity, not the amount of the enzyme protein, in various tissues. As described later, activity assay generally utilized for SOD measurement may lack specificity and may be subjected to interference from other factors, so that the results of different studies on SOD activity in various physiological and pathological stages are sometimes conflicting and are difficult to interpret. In addition, several excellent reviews on activity changes in various diseases already exist [22,23].

In the current review, first, we outline in brief the general properties and assays of SOD. Secondly, an attempt will be made to summarize former data on the effect of exercise on SOD activity in humans and animals. Thirdly, **putting stress on our work** with data on exercise and SOD isoenzyme levels (which were obtained mainly by enzyme-linked immunosorbent assays (ELISA) specific for each isoenzyme) will be introduced. Lastly, we will also summarize our recent data on Cu,Zn-SOD and Mn-SOD in diseases.

2 GENERAL PROPERTIES AND ASSAYS OF SOD

2.1 General Properties of SOD

Three types of SOD isoenzymes which are characterized by metal ions and their different localizations have been identified in mammals (Table 1). Cu,Zn-SOD is found in the cytosol and contains copper and zinc ions in a molecule, whereas Mn-SOD is located in the mitochondria with a manganese ion. For example, most of SOD activity in rat liver homogenates is present in the soluble fraction (84—92%), the rest being associated with mitochondria [24,25]. It has been estimated that 80% of the totally formed superoxide radicals in the mitochondria may be reduced by the mitochondrial SOD [26]. The remaining 20% will probably escape to the cytosol. Asanuma et al. [27] have shown that the regulation of Cu,Zn-SOD is independent of oxidative metabolism and is different from that of Mn-SOD, suggesting that the two isoenzymes scavenge superoxide from different subcellular sites of generation, one from cytosol and the other from mitochondria. Much is known about the biochemical and physical properties of the two isoenzymes [21,22,28,29]. In addition, there are a great many studies on Cu,Zn-SOD and Mn-SOD under a large variety of physiological and pathological conditions [20,22,23,28,29]. The third isoenzyme, copper and zinc containing extracellular SOD (EC-SOD), is a secretory glycoprotein [30—32] and is predominantly located in the extracellular space, such as plasma [33], however, it also occurs in tissues [34—36], this being unlike Cu,Zn-SOD and Mn-SOD. However, its clinical significance still remains to be elucidated. Furthermore, to our knowledge, there is no report about the effect of exercise on EC-SOD excepting our unpublished data.

Table 1. Properties of human SOD isoenzymes.

Property	Cu,Zn-SOD	Mn-SOD	EC-SOD
Distribution	Cytosol	Mitochondrial matrix	Extracellular
Molecular weight	32000	88000	135000
Subunit	Dimer	Tetramer	Tetramer
Metal/monomer	1 Cu, 1 Zn	1 Mn	1 Cu, 1 Zn
Inhibition by CN^-	+	−	++
Inhibition by H_2O_2	+	−	+
Inhibition by diethyldithiocarbamate	+	−	++
Inhibition by 2% sodium dodeyl sulfate	−	+	++
Inhibition by chloroform/ethanol	−	+	−
Rate constant for reaction with O_2^-	0.62×10^9	1.2×10^9	$0.72—1.0 \times 10^9$
Heterogeneity	Glycation, sulfhydryl	Sulfhydryl	Heparin binding

2.2 Assays of SOD

As already stated, many experiments have been conducted to determine SOD activity under various physiological or pathological conditions. It is difficult to measure the disappearance of the enzyme substrate or the formation of the products, as is routine, in enzymatic assays because the substrate and products are unstable. Therefore, routine assays for SOD activity employ the xanthine/ xanthine oxidase (XO) reaction for O_2^- generation and reduction of cytochrome c or nitroblue tetrazolium for O_2^- detection [21,37]. Reactions that have been useful in this way include the autoxidations of sulfite, epinephrine, hydroxyamine, and pyrogallol (for reviews see Fridovich [21] and Taniguchi [28]). Cu,Zn-SOD is sensitive to cyanide and H_2O_2, while Mn-SOD is resistant to these reagents [38]. The difference in the cyanide sensitivity of the two isoenzymes makes it possible to distinguish the enzymatic activities of the SODs. On the other hand, EC-SOD is thought to be the least abundant form of SOD in mammalian tissues. Although most species appear to have a relatively higher concentration of EC-SOD in the lung, the ratio of EC-SOD activity to the total SOD activity is only 5—10% even in the lungs [34,35]. Therefore, the SOD activities derived from intracellular Cu,Zn-SOD and Mn-SOD interfere greatly with the EC-SOD assay. A chromatography on gel-filtration [39] or concanavalin A-Sepharose [34] has thus, been employed to separate EC-SOD from other SODs, but these procedures are complicated and are difficult for a bulk assay.

As compared with enzymatic methods, immunochemical assay methods for SODs appear to be more reliable and reproducible because the determinations are specific to the protein moiety. Accordingly, activity may not always reflect the true amount of the enzyme protein, due to the presence or absence of cofactors, activators, and inhibitors. Indeed, our previous studies on γ-glutamyltransferase (γ-GT) in plasma [40] and liver [41] from physically trained subjects and rats, respectively, have indicated that the immunological level of γ-GT does not correlate well with the enzyme activity. Furthermore, when conventional enzymatic assays are used to determine SOD activities in tissues, nonspecific reactions due to other proteins or low molecular weight compounds possessing SOD-like activities in the tissues can cause erroneous results [38].

For the immunochemical assay of SOD, polyclonal or monoclonal antibodies are used. SOD protein levels can be determined by single radical immunodiffusion [42], radioimmunoassay [27], or ELISA [36,43—46]. In general, a sandwich-type ELISA is the most convenient method of immunochemical assay. Monoclonal antibodies are useful for this purpose. Monoclonal antibodies raised against human Cu,Zn-SOD [44] and Mn-SOD [45] have been employed in estimating the respective levels by a sandwich-type immunoassay (for a detailed explanation see Taniguchi [28]). Moreover, we have recently developed ELISA systems using polyclonal antibodies to mouse [36] and human [47] EC-SODs, as well as to rat Cu,Zn-SOD and Mn-SOD [46].

3   SOD IN EXERCISE

3.1 Effect of exercise on SOD activity in humans

3.1.1   *Acute exercise*

Table 2 compiles the former findings on the relationships between acute exercise and SOD activity in humans. Minami et al. [48] demonstrated a significantly increased plasma level of total SOD activity immediately after 10-min severe cycle of ergometer exercise. Conversely, as stated later, our pervious work showed a marked decrease in plasma level of Cu,Zn-SOD at 15 min after 15-min cycle ergometer exercise with almost the same load as the above study [49]. The discrepancy is probably due to the fact that even a trace of hemolysis affects serum level of Cu,Zn-SOD because Cu,Zn-SOD exists in large quantities in erythrocytes [50,51]. Accordingly, in the study of Minami et al. [48], consideration might not be given to the influence of hemolysis on SOD activity in plasma. Likewise, it would probably not be denied that the increased SOD activity was due in part to increased levels of plasma proteins and/or hemoconcentration [52]. For example, plasma ceruloplasmin reacts stoichiometrically with O_2^- [53]. Actually, a significant increase in ceruloplasmin concentration in human plasma has been observed immediately after cycle ergometer exercise [54].

It seems likely that the increased red blood cell SOD activity in the professional cyclists who covered 2,800 km in 20 days, was due to adaptation to aerobic endurance training, although the exercise period was not long [55]. Even marathon running had no effect on total SOD activity in skeletal muscle [56]. Likewise, loading of the athletes with L-carnitine for 10 days before running a marathon did not change the SOD activity substantially, resulting in no detectable improvement in performance of the marathon [56]. It appears, thus, that acute exercise has little effect on SOD activity in humans, although 20-min cycle ergometer exercise induced a small but significant increase in Cu,Zn-SOD activity in platelets [58].

Table 2. Acute exercise performance and SOD activity in humans.

Investigator	Subject	Tissue	Type of work	SOD	Change
Minami et al. [48]	Healthy student	Plasma	10 min bicycle, 182 W	Total	↑↑
Cooper et al. [56]	Marathon runners	Vastus lateralis m.	Marathon running	Total	→
	Marathon runner, carnitine-treated	Vastus lateralis m.	Marathon running	Total	→
Ohno et al. [57]	Untrained student	Red blood cells	30 min bicycle, 75% max	Cu,Zn	→
Mena et al. [55]	Professional cyclist	Red blood cells	5 h bicycle, race	Cu,Zn	→
	Professional cyclist	Red blood cells	6 days bicycle race	Cu,Zn	→
	Professional cyclist	Red blood cells	20 days bicycle race	Cu,Zn	↑
Kedziora et al. [58]	Healthy subjects	Platelet	20 min bicycle, 2W/kg BW	Cu,Zn	↑

3.1.2 Chronic exercise

Red blood cells may not accurately reflect muscle metabolism [59]. Nevertheless, red blood cell Cu,Zn-SOD activity increased significantly after long-term physical training [55,60], which is in agreement with the muscle study [61,62], as shown in Table 3. Lukaski et al. [60] indicated that the increases in red blood cell activity of Cu,Zn-SOD (a copper-dependent enzyme) without an increase in dietary copper were a functional adaptation of copper metabolism to aerobic training. Until a recent date the study by Jenkins et al. [61] was the only published work on a relationship between physical training and SOD in human skeletal muscle. There was a positive correlation between total SOD activity in the vastus lateralis muscle and $\dot{V}o_2$max. Quite recently Ørtenblad et al. [62] have also found that in resting muscle total SOD and Mn-SOD activities are significantly higher in jump-trained humans compared with untrained subjects. The intensity and/or duration of training employed by our group was insufficient to increase red blood cell Cu,Zn-SOD activity [63]. These findings suggest that adequate training increases the activity of SOD in humans, with resultant enhanced capacity for enzymatic scavenging of superoxide radical.

In future studies of SOD in human skeletal muscles it will be important to consider the fiber type profiles of skeletal muscles.

3.2 Effect of exercise on SOD activity in animals

3.2.1 Acute exercise

As shown in Table 4, the data related to the effect of acute running exercise on SOD activity in several tissues of rats and mice are different and sometimes conflicting. The different intensity of exercise may offer some explanation; that is, at heavy exercise the increases in SOD activity in skeletal muscle, heart, and liver appear to be greater. Even in the separate works of the same investigators on exhaustive exercise, however, total SOD activity in the red vastus lateralis muscle

Table 3. Chronic exercise performance and SOD activity in humans.

Investigator	Subject	Tissue	Type of work	SOD	Change
Jenkins et al. [61]	Healthy subjects, $\dot{V}_{O_2} \geqslant 60$ ml/kg/min	Vastus lateralis m.	Unexplained	Total	↑
Ohno et al. [63]	Healthy students	Red blood cells	10 weeks running	Cu,Zn	→
Lukaski et al. [60]	Varsity swimmers	Red blood cells	Swimming	Cu,Zn	↑↑
Mena et al. [55]	Amateur cyclist	Red blood cells	Bicycle	Cu,Zn	↑
	Professional cyclist	Red blood cells	Bicycle	Cu,Zn	↑
Ørtenblad et al. [62]	Volleyball players	Red blood cells	Volleyball	Cu,Zn	→
	Volleyball players	Vastus lateralis m.	Volleyball	Total	↑
	Volleyball players	Vastus lateralis m.	Volleyball	Mn	↑↑

Table 4. Acute exercise performance and SOD activity in animals.

Investigator	Subject	Tissue	Type of work	SOD	Change
Quintanilha	Untrained rats	Skeletal muscle	Exhaustive running	Cu, Zn	↑
and	Untrained rats	Skeletal muscle	Exhaustive running	Mn	↑↑
Packer [67]	Untrained rats	Heart	Exhaustive running	Cu, Zn	↑↑
	Untrained rats	Heart	Exhaustive running	Mn	↑↑
	Untrained rats	Liver	Exhaustive running	Cu, Zn	→
	Untrained rats	Liver	Exhaustive running	Mn	↑
	Untrained rats	Lung	Exhaustive running	Cu, Zn	→
	Untrained rats	Lung	Exhaustive running	Mn	→
	Trained rats	Skeletal muscle	Exhaustive running	Cu, Zn	→
	Trained rats	Skeletal muscle	Exhaustive running	Mn	→
	Trained rats	Heart	Exhaustive running	Cu, Zn	→
	Trained rats	Heart	Exhaustive running	Mn	↓↓
	Trained rats	Liver	Exhaustive running	Cu, Zn	→
	Trained rats	Liver	Exhaustive running	Mn	↑
	Trained rats	Lung	Exhaustive running	Cu, Zn	→
	Trained rats	Lung	Exhaustive running	Mn	→
Alessio	Untrained rats	Red vastus lateralis m.	20 min running	Total	→
and	Untrained rats	White vastus lateralis m.	20 min running	Total	→
Goldfarb	Untrained rats	Liver	20 min running	Total	→
[75]	Trained rats	Red vastus lateralis m.	20 min running	Total	→
	Trained rats	White vastus lateralis m.	20 min running	Total	→
	Trained rats	Liver	20 min running	Total	→
Ji et al.	Untrained rats	Skeletal muscle	1 h running	Cu, Zn	→
[76]	Untrained rats	Skeletal muscle	1 h running	Mn	→
	Untrained rats	Liver	1 h running	Cu, Zn	→
	Untrained rats	Liver	1 h running	Mn	→
	Trained rats	Skeletal muscle	1 h running	Cu, Zn	→
	Trained rats	Skeletal muscle	1 h running	Mn	→
	Trained rats	Liver	1 h running	Cu, Zn	→
	Trained rats	Liver	1 h running	Mn	→
	Se-deficient untrained rats	Skeletal muscle	1 h running	Cu, Zn	→
	Se-deficient untrained rats	Skeletal muscle	1 h running	Mn	→
	Se-deficient untrained rats	Liver	1 h running	Cu, Zn	↑
	Se-deficient untrained rats	Liver	1 h running	Mn	→
	Se-deficient trained rats	Skeletal muscle	1 h running	Cu, Zn	→
	Se-deficient trained rats	Skeletal muscle	1 h running	Mn	→
	Se-deficient trained rats	Liver	1 h running	Cu, Zn	→
	Se-deficient trained rats	Liver	1 h running	Mn	→

(Continued.)

Table 4. Continued.

Investigator	Subject	Tissue	Type of work	SOD	Change
Ji et al. [73]	4-month-old untrained rats	Vastus lateralis m.	1 h running	Cu, Zn	→
	4-month-old untrained rats	Vastus lateralis m.	1 h running	Mn	→
	4-month-old untrained rats	Liver	1 h running	Cu,Zn	→
	4-month-old untrained rats	Liver	1 h running	Mn	→
	26-month-old untrained rats	Vastus lateralis m.	1 h running	Cu,Zn	→
	26-month-old untrained rats	Vastus lateralis m.	1 h running	Mn	→
	26-month-old untrained rats	Liver	1 h running	Cu,Zn	→
	26-month-old untrained rats	Liver	1 h running	Mn	→
	31-month-old untrained rats	Vastus lateralis m.	1 h running	Cu,Zn	→
	31-month-old untrained rats	Vastus lateralis m.	1 h running	Mn	→
	31-month-old untrained rats	Liver	1 h running	Cu,Zn	→
	31-month-old untrained rats	Liver	1 h running	Mn	→
Spodaryk and Gaertner [77]	Untrained rats	Bone marrow	Exhaustive running	Total	→
Ji et al. [65]	4-month-old untrained rats	Heart	1 h running	Cu,Zn	↑
	26-month-old untrained rats	Heart	1 h running	Cu,Zn	↑
	31-month-old untrained rats	Heart	1 h running	Cu, Zn	↑↑
Ji and Fu [64]	Untrained rats	Red vastus lateralism.	Exhaustive running	Total	↑
	Untrained rats	Liver	Exhaustive running	Cu, Zn	↑
	Untrained rats	Liver	Exhaustive running	Mn	→
	Hydroperoxide-injected	Red vastus lateralis m.	Exhaustive running	Total	↑
	Untrained rats	Liver	Exhaustive running	Cu,Zn	↑
	Untrained rats	Liver	Exhaustive running	Mn	→
Ji et al. [65]	Untrained rats	Soleus m.	Light or exhaustive running	Total	→
	Untrained rats	Red vastus lateralis m.	Light or exhaustive running	Total	→
Ji [68]	Untrained rats	White vastus lateralis m.	Light or exhaustive running	Total	→
	Untrained rats	Heart	Exhaustive running	Total	↑
	Untrained rats	Liver	Exhaustive running	Cu,Zn	↑
	Untrained rats	Liver	Exhaustive running	Mn	→

(Continued.)

Table 4. Continued.

Investigator	Subject	Tissue	Type of work	SOD	Change
Mizunuma et al. [71]	Untrained rats	Soleus m.	Exhaustive running	Total	→
	Untrained rats	Gastrocnemius m.	Exhaustive running	Total	→
	Trained rats	Soleus m.	Exhaustive running	Total	↑
	Trained rats	Gastrocnemius m.	Exhaustive running	Total	↑↑
Lawler et al. [78]	4-month-old untrained rats	Soleus m.	40 min running, 70% max	Total	→
	4-month-old untrained rats	Red gastrocnemius m.	40 min running, 70% max	Total	→
	4-month-old untrained rats	White gastrocnemius m.	40 min running, 70% max	Total	→
	24-month-old untrained rats	Soleus m.	40 min running, 70% max	Total	→
	24-month-old untrained rats	Red gastrocnemius m.	40 min running, 70% max	Total	→
	24-month-old untrained rats	White gastrocnemius m.	40 min running, 70% max	Total	→
Lawler et al.[79]	4-month-old untrained rats	Costal diaphragm	40 min running, 75% max	Total	→
	4-month-old untrained rats	Crural diaphragm	40 min running, 75% max	Total	↑
	24-month-old untrained rats	Costal diaphragm	40 min running, 75% max	Total	→
	24-month-old untrained rats	Crural diaphragm	40 min running, 75% max	Total	→
Sen et al.[69]	Untrained rats	Red gastrocnemius m.	Exhaustive running	Mn	→
	Untrained rats	Mixed vastus lateralis m.	Exhaustive running	Mn	→
	Untrained rats	Longissimus dorsi m.	Exhaustive running	Mn	→
	Untrained rats	Liver	Exhaustive running	Mn	→
	Untrained rats	Heart	Exhaustive running	Mn	→
	Untrained rats	Kidney	Exhaustive running	Mn	→
	Untrained rats	Plasma	Exhaustive running	Mn	↑
	Trained rats	Red gastrocnemius	Exhaustive running	Mn	→
	Trained rats	Mixed vastus lateralis m.	Exhaustive running	Mn	→
	Trained rats	Longissimus dorsi m.	Exhaustive running	Mn	→
	Trained rats	Liver	Exhaustive running	Mn	→
	Trained rats	Heart	Exhaustive running	Mn	→
	Trained rats	Kidney	Exhaustive running	Mn	→
	Trained rats	Plasma	Exhaustive running	Mn	→
Somani et al. [80]	Untrained rats	Red blood cells	100% max running	Cu,Zn	↑
	Untrained rats	Heart	100% max running	Total	→
	Untrained rats	Heart, cytosol	100% max running	Cu,Zn	→
	Untrained rats	Heart, mitochondria	100% max running	Mn	↑
	Trained rats	Red blood cells	100% max running	Cu,Zn	↑↑
	Trained rats	Heart	100% max running	Total	↑
	Trained rats	Heart, cytosol	100% max running	Cu,Zn	↑
	Trained rats	Heart, mitochondria	100% max running	Mn	↑

(Continued.)

Table 4. Continued.

Investigator	Subject	Tissue	Type of work	SOD	Change
Leeuwenburgh et al.[81]	GSH-adequate mice	Liver	Exhaustive swimming	Total	→
	GSH-adequate mice	Kidney	Exhaustive swimming	Total	→
	GSH-adequate mice	Quadriceps m.	Exhaustive swimming	Total	→
	GSH-depleted mice	Liver	Exhaustive swimming	Total	→
	GSH-depleted mice	Kidney	Exhaustive swimming	Total	→
	GSH-depleted mice	Quadriceps m.	Exhaustive swimming	Total	→
Radák et al. [82]	Untrained rats	Hippocampus	Exhaustive running	Cu,Zn	→
	Untrained rats	Hippocampus	Exhaustive running	Mn	→
	Untrained rats	Cerebellum	Exhaustive running	Cu,Zn	→
	Untrained rats	Cerebellum	Exhaustive running	Mn	→
Leeuwenburgh et al.[83]	GSH-adequate mice	Heart	Exhaustive swimming	Total	↑
	GSH-depleted mice	Heart	Exhaustive swimming	Total	→
Leeuwenburgh et al. [66]	48-h unfed rats	Deep vastus lateralis m.	Exhaustive running	Total	→
	48-h unfed rats, refed at 24 h	Deep vastus lateralis m.	Exhaustive running	Total	→
	48-h unfed rats, refed at 48h	Deep vastus lateralis m.	Exhaustive running	Total	→
Oh-ishi et al. [84]	Untrained rats	Soleus m.	90 min running	Cu,Zn	↑
	Untrained rats	Soleus m.	90 min running	Mn	→
	Trained rats	Soleus m.	90 min running	Cu,Zn	→
	Trained rats	Soleus m.	90 min running	Mn	→
Oh-ishi et al. [85]	Untrained rats	Diaphragm	90 min running	Cu,Zn	→
	Untrained rats	Diaphragm	90 min running	Mn	→
	Trained rats	Diaphragm	90 min running	Cu,Zn	→
	Trained rats	Diaphragm	90 min running	Mn	→

of untrained rats has been reported to be increased [64] or unchanged [65,66]. Furthermore, in exhaustive exercise, the findings in liver for Cu,Zn-SOD and Mn-SOD are inconsistent [64,67—69].

It is known that SOD is induced by increased exposure to O_2 radicals in various organs and tissues [70]. It is also well known that strenuous exercise induces oxygen free radical generation [3,4,8,10—20]. The mechanism by which SOD can be activated within a relatively short period of time during exercise (less than 1 h) is largely unresolved [68].

Quintanilha and Packer [67] have demonstrated that, compared with untrained rats, the increases in both SOD isoenzyme activities in skeletal muscle and in the liver of trained rats are smaller after exhaustive running, suggesting a training effect. This finding on skeletal muscle is in sharp contrast to that by Mizunuma et al. [71]. From the facts that, at rest or after an acute bout of exercise at different intensities, SOD displayed little interfiber difference among the three muscle types, that is, its activities were similar, Ji et al. [65] have suggested that skeletal muscles probably have sufficient reserve in SOD activity and that the elimination of superoxide radicals may not be a limiting factor in muscle defense against O_2 free radicals.

Increased catecholamine values during stress have been reported to be significantly correlated to the severity of myocardial cell necrosis, through formation of strongly cytotoxic free radicals at the intracellular level [72]. Strenuous exercise markedly increases the blood levels for epinephrine and norepinephrine. Unexpectedly, Quintanilha and Packer [67] observed notable decreases in Mn-SOD activity in the heart of trained rats after exhaustive exercise. The physiological or pathological meaning of this decrease, therefore, should await further study. Sen et al. [69], however, failed to observe such a decrease in Mn-SOD activity in heart of trained rats after exhaustive running.

In skeletal muscle, on the other hand, Cu,Zn-SOD and Mn-SOD activities were significantly higher in 26- and 31-month-old rats, whereas the aged rats had significantly lower hepatic Cu,Zn-SOD activity than their young counterparts [73]. However, an acute bout of exercise had no overt effect on muscle or liver SOD activity, regardless of the animal's age. Meanwhile, in rats of the same age, Cu,Zn-SOD activity in the heart was increased after 1 h of running [74].

3.2.2 *Chronic exercise*

Endurance training may increase the resistance of skeletal muscle to injuries caused by lipid peroxidation [4,10,18,86]. So, endurance training would be expected to strengthen scavenger systems including antioxidant enzymes. Indeed, Jenkins [4] and Sjödin et al. [10] have indicated in each review that the data related to the effect of training on SOD are relatively more constant than those found for other antioxidant enzymes. As shown in Table 5, however, the findings for chronic exercise for SOD activity appear to be rather more conflicting than for acute exercise.

For example, significant increases in SOD activity in skeletal muscle [69,84,87—95] and heart [80,96—100] were noted after endurance training, but not in the other studies on skeletal muscle [68,75,76,101—104] or heart [68,69,88,95,105—108]. Such conflicting views on skeletal muscles were probably not due to the difference of either fiber types or SOD isoenzymes. In liver the same trend has also been shown [68,69,75,76,88,94,95,104—106,109,110]. The influence of physical training on liver SOD activity appeared to be dependent upon the regimen of exercise and animal model used; namely, swimming-trained mice had a significantly elevated level of SOD activity compared with running-trained rats [105,106,110]. It cannot be denied, however, that this swimming effect on hepatic SOD activity was attributable to cold acclimation rather than

Table 5. Chronic exercise performance and SOD activity in animals.

Investigator	Subject	Tissue	Type of work	SOD	Change
Reznick et al.	6-month-old mice	Heart	5 weeks running	Total	↑
[96]	22-month-old mice	Heart	5 weeks running	Total	→
	27-month-old mice	Heart	5 weeks running	Total	↓?
Jenkins [87]	Rats	Soleus m.	8 weeks running	Total	→
	Rats	Soleus m.	10 weeks running	Total	↑
Sohal et al.	Houseflies	Whole body	7 days flying	Total	→
[120]	Houseflies	Whole body	9 days flying	Total	→
	Houseflies	Whole body	14 days flying	Total	→
Kanter et al.	Mice	Whole blood	9 weeks swimming	Total	↑
[105]	Mice	Heart	9 weeks swimming	Total	→
	Mice	Liver	9 weeks swimming	Total	→
	Mice	Whole blood	21 weeks swimming	Total	↑↑
	Mice	Heart	21 weeks swimming	Total	→
	Mice	Liver	21 weeks swimming	Total	↑
Higuchi et al.	Rats	Soleus m.	3 months running	Cu,Zn	→
[88]	Rats	Soleus m.	3 months running	Mn	↑
	Rats	Red vastus lateralis m.	3 months running	Cu,Zn	→
	Rats	Red vastus lateralis m.	3 months running	Mn	↑
	Rats	White vastus lateralis m.	3 months running	Cu,Zn	→
	Rats	White vastus lateralis m.	3 months running	Mn	↑
	Rats	Heart	3 months running	Cu,Zn	→
	Rats	Heart	3 months running	Mn	→
	Rats	Liver	3 months running	Cu,Zn	→
	Rats	Liver	3 months running	Mn	→
Alessio and	Rats	Red vastus lateralis m.	18 weeks running	Total	→
Goldfarb [75]	Rats	White vastus lateralis m.	18 weeks running	Total	→
	Rats	Liver	18 weeks running	Total	→
Ji et al. [76]	Rats	Skeletal muscle	10 weeks running	Cu,Zn	→
	Rats	Skeletal muscle	10 weeks running	Mn	→
	Rats	Liver	10 weeks running	Cu,Zn	→
	Rats	Liver	10 weeks running	Mn	→
	Se-deficient rats	Skeletal muscle	10 weeks running	Cu,Zn	→
	Se-deficient rats	Skeletal muscle	10 weeks running	Mn	→
	Se-deficient rats	Liver	10 weeks running	Cu,Zn	→
	Se-deficient rats	Liver	10 weeks running	Mn	↑
Vani et al.	Rats	Liver	1 day swimming	Total	→
[109]	Rats	Liver	10 days swimming	Total	↑
	Rats	Liver	60 days swimming	Total	↑↑
Laughlin	Rats	Soleus m.	12 weeks running	Total	→
et al. [101]	Rats	Red gastrocnemius m.	12 weeks running	Total	→
	Rats	White gastrocnemius m.	12 weeks running	Total	→
	Rats	Red long head of triceps m.	12 weeks running	Total	→
	Rats	Medial head of triceps m.	12 weeks running	Total	→
	Rats, 1 h ischemia - 1 h reperfusion	Soleus m.	12 weeks running	Total	→
	Rats, (as above)	Red gastrocnemius m.	12 weeks running	Total	→
	Rats, (as above)	White gastrocnemius m.	12 weeks running	Total	→

(Continued.)

Table 5. Continued.

Investigator	Subject	Tissue	Type of work	SOD	Change
Cao and	Mice	Blood	6 weeks swimming	Cu,Zn	↑
Chen [110]	Mice	Liver	6 weeks swimming	Cu,Zn	↑
	Mice	Liver	6 weeks swimming	Mn	↑
	Zn-deficient mice	Blood	6 weeks swimming	Cu, Zn	→
	Zn-deficient mice	Liver	6 weeks swimming	Cu, Zn	→
	Zn-deficient mice	Liver	6 weeks swimming	Mn	→
Ji et al. [102]	25-month-old rats	Red vastus lateralis m.	10 weeks running	Total	→
Spodaryk and	Rats	Bone marrow	4 weeks running	Total	→
Gaertner [77]					
Kumar					
et al. [97]	Rats	Heart	60 days swimming	Total	↑
	Vit E-supplement	Heart	60 days swimming	Total	↓
Kramer et al.	rats				
[121]	Rats	Plasma	18 weeks running	Total	→
Ji [68]					
	Rats	Red vastus lateralis m.	12 weeks running	Cu, Zn	→
	Rats	Red vastus lateralis m.	12 weeks running	Mn	→
	Rats	Heart	12 weeks running	Total	→
	Rats	Liver	12 weeks running	Cu, Zn	→
Criswell	Rats	Liver	12 weeks running	Mn	→
et al.[89]	Rats	Mixed gastercnemius m.	12 weeks running, continuous	Total	→
	Rats	Rectus femoris m.	12 weeks running, continuous	Total	→
	Rats	Soleus m.	12 weeks running, continuous	Total	↑
	Rats	Mixed gasterocnemius m.	12 weeks running, interval	Total	→
	Rats	Rectus femoris m.	12 weeks running, interval	Total	→
	Rats	Soleus m.	12 weeks running, interval	Total	↑
Sen et al. [69]	Rats	Red gastrocnemius m.	8 weeks running	Mn	↑
	Rats	Mixed vastus lateralis m.	8 weeks running	Mn	→
	Rats	Longissimus dorsi m.	8 weeks running	Mn	→
	Rats	Liver	8 weeks running	Mn	→
	Rats	Heart	8 weeks running	Mn	→
	Rats	Kidney	8 weeks running	Mn	→
Powers et	Rats	Plasma	8 weeks running	Mn	→
al.[98]	Rats	R. ventricular myocardium	10 weeks running, 55% max, 30 min	Total	→
	Rats	L. ventricular myocardium	10 weeks running, 55% max, 30 min	Total	→
	Rats	R. ventricular myocardium	10 weeks running, 65% max, 30 min	Total	→
	Rats	L. ventricular myocardium	10 weeks running, 65% max, 30 min	Total	→

(Continued.)

Table 5. Continued.

Investigator	Subject	Tissue	Type of work	SOD	Change
Powers	Rats	R. ventricular myocardium	10 weeks running, 75% max, 30 min	Total	↑
et al. [98]	Rats	L. ventricular myocardium	10 weeks running, 75% max, 30 min	Total	↑
	Rats	R. ventricular myocardium	10 weeks running, 55% max, 60 min	Total	→
	Rats	L. ventricular myocardium	10 weeks running, 55% max, 60 min	Total	↑
	Rats	R. ventricular myocardium	10 weeks running, 65% max, 60 min	Total	→
	Rats	L. ventricular myocardium	10 weeks running, 65% max, 60 min	Total	↑
	Rats	R. ventricular myocardium	10 weeks running, 75% max, 60 min	Total	↑
	Rats	L. ventricular myocardium	10 weeks running, 75% max, 60 min	Total	↑
	Rats	R. ventricular myocardium	10 weeks running, 55% max, 90 min	Total	→
	Rats	L. ventricular myocardium	10 weeks running, 55% max, 90 min	Total	↑
	Rats	R. ventricular myocardium	10 weeks running, 65% max, 90 min	Total	↑
	Rats	L. ventricular myocardium	10 weeks running, 65% max, 90 min	Total	↑
	Rats	R. ventricular myocardium	10 weeks running, 75% max, 90 min	Total	↑
	Rats	L. ventricular myocardium	10 weeks running, 75% max, 90 min	Total	↑
Powers	Rats	Soleus m.	10 weeks running, 55% max, 30 min	Total	↑
et al. [90]	Rats	Red gastrocnemius m.	10 weeks running, 55% max, 30 min	Total	→
	Rats	White gastrocnemius m.	10 weeks running, 55% max, 30 min	Total	→
	Rats	Soleus m.	10 weeks running, 65% max, 30 min	Total	↑
	Rats	Red gastrocnemius m.	10 weeks running, 65% max, 30 min	Total	→
	Rats	White gastrocnemius m.	10 weeks running, 65% max, 30 min	Total	↓
	Rats	Soleus m.	10 weeks running, 75% max, 30 min	Total	↑
	Rats	Red gastrocnemius m.	10 weeks running, 75% max, 30 min	Total	→
	Rats	White gastrocnemius m.	10 weeks running, 75% max, 30 min	Total	↓
	Rats	Soleus m.	10 weeks running, 55% max, 60 min	Total	↑↑
	Rats	Red gastrocnemius m.	10 weeks running, 55% max, 60 min	Total	→
	Rats	White gastrocnemius m.	10 weeks running, 55% max, 60 min	Total	↓
	Rats	Soleus m.	10 weeks running, 65% max, 60 min	Total	↑↑
	Rats	Red gastrocnemius m.	10 weeks running, 65% max, 60 min	Total	→
	Rats	White gastrocnemius m.	10 weeks running, 65% max, 60 min	Total	↓
	Rats	Soleus m.	10 weeks running, 75% max, 60 min	Total	↑↑
	Rats	Red gastrocnemius m.	10 weeks running, 75% max, 60 min	Total	→
	Rats	White gastrocnemius m.	10 weeks running, 75% max, 60 min	Total	↓
	Rats	Soleus m.	10 weeks running, 55% max, 90 min	Total	↑↑
	Rats	Red gastrocnemius m.	10 weeks running, 55% max, 90 min	Total	→
	Rats	White gastrocnemius m.	10 weeks running, 55% max, 90 min	Total	↓↓
	Rats	Soleus m.	10 weeks running, 65% max, 90 min	Total	↑↑
	Rats	Red gastrocnemius m.	10 weeks running, 65% max, 90 min	Total	→
	Rats	White gastrocnemius m.	10 weeks running, 65% max, 90 min	Total	↓↓
	Rats	Soleus m.	10 weeks running, 75% max, 90 min	Total	↑↑
	Rats	Red gastricnemius m.	10 weeks running, 75% max, 90 min	Total	↑
	Rats	White gastrocnemius m.	10 weeks running, 75% max, 90 min	Total	↓↓
Powers	Rats	Costal diaphragm	10 weeks running, 55% max, 30 min	Total	↑
et al. [92]	Rats	Crural diaphragm	10 weeks running, 55% max, 30 min	Total	↑
	Rats	Plantaris m.	10 weeks running, 55% max, 30 min	Total	→
	Rats	Parasternal intercostal m.	10 weeks running, 55% max, 30 min	Total	→
	Rats	Costal diaphragm	10 weeks running, 65% max, 30 min	Total	↑
	Rats	Crural diaphragm	10 weeks running, 65% max, 30 min	Total	→
	Rats	Plantaris m.	10 weeks running, 65% max, 30 min	Total	→
	Rats	Parasternal intercostal m.	10 weeks running, 65% max, 30 min	Total	→
	Rats	Costal diaphragm	10 weeks running, 75% max, 30 min	Total	↑
	Rats	Crural diaphragm	10 weeks running, 75% max, 30 min	Total	→
	Rats	Plantaris m.	10 weeks running, 75% max, 30 min	Total	→
	Rats	Parasternal intercostal m.	10 weeks running, 75% max, 30 min	Total	→

(Continued.)

Table 5. Continued.

Investigator	Subject	Tissue	Type of work	SOD	Change
Powers et al.[92]	Rats	Costal diaphragm	10 weeks running, 55% max, 60 min	Total	↑
	Rats	Crural diaphragm	10 weeks running, 55% max, 60 min	Total	↑
	Rats	Plantaris m.	10 weeks running, 55% max, 60 min	Total	↑
	Rats	Parasternal intercostal m.	10 weeks running, 55% max, 60 min	Total	↑
	Rats	Costal diaphragm	10 weeks running, 65% max, 60 min	Total	↑
	Rats	Crural diaphragm	10 weeks running, 65% max, 60 min	Total	↑
	Rats	Plantaris m.	10 weeks running, 65% max, 60 min	Total	↑
	Rats	Parasternal intercostal m.	10 weeks running, 65% max, 60 min	Total	↑
	Rats	Costal diaphragm	10 weeks running, 75% max, 60 min	Total	↑
	Rats	Crural diaphragm	10 weeks running, 75% max, 60 min	Total	↑
	Rats	Plantaris m.	10 weeks running, 75% max, 60 min	Total	↑
	Rats	Parasternal intercostal m.	10 weeks running, 75% max, 60 min	Total	↑
	Rats	Costal diaphragm	10 weeks running, 55% max, 90 min	Total	↑
	Rats	Crural diaphragm	10 weeks running, 55% max, 90 min	Total	↑
	Rats	Plantaris m.	10 weeks running, 55% max, 90 min	Total	↑
	Rats	Parasternal intercostal m.	10 weeks running, 55% max, 90 min	Total	↑
	Rats	Costal diaphragm	10 weeks running, 65% max, 90 min	Total	↑
	Rats	Crural diaphragm	10 weeks running, 65% max, 90 min	Total	↑
	Rats	Plantaris m.	10 weeks running, 65% max, 90 min	Total	↑
	Rats	Parasternal intercostal m.	10 weeks running, 65% max, 90 min	Total	↑
	Rats	Costal diaphragm	10 weeks running, 75% max, 90 min	Total	↑
	Rats	Crural diaphragm	10 weeks running, 75% max, 90 min	Total	↑
	Rats	Plantaris m.	10 weeks running, 75% max, 90 min	Total	↑
	Rats	Parasternal intercostal m.	10 weeks running, 75% max, 90 min	Total	↑
Leeuwen-burgh et al.[91]	4.5-month-old rats	Deep vastus lateralis m.	10 weeks running	Total	↑
	4.5-month-old rats	Soleus m.	10 weeks running	Total	→
	14.5-month-old rats	Deep vastus lateralis m.	10 weeks running	Total	→
	14.5-month-old rats	Soleus m.	10 weeks running	Total	→
	26.5-month-old rats	Deep vastus lateralis m.	10 weeks running	Total	→
	26.5-month-old rats	Soleus m.	10 weeks running	Total	→
Pereira et al. [103]	Rats, standard diet	Mesenteric lymph nodes	8 weeks swimming	Cu,Zn	→
	Rats, standard diet	Mesenteric lymph nodes	8 weeks swimming	Mn	→
	Rats, standard diet	Thymus	8 weeks swimming	Cu,Zn	→
	Rats, standard diet	Thymus	8 weeks swimming	Mn	→
	Rats, standard diet	Spleen	8 weeks swimming	Cu,Zn	↓↓
	Rats, standard diet	Spleen	8 weeks swimming	Mn	→

(Continued.)

Table 5. Continued.

Investigator	Subject	Tissue	Type of work	SOD	Change
Pereira et al. [103]	Rats, standard diet	White gastrocnemius m.	8 weeks swimming	Cu,Zn	→
	Rats, standard diet	White gastrocnemius m.	8 weeks swimming	Mn	→
	Rats, standard diet	Soleus m.	8 weeks swimming	Cu,Zn	→
	Rats, standard diet	Soleus m.	8 weeks swimming	Mn	→
	Rats, polyunsaturated fatty-acid rich diet	Mesenteric lymph nodes	8 weeks swimming	Cu,Zn	↑↑
	Rats, polyunsaturated fatty-acid rich diet	Mesenteric lymph nodes	8 weeks swimming	Mn	↑
	Rats, polyunsaturated fatty-acid rich diet	Thymus	8 weeks swimming	Cu,Zn	↑↑
	Rats, polyunsaturated fatty-acid rich diet	Thymus	8 weeks swimming	Mn	↑
	Rats, polyunsaturated fatty-acid rich diet	Spleen	8 weeks swimming	Cu,Zn	↑
	Rats, polyunsaturated fatty-acid rich diet	Spleen	8 weeks swimming	Mn	→
	Rats, polyunsaturated fatty-acid rich diet	White gastrocnemius m.	8 weeks swimming	Cu,Zn	↓↓
	Rats, polyunsaturated fatty-acid rich diet	White gastrocnemius m.	8 weeks swimming	Mn	→
	Rats, polyunsaturated fatty-acid rich diet	Soleus m.	8 weeks swimming	Cu,Zn	→
	Rats, polyunsaturated fatty-acid rich diet	Soleus m.	8 weeks swimming	Mn	→
	Rats, saturated fatty-acid rich diet	Mesenteric lymph nodes	8 weeks swimming	Cu,Zn	↑
	Rats, saturated fatty-acid rich diet	Mesenteric lymph nodes	8 weeks swimming	Mn	→
	Rats, saturated fatty-acid rich diet	Thymus	8 weeks swimming	Cu,Zn	↑
	Rats, saturated fatty-acid rich diet	Thymus	8 weeks swimming	Mn	↑↑
	Rats, saturated fatty-acid rich diet	Spleen	8 weeks swimming	Cu,Zn	↑
	Rats, saturated fatty-acid rich diet	Spleen	8 weeks swimming	Mn	→
	Rats, saturated fatty-acid rich diet	White gastrocnemius m.	8 weeks swimming	Cu,Zn	↓↓
	Rats, saturated fatty-acid rich diet	White gastrocnemius m.	8 weeks swimming	Mn	↑
	Rats, saturated fatty-acid rich diet	Soleus m.	8 weeks swimming	Cu,Zn	→
	Rats, saturated fatty-acid rich diet	Soleus m.	8 weeks swimming	Mn	→
Pereira et al. [93]	Rats	Mesenteric lymph nodes	8 weeks swimming	Cu,Zn	→
	Rats	Mesenteric lymph nodes	8 weeks swimming	Mn	↓↓
	Rats	Thymus	8 weeks swimming	Cu,Zn	→
	Rats	Thymus	8 weeks swimming	Mn	→
	Rats	Spleen	8 weeks swimming	Cu,Zn	↓↓
	Rats	Spleen	8 weeks swimming	Mn	→
	Rats	White gastrocnemius m.	8 weeks swimming	Cu,Zn	↓↓
	Rats	White gastrocnemius m.	8 weeks swimming	Mn	↓↓
	Rats	Soleus m.	8 weeks swimming	Cu,Zn	→
	Rats	Soleus m.	8 weeks swimming	Mn	↑

(Continued.)

Table 5. Continued.

Investigator	Subject	Tissue	Type of work	SOD	Change
Shimojo et al. [106]	Mice	Brain	9 weeks swimming	Total	→
	Mice	Lung	9 weeks swimming	Total	→
	Mice	Heart	9 weeks swimming	Total	→
	Mice	Liver	9 weeks swimming	Total	↑
	Mice	Kidney	9 weeks swimming	Total	→
	Mice	Red blood cells	9 weeks swimming	Total	↑
Somani et al. [80]	Rats	Heart	10 weeks running	Cu,Zn	↑
	Rats	Heart	10 weeks running	Mn	↑
Hong et al. [94]	Normotensive rats	Outer wall of l. ventricle	10 weeks running	Total	→
	Normotensive rats	Longissimus dorsi m.	10 weeks running	Total	↑↑
	Normotensive rats	Quadriceps femoris m.	10 weeks running	Total	→
	Normotensive rats	Liver	10 weeks running	Total	↓
	Normotensive rats	Kidney	10 weeks running	Total	→
	Hypertensive rats	Outer wall of l. ventricle	10 weeks running	Total	→
	Hypertensive rats	Longissimus dorsi m.	10 weeks running	Total	→
	Hypertensive rats	Quadriceps femoris m.	10 weeks running	Total	↑
	Hypertensive rats	Liver	10 weeks running	Total	↓
	Hypertensive rats	Kidney	10 weeks running	Total	→
Oh-ishi et al. [117]	2-month-old mice	Diaphragm	6 weeks swimming	Cu,Zn	↑
	2-month-old mice	Diaphragm	6 weeks swimming	Mn	→
	26-month old mice	Diaphragm	6 weeks swimming	Cu,Zn	→
	26-month-old mice	Diaphragm	6 weeks swimming	Mn	→
Kim et al. [107]	Rats	Heart	18.5-month wheel running	Total	→
	Food-restricted rats	Heart	18.5-month wheel running	Total	→
Song et al. [104]	Rats, normal protein diet	Liver	12 weeks running	Cu,Zn	↑
	Rats, normal protein diet	Liver	12 weeks running	Mn	→
	Rats, normal protein diet	Gastrocnemius m.	12 weeks running	Cu,Zn	→
	Rats, normal protein diet	Gastrocnemius m.	12 weeks running	Mn	→
	Rats, casein protein diet	Liver	12 weeks running	Cu,Zn	→
	Rats, casein protein diet	Liver	12 weeks running	Mn	→
	Rats, casein protein diet	Gastrocnemius m.	12 weeks running	Cu,Zn	→
	Rats, casein protein diet	Gastrocnemius m.	12 weeks running	Mn	→
	Rats, soy protein diet	Liver	12 weeks running	Cu,Zn	→
	Rats, soy protein diet	Liver	12 weeks running	Mn	→
	Rats, soy protein diet	Gastrocnemius m.	12 weeks running	Cu,Zn	→
	Rats, soy protein diet	Gastrocnemius m.	12 weeks running	Mn	→
Somani et al. [99]	77-week-old rats	Heart	9 weeks running	Total	↑

(Continued.)

Table 5. Continued.

Investigator	Subject	Tissue	Type of work	SOD	Change
Husain and	Rats	Heart	6.5 weeks running	Total	↑
Somani [100]	Ethanol-treated rats	Heart	6.5 weeks running	Total	↑
Oh-ishi et al.	Rats	Soleus m.	9 weeks running	Cu,Zn	↑
[84]	Rats	Soleus m.	9 weeks running	Mn	↑
Oh-ishi et al.	Rats	Diaphragm	9 weeks running	Cu,Zn	↑
[85]	Rats	Diaphragm	9 weeks running	Mn	↑
Leeuwenburgh	Rats	Liver	10 weeks running	Cu,Zn	→
et al. [95]	Rats	Liver	10 weeks running	Mn	→
	Rats	Liver	10 weeks running	Total	→
	Rats	Heart	10 weeks running	Cu,Zn	→
	Rats	Heart	10 weeks running	Mn	→
	Rats	Heart	10 weeks running	Total	→
	Rats	Deep vastus lateralis m.	10 weeks running	Cu,Zn	↑
	Rats	Deep vastus lateralis m.	10 weeks running	Mn	→
	Rats	Deep vastus lateralis m.	10 weeks running	Total	↑
	Rats	Soleus m.	10 weeks running	Cu,Zn	→
	Rats	Soleus m.	10 weeks running	Mn	→
	Rats	Soleus m.	10 weeks running	Total	→
Libonati et	Rats	Heart	6 weeks sprint running	Total	→
al.[108]	Rats	Heart	6 weeks endurance running	Total	→
Toshinai	2-month-old mice	Kidney	6 weeks swimming	Cu,Zn	→
et al. [122]	2-month-old mice	Kidney	6 weeks swimming	Mn	→
	26-month-old mice	Kidney	6 weeks swimming	Cu,Zn	→
	26-month-old mice	Kidney	6 weeks swimming	Mn	↑

physical training, because the adaptive changes produced by swimming training were revealed more closely to resemble those produced by cold acclimation rather than those resulting from running exercise [111–115]. Actually, 4-week exposure to cold at 5°C definitely increased rat liver Mn-SOD level estimated by an ELISA [116]. On the other hand, the effect of physical training on diaphragmatic SOD activity appeared to be constant, namely, positive [85,92,117]. These data indicate that endurance training can cause tissue-specific adaptation of SOD.

Meanwhile, zinc has been reported to affect the free radical production in sedentary mice [118]. In the work of Cao and Chen [110], zinc deficiency eliminated the training-induced increases in blood and hepatic SOD activities which existed in zinc-adequate mice. However, a high amount of dietary zinc had even a harmful effect on both sedentary and exercised zinc-deficient animals. Physical training also increased SOD activity in blood [105,106,110], being in accord with human studies [55,60,119]; however, SOD activity in bone marrow was not increased after 4-week running training [77]. Finally, training effect on cardiac SOD activity was apparently reduced by aging [96].

Table 6. Acute exercise performance and SOD level in humans.

Investigator	Subject	Tissue	Type of work	SOD	Change
Ohno et al. [57]	Untrained students	Red blood cells	30 min bicycle, 75% max	Cu, Zn	→
Ohno et al. [49]	Volleyball players	Plasma	15 min bicycle, 75% max	Cu, Zn	→
	Volleyball players	Plasma	15 min bicycle, 75% max	Mn	→
Ohno et al. [123]	Soccer players	Serum	2 h soccer	Cu, Zn	↓↓
	Soccer players	Serum	2 h soccer	Mn	→
	Soccer players	Urine	2 h soccer	Cu, Zn	↑↑
	Soccer players	Urine	2 h soccer	Mn	→[a]
Ohno et al. [124]	Soldiers	Serum	93 h ranger training	Cu, Zn	→
	Soliders	Serum	93 h ranger training	Mn	↑↑
Haga et al.	Untrained students	Plasma	$\dot{V}_{O_2}$ max test, bicycle	EC	→
(unpublished data)	Trained students	Plasma	$\dot{V}_{O_2}$ max test, bicycle	EC	↑

[a]No immunoreactive Mn-SOD level in urine was detected before and after 2 h soccer training.

3.3 Effect of exercise on SOD level in humans

3.3.1 Acute exercise

Sedentary students were studied, using a bicycle ergometer, for 30 min at about 75% $\dot{V}_{O_2}$max [57]. As a result, red blood cell Cu,Zn-SOD level (which was measured by a single radial immunodiffusion technique) did not change substantially (Table 6).

On the other hand, Cu,Zn-SOD level (estimated by an ELISA) in plasma decreased markedly at 15 min and 24 h after 15-min cycle ergometer exercise, whereas the Mn-SOD level did not vary significantly (Table 7) [49]. The reduced plasma level of Cu,Zn-SOD, the molecular weight of which is 32,000 (smaller than that of Mn-SOD) (Table 1), could be the result of an increased glomerular permeability, although the mechanism remained obscure. Cu,Zn-SOD actually emerged into urine, in connection with the reduced plasma level of Cu,Zn-SOD after 2 h of soccer training [123]. Further investigations into the meaning of the

Table 7. Variations in plasma enzyme values and hematocrit level at ~ 75% $\dot{V}_{O_2}$ max on a cycle ergometer (n = 10) [49].

Variable	Initial control	Immediately after 15 min exercise	After 15 min rest	24 h after exercise
Mn-SOD (μg/l)	110 ± 6	113 ± 6	104 ± 9	109 ± 7
Cu,Zn-SOD (μg/l)	38.1 ± 5.1	30.2 ± 6.3	10.6 ± 2.9[a]	12.6 ± 4.5[a]
AST-m (IU/l)	5.73 ± 0.30	7.97 ± 0.62[a]	6.74 ± 0.70	5.62 ± 0.49
CK (IU/l)	91.2 ± 8.4	133 ± 14[a]	109 ± 19	78.1 ± 14.7
Hematocrit (%)	43.0 ± 0.8	46.6 ± 1.1[a]	44.1 ± 0.8	43.4 ± 0.7

Values are means ± S.E.M. SOD: superoxide dismutase; AST-m: mitochondrial aspartate aminotransferase; CK: creatine kinase. [a]$p < 0.05$ vs. initial control values.

changes in the renal clearance of Cu,Zn-SOD after physical exercise seem to be required.

Next, the ranger training was practiced for 93 h [124,125]. The soldiers moved about 80 km through a secluded place among the mountains, carrying 30–40 kg of equipment. Immediately after the ranger training there was a notable increase in Mn-SOD level in serum. The increased Mn-SOD seemed to be derived from skeletal muscles, since a positive correlation between Mn-SOD level and creatine kinase (CK) activity was noted (Fig. 1). CK is present mostly in the cytosolic fraction of cells. It is generally accepted, therefore, that the enzyme is released into the bloodstream even when there is a change in the cell membrane permeability [126]. Meanwhile, the increased serum Mn-SOD (which exists in the mitochondrial matrix) might reflect a disintegration of skeletal muscle in addition to increased O_2 radical species. Despite the fact that Cu,Zn-SOD is predominantly localized in the cytoplasm like CK, it was unaltered, possibly because of increased renal clearance. Furthermore, cytokines may offer a partial explanation for these changes. For example, interleukin-1 (IL-1) induces the mRNA for Mn-SOD, not for Cu,Zn-SOD [127]. It has actually been shown that IL-1 activity in human plasma is significantly elevated several hours after exercise on an cycle ergometer (1 h at 60% of aerobic capacity) [128], confirmed by the same group [129].

During the recovery period, Mn-SOD level in serum appeared to rise, while CK activity had returned to the pre-experiment value within 8 days after the ranger training. In view of the intimate interplay between Mn-SOD on the one hand, and aspartate aminotransferase (AST) and alanine aminotransferase (ALT) activities on the other after an 8-day rest (Fig. 2), along with the reduced activity of cholinesterase (Ch-E; a good index of hepatic function), one may deduce that the elevation of Mn-SOD level was derived mostly from the liver. In

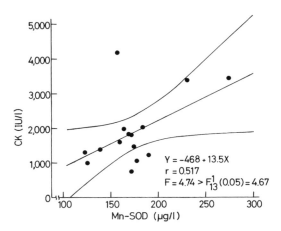

$$Y = -468 + 13.5X$$
$$r = 0.517$$
$$F = 4.74 > F_{13}^1 (0.05) = 4.67$$

Fig. 1. Correlation between Mn-SOD level and CK activity in serum immediately after 93 h strenuous ranger training. The 95% confidence limits for the predicted mean value of Y are shown.

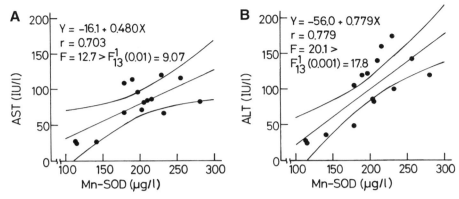

Fig. 2. Correlation between Mn-SOD level and AST activity (A) or Mn-SOD level and ALT activity (B) 8 days after 93 h strenuous ranger training. The 95% confidence limits are also shown in each panel.

the study of Ahlborg and Brohult [130], one week after prolonged physical exercise a significant increase in ornithine carbamoyltransferase activity in human serum has also been observed, suggesting inadequate maintenance of the hepatic circulation and a metabolic steady state. It, thus, seemed likely that marked increases in serum Mn-SOD level during an 8-day recovery period resulted mainly from skeletal muscle damage at the early stage and from liver damage at the later stage, respectively. Moreover, the subjects showing prominent leukocytosis (over 9,500 cells/μl) exhibited a lower activity of serum Ch-E than those who showed milder leukocytosis during and after the ranger training [125]. The degree of leukocytosis also showed a close correlation with the values of some serum parameters, such as those of AST, lactate dehydrogenase, blood urea nitrogen, CK, Mn-SOD, ALT, and uric acid, reflecting organ damage and restoration after strenuous exercise. These findings suggest that immunoreactive Mn-SOD level in human serum provides a reliable index of strenuous physical exercise.

As to immunological EC-SOD, a single bout of exhaustive cycle ergometer exercise induced a significant increase in its serum concentration in trained university students, but not in sedentary university students, although the precise physiological meaning remains to be clarified (Ookawara et al., unpublished data).

3.3.2 Chronic exercise

Effect of 10 weeks of running training on red blood cell Cu,Zn-SOD level was investigated in sedentary students [63]. There was no significant change in the Cu,Zn-SOD level after training, being in accord with that in the enzyme activity Table 8).

On the other hand, athletes had a significantly higher plasma level of Mn-SOD as compared to sedentary individuals, whereas there was no disparity of Cu,Zn-

Table 8. Chronic exercise performance and SOD level in humans.

Investigator	Subject	Tissue	Type of work	SOD	Change
Ohno et al. [63]	Healthy students	Red blood cells	10 weeks running	Cu, Zn	→
Ohno et al. [131]	Cross-country skiers	Plasma	Cross-country skiing	Cu, Zn	→
	Cross-country skiers	Plasma	Cross-country skiing	Mn	↑
Ookawara et al.	Healthy students	Plasma	3 months swimming	EC	→
(unpublished data)	Healthy students	Plasma	3 months swimming	EC	→

SOD level [131]. This was in approximate agreement with previous findings in skeletal muscles; that is, there was a significant increase in Mn-SOD activity in any fast-twitch, slow-twitch, and white types of muscle of rats after 3 months of running training, but not in Cu,Zn-SOD activity [88]. In addition, elevated total SOD activity was observed in vastus lateralis muscle of trained subjects [61]. These findings may indicate that the physical training induces an increased capacity for enzymatic scavenging of superoxide radical in skeletal muscle, especially in the mitochondria, which are probably faced with the elevated rate of oxygen utilization.

Lastly, no definite effect on 3-month swimming or running training was noted on plasma EC-SOD concentration in university students (Ookawara et al., unpublished data). Possible effects of physical exercise on EC-SOD, however, should await further study.

3.4 Effect of exercise on SOD level in animals

3.4.1 Acute exercise

A single bout of exhaustive running significantly increased the plasma level of immunoreactive Mn-SOD in both untrained and trained rats [69] (Table 9). In spite of the fact that the untrained rats could run for a shorter duration compared to their trained counterpart, the extent of the change was more prominent in the untrained rats compared to the trained rats; however, the difference was not significant. Meanwhile, in other six tissues of either rats the Mn-SOD level was unaffected by the acute exercise. Immediately after 90 min of running, either Cu,Zn-SOD content or Mn-SOD content was unchanged in soleus muscle [84] or diaphragm [85] from untrained and trained rats. After the acute exercise the expression of Mn-SOD mRNA was remarkably attenuated only in soleus muscle of untrained rats, whereas that of other mRNAs was not influenced definitely. This finding suggests that, compared with trained rats, the limb skeletal muscle of untrained rats would be subject to a more severe oxidative stress during exercise.

Table 9. Acute exercise performance and SOD level in animals.

Investigator	Subject	Tissue	Type of work	SOD	Change
Sen et al. [69]	Untrained rats	Red gastrocnemius m.	Exhaustive running	Mn	→
	Untrained rats	Mixed vastus lateralis	Exhaustive running	Mn	→
	Untrained rats	Longissimus dorsi m.	Exhaustive running	Mn	→
	Untrained rats	Heart	Exhaustive running	Mn	→
	Untrained rats	Liver	Exhaustive running	Mn	→
	Untrained rats	Kidney	Exhaustive running	Mn	→
	Untrained rats	Plasma	Exhaustive running	Mn	↑
	Trained rats	Red gastrocnemius m.	Exhaustive running	Mn	→
	Trained rats	Mixed vastus lateralis	Exhaustive running	Mn	→
	Trained rats	Longissimus dorsi m.	Exhaustive running	Mn	→
	Trained rats	Heart	Exhaustive running	Mn	→
	Trained rats	Liver	Exhaustive running	Mn	→
	Trained rats	Kidney	Exhaustive running	Mn	→
	Trained rats	Plasma	Exhaustive running	Mn	↑
Oh-ishi et al. [84]	Untrained rats	Soleus m.	90 min running	Cu,Zn	→
	Untrained rats	Soleus m.	90 min running	Mn	→
	Trained rats	Soleus m.	90 min running	Cu,Zn	→
	Trained rats	Soleus m.	90 min running	Mn	→
Oh-ishi et al. [85]	Untrained rats	Diaphragm	90 min running	Cu,Zn	→
	Untrained rats	Diaphragm	90 min running	Mn	→
	Trained rats	Diaphragm	90 min running	Cu,Zn	→
	Trained rats	Diaphragm	90 min running	Mn	→

3.4.2 *Chronic exercise*

Both Cu,Zn-SOD and Mn-SOD contents in diaphragm muscle of rats were significantly increased with running training [85]; however, the mRNA expressions of both forms of SOD did not show any significant change with endurance training. Therefore, the increases in SODs during training appears not to be controlled by a transcriptional process, but by some post-transcriptional mechanisms, i.e., by a translational and/or a post-translational process. It may also be possible that the expressions of SOD mRNAs were initially upregulated and then downregulated because oxidative stress is generated during exercise (especially at the early stage of training), which is known to activate nuclear factor-κB, and thereby induces transcription of SODs, in particular Mn-SOD [132]. The precise mechanism, however, must await further study. Similar findings (except for immunoreactive Cu,Zn-SOD content) were also found in soleus muscle [84]. The contents of Cu,Zn-SOD in soleus muscle of untrained and trained rats were not different at rest, although its activity was significantly higher in trained rats than in untrained rats, probably due to changes in the specific activity (activity/enzyme protein), possibly because of increased levels of effector(s) and/or decreased levels of inhibitor(s); the mechanism of the regulation also remains unclear (Table 10).

On the other hand, a 6-week swimming training failed to increase Cu,Zn-SOD and Mn-SOD contents in diaphragm of 2- and 26-month-old mice [117]. Likewise, no overt effect of endurance training was observed on Mn-SOD content in

Table 10. Chronic exercise performance and SOD level in animals.

Investigator	Subject	Tissue	Type of work	SOD	Change
Sen et al. [69]	Rats	Red gastrocnemius m.	8 weeks running	Mn	→
	Rats	Mixed vastus lateralis m.	8 weeks running	Mn	→
	Rats	Longissimus dorsi m.	8 weeks running	Mn	→
	Rats	Heart	8 weeks running	Mn	→
	Rats	Liver	8 weeks running	Mn	→
	Rats	Kidney	8 weeks running	Mn	→
	Rats	Plasma	8 weeks running	Mn	→
Oh-ishi et al. [117]	2-month-old mice	Diaphragm	6 weeks swimming	Cu,Zn	→
	2-month-old mice	Diaphragm	6 weeks swimming	Mn	→
	26-month-old mice	Diaphragm	6 weeks swimming	Cu,Zn	→
	26-month-old mice	Diaphragm	6 weeks swimming	Mn	→
Oh-ishi et al. [84]	Rats	Soleus m.	9 weeks running	Cu,Zn	→
	Rats	Soleus m.	9 weeks running	Mn	↑
Oh-ishi et al. [85]	Rats	Diaphragm	9 weeks running	Cu,Zn	↑
	Rats	Diaphragm	9 weeks running	Mn	↑
Toshinai et al. [122]	2-month-old mice	Kidney	6 weeks swimming	Cu,Zn	↓
	2-month-old mice	Kidney	6 weeks swimming	Mn	↓
	26-month-old mice	Kidney	6 weeks swimming	Cu,Zn	↓
	26-month-old mice	Kidney	6 weeks swimming	Mn	↓
Husain and Somani [100]	Rats	Heart	6.5 weeks running	Cu,Zn	→
	Ethanol-treated rats	Heart	6.5 weeks running	Cu,Zn	→
Ookawara et al. (unpublished data)	Lean rats	Serum	6 weeks swimming	EC	→
	Obese (ob/ob)mice	Serum	6 weeks swimming	EC	→

seven tissues of rats [69], or on Cu,Zn-SOD content in heart of rats [100]. Unexpectedly, on the other hand, the contents of Cu,Zn-SOD and Mn-SOD showed a downward trend in the kidney of young and old mice after a 6-week swimming training [122].

Very recently we have investigated the effect of a 6-week endurance swimming training on immunoreactive EC-SOD concentration (as judged by an ELISA) in serum from lean and obese (ob/ob) mice (Ookawara et al., unpublished data). As the result, serum EC-SOD concentration on either type of mouse was unaffected by the training. Meanwhile, interestingly, serum EC-SOD concentration was markedly higher in obese mice than in lean mice. Indeed, white adipose tissue had a high content of the enzyme and showed a relatively strong expression of the mRNA [36]. In addition, EC-SOD concentration in serum of lean mice increased significantly with age (Ookawara et al., unpublished data).

These disparate results may be due to differences in intensity, duration, and mode of physical exercise, subcellular distribution of SOD isoenzymes, and tissue-specific expression of these isoenzymes.

3.5 Combined effects of dietary calcium restriction and acute exercise on SOD in animals

A study was made of the combined effects of dietary calcium restriction and exhaustive exercise on Cu,Zn-SOD and Mn-SOD in rat soleus muscle [133].

Rats were assigned to the control rats or the calcium-restricted rats; they were restricted for 1 month or 3 months. Each group was subdivided into acutely exercised or nonexercised groups. Three-month dietary calcium restriction resulted in calcium deficiency, and upregulated both SOD isoenzymes (activity and content). Unlike glutathione peroxidase (GPX) and catalase activities, exhaustive exercise did not decrease either Cu,Zn-SOD or Mn-SOD activity. During the 3-month calcium restriction, on the other hand, the mRNA expressions of both forms of SOD showed an initial upregulation, followed by a downregulation. Exhaustive exercise significantly increased their mRNA expressions only in the 3-month calcium-restricted rats. Also, exhaustive exercise markedly increased the activity of myeloperoxidase (an index of the infiltration of neutrophils in tissues) in soleus muscle from the 1-month and 3-month calcium-restricted rats as compared with the control rats; this significantly enhanced the ability of neutrophils to generate superoxide only in the 3 month calcium-restricted rats. The results obtained demonstrate that dietary calcium restriction upregulates both SOD isoenzymes in rat soleus muscle, indicating the potential for improvement of the resistance to the increase in intracellular reactive oxygen species. The results also suggest that exhaustive exercise may cause oxidative damage in soleus muscle of calcium-deficient rats through the activation of neutrophils.

3.6 Combined effects of hypoxia and chronic exercise on SOD in animals

A number of studies have revealed that chronic hypoxia, by decreasing the total SOD activity [134,135] or Mn-SOD content [136,137], may lead to increased susceptibility to oxidant injury particularly in liver and soleus muscle. Thus, the oxidative stress-related consequences of physical training at high altitude were investigated [138]. As the result, the 4-week running training performed under hypobaric hypoxia, equivalent to an altitude of 4,000 m, increased the level of reactive carbonyl derivatives measured by anti-2,4-dinitrophenylhydrazone antibodies and spectrophotometry in both white and red types of skeletal muscle of rats compared with sea level trained rats and control groups. The altitude training also increased the activity of Mn-SOD in both types of muscle, whereas the Cu,Zn-SOD activity was not changed significantly (Table 11). Since GPX and catalase activities in either

Table 11. Cu,Zn-SOD and Mn-SOD activities in white (WQ) and red (RQ) portions of quadriceps muscles of rats [138].

Group (n = 6)	Cu,Zn-SOD (U/mg protein)		Mn-SOD (U/mg protein)	
	WQ	RQ	WQ	RQ
Control	9.06 ± 0.7	11.5 ± 0.5	5.24 ± 0.5	8.18 ± 0.3
Sea level	9.16 ± 0.4	14.9 ± 1.1	8.31 ± 0.7^a	10.3 ± 0.8
High altitude	9.46 ± 0.6	13.5 ± 1.3	8.48 ± 0.6^a	11.9 ± 1.1^a

Values are means $\pm$ S.E.M. [a]$p < 0.05$ vs. control group.

white or red type of muscle of altitude trained rats did not vary substantially, it was suggested that the oxidative modification of certain amino acids is due to the increasing gap between activity of SOD and peroxide scavenging enzymes, which results in an increase in the number of hydrogen peroxide molecules.

3.7 Combined effects of SOD treatment and acute exercise on oxidative stress in animals

An SOD derivative (SM-SOD), synthesized by covalently linking poly-(stylene-co-maleic acid) butyl ester to a Cu,Zn-SOD, which circulates and is bound to albumin with a halflife of 6 h [139] was injected intraperitoneally into the rats prior to exhaustive running [140]. The exercise induced a marked increase in the activity of XO (which utelizes molecular oxygen as an electron acceptor and thus, generates O_2^-) in plasma, and an increase in thiobarbituric-reactive substances (TBARS), an indicator of lipid peroxidation, in the plasma, as well as in the soleus and tibialis muscles from nonadministered rats immediately after the exercise, indicating massive free radical formation. The immunoreactive content and activity of both SOD isoenzymes (Cu,Zn-SOD and Mn-SOD) of nonadministered rats increased significantly in the soleus and tibialis muscles immediately after running; this also suggested an increased output of O_2^-. SM-SOD treatment definitely attenuated the degree of the increases in XO and TBARS in all the samples examined immediately after exercise. These findings suggest that a single bout of exhaustive exercise induces oxidative stress in skeletal muscle of rats, irrespective of its fiber type, and that this oxidative stress can be weakened by exogenous SM-SOD. Similar results were also given by the study on liver and kidney [141]. By contrast, Homans et al. [142] have shown that infusion of bovine serum SOD via the left atrial catheter in dogs affects neither the transient rebound function occurring early after exercise nor the prolonged period of stunning, indicating that the myocardial stunning that follows exercise induced ischemia is unlikely to be mediated by oxygen free radicals. The disparity noted between the studies by Radák et al. [140,141] and by Homans et al. [142] would probably be attributable to that in the half life of SODs administered (the former: 6 h and the latter: 5 min) [139]. Actually, a single injection of SM-SOD was effective under various oxidative stresses [143–146].

4   SOD IN DISEASES

It has been strongly suggested that many of the cell alterations seen in normal aging process and various diseases including cancer, are due to oxidative damage from active oxygen species. SODs scavenge O_2^-, and so, the study of these enzymes is of potential clinical interest. In this chapter we will attempt to summarize recent data on the clinical and pathological significance of Cu,Zn-SOD and Mn-SOD, especially in relation to neuronal degeneration, diabetes, cancer, and ischemia [28,29,147,148].

4.1 Knockout mice of SODs

To analyze roles of SODs, several mice lines with targeted inactivation of SODs have been generated. These data provide new insight into understanding the significance of SODs in vivo.

4.1.1 Cu, Zn-SOD-deficient mice

It has been reported that some cases of familial amyotrophic lateral sclerosis (FALS) are associated with mutations in the Cu,Zn-SOD gene (SOD1) and that Cu,Zn-SOD protects neuronal cells from various damages including ischemia or apoptosis. In order to analyze the role of Cu,Zn-SOD, two groups generated mouse lines with targeted inactivation of Cu,Zn-SOD [149, 150]. Contrary to their expectations these mice developed normally and showed no phenotypic abnormality under normal conditions. However, Cu,Zn-SOD knockout mice exhibited marked vulnerability to motor neuron loss after axonal injury [149], and showed a high level of blood brain barrier disruption soon after 1 h of middle cerebral artery occlusion and 100% mortality at 24 h after ischemia, while wild-type mice showed 11% mortality [150]. These results suggest that Cu,Zn-SOD is not necessary for normal development and function, but is required under stressful conditions following injury or ischemia.

4.1.2 Mn-SOD-deficient mice

Mn-SOD-deficient mice were also generated by another two groups [151,152]. One mouse line with a targeted inactivation of Mn-SOD (deletion of exon 3) showed dilated cardiomyopthy, accumulation of lipids in the liver and skeletal muscle, and metabolic acidosis [152]. These mice were exceedingly hypotonic, hypothermic, and paler compared with wild mice. And they died within or on the first 10 days. A severe reduction in succinate dehydrogenase (the complex II) and aconitase activities were also found. Another mouse line with targeted inactivation of Mn-SOD (deletion of exons 1 and 2) exhibit reduced growth rate and survival (up to 3 weeks) [152]. Likewise, they exhibited severe anemia, dilated heart, degeneration of neurons in the basal ganglia and brain stem, and progressive motor disturbance (weakness, rapid fatigue, and circling behavior). These finding indicate that Mn-SOD is important for maintaining the integrity of mitochondrial enzymes and that its deficiency causes increased susceptibility to oxidative mitochondrial injury in many tissues, such as cardiac myocytes, skeletal muscles, central nervous systems, hepatocytes, and the like.

4.1.3 EC-SOD-deficient mice

EC-SOD-deficient mice were also generated and developed normally and remained healthy up to the age of 14 months or more [153]. However, when they were exposed to almost 100% oxygen, they considerably reduced a survival time compared to wild mice.

4.2 Cu,Zn-SOD

4.2.1   Clinical significance of Cu,Zn-SOD

Recently many investigators try to use recombinant Cu,Zn-SOD as a therapeutics, e.g., to reduce the infarct size in acute myocardial infarction. Many modified Cu,Zn-SODs have also been made, but in this section we will discuss the clinical significance of endogenous Cu,Zn-SOD.

The role of Cu,Zn-SOD under various pathogenic conditions has been widely studied. For example, it is well known that there may be a correlation between the life span and the Cu,Zn-SOD activity [154]. Recently, it was reported that mutations of Cu,Zn-SOD are related to the pathogenesis of FALS and that Cu,Zn-SOD is glycated and inactivated in diabetes. In both cases decreased activity of Cu,Zn-SOD may result in accumulation of damages by reactive oxygen species. Such slow and continuous damages by reactive oxygen species should be further studied in addition to the acute damages.

As Cu,Zn-SOD is encoded by the human chromosome 21, it has been suggested that overexpression of Cu,Zn-SOD may play an important role in the neurobiological abnormalities of Down syndrome [155,156]. However, a partial trisomy 21 with overexpression of Cu,Zn-SOD was associated with none of the usual symptoms [157,158]. Therefore, this hypothesis seems unlikely.

Cu,Zn-SOD is widely and abundantly distributed in the cytosol of cells. Human liver samples contain approximately 0.65−1.5 mg/g of Cu,Zn-SOD in liver protein [159], whereas human erythrocytes contain 0.5−0.75 mg/g of Cu,Zn-SOD in hemoglobin. Therefore, particular attention must be paid to measure serum or tissue levels of Cu,Zn-SOD because hemolysis or contamination of erythrocytes leads to misinterpretation.

4.2.2 ALS

ALS is a degenerative disorder of motor neurons in the cortex, brain stem and spinal cord. About 10% of cases are familial (an autosomal dominant trait). FALS cannot be clinically distinguished from sporadic ALS. As already stated, it has recently been reported that there is a tight linkage between FALS and various SOD1 missense mutations in different FALS families [160, 161]. Almost 50 mutations were found in patients with FALS (Fig. 3). However, definite mutations could not be identified in the exon 3, which forms active site region of Cu,Zn-SOD. So, these mutations were assumed to alter interactions critical to the β-barrel fold and dimer contact rather than catalysis [161]. In addition, late onset progressive paralysis in the transgene mice was demonstrated [162]. The exact mechanism of motor neuron death, however, is still unclear and controversial

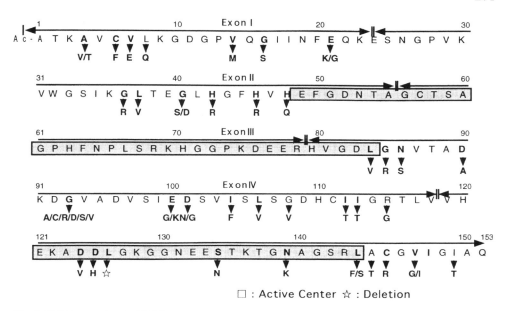

Fig. 3. SOD1 mutation in FALS.

because both suppression and overexpression of SOD activity induced normal cell death and several groups reported a gain in function of mutant Cu,Zn-SOD. For instance, we have actually produced wild-type and six mutant Cu,Zn-SODs related to FALS in a baculovirus/insect cell expression system and showed that mutant Cu,Zn-SODs have a lower scavenging activity and more vulnerability to glycation reaction than wild-type [163]. Decreased scavenging ability, vulnerability to glycation, and free copper release from the inactivated enzymes are all likely reasons why the mutant enzymes might produce hydroxy radicals which may be a potent causative factor of FALS via the Fenton reaction. On the other hand, several groups reported that FALS was due to a toxic gain of function of mutant Cu,Zn-SOD rather than to lower SOD activity. The mutant Cu,Zn-SODs associated with FALS were shown to catalyze the oxidation of a model substrate by hydrogen peroxide at a higher rate than wild-type, these oxidative reactions catalyzed by mutant enzymes initiating the neuropathologic changes of FALS [164]. Moreover, other gains in function have also been reported: the ability to catalyze nitration of neurofilaments by peroxynitraite [165] and the ability of free radical formation from H_2O_2 [166]. Since each mutant Cu,Zn-SOD may have different properties, all these observations may be true in each mutant Cu,Zn-SOD. Further investigation will be expected, including the pathogenesis of sporadic ALS which is indistinguishable from FALS clinically even though mutation of Cu,Zn-SOD was also reported in sporadic ALS, even though mutation of Cu,Zn-SOD was also reported in sporadic ALS.

4.2.3 Diabetes mellitus

4.2.3.1 Glycation of proteins. Many proteins undergo nonenzymatic glycosylation reactions under hyperglycemic conditions and some of their activities are modified. These reactions are known as glycation to distinguish them from enzymatic glycosylation catalyzed by glycosyltransferase. Glycation is a post-translational modification that occurs in vivo through the direct chemical reaction between glucose and the primary amino groups of proteins. The initial product is a labile Schiff base adduct, and then this adduct undergoes a slow Amadori rearrangement to a stable ketoamine derivative of the protein (Fig. 4). Glycation

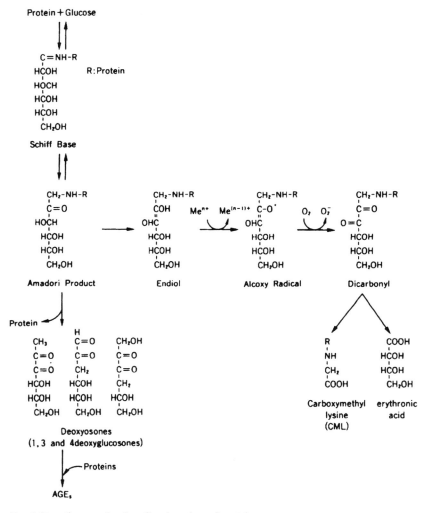

Fig. 4. Reaction mechanism for glycation of proteins.

is considered to be the first step in a complex series of browning, or Maillard, reactions that occur in the presence of reducing sugar. Increased glycation and the subsequent Maillard reaction are thought to be involved in the structural and functional changes in body proteins that occur during normal aging and at accelerated rates in diabetes [167—169]. The reaction was found in the browning reaction of food in the 19th century. Glycation has also been seen in various proteins and in several enzymes such as ribonuclease [170], carbonic anhydrase [171], Cu,Zn-SOD [172], and Na^+,K^+-ATPase [173].

4.2.3.2 Glycation of Cu,Zn-SOD. Erythrocytes are subjected to a continuous flux of O_2^- and H_2O_2 due to hemoglobin auto-oxidation [154,174—176] and also undergo oxidative stress from environmental agents [177]. Cu,Zn-SOD in the erythrocytes may have some physiologically important role in combating these processes. Human erythrocytes contain glycated and nonglycated Cu,Zn-SOD, which can be separated by boronate affinity chromatoghraphy [178,179]. Actually, 50% or more of the erythrocyte Cu,Zn-SOD from diabetic patients was found to be glycated. Although such a high percentage of the Cu,Zn-SOD in the erythrocytes of diabetic patients was glycated, the total Cu,Zn-SOD activity did not differ much between the diabetic patients and the controls. Nonetheless, the specific activity of Cu,Zn-SOD in the erythrocytes of patients with diabetes was always lower than in nondiabetics [180]. These facts indicate that the Cu,Zn-SOD is inactivated under hyperglycemic conditions. Indeed, when purified Cu,Zn-SOD was incubated with glucose under sterile conditions, the SOD activity showed a time- and dose-dependent decrease and the amount of ketoamine adduct increased simultaneously.

4.2.3.3 Inactivation and Fragmentation of Cu,Zn-SOD by Glycation. The mechanism by which Cu,Zn-SOD undergoes glycation and inactivation has been studied [179—182]. Human Cu,Zn-SOD undergoes glycation reaction at specific lysine residues such as Lys-122 and Lys-128 which comprise a positively charged channel track. The glycation of the lysine residues resulted in a relatively negative charge, which may interfere with the electrostatic guidance of the substrate superoxide anion to the active site. The computer image of spinach Cu,Zn-SOD indicates that Lys-122 and Lys-128 are located on the surface of the enzyme molecule and appear to be easily attacked by glucose.

In addition to the above mechanism, fragmentation of Cu,Zn-SOD was recently reported. Several groups reported that glycated proteins produce O_2^- in the presence of transition metal ions [183—186]. And it is well known that Cu,Zn-SOD is sensitive to H_2O_2 and undergoes random fragmentation after exposure to H_2O_2 [187—188]. Recently, both site-specific and random fragmentation of Cu,Zn-SOD was found following the glycation reaction [189]. The fragmentation proceeded in two steps. In the first step, Cu,Zn-SOD was cleaved at a peptide bond between Pro-62 and His-63, as judged by amino acid analysis and sequencing of fragment peptides, yielding a large (15 kDa) and a small (5 kDa) fragment (Fig. 5). In the second step, random fragmentation occurred. Electron spin resonance (ESR) spectra were also measured, the results suggesting that reactive oxygen species was implicated in both steps.

4.2.3.4 Increase of Glycated Cu,Zn-SOD in Diabetic Retinopathy and Cataracts.

The glycation of proteins may play an important role in diabetic complications [167]. Cu,Zn-SOD is located in the lens epithelium [190,191], as are most of the drug-metabolizing enzymes and antioxidant enzymes [192]. Glycation of Cu,Zn-SOD in the lens may play an important role in cataractogenesis. In general, glycated Cu,Zn-SOD level seems to correlate with the level of HbA1c. In patients with diabetic cataracts the correlation is not apparent, whereas the level of glycated Cu,Zn-SOD is rather high compared to that in diabetic patients with no complications. An aged persons with senile cataracts, also have relatively higher levels of glycated Cu,Zn-SOD in their erythrocytes. It is unclear, however, whether the increased amount of glycated Cu,Zn-SOD is really related to the senile cataracts or due to other minor atherosclerotic changes in aged persons. If one separates younger and older populations of normal erythrocytes by centrifugation and compares the activities of those populations, the activity of normal younger erythrocytes is higher than that of aged erythrocytes.

Stevens et al. [193] proposed that glycation might have a role in the browning and aging of lens crystallines associated with the development of senile and diabetic cataracts. Several investigators subsequently reported age-related increases in glycation of normal human [194—196], bovine [167], and rat lens [197], that is, they suggested that increased glycation of proteins with age could cause an age-related acceleration of glucose-dependent damage to protein. However, Patrick et al. [198] reported that glycation of human lens protein is essentially constant with age in normal lens.

Streptozotocin, a nitrosourea compound produced by *Streptomyces achromogenes*, has been used to induce experimental diabetes. The drug also induces DNA strand breakage in islet cells. Streptozotocin injection into rats has been

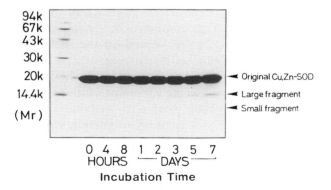

Fig. 5. Fragmentation of Cu,ZnSOD after incubation with glucose.

observed to decrease the Cu,Zn-SOD activity of retina cells, erythrocytes, and islet cells [199,200]. However, the mechanism by which the Cu,Zn-SOD activity decreases in experimental diabetes is not yet known.

Streptozotocin-induced diabetic rats also had high levels of glycated Cu,Zn-SOD in the erythrocytes [201] and lens, as judged by affinity chromatography on a boronate column. As described above, much of the glycated Cu,Zn-SOD is inactive. This is one of the reasons that Cu,Zn-SOD activity is decreased in rats with streptozotocin-induced diabetes. Even in normal rat lens, approximately 40% of the Cu,Zn-SOD undergoes glycation. Under diabetic conditions, over 80% of the enzyme was found to have undergone glycation (Kawamura et al., unpublished data).

Thus, under diabetic conditions, the glycated proteins produce O_2^- on one hand, and the Cu,Zn-SOD undergoes glycation and inactivation on the other hand. These events may enhance the accumulation of O_2^- in the microenvironment of the tissues and, as a result, tissue damage and diabetic complications would be accelerated (Fig. 6).

4.2.4 Werner's syndrome

Werner's syndrome is an autosomal recessive condition and is sometimes referred to as adult progeria. The disease is clinically characterized by accelerated aging and increased frequency of malignant tumors and diabetes [202]. At the cellular and molecular levels, cultured fibroblasts from patients with Werner's

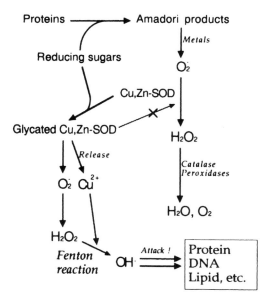

Fig. 6. A possible mechanism for accumulation of O_2^- in a microenviroment due to inactivation of SOD.

syndrome have a markedly decreased replicative life span [203]. In addition, increased proportions of several enzymes in the fibroblasts have been reported to be heat-labile [203,204], as found in old fibroblasts. The etiology of the disease is still unknown, but an involvement of the free-radical scavenging system has been suggested [205]. An age-related reduction in Cu,Zn-SOD has been reported [206,207]. In patients with Werner's syndrome, erythrocyte Cu,Zn-SOD undergoes nonenzymatic glycosylation at multiple lysine residues, irrespective of the glycemic state. The enzyme purified from the patient was found to be unstable and had a very low specific activity due to nonenzymatic glycosylation. As already described, accelerated glycation reactions appear to bring about the production and accumulation of O_2^- and it may cause tissue damage and relate to the clinical feature of the progeria.

4.3 Mn-SOD

4.3.1   Clinical significance of Mn-SOD

It is widely believed that Mn-SOD plays a role in various pathogenic conditions such as aging, carcinogenesis, inflammation, ischemia and others. Recently Mn-SOD-deficient mice showed that Mn-SOD gene (SOD2) is a lethal gene. Mn-SOD may protect mitochondria by protecting mitochondrial enzymes from reactive oxygen species. Moreover, very recently it has been reported that faulty localization of Mn-SOD may be related to progeria [208] and that Mn-SOD is inactivated by peroxynitrate (nitration), e.g., probably leading to chronic rejection of human renal allografts [209]. It is also widely known that Mn-SOD is induced by various cytokines, such as tumor necrosis factor (TNF)-α or IL-1, and that Mn-SOD is a protective enzyme against cytotoxicity of TNF [127,210]. This allows more interests to be focused on Mn-SOD. No direct evidence, however, has been presented linking Mn-SOD to these pathogenic conditions. Several laboratories found that, in cancer tissues or transformed cells, as well as in aged tissues, the activity of SOD decreased or disappeared as compared to that in uninvolved or younger tissues [211–217]. In a previous study [218] we found that the immunoreactive Mn-SOD levels in human lung cancer tissues are higher than those in uninvolved tissues from the same patients, whereas the level of the active enzyme does not increase. It still seems that the level of immunoreactive enzyme may provide a useful piece of information for monitoring cancer tissues. Recently we raised three monoclonal antibodies against human liver Mn-SOD. The epitope of one of these antibodies was found to be a COOH-terminal peptide, as judged by competitive inhibition assay using synthetic peptides [219]. Using this antibody we developed an ELISA method and found that the enzyme is also present in human serum [45]. Measurement of the serum immunoreactive Mn-SOD protein levels in various diseases revealed that the enzyme levels are increased in certain pathological conditions, such as acute myocardial infarction, primary biliary cirrhosis, primary hepatoma, gastric cancer, and acute myeloid leukemia. Mn-SOD levels were also increased in the sera of patients with epithelial type ovarian cancer.

In this section at first we will mention the induction mechanism of Mn-SOD in vitro and later explain linkages of each disease and Mn-SOD.

4.3.2 *Expression of Mn-SOD in vitro*

4.3.2.1 Expression of Mn-SOD in TNF-resistant and sensitive cell lines. TNF or IL-1 specifically induces mRNA for Mn-SOD, Mn-SOD is one of the protective proteins against TNF cytotoxicity [127,210,220]. This effect is blocked by actinomycin D, but not by cyclohexamide, indicating that the increase in Mn-SOD mRNA results from an increase in transcription of the Mn-SOD gene. Lipopolysaccharide (LPS) also induces Mn-SOD mRNA in pulmonary epithelial cells by a similar mechanism [221]. Recently it was reported that phorbol 12-myristate 13-acetate (TPA), a potent tumor promoter and protein kinase C activator, also induced Mn-SOD expression only in TNF-resistant cell lines and presented two hypothetical signal transducing pathways in this gene expression [222]. The importance of Mn-SOD for cellular resistance to TNF cytotoxicity has been reported [221]. However, no data were available regarding the levels of Mn-SOD protein after TNF treatment. The development of a monoclonal antibody and the ELISA technique made it possible to quantitatively determine Mn-SOD protein levels.

The effect of TNF on the expression of Mn-SOD protein in TNF-resistant cells was examined. In the case of WI-38 (fetal lung cells), Mn-SOD protein levels increased dramatically, approximately 80-fold, after TNF treatment (Fig. 7). On the other hand, TNF treatment did not cause any changes in Cu,Zn-SOD expression in most of the TNF-resistant cells [223]. Induction of Mn-SOD was also seen in A549 cells (a human adenocarcinoma cell line).

In ME-180, a human cervical epidermoid carcinoma cell line, and KYM-1, a human myosarcoma cell line, which are TNF sensitive, Mn-SOD levels are one order of magnitude lower than in TNF-resistant cells. However, ZR-75-1, a human breast cancer cell line, which is also TNF sensitive, contains a relatively high level of Mn-SOD, even though its level is not as high as that of TNF-resistant cells. The basal Mn-SOD protein levels in ME-180 and KYM-1 cells are very low, and even after treatment with TNF, no increase in Mn-SOD was observed. In ZR-75-1 cells, however, a tendency toward increased Mn-SOD levels was observed after TNF treatment. Therefore, in this cell line it seems likely that a different mechanism may control Mn-SOD expression.

4.3.2.2 Mechanism of Mn-SOD induction by TNF or TPA. Although several stimulators such as TNF, IL-1, and LPS have been reported to enhance Mn-SOD expression in some cell lines, the pathway that transduces a signal from corresponding receptors to Mn-SOD gene is not clearly understood. Recently, it was reported that phorbol ester (TPA), a protein kinase C activator, also induces

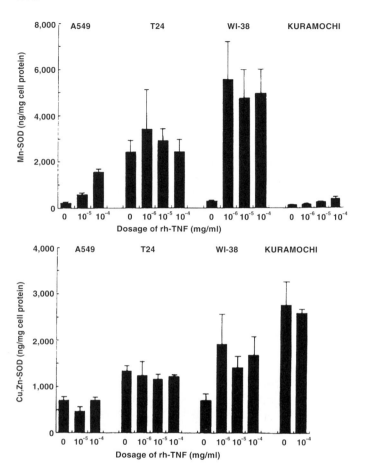

Fig. 7. Effect of TNF on MnSOD and Cu,ZnSOD levels in TNF-resistant cells.

Mn-SOD in various cell lines which are all resistant to TNF (Table 12) [222]. This gives us clue to investigate the intracellular signal transduction pathway. Since TPA enhanced Mn-SOD mRNA expression in TNF-resistant cell lines, in which other stimulators also induced the expression of the gene but did not affect TNF-sensitive cells, it is conceivable that protein kinase C is involved in this gene expression by TNF through phosphorylation of certain substrates.

One possibility would be that activator protein-1 (AP-1) is responsible for this gene expression. Ho et al. [224] found the consensus sequence for AP-1 enhancer binding protein in the 5′-flanking region of the rat Mn-SOD gene. TPA acts to both activate AP-1 protein and to enhance protooncogene Jun/AP-1 expression. However, there would be more than one pathway because TNF could induce Mn-SOD in the cells that were desensitized to TPA by TPA-pretreatment. Thus, at least two pathways participate in Mn-SOD expression. One is triggered by pro-

Table 12. Relative stimulation of Mn-SOD mRNA expression by TPA, TNF, IL-1 and LPS in various cell lines[a] [222].

Cell line	Control	TPA (10 ng/ml)	TNFα (100 ng/ml)	IL-1ß (1000 U/ml)	LPS (10 µg/ml)
HeLa[b]	1.0 ± 0.1	18.7 ± 1.0	7.8 ± 2.5	8.1 ± 1.2	3.0 ± 0.7
A549[b]	1.0 ± 0.2	9.0 ± 1.2	18.5 ± 1.4	25.3 ± 3.8	1.0 ± 0.1
Kuramochi[b]	1.0 ± 0.1	6.7 ± 0.1	2.7 ± 0.5	19.8 ± 2.7	1.4 ± 0.1
MCAS[b]	1.0 ± 0.1	11.2 ± 1.3	1.4 ± 0.8	6.0 ± 1.4	16.5 ± 0.7
ME180[c]	1.0 ± 0.3	1.2 ± 0.1	0.8 ± 0.4	1.3 ± 0.2	0.4 ± 0.2
HL60[c]	1.0 ± 0.2	0.4 ± 0.1	0.6 ± 0.1	0.7 ± 0.1	0.6 ± 0.4
K562[c]	1.0 ± 0.1	0.9 ± 0.1	1.0 ± 0.3	1.3 ± 0.1	1.0 ± 0.1

[a]Total RNA was prepared from various cells treated with 10 ng/ml TPA, 100 ng/ml TNF, 1000 units/ml IL-1, or 10 µg/ml LPS for 4 h. The amount of Mn-SOD mRNA was evaluated by scanning X-ray film exposed to Northern blot membrane filters. The mRNA levels relative to the control are presented as the means ± SD for three experiments. [b]TNF-resistant cell. [c]TNF-sensitive cell.

tein kinase C activation, itself in the absence of new protein synthesis, and the other can be activated by TNF without protein kinase C activation [222]

4.3.2.3 Induction and release into serum of Mn-SOD from endothelial cells.
Serum levels of Mn-SOD are elevated in patients with various diseases. However, the mechanism of serum increase of Mn-SOD was unclear. Recently we reported that Mn-SOD in human endothelial cells is also induced by TNF, TPA, IL-1 and LPS [225] these showed there is a possibility that Mn-SOD induced in endothelial cells is released into serum and thus, results in an increased serum levels of Mn-SOD in various diseases [226]. Mn-SOD in human endothelial cells, which were obtained from umbilical cords, is dramatically induced by TNF (Fig. 8) and this induction is partially blocked by H7, a protein kinase C inhibi-

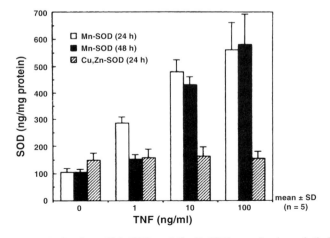

Fig. 8. Induction of MnSOD and Cu,ZnSOD proteins in endothelial cells.

tor, and dexamethasone. Meanwhile, Cu,Zn-SOD levels are unchanged. Similar to cancer cell lines, there are at least two pathways in Mn-SOD expression in endothelial cells: one is triggered by protein kinase C and the other is activated by TNF without protein kinase C activation [225]. Mn-SOD levels in culture medium of endothelial cells are elevated after treatment of TNF (Fig. 9) [226]. These facts suggest that Mn-SOD induced in endothelial cells is released into serum of patients with various diseases especially in which cytokines have a major roles in pathogenesis including inflammation and ischemia [227].

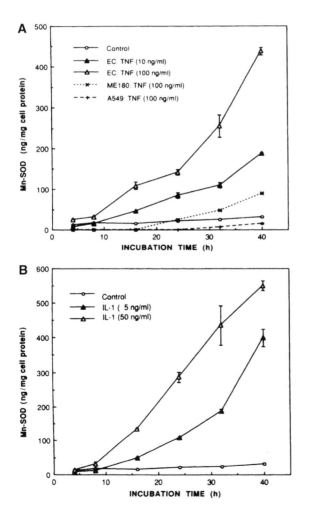

Fig. 9. The MnSOD levels in the culture medium of cells stimulated with TNF and IL-1.

4.3.3 Mn-SOD in diseases

4.3.3.1 Mn-SOD levels in normal healthy controls. The levels of Mn-SOD in sera from 194 males and 207 females who were healthy adult individuals were examined by an ELISA [45]. The frequency distribution of serum Mn-SOD levels for the normal adult male was found to follow a normal distribution pattern. The distribution for the normal female adult was found to be slightly skewed, but the plotting of the cumulative frequency using normal probability paper gave a near-straight line. The mean level and SD for male and female were 99.8 ng/ml ± 24.8 and 88.8 ± 20.8 ng/ml, respectively. Assuming the upper limit of the normal male to be 150 ng/ml (equivalent to the mean value for normal male subjects plus 2 SD), the percentage of false positives was 2.1%. Similarly, assuming the upper limit of the normal female to be 130 ng/ml, the percentage of false positives was 1.0%. In children, the serum Mn-SOD levels are slightly lower than in adults and gradually increase in proportion to age. By 10 years of age the Mn-SOD levels are nearly at the adult level. In various diseases, including cancer, Mn-SOD levels are relatively high (Fig. 10).

4.3.3.2 Acute myocardial infarction. A great deal of interest has developed in the role of SOD modifying the toxic effects of O_2^- arising in cardiac tissue during

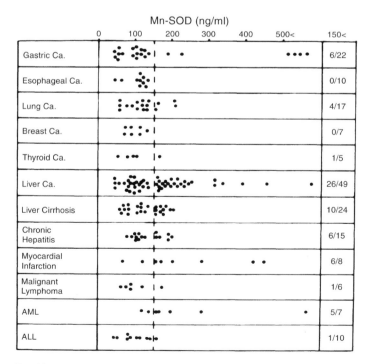

Fig. 10. Immunoreactive MnSOD contents of sera from various diseases.

reperfusion following an ischemic episode. Much of the interest has centered on the role of the widely distributed Mn-SOD. Very recently it was reported that induction of Mn-SOD by cytokines was effective to protect myocardium from ischemia in animal models [228,229].

The intravenous administration of SOD appears to be effective in reducing the size of experimentally induced infarct. There is still considerable controversy, however, regarding the salvage effects of SOD in the myocardium.

4.3.3.2.1 Serum levels of Mn-SOD in acute myocardial infarction. Serum Mn-SOD levels were determined in 29 patients with acute myocardial infarction by an ELISA using a monoclonal antibody [227]. Figure 11 shows typical changes in serum Mn-SOD in two patients following acute myocardial infarction. Case A is an example of a successful reperfusion of the infarcted vessel at an acute stage, and case B is a case without reperfusion. In both instances a biphasic ele-

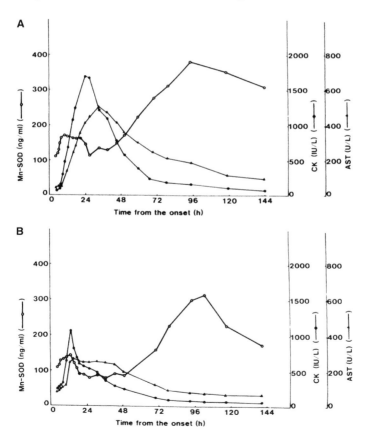

Fig. 11. Typical patterns of MnSOD release into serum for two patients with acute myocardial infarction: (**A**) a case with an unsuccessful reperfusion; (**B**) a successful case.

vation of Mn-SOD is noted: a small early one that is slightly higher than the levels seen in normal, healthy controls and a later phase elevation that is typically much larger. The initial rise follows a pattern similar to that of CK [230], whereas the later phase elevation occurs much later than increases in other enzymes.

The results of serial determinations of serum Mn-SOD for the 29 patients are shown in Fig. 12. Figure 12A shows results for 23 reperfused patients, whereas Fig. 12B depicts six cases without reperfusion. In four of the latter patients either intracoronary thrombolysis or percutaneous transluminal coronary angioplasty was unsuccessfully employed. In two cases, reocclusion occurred after reperfusion. This was confirmed later by coronary angiography during the convalescent stage. In most of these cases, irrespective of whether reperfusion was successful, two elevations of Mn-SOD were observed. The maximum levels (± SD) of serum Mn-SOD for the early and later stage elevations were 164 ± 84 and 248 ± 103 ng/ml, respectively. The time of appearance of the early elevation was 16.2 ± 7.3

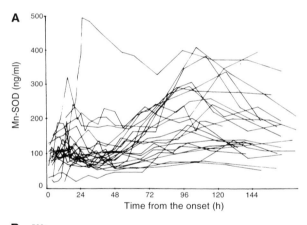

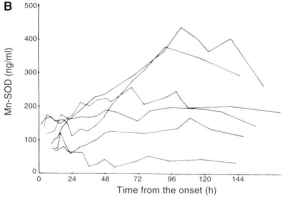

Fig. 12. Serial determination of serum MnSOD in 29 patients with acute myocardial infarction: (**A**) 23 cases with successful reperfusion; (**B**) six cases with unsuccessful reperfusion.

h, and the later elevation was at 108 ± 21 h. No significant correlation was found between the peak level of CK and the maximum level of the late elevation of Mn-SOD ($r = 0.26$). This indicates that different mechanisms are operating for the release of these two enzymes. Reperfusion did not affect the time required for the late elevation to occur, but the procedure shortened the time for appearance of the early rise. The appearance of the early elevation correlated with the time at which reperfusion was carried out.

4.3.3.2.2 Mechanism of Mn-SOD release into serum in patients with acute myocardial infarction. Immunoelectron microscopy of cardiac muscle revealed that immunogold was deposited on the mitochondria among the myofibrils, as well as on the mitochondria beneath the sarcoplasmic membrane (Fig. 13A) [225]. In addition, the mitochondria of the endothelial cells of the blood capillaries reacted with this antibody (Fig. 13B); it seems that more Mn-SOD existed in endothelial cells than in myocytes. Histochemical studies demonstrated that Mn-SOD is localized in the mitochondria of the myocardium and endothelial cells, suggesting that it is released from this organelle. The early elevation of Mn-SOD is probably simple leakage from cells like CK.

In myocardial infarction, neutrophils and macrophages could move to the necrotized tissues following the early elevation and thus, release the cytokines. This could induce Mn-SOD synthesis in mitochondria, from which the enzyme

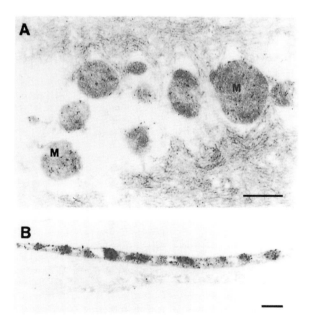

Fig. 13. Immunoreactive microscopy of cardiac muscle (**A**) and endothelial cells (**B**) treated with anti-human MnSOD IgG.

could be released due to cell damage at the later phase. In such an induction hypothesis, ischemic tissues would be thought of as inflammatory foci. Figure 14 shows that plasma levels of TNF are elevated in patients with acute myocardial infarction and that their peaks exist three or four days after the onset of infarction. As mentioned in previous section, Mn-SOD in endothelial cells is increased by TNF and released into the culture medium. These facts suggest that Mn-SOD in endothelial cells or myocardium is induced by TNF and released into serum through damaged membranes by ischemia.

4.3.3.3 Primary hepatoma and primary biliary cirrhosis. Approximately 60% of patients with primary hepatoma gave positive values for Mn-SOD estimated by the ELISA. Due to serum Mn-SOD levels were also elevated in various other diseases, including gastric cancer and primary biliary cirrhosis, however, whether the immunoreactive Mn-SOD can be used as a marker for the diagnosis and monitoring of primary hepatoma remains to be clarified.

Interestingly, 30 out of 31 patients with primary biliary cirrhosis had increased levels of serum Mn-SOD [231]. Mn-SOD levels at early stages of the disease were found to be higher than those at late stage. Primary biliary cirrhosis is an idiopathic liver disease characterized by spontaneous destruction of interlobular bile ducts [232,233]. The disorder is considered to be the result of an altered autoimmune response mediated by T cells or, though less likely, by disease-specific auto-antibodies against mitochondrial enzyme complexes [234—236]. The mechanism by which Mn-SOD is expressed in the early stages of the disease remains unclear. Cytokines such as IL-1 and TNF may be expressed in this tis-

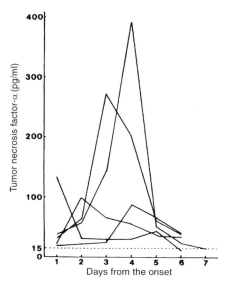

Fig. 14. Serial determination of plasma TNF in five patients with acute myocardial infarction.

sue, and these cytokines may stimulate the expression of Mn-SOD. In any case the early elevation of serum Mn-SOD in primary biliary cirrhosis appears to be a very interesting phenomenon.

4.3.3.4 Acute leukemia. We also found that nine out of 15 patients with acute myeloid leukemia and four out of 15 patients with acute lymphocytic leukemia had increased levels of serum Mn-SOD, whereas no increased value was observed in patients with chronic myeloid or chronic lymphocytic leukemias [237]. This suggests that acute leukemia cells, especially myeloid cells, synthesize Mn-SOD. As described above, the mRNA for Mn-SOD is induced by IL-1 or TNF. TNF has been reported to be expressed in human peripheral blood mononuclear cells [238]. Moreover, IL-1 has been reported to act as an autocrine factor in the acute myeloid cells [239] and hairy cell leukemia [240]. This suggests that the synthesis of IL-1 in acute myeloid cells induces Mn-SOD in the cells, thereby resulting in high levels of serum Mn-SOD in patients with acute myeloid leukemia.

4.3.3.5 Epithelial ovarian cancer and other gynecological malignancies. A difficult problem often encountered by gynecologists is in differentiating malignant tumors from benign ones in patients with pelvic masses. A monoclonal antibody (OC 125) reactive against an ovarian carcinoma antigen (CA 125) was prepared by Bast et al. [241]. The use of the antibody to estimate serum immunoreactive CA 125 levels has become a relatively effective method for evaluating such malignancies [241]. Approximately two-thirds of patients with adenocarcinoma of the ovary have elevated serum levels of this antigen [241,242].

Due to the insidious onset and progression of ovarian cancer, an early diagnosis is very difficult. Moreover, accurate monitoring of tumor status is also difficult because patients are often in clinical remission when a subclinical disease is present.

We used ELISA with a monoclonal antibody against human Mn-SOD to investigate the possibility of using this enzyme as a marker for epithelial ovarian carcinoma [243]. In our series of 308 patients, 158 proved to have invasive pelvic neoplasms. As already described, fewer than 1.4% of healthy adult females have serum Mn-SOD levels above 130 ng/ml. Only five of the 40 patients (13%) with benign ovarian tumors had Mn-SOD levels exceeding 130 ng/ml. In the nonovarian gynecological malignancy groups, eight out of 42 patients (19%) with uterine cervical cancer and nine of 41 patients (22%) with endometrial cancer had Mn-SOD levels above 130 ng/ml. Seventy-five patients had malignant ovarian tumors, 63 had epithelial and 12 had nonepithelial carcinomas. A serum Mn-SOD value greater than 130 ng/ml was utilized as the diagnostic criterion, the positive rate was 62% for patients with epithelial ovarian carcinomas and 0% for patients with nonepithelial carcinomas (Table 13). The mean value of serum Mn-SOD in patients with epithelial carcinomas was 195 ng/ml, compared with 92.4 ng/ml in patients with nonepithelial carcinomas. Statistical analysis showed a significant difference ($p = 0.01$) between these two groups.

Table 13. Positivity rate for serum Mn-SOD in patients with borderline and ovarian carcinomas.

Type	Total No. tested	No. (%) of positive cases above 150 ng/ml
Epithelial carcinomas	63	39 (62%)
Serous cystadenocarcinoma	33	22 (67%)
Clear cell adenocarcinoma	11	6 (55%)
Endometroid adenocarinoma	12	9 (75%)
Mucinous cystadenocarcinoma	7	2 (29%)
Germ-cell tumors	4	0
Sex cord stormal tumors	2	0
Metastatic tumors	4	0
Mucinous tumor of borderline malignancy	2	0

In one patient with serious cystadenocarcinoma (stage IIb), it was possible to monitor Mn-SOD levels on nine occasions over 30 months. After surgical cytoreduction and chemotherapy with a combination of cyclophosphamide, adriamycin, and cisplatin, i.e., CAP, Mn-SOD levels decreased from 266 to 66 ng/ml. Laparotomy failed to reveal residual tumor, and treatment was then continued with cisplatin. After 2 years the Mn-SOD level rose to 167 ng/ml, with CA 125 rising to 150 U/ml. At that time, abdominal computerized tomography (CT) revealed a small pelvic mass and ascites. Thus, increases in Mn-SOD and CA 125 were observed upon recurrence of disease. In rats, experimental serous cystadenocarcinomas induced by a carcinogen, dimethylbenz[a]anthrachene, were also found to have increased Mn-SOD [244].

In patients with epithelial ovarian carcinomas, serum Mn-SOD levels increased in accordance with the clinical progression of disease. At the early stage, however, the incidence of cases with elevated serum levels was low. Therefore, measurements of serum Mn-SOD may not always be useful for the early diagnosis of epithelial ovarian carcinoma. The decline in serum Mn-SOD levels following effective therapy seems to reflect the disappearance of lesions. Decreases occurred after therapy and increases occurred with recurrence. Thus, it appears that the measurement of this enzyme in serum can provide useful data for monitoring epithelial ovarian cancer following therapy, and for the early diagnosis of recurrence of the disease.

4.3.3.6 Adult respiratory distress syndrome. Adult respiratory distress syndrome (ARDS) is an acute inflammatory process characterized by neutrophil accumulation and edema in the lungs and progressive hypoxemia. ARDS occurs unpredictably as a complication in patients with sepsis and several other predisposing disorders. Recently, Leff et al. [245] reported that 6–12 h before the development of ARDS, Mn-SOD and catalase levels were increased in sepsis patients who later developed ARDS compared with patients who did not develop ARDS. Table 14 shows sensitivity and specificity of blood markers as predictors of ARDS in

Table 14. Sensitivity and specificity of blood makers as predictors of ARDS in patients with sepsis [245].

Cell line	Cutoff	Value (%) and 95% Cl				
		Sensitivity	Specificity	Positive predictive value	Negative predicted value	Efficiency[a]
Mn-SOD	⩾ 450 ng/ml	67 (42—94)	88 (75—98)	67 (42—49)	88 (75—98)	83 (70—94)
Catalase	⩾ 30 U/ml	83 (61—99)	65 (49-82)	42 (25—68)	93 (81-100)	69 (55—84)
GPX	⩾ 0.72 U/ml	50 (27-85)	47 (31—69)	25 (21—53)	73 (53—92)	48 (34—66)
LDH	⩾ 250 U/l	67 (42—94)	78 (62-92)	50 (29-81)	88 (74—98)	75 (61—89)
Factor VIII	⩾ 455% control	83 (61-99)	67 (42—94)	45 (27—73)	92 (80—100)	71 (57—85)
α₁Pi-elastase	⩾ 940 ng/ml	67 (37—98)	64 (50-80)	18 (8—47)	94 (84-100)	64 (51—79)

[a]True results as a percentage of all results.

patients with sepsis. High concentrations of TNF, IL-1, and endotoxin have been found in ARDS patients [246] and can cause an increase in Mn-SOD and catalase.

5   SUMMARY

1. Both Cu,Zn-SOD and Mn-SOD are widely and abundantly distributed in various tissues and play the important role in the cellular defense against O^-_2. So, it is not surprising that changes in the SODs are associated with a large variety of physiological or pathological conditions.

2. EC-SOD is mainly located in the extracellular space; however, unlike Cu,Zn-SOD and Mn-SOD, its physiological or clinical significance still remains vague.

3. The recent development of ELISAs for the three SOD isoenzymes has facilitated accurate and reproducible determination of their protein levels in serum and other tissues. The ELISA is preferable to enzymatic assays for SOD because SOD-like activities in tissues can interfere with the quantitation of SOD activity.

4. Modifications of SOD (such as glycation of Cu,Zn- and EC-SODs and nitration of Mn-SOD) can result in inactivation, thereby precluding accurate determination of enzyme levels by activity assay.

5. Thus, it is by no means an infrequent sight to see the conflicting data related to the effect of physical exercise on SOD activity in humans or animals. On the other hand, immunoreactive Mn-SOD level in human serum appears to provide a reliable index of strenuous exercise and/or physical training. These findings have been confirmed by the studies on rat skeletal muscle.

6. Measurement of serum immunoreactive SOD levels shows promise as a diagnostic tool, and assessment of changes in tissue levels of the enzymes will likely provide insight into the biochemical processes involved in a number of diseases, including exercise stress.

6   PERSPECTIVES

A relationship between FALS and mutant Cu,Zn-SOD is one of the most dispu-
table subjects in radical-induced pathological conditions. Both mutant Mn-SOD
and EC-SOD may also participate in such pathological conditions. Of additional
interest are studies regarding the mechanism by which SOD isoenzyme, particularly Mn-SOD, is changed during physical exercise.

7   ABBREVIATIONS

ALT:	alanine aminotransferase
AP-1:	activator protein-1
ARDS:	adult respiratory distress syndrome
AST:	aspartate aminotransferase
Ch-E:	cholinesterase
CK:	creatine kinase
CT:	computerized tomography
EC-SOD:	extracellular SOD
ELISA:	enzyme-linked immunosorbent assays
ESR:	electron spin resonance
FALS:	familial amyotrophic lateral scleosis
GPX:	glutathione peroxidase
γ-GT:	γ-glutamyltransferase
IL-1:	interleukin-1
LPS:	lipopolysaccharide
O_2^-:	superoxide anion
SOD:	superoxide dismutase
SOD1:	Cu,Zn-SOD gene
SOD2:	Mn-SOD gene
SM-SOD:	synthesized by covalently linking poly-(stylene-co-maleic acid) butyl ester to a Cu,Zn-SOD
TBARS:	thiobarbituric-reactive substances
TNF:	tumor necrosis factor
TPA:	12-*O*-tetradecanoylphorbol 13-acetate (phorbol 12-myristate 13-acetate)
XO:	xanthine oxidase

8   REFERENCES

1. Spitzer JA. Proc Soc Exp Biol Med 1995;209:102−103.
2. Halliwell B, Gutteridge MC. Biochem J 1984;219:1−14.
3. Clark IA, Cowden WB, Hunt NH. Med Res Rev 1985;5:297−332.
4. Jenkins RR. Sports Med 1988;5:156−170.
5. Cadenas E. Annu Rev Biochem 1989;58:79−110.
6. Jenner P. Lancet 1994;344:796−798.

7. Jaeschke H. Proc Soc Exp Biol Med 1995;209:104—111.
8. Aruoma OI, Halliwell B. In: Kies CV, Driskell JA (eds) Sports Nutrition: Minerals and Electro-lytes. Boca Raton: CRC Press, 1995;317—324.
9. Dean RT, Fu S, Stocker R, Davies MJ. Biochem J 1997;324:1—18.
10. Sjödin B, Westing YH, Apple FS. Sports Med 1990;10:236—254.
11. Gerster H. Z Ernährungswiss 1991;30:89—97.
12. Witt EH, Reznick AZ, Viguie CA, Starke-Reed P et al. J Nutr 1992;122:766—773.
13. Jenkins RR, Goldfarb A. Med Sci Sports Exerc 1993;25:210—212.
14. Jenkins RR. Int J Sport Nutr 1993;3:356—375.
15. Aruoma OI. J Nutr Biochem 1994;5:370—381.
16. Jackson MJ. In: Sen CK, Packer L, Hänninen O. (eds) Exercise and Oxygen Toxicity. Amster-dam: Elsevier, 1994:49—57.
17. Ji LL. In: Holloszy JO. (ed) Exercise and Sport Sciences Reviews. vol 23. Baltimore: Williams and Wilkins, 1995:135—166.
18. Sen CK. J Appl Physiol 1995;79:675—686.
19. Powers SK, Criswell D. Med Sci Sports Exerc 1996;28:1115—1122.
20. Ohno H, Oh-ishi S, Ookawara T, Kizaki T et al. Med Sportiva 1998; 2:219—229.
21. Fridovich I. Ann Rev Biochem 1975;44:147—159.
22. Fridovich I. Ann Rev Pharmacol Toxicol 1983;23:239—257.
23. Bannister JV, Bannister WH, Rotilio G. CRC Crit Rev Biochem 1987;22:111—180.
24. Tyler DD. Biochem J 1975;147:493—504.
25. Peeters-Joris C, Vandervoorde A-M, Baudhuin P. Biochem J 1975;150:31—39.
26. Nohl H, Hegner D. Eur J Biochem 1978;82:563—567.
27. Asanuma K, Dobashi K, Hayashibe H, Megata Y et al. Endocrinology 1987;121:2112—2118.
28. Taniguchi N. Adv Clin Chem 1992;29:1—59.
29. Fridovich I. J Biol Chem 1997;272:18515—18517.
30. Marklund SL. Proc Natl Acad Sci USA 1982;79:7634—7638.
31. Hjalmarsson K, Marklund SL, Engström A, Edlund T. Proc Natl Acad Sci USA 1987;84:6340—6344.
32. Tibell L, Hjalmarsson K, Edlund T, Skogman G et al. Proc Natl Acad Sci USA 1987;84:6634—6638.
33. Marklund SL, Holme E, Hellner L. Clin Chim Acta 1982;126:41—51.
34. Marklund SL. Biochem J 1984;222:649—655.
35. Ookawara T, Kizaki T, Oh-ishi S, Yamamoto M et al. Arch Biochem Biophys 1997;340:299—304.
36. Ookawara T, Imazeki N, Matsubara O, Kizaki T et al. Am J Physiol 1998;275:C840—C847.
37. Beauchamp C, Fridovich I. Anal Biochem 1971;44:276—287.
38. Elstner EF, Heupel A. Anal Biochem 1976;70:616—620.
39. Karlsson K, Marklund SL. Biochem J 1988;255:223—228.
40. Ohno H, Yahata T, Yamashita K, Yamamura K et al. Enzyme 1988;39:110—114.
41. Ohno H, Gasa S, Habara Y, Kuroshima A et al. Biochim Biophys Acta 1990;1033:19—22.
42. Stansell MJ, Deutsch HF. Clin Chim Acta 1966;14:598—607.
43. Adachi T, Usami Y, Kishi T, Hirano K et al. J Immunol Meth 1988;109:93—101.
44. Oka S, Ogino K, Matsuura S, Yoshimura S et al. Clin Chim Acta 1989;182:209—220.
45. Kawaguchi T, Suzuki K, Matsuda Y, Nishiura T et al. J Immunol Meth 1990;127:249—254.
46. Suzuki K, Nakata T, Seo HG, Miyazawa N et al. In: Mori M, Yoshida MC, Takeuchi N, Taniguchi N (eds) The LEC Rats. Tokyo: Springer-Verlag, 1991:142—148.
47. Ookawara T, Nakao C, Kizaki T, Oh-ishi S et al. (In preparation).
48. Minami M, Mori K, Nagatsu T. Ind Health 1981;19:133—138.
49. Ohno H, Yamashita H, Ookawara T, Saitoh D et al. Tohoku J Exp Med 1992;167:301—303.
50. Ohno H, Iizuka S, Kondo T, Yamamura K et al. Klin Wochenschr 1984;62:287—288.
51. Ohno H, Doi R, Yamamura K, Yamashita K et al. Blut 1985;50:113—116.
52. Ohno H, Yamashita K, Doi R, Yamamura K et al. J Appl Physiol 1985;58:1453—1458.

53. Goldstein IM, Kaplan HB, Edelson HS, Weissmann G. J Biol Chem 1979;254:4040–4045.
54. Ohno H, Doi R, Yamashita K, Yamamura K et al. J Sports Med Phys Fit 1985;25:65–68.
55. Mena P, Maynar M, Gutierrez JM, Maynar J et al. Int J Sports Med 1991;12:563–566.
56. Cooper MB, Jones DA, Edwards PHT, Corbucci GC et al. J Sports Sci 1986;4:79–87.
57. Ohno H, Sato Y, Yamashita K, Doi R et al. Can J Physiol Pharmacol 1986;64:1263–1265.
58. Kedziora J, Buczynski A, Kedziora–Kornafowska K. Int J Occup Med Env Health 1995;8 33–39.
59. Burr IM, Asayama K, Fenichel GM. Muscle Nerve 1987;10:150–154.
60. Lukaski H, Hoverson BS, Gallagher SK, Bolonchuk WW. Am J Clin Nutr 1990;51:1093–1099.
61. Jenkins RR, Friedland R, Howald H. Int J Sports Med 1984;5:11–14.
62. Ørtenblad N, Madsen K, Djurhuus MS. Am J Physiol 1997;272:R1258–R1263.
63. Ohno H, Yahata T, Sato Y, Yamamura K et al. Eur J Appl Physiol 1988;57:173–176.
64. Ji LL, Fu R. J Appl Physiol 1992;72:549–554.
65. Ji LL, Fu R, Mitchell EW. J Appl Physiol 1992;73:1854–1859.
66. Leeuwenburgh C, Ji LL. J Nutr 1996;126:1833–1843.
67. Quintanilha AT, Packer L. In: Porter R, Whelan J (eds) Biology of Vitamin E: Ciba Foundation Symposium 101. London: Pitman, 1983;56–69.
68. Ji LL. Med Sci Sports Exerc 1993;25:225–231.
69. Sen CK, Ookawara T, Suzuki K, Taniguchi N et al. Pathophysiology 1994;1:165–168.
70. Stevens JB, Autor AP. J Biol Chem 1977;252:3509–3514.
71. Mizunuma T, Kajikawa T, Kishino Y. Jpn J Phys Fit Sports Med 1993;42:69–81.
72. Häggendal J, Jönsson L, Johansson G, Bjurström S et al. Acta Physiol Scand 1987;131: 447–452.
73. Ji LL, Dillon D, Wu E. Am J Physiol 1990;258:R918–R923.
74. Ji LL, Dillon D, Wu E, Am J Physiol 1991;261:R386–392.
75. Alessio HM, Goldfarb AH. J Appl Physiol 1988;64:1333–1336.
76. Ji LL, Stratman FW, Lardy HA. Arch Biochem Biophys 1988;263:150–160.
77. Spodaryk K, Gaertner H. In: Program and Abstracts of the 8th International Biochemistry of Exercise Conference. Nagoya: Nagoya University; 1991;168.
78. Lawler JM, Powers SK, Visser T, Van Dijk H et al. Am J Physiol 1993;265:R1344–R1350.
79. Lawler JM, Powers SK, Van Dijk H, Visser T et al. Respir Physiol 1994;96:139–149.
80. Somani SM, Frank S, Rybak LP. Pharmacol Biochem Behav 1995;51:627–634.
81. Leeuwenburgh C, Ji LL. Arch Biochem Biophys 1995;316:941–949.
82. Radák Z, Asano K, Kizaki T, Oh-ishi S et al. Pathophysiology 1995;2:243–245.
83. Leeuwenburgh C, Leichtweis S, Hollander J, Fiebig R et al. Molec Cell Biochem 1996;156: 17–24.
84. Oh-ishi S, Kizaki T, Nagasawa J, Izawa T et al. Clin Exp Pharmacol Physiol 1997;24:326–332.
85. Oh-ishi S, Kizaki T, Ookawara T, Sakurai T et al. Am J Respir Crit Care Med 1997;156: 1579–1585.
86. Salminen A, Vihko V. Acta Physiol Scand 1983;117:109–113.
87. Jenkins RR. In: Knuttgen HG, Vogel JA, Poortmans J (eds) Biochemistry of Exercise. vol 13. Champaign: Human Kinetics Publishers; 1983;467–471.
88. Higuchi M, Cartier L-J, Chen M, Holloszy JO. J Gerontol 1985;40:281–286.
89. Criswell D, Powers S, Dodd S, Lawler J et al. Med Sci Sports Exerc 1993;25:1135–1140.
90. Powers SK, Criswell D, Lawler J, Ji LL et al. Am J Physiol 1994;266:R375–R380.
91. Leeuwenburgh C, Fiebig R, Chandwaney R, Ji LL. Am J Physiol 1994;267:R439–R445.
92. Powers SK, Criswell D, Lawler J, Martin D et al. Respir Physiol 1994;95:227–237.
93. Pereira B, Costa Rosa LFB, Safi DA, Medeiros MHG et al. Physiol Behav 1994;56:1095–1099.
94. Hong H, Johnson P, Int J Biochem Cell Biol 1995;27:923–931.
95. Leeuwenburg C, Hollander J, Leichtweis S, Griffiths M et al. Am J Physiol 1997;272: R363–R369.
96. Reznick AZ, Steinhagen-Thiessen E, Gershon D. Biochem Med 1982;28:347–352.

97. Kumar CT, Reddy VK, Prasad M, Thyagaraju K et al. Molec Cell Biochem 1992;111:109−115.
98. Powers SK, Criswell D, Lawler J, Martin D et al. Am J Physiol 1993;265:H2094−H2098.
99. Somani SM, Rybak LP, Ind J Physiol Pharmacol 1996;40:205−212.
100. Husain K, Somani SM. Alcohol 1997;14:301−307.
101. Laughlin MH, Simpson T, Sexton WL, Brown OR et al. J Appl Physiol 1990;68:2337−2343.
102. Ji LL, Wu E, Thomas DP. Gerontology 1991;37:317−325.
103. Pereira B, Costa Rosa LFBP, Safi DA, Guimarâes ARP et al. Physiol Behav 1994;56: 1049−1955.
104. Song YJ, Igawa S, Horii A. Appl Hum Sci 1996;15:219−225.
105. Kanter NM, Hamlin RL, Unverferth DV, Davis HW et al. J Appl Physiol 1985;59:1298−1303.
106. Shimojo N, Arai Y. Hum Exp Toxicol 1994;13:524−528.
107. Kim JD, Yu BP, McCarter RJM, Lee SY et al. Free Rad Biol Med 1996;20:83−88.
108. Libonati JR, Gaughan JP, Hefner CA, Gow A et al. Hed Sci Spots Exerc 1997;29:509−516.
109. Vani M, Reddy GP, Reddy GR, Thyagaraju K et al. Biochem Int 1990;21:17−26.
110. Cao G, Chen J. Arch Biochem Biophys 1991;291:147−153.
111. Harri M, Kuusela P. Acta Physiol Scand 1986;126:189−197.
112. Ohno H, Yahata T, kuroshima A, Gasa S et al. In: Ueda G, Kusama S, Voelkel NF (eds) High-altitude Medical Science. Matsumoto: Shinshu University, 1988;431−435.
113. Ohno H, Kizaki T, Oh-ishi S, Yamashita H et al. Acta Physiol Scand 1995;155:333−334.
114. Oh-ishi S, Kizaki T, Toshinai K, Haga S et al. Mech Ageing Devel 1996;89:67−78.
115. Ueno N, Oh-ishi S, Kizaki T, Nishida M et al. Res Commun Mol Pathol Pharmacol 1997; 95:92−104.
116. Ookawara T, Kizaki T, Yamashita H, Oh-ishi S et al. Pathophysiology 1995;2:161−166.
117. Oh-ishi S, Toshinai K, Kizaki T, Haga S et al. Respir Physiol 1996;105:195−202.
118. Burke JP, Fenton MR. Proc Soc Exp Biol Med 1985;179:187−191.
119. Ohno H, Sato Y, Kizaki T, Yamashita H et al. In: Kies CV, Driskell JA (eds) Sports Nutrition: Minerals and Electrolytes. Boca Raton: CRC Press, 1995;129−138.
120. Sohal RS, Allen RG, Farmer KJ, Procter J. Mech Ageing Devel 1984;26:75−81.
121. Kramer K, Dijkstra H, Bast A. Physiol Behav 1993;53:271−276.
122. Toshinai K, Oh-ishi S, Kizaki T, Ookawara T et al. Res Commun Mol Pathol Pharmacol 1997; 95:259−274.
123. Ohno H, Yamashita H, Ookawara T, Kizaki T et al. Acta Physiol Scand 1993;148:353−355.
124. Ohno H, Kayashima S, Nagata N, Yamashita H et al. Clin Chim Acta 1993;215:213−219.
125. Kayashima S, Ohno H, Fujioka T, Taniguchi N et al. Eur J Appl Physiol 1995;70:413−420.
126. Schmidt E, Schmidt FW. In: Poortmans JR (ed) Medicine and Sport. vol 3. Biochemistry of Exercise. Basel: Karger; 1969;216−238.
127. Wong GHW, Goeddel DV. Science 1988;242:941−944.
128. Cannon JG, Evans WJ, Hughes VA, Meredith CN et al. J Appl Physiol 1986;61:1869−1874.
129. Cannon JG, Meydani SN, Fielding RA, Fiatarone MA et al. Am J Physiol 1991;260:R1235−R1240.
130. Ahlborg B, Brohult J. Acta Med Scand 1967;182:41−54.
131. Ohno H, Yamashita H, Ookawara T, Saitoh D et al. Acta Physiol Scand 1992;146:291−292.
132. Sen CK, Packer L. FASEB J 1996;10:709−720.
133. Oh-ishi S, Kizaki T, Ookawara T, Toshinai K et al. Pflügers Arch 1998;435:767−774.
134. Liu J, Simon LM, Phillips JR, Robin ED. J Appl Physiol 1997;42:107−110.
135. Costa LE. Am J Physiol 1990;259:C654−C659.
136. Radák Z, Lee K, Choi W, Sunoo S et al. Eur J Appl Physiol 1994;69:392−395.
137. Nakanishi K, Tajima F, Nakamura A, Yagura S et al. J Physiol 1995;489:869−876.
138. Radák Z, Asano K, Lee KC, Ohno H et al. Free Rad Biol Med 1997;22:1109−1114.
139. Inoue M, Ebashi I, Watanabe N, Morino Y. Biochemistry 1989;28:6619−6624.
140. Radák Z, Asano K, Inoue M, Kizaki T et al. J Appl Physiol 1995;79:129−135.
140. Radák Z, Asano K, Inoue M, Kizaki T et al. Eur J Appl Physiol 1996;72:189−194.

142. Homans DC, Asinger R, Pavek T, Crampton M et al. Am J Physiol 1992;263:H392—H398.
143. Ando Y, Inoue M, Morino Y, Araki S. Brain Res 1989;477:286—291.
144. Hasuoka H, Sakagami K, Takasu S, Morisaki F et al. Transplant Proc 1989;50:164—165.
145. Watanabe N, Inoue M, Morino Y. Biochem Pharmacol 1989;38:3477—3483.
146. Saitoh D, Kadota T, Senoh A, Takahara T et al. Am J Emerg Med 1993;11:355—359.
147. Taniguchi N, Fujii J, Kaneto H, Asahi M et al. In: Montagnier L, Oliver R, Pasquier C (eds) Oxidative Stress in Cancer, AIDS, and Neurodegenerative Diseases. New York: Marcel Dekker, 1998;497—502.
148. Siddique T. Cold Spring Harbour Symp Quant Biol 1996;61:699—708.
149. Reaume AG, Elliott JL, Hoffman EK, Kowall NW et al. Nature Genet 1996;13:43—47.
150. Kondo T, Reaune AG, Huang TT, Carison E et al. J Neurosci 1997;17:4180—4189.
151. Li Y, Huang TT, Carlson EJ, Melov S et al. Nature Genet 1995;11:376—381.
152. Lebovitz RM, Zhang H, Vogel H, Cartwright Jr J et al. Proc Natl Acad Sci USA 1996;93: 9782—9789.
153. Carlsson LM, Jonsson J, Edlund T, Marklund SL. Proc Natl Acad Sci USA 1995;92: 6264—6268.
154. Tolmasoff JM, Ono T, Culter RG. Proc Natl Acad Sci USA 1980;77:2777—2781.
155. Sinet PM. Ann NY Acad Sci 1982;396:83—95.
156. Epstein CJ, Avraham KB, Lovett M, Smith S et al. Proc Natl Acad Sci USA 1987;84: 8044—8048.
157. Leschot NJ, Slater RM, Joenje H, Becker-Bloemkolk MJ et al. Hum Genet 1981;57:220—223
158. Torre DL, Casado A, Lopez-Fernandez E, Carrascosa D et al. Experientia 1996;52:871—873.
159. Deutsch HF, Hoshi S, Matsuda Y, Suzuki K et al. J Molec Biol 1991;219:103—108.
160. Rosen DR, Siddique T, Patterson D, Figlewicz DA et al. Nature 1993;362:59—62.
161. Dong H-X, Hentani A, Tainer JA, Iqbal Z et al. Science 1993;261:1047—1051.
162. Tu PH, Raju P, Robinson KA, Gurney ME et al. Proc Natl Acad Sci USA 1996;93:3155—3160.
163. Fujii J, Myint T, Seo HK, Kayanoki Y et al. J Neurochem 1995;64,1456—1461.
164. Wiedau-Pazos M, Goto JJ, Rabizadeh S, Gralla EB et al. Science 1996;271:515—518.
165. Beckman JS. Chem Res Toxicol 1996;9:836—844.
166. Yim MB, Kang JH, Yim H-S, Kwak H-S et al. Proc Natl Acad Sci USA 1996;93:5709—5714.
167. Bernstein RE. Adv Clin Chem 1978;26:1—78.
168. Cerami A, Stevens VJ, Monnier UM. Metab Clin Exp 1979;28:431—437.
169. Monnier VM. In: Baynes JW, Monnier VM (eds) The Maillard Reaction in Aging, Diabetes and Nutrition. New York: Alan R Liss, 1988;1—22
170. Waltkins NG, Thorpe SR, Baynes JW. J Biol Chem 1985;260:10629—10636.
171. Kondo T, Murakami K, Ohtsuka Y, Tsuji M et al. Clin Chim Acta 1987;166:227—236
172. Arai K, Iizuka S, Makita A, Oikawa K et al. J Immunol Meth 1986;91:139—140.
173. Garner MH, Bahador A, Sachs G. J Biol Chem 1990;265:15058—15066.
174. Hebbel RP, Eaton JW, Balasingam M, Steinberg MH. J Clin Invest 1982;70:1253—1259.
175. Mirsa HP. J Biol Chem 1984;259:12678—12684.
176. Watkins JA, Kawanishi S, Caughey WS. Biochem Biophys Res Commun 1985;132:742—748.
177. Cohen G, Hochstein P. Biochemistry 1964;3:895—900.
178. Arai K, Iizuka S, Tada Y, Oikawa K et al. Biochim Biophys Acta 1987;924:292—296.
179. Taniguchi N, Arai K, Kinoshita N. In: Wassarman PM, Kornberg RD (eds) Methods in Enzymology. vol 170. San Diego: Academic Press, 1989;397—408.
180. Kawamura N, Ookawara T, Suzuki K, Konishi K et al. J Clin Endocrinol Metab 1992;74: 1352—1354.
181. Arai K, Maguchi S, Fujii S, Ishibashi S et al. J Biol Chem 1987;262:16969—16972.
182. Taniguchi N, Kinoshita N, Arai K, Iizuka S et al. In: Baynes JW, Monnier VM (eds) The Maillard Reaction in Aging, Diabetes and Nutrition. New York: Alan R Liss; 1988;277—290.
183. Hunt JV, Dean RT, Wolff SP. Biochem J 1988;256:205—212.
184. Morita J, Kashimura N. In: Finot PA (ed) The Maillard Reaction: Advances in Life Sciences.

Basel: Birkhäuser Verlag, 1990;505–510.
185. Sakurai T, Sugioka K, Nakano M. Biochim Biophys Acta 1990;1043:27–33.
186. Salin ML, McCord JM. J Clin Invest 1974;54:1005–1009.
187. Davies KJ. Free Rad Biol Med 1986;2:155–173.
188. Salo DC, Pacifici RE, Lin SW, Giulivi C et al. J Biol Chem 1990;265:11919–11927.
189. Ookawara T, Kawamura N, Kitagawa Y, Taniguchi N. J Biol Chem 1992;267:18505–18510.
190. Bhuyan KC, Bhuyan DK. Biochim Biophys Acta 1978;542:28–38.
191. Scharf J, Dovrat A. Ophthalmic Res 1986;18:332–337.
192. Hesketh JE, Virmaux N, Mandel P. Biochim Biophys Acta 1978;542:39–46.
193. Stevens VJ, Rouzer CA, Monnier VM, Cerami A. Proc Natl Acad Sci USA 1978;75:2918–2922.
194. Garlick RL, Mazer JS, Chylack LT Jr, Tung WH et al. J Clin Invest 1984;74:1742–1749.
195. Oimomi M, Maeda Y, Hata F, Kitamura Y et al. Exp Eye Res 1988;46:415420.
196. Vidal P, FernandezVigo J, CabezasCerrato J. Acta Ophthalmol 1988;66:220–222.
197. Swamy MS, Abraham EC. Invest Ophthalmol Vis Sci 1987;28:1693–1701.
198. Patrick JS, Thorpe SR, Baynes JW. J Gerontol 1990;45:B18–B23.
199. Crouch RK, Gandy SE, Kimsey G, Galbraith RA et al. Diabetes 1981;30:235–241.
200. Gandy SE, Buse MG, Crouch RK. J Clin Invest 1982;70:650–658.
201. Kinoshita N, Tada Y, Arai K, Matsuda Y et al. In: Hayaishi O, Niki E, Kondo M, Yoshikaw T (eds) Medical, Biochemical and Chemical Aspects of Free Radicals: proc of the 4th Biennial General Meeting of the Society for Free Radical Research. Amsterdam: Elsevier, 1989; 719–722.
202. Fleischmajer R, Nedwick A. Am J Med 1973;54:111–118.
203. Goldstein S, Moerman EJ. Nature 1975;255:159.
204. Holliday R, Porterfield JS. Nature 1974;248:114–124.
205. Nordenson I. Hereditas 1977;87:151–154.
206. Glass GA, Gershon D. Biochem Biophys Res Commun 1981;103:1245–1253.
207. Reiss U, Gershon D. Biochem Biophys Res Commun 1976;73:255–262.
208. Rosenblum JS, Gilula NB, Lerner RA. Proc Natl Acad Sci USA 1996;93:4471–4473.
209. MacMillanCrow LA, Crow JP, Kerby JD, Beckman JS et al. Proc Natl Acad Sci USA 1996; 93:11853–11858.
210. Masuda A, Longo DL, Kobayashi Y, Appella E et al. FASEB J 1988;2:3087–3090.
211. Danh HC, Benedetti MS, Dostert P. J Neurochem 1974;40:1003–1007.
212. Dovrat A, Gershon D. Exp Eye Res 1981;33:651–661.
213. Marlhens F, Nicole A, Sinet PM. Biochem Biophys Res Commun 1985;129:300–305.
214. Nagai R, Chiu CC, Yamaoki K, Ohuchi Y et al. Am J Physiol 1983;245:H413–H419.
215. Nakada T, Akiya T, Koike H, Katayama T. Eur Urol 1988;14:50–55.
216. Nakamura Y, Gindhart TD, Winterstein D, Tomita I et al. Carcinogenesis 1988;9:203–207.
217. Oberley LW, Buettner GR. Cancer Res 1979;39:1141–1149.
218. Iizuka S, Taniguchi N, Makita A. J Natl Cancer Inst 1984;72:1043–1049.
219. Kawaguchi T, Noji S, Uda T, Nakashima Y et al. J Biol Chem 1989;264:5762–5767.
220. Wong GHW, Elwell JH, Oberley LW, Goeddel DV. Cell 1989;58:923–931.
221. Visner GA, Dougall WC, Wilson JM et al. J Biol Chem 1990;265:2856–2864.
222. Fujii J, Taniguchi N. J Biol Chem 1991;266:23142–23146.
223. Kawaguchi T, Takeyasu A, Matsunobu K, Uda T et al. Biochem Biophys Res Commun 1990;171: 1378–1386.
224. Ho YS, Howard AJ, Crapo JD. Am J Respir Cell Mol Biol 1991;4:278–286.
225. Suzuki K, Tatsumi H, Satoh S, Senda T et al. Am J Physiol 1993;265:H1173–H1178.
226. Nakata T, Suzuki K, Fujii J, Ishikawa M et al. Int J Cancer 1993;55:646–650.
227. Suzuki K, Kinoshita N, Matsuda Y, Higashiyama S et al. Free Rad Res Comms 1992;15: 325–334.
228. Yamashita N, Nishida M, Hoshida S, Kuzuya T et al. J Clin Invest 1994;94:2193–2199.
229. Nogae C, Makino N, Hata T, Nogae I et al. J Mol Cell Cardiol 1995;27:2091–2099.

230. Wagner GS, Roe CR, Limbird LE, Rosati RA et al. Circulation 1973;47:263–269.
231. Ono M, Sekiya M, Ohhira, M, Ohhira M et al. J Lab Clin Med 1991;118:476–483.
232. James SP, Hoofnagle JH, Strober W, Jones EA. Ann Int Med 1983;99:500–512.
233. Rubin E, Schaffer F, Popper H. Am J Pathol 1965;46:387–407.
234. Berg PA, Klein R, Lindenborn Fotinos J, Kloppel W. Lancet 1982;2:1243–1245.
235. Coppel RL, McNeilage LJ, Surh CD, Van de Water J et al. Proc Natl Acad Sci USA 1988;85:
    7317–7321.
236. Gershwin ME, Mackay IR, Sturgess A, Coppel RL. J Immunol 1987;138:3525–3531.
237. Nishiura T, Suzuki K, Kawaguchi T, Nakao H et al. Cancer Lett 1992;62:211–215.
238. Kasid A, Director EP, Stovroff MC, Lotze MT et al. Cancer Res 1990;50:5072–5076.
239. Cozzolino F, Rubartelli A, Aldnucci D, Sitia R. Proc Natl Acad Sci USA 1989;86:2369–2373.
240. Cordingley FT, Bianchi A, Hoftbrand AV, Reittie JE et al. Lancet 1988;1:969–971.
241. Bast RC, Feeney M, Lazarus H, Nadler LM et al. J Clin Invest 1981;68:1331–1337.
242. Canney PA, Moore M, Wilkinson PM, James RD. Br J Cancer 1984;50:765–769.
243. Ishikawa M, Yaginuma Y, Hayashi H, Shimizu T et al. Cancer Res 1990;50:2538–2542.
244. Nakata T, Suzuki K, Fujii J, Ishikawa M et al. Carcinogenesis 1992;13:1941–1943.
245. Leff JA, Parsons PE, Day CE, Taniguchi N et al. Lancet 1993;341:777–780.
246. Suter PM, Suter S, Girardin E, RouxLombard P et al. Am Rev Respir Dis 1992;145:
    1016–1022.

© 2000 Elsevier Science B.V. All rights reserved.
Handbook of Oxidants and Antioxidants in Exercise.
C.K. Sen, L. Packer and O. Hänninen, editors.

Part IV • Chapter 12

Antioxidants and physical exercise

Chandan K. Sen[1] and Allan H. Goldfarb[2]

[1]*Lawrence Berkeley National Laboratory, University of California, One Cyclotron Road, Building 90, Room 3031, Berkeley, CA 94720-3200, USA. Fax: +1-510-644-2341.*
E-mail: cksen@socrates.berkely.edu
[2]*Department of Exercise and Sports Science, The University of North Carolina, Greensboro, 250 HHP Building, Greensboro, North Carolina 27402-6169, USA*

1   INTRODUCTION
2   ANTIOXIDANT NUTRIENTS
     2.1   Vitamin E
     2.2   Carotenoids
     2.3   Ubiquinone
     2.4   Vitamin C
     2.5   Glutathione
     2.6   α-Lipoic acid
     2.7   Selenium
     2.8   Recommended daily allowances
3   ANTIOXIDANT DEFICIENCY IN EXERCISE
4   ANTIOXIDANT SUPPLEMENTATION IN EXERCISE
     4.1   Vitamin E
     4.2   Vitamin C
     4.3   Coenzyme Q_{10}
     4.4   Glutathione
     4.5   N-acetyl-L-cysteine
     4.6   α-Lipoic acid
     4.7   Other nutrients
     4.8   Antioxidant interaction
5   PERSPECTIVES
6   SUMMARY
7   ABBREVIATIONS
8   REFERENCES

1   INTRODUCTION

Physical exercise may be associated with oxidative stress [1]. Elevated levels of oxidative stress markers have been observed in several studies. Endogenous antioxidant defense mechanisms work in concert with nutritional antioxidants to provide protection against oxidative damage. Manipulation of tissue antioxidant defense status by gene therapy-dependent techniques has been proposed to be valuable in treating various clinical disorders [2]. Physical training strengthens antioxidant defense mechanisms in several tissues including the skeletal muscle (see Chapter 10 by Powers and Sen in this volume, 219—242). To evaluate the possible protective role of endogenous and exogenous antioxidants against exercise-induced oxidative stress studies involving antioxidant-supplementation and deficiency have been carried out. The aim of this chapter is to summarize our current understanding of the role of antioxidants in exercise-induced oxidative stress.

2   ANTIOXIDANT NUTRIENTS

The Food and Nutrition Board of the National Institute of Medicine USA, has recently formulated the following definition for dietary antioxidants: "a dietary antioxidant is a substance in foods that significantly decreases the adverse effects of reactive oxygen species, reactive nitrogen species, or both on normal physiological function in humans." This proposed definition is based on several criteria:

1) the substance is found in human diets;
2) the content of the substance has been measured in foods commonly consumed; and
3) in humans, the substance decreases the adverse effects of reactive oxygen and nitrogen species in vivo.

In order to meet the definition of a dietary antioxidant proposed here, nutrients and food components must be found in typical human diets. Many substances have been shown to have antioxidant activity *in vitro*. However, *in vitro* findings are of uncertain relevance to the *in vivo* situation in healthy humans. The definition of a dietary antioxidant focuses on antioxidant effects of substances when consumed by humans. Therefore, dietary antioxidants are substances that have been shown to decrease the effects of reactive oxygen and nitrogen species in humans.

The chemical nature of any antioxidant determines its solubility, and thus its localization in biological tissues (Fig. 1). For example, lipid soluble antioxidants are localized in membranes and function to protect against oxidative damage of membranes. Water-soluble antioxidants, located for example in the cytosol, mitochondrial matrix or extracellular fluids, may not have access to ROS generated in membranes. Vitamin C, glutathione, uric acid and lipoic acid are the most commonly known water-soluble antioxidants (Fig. 2). Vitamins E and A, co-enzyme Q, carotenoids, flavonoids, and polyphenols represent the most extensively studied naturally occurring fat-soluble antioxidants (Fig. 3). The antioxidants that have been tested in exercise-related studies are briefly introduced in the following section.

2.1 Vitamin E

Vitamin E refers to all tocol and tocotrienol derivatives which exhibit the biological activity of α-tocopherol [3]. The form of vitamin E that has the most biological activity is RRR-α-tocopherol, previously known as d-α-tocopherol (see Chapter 14 by Traber in this volume, 359–371). Vitamin supplements are marketed as

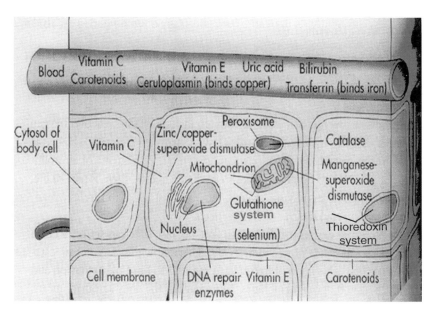

Fig. 1. Distribution of various major antioxidants. Vitamins E, C, uric acid, cartenoids, bilirubin and metal binding proteins such as caeruloplasmin and transferrin are found in the blood. In the cell, lipophilic antioxidants such as vitamin E and cartenoids are found in the membranes. Antioxidant defense mechanisms in the aqueous phase (e.g., cytosol) include the GSH system (GSH, related enzymes and selenium), thioredoxin system (thioredoxin, related enzymes and selenium; selenium facilitates thioredoxin reductase activity), superoxide dimutases and vitamin C. Catalase is mostly found in peroxisomes. The form of superoxide dimutase mostly found in the cystol is Cu,Zn-superoxide dimutase. Mn-superoxide dimutase is mostly a mitochondrial antioxidant. In the nucleus, DNA repair enzymes facilitate repair of oxidatively damaged DNA.

mixed tocopherols, α-tocopherol or esterified derivatives e.g., α-tocopheryl-acetate, -nicotinate or -succinate. Edible vegetable oils are the richest natural source of vitamin E. Unprocessed cereal grains and nuts are also good sources of vitamin E. Animal source of vitamin E includes meat, especially fat. One of the most significant properties of vitamin E is that it is an antioxidant. Vitamin E especially protects polyunsaturated fatty acids within phospholipids of biological membranes and in plasma lipoproteins [4]. The phenolic moiety of tocopherol reacts with peroxyl ($ROO^{\cdot}$, where R = alkyl residue) radicals to form the corresponding organic hydroperoxide and the tocopheroxyl radical. In this radical form vitamin E is not anymore an effective antioxidant, and when sufficiently accumulated may even have toxic pro-oxidant effects. The effects of vitamin E on oxidation of various biological molecules, membranes and tissues have been extensively studied. Vitamin E suppresses the oxidative damage of biological membranes, lipoproteins and tissues. Tocopherols are unstable and are readily oxidized by air, especially in the presence of iron and other transition metal ions. The resulting tocopherylquinone has no biological activity. To prevent this loss of biological potency in nutritional

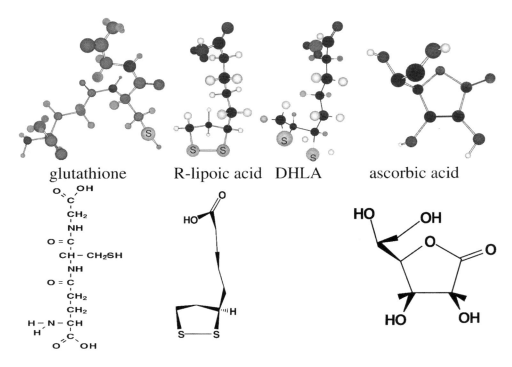

Fig. 2. Water soluble antioxidants. DHLA: dihydrolipoic acid. Black balls: carbon; light shaded balls: hydrogen.

supplements vitamin E is presented in the esterified form. In the gastrointestinal tract the ester is enzymatically hydrolyzed and free tocopherol is absorbed [5].

2.2 Carotenoids

Carotenoid designates a long chain molecule with 40 carbon atoms and an extensive conjugated system of double bonds. Plant and microorganism-derived carotenoids are efficient scavengers of several forms of ROS [6]. The major forms of carotenoids that have been studied for their antioxidant properties include α-, β- and γ-carotene, lycopene, β-cryptoxanthin, lutein, zeaxanthin, astaxanthin, canthaxanthin, violaxanthin, and β-carotene-5,6-epoxide. Leaves of photosynthetic plant are rich in carotenoids containing predominantly β-carotene, lutein, and epoxycarotenoids e.g., violaxanthin. Storage bodies such as carrot, papaya or squash contain mostly β-carotene, α-carotene and β-cryptoxanthin. Tomatoes are rich in lycopene because the β-carotene biosynthetic pathway terminates prior to the formation of the terminal rings. Chemically, carotenoids are highly unstable and are susceptible to auto-oxidation [7]. Although most reports indicate that carotenoids do have effective antioxidant functions in biological systems, some studies show that carotenoids may also show toxic pro-oxidant effects [8,9].

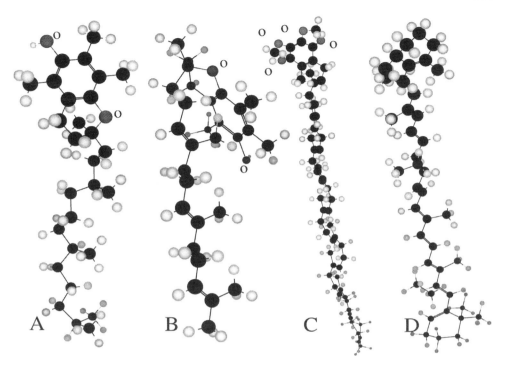

Fig. 3. Fat soluble antioxidants. **A:** tocopherol. **B:** tocotrienol. **C:** ubiquinone 10. **D:** β-carotene. Black balls: carbon; light shaded balls: hydrogen; oxygen is represented by dark shaded balls labelled as "O".

2.3 Ubiquinone

Coenzyme Q_{10}, also called ubiquinone, is an integral component of the mitochondrial electron transport chain. Coenzyme Q_{10} is found partitioned within phospholipid bilayer of plasma membranes, all intracellular membranes and also in low-density lipoproteins. The actual mechanism of antioxidant action of ubiquinones is still conjectural. One possibility is that ubiquinols act independently as lipid peroxidation chain breaking antioxidants. Alternatively, a redox interaction of ubiquinol with vitamin E has been suggested in which ubiquinol mainly acts by regenerating vitamin E from its oxidized form [10]. The serum levels of ubiquinone depend mostly on the amount of ubiquinone-containing lipoproteins in the circulation. Physical activity markedly affects muscle tissue levels of ubiquinone. It has been observed that serum and muscle tissue ubiquinone levels do not correlate with each other, suggesting that they are independently regulated [11].

2.4 Vitamin C

Vitamin C or ascorbate is an excellent water-soluble antioxidant. Although in most higher organisms it is synthesized from abundant glucose precursors, others including humans solely depend on nutritional supply. Because of its strong reducing properties ascorbate readily reduces Fe^{3+} and Cu^{2+} to Fe^{2+} and Cu^+, respectively. In this way, ascorbate can contribute to the redox cycling of these metals generating transition metal ions that can stimulate free radical chemistry. Thus, in the presence of free metals ascorbate may have pro-oxidant effects [12,13]. Apart from direct free radical scavenging activity, ascorbate may also enhance the antioxidant action of vitamin E. The phenol group of tocopherol, which is the basis of its antioxidant action, appears to be located at the water-membrane interface of biological membranes. Such localization facilitates ascorbate-vitamin E interaction. Dehydroascorbate, the two-electron oxidation product of ascorbate, is reduced to ascorbate by reduced glutathione. Thus, ascorbate plays a central role in the antioxidant network.

2.5 Glutathione

Glutathione (L-γ-glutamyl-L-cysteinylglycine) is implicated in the circumvention of cellular oxidative stress and maintenance of intracellular thiol redox status [14−17]. Glutathione peroxidase is specific for its hydrogen donor, reduced glutathione, but may use a wide range of substrates extending from H_2O_2 to organic hydroperoxides. The cytosolic and membrane-bound monomer GSH phospholipid hydroperoxide-glutathione peroxidase and the distinct tetramer plasma glutathione peroxidase are able to reduce phospholipid hydroperoxides without the necessity of prior hydrolysis by phospholipase A_2. The protective action of phospholipid hydroperoxide-glutathione peroxidase against membrane damaging lipid peroxidation has been directly demonstrated [18]. Reduced glutathione GSH is a major cellular electrophile conjugator as well. Glutathione S-transferases catalyze the reaction between the -SH group of GSH and potential alkylating agents thereby neutralizing their electrophilic sites and rendering them more water soluble. Glutathione S-transferases represent a major group of phase II detoxification enzymes [19].

Intracellular synthesis of GSH is a tightly regulated two-step process, both of which are ATP-dependent. γ-Glutamylcysteine synthetase (also referred to as glutamate-cysteine ligase) catalyses the formation of the dipeptide γ-glutamylcysteine [20] and subsequently the addition of glycine is catalyzed by glutathione synthetase. Substrates for such synthesis are provided both by direct amino acid transport and by γ-glutamyl transpeptidase (also known as glutamyl transferase) that couples the γ-glutamyl moiety to a suitable amino acid acceptor for transport into the cell. GSH is also generated intracellularly from its oxidized form glutathione disulfide (GSSG) by glutathione disulfide reductase activity in the presence of NADPH. Under normal conditions the rate-limiting factor in cellular GSH synthesis is the availability of the constituent amino acid cysteine. Thus, given that the GSH synthesizing enzymes are normal in their activity improving cysteine delivery to cells is often effective to increase cell GSH. Cysteine per se is highly unstable in its reduced form. As a result considerable research has been focused on alternative strategies for cysteine delivery to cells.

Administered GSH per se is not effectively transported into cells [21] except in the small intestine [22–25]. It is mostly degraded in the extracellular compartment. The degradation products, i.e., the constituent amino acids, may be used as substrates for GSH neosynthesis inside the cell. Two clinically relevant pro-GSH agents that have been most extensively studied so far are N-acetyl-L-cysteine (NAC; 2-mercapto-propionyl glycine) and α-lipoate [26–38]. In addition to its reactive oxygen detoxifying properties [30,39], NAC is thought to function as a cysteine delivery compound [36,40]. After free NAC enters a cell, it is rapidly hydrolyzed to release cysteine. NAC, but not N-acetyl-D-cysteine or the oxidized disulfide form of NAC, is deacetylated in several tissues to release cysteine [41]. NAC is safe for human use and has been used as a clinical mucolytic agent for many years.

2.6 α-Lipoic acid

α-Lipoic acid is also known as thioctic acid, 1,2-dithiolane-3-pentanoic acid, 1,2-dithiolane-3-valeric acid or 6,8-thioctic acid [27,28,37]. At physiological pH, lipoic acid is anionic and is referred to as lipoate. In human cells, α-lipoic acid is present in a bound lipoyllysine form in mitochondrial proteins that play a central role in oxidative metabolism. Lipoate exists as lipoamide in at least five proteins where it is covalently linked to a lysyl residue. Four of these proteins are found in α-ketoacid dehydrogenase complexes, the pyruvate dehydrogenase complex, the branched chain keto-acid dehydrogenase complex and the α-ketoglutarate dehydrogenase complex. Three lipoamide- containing proteins are present in the E2 enzyme dihydrolipoyl acyltransferase, which is different in each of the complexes and specific for the substrate of the complex. One lipoyl residue is found in protein X, which is the same in each complex. The fifth lipoamide residue is present in the glycine cleavage system [42]. Although it has been indicated that lipoate supplementation may improve mitochondrial function by facilitating the activity of lipoyllysine containing enzymes [43], there is no evidence to support this contention. The first study testing the possible effects of oral α-lipoic acid supplementation, a single bout of strenuous exercise and endurance exercise training on the lipoyllysine content in skeletal muscle and liver tissues of rat was recently reported [44]. Incorporation of lipoyl moiety to tissue protein was not increased by dietary lipoate. Interestingly, endurance exercise training markedly increased lipoyllysine content in the liver. A bout of exhaustive exercise also increased hepatic lipoyllysine content. A significant interaction of exhaustive exercise and training to increase tissue lipoyllysine content was evident. In vastus lateralis skeletal muscle, training did not influence tissue lipoyllysine content. A single bout of exhaustive exercise, however, clearly increased the level of lipoyllysine in the muscle. Comparison of tissue lipoyllysine data with that of free or loosely bound lipoate results showed a clear lack of association between the two apparently related parameters. Thus, the tightly protein-bound lipoyllysine pool in tissues is independent of the loosely bound or free lipoate status in the tissue [44].

Lipoic acid has been detected in the form of lipoyllysine in various natural sources. In the plant material studied, lipoyllysine content was highest in spinach (3.15 µg/g dry weight; 92.51 µg/mg protein). When expressed as weight per dry weight of lyophilized vegetables, the abundance of naturally existing lipoate in spinach was over 3- and 5-fold higher than that in broccoli and tomato, respectively. Lower concentration of lipoyllysine were also detected in garden pea, brussel sprouts and rice bran. Lipoyllysine concentration was below detection limits in acetone powders of banana, orange peel, soybean and horseradish, however. In animal tissues, the abundance of lipoyllysine in bovine acetone powders can be represented in the following order: kidney > heart > liver > spleen > brain > pancreas > lung. The concentration of lipoyllysine in bovine kidney and heart were 2.64 ± 1.23 and 1.51 ± 0.75 µg/g dry weight, respectively [Lodge, 1997; see 37]

Studies with human Jurkat T cells have shown that when added to the culture medium, lipoate readily enters the cell where it is reduced to its dithiol form, dihydrolipoate (DHLA). DHLA accumulated in the cell pellet, and when monitored over a 2 h interval the dithiol was released to the culture medium [45]. As a result of lipoate treatment to the Jurkat T cells and human neonatal fibroblasts, accumulation of DHLA in the culture medium was observed. The redox potential of the lipoate-DHLA couple is −320 mV. Thus, DHLA is a strong reductant capable of chemically reducing GSSG to GSH. Following lipoate supplementation, extracellular DHLA reduces cystine outside the cell to cysteine. The cellular uptake mechanism for cysteine by the ASC system is approximately 10 times faster than that for cystine by the x_c^- − system [46]. Thus, DHLA markedly improves cysteine availability within the cell resulting in accelerated GSH synthesis [28,47]. Both lipoate and DHLA have remarkable reactive oxygen detoxifying properties [37]. Recent studies show that lipoic acid can potently stimulate glucose uptake in differentiated skeletal muscle-derived L6 myotubes. Glucose uptake in cytokine-treated insulin-resistant cells was enhanced by lipoic acid treatment suggesting that lipoic acid treatment may help in conditions such as infection-related disorders in glucose metabolism [48].

α-Lipoic acid is taken up by cells and reduced to its potent dithiol form, dihydrolipoate (DHLA), much of which is rapidly effluxed out from cells. To improve retention in cells, the lipoic acid molecule has been recently modified to confer a positive charge at physiological pH. This novel protonated form of lipoic acid is known as lipoic acid − plus or LA-Plus [49]. Structurally, compared to lipoic acid, LA-Plus more closely resembles the naturally occurring form of lipoic acid i.e., lipoyllysine. The uptake and reduction of LA-Plus by human Wurzburg T cells was higher compared to that of lipoic acid. Several-fold higher amounts of DHLA-Plus, the corresponding reduced form of LA-Plus, were detected in LA-Plus treated cells compared to the amount of DHLA found in cells treated with lipoic acid. On a concentration basis, LA-Plus has been observed to be much more cytoprotective than native lipoic acid [49].

2.7 Selenium

Forty years ago traces of dietary selenium was observed to prevent nutritional liver necrosis in vitamin E deficient rats [50]. At present, selenium is widely used in agriculture to prevent a variety of selenium- and vitamin E-sensitive conditions in livestock and poultry [51]. In animal tissues, selenium is either present as selenocysteine in selenoproteins such as glutathione peroxidase, selenoprotein P or thioredoxin reductase. Additionally, selenium may be present in animal tissues as selenomethionine that is incorporated in place of methionine in a variety of proteins. Selenomethionine containing proteins serve as a reservoir of selenium that provides selenium to the organism when dietary supply of selenium is interrupted. Selenocysteine is the form of selenium that accounts for its biological activity. Perhaps the most prominent biological activity of selenium is that it is an essential cofactor for the critical hydroperoxide metabolizing enzyme glutathione peroxidase [52]. It has been suggested that selenium may also have direct antioxidant effects in biological systems [53]. Selenium content in food sources may markedly vary depending on the selenium content of the feed for animals, or selenium content in the agricultural soil. Organ meats, seafoods and muscle meat are considerable sources of selenium. Dairy products, and cereal and grains may also provide significant amounts to meet the RDA value of 70 and 55 µg/day calculated for adult men and women respectively [54].

2.8 Recommended daily allowances

The Food and Nutrition Board of the National Academy of Science and the National Research Council have developed guidelines for several dietary factors. These recommended daily allowances (RDA) were last revised in 1989 and at the time this work was written another process of revision was in progress. The allowances are intended to supply adequate amounts of these substances for an average daily intake over time and takes into account individual variations for most normal individuals who live in the US under usual environmental stresses. The RDAs can vary for infants, children, adults, elderly as well as for lactating women. According to values of 1989, the RDA for vitamin E is 10 mg for adult males and 8 mg for adult females. β-Carotene is not identified directly but its RDA is thought to be 1/6 the amount recommended for vitamin A (RDA 1 mg and 0.8 mg for men and women, respectively). Selenium has a suggested RDA of 0.07 mg for adult males and 0.055 mg for adult females. Vitamin C has a RDA of 60 mg for adults. There are no particular guidelines established for glutathione. However, glutathione is composed of three amino acids, glycine, cysteine and glutamine. Adequate protein intake in the diet is needed but this does not guarantee glutathione synthesis as indicated previously [41].

3   ANTIOXIDANT DEFICIENCY IN EXERCISE

The antioxidant deficiency model has been used to test the significance of various antioxidants in exercise-induced oxidative stress. Several studies have consistently indicated that vitamin E deficiency can lead to enhanced free radical formation resulting in compromised exercise performance and increased tissue lipid peroxidation [55—61]. These studies suggest that inadequate amounts of dietary vitamin E may decrease endurance performance by as much as 40% and lead to enhanced oxidative lipid damage of several tissues [57,62—64]. Also, vitamin E deficiency was associated with increased fragility of lysosomal membranes and greater hemolysis of red blood cells [57,62]. Vitamin E deficiency also decreased oxidative phosphorylation [59,63] in skeletal muscle, liver and adipose tissues. In female rats, however, vitamin E deficiency does not appear to influence the ability to run nor does it enhance tissue lipid peroxidation [65]. It has been suggested that female rats may be less susceptible to free radical damage compared to male rats because of higher levels of estrogen, a potential antioxidant, in circulation [61,62,66]. The effects of an ascorbate depleting diet on run time was examined in guinea pigs which do not synthesize vitamin C. Run time of ascorbate-depleted guinea pigs was significantly less than ascorbate-adequate animals [67].

Dietary selenium deficiency impairs tissue antioxidant defenses by markedly downregulating glutathione peroxidase activity in tissues such as the liver and muscle. This effect on the antioxidant enzyme did not influence endurance to a treadmill run, however. This suggests that muscle glutathione peroxidase activity is not a limiting factor in physical performance (Lang et al., 1987). Selenium deficiency has been also found to enhance lipid peroxidation in skeletal muscle mitochondria of rats that were exercised for 1 h [68]. Activity of antioxidant enzymes in both liver and skeletal muscle have been observed to adapt in response to selenium deficiency suggesting that the organs may have encountered and responded to an enhanced oxidative challenge. The relative role of endogenous GSH in the circumvention of exhaustive exercise-induced oxidative stress has been investigated using GSH deficient rats. GSH synthesis was inhibited by intraperitoneally administered L -buthionine-sulfoximine (BSO) to produce glutathione deficiency. The BSO treatment resulted in:

1)   ~ 50% decrease in the total glutathione pools of the liver, lung, blood and plasma, and
2)   80—90% decrease in the total glutathione pools of the skeletal muscle and heart.

Compared to controls, glutathione deficient rats had remarkably higher levels of tissue lipid peroxides. A significant effect of glutathione deficiency on endurance to exhaustion was observed. Glutathione deficient rats could run for only about half the interval when compared to the saline injected controls. This observation underscores the critical role for tissue glutathione in the circumvention of exercise-induced oxidative stress and as a determinant of exercise performance [69]. Increased susceptibility to oxidative stress was also observed in muscle-derived cells pretreated with BSO [70].

Leeuwenburgh et al. [71] studied the effect of chronic *in vivo* glutathione depletion by BSO on intracellular and interorgan GSH homeostasis in mice both at rest and after an acute bout of exhaustive swim exercise. BSO treatment for 12 days decreased concentrations of GSH in the liver, kidney, quadriceps muscle, and plasma to 28, 15, 7, and 35%, respectively, compared to GSH-adequate mice. GSH depletion was associated with adaptive changes in the activities of several enzymes related to GSH metabolism. Exhaustive exercise in the GSH-adequate state severely depleted GSH content in the liver (−55%) and kidney (−35%), whereas plasma and muscle GSH levels remained constant. However, exercise in the GSH-depleted state exacerbated GSH deficit in the liver (−57%), kidney (−33%), plasma (−65%), and muscle (−25%) in the absence of adequate reserves of liver GSH. Hepatic lipid peroxidation increased by 220 and 290%, respectively, after exhaustive exercise in the GSH-adequate and -depleted mice. It was concluded that GSH homeostasis is an essential component of the pro-oxidant-antioxidant balance during prolonged physical exercise.

4   ANTIOXIDANT SUPPLEMENTATION IN EXERCISE

4.1 Vitamin E

Venditti et al. [72] observed that free radical-induced damage in muscle could be one of the factors terminating muscle effort. They suggested that greater antioxidant levels in the tissue should allow trained muscle to withstand oxidative processes more effectively, thus lengthening the time required so that the cell function is sufficiently damaged as to make further exercise impossible. Whether oxidative stress is the single most important factor determining muscle performance is certainly a debatable issue. The contention that strengthened antioxidant defense of the muscle may protect against exercise-induced oxidative stress-dependent muscle damage is much more readily acceptable [73]. Animal experiments studying the effect of vitamin E have shown mixed results on the prevention of lipid peroxidation [1] with the general trend that such supplementation may diminish oxidative tissue damage. Brady and coworkers [74] examined the effects of vitamin E supplementation (50 IU/kg diet) on lipid peroxidation in liver and skeletal muscle at rest and following exhaustive swim exercise. Vitamin E effectively decreased lipid peroxidation in liver independent of selenium supplementation, whereas skeletal muscle lipid peroxidation response was unaffected by the supplementation. Goldfarb et al. [75] observed that vitamin E supplementation can protect against run-induced lipid peroxidation in the skeletal muscle and blood. The effect in skeletal muscle was muscle fiber type-dependent. The protective effect of vitamin E was more clearly evident when the animals were exposed to an additional stressor, dehydroepiandrosterone.

Jackson et al. [76] examined the effect of both vitamin E deficiency and supplementation on the contractile activity of muscle. Male rats and female mice were given either a standard diet, a vitamin E-deficient diet with 0.5 mg/kg selenium or a diet supplemented with 240 mg α-tocopherol acetate/kg diet. The animals were given this diet for 42 to 45 days. Vitamin E deficiency, in both mice and rats, was associated with increased susceptibility to contractile damage. Vitamin E supplementation clearly protected against such damage. Despite the fact that vitamin E supplementation protected the muscles from damage as indicated by creatine kinase and lactate dehydrogenase leakage there was no apparent effect on muscle lipid peroxidation. Kumar et al. [77] noted that vitamin E supplementation for 60 days in female adult albino rats completely abolished the increase in free radical mediated lipid peroxidation in the myocardium as a result of exhaustive endurance exercise. They reported that exercise-induced lipid peroxidation in heart tissue increased in control rats but did not increase in the vitamin E supplemented rats. Consistently, it has been also observed that vitamin E supplementation for 5 weeks attenuated exercise-induced increase in myocardial lipid peroxidation [75,78,79].

McIntosh et al. [80,81] observed that vitamin E supplemented diets protect against peroxisomal fatty acid oxidation-dependent leakage of hepatic enzymes into the plasma in response to physical exercise and dehydroepiandrosterone treatment. Vitamin E prevented dehydroepiandrosterone-induced increase of peroxisomal fatty acid oxidation and leakage of alanine aminotransferase and aspartate aminotransferase into the plasma. Exercised animals on a normal diet demonstrated similar peroxisomal fatty acid oxidation profile and plasma enzyme levels as the vitamin E supplemented group. Novelli et al. [82] examined the effects of intramuscular injections of three spin-trappers and vitamin E on endurance swimming to exhaustion in mice. Mice were injected on 3 successive days. It was observed that compared to either the control or placebo saline injected animals the spin-trap and vitamin E injected group had significantly increased swim endurance. In a study reported by Quintanilha and Packer [60] rats were given one of the following three diets and compared for liver mitochondrial respiration and lipid peroxidation: a diet deficient of vitamin E, a diet with 40 IU vitamin E/kg, or a diet with 400 IU vitamin E/kg. Hepatic mitochondrial respiratory control ratio were highest in the group supplemented with 400 IU/ kg. Additionally, liver lipid peroxidation in nuclei and microsomes was lowest in the vitamin E supplemented group especially when NADPH was present. Warren et al. [83] studied the effects of vitamin E supplementation, 10,000 IU/kg diet for 5 weeks, on muscle damage and free radical damage to membranes as indicated by alterations in plasma enzymes. Susceptibility of the skeletal muscles to oxidative stress was markedly decreased in response to vitamin E supplementation but this did not attenuate muscle injury triggered by eccentric contractions. It was concluded that vitamin E supplementation may be beneficial in protecting against free radical damage, but that the injury caused by eccentric exercise may not be ROS mediated. The effect of dietary vitamin E on exercise-induced oxidative protein damage has been investigated in the skeletal muscle of rats. For a period of 4 weeks rats were fed with high vitamin E diet (10,000 IU/kg diet), a α-tocopherol and tocotrienol (7000 mg tocotrienol/kg diet) rich palm oil diet or control diet with basal levels of α-tocopherol (30 IU/kg body weight). Uphill exhaustive treadmill exercise caused oxidative protein damage in skeletal muscles. A protective effect of vitamin E supplementation against exercise-induced protein oxidation in skeletal muscles was clearly evident [84]. α-Tocopherol level and fluidity has been studied in the neuronal membrane of rat brain after exhaustive exercise. The order parameter, 5-doxyl-stearic acid (5-DS), which is utilized for assessing the fluidity of the lipid bilayer closer to the hydrophilic face of the membrane, decreased in the pons-medulla oblongata; and the motion parameter, 16-doxyl-stearic acid (16-DS) for the study of the lipid bilayer core, decreased in the cortex, hippocampus, hypothalamus and striatum, whereas it increased in the cerebellum after exercise. The w/s ratio of n- (1-oxyl-2,2,6,6-tetramethyl-4-piperidinyl) -maleimido, used for the study of sulfhydryl protein conformation, also decreased in the hippocampus and midbrain after exercise. These exercise-dependent changes were prevented by α-tocopheryl acetate supplementation (10,000 IU vitamin E /kg diet) [85].

Fish oils have been shown to have a beneficial effect on cardiovascular mortality based on numerous epidemiological studies [86], presumably *via* effects on triglyceride levels, membrane fluidity and platelet and leukocyte function [87]. Not all studies show beneficial effects, however [88]. Because the (n–3) fatty acids making up fish oil are highly polyunsaturated, concerns have been raised regarding increased oxidative stress from fish oil intake [89—93]. Furthermore, fish oils induce peroxisomal β-oxidation, in which fatty-acyl oxidation yields hydrogen peroxide (H_2O_2) as a normal byproduct, and upregulate the activity of the H_2O_2 decomposing enzyme catalase [89,90,94]. Under normal conditions up to 20% of cellular O_2 consumption has in fact been estimated to occur in the peroxisome [95]. The beneficial effects of regular exercise on cardiovascular and overall mortality [96] may be decreased by uncontrolled exercise-induced oxidative stress. This may be particularly concerning in groups predisposed to oxidative stress, including that induced by fish oil [91—93]. Sen et al. examined the effect of fish oil and vitamin E supplementation compared to placebo soy oil and vitamin E supplementation on physiological antioxidant defenses and resting and exercise-induced oxidative stress in rat liver, heart and skeletal muscle [97]. The effects of 8 week vitamin E and fish oil supplementation on resting and exercise-induced oxidative stress was examined. Lipid peroxidation was 33% higher in fish oil fed rats compared to the placebo group in the liver, but oxidative protein damage remained similar in both liver and red gastrocnemius muscle. Vitamin E supplementation markedly decreased liver and muscle lipid peroxidation induced by fish oil diet. Vitamin E supplementation also markedly decreased oxidative protein damage in the liver and muscle. Exhaustive treadmill exercise increased liver and muscle lipid peroxidation, and muscle oxidative protein damage. Vitamin E effectively decreased exercise-induced lipid peroxidation and protein oxidation [97].

A limited number of studies have examined the effect of vitamin E supplementation in humans. Exercise performance and physical fitness have multifactorial determinants and may not serve as reasonable end points to test the efficacy of antioxidant supplementation. Vitamin E supplementation (900 IU·d^{-1} for 6 months) in trained swimmers did not alter their swim performance nor their lactate response in plasma [98]. Neither did vitamin E supplementation (800 IU·d^{-1} for 4 weeks) alter the work load needed to run at 80% VO$_2$ max in trained and untrained men [99]. Volunteers given 400 IU·d^{-1} of vitamin E for 6 weeks showed no influence on cycle time, swim time, or step time [100]. Additionally no changes in VO$_2$ max, a marker of physical fitness, was noted in humans following vitamin E supplementation [99,101,102]. However, Cannon et al. (1990) reported that 400 IU·d^{-1} of vitamin E supplementation for 48 days decreased the amount of creatine kinase leakage from muscles during recovery from a downhill run. Sumida et al. [101] examined the effects of 4 weeks of vitamin E supplementation in 21 healthy college-aged males. The subjects ingested 300 mg of vitamin E daily and blood levels of several enzymes and lipid peroxides were determined before and for up to 3 h after cycling exercise to exhaustion. Exercise increased the level of lipid peroxidation byproducts in plasma immediately after the cycling. Such levels returned to normal at 1 and 3 h of recovery. Vitamin E supplementation significantly decreased the resting level of plasma lipid peroxides. Meydani et al. [103] reported that urinary excretion of lipid peroxidation byproducts tended to be lower in vitamin E supplemented individuals (400 IU doses, twice daily, for 48 days) compared to the corresponding placebo group. This effect was only significant 12 days after downhill running. The subjects ran 16% downhill at 75% of their maximum heart rate for three 15 min periods. Muscle biopsies were obtained from the vastus lateralis of young subjects. It was observed that exercise increased the level of lipid peroxidation byproducts increased in muscle of placebo group whereas in the muscle of the vitamin E supplemented group no such oxidative lipid damage was evident. Another study examined the effect of vitamin E supplementation (800 ·d^{-1} for 4 weeks) and compared that to a placebo treatment in the same individuals at a specific exercise intensity [99]. Subjects were randomly assigned to either a placebo or vitamin E treatment group in a counter-balanced design. Subjects were exercised for 30 min at 80% VO$_2$ max and blood samples were collected before and after the run. Vitamin E treatment attenuated the level of resting plasma lipid peroxidation byproducts and also protected against the exercise response. The effects of 5 months of α-tocopherol supplementation have been studied in 30 top class cyclists. Although the supplementation did not improve physical performance, it was evident that exercise-induced muscle damage was less in response to antioxidant supplementation [104]. In humans it has been observed that a combination of vitamin E and fish oil supplement delays oxidative modification of low density lipoprotein [105].

In 1980, the US recommended daily allowance for vitamin E was reduced from 30 IU (recommended in 1968) to 15 IU. In the same year it was estimated that in the US, the amount of vitamin E supplied by a "normal" diet was about 11 IU (7.4 mg). Packer et al. have discussed that such dosages are insufficient for active athletes and that dosages of up to 400 IU/day may be reasonable recommendation for active athletes engaged in moderate to heavy exercise [106]. Vitamin E is proven to be safe at levels of intake up to approximately 3000 mg for prolonged periods of time [107]. However, individuals taking anticoagulants should refrain from taking very high doses (> 4000 IU) of vitamin E because vitamin E can act synergistically with this class of drug [108]. Long-term studies are necessary to determine safety issues related to vitamin E supplementation in humans.

4.2 Vitamin C

Levels of vitamin C in the plasma has been shown to decrease in response to acute swim exercise [109]. Such effect as been noted to be proportional to the duration of exercise. This observation suggests that prolonged physical exercise is associated with enhanced consumption of vitamin C in the circulation [109]. Vitamin C supplements (3 g/kg diet) given to rats who were placed on a vitamin E deficient diet did not alter the run time to exhaustion in the vitamin E deficient animals. Vitamin C was also unable to counter the deleterious effects of vitamin E deficiency [57]. Oral vitamin C, however, did prevent exercise-induced blood GSH oxidation in rats [110]. In a preliminary report the effect of vitamin C supplementation in humans was documented. A mild protective effect of vitamin C supplementation, based on elevated total antioxidant capacity of the plasma, was observed [111]. In a double-blind, randomized crossover study, 19 healthy subjects (men and women) mean 35 years of age were given two separate bouts of eccentric work on their plantar flexors on separate legs 3 weeks apart [112]. Vitamin C (3 g/day) was supplemented for 3 days preceding exercise, and continued for 1 week. Vitamin C supplementation attenuated muscle soreness compared to placebo. In another study it was also noted that 400 mg of vitamin C supplement improves recovery from eccentric muscle damage [113]. Whether this effect of vitamin C was related to its antioxidant property is not clear.

4.3 Coenzyme Q_{10}

A few studies have examined the effects of coenzyme Q_{10} to determine if additional amounts of this factor in the electron transport chain would be beneficial in preventing free radical damage [114–116]. Dietary coenzyme Q_{10} supplementation protected against leakage of creatine kinase and lactate dehydrogenase from the muscles to serum following downhill run [114]. In two human studies, however, this beneficial effect of coenzyme Q_{10} could not be observed [115,116].

The effects of ubiquinone supplementation (120 mg/day for 6 weeks) on aerobic capacity and lipid peroxidation during exercise has been investigated in 11 young (aged 22—38 years) and 8 older (aged 60—74 years), trained men. This crossover study was double-blind and placebo-controlled. Ubiquinone supplementation effectively increased serum ubiquinone concentration in both age groups but did not influence maximal aerobic capacity. Consistent with previous reports, oral ubiquinone supplementation was ineffective as an ergogenic aid in both the young and older, trained men [117]. Kamikawa et al [118] noted, however, that 150 mg/day of ubiquinone supplementation for 28 days increases maximal exercise tolerance in angina pectoris patients. Karlsson and co-workers have also investigated the potential beneficial effects of ubiquinone on several physiological parameters and its relationship to other antioxidants [119—122]. They reported that 100 mg/day of ubiquinone supplementation for 6 weeks was beneficial in improving exercise capacity [122]. Swedish downhill skiers were noted to have decreased ubiquinone levels in their muscles and plasma following 3 days of skiing. A relationship with the amount of ubiquinone in muscle and exercise capacity in hypertensive and ischemic heart diseased individuals compared to age matched controls was suggested [120]. Ubiquinone supplementation may be beneficial but it may have certain limitations too. In one study it has been evident that supplementation of ubiquinone may enhance cellular damage during intense exercise [123]. Optimization of a proper ubiquinone supplementation regimen that would provide beneficial effects with minimum risk requires further research.

4.4 Glutathione

Two brief rodent studies have shown that exogenous GSH may remarkably increase endurance to physical exercise [124,125]. Compared to placebo treated controls 0.5, 0.75 and 1 g/kg intraperitoneal doses of GSH increased endurance to swimming by a marked 102.4%, 120% and 140.7%, respectively [125]. At a dose 0.25 g/kg, GSH did not affect endurance when injected once but such a dose could significantly increase endurance when injected once a day for 7 consecutive days. In another study, oral GSH at dosages 0.25 to 1 g/kg caused a dose-dependent significant improvement in swim endurance [124]. Both abovementioned studies employed brief bursts of swimming as the exercise challenge and did not report any biochemical data related to either glutathione metabolism or other indices of oxidative stress. Sen et al. [69] attempted to clarify the possible mechanism of such beneficial effect of GSH supplementation. Almost all evidence supporting the contention that a single bout of exercise may induce oxidative stress have been obtained from studies using exercise types that were long in duration, and mostly running or cycling in nature. Intraperitoneal injection of GSH solution (1 g/kg body weight) resulted in a rapid appearance of GSH in the plasma and was followed by a rapid clearance of the thiol. Following the injection excess plasma GSH was rapidly oxidized. GSH injection did not influence GSH status of other tissues studied. Following the repeated administration of GSH, blood and kidney total glutathione levels were increased. Plasma total glutathione of GSH supplemented animals was rapidly cleared during exhaustive exercise. The GSH administration protocol, as used in this study, did not influence the endurance to exhaustive physical exercise of rats. It has been shown that following a treadmill run to exhaustion levels of immunoreactive Mn-SOD (manganese superoxide dismutase, a mitochondrial protein) remarkably increases in the plasma. Glutathione supplementation (500 mg/kg body weight) marginally suppressed such release of the mitochondrial protein to the plasma [126]. The inability of exogenous GSH to provide added antioxidant protection to tissues may be largely attributed to the poor availability of exogenous administered GSH to the tissues. In another part of this study, Atalay et al. [31] tested the effect of GSH supplementation on exercise-induced leukocyte margination and neutrophil oxidative burst activity. Exercise-associated leukocyte margination was prevented by GSH supplementation. Peripheral blood neutrophil counts were significantly higher in GSH-supplemented groups compared to the placebo control groups. Also, exercise-induced increase in peripheral blood neutrophil oxidative burst activity as measured by luminol-enhanced chemiluminescence per volume of blood tended to be higher in the GSH-supplemented group, and lower in the GSH-deficient rats suggesting high plasma GSH may have augmented exercise-dependent neutrophil priming. In these experiments, for the first time it was shown that GSH supplementation can induce neutrophil mobilization and decrease exercise-induced leukocyte margination, and that exogenous and endogenous GSH can regulate exercise-induced priming of neutrophil for oxidative burst response [31].

4.5 N-acetyl-L-cysteine

Blood glutathione homeostasis has been suggested to be a determinant of resting and exercise-induced oxidative stress in young men [127]. The effect of oral N-acetyl-L-cysteine (NAC) on exercise-associated rapid blood GSH oxidation in healthy adult males who performed two identical maximal bicycle ergometer exercises 3 weeks apart has been investigated. Before the second maximal exercise test, men took effervescent NAC tablets (200 mg × 4 /day) for 2 days, and an additional 800 mg in the morning of the test. The NAC supplementation protocol used in the study 1) increased the net peroxyl radical scavenging capacity of the plasma, and 2) spared exercise-induced blood glutathione oxidation [39]. The ability of oral N-acetyl-L-cysteine to prevent exercise-induced oxidation of blood GSH has been also observed in rats [110].

Reid and associates have tested the effect of NAC on muscle fatigue [128,129]. Fiber bundles were removed from diaphragms and stimulated directly using supramaximal current intensity. Studies of unfatigued muscle showed that 10 mM NAC reduced peak twitch stress, shortened time to peak twitch stress, and shifted the stress-frequency curve down and to the right. Fiber bundles incubated in 0.1−10 mM NAC exhibited a dose-dependent decrease in relative stresses developed during 30 Hz contraction with no change in maximal tetanic (200 Hz) stress. NAC (10 mM) also inhibited acute fatigue. In a later experiment, this effect of NAC was tested in humans. Healthy volunteers were studied on two occasions each. Subjects were pretreated with NAC 150 mg/kg or 5% dextrose in water by intravenous infusion. It was evident that NAC pretreatment can improve performance of human limb muscle during fatiguing exercise, suggesting that oxidative stress plays a causal role in the fatigue process and identifying antioxidant therapy as a novel intervention that may be useful clinically [128,129].

4.6 α-Lipoic acid

The first study testing the efficacy of α-lipoate supplementation in exercise-induced oxidative stress has been just reported. Khanna et al. [130] studied the effect of intragastric lipoate supplementation (150 mg/kg body weight for 8 weeks) on lipid peroxidation and glutathione-dependent antioxidant defenses in liver, heart, kidney and skeletal muscle of male Wistar rats. Lipoate supplementation significantly increased total glutathione levels in liver and blood. This information is consistent with results from previous *in vitro* experiments [41], and shows that indeed lipoate supplementation may increase glutathione levels of certain tissues *in vivo*. Lipoate supplementation, however, did not affect the total glutathione content of organs such as the kidney, heart and skeletal muscles. Lipoate supplementation-dependent increase in hepatic glutathione pool was associated with increased resistance to lipid peroxidation. This beneficial effect against oxidative lipid damage was also observed in the heart and red gastrocnemius skeletal muscle. Lower lipid peroxide levels in certain tissues of lipoate fed rats suggest strengthening of the antioxidant defense network in these tissues [130].

4.7 Other nutrients

Other nutrients that have been ascribed to be beneficial as antioxidants such as selenium and ß-carotene have not been examined individually but have been assessed in conjunction with either vitamin E deficiency or in combination with other antioxidants. The effects of selenium supplementation (0.5 ppm diet) or deprivation have been tested in liver, muscle and blood of swim exercised rats [74]. Some rats were additionally supplemented with vitamin E (50 $\cdot d^{-1}$). Selenium supplementation increased the activity of the hydroperoxide metabolizing enzyme glutathione peroxidase in the liver. A tight regulation of tissue glutathione peroxidase activity by dietary selenium was observed because selenium-deficient diet markedly downregulated the activity of the enzyme. Muscle glutathione peroxidase activity demonstrated similar responses to selenium intervention compared to the liver. Increased tissue lipid peroxidation was evident when both selenium and vitamin E were deficient. However, selenium deficiency had little effect when vitamin E was present. Selenium appeared to have minimal effects on swim-induced lipid peroxidation in the liver or muscle. Dietary selenium supplementation in horses (0.15 ppm daily for 4 weeks) had minimal effects on exercise-induced lipid peroxidation as indicated by blood level of lipid peroxidation byproducts [131]. In a double blind human study no effect of selenium supplementation on human physical performance was observed [132]. Selenium poisoning is rare in the US, but the case of a man who was poisoned by selenium containing vitamin tablets has been described [133]. Strenuous physical exercise has been shown to decrease β-carotene levels in the serum. In a study of 574 women and 57 men from a rural city in Japan it was noted that the serum β-carotene lowering effect of exercise was independent of dietary factors, smoking and cholesterol intake as indicated by 3-day food records [134].

4.8 Antioxidant interaction

From the biochemistry of antioxidant action it is evident that antioxidants function in a network (see Chapter 10 by Sen and Powers in this volume, 219–242) and interaction between several major antioxidants have been clearly evident [1]. As a result, some studies have attempted to investigate the efficacy of a combination of several antioxidants as supplements [135–137]. Supplementation of individuals with a vitamin mixture containing 37.5 mg ß-carotene, 1250 mg vitamin C and 1000 IU of vitamin E for 5 weeks decreased the level of lipid peroxidation byproducts in the serum and breath, both at rest and following exercise at both 60 and 90% VO_2 max [136]. In contrast, a previous study which used a similar mixture of antioxidants and exercised the subjects at 65% of maximal heart rate in a downhill run was unable to demonstrate any positive effects [135]. This inconsistency in observation was explained by differences in the nature and intensity of the exercise in the two studies. The effects of an antioxidant mixture (10 mg ß-carotene, 1000 mg vitamin C and 800 IU of vitamin E) on human blood glutathione system and muscle damage has been determined [137]. A protective effect on the blood glutathione system and muscle damage was evident. A randomized and placebo-controlled study has been carried out on 24 trained long-distance runners who were supplemented with α-tocopherol (400 IU /day) and ascorbic acid (200 mg /day) for 4.5 weeks before a marathon race. Serum content of ascorbic acid as well as α-tocopherol were elevated in supplemented individuals. In this study, the antioxidant supplementation protocol was observed to significantly protect against exercise-induced muscle damage as manifested by the loss of creatine kinase from the muscle to the serum [138].

5   PERSPECTIVES

Several lines of evidence consistently show that physical exercise may induce oxidative stress. The relationship between physical activity, physical fitness and total radical trapping antioxidant potential was examined in the Northern Ireland Health and Activity Survey. This was a large cross-sectional population study (n = 1600) using a two-stage probability sample of the population. A necessity for antioxidant supplementation, especially in physically active and fit individuals, was indicated [139]. Depending on nutritional habits and genetic disposition susceptibility to oxidative stress may vary from person to person. Determination of tissue antioxidant status of individuals is thus recommended. Such information will be necessary to identify specific necessities and formulate effective strategies for antioxidant therapy. Nutritional antioxidant supplements are known to be bio-available to tissues and may strengthen defense systems against the ravages of reactive species. Results from antioxidant supplementation studies considerably vary depending on the study design and measures of outcome. Physical performance is regulated by multifactorial processes and may not serve as a good indicator to test the effect of antioxidant supplementation. The general trend of results shows no effect of antioxidant supplementation on physical performance. However, in a large number of studies it has been consistently evident that antioxidant supplementation protects against exercise-induced tissue damage. Diet of laboratory animals are often heavily enriched with antioxidant vitamins, particularly vitamin E. This may be one reason why antioxidant supplementation to animals fed a regular diet does not influence several measures of outcome. At present there is a growing trend among people to cut down the amount of fat in their diets. While this does markedly decrease caloric intake, in many cases this may also contribute to a marked decrease in the intake of fat-soluble essential nutrients including antioxidant vitamins. From available information we know that under regular circumstances antioxidants such as α-tocopherol, ascorbic acid and β-carotene are well tolerated and free from toxicity even when consumed at doses several-fold higher than the recommended dietary allowances [140]. In view of this and the potential of antioxidant therapy, consumption of a diet rich in a mixture of different antioxidants may be expected to be a prudent course.

6   SUMMARY

1. The chemical nature of any antioxidant determines its solubility, and thus its localization in biological tissues. For example, lipid soluble antioxidants are localized in membranes and function to protect against oxidative damage of membranes. Water-soluble antioxidants, located for example in the cytosol, mitochondrial matrix or extracellular fluids, may not have access to ROS generated in membranes.
2. Studies with antioxidant deficient animals show that such deficiency may enhance exercise-induced tissue damage and may compromise work performance.
3. Results from antioxidant supplementation studies considerably vary depending on the study design and measures of outcome. Physical performance is regulated by multifactorial processes and may not serve as a good indicator to test the effect of antioxidant supplementation. The general trend of results shows no effect of antioxidant supplementation on physical performance.

However, in a large number of studies it has been consistently evident that antioxidant supplementation protects against exercise-induced tissue damage.

4. While further studies are needed to establish which antioxidant supplement regimen is appropriate for the physically active individual, consumption of a diet rich in a mixture of different natural antioxidants may be expected to be a prudent course.

7   ABBREVIATIONS

BSO: L-buthionine-sulfoximine
DHLA: dihydrolipoate
GSH: reduced glutathione
GSSG: glutathione disulfide
IU: international unit
NAC: N-acetyl-L-cysteine
ppm: parts per million
RDA: recommended daily allowances
SOD: superoxide dismutase

8   REFERENCES

1. Sen CK. J Appl Physiol 1995;79,675—686.
2. Engelhardt JF. Antiox Redox Signal 1999;1:5—27.
3. Sheppard AJ, Pennington, JAT and Weihrauch, JL. In: Packer L, Fuchs J (eds) Vitamin E in Health and Disease. New York: Marcel Dekker, 1993;9—31.
4. Burton GW, Joyce A, Ingold KU. Archives of Biochemistry and Biophysics 1983;221:281—290.
5. Traber MG, Sies H. Annu Rev Nutr 1996;16:321—347.
6. Handelman GJ. In: Cadenas E, Packer L (eds) Handbook of Antioxidants. New York: Marcel Dekker, 1996;259—314.
7. Handelman GJ, van Kuijk FJ, Chatterjee A, Krinsky NI. Free Radic Biol Med 1991;10: 427—437.
8. Burton GW, Ingold KU. Science 1984;224:569—573.
9. Andersen HR, Andersen O. Pharmacol Toxicol 1993;73:192—201.
10. Kagan V, Nohl H, Quinn PJ. In: Cadenas C, Packer, L (eds) Handbook of Antioxidants. New York: Marcel Dekker, 1996.
11. Laaksonen R, Riihimaki A, Laitita J, Martensson K, Tikkanen MJ, Himberg JJ. Journal of Laboratory and Clinical Medicine 1995;125:517—521.
12. Aust SD, Morehouse LA and Thomas CE. Free Radic Biol Med 1985;1:3—25.
13. Buettner GR. Free Radic Res Commun 1986;1:349—353.
14. Meister A. Methods Enzymol 1995;251:3—7.
15. Meister A. Biochem Pharmacol 1992;44:1905—1915.
16. Meister A. J Nutr Sci Vitaminol. Tokyo 1992;Spec No:1—6.
17. Sen CK, Hanninen O In: Sen CK, Packer L, Hanninen O (eds) Exercise and oxygen toxicity. Amsterdam: Elsevier Science Publishers BV, 1994:89—126.
18. Thomas JP, Maiorino M, Ursini F, Girotti AW. J Biol Chem 1990;265:454—461.
19. Hayes JD, Pulford DJ. Crit Rev Biochem Mol Biol 1995;30:445—600.
20. DeLeve LD, Kaplowitz N. Semin Liver Dis 1990;10:251—266.
21. Meister A. Pharmacol Ther 1991;51:155—194.

22. Vina J, Perez C, Furukawa T, Palacin M, Vina JR. Br J Nutr 1989;62:683—691.
23. Martensson J, Jain A, Meister A. Proc Natl Acad Sci USA 1990;87:1715—1719.
24. Hagen TM, Wierzbicka GT, Bowman BB, Aw TY, Jones DP. Am J Physiol 1990;259:G530—535.
25. Aw TY, Wierzbicka G, Jones DP. Chem Biol Interact 1991;80:89—97.
26. Packer L, Witt EH, Tritschler HJ. Free Radic Biol Med 1995;19:227—250.
27. Sen CK, Roy S, Packer L In: Montagnier L, Olivier R, Pasquier C (eds) Oxidative Stress Cancer, AIDS and Neurodegenerative Diseases. New York: Marcel Dekker Inc, 1997;251—267.
28. Sen CK, Roy S, Han D, Packer L. Free Radical Biology and Medicine 1997;22:1241—1257.
29. Akerlund B, Jarstrand C, Lindeke B, Sonnerborg A, Akerblad AC, Rasool O. Eur J Clin Pharmacol 1996;50:457—461.
30. Aruoma OI, Halliwell B, Hoey BM, Butler J. Free Radic Biol Med 1989;6:59359—59357.
31. Atalay M, Marnila P, Lilius EM, Hanninen O, Sen CK. Eur J Appl Physiol 1996;74:342—347.
32. Borgstrom L, Kagedal B, Paulsen O. Eur J Clin Pharmacol 1986;31:217—222.
33. Ferrari G, Yan CY, Greene LA. J Neurosci 1995;15:2857—2866.
34. Holdiness MR. Clinical Pharmacokinetics 1991;20:123—134.
35. Huupponen MR, Makinen LH, Hyvonen PM, Sen CK, Rankinen T, Vaisanen S, Rauramaa R. Int J Sports Med 1995;16:399—403.
36. Issels RD, Nagele A, Eckert KG, Wilmanns W. Biochem Pharmacol 1988;37:881—888.
37. Packer L, Roy S, Sen CK. Adv Pharmacol 1997;38:79—101.
38. va Zandwijk N. J Cell Biochem Suppl 1995;22:24—32.
39. Sen CK, Rankinen T, Vaisanen S, Rauramaa R. J Appl Physiol 1994;76:2570—2577.
40. Sjodin K, Nilsson E, Hallberg A, Tunek A. Biochem Pharmacol 1989;38:3981—3985.
41. Sen CK. J Nutr Biochem 1997;8:660—672.
42. Fujiwara K, Okamura-Ikeda K, Motokawa Y. FEBS Letters 1991;293:115—118.
43. Bustamante J, Lodge JK, Marcocci L, Tritschler HJ, Packer L, Rihn BH. Free Radic Biol Med 1998;24:1023—1039.
44. Khanna S, Atalay M, Lodge JK, Laaksonen DE, Roy S, Hanninen O, Packer L, Sen CK. Biochem Mol Biol Int 1998;46:297—306.
45. Handelman GJ, Han D, Tritschler H, Packer L. Biochem Pharmacol 1994;47:1725—1730.
46. Watanabe H, Bannai S. J Exp Med 1987;165:628—640.
47. Han D, Handelman G, Marcocci L, Sen CK, Roy S, Kobuchi H, Flohe L, Packer, L. Biofactors 1997;6:321—338.
48. Khanna S, Roy S, Packer L, Sen CK. Am J Physiol 1999;276:R1327—R1333.
49. Sen CK, Tirosh O, Roy S, Kobayashi MS, Packer L. Biochem Biophys Res Commun 1998;247: 223—228.
50. Schwarz K, Foltz CM. Journal of American Chemical Society 1957;79:3292—3293.
51. Board on Agriculture, CoAN National Research Council, National Academy of Sciences, Washington DC 1983.
52. Rotruck JT, Pope AL, Ganther HE, Swanson AB, Hafeman DG, Hoekstra WG. Science 1973; 179:588—590.
53. Burk RF, Lawrence RA, Lane JM. J Clin Invest 1980;65:1024—1031.
54. Safety IPoC. In: Environmental Health Criteria, vol 58. Geneva: World Health Organization, 1987.
55. Amelink GJ, van der Wal WA, Wokke JH, van Asbeck BS, Bar PR. Pflugers Arch 1991;419: 304—309.
56. Dillard CJ, Litov RE, Savin WM, Dumelin EE, Tappel AL. J Appl Physiol 1978;45:927—932.
57. Gohil K, Packer L, de Lumen B, Brooks GA, Terblanche SE. J Appl Physiol 1986;60: 1986—1991.
58. Jackson MJ. Proc Nutr Soc 1987;46:77—80.
59. Quintanilha AT, Packer L, Davies JM, Racanelli TL, Davies KJ. Ann N Y Acad Sci 1982;393: 32—47.
60. Quintanilha AT, Packer L. Ciba Found Symp 1983;101:56—69.

61. Salminen A, Kainulainen H, Arstila AU, Vihko V. Acta Physiol Scand 1984;122:565—70.
62. Davies KJ, Quintanilha AT Brooks GA, Packer L. Biochem Biophys Res Commun 1982;107: 1198—1205.
63. Gohil K, Henderson S, Terblanche SE, Brooks GA, Packer L. Biosci Rep 1984;4:987—993.
64. Dillard CJ, Dumelin EE, Tappel AL. Lipids 1977;12:109—114.
65. Tiidus PM, Behrens WA, Madere R, Kim JJ, Houston ME. Nutritional Research 1993;13: 219—224.
66. Bar PR, Amelink GJ. Biochem Soc Trans 1997;25:50—54.
67. Packer L, Gohil K, deLumen B, Terblanche SE. Comp Biochem Physiol (B) 1986;83:235—240.
68. Ji LL, Stratman FW, Lardy HA. Arch Biochem Biophys 1988;263:150—160.
69. Sen CK, Atalay M, Hanninen O. J Appl Physiol 1994;77:2177—2187.
70. Sen CK, Rahkila P, Hanninen O. Acta Physiol Scand 1993;148:21—26.
71. Leeuwenburgh C, Ji LL. Arch Biochem Biophys 1995;316:941—949.
72. Venditti P, Di Meo S. Arch Biochem Biophys 1996;331:63—68.
73. Dekkers JC, van Doornen LJ, Kemper HC. Sports Med 1996;21:213—238.
74. Brady PS, Brady LJ, Ullrey DE. J Nutr 1979;109:1103—1109.
75. Goldfarb AH, McIntosh MK, Boyer BT, Fatouros J. J Appl Physiol 1994;76:1630—1635.
76. Jackson MJ, Jones DA, Edwards RHT. In: Porter R, Wheelan J (eds) Biology of Vitamin E. Proceedings of a Ciba Foundation Symposium: London: Pitman Medical Ltd 1983;224—239.
77. Kumar CT, Reddy VK, Prasad M, Thyagaraju K, Reddanna P. Mol Cell Biochem 1992;111: 109—115.
78. Goldfarb AH, McIntosh MK, Boyer BT. Med Sci Sports Exe 1993; 25:S129.
79. Goldfarb AH, McIntosh MK, Boyer BT. J Appl Physiol 1996;80:486—490.
80. McIntosh MK, Goldfarb AH, Cote PS, Griffin K. Nutr Biochem 1993;4:298—303.
81. McIntosh MK, Goldfarb AH, Curtis LN, Cote PS. J Nutr 1993;123:216—224.
82. Novelli GP, Braccitiotti G, Falsini S. Free Radical Biology and Medicine 1990;8:9—13.
83. Warren JA, Jenkins RR, Packer L, Witt EH, Armstrong RB. J Appl Physiol 1992;72:2168—2175.
84. Reznick AZ, Witt E, Matsumoto M, Packer L. Biochem Biophys Res Commun 1992;189: 801—806.
85. Hiramatsu M, Edamatsu R, Velasco RD, Ooba S, Kanakura K, Mori A. Neurochem Res 1993; 18:313—316.
86. Kromhout D, Bosschieter EB, de Lezenne Coulander C. N Engl J Med 1985;312:1205—1209.
87. Schmidt EB, Dyerberg J. Drugs 1994;47:405—424.
88. Ascherio A, Rimm EB, Stampfer MJ, Giovannucci EL, Willett WC. N Engl J Med 1995;332: 977—982.
89. Demoz A, Willumsen N, Berge RK. Lipids 1992;27:968—971.
90. Demoz A, Asiedu DK, Lie O, Berge RK. Biochim Biophys Acta 1994;1199:238—244.
91. Hu ML, Frankel EN, Leibovitz BE, Tappel AL. J Nutr 1989;119:1574—1582.
92. Leibovitz BE, Hu ML, Tappel AL. Lipids 1990;25:125—129.
93. Nalbone G, Leonardi J, Termine E, Portugal H, Lechene P, Pauli AM, Lafont H. Lipids 1989;24: 179—186.
94. Aarsland A, Lundquist M, Borretsen B, Berge RK. Lipids 1990;25:546—548.
95. Chance B, Sies H, Boveris A. Physiol Rev 1979;59:527—605.
96. Paffenbarger RS Jr. Hyde RT, Wing AL, Steinmetz CH. JAMA 1984;252:491—495.
97. Sen CK, Atalay M, Agren J, Laaksonen DE, Roy S, Hanninen O. App Physiol 1997;83:189—195.
98. Lawrence JD, Bower RC, Riehl WP, Smith JL. Am J Clin Nutr 1975;28:205—208.
99. Goldfarb AH, Todd MK, Boyer BT, Alessio HM, Cutler RG. Medicine and Science in Sports and Exercise 1989;21:S16.
100. Sharman IM, Down MG, Norgan NG. J Sports Med Phys Fitness 1976;16:215—225.
101. Sumida S, Tanaka K, Kitao H, Nakadomo F. Int J Biochem 1989;21:835—838.
102. Watt T, Romet TT, McFarlane I, McGuey D, Allen C, Goode RC. Lancet 1974;2:354—355.

103. Meydani M et al. Am J Physiol 1993;264:R992—998.
104. Rokitzki L, Logemann E, Huber G, Keck E, Keul J. Int J Sport Nutr 1994;4:253—264.
105. Oostenbrug GS, Mensink RP, Hardeman MR, De Vries T, Brouns F, Hornstra G. J Appl Physiol 1997;83:746—752.
106. Packer L, Reznick AZ. In: Fuchs J, Packer L (eds) Vitamin E in Health and Disease. New York: Marcel Dekker 1992;465—471.
107. Bendich A, Machlin LJ. Am J Clin Nutr 1988;48:612—619.
108. Corrigan JJ Jr. Am J Pediatr Hematol Oncol 1979;1:169—173.
109. Koz M, Erbas D, Bilgihan A, Aricioglu A. Can J Physiol Pharmacol 1992;70:1392—1395.
110. Sastre J, Asensi M, Gasco E, Pallardo FV, Ferrero JA, Furukawa T, Vina J. Am J Physiol 1992;263:R992—995.
111. Alessio HM, Goldfarb AH, Cao G, Cutler RG. Medicine and Science in Sports and Exercise 1993;25:S79.
112. Kaminski M, Boal R. Pain 1992;50:317—321.
113. Jakeman P, Maxwell S. Eur J Appl Physiol 1993;67:426—430.
114. Shimomura Y, Suzuki M, Sugiyama S, Hanaki Y, Ozawa T. Biochem Biophys Res Commun 1991;176:349—355.
115. Snider IP, Bazzarre TL, Murdoch SD, Goldfarb A. Int J Sport Nutr 1992;2:272—286.
116. Zuliani U, Bonetti A, Campana M, Cerioli G, Solito F, Novarini A. J Sports Med Phys Fitness 1989;29:57—62.
117. Laaksonen R, Fogelholm M, Himberg JJ, Laakso J, Salorinne Y. Eur J Appl Physiol 1995;72: 95—100.
118. Kamikawa T, Kobayashi A, Yamashita T, Hayashi H, Yamazaki N. Am J Cardiol 1985;56: 247—251.
119. Karlsson J. World Rev Nutr Diet 1997;82:81—100.
120. Karlsson J, Lin L, Sylven C, Jansson E. Mol Cell Biochem 1996;156:169—172.
121. Karlsson J, Diamant B, Folkers K. Respiration 1992;59:18—23.
122. Karlsson J, Diamant B, Folkers, K, Lund B. Ann Med 1991;23:339—344.
123. Malm C, Svensson M, Sjoberg B, Ekblom B, Sjodin B. Acta Physiol Scand 1996;157:511—512.
124. Cazzulani P, Cassin M, Ceserani R. Medical Science Research 1991;19:543—544.
125. Novelli GP, Falsini S, Bracciotti G. Pharmacological Research 1991;23:149—156.
126. Sen CK, Ookawara T, Suzuki K, Taniguchi N, Hanninen O, Ohno H. Pathophysiology 1994;1: 165—168.
127. Laaksonen DE, Atalay M, Niskanen L, Uusitupa M, Hanninen O, Sen CK. Redox Report 1999;4:(In press).
128. Reid MB, Stokic DS, Koch SM, Khawli FA, Leis AA. J Clin Invest 1994;94:2468—2474.
129. Khawli FA, Reid MB. Journal of Applied Physiology 1994;77:317—324.
130. Khanna S, Atalay M, Laaksonen DE, Gul M, Roy S, Sen CK. J. Appl. Physiol. 1999;86:1191—1196.
131. Brady PS, Ku PK, Ullrey DE. J Anim Sci 1978;47:492—496.
132. Tessier F, Margaritis I, Richard MJ, Moynot C, Marconnet P. Med Sci Sports Exerc 1995;27: 390—396.
133. Clark RF, Strukle E, Williams SR, Manoguerra AS. JAMA 1996;275:1087—1088.
134. Takatsuka N, Kawakami N, Ohwaki A, Ito Y, Matsushita Y, Ido M, Shimizu H. Tohoku J Exp Med 1995;176:131—135.
135. Kanter MM, Eddy DE. Medicine and Science in Sports and Exercise 1992;24:S17.
136. Kanter MM, Nolte LA, Holloszy JO. J Appl Physiol 1993;74:965—969.
137. Viguie CA, Packer L, Brooks GA. Medicine and Science in Sports and Exercise 1989;21:S16.
138. Rokitzki L, Logemann E, Sagredos AN, Murphy M, Wetzel-Roth W, Keul J. Acta Physiol Scand 1994;151:149—158.
139. Sharpe PC et al. Qjm 1996;89:223—228.
140. Garewal HS, Diplock AT. Drug Saf 1995;13:8—14.

Part V

Nutrition

©2000 Elsevier Science B.V. All rights reserved.
Handbook of Oxidants and Antioxidants in Exercise.
C.K. Sen, L. Packer and O. Hänninen, editors.

Part V • Chapter 13

Dietary sources and bioavailability of essential and nonessential antioxidants

Eric A. Decker[1] and Priscilla M. Clarkson[2]

[1]*Department of Food Science, Chenoweth Lab, University of Massachusetts, Amherst, MA 01003, USA.
Tel.: +1-413-545-1026 2. Fax: +1-413-545-1262. E-mail: edecker@foodsci.umass.edu*
[2]*Department of Exercise Science, Totman Building, University of Massachusetts, Amherst, MA 01003,
USA. Tel.: +1-413-545-6069. Fax: +1-413-545-2906. E-mail: clarkson@excsci.umass.edu*

1   INTRODUCTION
2   ESSENTIAL ANTIOXIDANTS
     2.1   Vitamin E
            2.1.1 Sources
            2.1.2 Absorption
            2.1.3 Transport
            2.1.4 Storage
            2.1.5 Interactions with other nutrients
     2.2 Carotenoids
            2.2.1 Sources
            2.2.2 Absorption
            2.2.3 β Carotene *trans* and *cis* isomers
            2.2.4 Transport and storage
            2.2.5 Factors that influence carotenoid status
     2.3 Vitamin C
            2.3.1 Sources
            2.3.2 Absorption
            2.3.3 Transport and storage
            2.3.4 Interactions with other nutrients
3   NONESSENTIAL ANTIOXIDANTS
     3.1 Synthetic and plant phenolics
            3.1.1 Sources
            3.1.2 Absorption, storage and transport
            3.1.3 Interaction with other nutrients
     3.2 Pyrroloquinoline quinone
     3.3 Ubiquinone (coenzyme Q)
     3.4 Conjugated linoleic acid
     3.5 Histidine-containing dipeptides
            3.5.1 Absorption, transport and storage
     3.6 Polyamines, nucleotides and related compounds
     3.7 Thiols
     3.8 Phytic acid
4   ANTIOXIDANTS FROM FOOD SOURCES VS. DIETARY SUPPLEMENTS
5   SUMMARY
6   PERSPECTIVES
7   ABBREVIATIONS
8   REFERENCES

1   INTRODUCTION

Dietary antioxidants have been associated with the modulation of numerous bio-chemical and physiological functions, as well as with a decreased risk of diseases such as atherosclerosis and cancer. Due to their role in health, there is wide-spread interest in antioxidant composition of foods and how the body derives antioxidants from food. Dietary antioxidants can be classified as those which are essential to health (vitamins A, C and E and other compounds which may be converted into the antioxidant vitamins *in vivo*) and others, which while not essential, may be beneficial to health.

The nonessential antioxidants consist of a vast array of compounds which inhibit oxidative reactions by a variety of mechanisms. These nonessential antioxidants are found in both plant- and animal-based foods and are often consumed in quantities far exceeding the essential antioxidants. However, nonessential antioxidants are less likely to be stored in the body and, therefore, may only increase the oxidative stability of tissues for a short period of time. This chapter will review sources, stability, bioavailability, transport, storage and interaction with other nutrients of both essential and nonessential antioxidants which are common components of the diet.

2   ESSENTIAL ANTIOXIDANTS

2.1 Vitamin E

Tocopherols and Tocotrienols are two groups of compounds with vitamin E biological activity, whose basic structure is a hydroxylated ring system (chromanol ring) and isoprenoid side chain. The four members of each group, α (Fig. 1), β, γ, and δ, differ in the number and position of the methyl groups on the chromanol ring. The difference in structure between the tocopherols and the tocotrienols is that the tocotrienols have an unsaturated side chain. Compared with α-tocopherol, β-tocopherol is only 25–50% as active, γ-tocopherol is only 10–35% as active, and α-tocotrienol is only 30% as active [1].

There are eight possible stereoisomers from each tocopherol [2]. The RRR isomer (D-α-tocopherol) is most abundant in nature and the most biologically active. However, when vitamin E is synthesized, an equal mixture of the eight stereoisomers is obtained and this mixture is called all-racemic α-tocopherol (all-rac α-tocopherol). Nomenclature can be confusing, but it is generally accepted that the natural form is designated as D-RRR-α-tocopherol and the synthetic forms as DL-all rac α-tocopherol [3]. Also, for stability, synthetic forms are often an ester of α-tocopherol with acetate or succinate, available both as D and DL [3]. α-tocopherol esters are more resistance to oxidation than α-tocopherol [4]. Biopotency of these esterified forms is computed from their α-tocopherol content [3].

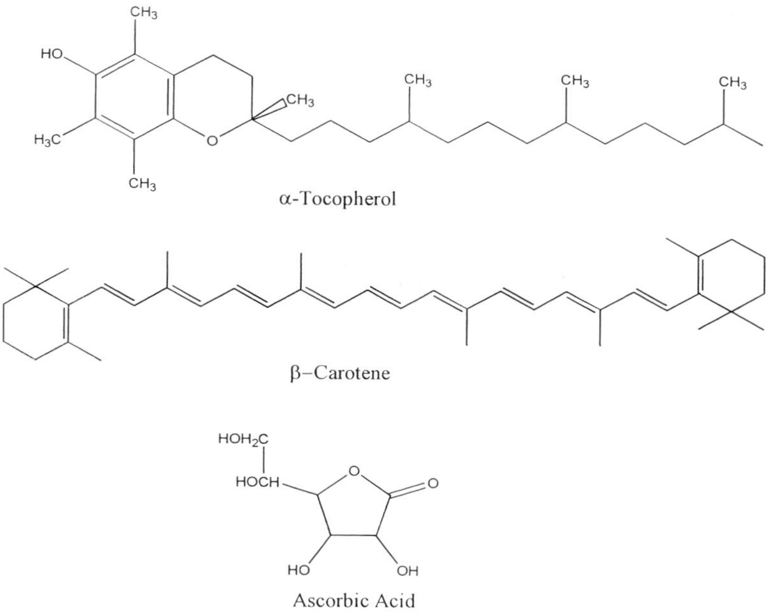

α-Tocopherol

β–Carotene

Ascorbic Acid

Fig. 1. Structures of the antioxidant vitamins.

2.1.1 *Sources*

Tocopherols are found mostly in plant oils because only plants can synthesize tocopherols. There are only moderate amounts in meat and dairy products [5]. Soybean, corn, safflower, and cottonseed oils are rich in tocopherols and grains contain some vitamin E activity (Table 1). Leaves and other green chloroplast parts of plants contain mostly α-tocopherol while nongreen parts contain β, γ, and δ-tocopherols [6]. Tocotrienols are found in bran and germ parts of some plants; wheat germ oil and palm oil contains a significant source of tocotrienols [6]. Soybean oil contains a significant amount of γ-and δ-tocopherols.

The content of tocopherols in food varies widely because it can be altered by processing, storage and preparation [1]. Due to tocopherols being antioxidants, they are destroyed by oxidizing conditions such as air and light exposures, heat, and the presence of copper [5]. However, canned and frozen vegetables maintain levels of vitamin E fairly well [7].

A recent epidemiological study of a large Finnish population showed that α-tocopherol accounted for about 85% of the total dietary vitamin E intake [8]. The intakes of the various tocopherols and tocotrienols were derived from consumption cereal products and/or margarines and oils. Cereals were the main food source of α-tocotrienol, β-tocopherol, and β-tocotrienol. γ-tocopherol and small amounts of δ-tocopherol and δ-tocotrienol were mainly derived from margarine.

Table 1. Vitamin E content of food (expressed as α-tocopherol equivalents) [6,7].

Food	mg/100 g
Oil	
Wheat germ	156.9
Corn	15—20
Peanut	15—20
Safflower	25—40
Soybean	10—17
Sunflower	49—50
Olive	5
Cod liver	20
Butter	2
Low fat spread	6
Animal fat	trace
Cheeses and milk	< 1
Peanuts	7—10
Vegetables	0.1—1
Fruits	0.1—0.3
Meat/fish	0.2—0.6
Pasta/rice	< 1
Breads	trace
Cereals	
All-bran	2
Corn flakes	0.4
Rice krispies	0.6
Shredded wheat	1
Pizza	1

2.1.2 Absorption

Once ingested, vitamin E is absorbed in the small intestine similar to dietary fat [2]. Tocopherol is found free in foods, but tocotrienols and synthetic forms of α-tocopherol (acetate and succinate) are esterified so they must be hydrolyzed [6]. Bile salts secreted from the liver and lipases secreted from the pancreas solubilize α-tocopherol so it can traverse the intestinal lumen by passive diffusion [2]. Vitamin E supplements given to cystic fibrosis patients with exocrine pancreatic insufficiency are not well absorbed, and the mean α-tocopherol levels in their blood are low [9]. Therefore, these patients are given vitamin E supplements along with appropriate amount of pancreatic enzymes [10]. Also patients with liver disease show evidence of impaired absorption of vitamin E [2].

Little is known about absorption efficiency, but in rats it appears to be about 40—65% and in humans about 21—86% [5]. The large variability could be attributed to different experimental approaches, especially in humans. Also, many factors can affect the absorption of vitamin E. When oral RRR-α-tocopherol was administered to healthy humans, the extent of absorption varied considerably among subjects [11]. Munro et al. [12] examined plasma kinetics of α-tocopherol after oral ingestion of deuterium-labeled α-tocopherol and found that both the free phenol and the acetate ester concentrations were lower in smokers compared with non-smokers. Smokers demonstrated preferential uptake of the phenol form. Thus, smoking either reduced the ability to absorb α-tocopherol, particularly the acetate ester, or it increased the clearance of the newly absorbed tocopherol. Ingestion of graded levels of RRR-γ-tocopherol along with constant levels of RRR-α-tocopherol in rats resulted in an increase in α-tocopherol concentrations in the blood and in many tissue including skeletal muscle, heart and liver compared to rats fed a control diet containing RRR-α-tocopherol alone [13]. Furthermore, as vitamin E intake increases, the absorption decreases such that for pharmacological doses of 200 mg the absorption rate may be less than 10% [6].

Information on the absorption of vitamin E from foods is lacking [5]. Brink et al. [14] examined the effect of a low-fat diet in rats on the absorption of vitamin E. Different concentrations of vitamin E were incorporated into a low-fat meal for 3 weeks. The magnitude of vitamin E absorption was not significantly different from that of meals containing high amounts of fat. These data suggest that low-fat diets will not have an impact on the absorption of vitamin E supplements.

β- and δ-tocopherols are poorly absorbed compared with α-and γ-tocopherol which are initially absorbed in a similar manner. However, γ-tocopherol is preferentially excreted in the bile which lowers its concentration in the blood [5]. Ikeda et al. [15] reported that there was a preferential absorption of α-tocotrienol compared to the other tocotrienols and α-tocopherol. The absorption of γ- and δ-tocotrienols and α-tocopherol were similar. This study examined the concentration of tocotrienols and tocopherols in the lymph of rats after administration of a test emulsion containing a mixture of tocopherols and tocotrienols.

Studies of both rodents and humans have found that the bioavailability of dietary α-tocopherol and the synthetic tocopheryl esters are similar [4,11,16]. However, not all studies found this [3]. Kiyose et al. [17] examined biodiscrimination of natural and synthetic forms of α-tocopherol acetate after oral administration in healthy adult women. Subjects either ingested a daily dose of 100 mg RRR-α-tocopherol, 100 mg all-rac-α-tocopheryl acetate, or 300 mg all-rac-α-tocopheryl acetate for 28 days. The bioavailability of the RRR-α-tocopherol was greater than that of either of the acetate forms when α-tocopherol stereoisomer concentrations were examined in serum and lipoproteins. The increase in concentration of RRR- or all-rac-α-tocopherol in serum was similar for the 100 mg RRR-α-tocopherol and the 300 mg all-rac-α-tocopheryl acetate. The authors suggested that the tocopherol-binding protein in the liver cytosol could discriminate between the two isomers, preferentially incorporating the RRR isomers into very low-density lipoproteins (VLDL).

2.1.3 Transport

Once absorbed into the intestine wall, vitamin E is incorporated into chylomicrons and transported into the lymph [2]. The enzyme lipoprotein lipase in the circulation hydrolyzes the triglyceride content of chylomicrons and the remnants containing mostly α- and γ-tocopherol are taken-up by the liver [5]. Some vitamin E may also be taken up by tissues or incorporated into high-density lipoproteins (HDL) [2].

Vitamin E, preferentially the RRR stereoisomer of α-tocopherol, in the liver is incorporated into very low-density lipoproteins (VLDL) [2,18]. Papas [3] reported that subjects given either RRR α-tocopheryl acetate or all rac α-tocopherol acetate, had greater plasma levels of the RRR form. The RRR-α-tocopherol was found to be preferentially secreted in VLDL in the liver and was the predominant form in HDL and low-density lipoproteins (LDL) [3]. Thus, the liver is the source for biodiscrimination of tocopherol stereoisomers and not during absorption in the small intestine [19,20]. The liver cells contain a tocopherol transport protein that discriminates between the isomers and transfers the RRR stereoisomer into the VLDL [2,21,22]. This transport protein carries the RRR form in the remnants of the chylomicrons to the endoplasmic reticulum or Golgi where they are packaged into VLDL. A condition called familial vitamin E deficiency that causes ataxia and peripheral neuropathy, has recently been associated with a genetic defect in the production of this protein [21−23]. However, this transport protein is specific for α-tocopherol, other stereoisomers of α-tocopherol and γ-tocopherol are not found to a significant extent in VLDLs [2].

The lipolysis of VLDLs in the circulation results in α-tocopherol transfer to HDLs and LDLs [5]. With the action of lipoprotein lipase, the lipolysis of VLDLs can transfer tocopherol to tissues [2]. Also the binding of LDLs to tissues may allow the transfer of tocopherol [2]. Transfer proteins have been identified whose function is to catalyze the exchange between different lipoproteins [24].

2.1.4 Storage

The RRR-α-tocopherol form is found in most tissues due to biodiscrimination by the liver for this form to distribute to the lipoproteins [4]. α-Tocopherol is mostly stored in adipose tissue, where accumulation and release occur slowly [2,5]. The liver serves as a rapid turnover store of vitamin E, but never accumulates large amounts [2]. When doses of varying concentrations of D-α-tocopherol were administered to sheep, after 7 days, the highest tocopherol concentrations were found in the pancreas and adrenal glands, lowest in neck muscle and intermediate amounts in the kidneys [25]. Most tissues store some vitamin E in their membranes including the plasma, mitochondrial, and microsomal membranes [5,6]. The orientation of vitamin E in the membrane occurs with the chromanol group toward the surface of the membrane near the phosphate region of phospholipids, and the phytyl region located within the hydrocarbon area [6]. The phytyl side chain may function in placing tocopherol at an optimal position in the membrane for scavenging free radicals [26].

When there is insufficient vitamin E in the diet, vitamin E will be released rapidly from liver and is also released from heart and skeletal muscle [6]. For example, inhalation exposure to ozone increases pulmonary α-tocopherol content which is thought to represent a mobilization of α-tocopherol from other tissue stores to the lung [4]. Also, exposure of rats to chemical oxidative stress resulted in a depletion of liver α-tocopherol which was thought to be due to mobilization of α-tocopherol out of the liver tissues to other tissues [4]. In preliminary studies, physical exercise that produced an oxidative stress also resulted in mobilization of tocopherol [27].

Transport of vitamin E in tissues is likely to occur with the help of specific tocopherol binding proteins, as is the case of the liver [5]. Several binding proteins have been identified and are probably involved in intracellular transport and metabolism [5,28]. Knowledge of how tocopherols are transported into tissue may help improve delivery of supplements. For example, Bonina et al. [29] have shown that a monocarboxylate transport protein and a glucose transport protein were involved in the uptake of tocopherol succinate and a newly synthesized tocopherol ester (tocopherol succinate-3-glucose), respectively, into erythrocyte membranes. These tocopherol derivatives showed greater intracellular accumulation than tocopherol alone.

2.1.5 *Interactions with other nutrients*

Large doses of vitamin E may inhibit β carotene absorption or its conversion to retinol in the intestine [6]. However, cleavage of β carotene into retinal requires the use of vitamin E [6]. Also, very high-dietary levels of vitamin A can depress vitamin E utilization [30]. There appears to be an optimal intake and balance needed of these two vitamins. Also, high vitamin E intake can interfere with vitamin K absorption and affect blood clotting [2].

Several dietary compounds can affect vitamin E. Sesamin, a compound derived from sesame oil, was found to increase the bioavailability of γ-tocopherol in rats, fed diets that were adequate in α-tocopherol but high in γ-tocopherol [31]. Stimulated lipid peroxidation was examined in the bovine retina after treatment with various flavonoids and vitamin E [32]. When vitamin E and epigallocatechin or quercetin were combined, the antioxidant effects were enhanced. In another study [33], rats were fed for 6 weeks a diet containing oxidized frying oil (OFO), or a controlled diet (stripped of vitamin E) and then they received all-rac-α-tocopheryl acetate supplements. The rats ingesting the OFO diet had significantly higher amounts of tissue peroxidation products and lower levels of α-tocopherol in most tissues compared with rats ingesting the control diet. After supplementation with normal amounts (50 mg/kg diet) of all rac-α-tocopherol, those on the OFO diet still had lower levels of α-tocopherol in tissues. However, supplementation with high amounts (500 mg/kg diet) produced similar tissue levels as the normal vitamin E supplemented controlled diet. Thus, OFO diets may affect the absorption and/or catabolism or turnover of vitamin E resulting in low tissue levels of α-tocopherol.

2.2 Carotenoids

Over 500 different carotenoids have been identified, and these are characterized by a long hydrocarbon chain containing conjugated double bonds and flanked by 2 β-ionone rings [5]. About 50 carotenoids, especially β carotene (Fig. 1), have provitamin A activity. Carotenes in the diet can be taken into the intestine mucosal cells and converted to retinol, the active form of vitamin A. Initially the importance of carotenes was linked mainly to their action regarding vitamin A activity. Due to β carotene having the greatest provitamin A activity, it has been the vitamin that has been the most studied. However, recent attention has been given to the role carotenoids playing a part as antioxidants, independent of their role in vitamin A activity. For example, carotenoids lutein and lycopene have no vitamin A activity but may serve in reducing oxidative stress [34,35]. The conjugated double bonds of carotenoids make then highly efficient as quenchers of singlet oxygen [5].

2.2.1 Sources

Carotenoids are found in all vegetables that contain chlorophyll. Yellow, red, or orange vegetables provide significant amounts of carotenoids [6] (Table 2). The major source of carotenes in various countries include carrots in North America, yellow and green vegetables in Japan, red palm oil in West Africa, and dark green leafy vegetables in China [6]. In a study of a Finnish population, carrots provided 54% of total β carotene for men and up to 70% for women [8]. Vegetables provided α-carotene and γ-carotene. Major sources of lycopene are tomatoes and tomato products [36], sources of β-cryptoxanthin are oranges, orange juice, tangerines and peaches, and sources of lutein are spinach and other greens, broccoli, corn green beans and green peas [37]. Diets high in fruits and vegetables can increase plasma carotenoids in a relatively short period of time (15 days) [38]. Naturally occurring β carotene is in the form of all-*trans* β carotene [35]. When in solution and exposed to light and oxygen, carotenes are sensitive to oxidation, isomerization, and polymerization [35].

2.2.2 Absorption

Carotenes are found in combination with protein and are released from protein by the action of pepsin in the stomach and proteolytic enzymes in the small intestine [5]. They are then solubilized into micelles through bile salts and traverse the intestinal wall. Of the total β carotene consumed, only about 5–50% is absorbed [5]. Several factors have been found to influence absorption. For example, absorption is enhanced by cooking vegetables. The bioavailability of lycopene was found to be greater from tomato paste than from fresh vegetables and higher in processed (boiled) tomato juice than unprocessed tomato juice [39,40]. However, cooking can reduce the concentration of β carotene [41]. Increasing doses,

Table 2. Carotene content of foods [7].

Food	μg/100 g
Breads/cereals	trace
Milk, whole	21
Milk, skim	trace
Cheeses	100—400
Rice/pasta	trace
Meat/fish	trace
Potatoes	trace
Beansprouts, mung	40
Tofu	2
Vegetables	
Peas, cooked	250—450
Asparagus, cooked	530
Broccoli, cooked	575
Carrots, raw	4300—11000
Kale, cooked	3375
Green pepper	175—265
Red pepper	3780—3840
Pumpkin, cooked	955
Spinach	3840
Sweet potato, cooked	3960
Corn	71—110
Tomato puree	1300
Tomato raw	640
Tomato juice	200
Fruits	
Apples	12—18
Apricots	200—3370
Bananas	21
Grapefruit	17
Pink grapefruit	280
Guava with skin	435
Mangoes	300—3000
Canteloupe	1000
Honeydew melon	48
Oranges	28
Blood oranges	155
Peaches	58

decreases absorption [5]. High gastric pH appears to slow down movement of micelles containing carotenes [42].

Dietary fat is also important as it has been reported that absorption is decreased to only 5% on a low-fat diet (7% of total energy intake) [5]. β Carotene supplements ingested without dietary fat resulted in no change in serum β carotene levels [37]. Zhi et al. [43] examined absorption of β carotene in patients taking orlistat, a lipase inhibitor, and found that absorption was reduced by about one third. Also, dietary fiber appears to exert an inhibitory effect on β carotene absorption [37].

In the intestinal mucosa some of the carotenes are converted into retinol. Other carotenoids are absorbed unchanged and incorporated into chylomicrons, along with cholesterol esters, phospholipids, triacylglycerols, and apoproteins. Novotny et al. [44] reported that 22% of β carotene was absorbed, and of this, 17.8% was absorbed as intact β carotene and 4.2% as retinoid. The composition of the diet may affect which pathway is used. Lakshman et al. [45] found that in ferrets dietary taurocholate, high-fat and high-protein increased exposure of β carotene to cleavage enzymes converting it into retinol.

Major carotenoids in plasma are zeaxanthin, lutein, lycopene, cryptoxanthin, α carotene, and β carotene with trace amounts of other species [34]. However, Wingerath et al. [46] reported that ingestion of tangerine juice (rich in β cryptoxanthin esters) increased free β cryptoxanthin in chylomicrons and serum. No β cryptoxanthin esters were detected, indicating that the cleavage of carotenoid esters occurred in the intestine before being incorporated into lipoproteins by the liver. Free β cryptoxanthin in chylomicrons peaked at 6 h and returned to baseline by 9 h. Bierer et al. [47] found that oral administration of β carotene, canthaxanthin, lutein, lycopene, and α carotene to calves resulted in absorption of all carotenoids. Canthaxanthin and lutein peaked earlier in the serum and were cleared more quickly [47]. Carotenoids interact with each other during intestinal absorption, metabolism, and serum clearance [48].

2.2.3 β Carotene trans and cis isomers

Carotenoids can exist in *cis* and *trans* forms. The all-*trans* configuration has an extended conjugated double bond system and is a linear, rigid molecule [49], whereas the *cis*-configuration is not a simple linear molecule. These different forms provide a different shape and ability to fit into subcellular structures. *Cis* isomers may be more easily solubilized, absorbed, and transported than the all-*trans* forms. However, little is known about these properties of isomers and how they impart specific functions in tissues.

Johnson et al. [50] and Stahl et al. [51] examined serum levels of β carotene after ingestion of all-*trans* β carotene or a naturally occurring mixture of isomers with 80% 9-*cis* β carotene (algae product, Dunaliella salina), finding that the all-*trans* form resulted in greater serum levels. Subjects supplemented with the mixture of all-*trans* and 9-*cis* isomers showed that the resulting 9-*cis* isomer in the blood was only a small fraction of the total plasma β carotene [52]. These data could indicate poor absorption of 9-*cis* β carotene, rapid isomerization to the all-*trans* form, or rapid tissue uptake. In another study, all-*trans* β carotene, or a naturally occurring mixture of isomers (Dunaliella bardawil), resulted in the all-*trans* form showing greater blood levels of both all-*trans* and 9-*cis* compared to the mixture. It was suggested that isomerization of the all-*trans* form to the 9-*cis* form can occur during or after absorption [53]. Levin and Mokady [54] reported that the presence of 9-*cis* isomers enhanced the incorporation of carotenes into micelles and thereby increased carotene bioavailability. Using ^{13}C labeled *9-cis* β carotene, You et al. [55] found that *9-cis* β carotene was isomerized into all-*trans*, and that isomerization did not exclusively occur before uptake in the intestinal mucosa.

The benefits of *9-cis* β carotene are still controversial. Ben-Amotz and Levy [56] reported that supplementation of Dunaliella bardawil, containing equal amounts of all-*trans* and *9-cis* isomers, resulted in low levels of serum-oxidized dienoic products than did supplementation with only all-*trans* β carotene. *9-cis* isomers appear to have greater antioxidant capabilities than the all-*trans* β isomers [57].

2.2.4 *Transport and storage*

The chylomicrons are carried to the liver where they have 3 possible fates [5]. Some carotenes may be incorporated into VLDL, some may be stored in the liver, and some converted to retinol [5]. When incorporated into VLDLs, they are released into the circulatory system and transported to fatty tissues. Hydrocarbon carotenoids (e.g., β carotene) are associated primarily with low-density lipoproteins in plasma while more polar ones (e.g., lutein+zeaxanthin) are distributed evenly among HDLs and LDLs [34,58]. About 15—30% of total plasma carotenes are in the β form [34]. The mechanisms to explain how carotenoids move between intracellular organelles or how they are incorporated into lipoproteins is not known, but it is thought that unlike other lipids, these processes are not mediated by cytosolic transport proteins [59]. Although still not identified, the transport may take place by vesicular transport or by membrane-bound proteins [59].

Storage of β carotene is not fully known, but is thought to occur in lipids throughout the body. After injection of β carotene in rats, β carotene appeared quickly in the lungs (5 min), then appeared in adipose tissue (after 1 week), pancreas (2 weeks), and muscle or testes (3 weeks) [60]. Oral administration of radio-labeled β carotene in pigs showed that high levels appeared in the lungs and liver; assessment was made at 24 h postinjection. Redlich et al. [61] suggested that β carotene may have an important protective effect in the lungs. However, the high concentration of β carotene in the lungs remains speculative [62]. In humans, adipose tissue is the primary storage area, but liver, adrenal glands, and testes contain relatively high amounts of carotenoids with β carotene making up most of the carotenoids in liver and adrenal glands and lycopene in testes [63]. Zeaxanthin and lutein and not β carotene are found in the macula area [63]. Thus, the selective occurrence of carotenoids suggests that they may have specific functions in various tissues.

2.2.5 *Factors that influence carotenoid status*

Vitamin E has been suggested to inhibit β carotene absorption [6]. However, a study in ferrets showed that after perfusion of the small intestine with β carotene and varying levels of α-tocopherol, the lymphatic transport of β carotene was enhanced 4-fold by α-tocopherol at a physiological dose and 12— to 21-fold with a pharmacological dose. The authors concluded that α-tocopherol had a positive effect on intestinal absorption of β carotene [64].

Van Vliet et al. [65] found that vitamin A status could affect β carotene absorption. They reported that in rats, intestinal β carotene cleavage activity was higher in rats who were vitamin A deficient compared to rats with high intake of vitamin A or β carotene. Thus, low vitamin A status may enhance the conversion of β carotene to retinol at the expense of direct absorption of β carotene for use as an antioxidant. While zinc, iron, and protein intakes affect vitamin A status, metabolism or transport, their effect on carotenoids is not clear.

Smoking is associated with low serum carotene levels, and there appears to be a strong dose-responsive relationship; the greater the number of cigarettes smoked, the lower the serum carotene levels [5,66]. In another study, although lower serum concentrations of α carotene, β carotene, β cryptoxanthin, and lutein+zeaxanthin were associated with smoking, the relationship was attributed to dietary intake of carotenoids [67]. However, Handelman et al. [68] found that when plasma was exposed in vitro to cigarette smoke, there was a depletion of most of the lipophilic antioxidants. Conditions of impaired lipid absorption, such as jaundice, cirrhosis of the liver, and cystic fibrosis, also result in low carotene status. Winklhofer-Roob et al. [69] reported that oral β carotene supplements were effective in normalizing β carotene status of cystic fibrosis patients.

2.3 Vitamin C

Vitamin C exists in two forms, L-ascorbic acid (Fig. 1), the strong reducing agent, and the oxidized form, L-dehydroascorbic acid (DHAA) [5]. The reason ascorbic acid is a good reducing agent is that it can lose electrons easily and thus, is an effective electron donor [70]. Ascorbic acid (AA) is soluble in water but in an aqueous solution is easily oxidized to DHAA [71]. The reaction between AA and DHAA is reversible but oxidation of DHAA into other products (di-ketogulonic acid, oxalic and threonic acids) is not [71]. The latter products, except for erythorbic acid, have no vitamin C activity [71]. The role AA plays as antioxidant is due to its ability to provide electrons to chemical compounds that are oxidants [72]. Erythorbic acid is widely used as a food preservative because of its antioxidant activity [5].

2.3.1 Sources

Most of the vitamin C in western diets comes from green vegetables, citrus fruits, tomatoes, berries and potatoes [71]. Those foods with vitamin C concentrations of over 50 mg/100 g are black currants, brussel sprouts, cauliflower, strawberries, lemons, cabbage and oranges [71] (Table 3). However, the richest sources of vitamin C are found in the West Indian cherry and the rose hip [5]. Fortified dairy products and some meat and fish have minor amounts of vitamin C [71]. Cooking causes a dramatic loss in vitamin C because of its water solubility and destruction by heat [5]. Different parts of the same vegetable can be affected differently by cooking. For example, the broccoli head contains more vitamin C (158 mg /g) than then stem (110 mg/g), but during 10 min of cooking, the head loses 40% or more of vitamin C but the stem only loses about 20% [5]. Copper in cooking utensils can promote the loss of vitamin C during cooking [5].

Also storage of food will result in a loss in vitamin C [5]. For example, when potatoes are fresh, the vitamin C content is 30 mg/100 g, but when they are stored for several months, the content can be reduced to 7—8 mg/100 g [5]. Vitamin C accumulates in fruits whilst they are ripening on the vine, therefore, a ripe fruit has more vitamin C than one that is not ripe [5]. Exposure to air enhances the breakdown of vitamin C such that chopped or shredded vegetables retain less vitamin C than whole vegetables [5]. Vitamin C in foods or beverages is stable in acidic conditions.

Table 3. Vitamin C content of foods [7].

Food	mg/100 g
Cereals	< 30
Breads	0
Rice/Pasta	0
Milk	1
Cheeses	trace
Oils, butter	0
Meats	0
Fish	trace
Vegetables	
Potatoes, cooked	5—14
Bean/lentils	trace
Peas, cooked	4.5—5.1
Broccoli, cooked	44
Asparagus, cooked	10
Carrots, raw	6
Kale, cooked	71
Green peppers, raw	120
Red peppers, raw	140
Tomato puree	38
Tomato raw	17
Fruits	
Apples	3—20
Bananas	11
Black currants	150—230
Grapefruit	36
Mangoes	37
Nectarines	37
Oranges	44—79

2.3.2 Absorption

Vitamin C can be absorbed by mucosal cells in the mouth through passive diffusion [5]. In the intestines, vitamin C is absorbed through an active carrier mediated process that is dose-dependent [5,71]. Absorption becomes saturated when the mucosal concentration of vitamin C is greater than 6 mmol/l, possibly explaining why vitamin C absorption decreases with increasing ingestion [5]. Absorption is about 70—90% at ingested amounts of 30—180 mg/day; 50% at amounts of 1.5 g; and 16% with 12 g/day [71]. Larger doses result in greater postabsorptive degradation [71]. With large ingested amounts, a greater concentration of vitamin C remains in the intestines which can produce osmotic diarrhea [71]. DHAA may be absorbed more quickly than AA, so it is speculated that some conversion from AA to DHAA occurs, and once absorbed into the intestinal epithelium, DHAA is then reduced back to AA [71].

Levine et al. [73] studied seven volunteers who were hospitalized for 4—6 months and consumed a diet containing < 5 mg vitamin C per day with supplemental doses of 30—2500 mg vitamin C. Single doses of 500 mg and higher resulted in a decline in bioavailability and increased excretion. In fact, bioavailability was complete for the 200 mg doses indicating that doses higher than this are inefficient and not necessary.

Bioavailability is increased when doses of less than 1 g are spaced throughout the day [71]. Also, sustained release supplements improve bioavailability [71]. Comparison of the bioavailability of pure synthetic AA vs. natural forms have produced equivocal results [71]. However, the weight of the data suggest that there is no difference [71]. Erythorbic acid, an epimere of L-AA, is found in many foods but does not seem to either have a beneficial or a deleterious effect on vitamin C status [74]. Sauberlich et al. [74] found that increased erythorbic acid intake over a prolonged period did not affect the absorption of AA.

Smokers have lower plasma and leukocyte AA levels compared with nonsmokers, which is not attributed entirely to lower vitamin C ingestion [71,75]. Smokers must increase their vitamin C intake to maintain plasma levels. The recommended intake for smokers is 100 mg/day compared with the 60 mg/day RDA (1). Unlike the lower vitamin E and carotene levels found in smokers that could be associated with a decreased absorption, the lower AA levels in smokers appears to be due to an increased turnover of AA, as well. It has been suggested that the oxidative stress of smoking increases catabolism of AA, but this has not been proven [71].

2.3.3 Transport and storage

AA is mostly transported free in the plasma [6]. Some transported AA is associated with albumen, and 5% is in the DHAA form [6]. The concentration of AA is higher in cells than in the blood (by about 3- to 10-fold) indicating an energy driven transport into cells [71]. Transport of AA into leukocytes, neutrophils or other cells has been used as a model to study cellular uptake mechanisms [71]. Welch et al. [76] reported that AA and DHAA are transported into neutrophils and fibroblasts by two different mechanisms. Transport of DHAA is mediated by a facilitated mechanism involving glucose transporters and is not sodium-dependent [77], while transport of AA involves a sodium-AA mediated transporter [78]. Thus, high blood levels of glucose, such as those that occurs in diabetes, may impair DHAA uptake [79). Once in the cell, DHAA is immediately converted to AA [76]. Ascorbate is localized in the cytosol in lymphocytes and is not protein bound [80].

Highest concentrations of vitamin C are found in the adrenal glands (30—40 mg/100 g wet tissue), pituitary, leukocytes, and eye lens [6,70, 71]. Intermediate amounts are found in the liver, pancreas, and heart muscle and lesser amounts (< 15 mg/100 g wet tissue) are found in other tissues such as skeletal muscle [5,6]. Using isotopic techniques, the total body pool of AA was estimated to be about 20 mg/kg of body weight [71].

2.3.4 Interactions with other nutrients

Vitamin C enhances the absorption of nonheme-iron [5,81]. It is thought that AA in the gut maintains iron in its reduced form which prevents the formation of insoluble ferric hydroxide [5]. AA can serve as a soluble ligand for iron [5]. Vitamin C may maintain folate in a reduced state which maintains the active form of folate and keeps nitrite from reacting with amines to form hepatotoxic and carcinogenic nitroso compounds [5]. Vitamin C intakes of 1.5 g for about 2 months, result in a decrease in serum copper and ceruloplasmin, but not below normal ranges [6]. Animal studies have reported that high amounts of AA decrease intestinal absorption of copper.

α-Tocopherol and AA appear to act synergistically to inhibit oxidation [82]. α-Tocopherol scavenges free radicals in membranes and lipoproteins, producing an α-tocopheroxyl radical [82]. AA then reduces the α-tocopheroxyl radical to regenerate α-tocopherol and inhibit further oxidation by the α-tocopheroxyl radical [82].

3   NONESSENTIAL ANTIOXIDANTS

3.1 Synthetic and plant phenolics

Phenolics represent a vast array of both naturally occurring and synthetic compounds. These compounds inhibit lipid oxidation through their ability to scavenge free radicals, chelate prooxidative metals and inhibit lipoxygenases [83—85]. Synthetic phenolics such as butylated hydroxyanisole, butylated hydroxytoluene (Fig. 2), propyl gallate and tertiary butylated hydroxyquinone are commonly used in food products to inhibit oxidative rancidity. Addition of synthetic phenolic antioxidants to foods is strictly regulated with legal concentration limits of 200 ppm or less [86].

Numerous studies have evaluated the safety of synthetic phenolics. Consumption of extremely high concentrations (>2 g/day) of synthetic phenolics for several months can produce carcinoma in the rat forestomach. These high levels of synthetic antioxidants can inhibit archadonic acid metabolism and can be prooxidative leading to the depletion of glutathione. However, lower levels of synthetic antioxidants are capable of altering phase II enzymes in the liver and thus, can reduce the carcinogenic activity of several known carcinogens. These lower level of synthetic phenolic, which reflect typical human exposure, are not believed to be harmful to health and may actually be beneficial through their ability to inactivate free radicals in vivo [87,88].

Naturally occurring plant phenolics are much more prevalent in the diet than synthetic phenolics since they are found in a wide range of plant foods. The plant phenolics can be classified as simple phenolics and phenolic acids, hydroxycinnamic acid derivatives, and flavonoids. In addition to the basic hydroxylated benzene ring structure of these compounds, plant phenolics are often associated with sugars and organic acids. Many natural phenolics are capable of inhibiting oxidative reactions. However, due to the chemical diversity of these compounds, it is not surprising that antioxidant activities vary greatly. Under certain conditions, some plant phenolics accelerate oxidative reactions,this can be seen with phenolics from soybeans (chlorogenic acid, gallic acid and caffeic acid) and rosemary (carnosol and carnosic acid) which promote iron-catalyzed oxidation

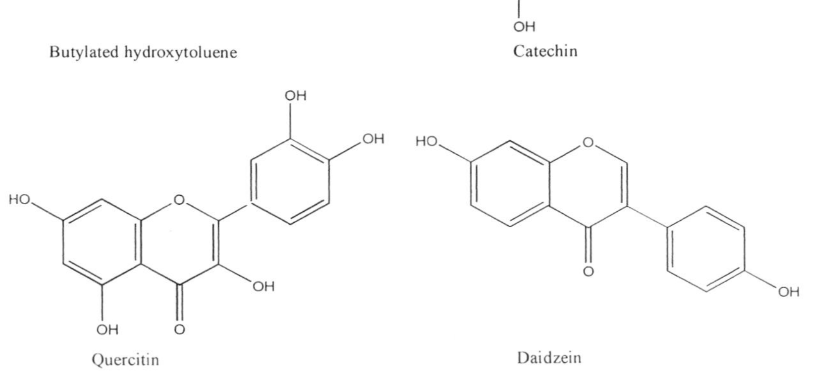

Butylated hydroxytoluene

Catechin

Quercitin

Daidzein

Fig. 2. Structures of phenolics commonly found in foods.

of DNA [85,89]. Despite the fact that phenolics are sometimes prooxidative, their presence in the diet has been positively associated with prevention of diseases such as cancer and atherosclerosis [88,90].

3.1.1 Sources

Phenolics are found in the majority of plants from which foods are derived. Consumption quantities of plant phenolics have been estimated to be up to 1 g per day [88]. Most dietary phenolics come directly from plant foods since their use as food additives are limited by associated flavors, colors, ability to participate in enzymic browning reactions and their complexation with other food components such as proteins and minerals. Table 4 and Fig. 2 show sources and structures of some common phenolics in foods. Plant foods that are high in phenolics include seeds and seed hulls (e.g., sesame, oats, soybeans and coffee), red and blue colored fruits (e.g., grapes, strawberries and plums) and the leaves of certain plants (e.g., tea, rosemary and thyme). Due to the huge diversity of this group of

Table 4. Phenolic antioxidative compounds in foods.

Antioxidant	Source	Concentration	Reference
Phenolics			
Quercetin derivatives[a]	Onions	1096 mg/kg	[194]
	Raspberries	118 mg/kg	[195]
	Apple	36 mg/kg	[196]
	Kale	110 mg/kg	[196]
	Red wine	15 mg/l	[94]
	White wine	1 mg/l	[94]
Catechin derivatives[b]	Green tea	34 mg/g dried extract	[91]
	Black tea	4.2 mg/g dried extract	[91]
	Red wine	200–530 mg/l	[197]
Isoflavones[c]	Roasted Soybeans	1.63 mg/g	[96]
	Tofu	0.35 mg/g	[96]
	Tempeh	0.63 mg/g	[96]
	Miso	0.29 mg/g	[96]
Pyrroloquinoline quinone	Milk	3.4 µg/l	[198]
	Soybeans	9.3 µg/kg	[199]
	Apple	6.1 µg/kg	[199]
	Kiwi	27.4 µg/kg	[199]
	Green tea	29.6 µg/l	[199]
	Miso	16.7 µg/kg	[199]

[a]Quercetin and rutin combined.
[b]Catechin, epicatechin, epicatechin gallate, gallocatechin, epigallocatechin gallate and epigallocatechin combined.
[c]Catechin and epicatechin.

dietary components, this review will focus on several of the best studied dietary phenolics.

Tea has recently gained much attention as a source of dietary phenolics because it is one of the most common beverages in the world with annual consumption of over 40 liters/person/year [91]. Tea contains a variety of catechin derivatives, including catechin (Fig. 2), epicatechin, epicatechin gallate, gallocatechin, epigallocatechin gallate and epigallocatechin, which have been associated with cancer prevention [88]. Tea originates from the leaves of the bush, *Camellia sinensis*. After harvesting, the tea leaves are either rapidly heated to produce green tea or fermented to produce oolong or black tea. The fermentation process allows endogenous enzymes to react with phenolics such as the catechins resulting in the formation of condensed polyphenols which contribute to the typical color and flavor of black teas. Green tea leaf extracts contain 38.8% phenolics on a dry weight basis with catechins contributing over 85% of the total phenolics. Black tea extracts contain 24.4% phenolics of which 17% are catechins and 70% are condensed polyphenols (thearubigens) [91]. Extraction of phenolics with water from the leaves of Rooibos (*Aspalathus linearis*) resulted in increased antioxidant activity with increasing extraction temperature and time [92] suggesting that brewing techniques could influence the antioxidant phenolic content of teas.

Grapes and wines are also significant sources of phenolic antioxidants. Grapes contain a large number of different phenolics including anthocyanins, flavan-3-ols (catechin), flavonols (quercetin and rutin) and cinnamates (S-glutathionylcaftaric acid) [93]. The majority of phenolics in grapes are found in the skin, seeds and stems (collectively termed pomace). During extraction of juice, the pomace is left in contact with the juice for varying times. Increasing contact time results in increased extraction of phenolics into the juice and thus, formation of a darker color. Therefore, while white grape juices and wines contain phenolics, their total phenolic concentrations (119 mg of gallic acid equivalents/liter) and antioxidant activity is significantly lower than red wines (2057 mg of gallic acid equivalents/liter) [93,94]. Processing conditions will influence the phenolic concentration and compositions of grape juices with processes such as the crushing of seeds resulting in increased phenolic content and antioxidant activity [93]. Both grape juice and wines have been suggested to have positive heath benefits, however, their phenolic compositions are not the same due to differences in juice preparation and changes in phenolic composition which occurs during both fermentation and storage [95].

Soybeans contain a group of anticarcinogenic phenolics known as isoflavones. The major isoflavones in soybeans are daidzein (Fig. 2), genistein and glycitein and the glycosolated counterparts daidzin, genistin and glycitin [96]. Soybean isoflavones are often associated with proteins and, therefore, are found in soy flour and not in soybean oil. The concentrations of these compounds vary with soybean variety and the environmental conditions under which the beans were grown. Isoflavone concentrations and composition are altered during food processing operations such as heating and fermentation. Besides whole soybeans, isoflavones are found in soy-based foods including roasted soybeans, soy milk, tempeh, miso and tofu at concentrations ranging from 294—1625 µg/g (Table 1) [96].

3.1.2 Absorption, storage and transport

Many studies have been conducted to show that dietary phenolics are bioactive in different tissues, thus indirectly suggesting that they or their derivatives are absorbed into the blood. Unfortunately, the mechanisms and efficiency of phenolic absorption and the in vivo stability of most of these compounds is poorly understood. Catechins from tea and isoflavonoids from soybeans are two examples of phenolics whose bioavailability has been studied extensively. Dietary epicatechin, epigallocatechin, epicatechin gallate and epigallocatechin gallate are all absorbed into rat blood with maximum concentrations occurring approximately 30—60 min after ingestion after which concentrations decreased rapidly [97,98]. Consumption of green or black tea increased the antioxidant activity of human blood plasma [99]. Green tea increases the total phenolic concentrations of blood greater than black tea and decaffeinated black tea [100]. However, in terms of antioxidant activity, both green and black teas increase the oxidative stability of blood at similar rates [99].

The soybean isoflavones, genistein and daidzein, are absorbed into human blood from dietary sources such as tofu, textured vegetable protein and soy protein beverages [101,102]. The bioavailability of daidzein and genistein have been estimated to be approximately 21 and 9%, respectively. Absorbed isoflavones are rapidly removed from the blood with less then 10% of the isoflavones present 24 h after ingestion [103]. The majority of dietary isoflavones (85%) are believed to be degraded in the intestine by endogenous enzymes or by gastrointestinal microorganisms [103].

Several other phenolics have also been shown to be bioavailable. Phenolic acids such as homovanillic acid, benzoic acid and hippuric acid have been detected in the blood of rats after oral administration of *Ginkgo biloba* extract [104]. Dietary quercetin in rats [105] and naringein in humans [106] are also absorbed into the blood. However, these phenolics are often found in foods conjugated to sugar molecules (rutin and naringin). Before these glycosolated phenolics can be absorbed, the sugar molecules must be removed by enzymes originating from intestinal microorganisms [105].

While many phenolics are known to be absorbed into the blood, their transport mechanism are unknown. Since the phenolics exhibit a wide range of solubility characteristics, from highly water-soluble (e.g., catechins) to highly lipid-soluble (e.g., carnosol from rosemary), they may be transported within the plasma, blood lipids or both. More research is needed on transportation mechanisms of phenolics in vivo in order to better understand the antioxidant activity of phenolics in biological systems.

3.1.3 Interaction with other nutrients

Phenolics interact strongly with other nutrients such as proteins and minerals. Phenolics are commonly found in foods complexed with proteins resulting in low water solubility and bioavailability. For instance, ingestion of tea increases the antioxidant activity of blood plasma. However, addition of milk to tea prior to ingestion results in no changes in plasma antioxidant activity [99]. Formation of insoluble protein-phenolic complexes results in haze formation in juices, wines, beer and teas. Due to low consumer acceptance of cloudy beverages, phenolics and/or protein concentrations in these beverages are often reduced during commercial production. Phenolics also form strong complexes with minerals. The ability of phenolics, especially tannins, to inhibit iron absorption is well-documented [107].

Epicatechin and epigallocatechin have been shown to decrease cholesterol absorption in rats presumably by forming cholesterol complexes with reduced solubility [108]. Absorption of the isoflavones, daidzein and genistein, is inhibited by dietary fiber through direct binding or by altering gut microflora and thus, increasing isoflavone degradation [102]. In general, plant phenolics are stable components in stored foods, however, they can be degraded by metals and light which are capable of accelerating oxidative reactions.

3.2 Pyrroloquinoline quinone

Pyrroloquinoline quinone (PQQ), also known as methoxatin, is a water-soluble compound widely distributed in microorganisms, plants, and animals in both free and protein-bound forms [109]. PQQ seems to be an essential nutrient since mice that were fed chemically defined diets devoid of PQQ grew poorly, failed to reproduce, became osteolathyritic, and had friable skin. Administration of low concentrations of dietary PQQ (0.5–1.0 nmol) were capable of reversing these effects [110]. The exact physiological role of PQQ is not clear, however, several authors have suggested that PQQ either acts as a cofactor for enzymes [111,112] or protects tissues from oxidative stress [113]. PQQ inhibits lipid oxidation in rat brain homogenate and in heart and brain tissue subjected to ischemic reperfusion [114–116]. The antioxidant mechanisms of PQQ has been postulated to be due to metal chelation and/or free radical scavenging. The reducing potential of PQQ (+90 mV at pH 7.0) also suggests that it could regenerate oxidized tocopherol in a manner similar to ascorbic acid.

Since eukaryotic organisms are not thought to produce PQQ, in animals PQQ is most likely obtained either from enteric bacteria or foods via absorption through the large intestine [117]. Human blood plasma and lung tissue have been reported to contain from 1.7 to 3.0 ng free PQQ/g wet tissue [118]. Foods containing free PQQ include dairy products, fruits and various beverages where concentrations range from 3–30 µg/kg or L (Table 1).

3.3 Ubiquinone (coenzyme Q)

Ubiquinone (Fig. 3) is an important electron carrier found in mitochondria, plasma membranes and the Golgi apparatus. Ubiquinone contains a benzoquinone ring with an isoprenoid side chain which helps anchor the molecule into the membrane (Fig. 3). The side chain of ubiquinones ranges from 2–10 (Q_{2-10}) isoprenoid units with 10 being the most common [119]. In LDL, biological membranes and liposomes, ubiquinone inhibits lipid oxidation presumably through free radical scavenging mechanisms [120].

Since ubiquinones are found in biological membranes, these compounds are a common component of the diet. Diet can increase ubiquinone concentrations in the blood and liver of rats but not in kidney, heart, skeletal muscle and brain [121]. In the liver, dietary ubiquinone was deposited mainly in the mitochondria, lysosomes, Golgi apparatus and plasma membranes. The mechanism of ubiquinone absorption is poorly understood. In studies with rats, only a small proportion of dietary ubiquione was absorbed (2–3%) [122]. Absorbed ubiquinone increased blood levels continuously during six weeks of dietary supplementation,

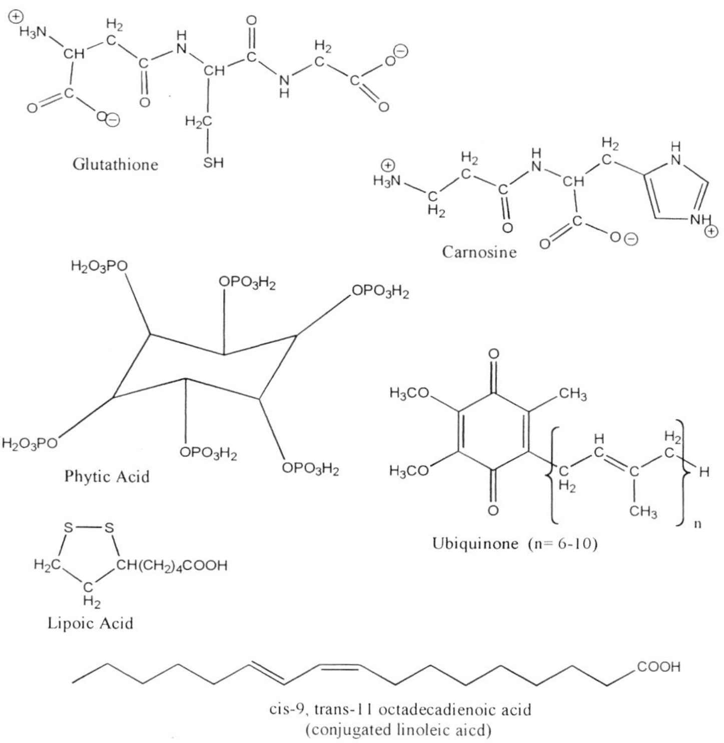

Fig. 3. Examples of several nonessential antioxidants found in foods.

but disappeared rapidly from the liver and plasma after withdrawal of this lipid from the diet [121]. Dietary deficiency of α-tocopherol did not alter ubiquinone concentrations in the plasma and liver, but α-tocopherol supplementation increased liver and plasma ubiquinone incorporation. Supplementation of 90 mg ubiquinone Q_{10} for 9 months increased plasma concentrations from 1 to 2 mg/l in 21 human subjects. Plasma concentrations returned to baseline levels 3 months after withdraw of the ubiquinone supplementation [123]. Ubiquinone supplementation to men resulted in increased plasma concentrations but did not affect exercise capacity [124]. Data on ubiquinone concentrations in raw, processed and stored foods are severely lacking. As with most phenolic antioxidants, ubiquinones are known to be destroyed by oxidative reactions and thus, are susceptible to light and metal degradation.

3.4 Conjugated linoleic acid

The two double bonds of linoleic acid are normally in a methylene interrupted system where two single bonds separate the double bonds. However, the double bond system is sometimes altered resulting in isomerization of the double bonds to a conjugated configuration. These isomers, known as conjugated linoleic acid (CLA; Fig. 3), have gained widespread interest due to their ability to inhibit cancer [125,126], lower blood cholesterol [127,128] and influence weight gain [129]. CLA also inhibits lipid oxidation in vitro and in biological membranes although the mechanism by which CLA inhibits oxidation is unknown. In linoleic acid micelles, CLA inhibits oxidation as determined by lipid peroxides 130]. CLA incorporated into biological membranes via the diet also decreased oxidation rates [131], but physical incorporation of CLA into phospholipid liposomes has no effect on oxidation [132]. Recent unpublished data from our laboratory [133] shows that dietary CLA increases the oxidative stability of isolated rat liver microsomes. However, dietary CLA also altered membrane fatty acid compositions. Therefore, it is unknown whether the ability of CLA to decrease oxidation in biological membranes was truly due to antioxidant activity or is due to alterations in oxidizable substrate concentrations. Obviously more research is needed to elucidate the exact antioxidant mechanism of CLA.

Formation of conjugated linoleic acid isomers can be catalyzed by microorganisms found in the rumen or by chemical pathways such as hydrogenation. The major dietary sources of CLA are beef, lamb and dairy products with CLA concentrations in nonuruminants, (chicken, pork and fish), and vegetable oils being 5—20 times lower than ruminant-derived fats [134] (Table 5). Typical CLA concentrations in beef and dairy fat are in the order of 4—8 mg/g fat [135,136] (Table 2). Recent advances in animal nutrition have been able to increase CLA concentrations in milk fat 2- to 5-fold [137]. Since CLA is a fatty acid, it is associated with the lipids and is, therefore, found in lower concentrations in low fat foods. However, since CLA is found in phospholipids, it is present in virtually all beef and dairy products. CLA is remarkably stable in foods and is not noticeably

Table 5. Miscellaneous nonessential antioxidants in foods.

Antioxidant	Source	Concentration	Reference
Conjugated linoleic acid	Ground beef	7.0 mg/g fat	[135]
	Lamb	5.6 mg/g fat	[134]
	Butter	8.0 mg/g fat	[136]
	Mozzarella cheese	5.0 mg/g fat	[136]
Carnosine	Chicken breast	2.7 g/kg	[140]
	Chicken thigh	0.5 g/kg	[140]
	Beef	1.5 g/kg	[140]
	Pork	2.8 g/kg	[140]
	Salmon	0.0 g/kg	[140]
Polyamines			
Spermine	Cooked pork	31.9 mg/kg	[200]
	Trout	100 mg/kg	[201]
	Mushrooms	3.0 mg/kg	[202]
	Soybeans	78 mg/kg	[202]
Spermidine	Cooked beef	18.7 mg/g	[200]
	Trout	30 mg/kg	[201]
	Mushrooms	192 mg/kg	[202]
	Soybeans	226 mg/kg	[202]
Glutathione	Mackerel	0.7 mg/kg	[177]
	Bluefish	0.6 mg/kg	[177]
	Turkey thigh	0.9 mg/kg	[176]
Phytate	Wheat	11.0 g/kg	[184]
	Oats	8.0 g/kg	[184]
	Soybeans	14.0 g/kg	[184]
	Sesame seeds	53.0 g/kg	[184]

altered by food processing and storage even in situations where other fatty acids are oxidizing rapidly [135].

Dietary CLA is readily absorbed along with other fatty acids into the blood. Cheddar cheese (112 g/day) increased plasma CLA 19–27% in men, after removal of cheese from the diet, plasma CLA concentrations decreased back to baseline levels within 4 weeks [138]. Dietary CLA is incorporated into numerous tissue sources of rats with the diet providing the majority of CLA source since nonruminants only have a limited ability to isomerize linoleic acid in the gastro-intestinal tract [139]. The exact amount of CLA consumed by humans is not well-understood, however, it has been estimated to be in the order of several hundred mg/person/day [130].

3.5 Histidine-containing dipeptides

Carnosine and anserine are *N*-ß-alanyl-L-histidine and *N*-ß-alanyl-3-methyl-L-histidine dipeptides (Fig. 3), respectively, endogenous to skeletal muscle (Table 2). Carnosine and anserine are found exclusively in the muscle and nervous tissues of animals. White muscle fibers generally have higher anserine and carnosine concentrations than red muscle with chicken breast and leg muscle having combined dipeptide concentrations of 1.2% (71 mM) and 0.2% (12.2 mM), respectively, of the wet weight of the muscle [140]. Since the pK_a's of the imidazole ring of carnosine and anserine are 6.83 and 7.04, respectively, these histidine-containing dipeptides exhibit excellent buffering capacity at physiological pH values. Anserine and carnosine have been estimated to provide up to 40% of pH-buffering capacity of skeletal muscle [141] and the buffering capacity of muscle has been correlated with carnosine concentrations in horse, dog and man [142]. The role of carnosine and anserine as buffers could explain why higher concentrations are found in white muscle fibers where anaerobic metabolism is common.

Boldyrev and co-workers [143,144] were the first to report the antioxidant activity of carnosine and anserine by demonstrating that carnosine and anserine could decrease lipid oxidation rates in sarcoplasmic reticulum as determined by thiobarbituric acid reactive substances. The antioxidant activity of carnosine and anserine has since been demonstrated in numerous model systems (for review see [26]). The antioxidant mechanism of carnosine and anserine involves both metal chelation and free radical scavenging. Carnosine chelates copper much more strongly than iron [145,146]. Carnosine also inactivates hydroxyl radicals generated from hydrogen peroxide by either iron or radiation [147,148]. Carnosine and anserine can quench singlet oxygen [149,150] but do not scavenge superoxide anions [151,152].

3.5.1 Absorption, transport and storage

Carnosine, but not anserine, is absorbed intact by a specific active transport system in brush border membranes from the small intestine [153,154]. Absorbed carnosine is transported through the blood where it is either utilized by peripheral tissue or is hydrolyzed into β-alanine and histidine by carnosinase, which is present in the blood, kidney, and liver [155,156], although the kidney seems to be the main organ responsible for the catabolism and excretion of the dipeptide [157]. Even though 0.05–0.25 g of carnosine are consumed daily (based on a diet containing 100 g pork, beef, or chicken/day), very little data are available about the dynamics of carnosine absorption, transport, and catabolism in humans.

Histidine deficiency in rats reduces skeletal muscle carnosine concentration [158,159]. Skeletal muscle carnosine concentrations in pigs are unaffected by low levels of histidine supplementation ($< 1\%$) [160,161] but can be increased

2.8-fold in rats supplemented with 5% histidine [159]. Low concentrations of dietary carnosine (0.9%) did not increase skeletal or heart muscle carnosine concentrations but did increase carnosine in the liver [162]. A higher dietary carnosine concentration (5%) was capable of doubling rat skeletal muscle carnosine concentrations [159]. Even though carnosine does not regenerate the α-tocopherol radical [163], an indirect relationship between carnosine and α-tocopherol seems to exist in vivo since α-tocopherol deficiency results in decreased rabbit skeletal muscle carnosine concentrations [164].

Carnosine and anserine concentrations vary as both a function of animal species and muscle type (Table 2). White (fast twitch) muscles generally have greater anserine and carnosine concentrations with chicken breast muscle containing 6-fold higher concentrations of the dipeptides than thigh muscle [140] and porcine Longissimus dorsi (high in white muscle fibers) having 1.5-fold higher anserine and carnosine concentrations than Vastus intermedius (high in red muscle fibers) muscle [161]. Animal species variations in anserine and carnosine include chicken, salmon and rabbits where anserine is predominant, whereas in humans, pigs, beef and turkey carnosine is predominant [165]. Anserine and carnosine concentrations in muscle foods are not only dependent on muscle type and species but also on fat content since the dipeptides are primarily a component of lean muscle tissue. Heat processing has little effect on anserine and carnosine concentrations, however, their concentrations will decrease during the oxidation of the muscle [133].

The ability of anserine and carnosine to inhibit oxidation at in vivo concentrations suggests that they are involved in the inactivation of prooxidant metals and free radicals in the aqueous phase of tissue. The higher concentrations of anserine and carnosine found in fast twitch (white) muscle fibers where anaerobic metabolism and reperfusion injury are more common suggests that the dipeptides could provide a crucial line of defense against oxidatively-induced tissue damage. Carnosine (2 mM) is capable of inhibiting copper-catalyzed oxidation of LDL and dietary carnosine (0.825%) inhibits 7,12-dimethylbenz(a)anthracene-induced breast cancer in vitamin E-deficient rats [166]. The ability of carnosine to inhibit factors involved with both atherosclerosis and cancer suggests that the dipeptide could be an important nonessential dietary antioxidant.

3.6 Polyamines, nucleotides and related compounds

The polyamines, putrescine [$NH_2(CH_2)_4NH_2$], spermidine [$NH_2(CH_2)_4NH-(CH_2)_3NH_2$] and spermine [$NH_2(CH_2)_3NH(CH_2)_4NH(CH_2)_3NH_2$] are found in numerous biological tissues. These polyamines have been postulated to play a role in membrane stabilization and antioxidant protection [167]. The polyamines inhibit lipid oxidation by free radical inactivation [168] and inhibition of iron-catalyzed reactions [167]. Antioxidant activity of the polyamines increases with increasing numbers of amine groups (e.g., spermine > spermidine > putrescine). The concentration of spermidine and spermine in plant foods and skeletal muscle (Table 2) are similar to those found to inhibit lipid oxidation in vitro.

Nucleotides including adenosine, xanthine, hypoxanthine and uric acid are capable of inhibiting lipid oxidation [169]. These compounds are produced from the anaerobic decomposition of ATP (ATP 6 hypoxanthine) [170] and the conversion of hypoxanthine to uric acid,through xanthine oxidase upon reoxygenation of anaerobic muscle [171]. The antioxidant activity of uric acid (Fig. 3) is the most widely recognized and best described of these compounds. Uric acid inhibits oxidative reactions by both iron chelation and free radical scavenging [172]. Its concentration in blood ranges from 320–470 μM [172–174]. While nucleotides derivatives are commonly found in foods, little is known about their concentrations, stability and bioactivity.

3.7 Thiols

Glutathione (Fig. 3) is a tripeptide consisting of γ-Glu-Cys-Gly where cysteine can be in either the reduced (GSH) or oxidized glutathione (GSSG) state. Reduced glutathione inhibits lipid oxidation directly (nonenzymically) by interacting with free radicals to form a relatively unstable sulfhydryl radical or by providing a source of electrons which allows glutathione peroxidase to enzymically decompose hydrogen and lipid peroxides [175]. Total glutathione concentrations in muscle foods range from 0.7–0.9 μg/kg (Table 2). Both total and reduced glutathione concentrations do not decrease during the cooking of turkey thigh muscle [176] but do decrease during the storage of mackerel and bluefish [177]. Oral administration of 3.0 g of glutathione to 7 healthy adults did not result in any increases in plasma glutathione, or cysteine concentrations after 270 min [178]. The bioavailability of glutathione in rats has also been reported to be low [179]. Lack of, or low absorption of glutathione may be due to the hydrolysis of the tripeptide by gastrointestinal proteases.

Lipoic (thioctic) acid (Fig. 3) is a cofactor for many plant and animal enzymes. In biological systems, the thiol groups are found in both reduced (dihydrolipoic acid) and oxidized (lipoic acid) forms. Both the oxidized and reduced forms of the molecule are capable of acting as antioxidants through their ability to quench singlet oxygen, scavenge free radicals, chelate iron and possibly regenerate other antioxidants such as ascorbate and tocopherols [180]. Lipoic and dehydrolipoic acids can protect LDL, erythrocytes and cardiac muscle from oxidative damage [181].

While lipoic acid has been found in numerous biological tissues, reports on its concentrations in foods are scarce. Lipoic acid is detectable in wheat germ (0.1 ppm) but not in wheat flour [182] and it has been detected in bovine liver kidney and skeletal muscle [183]. Oral administration of lipoic acid (1.65 g/kg fed) to rats for 5 weeks resulted in elevated levels of the thiol in the liver, kidney, heart and skin. When lipoic acid was added to diets lacking in vitamin E, symptoms typical of tocopherol deficiency were not observed suggesting that lipoic acid acts as an antioxidant in vivo. However, lipoic acid was not capable of recycling vitamin E in vivo as determined by the fact that α-tocopherol concentrations are not elevated by dietary lipoic acid in vitamin E deficient rats [180].

3.8 Phytic acid

Phytic acid or myoinositol hexaphosphate (Fig. 3) is the major phosphorous storage component of seeds, where it can be found at concentrations ranging from 0.8—5.3% [184]. Phytic acid is not readily digested by endogenous enzymes in the human gastrointestinal tract but can be digested by dietary plant phytases and by phytases originating from enteric microorganisms [185]. This highly phosphorylated compound forms strong chelates with iron which reduces iron's catalytic activity and thereby inhibits iron-catalyzed oxidative reactions [184]. The antioxidant properties of phytic acid are thought to help minimize oxidation in legumes and cereal grains, as well as in foods which may be susceptible to oxidation in the digestive tract. Phytic acid has been cited as a preventative agent in iron-mediated colon cancer. While phytate may be beneficial towards colon cancer, it should be noted that it can potentially have deleterious health effects because of its ability to dramatically decrease the bioavailability of minerals including iron, zinc and calcium [185].

4 ANTIOXIDANTS FROM FOOD SOURCES VS. DIETARY SUPPLEMENTS

Antioxidants are normal constituents of the biological tissues we use for foods. A well balanced diet will provide a variety of both essential and nonessential antioxidants from both plant and animal foods. In most cases the amount and diversity of antioxidants in plant foods is much greater than animal foods. This fact is supported by epidemiological studies which show that consumption of high amounts of plant foods, and in particular fruits and vegetables, are beneficial against diseases such as cancer and atherosclerosis. The potential health benefits of fruits and vegetables could be partially due to their antioxidant content. This was observed in a study where vegetarians had higher plasma vitamin C, β-carotene, vitamin E/triacylglycerol ratio and glutathione peroxidase activity than nonvegetarians [186].

Animal-based foods also contain both essential and nonessential antioxidative nutrients, however, in most cases concentrations of vitamins A, C and E are low (with the exception of Vitamin A in liver and fortified dairy products). Since skeletal muscle tissue is very susceptible to oxidative reactions due to its high concentrations of lipid oxidation catalysts and polyunsaturated cellular membrane lipids, muscle contains a variety of antioxidants besides the antioxidant vitamins including carnosine, glutathione, polyamines and nucleotide metabolites. These muscle antioxidants are primarily cytosolic and thus, can be obtained from lean meat sources, thereby avoiding the potential problems associated with consumption of large amounts of animal fats. Unfortunately, the ability of muscle foods to influence the oxidative stability of different tissues by providing antioxidative nutrients is poorly understood.

A potential problem with obtaining antioxidative nutrients from the diet is that many of these compounds are lipid soluble. With increasing trends of low-fat diets, it is possible (although not well-documented) that the consumption and absorption of both essential and nonessential antioxidative lipids in some populations could be low. This potential problem, plus consumer desire to capitalize on the health benefits of antioxidants, has increased the availability of antioxidants in the forms of both fortified foods and nutritional supplements. Consumption of large amounts of the antioxidants can be impractical (because excess antioxidants are simply excreted from the body) and even dangerous.

High levels of vitamin E intake have not been associated with any deleterious health effects although in vitro α-tocopherol has been shown to be prooxidative at high concentrations [86]. In normal individuals, the long-term intake of excess vitamin C can result in decreased absorption and increased excretion of ascorbate [187]. In individuals who have large amounts of iron in their blood, vitamin C may actually increase oxidative reactions instead of acting as an antioxidant. In these cases, ascorbate causes reduction of iron from the ferric to ferrous form which results in its release from proteins such as transferrin and ferritin [188]. The released ferrous iron can catalyze scission of lipid and hydrogen peroxide into free radical species which can oxidize lipids, proteins and nucleic acids. Over consumption of vitamin A can also be dangerous and result in blurred vision, lack of muscle coordination, birth defects and even comas and death [187]. An additional risk could also occur in different tissue types since high concentrations of β carotene in high oxygen environments can be prooxidative [189]. Dietary β carotene might be deleterious to health in tissues such as the lung where, in high amounts it has been found to increase cancer risk [190].

In recent years the number of nonessential antioxidant available as supplements has increase dramatically. Many of these supplements contain specific antioxidant compounds at concentrations which would be difficult if not impossible to obtain from dietary sources. The problem with nonessential antioxidant supplements is that very little is known about their overall health effects. While the evidence that dietary phenolics are beneficial to health is strong, whether their bioactivity is always related to their antioxidant activity needs further study. Many antioxidants can be both prooxidative (especially at high concentrations) and antioxidative [86,191], indicating that under certain conditions and in certain tissues the antioxidants could be more of an oxidative risk than a benefit. In addition, many nonessential antioxidants are known to influence the activity of a large number of biological functions through their ability to inhibit enzymes, inflammatory response, platelet aggregation and arachidonic acid metabolism. The ability of the nonessential antioxidants to influence biochemical pathways could explain why some phenolics such as catechins, caffeic acid, and sesamol sometimes promote cancer in animal tissues [192,193]. Due to the lack of knowledge of the exact mechanisms and magnitude by which nonessential antioxidants may effect health, consumption of large amounts of these compounds, in the form of either foods or supplements, may not be prudent until the bioactivity of these compounds is better understood.

5   SUMMARY

1. The diet provides both essential and nonessential antioxidants which may be beneficial to health. The essential antioxidants (Vitamins A, C and E) are found primarily in plant foods since animals are unable to synthesize these compounds.
2. Tocopherols consist of four isomers of varying vitamin E activity. Because tocopherols are lipid soluble compounds synthesized by plants, significant dietary sources include plant oils and plant foods that are either high in fat or lipid-containing organelles (e.g., chloroplasts). Once absorbed and transported, α-tocopherol is stored predominantly in adipose tissue where the turnover is slow and in the liver where turnover is fast so that tocopherol can be mobilized if needed.
3. Carotenoids consists of over 500 compounds of which several have Vitamin A activity. Dietary carotenoids are obtained from red, yellow and orange plant foods and also from foods high in chlorophyll. Carotenoids exist in *cis* and *trans* form, however, little is known about the properties of these isomers and how they affect specific functions. Storage of carotenoids occurs in lipids throughout the body.
4. Vitamin C is a water soluble antioxidant found in significant concentrations in plant food including berries, citrus fruits, broccoli and potatoes. Concentrations in foods can vary greatly since vitamin C degrades rapidly during cooking and storage. The transportation of vitamin C from the blood into tissues requires transporter proteins which are specific for the two vitamin C forms: ascorbic acid and dehydroascorbic acid. Vitamin C is stored predominantly in the adrenal glands.
5. Phenolics are nonessential antioxidants found in foods such as soybeans, tea, onions and fruits. Consumption of phenolics has been estimated to be up to 1 g per day due to the widespread existence of these compounds in plant foods.
6. Carnosine is a histidine-containing dipeptide found in high concentrations in muscle foods. Absorption of carnosine through the small intestine and its ability to inhibit cancer and LDL oxidation, suggests that it may be an important nonessential antioxidant.
7. Although nonessential antioxidants such as phenolics and carnosine are often consumed in higher quantities than the antioxidant vitamins, they are often absorbed and retained much less efficiently.
8. Antioxidants can modify numerous biochemical pathways and physiological functions besides oxidative reactions. Under certain circumstances, antioxidants can accelerate oxidative reactions. Since the chemical reactivity of anti-

oxidants can vary greatly, it may not be wise to consume large quantities of these dietary components until their physiological role is better understood.

6   PERSPECTIVES

The absorption, transport, and/or storage of many essential and nonessential antioxidants is just beginning to be understood. Information on the interaction of the various antioxidants with each other and with other nutrients is scant. Some antioxidants, like the carotenoids, occur in various isomers, and the advantages of different isomers are controversial. Many of the phenolic antioxidants have gained recent attention due to their presence in tea and wine, but the health benefits from ingesting tea and wine are not well-understood and many of the phenolics have been shown to be prooxidative in vitro. Data on the physiological functions and/or food concentrations of many other nonessential antioxidants such as ubiquinone, carnosine, polyamines, nucleotides and thiols is lacking so their role in the diet cannot be fully ascertained at this time.

The paucity of data regarding various antioxidant concentrations in foods or their action in the body, along with their purported health benefits, led to the concern that people are not ingesting sufficient amounts. This concern has fueled interest in supplements, and a wealth of antioxidant supplements, both essential and nonessential, have appeared on the market. Taking these supplements, especially in high amounts, may pose a greater risk than they do a benefit. Until more information is generated on food composition, bioavailability and function of various antioxidants, the public should be cautioned against their indiscriminate use.

7   ABBREVIATIONS

all-rac α-tocopherol:
   all-racemic alpha tocopherol
AA: ascorbic acid
ATP: adenosine 5' -triphosphate
CLA: conjugated linoleic acid
DHAA: 1-dehydroascorbic acid
DNA: deoxyribonucleic acid
GSH: glutathione (reduced)
GSSH: glutathione (oxidised)
HDL: high-density lipoprotein
LDL: low-density lipoprotein
OFO: oxidised frying oil
ppm: parts per million
PQQ: pyrroloquinoline quinone
RDA: recommended dietary allowance
VLDL: very low-density lipoprotein

8   REFERENCES

1. National Research Council. Recommended Dietary Allowances, 10th ed. National Academy Press: Washington DC, 1989.
2. Sokol RJ. In: Ziegler EE, Filer LJ Jr (eds). Present Knowledge In Nutrition. Washington DC:ILSI Press, 1996;130—136.
3. Papas AM. In: Simopoulos AP (ed) World Review of Nutrition and Dietetics: Nutrition and Fitness and Health and Disease. Basel, Switzerland: S. Karger, 1993;72:165—176.
4. Liebler DC. Crit Rev Toxicol 1993;23(2):147—169.
5. Basu TK, Dickerson JWT. Vitamins in human health and disease. UK:CAB International, 1996.
6. Groff JL, Gropper SS, Hunt SM. Advanced nutrition and human metabolism. 2nd edn. Minneapolis/St. Paul: West Publishing Company, 1995.
7. Holland B, Welch AA, Unwin ID, Buss DH, Paul AA, Southgate DAT. McCance and Widdowson's The Composition of Foods. 5th edn. UK: Royal Society of Chemistry, 1991.
8. Järvinen R. Int J Uit Nutr Res 1995;65(1):24—30.
9. Nakamura T, Takebe K, Imamura K, Tando Y, Yamada N, Arai Y, Terada A, Ishii M, Kikuchi H, Suda T. Acta Gastroenterol Belg 1996;59(1):10—14.
10. Winklhofer-Roob BM, Tuchschmid PE, Molinari L, Shmerling DH. Am J Clin Nutr 1996;63(5): 717—721.
11. Cheeseman KH, Holley AE, Kelly FJ, Wasil M, Hughes L, Burton G. Free Radic Biol Med 1995;19(5):591—598.
12. Munro LH, Burton G, Kelly FJ. Clin Sci (Colch) 1997;92(1):87—93.
13. Clément M, Bourre JM. Biochim Biophys Acta 1997;1334(2—3):173—181.
14. Brink EJ, Haddeman E, Tijburg LB. Br J Nutr 1996;75(6):939—948.
15. Ikeda I, Imasato Y, Sasaki E, Sugano M. Int J Vitam Nutr Res 1996;66(3):217—221.
16. Eicher SD, Morrill JL, Velazco J. J Dairy Sci 1997;80(2):393—399.
17. Kiyose C, Muramatsu R, Kameyama Y, Ueda T, Igarashi O. Am J Clin Nutr 1997;65(3): 785—789.
18. Cohn W. Eur J Clin Nutr 1997;51(Suppl1):S80—S85.
19. Kiyose C, Muramatsu R, Fujiyama-Fujiwara Y, Ueda T, Igarashi O. Lipids 1995;30(11):1015—1018.
20. Kiyose C, Muramatsu R, Ueda T, Igarashi O. Biosci Biotechnol Biochem 1995;59(5):791—795.
21. Hentati A, Deng HX, Hung WY, Nayer M, Ahmed MS, He X, Tim R, Stumpf DA, Siddique T, Ahmed. Ann Neurol 1996;39(3):295—300.
22. Traber MG, Sies H. Annu Rev Nutr 1996;16:321—347.
23. Hosomi A, Arita M, Sato Y, Kiyose C, Ueda T, Igarashi O, Arai H, Inoue K. FEBS Lett 1997; 409(1):105—108.
24. Kostner GM, Oettl K, Jauhiainen M, Ehnholm C, Esterbauer H, Dieplinger H. Biochem J 1995;305(Part2):659—667.
25. Toutain PL, Hidiroglou M, Charmley E. J Dairy Sci 1995;78(7):1561—1566.
26. Chan KM, Decker EA. Crit Rev Food Sci Nutr 1994;34(4):403—426.
27. Camu G, Pincemail J, Roesgen A, Dreezen E, Sluse FE, Deby C. Arch Int Physiol Biochem 1990;98:121—126.
28. Gordon MJ, Campbell FM, Duthie GG, Dutta-Roy AK. Arch Biochem Biophys 1995;318(1): 140—146.
29. Bonina F, Lanza M, Montenegro L, Salerno L, Smeriglio P, Trombetta D, Saija A. Pharmacol Res 1996;13(9):1343—1347.
30. Schelling GT, Roeder RA, Garber MJ, Pumfrey WM. J Nutr 1995;125(6,Suppl):1799S—1803S.
31. Kamal-Eldin A, Pettersson D, Appelqvist LA. Lipids 1995;30(6):499—505.
32. Ueda T, Ueda T, Armstrong D. Ophthalmic Res 1996;28(30):184—192.
33. Liu JF, Huang CJ. J Nutr 1995;125(120):3071—3080.

34. Olson JA. Vitamin A. In: Ziegler EE, Filer Jr LJ (eds) Present Knowledge In Nutrition. Washington, DC: ILSI Press, 1996:109—119.
35. Olson JA. In: Shils ME, Olson JA, Shike M. Modern Nutrition in Health and Disease. 8th edn. Philadelphia:Lea & Febiger, 1994:287—307.
36. Stahl W, Sies H. Arch Biochem Biophys 1996;336(1):1—9.
37. Rock CL, Jacob RA, Bowen PE. J Am Diet Assoc 1996;96(7):693—702.
38. Yeum KJ, Booth SL, Sadowski JA, Liu C, Tang G, Krinsky NI, Russell RM. Am J Clin Nutr 1996;64(4):594—602.
39. Gärtner C, Stahl W, Sies H. Am J Clin Nutr 1997:66(1):116—122.
40. Stahl W, Sies H. J Nutr 1992;122(11):2161—2166.
41. Yadav SK, Sehgal S. Plant Foods Hum Nutr 1995;47(2):125—131.
42. Tang G, Serfaty-Lacrosniere C, Camilo ME, Russell RM. Am J Clin Nutr 1996;64(4):622—626.
43. Zhi J, Melia AT, Koss-Twardy SG, Arora S, Patel IH. J Clin Pharm 1996;36(2):152—159.
44. Novotny JA, Dueker SR, Zech LA, Clifford AJ. J Lipid Res 1995;36(8):1825—1838.
45. Lakshman MR, Liu QH, Sapp R, Somanchi M, Sundaresan PR. Nutr Cancer 1996;26(1):49—61.
46. Wingerath T, Stahl W, Sies H. Arch Biochem Biophys 1995;324(2):385—390.
47. Bierer TL, Merchen NR, Erdman JW Jr. J Nutr 1995;125(6):1569—1577.
48. Kostic D, White WS, Olson JA. Am J Clin Nutr 1995;62(3):604—610.
49. Britton G. FASEB J 1995;9(15):1551—1558.
50. Johnson EJ, Krinsky NI, Russell RM. J Am Coll Nutr 1996;15(6):620—624.
51. Stahl W, Schwarz W, Sies H. J Nutr 1993;123(5):847—851.
52. Gaziano JM, Johnson EJ, Russell RM, Manson JE, Stampfer MJ, Ridker PM, Frei B, Hennekens CH, Krinsky NI. Am J Clin Nutr 1995;61(6):1248—1252.
53. Amai H, Morinobu T, Murata T, Manago M, Mino M. Lipids 1995;30(6):493—498.
54. Levin G, Mokady S. Lipids 1995;30(2):177—179.
55. You CS, Parker RS, Goodman KJ, Swanson JE, Corso TN. Am J Clin Nutr 1996:64(2):177—183.
56. Ben-Amotz A, Levy Y. Am J Clin Nutr 1996;63(5):729—734.
57. Levin G, Yeshurun M, Mokady S. Nutr Cancer 1997;27(3):293—297.
58. Ziouzenkova O, Winklhofer-Roob BM, Puhl H, Roob JM, Esterbauer H. J Lipid Res 1996;37(9):1936—1946.
59. Gugger ET; Erdman JW Jr. J Nutr 1996;126:1470—1474.
60. Yamanushi T, Igarashi O. J Nutr Sci Vitaminol (Tokyo) 1995;41(2):169—177.
61. Redlich CA, Grauer JN, Van Bennekum AM, Clever SL, Ponn RB, Blaner WS. Am J Respir Crit Care Med 1996;154(50);1436—1443.
62. Schweigert FJ, Rosival I, Rambeck WA, Gropp J. Int J Uit Nutr Res1995;65(2):95—100.
63. Sies H, Stahl W. Am J Clin Nutr 1995;62:1315S—1321S.
64. Wang XD, Marini RP, Hebuterne X, Fox JG, Krinsky NI, Russell RM. Gastroenterology 1995;108(3):719—726.
65. van Vliet T, van Vlissingen MF, van Schaik F, van den Berg H. J Nutr, 1996 Feb,126:(2);499—508
66. Ross MA, Crosley LK, Brown KM, Duthie SJ, Collins AC, Arthur JR, Duthie GG. Eur J Clin Nutr 1995;49(11):861—865.
67. Brady WE, Mares-Perlman JA, Bowen P, Stacewicz-Sapuntzakis M. J Nutr 1996;126(1):129—137.
68. Handelman GJ, Packer L, Cross CE. Am J Clin Nutr 1996:63(4):559—565.
69. Winklhofer-Roob BM; van't Hof MA; Shmerling DH. Acta Paediatrica 1995;84:132—1136.
70. Levine M, Rumsey S, Wang Y, Park J, Kwon O, Xu W, Amano N. In: Ziegler EE, Filer LJ Jr.(eds) Present Knowledge In Nutrition. Washington, DC: ILSI Press, 1996:146—159.
71. Jacob RA. In: Shils ME, Olson JA, Shike M. Modern Nutrition in Health and Disease. 8th edn. Philadelphia: Lea & Febiger, 1994:432—448.

72. Levine M, Dhariwal KR, Welch RW, Wang Y, Park JB. Am J Clin Nutr 1995;62:1347S—1356S.
73. Levine M, Conry-Cantilena C, Wang Y, Welch RW, Washko PW et al. Proc Natl Acad Sci USA 1996;93(8):3704—3709.
74. Sauberlich HE, Tamura T, Craig CB, Freeberg LE, Liu T. Am J Clin Nutr 1996;64(3):336—346.
75. Weber P, Bendich A, Schalch W. Int J Vitam Nutr Res 1996;66(1):19—30.
76. Welch RW, Wang Y, Crossman A Jr, Park JB, Kirk KL, Levine M. J Biol Chem 1995;270(21): 12584—12592.
77. Vera JC, Rivas CI, Velásquez FV, Zhang RH, Concha II, Golde DW. J Biol Chem 1995;270(40): 23706—23712.
78. Spielholz C, Golde DW, Houghton AN, Nualart F, Vera JC. Cancer Res 1997;57(12): 2529—2537.
79. Ngkeekwong FC, Ng LL. Biochem J 1997;324(1):225—230.
80. Bergsten P; Yu R; Kehrl J; Levine M. Arch Biochem Biophys 1995;317(1):208—214.
81. Lynch SR. Nutr Rev 1997;55(4):102—110.
82. Niki E, Noguchi N, Tsuchihashi H, Gotoh N. Am J Clin Nutr 1995;62(6)(Suppl):1322S—1326S.
83. Shahidi F, Wanasundara JPK. Crit Rev Food Sci Nutr 1992;32:67.
84. Laughton M J, Evans PJ, Moroney MA, Hoult JRS et al. Biochem Pharmacol, 1991;42(9):1673.
85. Morgan JF, Klucas RV, Grayer RJ, Abian J et al. Free Radic Biol Med 1997;22(5):861—870.
86. Nawar WW. In: Fennema O (ed) Lipids, Food Chemistry, 3rd edn. NY Marcel Dekker, 1996;225.
87. Iverson F. Cancer Lett 1995;93:49—54.
88. Huang MT, Ferraro T. In: Ho CT, Lee CY, Huang MT (eds) Phenolic compounds in food and their effects on health. Vol 2. Antioxidants and Cancer Prevention. Am Chem Soc 1992;8—34.
89. Aruoma OI, Halliwell B, Aeschbach R, Löligers J. Xenobiotica 1992;22(2):257.
90. Kinsella JE, Frankel E, German B, Kanner J. Food Sci Technol Today 1993:85—89.
91. Balentine DA. In: Ho C-T, Lee CY, Huang M-T (eds) Phenolic compounds in foods and their effects on health. Vol 1. Analysis, occurrence, and Chemistry. Am Chem Soc, Washington, DC 1992;102—17.
92. von Gadow A, Joubert E, Hansmann CF. J Agricul Food Chem 1997;45:1370—1374.
93. Meyer AS, Yi O-S, Pearson DA, Waterhouse et al. J Agricul Food Chem 1997;45:1638—1643.
94. Simonetti P, Pietta P, Testolin G. J Agricul Food Chem 1997;45:1152—1155.
95. Singleton VL. Am J Enol Vittic 1987;38:69-77.
96. Wang HJ, Murphy PA. J Agricul Food Chem 1994;42:1666—1673.
97. Unno T, Takeo T. Biosci Biotechnol Biochem 1995;59(8):1558—1559.
98. Okushio K, Matsumoto N, Kohri T, Suzuki M et al. Biol Pharm Bull 1996;19(2):326—329.
99. Serafini M, Ghiselli A, Ferro-Luzzi A. Eur J Clin Nutr 1996;50(1):28—32.
100. He YH, Kies C. Plant Foods Hum Nutr 1994;46(3):221—228.
101. Gooderham MJ, Herman A, Ojala ST, Wähälä K et al. J Nutr 1996;126:2000—2006.
102. Tew B-Y, Xu X, Wang H-J, Murphy PA et al. J Nutr 1996;126:871—877.
103. Xu X, Wang H-J, Murphy PA, Cook L et al. J Nut 1994;124:825—832.
104. Pietta PG, Gardana C, Mauri PL, Maffei-Facino R et al. J Chromatogr 1995;673:75—80.
105. Manach C, Morand C, Texier O, Favier M-L et al. J Nutr 1995;125:1911—1922.
106. Fuhr U, Kummert AL. Clin Pharmacol Ther 1995;58(4):365—373.
107. Miller DD. In: Fennema O,(ed). Food Chemistry 3rd edn. Marcel Dekker, NY, 1996;617.
108. Ikeda I, Imasato Y, Sasaki E, Nakayama M et al. Biochim Biophys Acta 1992;1127(2):141—146.
109. Paz M A, Fluckiger R, Gallop PM. The Biomedical Significance of PQQ, Principles and Applications of Quinoproteins. Marcel Dekker, Inc, New York, 1992.
110. Killgore J, Smidt L, Dutch et al. Science 1989;245:850—851.
111. Van Der Meer RA, Van Wassenaar PD, Van Brouwershaven JH, Duine JA. Biochem Biophys Res Commun 1989;159(2):726—733.
112. Lobenstein-Verbeek CL, Jongejan JA, Frank J, Duine JA. FEBS Lett 1984; 170(2):305—309.
113. Smidt CR, Steinberg FM, Rucker RB. Proc Soc Exp Biol Med 1991;197:19—26.

114. Hamagishi Y, Murata S, Kamei H, Oki T, Adachi O et al. J Pharmacol Exp Ther 1990;255(3): 980–985.
115. Xu F, Mack CP, Quandt KS, Schlafer M, Massey V, Hultquist DE. Biochem Biophys Res Commun 1993;193:434–439.
116. Jensen FE, Gardner GJ, Williams AP, Gallop PM et al. Neuroscience 1994;62(2):399–406.
117. Smidt CR, Unkefer CJ, Houck DR, Rucker RB. Proc Soc Exp Biol Med 1991;197:27–31.
118. Kumazawa T, Seno H, Urakami T, Matsumoto T et al. Biochimica Biophys Acta 1992;1156: 62–66.
119. Zubay G. In: Rogers B (ed) Biochemistry. Reading: Addison-Wesley Publishing Company, MA, 1984.
120. Cabrini L, Pasquali P, Tadolini B, Sechi AM, Landi L. Free Rad Res Commun 1986;2:85.
121. Zhang Y, Turunen M, Appelkvist E-L. J Nutr 1996;126:2089–2097.
122. Zhang Y, Åberg F, Appelkvist E-L, Dallner G et al. J Nutr 1995;125:446–453.
123. Folkers K, Moesgaard S, Morita M. Molec Aspect Med 1994;15(Suppl):s281–s285.
124. Laaksonen R, Fogelhom M, Himberg J-J, Laakso J, Salorinne Y. Eur J Appl Physiol 1995; 72:95–100.
125. Ha YL, Grimm NK, Pariza MW. Carcinogenesis 1987;8:1881–1887.
126. Ip C, Singh M, Thomspon HJ, Scimeca JA. Cancer Res 1994;54:1212–1215.
127. Nicolosi RJ, Rogers EJ, Kritchevsky D, Scimeca JA et al. Artery 1997;22(5):266–277.
128. Lee KN, Kritchevsky D, Pariza MW. Atherosclerosis 1994;108(1):19–25.
129. Chin SF, Storkson JM, Liu W, Albright KJ et al. Am Inst Nutr 1994:1–8.
130. Ha YL, Storkson J, Pariza MW. Cancer Res 1990;50:1097–1101.
131. Ip C, Chin SF, Scimeca JA, Pariza MW. Cancer Res 1991;51:6118–6124.
132. van den Berg JJM, Cook NE, Tribble DL. Lipids 1995;30(7)599–605.
133. Livisay SA. Ph.D. Dissertation, University of Massachusetts, Amherst, 1998.
134. Chin SF, Liu W, Storkson JM, Ha YL et al. J Food Comp Anal 1992;5:185–197.
135. Shantha NC, Crum AD, Decker EA. J Agricul Food Chem 1994;42:1757–1760.
136. Shantha NC, Ram LN, O'Leary J, Hicks CL. J Food Sci 1995;60:695–697,720.
137. Jiang J, Bjoerck L, Fonden R, Emanuelson M. J Dairy Sci 1996;79(3):438–445.
138. Huang Y-C, Luedecke LO, Shultz TD. Nutr Res 1994;14(3):373–386.
139. Chin SF, Storkson JM, Liu W, Albright KJ et al. J Nutr 1994;124:694–701.
140. Crush KG. Comp Biochem Physiol 1970;34:3.
141. Davey CL. Arch Biochem Biophys 1960;89:303.
142. Harris RC, Marlin DJ, Dunnett M, Snow DH et al. Comp Biochem Physiol 1990;97A:249.
143. Boldyrev AA, Dupin AM, Bunin AY, Babizhaev MA et al. Biochem Int 1987;15:1105–1113.
144. Boldyrev AA, Dupin AM, Pindel E, Severin SE. Comp Biochem Physiol 1988;89B(2):245.
145. Kohen R, Yamamoto Y, Cundy KC, Ames B. Proc Natl Acad Sci USA 1988;85:3175.
146. Decker EA, Crum AD, Calvert JT. J Agric Food Chem 1992;40:756
147. Rubtsov AM, Schara M, Sentiurc M, Boldyrev AA. Acta Pharm Jugosl 1991;41:401.
148. Chan KM, Decker EA, Lee JB, Butterfield DA. J Agric Food Chem 1994;42:461.
149. Dahl TA, Midden WR, Hartman PE. Phytochem Phytobiol 1988;47:357.
150. Egorov SY, Kurella EG, Boldyrev AA, Krasnovskii AA. Bioorg Khim 1992;19(1):169–172.
151. Aruoma OI, Laughton MJ, Halliwell B. Biochem J 1989;264(3):863.
152. Yoshikawa T, Naito Y, Tanigawa T, Yoneta T et al. Free Rad Res Commun 1991;14(4):289.
153. Ferraris RP, Diamond J, Kwan WW. Am J Physiol 1988;225(2):G143–G150.
154. Gardner MLG, Illingworth KM, Kelleher J, Wood D. J Physiol 1991;439:411–418.
155. Jackson MC, Kucera CM, Lenney JF. Clin Chim Acta, 1991;196:193–206.
156. Wolos A, Jablonowska C, Faruga A, Jankowski J. Comp Biochem Physiol 1982;71A:145–148.
157. Abe H. Comp Biochem Physiol 1991;100B(4):717–720.
158. Fuller AT, Neuberger A, Webster TA. Biochem J 1947;41:11–18.
159. Tamaki N, Funatsuka A, Fujimotot S, Hama T. J Nutr Sci Vitaminol 1984;30:541–551.
160. Easter RA, Baker DH. J Nutr 1977;107:120–125.

161. Mei L, Cromwell GL, Crum AD, Decker EA. Meat Sci 1997;(in press).
162. Chan WKM, Decker EA, Chow CK, Biossonneault GA. Lipids 1994;29:461—466.
163. Gorbunov N, Erin A. Bull Exp Biol Med 1991;11:111—116.
164. McManus IR. J Biol Chem 1960;235:1398—1403.
165. Decker EA, Mei L. Reciprocal Meat Conference Proceedings 1996;49:64—72.
166. Decker EA. Nutr Rev 1995;53(3):49—58.
167. Lovaas E, Carlin G. Free Rad Biol Med 1991;11:455.
168. Droplet GL, Dumbroff EB, Legge RL, Thompson JE. Phytochem 1986;25:367.
169. Matsushita S, Ibuki F, Aoki A. Arch Biochem Biophys 1963;102:446.
170. Hultin HO. In: Fennema O,(ed). Food Chemistry 2nd edn. Marcel Dekker, NY, 1985;725.
171. Tzeng E, Billiar TR. In: Fantini GA (ed) Ischemia-Reperfusion Injury of Skeletal Muscle. RG Landes Co, Austin, TX 1994;103.
172. Hochstein P, Hatch L, Sevanian A. Meth Enzymol 1984;105:162.
173. Wayner DDM, Burton GW, Ingold KU, Barclay LRC et al. Biochim Biophys Acta 1987;924:408.
174. Frei B, Stocker R, Ames BN. Proc Natl Acad Sci USA 1988;85:9748.
175. Buettner G R. Arch Biochem Biophys 1993;300(2)535.
176. Lee SK, Mei L, Decker EA. J Food Sci 1996;61:726—728,795.
177. Jia T-D, Kelleher S, Hultin HO, Petillo D et al. J Agricul Food Chem 1996;44:1195.
178. Witschi A, Reddy S, Stofer B, Lauterburg BH. Eur J Clin Pharmacol 1992;43(6):667—669.
179. Grattagliano I, Wieland P, Schranz C, Lauterburg BH. Pharmacol Toxicol 1994;75(6):343—347.
180. Podda M, Tritschler HJ, Ulrich H, Packer L. Biochem Biophys Res Commun 1994;204(1): 98—104.
181. Constantinescu A, Pick U, Handelsman GJ, Haramaki N et al. Biochem Pharmacol 1995;50(2): 253—261.
182. Vianey-Liaud N, Kobrehel K, Sauvaire Y, Wong JH. J Agricul Food Chem 1994;42:1110—1114.
183. Mattulat A, Baltes W. Z Lebensm Uters Forsch 1992;194(4):326—329.
184. Graf E, Eaton JW. Free Rad Biol Med 1990;8:61.
185. Zhou JR, Erdman JW. Crit Rev Food Sci Nutr 1995;35(6):495—508.
186. Krajcovicova-Kudlackov M, Simoncic R, Bederova A, Klvanova J. et al. Nahrung 1996;40(1): 17—20.
187. Smolin LA, Grosvenor MB. Nutrition science and applications. Saunders College Publishing, 1994.
188. Herbert V. Nutr Today 1993;28:28—32.
189. Burton GW, Ingold KU. Science 1984;224:569.
190. Omenn GS, Goodman GE, Thornquist MD, Balmes J et al. N Engl J Med 1996;334:1150—1155.
191. Decker, EA. Nutr Rev 1997;55(10):(in press).
192. Hirose M, Kawabe M, Shibata M, Takahashs et al. Carcinogenesis 1992;13:1825—1928.
193. Ito N, Hirose M, Shirai T. In: Ho C-T, Lee CY, Huang M-T (eds) Phenolic compounds in food and their effects on health. Vol 2. Antioxidants and Cancer Prevention. Am Chem Soc 1992; 269—283.
194. Leighton T, Ginther C, Fluss L, Harter WK et al. In: Huang M-T, Ho C-T, Lee C Y,(eds). Phenoloic compounds in food and their effects on health 2. Antioxidants and cancer prevention. American Chemical Society, Washington, DC 1991;507:220—238.
195. Rommel A, Wrolstad RE, Durst RW. In: Huang M-T, Ho C-T, Lee C Y (eds) Phenoloic compounds in food and their effects on health 1. Analysis, occurence, and chemistry. American Chemical Society, Washington, DC 1991;506:259—286.
196. Hertog MGL, Hollman PCH, Katan MB. J Agricul Food Chem 1992;40:2379—2383.
197. Kovac V, Alonso E, Bourzeix M, Revilla E. J Agricul Food Chem 1992;40:1953—1957.
198. Kumazawa T, Seno H, Suzuki O. Biochem Biophys Res Commun 1993;193(1):1—5.
199. Kumazawa T, Sato K, Seno H, Ishii A et al. Biochem J 1995;307:331—333.

200. Hernández-Jover T, Izquierdo-Pulido M, Veciana-Nogués T, Vidal-Carou MC. J Agricul Food Chem 1996;44:2710—2715.
201. Yamanaka H, Shinakura K, Shiomi K, Kikuchi T et al. Nippon Suisan Gakkaishi 1987;53:2041.

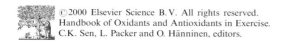
©2000 Elsevier Science B.V. All rights reserved.
Handbook of Oxidants and Antioxidants in Exercise.
C.K. Sen, L. Packer and O. Hänninen, editors.

Part V • Chapter 14

Vitamin E

Maret G. Traber

Department of Nutrition and Food Management, Linus Pauling Institute, Oregon State University,
Corvallis Dr 97331; Department of Internal Medicine, University of California, Davis, USA.
Tel.: +1-541-737-7977. Fax: +1-541-737-5077. E-mail: maret.traber@orst.edu

1   INTRODUCTION
2   WHAT IS VITAMIN E AND WHAT DOES IT DO?
    2.1   Vitamin E structures
    2.2   Antioxidant activity
3   HISTORY
4   VITAMIN E ABSORPTION, TRANSPORT AND METABOLISM
    4.1   Intestinal absorption
    4.2   Secretion of α-tocopherol from the liver
    4.3   Hepatic α-tocopherol transfer protein and other tocopherol binding proteins
    4.4   Plasma vitamin E kinetics
    4.5   Vitamin E delivery to tissues
    4.6   Metabolism
5   REQUIREMENTS AND RECOMMENDED INTAKES
    5.1   Vitamin E units
    5.2   Recommended intakes
    5.3   Dietary vitamin E
6   SUMMARY
7   ABBREVIATIONS
8   REFERENCES

1   INTRODUCTION

Vitamin E is a chain-breaking antioxidant, which means that once lipid peroxidation begins, vitamin E stops it from progressing further. This antioxidant function is quite important with relationship to exercise because exercise increases the throughput of energy in the mitochondria and thereby increases the number of radicals escaping the electron transport chain.

Vitamin E requirements are dependent upon the degree of oxidative stress, the dietary polyunsaturated fatty acid (PUFA) intake and the intake of other antioxidants. Furthermore, vitamin E activity is dependent upon an "antioxidant network" involving a wide variety of antioxidants and antioxidant enzymes, which functions to maintain vitamin E in its unoxidized state, ready to intercept and scavenge radicals [1].

This chapter will describe the antioxidant properties of vitamin E, its lipoprotein transport and delivery to tissues, and illustrate functional aspects with relationship to vitamin E in exercise.

2   WHAT IS VITAMIN E AND WHAT DOES IT DO?

2.1 Vitamin E structures

Vitamin E is a fat soluble vitamin; the most biologically potent form of which is α-tocopherol. There are eight different naturally occurring forms which display the biologic activity of α-tocopherol. These include four tocopherols and four tocotrienols; tocotrienols differ from tocopherols in that they have an unsaturated side chain; Greek symbols describe their chromanol structures. The α-form has three methyl groups, β- or γ-forms have 2 and the δ-forms have one (Fig. 1).

Synthetic vitamin E, all-rac-α-tocopherol (incorrectly called d,l-α-tocopherol), is not identical to the naturally occurring form, RRR-α-tocopherol (also called

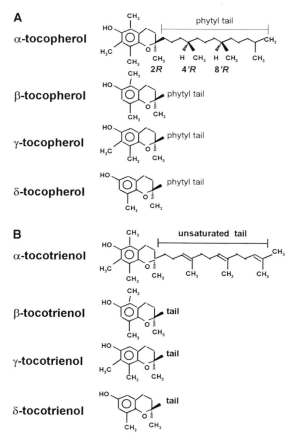

Fig. 1. Vitamin E structures. There are eight naturally occurring forms of vitamin E, the four tocopherols are shown in **A** and the four tocotrienols in **B**. Shown is the natural RRR-α-tocopherol stereochemistry; the three chiral centers give rise to eight different stereoisomers in synthetic vitamin E (all rac–α-tocopherol). These are: RRR-, RRS-, RSR-, RSS-, SRR-, SSR-, SRS-, SSS-.

d-α-tocopherol). all-rac-α-Tocopherol contains eight stereoisomers, arising from the three chiral centers in the phytyl tail (Fig. 1: 2R,4′R,8′R). The naturally occurring and most biologically active vitamin E form is only one of the eight stereoisomers present in all rac-α-tocopherol. In general, the 2S-forms have lower activity than the 2R-forms [2,3].

Vitamin E supplements often contain esters of α-tocopherol, such as α-tocopheryl acetate, succinate or nicotinate. The ester forms prevent oxidation of vitamin E during storage. The esters are readily hydrolyzed in the gut and unesterified tocopherol is absorbed [4].

2.2 Antioxidant activity

Vitamin E functions in vivo as a chain-breaking antioxidant that prevents the propagation of free radical damage in biological membranes [5—8]. When lipid hydroperoxides are oxidized to peroxyl radicals (ROO·), vitamin E reacts 1000 times faster with these than do polyunsaturated fatty acids in membrane or lipoprotein lipids [1]. Further information concerning the antioxidant reactions of tocopherols and tocotrienols in vivo and in vitro can be found in the extensive review by Kamal-Eldin and Appelqvist [9].

The vitamin E radical formed during lipid peroxidation readily reacts with other antioxidants and is reduced itself to the unoxidized form. Vitamin E reductants, which have been demonstrated in vitro to regenerate tocopherol from the tocopheroxyl radical, include ubiquinol [10], ascorbate (vitamin C), and thiols [11], especially glutathione [12—15]. Subsequently, ubiquinone, vitamin C, and thiyl radicals can be reduced by various metabolic processes. This process has been termed "vitamin E recycling", where the antioxidant function of the one electron oxidized form of vitamin E is continuously restored by other antioxidants [1]. This antioxidant network depends upon the continuous supply of aqueous antioxidants and the metabolic activity of cells.

3   HISTORY

Vitamin E deficiency was first described by Evans and Bishop [16] at the University of California in Berkeley in 1922 during their investigations of infertility in rancid lard-fed rats. In 1936, Evans et al. [17] isolated a factor from wheat germ with the biologic activity of vitamin E. They named this factor, "α-tocopherol" a name derived from the Greek "tokos" (offspring) and "pherein" (to bear) with an "ol" to indicate that it was an alcohol. Two other tocopherols, β- and γ-, were isolated from vegetable oils in the subsequent year and it was noted that these had lower biologic activities than α-tocopherol [18].

Vitamin E biologic activity was defined by Machlin [19], as the ability to prevent or reverse specific vitamin E deficiency symptoms (e.g., fetal resorption, muscular dystrophy and encephalomalacia). The most popular, though most tedious and time consuming, assay for the biologic activity of vitamin E is the fetal resorption assay [19]. Here, the vitamin E biologic activity depends on the amount necessary to maintain the maximum number of live fetuses.

Vitamin E deficiency symptoms in various animal species were described by Machlin [19] in his comprehensive book on vitamin E. Necrotizing myopathy, anemia and the accumulation of lipofuscin (a fluorescent pigment of "aging") in tissues of vitamin E-deficient animals are signs of vitamin E deficiency in animals. Horwitt [20,21] attempted to induce vitamin E deficiency in men by feeding a diet low in vitamin E for 6 years to volunteers at the Elgin State Hospital in Illinois. After about 2 years, their serum vitamin E levels decreased into the deficient range. Although their erythrocytes were more sensitive to peroxide-induced hemolysis, anemia did not develop.

It was not until the mid 60s that vitamin E deficiency was described in children with fat malabsorption syndromes, principally abetalipoproteinemia and cholestatic liver disease, as reviewed by Sokol [22]. By the mid 80s, it was clear that in humans the major vitamin E deficiency symptom was a peripheral neuropathy characterized by the degeneration of the large caliber axons in the sensory neurons [22]. Subsequently, patients with peripheral neuropathies without fat malabsorption, who were vitamin E-deficient, were described [23]. Studies in such patients have now opened new avenues in vitamin E investigations because these patients were found to have a genetic defect in the hepatic α-tocopherol transfer protein [24].

4 VITAMIN E ABSORPTION, TRANSPORT AND METABOLISM

4.1 Intestinal absorption

Vitamin E absorption from the small intestine is dependent upon processes necessary for fat digestion and uptake into enterocytes. Pancreatic esterases are required for release of free fatty acids from dietary triglycerides. Generally, these esterases are quite effective; the apparent absorption of deuterated RRR-α-tocopherol was similar whether administered as α-tocopherol, α-tocopheryl acetate or α-tocopheryl succinate [4]. Bile acids are also required for vitamin E absorption [25,26] because they along with monoglycerides and free fatty acids are important components of mixed micelles [27].

Vitamin E is absorbed into the intestinal mucosa. It is here that chylomicrons containing triglycerides, free and esterified cholesterol, phospholipids, and apolipoproteins (especially apolipoprotein (apo) B48) are synthesized and secreted into the lymph [28]. Chylomicrons also contain vitamin E, along with other fat-soluble vitamins, carotenoids and other fat-soluble dietary components.

Fractional vitamin E absorption has been estimated in humans. In the early 70s, vitamin E absorption was estimated to be 51−86%, measured as fecal radioactivity following ingestion of [³H]-α-tocopherol [29,30]. However, when Blomstrand and Forsgren [31] cannulated the thoracic lymph ducts in two subjects with gastric carcinoma and lymphatic leukemia, respectively, and measured vitamin E absorption, they found fractional absorption to be only 21 and 29% of [^{3}H]-α-tocopherol and [^{3}H]-α-tocopheryl acetate, respectively. Although these estimates are quite disparate, it is likely that only a fraction of a given amount of vitamin E ingested is absorbed.

Often it is assumed that differences in plasma concentrations of various forms of vitamin E result from differences in the degree of intestinal absorption. But, this is not the case. Various forms of vitamin E, such as α- and γ-tocopherols [32,33], or RRR- and SRR-α-tocopherols [34,35], were absorbed, similarly secreted in chylomicrons and appeared in the plasma in equal concentrations.

During chylomicron catabolism in the circulation, the size of the chylomicron triglyceride core is reduced and excess surface is created. This excess surface is transferred to high density lipoproteins (HDL) [34]. During this process, vitamin E is also transferred to HDL. Because HDL readily transfer vitamin E to other lipoproteins [37–41], vitamin E is distributed to all of the circulating lipoproteins (Fig. 2). Kostner et al. [42] have demonstrated that the plasma phospholipid transfer protein (PLTP) potentiates this process.

4.2 Secretion of α-tocopherol from the liver

Following partial delipidation, chylomicron remnants are taken up by the liver. These remnants likely contain a major portion of absorbed vitamin E. The dietary fats contained in the remnants are then repackaged and secreted into the plasma in very low density lipoproteins (VLDL) [34]. Like chylomicrons, VLDL have a triglyceride-rich core, but they have apolipoprotein β-100 (apoB 100) as a major apolipoprotein instead of apoB 48 [34]. Vitamin E is secreted from the liver in VLDL, as demonstrated in rats [43] and in isolated rat hepatocytes [43,44]. In the circulation, VLDL are delipidated to form LDL, which retain apoB 100. LDL then interact with receptors for apoB 100 in peripheral tissues, as well as in the liver. During VLDL delipidation, similarly to that described above for chylomicron catabolism, vitamin E is transferred to HDL, which can transfer vitamin E to all of the circulating lipoproteins. Unlike other fat-soluble vitamins, which have specific plasma transport proteins, vitamin E is nonspecifically transported in plasma lipoproteins.

Plasma vitamin E concentrations do depend upon liver vitamin E secretion [34,44,45]. Remarkably, only one form of vitamin E, RRR-α-tocopherol, is preferentially secreted from the liver, as illustrated in Fig. 3. In nascent VLDL, isolated from perfusates of livers from cynomolgus monkeys fed 24 h previously with various deuterated tocopherols, RRR-α-tocopherol represented about 80% of the total secreted deuterated tocopherols [47]. Thus the liver, not the intestine, discriminates between tocopherols. The liver contains the α-tocopherol transfer protein (α-TTP), which is a likely candidate for this function.

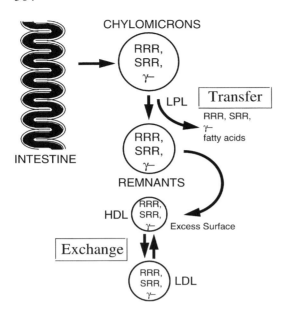

Fig. 2. Pathways for absorption of vitamin E and its delivery to tissues during chylomicron catabolism. Vitamin E absorption requires bile acids (secreted from the liver) and fatty acids and monoglycerides (released from dietary fat by pancreatic enzymes) for micelle formation. Following uptake into enterocytes of the intestine, all forms of dietary vitamin E are incorporated and secreted into the lymph in chylomicrons. These triglyceride-rich lipoproteins are secreted into the circulation where lipolysis by lipoprotein lipase (LPL) bound to the endothelial lining of capillary walls takes place. Chylomicron remnants are formed in the circulation by this process. During lipolysis, the various forms of vitamin E are transferred to tissues or to high density lipoproteins (HDL). Vitamin E can exchange between HDL and other circulating lipoproteins, which can also deliver vitamin E to peripheral tissues. This process is important for the delivery of dietary and supplemental vitamin E to the circulating lipoproteins. However, it is insufficient to maintain normal plasma vitamin E concentrations because patients who lack the α-tocopherol transfer protein become vitamin E deficient. Thus, secretion of α-tocopherol from the liver shown in Fig. 3 is essential. Figure modified from [84].

4.3 Hepatic α-tocopherol transfer protein and other tocopherol binding proteins

α-TTP (∼ 32 kDa) was first identified [48], purified and characterized [49,50] from rat liver cytosol. It has also been isolated from human liver cytosol [51] and its cDNA sequence reported [52]. The human protein has 94% homology to the rat protein, and some homology both to the retinaldehyde binding protein in the retina and to sec14, a phospholipid transfer protein [52]. The gene has been localized to the 8q13.1-13.3 region of chromosome 8 [52,53]. It has only been identified in hepatocytes [50].

Purified α-TTP preferentially transfers α-tocopherol between liposomes and microsomes [49]. Both α- and β-tocopherols are effective competitors, γ-tocopherol is about half as effective and Δ-tocopherol is about 1/3 as effective; α-tocopheryl acetate, tocopherol quinone and cholesterol were ineffective competi-

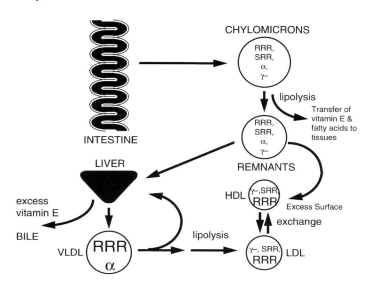

Fig. 3. Pathways for the preferential delivery of α-tocopherol to peripheral tissues. Chylomicron remnants containing various forms of vitamin E are taken up by the liver. In the liver, the α-tocopherol transfer protein is involved in the incorporation α-tocopherol into nascent very low density lipoproteins (VLDL). Following VLDL secretion into plasma, lipolysis of VLDL by lipoprotein lipase and hepatic triglyceride lipase results in the preferential enrichment of circulating lipoproteins with RRR-α-tocopherol. The catabolism of these lipoproteins results in the delivery of RRR-α-tocopherol to peripheral tissues. It has been estimated that the process shown in this figure results in the replacement of all of the circulating vitamin E [57]. Figure modified from [84].

tors [49]. Hypothetically, this ability to preferentially transfer RRR-α-tocopherol is necessary for the biologic activity of RRR-α-tocopherol [47,54].

Dutta-Roy et al. [54,55] have reported that both the liver and the heart contain an α-tocopherol-binding protein with a mass of 14.2 kDa. This protein is present in the liver in addition to α-TTP. The 14.2 kDa protein also transfers α-tocopherol in preference to γ- or δ-tocopherols. They suggest that the 14.2 kDa tocopherol binding protein might regulate cellular α-tocopherol concentrations.

4.4 Plasma vitamin E kinetics

Vitamin E turnover has been estimated from a kinetic model using data from studies with deuterium-labeled stereoisomers of α-tocopherol (RRR- and SRR-) [57]. The mathematical model assumes that the intestinal absorption and secretion of the two deuterated tocopherols (RRR- and SRR-α-tocopherols) into chylomicrons are similar and that the initial inputs into the plasma occur simultaneously for the two labels. In three patients with ataxia and vitamin E deficiency (abbreviated AVED), who have genetically defective α-TTP [24], the fractional disappearance rates of deuterium-labeled RRR- and SRR-α-tocopherols in plasma were measured. The disappearance rates were similar for the two stereoisomers (1.4 ± 0.6 and 1.3 ± 0.3 pools per day, respectively), with a half-life of approximately 13 h for each. Thus, in AVED patients both RRR- and SRR-α-tocopherols leave the plasma rapidly. In control subjects, the fractional disappearance rate of deuterium-labeled RRR-α-tocopherol (0.4 ± 0.1 pools per day) was significantly (p < 0.01) slower than for SRR- (1.2 ± 0.6). The apparent half-life of RRR-α-tocopherol in normal subjects was approximately 48 h, consistent with the "slow" disappearance of RRR-α-tocopherol from the plasma [57].

The similarity in the fractional disappearance rates for RRR- and SRR-α-tocopherols in the nondiscriminator patients, along with the similarity in SRR-α-tocopherol fractional catabolic rates between patients and controls, support the idea that SRR-α-tocopherol can be used in normal subjects to trace the irreversible loss of vitamin E from the plasma. The differences (0.8 ± 0.6 pools/day) between the RRR- and SRR-α-tocopherol rates in controls estimate the rate that RRR-α-tocopherol, which had left the plasma, was returned to the plasma. Although plasma labeled RRR-α-tocopherol concentrations in controls appear to change slowly, both RRR- and SRR-α-tocopherols leave the plasma rapidly. Because RRR-α-tocopherol is returned to the plasma, its apparent turnover is slow. This recirculation of RRR-α-tocopherol results in the daily replacement of nearly all of the circulating RRR-α-tocopherol.

α-TTP function is important during exercise because free fatty acids released from the periphery are taken up by the liver and resecreted as VLDL. Presumably this increased output of VLDL increases the output of liver vitamin E. This hypothesis fits with the observation that plasma vitamin E increases during exercise [41–58] and that this is not a result of lipolysis inhibitable by propranolol [59].

4.5 Vitamin E delivery to tissues

Vitamin E is transported in plasma lipoproteins and, therefore, it is likely that the mechanisms of lipoprotein metabolism determine the delivery of vitamin E to tissues. There are at least three major routes by which tissues are likely to acquire vitamin E:
1. via lipoprotein lipase mediated triglyceride-rich lipoprotein catabolism [62];
2. via the LDL receptor [63,64]; and
3. via vitamin E exchange between vitamin E-rich lipoproteins and vitamin E-poor membranes.

Lipoprotein lipase-mediated vitamin E delivery may be important during exercise for delivery of vitamin E, along with fatty acids to muscles.

Deuterated α-tocopherol has been used to assess the kinetics and distribution of α-tocopherol into various tissues both in rats and in guinea pigs [65,66]. From these studies it is apparent that a group of tissues is in rapid equilibrium with the plasma α-tocopherol pool. Tissues, such as erythrocytes, liver, and spleen, quickly replace "old" with "new" α-tocopherol [67]. Other tissues such as heart, muscle and spinal cord have slower α-tocopherol turnover times. The tissues with by far the slowest α-tocopherol turnover times appear to be the spinal cord and the brain.

The mechanisms for the release of tocopherols from tissues are unknown — no organ functions as a storage organ for α-tocopherol releasing it on demand. The bulk of vitamin E in the body is localized in the adipose tissue [68]. More than 90% of the human body pool of α-tocopherol is located in the adipose tissue, and more than 90% of adipose tissue α-tocopherol is in fat droplets, not membranes [68]. Handelman et al. [69] estimated that ⩾ 2 years are required for ratios of α-/γ-tocopherols to reach new steady state levels in response to changes in dietary intake.

4.6 Metabolism

As discussed in section 2.2, the vitamin E radical can be reduced back to the unoxidized form by other antioxidants; therefore, the degree to which vitamin E is partially oxidized and then reduced to its unoxidized state in vivo is unknown. Liebler and Burr et al. [70,71] suggest that biologically relevant oxidation products include 4α,5-epoxy- and 7,8-epoxy-8α(hydroperoxy)tocopherones and their respective hydrolysis products, 2,3-epoxy-tocopherol quinone and 5,6-epoxy-α-tocopherol quinone. The primary oxidation product of α-tocopherol is the two-electron oxidation product, α-tocopheryl quinone. This can be reduced to the hydroquinone and conjugated with glucuronate. The glucuronate can be excreted into bile or further degraded in the kidneys to α-tocopheronic acid, which is excreted in the urine [72]. Further oxidation products, including dimers and trimers, as well as other adducts have also been described [9].

Schultz et al. [73] have described an unoxidized metabolite of α-tocopherol (2,5,7,8-tetramethyl-2(2'carboxyethyl)-6-hydroxychromane), α-CEHC), which is excreted in the urine when large supplemental doses of RRR-α-tocopherol are fed to humans. Doses in excess of 50 mg vitamin E result in α-CEHC excretion. Thus, the excretion of this metabolite may indicate saturation of the plasma binding capacity for α-tocopherol [73]. A similar metabolite of γ-tocopherol has been proposed as a natriuretic factor and has been given the name, LLU-α [74].

The major route of excretion of ingested vitamin E is fecal elimination, due to its low intestinal absorption.

Skin may also be an important route for vitamin E excretion. In the early 70s, Shiratori [75] infused chylomicrons labeled with [³H] α-tocopherol into rats and found that nearly 40% was associated with the pelt. The application of these data to humans seemed questionable since humans do not have fur. However, recent studies in hairless mice have demonstrated that skin contains various forms of vitamin E, similar to those in the diet, while the brain has virtually only α-tocopherol [74]. Thus, skin vitamin E may be derived from chylomicrons containing dietary vitamin E. Furthermore, skin sebaceous glands may secrete vitamin E to provide antioxidants to protect cutaneous lipids. If so, this route could be important for vitamin E excretion in humans. It is also unknown how much vitamin E might be excreted during profuse sweating as occurs during exercise. Certainly, sweat will increase sebaceous gland secretion.

5. REQUIREMENTS AND RECOMMENDED INTAKES

5.1 Vitamin E units

A vitamin E international unit (IU) is equivalent to 1 mg of all rac-α-tocopheryl acetate. One milligram of RRR-α-tocopherol is equal to 1.49 IU. International units are used for calculation of daily value percentages (%DV) on nutritional labels and for labeling of products meeting requirements of the US Pharmacopeia (USP). Such products include vitamin pills and other pharmaceuticals containing vitamin E.

5.2 Recommended intakes

In 1968, the Food and Nutrition Board of the US National Academy of Sciences set for the first time a recommended daily allowance (RDA) for vitamin E; namely, 30 mg for adult males and 25 mg for adult females. Subsequently, the RDA was reduced, based on the observations that vitamin E intakes for most of the US population were lower than this amount and that PUFA fatty acid intakes were not as high as in experimental diets [19].

The current recommended dietary allowance (RDA) for vitamin E is 8 mg for women and 10 mg for men of RRR-α-tocopherol or RRR-α-tocopherol equivalents (α-TEs) [78]. These are based on subjects consuming a variety of foods. It has been assumed for the purpose of calculating vitamin E intakes in α-TEs that γ-tocopherol can substitute for α-tocopherol with an efficiency of 10%, β-tocopherol of 50% and α-tocotrienol of 30%. However, functionally these forms of vitamin E are not equivalent to α-tocopherol. α-TTP does not recognize γ-tocopherol very well [54] and the metabolic fate of γ-tocopherol is quite unlike that of α-tocopherol [35,79]. Thus, sources of polyunsaturated fatty acids (PUFA), such as corn or soybean oils, which have high concentrations of γ-tocopherol and lower concentrations of α-tocopherol, may increase the potential for in vivo lipid peroxidation. That is, the PUFA, which are protected from lipid peroxidation by γ-tocopherol in the oil, are not protected once they have been consumed because γ-tocopherol is not retained by the body [79]. Thus, PUFA may more easily "turn rancid" in the body.

5.3 Dietary vitamin E

The richest dietary sources of vitamin E are edible vegetable oils [80]. RRR-α-Tocopherol is especially high in wheat germ oil, safflower oil and sunflower oil. Soybean and corn oils contain predominantly γ-tocopherol, as well as some tocotrienols. Cottonseed oil, as well as palm oil, contain both α- and γ-tocopherols in equal proportion. In addition, palm oil contains large amounts of α-and γ-tocotrienols [81]. Unprocessed cereal grains and nuts are also good sources of vitamin E; fruits and vegetables contain smaller amounts. Meats, especially animal fat, also contain vitamin E.

Supplemental vitamin E may be recommended to prevent inadequate intakes in patients with chronic diseases that are associated with free radical damage due to oxidative stress. Doses of 400 IU have been shown to provide protection against oxidative stress during in vitro tests [82].

Currently many health conscious individual limit their fat intake by consuming reduced fat or fat-free products or just avoiding intake of visible fat. These changes in dietary habits may have deleterious effects on vitamin E intakes because most dietary vitamin E is present in fats [80]. This is especially true in subjects who have changed their diets to lower serum cholesterol by decreasing intake of saturated fats and increasing intake of PUFα-containing fats, usually corn oil or soybean oil, which contain high levels of γ-tocopherol, but much less α-tocopherol [80]. Intake of oxidizable lipids is thus increased, while intake of α-tocopherol is decreased. To avoid excessive intakes of PUFA, the ingestion of monounsaturated fats, such as olive or canola oils, is currently recommended [83].

6   SUMMARY

This chapter has focused on the dependence of the biologic activity of vitamin E on the normal transport and distribution of vitamin E in human plasma and tissues. Largely the discussion of antioxidant supplement on exercise performance and recovery are discussed in chapter 12 by Sen and Goldfarb in this volume, pp. 297–320.

7   ABBREVIATIONS

apo: apolipoprotein
AVED: ataxia and vitamin E deficiency
CEHC: 2′ carboxyethyl-6-hydroxychromane
DV: daily value
HDL: high-density lipoprotein
LDL: low-density lipoprotein
PLTP: phospholipid transfer protein
PUFA: polyunsaturated fatty acid
RDA: recommended dietary allowance
ROO·:   peroxyl radical
TTP: tocopherol transfer protein
USP: United States Pharmacopeia
Vitamin C: ascorbate
VLDL: very-low-density lipoprotein

8   REFERENCES

1. Packer L. Sci Am Sci Med 1994;1:54—63.
2. Weiser H, Vecchi M, Schlachter M. Int J Vit Nutr Res 1986;56:45—56.
3. Weiser H, Vecchi M, Internat J. Vit Nutr Res 1982;52:351—370.
4. Cheesemen KH, Holley AE, Kelly FJ, Wasil M et al. Free Rad Biol Med 1995;19:591—598.
5. Tappel AL. Vitam Horm (US) 1962;20:493—510.
6. Burton GW, Ingold KU. Acc Chem Res 1986;19:194—201.
7. Burton GW, Joyce A, Ingold K. Arch Biochem Biophys 1983;221:281—290.
8. Ingold KU, Webb AC, Witter D, Burton GW et al. Arch Biochem Biophys 1987;259:224—225.
9. Kamal-Eldin A, Appelqvist LA. Lipids 1996;31:671—701.
10. Stoyanovsky DA, Osipov AN, Quinn PJ, Kagan VE. Arch Biochem Biophys 1995;323:343—351.
11. Wefers H, Sies H. Eur J Biochem 1988;174:353—357.
12. McCay PB. Ann Rev Nutr 1985;5:323—340.
13. Niki E. Chem Phys Lipids 1987;44:227—253.
14. Sies H, Murphy ME. Photochem Photobiol 1991;8:211—224.
15. Sies H, Stahl W, Sundquist AR. Ann N.Y Acad Sci 1992;669:7—20.
16. Evans HM, Bishop KS. Science 1922;56:650—651.
17. Evans HM, Emerson OH, Emerson GA. J Biol Chem 1936;113:319—332.
18. Emerson OH, emerson GA, Mohammed A, Evans HM. J Biol Chem 1937;122:99—107.
19. Machlin LJ. In: Machlin LJ (ed) Handbook of Vitamins. New York: Marcel Dekker, 1991: 99—144.
20. Horwitt MK, Harvey CC, Duncan GD, Wilson WC. Am J Clin Nutr 1956;4:408—419.
21. Horwitt MK. Am J Clin Nutr 1960;8:451—461.
22. Sokol RJ. Annu Rev Nutr 1988;8:351—373.
23. Sokol RJ,. In: Packer L and Fuchs J (eds) Vitamin E in Health and Disease. New York: Marcel Dekker Inc.,1993:815—849.
24. Ouahchi K, Arita M, Kayden H, Hentati F et al., Nat Genet 1995;9:141—145.
25. Gallo—Torres H. Lipids 1970;5:379—384.
26. Sokol RJ, Heubi JE, Iannaccone S, Bove KE et al. Gastroenterology 1983;85:1172—1182.
27. Traber MG, Goldberg I, Davidson E, Lagmay N et al. Gastroenterology 1990;98:96—103.
28. Cohn JS, McNamara JR, Cohn SD, Ordovas JM et al. J Lipid Res 1988;29:925—936.
29. MacMahon MT, Neale G. Clin Sci 1970;38:197—210.
30. Kelleher J, Losowsky MS. Br J Nutr 1970;24:1033—1047.
31. Blomstrand R, Forsgren L. Int J Vit Nutr Res 1968;38:328—344.
32. Traber MG, Kayden HJ. Am J Clin Nutr 1989;49:517—526.
33. Meydani M, Cohn JS, Macauley JB, McNamara JR et al. J Nutr 1989;119:1252—1258.
34. Traber MG, Burton GW, Ingold KU, Kayden HJ. J Lipid Res 1990;31:675—685.
35. Traber MG, Burton GW, Hughes L, Ingold KU et al. J Lipid Res 1992;33:1171—1182.
36. Havel R. Am J Clin Nutr 1994;59:795—799.
37. Kayden HJ, Bjornson LK. Ann NY Acad Sci 1972;203:127—140.
38. Bjornson LK, Gniewkowski C, Kayden HJ. J Lipid Res 1975;16:39—53.
39. Massey JB. Biochim Biophys Acta 1984;793:387—392.
40. Granot E, Tamir I, Deckelbaum RJ. Lipids 1988;23:17—21.
41. Traber MG, Lane JC, Lagmay N, Kayden HJ. Lipids 1992;27:657—663.
42. Kostner GM, Oettl K, Jauhiainen M, Ehnholm C et al. Biochem J 1995;305:659—667.
43. Cohn W, Loechleiter F, Weber F. J Lipid Res 1988;29:1359—1366.
44. Bjørneboe A, Bjørneboe G-EA, Hagen BF, Nossen JO et al. Biochim Biophys Acta 1987;922: 199—205.
45. Traber MG, Sokol RJ, Burton GW, Ingold KU et al. J Clin Invest 1990;85:397—407.
46. Traber MG, Sokol RJ, Kohlschütter A, Yokota T et al. J Lipid Res 1993;34:201—210.
47. Traber MG, Rudel LL, Burton GW, Hughes L et al. J Lipid Res 1990;31:687—694.

48. Catignani GL, Bieri JG. Biochim Biophys Acta 1977;497:349—357.
49. Sato Y, Hagiwara K, Arai H, Inoue K. FEBS Lett 1991;288:41—45.
50. Yoshida H, Yusin M, Ren I, Kuhlenkamp J et al. J Lipid Res 1992;33:343—350.
51. Kuhlenkamp J, Ronk M, Yusin M, Stolz A et al. Prot Exp Purific 1993;4:382—389.
52. Arita M, Sato Y, Miyata A, Tanabe T et al. Biochem J 1995;306:437—443.
53. Doerflinger N, Linder C, Ouahchi K, Gyapay G et al. Am J Hum Genet 1995;56:1116—1124.
54. Hosomi A, Arita M, Sato Y, Kiyose C et al. FEBS Letters 1997;409:105—108.
55. Dutta—Roy A, Gordon M, Leishman D, Paterson BJ et al. Mol Cell Biochem 1993;123:139—144.
56. Dutta—Roy AK, Leishman DJ, Gordon MJ, Campbell FM et al. Biochem Biophys Res Comm 1993;196:1108—1112.
57. Traber MG, Ramakrishnan R, Kayden HJ. Proc Natl Acad Sci USA 1994;91:10005—10008.
58. Ouahchi K, Arita M, Kayden H, Hentati F et al. Nature Genetics 1995;9:141—145.
59. Pincemail J, Deby C, Camus G, Pirnay F et al. Eur J Appl Physiol 1988;57:189—191.
60. Camus G, Pincemail J, Roesgen A, Dreezen E et al. Arch Int Physiol Biochim 1990;98:121—126.
61. Vasankari TJ, Kujala UM, Vasankari TM, Vuorimaa T et al. Am J Clin Nutr 1997;65:1052—1056.
62. Vasankari TJ, Kujala UM, Vasankari TM, Vuorimaa T et al. Free Radic Biol Med 1997;22:509—513.
63. Traber MG, Olivecrona T, Kayden HJ. J Clin Invest 1985;75:1729—1734.
64. Traber MG, Kayden HJ. Am J Clin Nutr 1984;40:747—751.
65. Cohn W, Goss—Sampson M, Grun H. Biochem J 1992;287:247—254.
66. Ingold KU, Burton GW, Foster DO, Hughes L et al. Lipids 1987;22:163—172.
67. Burton GW, Wronska U, Stone L, Foster DO et al. Lipids 1990;25:199—210.
68. Burton GW, Traber MG. Annu Rev Nutr 1990;10:357—382.
69. Traber MG, Kayden HJ. Am J Clin Nutr 1987;46:488—495.
70. Handelman GJ, Epstein WL, Peerson J, Spiegelman D et al. Am J Clin Nutr 1994;59:1025—1032.
71. Liebler DC, Burr JA. Lipids 1995;30:789—793.
72. Liebler DC, Burr JA, Philips L, Ham AJ. Anal Biochem 1996;236:27—34.
73. Drevon CA. Free Rad Res Comm 1991;14:229—246.
74. Schultz M, Leist M, Petrzika M, Gassmann B et al. Am J Clin Nutr 1995;62 (Suppl):1527S—1534S.
75. Wechter WJ, Kantoci D, Murray EDJ, D'Amico DC et al. Proc Natl Acad Sci USA 1996;93:6002—6007.
76. Shiratori T. Life Sci 1974;14:929—935.
77. Podda M, Weber C, Traber MG, Packer L. J Lipid Res 1996;37:893—901.
78. Food and Nutrition Board NRC Recommended Dietary Allowances, 10th edn. Washington DC: National Academy of Sciences Press, 1989;285.
79. Traber MG, Carpentier YA, Kayden HJ, Richelle M et al. Metabolism 1993;42:701—709.
80. Sheppard AJ, Pennington JAT, Weihrauch JL. In: Packer L, Fuchs J (eds) Vitamin E in Health and Disease. New York: Marcel Dekker Inc, 1993:9—31.
81. Dial S, Eitenmiller RR. In: Ong ASH, Niki E, Packer L (eds) Nutrition Lipids Health and Disease. Champaign IL: AOCS Press, 1995:327—342.
82. Jialal I, Fuller CJ, Huet BA. Arterioscler Thromb Vasc Biol 1995;15:190—198.
83. Reaven P, Parthasarathy S, Grasse BJ, Miller E et al. Am J Clin Nutr 1991;54:701—706.
84. Kayden HJ, Traber MG. J Lipid Res 1993;34:343—358.

Part VI

Cellular and molecular mechanisms

©2000 Elsevier Science B.V. All rights reserved.
Handbook of Oxidants and Antioxidants in Exercise.
C.K. Sen, L. Packer and O. Hänninen, editors.

Part VI • Chapter 15

Biological thiols and redox regulation of cellular signal transduction pathways

Chandan K. Sen

Lawrence Berkeley National Laboratory, University of California, One Cyclotron Road, Building 90, Room 3031, Berkeley, CA 94720-3200, USA. Fax: +1-510-644-2341. E-mail: cksen@socrates.berkely.edu

1   BIOLOGICAL THIOLS
2   THIOREDOXIN AND GLUTATHIONE SYSTEMS
    2.1   The thioredoxin system
    2.2   The glutathione system
3   PROTEIN PHOSPHORYLATION
    3.1   Protein tyrosine kinases
    3.2   JAK-STAT regulation of tyrosine kinases
    3.3   Protein tyrosine phosphatases
    3.4   Tyrosine phosphorylation and PKC activation
    3.5   BMK-1 and SOK-1
    3.6   Cell proliferation
    3.7   Reactive nitrogen species
    3.8   Antioxidant sensitivity
4   PROTEIN-DNA INTERACTION
    4.1   NF-κB
    4.2   AP-1
    4.3   PEBP2/CBF, Pax-8 and TTF-1
    4.4   Ah gene battery
    4.5   NF-Y
    4.6   Zinc-finger and iron-sulfur proteins
    4.7   GA-binding protein
5   CELL CALCIUM
    5.1   NF-κB
6   MANIPULATION OF CELL REDOX
    6.1   N-acetyl-L-cysteine and α-Lipoic Acid
    6.2   Thioredoxin
7   SUMMARY
8   ABBREVIATIONS
9   REFERENCES

1   BIOLOGICAL THIOLS

Thiols refer to a class of organic sulfur derivatives that are characterized by the presence of sulfhydryl residues (–SH) at their active site. Chemically, thiols are mercaptans (C–SH) and biological mercaptans are often referred to as biological thiols or biothiols [1]. Biothiols can be classified as large molecular weight protein thiols and low molecular weight free thiols. Side chain functional CH_2–SH group of cysteinyl residues act as active sites for most biologically important thiols. Disulfide linkages (–S–S–) between two SH residues are important determinants of protein structure such as in insulin. Another characteristic feature of most thiols is that they can act as reducing agents. Reactive oxygen species (ROS) have a strong tendency to transfer electrons to other species or oxidise. Reducing agents such as thiols have negative standard reduction potentials and thus, act as prompt electron acceptors. Thus, in the case of an oxidant-thiol interaction the oxidant is neutralised to a relatively less toxic byproduct at the expense of the reducing power of thiol which itself gets oxidized to a disulfide (C–S–S–C). A thiyl radical (C–S˙) is produced when a thiol (C–SH) loses the H-atom from the –SH group, or loses an electron from the sulfur followed by a proton. Under conditions of physiological pH, thiyl radicals are unstable and may recombine to form the corresponding disulfide. In biological systems, there are specific reductases that recycle disulfides to reduced thiols at the expense of cellular reducing equivalents such as NADPH or NADH. In this way cell metabolism contributes to maintain a favorable oxidoreductive (or redox) *milieu* of thiols.

Recent work from several laboratories have led to the unfolding of one of the most exciting areas in biomedical research — antioxidant and redox regulation of cell signaling [2,3]. In contrast to the conventional idea that reactive oxygen is mostly a trigger for oxidative damage of biological structures, now we know that low physiologically relevant concentration of ROS can regulate a variety of key molecular mechanisms that may be linked with important processes such as immune response, cell-cell adhesion, cell proliferation, inflammation, metabolism, aging and programmed cell death [4—13]. Oxidation-reduction (redox) based regulation of gene expression appears to be a fundamental regulatory mechanism in cell biology.

Several proteins, with apparent redox-sensing activity, have been described. Electron flow through side chain functional CH_2–SH groups of conserved cysteinyl residues in these proteins account for their redox-sensing properties. From *in vitro* information presented so far this mechanism appears to account for most of the major redox-driven signal transduction. It has been shown that formation of protein-disulfide bonds following oxidant challenge may lead to protein destabilization and exposure of hydrophobic domains. Most intracellular proteins thiol groups are strongly "buffered" against oxidation by the highly reduced environment inside the cell mediated by high amounts of glutathione, thioredoxin and associated systems. Thus, only accessible protein thiol groups with high thiol-disulfide oxidation potentials are likely to be redox sensitive.

2 THIOREDOXIN AND GLUTATHIONE SYSTEMS

The ubiquitous endogenous thiols thioredoxin and glutathione are of central importance in redox signaling [14,15].

2.1 The thioredoxin system

Thioredoxin, also known as adult T cell leukemia-derived factor, is a pleiotropic NADPH-dependent disulfide oxidoreductase that catalyzes the reduction of exposed protein S–S bridges. Because of its dithiol/disulfide exchange activity, thioredoxin determines the oxidation state of protein thiols. This small (~ 12 kDa) protein is evolutionarily conserved between prokaryotes and eukaryotes from yeast to animals and plants. A characteristic feature of most thioredoxins is the presence of a conserved catalytic site Trp-Cys-Gly-Pro-Cys-Lys in a protrusion of the three-dimensional structure of the protein. The two cysteine residues of the site can be reversibly oxidized to form a disulfide bridge and thereafter reduced by action of the selenoenzyme thioredoxin reductase in the presence of NADPH ($\{$NADPH $+ $ H$^+$ $+$ thioredoxin-S$_2$ $\rightarrow$ NADP$^+$ $+$ thioredoxin-(SH)$_2\}$). Thioredoxin reductase from human placenta reacts with only a single molecule of NADPH, which leads to a stable intermediate similar to that observed in titrations of lipoamide dehydrogenase or glutathione reductase. Experiments related to the titration of thioredoxin reductase from human placenta with dithionite suggested that the penultimate selenocysteine of the protein is in redox communication with the active site disulfide/dithiol [16]. In addition to the two active site cysteine residues indicated above, two or three additional structural cysteine residues exist in the C-terminal half of the thioredoxin molecule. Oxidation of these residues result in loss of the enzymatic activity of thioredoxin [17]. Thioredoxin serves as the endogenous glucocorticoid receptor-activating factor, and thioredoxin reductase is required for generating the steroid-binding conformation of the glucocorticoid receptor by the endogenous receptor-activating system [18].

Thioredoxin peroxidase is a cytosolic protein that catalyzes the conversion of hydroperoxide and alkyl hydroperoxides into water and corresponding alcohols. Originally, thioredoxin peroxidase was identified as thiol-specific antioxidant or protector protein from yeast [19]. During the course of antioxidant protection, thiols (RSH) react with free radical species (A·) to neutralize (AH) the radical. As a result of such reaction thiyl radicals (RS·) are generated. Thiyl radicals are capable of triggering oxidative damage to several biological macromolecules, e.g., lipids and DNA. It appears that thioredoxin peroxidase detoxifies thiyl radicals or oxidized thiyl radical anions [20]. Antioxidant properties of thioredoxin peroxidase also include the removal of hydrogen peroxide by the overall reaction: 2RSH $+$ H$_2$O$_2$ $\rightarrow$ RSSR $+$ H$_2$O [21].

Antioxidant properties of thioredoxin (Fig. 1) include removal of hydrogen peroxide [22], free radical scavenging [23] and protection of cells against oxidative stress [24,25]. Recycling of ascorbate from its oxidized forms is essential to maintain stores of the vitamin in human cells. Previous works have shown that reduction of dehydroascorbate to ascorbate is largely GSH-dependent. Recently it has been shown that the selenium-dependent thioredoxin reductase system may contribute to ascorbate regeneration. It has been observed that purified rat liver

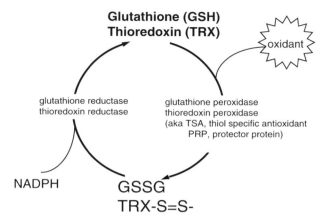

Fig. 1. Glutathione and thioredoxin redox cycles. aka, also known as.

thioredoxin reductase functions as an NADPH-dependent dehydroascorbate reductase. GSH-dependent dehydroascorbate reductase activity in liver cytosol was variable, but typically 2- to 3-fold that of NADPH-dependent activity [26]. The thioredoxin system can reduce dehydroascorbate and may thus, be counted in as a significant component of the antioxidant defense network [27,28]. Under conditions of L -cystine and glutathione depletion the antioxidant defenses of lymphoid cells are impaired. This results in apoptosis most likely *via* an oxidant-dependent mechanism. Thioredoxin has been observed to be protective under such conditions perhaps by virtue of its antioxidant properties [29]. Ultraviolet B (UVB) radiation is known to induce the generation of ROS in skin. Thioredoxin has been shown to be efficiently produced in and released from cultured normal human keratinocytes after UVB irradiation. When stored in the absence of reducing agents, human recombinant thioredoxin undergoes spontaneous oxidation, losing its ability to stimulate cell growth, but is still a substrate for NADPH-dependent reduction by human thioredoxin reductase. There is a slower spontaneous conversion of thioredoxin to a homodimer that is not a substrate for reduction by thioredoxin reductase and that does not stimulate cell proliferation. Both conversions can be induced by chemical oxidants and are reversible by treatment with the thiol reducing agent dithiothreitol [30].

Interaction of NO generated in cells with thiols result in the formation of nitrosothiols. The NO generating enzyme NO synthase itself is a target of such NO-dependent modification. Interaction of NO with vicinal dithiols in the regulatory domain of NO synthase protein is responsible for post-translational reduction of its catalytic activity. Thioredoxin has been observed to be able to reverse such NO-dependent functional inactivation of NO synthase [31]. In activated human neutrophils a burst of NO converts intracellular GSH to S-nitrosoglutathione (GSNO) which is subsequently cleaved to restore GSH by a yet unknown mechanism. Recently it has been observed that GSNO is an NADPH oxidizing substrate for human or calf thymus thioredoxin reductase. Addition of human thioredoxin stimulated the initial NADPH oxidation rate several-fold but was accompanied by progressive inactivation of thioredoxin reductase. Thioredoxin facilitates a homolytic cleavage mechanism of GSNO, giving rise to GSH and NO [32]. This ability of the thioredoxin system to process nitrosothiols suggest novel mechanisms for redox signaling.

2.2 The glutathione system

Glutathione has emerged to be one of the most fascinating endogenous molecules virtually present in all animal cells often in quite high (mM) concentrations. It is known to have multifaceted physiological functions including antioxidant defense, detoxification of electrophilic xenobiotics, modulation of redox regulated signal transduction, storage and transport of cysteine, regulation of cell proliferation, synthesis of deoxyribonucleotide synthesis, regulation of immune response, and regulation of leukotriene and prostaglandin metabolism [33—40]. A key mechanism that accounts for much of the metabolic and cell regulatory properties of glutathione is thiol-disulfide exchange equilibria. The function of several physiological proteins, including enzymes and signaling molecules, is regulated by thiol-disulfide exchange between protein thiols and low molecular weight disulfides. Thus, the side chain sulfhydryl (–SH) residue in cysteine of glutathione accounts for most of its physiological properties. It has been suggested that the secretion of low molecular weight thiols, e.g., cysteine and glutathione from the endoplasmic reticulum might link disulfide bond formation in the organelle to intra- and intercellular redox signaling [41]. Protein folding in the endoplasmic reticulum often involves the formation of disulfide bonds. The oxidizing conditions required within the endoplasmic reticulum is maintained through the release of small thiols, mainly cysteine and glutathione [41].

The antioxidant function of reduced glutathione (GSH) is implicated through two general mechanisms of reaction with ROS: direct or spontaneous, and glutathione peroxidase catalyzed. As a major by-product of such reactions glutathione disulfide (GSSG) is produced. Intracellular GSSG thus, formed may be reduced back to GSH by glutathione reductase activity (Fig. 1) or released to the extracellular compartment.

3   PROTEIN PHOSPHORYLATION

3.1 Protein tyrosine kinases

Signals are transduced from the cell surface to the nucleus through phosphorylation and dephosphorylation chain reaction of cellular proteins at tyrosine and serine/threonine. Protein phosphorylation, one of the most fundamental mediators of cell signaling, is redox sensitive. Treatment of cells with peroxide results in rapid and marked protein tyrosine phosphorylation (Fig. 2). The pattern of protein tyrosine phosphorylation following ROS treatment has striking similarity with that following surface immunoglobulin(sIg)-dependent physiological stimulation [42]. Src-family protein tyrosine kinases, e.g., lck, fyn, and lyn are activated following sIg stimulation. At least two members of the src family, $p56^{lck}$ and $p59^{fyn}$, have been found to be activated by hydrogen peroxide and also by the thiol oxidizing agent diamide [43—45]. In addition, ROS produced by adherent neutrophils are known to increase the activity of p58c-fgr and p53/56lyn tyrosine kinases of the Src family [46]. Sulfhydryl-based protein structural modification of Src kinases is thought to be a mechanism that contributes to the redox-dependent functional alteration of the enzyme [47].

Another member of the protein tyrosine kinase family that has been observed to be highly responsive to treatment of B-cells with hydrogen peroxide is syk [43]. Syk is responsive to hydrogen peroxide, ultraviolet light, as well as sIg stimulations suggesting a common pathway of signal transduction. Sulfhydryl oxidation in response to oxidative stress has been associated with protein tyrosine phosphorylation. Following the sulfhydryl oxidation-induced tyrosine phosphorylation of $p56^{lck}$, the kinase associates with phosphatidylinositol 3-kinase p85 subunit *via* binding of the C-terminal SH2 domain of p85 to the tyrosine-phosphorylated $p56^{lck}$. This is in contrast to the association of these two molecules in the case of CD4-$p56^{lck}$ cross-linking or interleukin-2 stimulation, where phosphatidylinositol 3-kinase p85 subunit binds to the SH3 or SH3/SH2 domain(s) of p56lck [48]. This suggests that T cells may utilize an alternative signaling machinery upon an oxidative stress-induced activation of a src family protein tyrosine kinase, $p56^{lck}$. The thiol antioxidant N-acetyl-L-cysteine (NAC) inhibits antigen mediated syk activation in mast cells [49]. In macrophages, phorbol ester,

100X

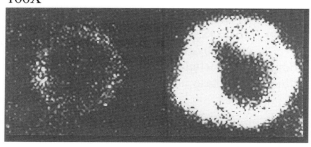

control   0.25 mM H_2O_2, 3 min

Fig. 2. H_2O_2 induced protein tyrosine phosphorylation in Jurkat T cells. Cells were challenged with 0.25 mM H_2O_2 in phosphate buffered saline (pH 7.4) containing 0.1 mM sodium orthovanadate for 3 min. Control cells were maintained in phosphate buffered saline containing 0.1 mM sodium orthovanadate for the same duration. Cells were fixed, permeabilized and immunostained with antiphosphotyrosine antibody coupled with fluorescein isothiocyanate.

zymosan and β-glucan induces tyrosine phosphorylation and all have been shown to be ROS mediated [50,51]. In fibroblasts, tumor necrosis factor and IL-1 rapidly induces the formation of ROS, as well [52]. In T cells, a syk-related tyrosine kinase ZAP 70, associated with the T cell receptor (TCR), is highly responsive to hydrogen peroxide [53]. Both syk and ZAP 70 contain SH2-domains and are, therefore, expected to participate in the complex SH2-mediated signaling cascade.

3.2 JAK-STAT Regulation of Tyrosine Kinases

$p56^{lck}$ is associated with CD4-CD8 surface molecules and IL-2 receptor β-chains, and $p59^{fyn}$ is associated with the T cell receptor/CD3 complex. Ligand-dependent activation of a particular class of surface receptor-associated tyrosine kinases, the Janus kinases or JAK, phosphorylate JAK proteins and receptor components, creating recruitment sites for STAT (signal transducers and activators of transcription) factors [54—56]. The STATs are phosphorylated, they dissociate from the receptor-JAK complex and translocate to the nucleus where they participate in transcriptional gene activation [57,58]. Recent findings have suggested that the interdependence of JAKs and STATs might not be absolute as originally thought [54]. The JAK-STAT system is known to activate the ROS sensitive tyrosine kinases. It has been shown that JAK1, JAK2 and JAK3, and STAT3 and STAT5 are involved in the cytokine receptor mediated activation of lck, fyn and syk tyrosine kinases [59].

3.3 Protein tyrosine phosphatases

Immunoprecipitated syk-family kinases were not responsive to oxidants or anti-oxidants indicating that these kinases may not be directly regulated by ROS [43]. It may thus, be hypothesized that only certain cellular syk-family kinase regulatory components are sensitive to ROS. For example, ZAP 70 may be activated following phosphotyrosine-phosphatase inhibition [60]. Reactive cysteinyl residues in the active site of protein-tyrosine phosphatases confer oxidant sensitivity to the activity of these enzymes [61]. This family of enzymes feature an essential nucleophilic thiol group which attacks the phosphorous atom in a substrate. The nucleophilic attack by Cys-12 in low molecular weight phosphotyrosine phosphatase is carried out by a thiolate anion form of this residue [62]. It has been shown that a single S to O atom substitution in the nucleophile, via Cys to Ser mutation, results in structural/conformational and functional changes that render phosphotyrosine phosphatases catalytically inactive [63]. *In vitro* studies [64—66] show that comparable to vanadate, hydrogen peroxide selectively inhibits phosphotyrosine phosphatase activity. Dephosphorylation of receptor tyrosine kinases has been identified as target of regulation by radiation, oxidants or alkylating agents [61]. Treatment of erythrocytes with the thiol-oxidizing agent diamide has been shown to lead to the formation of phosphotyrosine phosphatase disulfides [67]. Such inactivation of the enzyme inhibits dephosphorylation and thus, drives protein tyrosine phosphorylation [61].

3.4 Tyrosine phosphorylation and PKC activation

Protein tyrosine phosphorylation induced by ROS may be implicated in the activation of the other most prominent protein phosphorylation signaling cascade involving protein kinase C (PKC). PKC isoforms, α, βI, and γ of cPKC subgroup, δ and epsilon of nPKC subgroup, and zeta of aPKC subgroup, has been observed to be tyrosine phosphorylated in COS-7 cells in response to H_2O_2. These isoforms isolated from the H_2O_2-treated cells showed enhanced enzyme activity to various extents. Analysis of mutated molecules of PKC δ showed that tyrosine residues, which are conserved in the catalytic domain of the PKC family, are critical for PKC activation induced by H_2O_2 suggesting that PKC isoforms can be activated through tyrosine phosphorylation in a manner unrelated to receptor-coupled hydrolysis of inositol phospholipids [68].

3.5 BMK1 and SOK-1

Mitogen-activated protein (MAP) kinases represent a multigene tyrosine phosphoprotein family activated by many extracellular stimuli. There are three groups of MAP kinases based on their dual phosphorylation motifs, TEY, TPY, and TGY, which are termed extracellular signal-regulated protein kinases (ERK1/2), c-Jun N-terminal kinases (JNK), and p38, respectively. A new MAP kinase family member termed Big MAP kinase 1 (BMK1) or ERK5 has been recently cloned. BMK1 has a TEY sequence similar to ERK1/2 but has unique COOH-terminal and loop-12 domains. Angiotensin II, phorbol ester, platelet-derived growth factor, and tumor necrosis factor-α were the strongest activation stimuli for ERK1/2 but could only weakly activate BMK1 in cultured rat vascular smooth muscle cells. In contrast, H_2O_2 caused concentration-dependent activation of BMK1 but not ERK1/2. BMK1 activation by H_2O_2 is calcium-dependent and appears ubiquitous as shown by stimulation in human skin fibroblasts, human vascular smooth muscle cells, and human umbilical vein endothelial cells. These findings show that activation of BMK1 is different from ERK1/2 and suggest an important role for BMK1 as a redox-sensitive kinase [69]. More recently it has been shown that Src tyrosine kinase family members (c-Src and Fyn) play a central role in the activation of BMK1 by H_2O_2 in mouse fibroblasts. H_2O_2 stimulates c-Src activity which leads to events resulting in the activation of BMK1 [70]. Another mammalian stress-responsive kinase, SOK-1, has been observed to be activated 3- to 7-fold by ROS again suggesting that oxidant sensitive kinases do exist in mammalian cells. SOK-1 is not activated by growth factors, alkylating agents, cytokines or environmental stresses including heat shock and osmolar stress. The activation of SOK-1 is relatively specific for oxidant stress [71].

3.6 Cell proliferation

Activator protein-1 (AP-1) is an important mediator of cell proliferation [72,73]. Interaction between cJun and cFos proteins, products of *c-jun* and *c-fos* protoncogenes, *via* a "leucine-zipper" domain has been observed to have crucial regulatory implications on the expression of a wide variety of genes, especially those that are growth factor inducible [72]. cJun allows cFos to regulate gene expression by serving as an anchor that allows the Fos-Jun heterodimer to bind to a cognate DNA site. In addition, cJun contains three short region in its N-terminal half that are important for transcriptional activation *in vivo*. cJun expression is regulated by its own gene product *via* phosphorylation by JNKs. The involvement of ROS in the induction of cJun expression *via* upregulation of JNK activity has been evident [74].

The most compelling evidences suggesting that oxidation-reduction (redox) reactions participate in intracellular signal transduction come from studies of cell proliferation. Superoxide anion is suspected to mediate Ras(p21)-induced cell cycle progression [75]. Induction of Ras by ROS has been shown [76]. Another contention is that Ras mediates ROS signaling. In support of this inhibition of Ras activity impaired signaling by oxidants such as hydrogen peroxide and nitric oxide [77].

Oxidant-dependent signaling is involved in the regulation of early changes in gene expression during the G0 to G1 phase transition of lymphocytes. ERK2, a key element of MAP kinase, has been identified as a oxidant-sensitive molecule signaling during lymphocyte activation [78]. Activation of ERK2 and p54 JNK by oxidants has been also shown in human glomerular mesangial cells [79]. Superoxides mediate cell proliferation *via* activation of the p44 MAP kinase in the p21(Ras)/Raf-1/MEK2 pathway that leads to expression of the transcription factor c-fos downstream to the p44 MAP kinase signaling cascade. This has been shown in a lactosylceramide stimulated human aortic smooth muscle cell proliferation model [80]. Lactosylceramide stimulated endogenous superoxide production in human aortic smooth muscle cells specifically by activating membrane-associated NADPH oxidase. That ROS may play a role in growth regulatory signals has been also evident in baby hamster kidney fibroblasts [81]. ROS-dependent alteration in levels of intracellular GSH was thought to be critical in this respect. The MAP kinase signaling cascade is not only regulated by ROS but in the central nervous system-derived neuronal cell line it has been shown that the MAP kinase cascade may even contribute to the generation of ROS under conditions of nerve growth factor deprivation [82].

3.7 Reactive nitrogen species

Protein phosphorylation is not only sensitive to reactive oxygen but also to reactive nitrogen species. Critical signaling kinases, such as ERK, p38, and JNK, are activated by NO-related species and thus, participate in NO signal transduction [74,83]. Nitric oxide and related species (NOx) activate the extracellular sig-nal-regulated kinase (ERK), p38, and JNK subgroups of MAP kinases in human Jurkat T cells. JNK was found to be 100-fold more sensitive to NOx stimulation than p38 and ERK. In addition, the activation of JNK and p38 by NOx was more rapid than ERK activation. The site of molecular interaction between NO and Ras (p21) responsible for initiation of signal transduction has been identi-fied. Cys118 on Ras is a critical site of redox regulation. S-nitrosylation of this cysteine residue triggers guanine nucleotide exchange and downstream signaling. Following interaction with NO, Ras (p21) is singly S-nitrosylated at Cys118. A mutant form of Ras, in which Cys118 was changed to a serine residue (RasC118S), was not S-nitrosylated. NO-related species stimulated guanine nucleotide exchange on wild-type Ras, resulting in an active form, but not on RasC118S. Furthermore, in contrast to parental Jurkat T cells, NO-related spe-cies did not stimulate mitogen-activated protein kinase activity in cells trans-fected with RasC118S [84].

3.8 Antioxidant sensitivity

Under certain conditions protein phosphorylation has been also observed to be sensitive to antioxidants. The redox active protein thioredoxin regulates cell pro-liferation-related signal transduction [85]. Reduced thioredoxin activates protein kinase C through its translocation to the membrane. Structurally unrelated anti-oxidant agents pyrrolidine dithiocarbamate (PDTC), butylated hydroxyanisole, and N-acetylcysteine has been observed to activate JNK in Jurkat T cells. Such antioxidant-induced activation differed substantially from that mediated by phorbol 12-myristate 13-acetate (PMA) and Ca^{2+} ionophore or produced by costimulation with antibodies against the T cell receptor-CD3 complex and to CD28. The activation of JNK by classical T cell stimuli was transient, whereas that mediated by PDTC and butylated hydroxyanisole, but not NAC, was sus-tained [86]. The study of cell cycle arrest in thiol-deprived interleukin-2 stimu-lated natural killer cells has shown that under in vitro conditions the activities of the cyclin-dependent kinases (CDK) CDK6 and CDK2 are increased by thiol deprivation. This enhancement in kinase activity was associated with CDK hyperphosphorylation and prolonged phosphorylation, and could be observed before and beyond interleukin-2 stimulation. This premature and pro-longed enhancement of CDK activity in thiol-deprived natural killer cells is likely to be associated with, and, therefore, may contribute to, the reduced expression and phosphorylation of retinoblastoma gene product, a substrate for CDK [87].

4   PROTEIN-DNA INTERACTION

DNA binding proteins are involved in the regulation of cellular processes such as replication, recombination, viral integration and transcription. Several studies show that the interaction of certain transcription regulatory proteins with their respective cognate DNA sites is redox regulated.

4.1 NF-κB

Reduced thiols, e.g., dithiothreitol, cysteine, dihydroplipoate and reduced thioredoxin, enhance the DNA binding of activated NF-κB [2]. In response to oxidative stress-related stimuli such as UV irradiation, thioredoxin translocates from the cytosol to the nucleus to participate in the regulation of DNA binding of proteins [88]. A highly conserved Rel homology domain is responsible for DNA binding of NF-κB proteins. A short stretch of amino acids, the RxxRxRxxC motif (R = arginine, C = cysteine, x = other amino acid), at the beginning of the domain is essential to contact DNA directly [89–91]. The presence of cysteine residue in the motif is critical and it must be maintained in a reduced state to allow DNA binding because oxidation of this cysteine residue interferes with DNA binding of NF-κB [44,89–92]. Another cellular redox mechanism that may independently or in synergism with the thioredoxin system contribute to enhance NF-κB DNA binding is the apurinin/apyrimidinic endonuclease system or APEX nuclease [93], also known as redox factor-1 or Ref-1 [94,95]. Apurininc/apyrimidinic sites are generated in DNA as result of spontaneous hydrolysis or oxidative damage, and the subsequent action of DNA glycosylases removing the modified DNA bases. Such sites are the most frequent lesion found in cellular DNA and amount to over 10^4 residues per mammalian cell per day. The nuclease activity of Ref-1 is specific for the initial repair of DNA templates that are damaged by various noxious stimuli, e.g., ROS, UV light and ionizing radiation nucleases.

4.2 AP-1

Similar to NF-κB proteins, the DNA binding of AP-1 proteins is also redox sensitive. The DNA binding of Fos and Jun proteins *in vitro* is regulated by the reduction-oxidation of a single conserved cysteine residue (Lys-Cys-Arg) in the DNA-binding domains of the two proteins. The requirement of a single cysteine residue and the sensitivity of Fos and Jun to the -SH alkylating agent N-ethylmaleimide excludes the possibility that oxidation of the cysteine residue involves intra- and intermolecular disulfide bond formation. Conversion of the cysteine to reversible oxidation products such as sulfenic (RSOH) or sulfinic (RSO_2H) acids could contribute to the regulation of DNA binding [96]. The involvement of Ref-1 in the redox regulation of the DNA binding of AP-1 proteins has been also evident. Initially a hepatic nuclear protein was recognised to reduce Fos and Jun and stimulate AP-1 DNA binding. The effect of this nuclear protein could be considerably stimulated by reduced thioredoxin [96]. Further studies with HeLa nuclear extracts identified Ref-1 in the nuclear extract was actually responsible for the effects [94]. Ref-1, the protein product of the *Ref-1* gene, and other chemical reducing agents stimulate AP-1 DNA binding *in vitro* by acting on the regulatory cysteine residue of Lys-Cys-Arg. Replacement of the critical cysteine residue of a truncated Fos protein by serine resulted in a 3-fold increase in AP-1 DNA binding activity that was no longer redox regulated. Such observations indicate that redox regulation of AP-1 DNA binding limits the total level of Fos-Jun *in vivo* and that release from this control enhances transforming activity [97]. Oxidized thioredoxin and GSSG inhibit AP-1 DNA binding *in vitro*, the effect being most pronounced in response to the former.

4.3 PEBP2/CBF, Pax-8 and TTF-1

PEBP2/CBF is a heterodimeric transcription factor composed of α and β subunits. There are at least three closely related genes, *PEBP2αA/Cbfa1*, *AML1/PEBP2αB/Cbfa2* and *PEBP2αC/Cbfa3*, encoding the DNA-binding α subunit and one β subunit encoding gene. *PEBP2/CBF* is implicated in osteogenesis, muscle differentiation, T cell receptor gene arrangement and myeloperoxidase gene regulation. The 128-amino acid long, evolutionarily conserved Runt domain of the α subunit of the transcription factor PEBP2/CBF is responsible for both DNA binding, as well as heterodimerization with the regulatory subunit, β. The Runt domain contains two conserved cysteinyl residues, Cys-115 and Cys-124, that confers redox sensitivity to DNA binding of the proteins. Substitution of Cys-115 to serine partially impairs DNA binding. Substitution of Cys-124, however, increases DNA binding suggesting that both cysteine residues were responsible for the redox regulation in their own ways [98]. Thyroid-enriched transcription factors, Pax-8 and TTF-1, are involved in the thyroid-specific expression of the thyroglobulin gene. Reduction of the nuclear proteins is required for complete DNA binding of Pax-8 and TTF-1 *in vitro*. Electrophoretic mobility shift assay show that oxidation with diamide abolishes the DNA binding of Pax-8 and that subsequent reduction of the nuclear protein with dithiothreitol restores the binding. thioredoxin was more effective in restoring the DNA binding compared to dithiothreitol [99]. Similar redox regulation of DNA binding was observed with TTF-1. Oxidation of TTF-1 with diamide decreased its binding with DNA and the TTF-1-DNA complex migrated faster when electrophoretic mobility shift was studied. Also in this case dithiothreitol reversed these effects [99].

4.4 *Ah* gene battery

In animals, the Ah (aryl hydrocarbon) receptor is a transducer pathway for detecting toxic chemical stress and providing a defense response *via* induction of appropriate metabolic enzymes [100–104]. A group of six genes has been defined as the (*Ah*) gene battery. There are two Phase I (almost exclusively cytochrome P-450) genes, cytochrome P_1-450 (*CYP1A1*) and cytochrome P_3-450 (*CYP1A2*), and four Phase II (enzymes that act on oxygenated intermediates) genes, NAD(P)H:menadione oxidoreductase (*Nmo-1*), aldehyde dehydrogenase

(*Aldh-1*), UDP-glucuronosyltransferase (*Ugt-1*), and glutathione transferase (*Gt-1*). The inducer-receptor complex undergoes a temperature-dependent modification before gaining chromatin binding capacity. As a result, Ah receptor-mediated positive transcriptional activation of each of the genes in the (*Ah*) gene battery takes place. Ligand binding of cytosolic Ah receptor is followed by the transloca-tion of the complex to the nucleus where it heterodimerizes with the Ah receptor nuclear translocator (ARNT) protein [105—107]. In the form of a heterodimeric complex AhR and ARNT is transcriptionally active and binds to enhancer sequences termed aromatic hydrocarbon responsive elements (AhREs) or xeno-biotic responsive elements which are located in the 5'-flanking region of cyto-chromes P4501A1 (*CYP1A1*) and P4501A2 (*CYP1A2*) and several phase II genes. The purified DNA-binding form of rat liver Ah receptor contains three major components, with estimated molecular masses of 108, 98, and 96 kDa. Ah receptor itself and two forms of the ARNT protein are the major components of the purified DNA-binding form of receptor. DNA binding of the purified het-erodimer is redox sensitive. The binding is substantially decreased under oxidiz-ing conditions. Oxidation inhibits receptor DNA binding without greatly altering the size of the purified heterodimer. This sediments at 5.9S in its reduced form and at 6.5S in its oxidized form. Dithiothreitol, a strong reducing thiol, restores the xenobiotic responsive element binding of oxidized receptor, with similar effects on both of the receptor-xenobiotic responsive element complexes. In the presence of nuclear extract, reduced thioredoxin also restores the xenobiotic responsive element binding of the oxidized receptor [108].

4.5 NF-Y

NF-Y is a sequence-specific DNA-binding protein (nuclear factor) that interacts with the conserved Y motif or Y box of the major histocompatibility complex class II gene, Eα. It is a heterotrimeric transcription factor that specifically recognizes a CCAAT box motif found in a variety of eukaryotic promoter and enhancer elements. NF-Y activation is implicated in several cellular responses including hepatitis B viral activation, multidrug resistance, and the activation of Fas and aldehyde dehydrogenase two genes. Using recombinant NF-YA, NF-YB, and NF-YC subunits the subunit association and DNA binding properties of the NF-Y complex has been tested. Cell redox state is an important post-tran-scriptional determinant of NF-Y subunit association and DNA binding activities. The reduction of NF-YB by dithiothreitol is essential for reconstitution of spe-cific NF-Y CCAAT box DNA binding activity *in vitro*. NF-YB mutants in which the highly conserved Cys85 and Cys89 were substituted by serines existed only as monomers and escaped redox sensitivity suggesting a critical role of these cysteine residues in conferring redox sensitivity to the protein. Ref-1 and thio-redoxin, two endogenous reducing agents, stimulated the DNA binding activity of recombinant NF-Y. In cells where the redox cycling of thioredoxin was impaired by treatment with 1-chloro-2,4-dinitrobenzene, an irreversible inhibitor of thioredoxin reductase, decreased endogenous NF-Y DNA binding activity was observed [109].

4.6 Zinc-finger and iron-sulfur proteins

Both *in vitro* and *in vivo* evidence show that zinc-finger DNA-binding proteins, e.g., members of the Sp-1 family are redox sensitive. Thiol-groups confer redox-susceptibility to the zinc-finger transcription factor Sp1 and this redox-susceptibility is prevented by DNA-binding and depends on zinc-coordination of the protein. Apo-Sp1 contained in metal depleted nuclear extracts of human K562 cells exhibited a markedly increased susceptibility towards oxidizing and alkylating agents, as compared to holo-Sp 1. Moreover, DNA binding of apo-Sp1, but not of the holo-protein, is dramatically decreased in the presence of GSH/GSSG ratios within the physiological range [110]. A Sp-1 site mediated hyperoxidative repression of transcription from promoters with essential Sp-1 binding sites, including simian virus 40 early region, glycolytic enzyme, and dihydrofolate reductase genes has been observed [111]. ROS affect the interaction of the Sp1 transcription factor with its consensus sequence and subsequently regulate glycolytic gene expression [112]. Binding of the transcription factor early growth response-1 (Egr-1) to its specific DNA-binding sequence GCGGGGGCG occurs through the interaction of three zinc-finger motifs with demonstrated redox sensitivity [113,114]. Proteins with iron-sulfur prosthetic groups have been also identified to have remarkable redox sensing properties. The assembly and disassembly of (4Fe-4S) clusters is the key to redox sensing in these proteins [115]. The Fe−S containing proteins acquire their clusters by posttranslational assembly under the direction of L-cysteine/cystine C-S-lyase activity [116].

4.7 GA-binding protein

GA-binding protein (GABP) is a heteromeric transcription factor. GABP, also known as nuclear respiratory factor 2, regulates the expression of nuclear encoded mitochondrial proteins involved in oxidative phosphorylation, including cytochrome c oxidase subunits IV and Vb, as well as the expression of mitochondrial transcription factor 1. GABP is composed of two subunits, the Ets-related GABP-α, which mediates specific DNA binding, and GABP-β, which forms heterodimers and heterotetramers on DNA sequences containing the PEA3/Ets motif ((C/A)GGA(A/T)(G/A)). GABP DNA binding activity is redox-regulated *in vivo*, possibly by thioredoxin-mediated reduction and by GSSG-mediated oxidation of the GABP-α subunit. The DNA binding activity of GABP and GABP-dependent gene expression are inhibited in the presence of oxidizing conditions. Reducing agents, e.g., dithiothreitol and thioredoxin facilitates the DNA binding of recombinant GABP-α. The regulation of GABP DNA binding activity by cellular redox changes provides an important link between mitochondrial and nuclear gene expression, and redox state of the cell [117].

5   CELL CALCIUM

Changes in the concentration of intracellular calcium ion ($[Ca^{2+}]i$) control a wide variety of cellular functions including transcription and gene expression. Ca^{2+} driven protein phosphorylation and proteolytic processing of proteins are two major intracellular events that are implicated in signal transduction from the cell surface to the nucleus. Intracellular calcium homeostasis is regulated by the redox state of cellular thiols [118]. For example, ROS decrease NMDA-induced changes in intracellular free Ca^{2+} concentrations and NMDA-evoked cation currents in cortical neurons in culture [119]. The calcium release channel/ryanodine receptor complex of skeletal muscle sarcoplasmic reticulum has been shown to contain reactive thiols that are sensitive to glutathione [120]. In addition, the presence of an allosteric thiol-containing redox switch on the L-type calcium channel subunit complex has been described [121]. Thus, changes in cellular thiol redox state is expected to influence calcium sensitive signaling processes [2,121–123]. Activity of the capacitative Ca^{2+} influx channel has been found to be sensitive to thiol reagents formed endogenously within the cell. Cytosolic GSSG, produced within the endothelial cell, has been shown to decrease luminal Ca^{2+} content of $Ins(1,4,5)P_3$-sensitive Ca^{2+} stores. Depletion of internal Ca^{2+} stores by GSSG may represent a mechanism by which some forms of oxidant stress inhibit signal transduction in the vascular tissue. [124].

5.1 NF-κB

ROS disrupt the calcium homeostasis of cells at concentrations that do not lead to immediate cell death. The resulting elevation in cytosolic free calcium may activate a variety signaling pathways [125]. The following section focuses on the discussion of the involvement of $[Ca^{2+}]i$ in the activation of the redox sensitive transcription factor NF-κB. Although ROS have been suggested to function as a common intracellular messenger in the NF-κB activation cascade in response to a variety of stimuli [2,3], little is known about the precise mode of action. Different cell systems have been used as tool to address this issue. Jurkat T cells are not responsive to hydrogen peroxide with respect to NF-κB activation, however, in a subclone of these cells developed by P.A. Baeuerle (Frieburg, Germany) and named Würzburg cells hydrogen peroxide treatment results is marked activation of NF-κB [122,126]. These two related cell lines with contrasting peroxide sensitivity have been studied to reveal the possible factors that are responsible for oxidant-sensitivity of Würzburg cells (Fig. 3).

   Flow cytometric determination of intracellular Ca^{2+} concentration ($[Ca^{2+}]i$) revealed that 0.25 mM hydrogen peroxide treatment results in a marked calcium flux within the cell [122]. Using extracellular calcium chelators it has been observed that this flux is mainly contributed by calcium released from intracellular stores. In a more recent study with intestinal smooth muscle cells it has been shown that even in the absence of external calcium or in the presence of the cal-

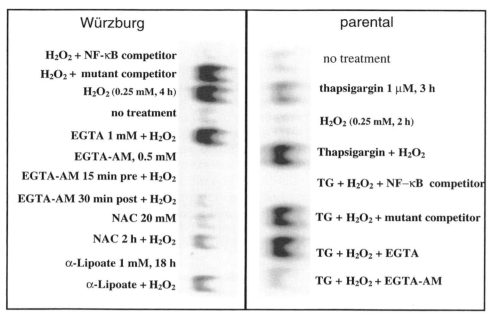

Fig. 3. Electrophoretic mobility shift assay showing the involvement of intracellular calcium in H_2O_2-induced NF-κB activation in Jurkat T cells. To test the specificity of the NF-κB band, nuclear extracts from activated cells were treated with an excess of unlabelled consensus NF-κB oligonucleotide or with an excess of cold mutant NF-κB oligonucleotide before incubation with ^{32}P-labelled consensus NF-κB probe. Würzburg Cells (from top): lanes 3 and 4, cells were either treated or not treated with 0.25 mM H_2O_2, respectively; lane 5, cells treated with 1 mM EGTA 10 min before H_2O_2 challenge; lane 6, cells treated with 0.5 mM EGTA-AM; lane 7, cells treated with 0.5 mM EGTA-AM (aceto-methoxyl ester of EGTA) 15 min before H_2O_2 challenge; lane 8, cells treated with 0.5 mM EGTA-AM 30 min after H_2O_2 challenge; lane 9, cells treated with 20 mM NAC (N-acetyl-L -cysteine) for 6 h; lane 10, cells pretreated with 20 mM NAC for 2 h before H_2O_2 treatment for 4 h; lane 11, cells treated with 1 mM α-lipoate for 22 h; lane 12, cells pretreated with α-lipoate for 18 h followed by H_2O_2 treatment for 4 h. Parental Jurkat cell (from top): Lane 1, no treatment; lane 2, cells treated with 1 µM thapsigargin for 3 h; lane 3, cells treated with 0.25 mM H_2O_2 for 2 h; lane 4, thapsigargin (1 µM) was added to the cells 1 h before H_2O_2 treatment; lane 5, nuclear extracts as of lane 4 were treated with an excess of unlabelled NF-κB consensus oligonucleotide before incubation with labelled NF-κB probe; lane 6, nuclear extracts as of lane 4 were treated with an excess of unlabelled NF-κB mutant oligonucleotide before incubation with labelled NF-κB probe; lane 7, thapsigargin and H_2O_2 treatment as in lane 4 was carried out in the presence of 1 mM EGTA added to the cells 10 min before H_2O_2 challenge; lane 8, thapsigargin and H_2O_2 treatment as in lane 4 was carried out in cells that were loaded with 0.5 mM EGTA-AM 15 min before H_2O_2 challenge. For more information, see [122].

cium channel blocker nifedipine, ROS increases intracellular free calcium level suggesting that calcium release from internal stores contributes to ROS-induced increase in cytosolic calcium [127]. Although Würzburg cells are derived from Jurkat T cells, there is a marked difference in the nature of oxidant-induced cell calcium response in these two cell types. In Jurkat, the calcium flux was rapid and transient. Within 10—15 min after oxidant treatment, intracellular calcium concentration was restored to pretreatment levels. In contrast, the calcium response in Würzburg cells was slower in kinetics and sustained for a longer time [122].

Two major steps in the activation of NF-κB are the phosphorylation and degradation of IκΒ. Currently there is limited information regarding the properties of the putative IκΒ kinase. It is unknown whether the kinase activity in vivo is calcium sensitive. However, as a general rule calcium is known to be required for most protein phosphorylation reactions. IκΒ contains a PEST sequence of amino acid and is thus, highly susceptible to proteolytic cleavage [128]. The degradation of such PEST containing sequence may be catalyzed by proteases such as m-calpain [129], the activity of which is calcium-dependent. Because intracellular calcium could potentially influence both phosphorylation and degradation of IκΒ the hypothesis that peroxide-induced differential calcium response in Jurkat and Würzburg cells is linked to their respective NF-κB responses was tested [122].

In Wurzburg cells that were loaded with the lipophilic esterified calcium chelator EGTA-AM, hydrogen peroxide failed to activate NF-κB. This observation provided the first clue that intracellular calcium flux in response to hydrogen peroxide treatment may be involved in the NF-κB activation process (Fig. 3). Slow and sustained flux of calcium within the cell in response to oxidant treatment appears to be a significant factor in oxidant-induced NF-κB activation [122]. In order to substantiate this conclusion we tested whether hydrogen peroxide would be able to trigger NF-κB activation under conditions where intracellular free calcium level were maintained high on a sustained basis. Such manipulation of the intracellular calcium level was possible by treating the cells with 1 μM of the sarco-endoplasmic reticulum calcium pump inhibitor thapsigargin. The sarco-endoplasmic reticulum serves as a major store-house of intracellular calcium. Calcium is sequestered from the cytosol and retained in this organelle against a high concentration gradient by the active function of the sarco-endoplasmic reticular calcium pumps. Inhibition of these pumps resulted in a release of stored calcium to the cytosol resulting in a high level of intracellular free calcium for at least 1 h. Thapsigargin treatment only weakly activated NF-κB. This activation was markedly potentiated by hydrogen peroxide treatment of the Jurkat cells (Fig. 3). Thus, NF-κB activation in Jurkat T cells did respond to hydrogen peroxide under conditions of elevated intracellular free calcium levels. This activation could be completely inhibited by the intracellular calcium chelator EGTA-AM. Thus, for the first time the involvement of intracellular calcium in oxidant-induced NF-κB activation was evident [122]. A later report showed that calpains indeed regulate gene expression through processing of NF-κB proteins. The C-terminal domain NF-κB proteins is sensitive to mu- and m-calpains *in vitro* [130].

Several later reports have associated cell calcium with the NF-κB activation cascade. For example, the activation of NF-κB by endoplasmic reticulum (ER) stress requires an increase in the intracellular levels of both ROS and Ca^{2+} [131]. Two distinct intracellular Ca^{2+} chelators prevented NF-κB activation by various ER stress-eliciting agents. Consistent with an involvement of calcium, the ER-resident Ca^{2+}-ATPase inhibitors thapsigargin and cyclopiazonic acid, which trigger a rapid efflux of Ca^{2+} from the ER, also potently activated NF-κB. Pretreatment with a Ca^{2+} chelator abrogated this induction. The lipophilic Ca^{2+} chelator BAPTA-AM inhibited ROS formation in response to thapsigargin and cyclopiazonic treatment, suggesting that the Ca^{2+} increase preceded ROS formation during NF-κB activation in this experimental system. The selective inhibitory effect of the drug tepoxalin suggested that the peroxidase activity of cyclooxygenases or lipoxygenases may have been responsible for the increased ROS production in response to Ca^{2+} release by thapsigargin [131]. CD18/ICAM-1-dependent cell-to-cell interaction with hepatoma cells causes NF-κB activation in Kupffer cells. This activation process has been also linked with cell calcium mobilization [132]. A short synthetic peptide (Pa) present in a number of human extracellular matrix proteins was found to elevate intracellular Ca^{2+} and stimulate NF-κB activation [133].

Signals transduced via the TCR activate NF-κB, which in turn, is critical to the transcriptional induction of many genes important for the proliferation and expression of a differentiated phenotype. Ligands binding to the CD4 molecule inhibit TCR mediated T cell activation. Binding of CD4 mAb to the CD4+ T cells prior to TCR/CD3 activation inhibits intracellular calcium elevation and also NF-κB activation suggesting a possible involvement of intracellular calcium in the NF-κB activation cascade [134]. A more clear-cut contribution of cell calcium to TCR-induced NF-κB activation has been observed in another study. TCR signaling was triggered by treating Jurkat T cells with phytohemagglutinin or anti-CD3 antibody, and NF-κB activation was monitored. Protein kinase C was not involved in this NF-κB activation cascade. TCR-mediated activation of NF-κB was dependent on Ca^{2+} influx, because Ca^{2+} channel blockers, as well as other agents that prevented the Ca^{2+} influx, inhibited NF-κB activation [135]. More recently, it has been shown that in B-lymphocytes the amplitude and duration of calcium signals controls the differential activation of NF-κB [125].

6   MANIPULATION OF CELL REDOX

Among the several thiol agents tested for their efficacy to modulate cellular redox status, N-acetyl-L-cysteine (NAC) and α-lipoic acid hold most promise for clinical use [39,136,137]. Some fundamental criteria that the use of such drugs should satisfy for clinical use are:
1. safety, i.e., nontoxic in humans;
2. elevate cell GSH; and
3. favorably modulate molecular responses that are implicated in disease pathogeneses, e.g., inhibition of NF-κB in HIV infection.

Both NAC and lipoate meet the aforementioned criteria.

A common limiting factor in GSH synthesis is the bio-availability of cysteine inside the cell. In the extracellular compartment, 90% of cysteine is estimated to be present as oxidized cystine [15,136]. In tissue culture media all of cysteine is present as cystine. Cells such as T lymphocytes have a weak membrane x_c^- transport system for cystine. However, the cysteine transporting ASC system is estimated to be ten times more efficient than x_c^-. Thus, delivery of the amino acid in its reduced form outside the cell should facilitate the availability of this GSH precursor inside the cell. Both NAC and lipoate facilitate cysteine delivery to the cell in their own unique ways [39].

6.1 N-acetyl-L-cysteine and α-lipoic acid

Cysteine *per se* is highly unstable in its reduced form. As a result considerable research has been focused on alternative strategies for cysteine delivery. In the N-acetylated form, i.e., NAC, the redox state of cysteine is markedly stabilized. After free NAC enters a cell, it is rapidly hydrolyzed to release cysteine. NAC, but not N-acetyl-D-cysteine or the oxidized disulfide form of NAC, is deacetylated in several tissues to release cysteine [39]. Lipoate functions as the prosthetic group for several redox reactions catalyzed by cellular α-keto-acid-dehydrogenases such as the pyruvate dehydrogenase complex. When treated to cells, lipoate is rapidly reduced to dihydrolipoate and released outside the cell. Members of the pyridine nucleotide-disulfide oxidoreductase family of dimeric flavoenzymes, e.g., lipoamide dehydrogenase, thioredoxin reductase, and glutathione reductase reduce intracellular lipoate to dihydrolipoate in the presence of cellular reducing equivalents NADH or NADPH. Thus, a unique advantage of lipoate is that it is able to utilize cellular reducing equivalents, and thus, harnesses the metabolic power of the cell, to continuously regenerate its reductive vicinal dithiol form. Because of such a recycling mechanism, the lipoate-dihydrolipoate couple can be continuously maintained in a favorable redox state at the expense of the cell's metabolic power. Dihydrolipoate released from cells reduces extracellular cystine to cysteine, and thus, promotes cellular cysteine uptake via the ASC system. The dihydrolipoate/lipoate redox couple has a strong reducing power with the standard reduction potential estimated to be –0.32 V. The ability of this couple to reduce protein thiols, e.g., thioredoxin [138–140] has been evident suggesting that lipoate may be effective in modulating redox sensitive signal transduction. Redox modulatory properties and implications of both lipoate and NAC have been recently reviewed [3,141]. The observed favorable effects of both lipoate and NAC on the molecular biology of HIV infection suggest a strong potential of these drugs for AIDS treatment [136,137].

6.2 Thioredoxin

The therapeutic potential of exogenous recombinant human thioredoxin (erTRX) has been also investigated in a few studies. erTRX inhibited the expression of human immunodeficiency virus in human macrophages (M Ø) by 71%, as evaluated by p24 antigen production and the integration of provirus at 14 days after infection. On a concentration basis, thioredoxin was 30,000-fold more effective in inhibiting HIV production compared to the reducing agent NAC. erTRX is cleaved by M $\emptyset$ to generate the inflammatory cytokine, eosinophil cytotoxicity-enhancing factor. In contrast to the effect of thioredoxin, eosinophil cyto-toxicity-enhancing factor enhances the production of HIV by 67%. Thus, whereas thioredoxin is a potent inhibitor of the expression of HIV in human M $\emptyset$, cleav-age of thioredoxin to eosinophil cytotoxicity-enhancing factor creates a mediator with opposite effect. Thioredoxin also inhibited the expression of integrated pro-virus in chronically infected cells indicating that it can act at a step subsequent to viral infection and integration [142]. Thioredoxin has been shown to be defi-cient in tissues but high in the plasma of AIDS patients. Approximately 25% of the HIV-infected individuals studied had plasma thioredoxin levels greater than the highest level found in controls (37 ng/ml). Interestingly, AIDS patients with higher plasma thioredoxin levels (37 ng/ml or greater) tended to have lower over-all CD4 counts. In addition, increase in plasma thioredoxin levels correlated with decreased cellular thiols and with changes in surface antigen expression (CD62L, CD38 and CD20) that occur in the later stages of HIV infection. Thus, it is apparent that elevation of plasma thioredoxin levels may be an impor-tant component of advanced HIV disease, perhaps related to the oxidative stress that is suspected to occur at this stage [143]. Thus, strategies involving modula-tion of the cell redox state appear to have a strong potential in the management of the HIV disease [15,137,144].

Human thioredoxin also contributes to cellular drug resistance. Thus, an effec-tive strategy to sensitize cancer cells to anticancer drugs is to downregulate cellu-lar thioredoxin activity pharmacologically or using molecular biology tools such as thioredoxin antisense constructs. The expression and activity of thioredoxin in Jurkat cells was dose-dependently enhanced by exposure to cisplatin. Treat-ment of Jurkat cells with cisplatin caused transcriptional activation of the human thioredoxin gene through increased generation of intracellular reactive oxygen intermediates. Cells overexpressing exogenous human thioredoxin displayed increased resistance to cisplatin-induced cytotoxicity, compared with the control clones. After exposure to cisplatin, the control cells showed a significant increase in the intracellular accumulation of peroxides, whereas the thioredoxin trans-fected cells did not. Thus, overexpressed human thioredoxin was observed to be responsible for the development of cellular resistance to cisplatin, possibly by scavenging intracellular toxic oxidants generated by this anticancer agent [145]. Thioredoxin-dependent increased resistance to adriamycin has been also reported. Adult T cell leukemia cell lines expressing thioredoxin at levels 2.8 to 12 times those of other T cell acute lymphocytic leukemia cell lines, were 2 to 15 times more resistant to adriamycin than other T cell acute lymphocytic leuke-mia cell lines. Diamide and sodium selenite, which have been reported to inhibit thioredoxin, restored the sensitivity to adriamycin in adult T cell leukemia cell lines [146].

Nitrosoureas of the carmustine type inhibit only the NADPH reduced form of human thioredoxin reductase and thereby impair thioredoxin activity. Because these compounds are widely used as cytostatic agents, it has been suggested that thioredoxin reductase should be studied as a target in cancer chemotherapy [16]. In thioredoxin antisense transfectants enhanced sensitivity of cancer cells to drugs such as cisplatin and also other superoxide-generating agents, e.g. doxorubicin, mitomycin C, etoposide, and hydrogen peroxide, as well as to UV irradiation has been observed [147]. Thioredoxin also plays an important role in the growth and transformed phenotype of some human cancers. The inhibition of tumor cell growth by a dominant negative redox-inactive mutant thioredoxin suggests that thioredoxin could be a novel target for the development of drugs to treat human cancer [148].

The distribution of thioredoxin in the brain implicates an important function in nerve cell metabolism, especially in regions with high energy demands and indicates a role of the choroid plexus in nerve cell protection from environmental influences. After mechanical injury induced by partial unilateral hemitransection, the thioredoxin mRNA expression is upregulated in the lesioned area and spreads to the cortical hemispheres at the lesioned level. Such response suggests a function of thioredoxin in the regeneration machinery of the brain following mechanical injury and oxidative stress [149]. Mouse thioredoxin peroxidase has a broad tissue distribution, but its expression is especially marked in cells that metabolize oxygen molecules at high levels such as erythroid cells, renal tubular cells, cardiac and skeletal muscle cells, and certain type of neurons. Levels of increased expression of thioredoxin peroxidase in the brain has been observed to be coincident with regions known to be especially sensitive to hypoxic and ischemic injury in humans. Expression of mouse thioredoxin peroxidase in PC12 pheochromocytoma cells prolonged survival of the cells in the absence of nerve growth factor and serum, indicating that thioredoxin peroxidase is able to promote neuronal cell survival. It has thus been proposed that thioredoxin peroxidase contributes to antioxidant defense in erythrocytes and neuronal cells by limiting the destructive capacity of oxygen radicals [150]. These findings have identified a novel gene that appears to be relevant to hypoxic brain injury and may be of importance in development of new approaches to abrogate the effects of ischemic- and hypoxic-related injury in the central nervous system.

7   SUMMARY

1. In contrast to the conventional notion that reactive oxygen is mostly a trigger for oxidative damage of biological structures, now we know that low physiologically relevant concentration of ROS can regulate a variety of key molecular mechanisms that may be linked with important cell functions (Fig. 4).
2. Oxidation-reduction (redox) based regulation of gene expression has emerged to be a fundamental regulatory mechanism in cell biology. Several proteins, with apparent redox-sensing activity, have been described. Electron flow

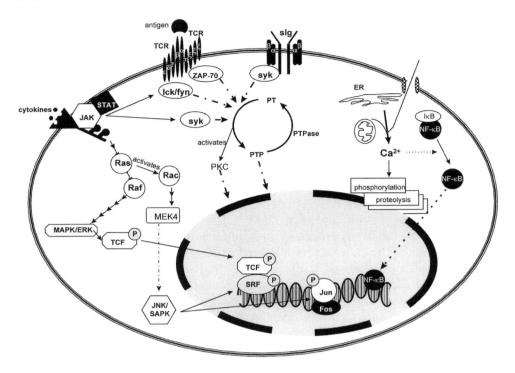

Fig. 4. Overview of the intercellular signaling pathways that are known to be regulated by redox dependent mechanisms. ER, endoplasmic reticulum; ERK, extracellular signal-regulated kinase;
JAK, janus kinases; JNK, c-Jun N-terminal kinases; MAPK, mitogen activated protein kinase;
MEK, MAPK kinase; PKC, protein kinase C; PT, protein tyrosine; PTP, phosphoprotein tyrosine;
PTPase, protein tyrosine phosphatase; SAPK, stress activated protein kinases; sIg, surface immunoglobulin; SRF, serum response factor; STAT, signal transducers and activators of transcription; TCF,
ternary complex factor; TCR, T cell receptor.

   through side chain functional CH_2-SH groups of conserved cysteinyl residues
   in these proteins account for the redox-sensing properties. Protein thiol
   groups with high thiol-disulfide oxidation potentials are likely to be redox
   sensitive.
3. The ubiquitous endogenous thiols thioredoxin and glutathione are of central
   importance in redox signaling.
4. Signals are transduced from the cell surface to the nucleus through phosphorylation and dephosphorylation chain reactions of cellular proteins at tyrosine
   and serine/threonine. Protein phosphorylation, one of the most fundamental
   mediators of cell signaling, is redox sensitive.
5. DNA binding proteins are involved in the regulation of cellular processes such
   as replication, recombination, viral integration and transcription. Several
   studies show that the interaction of certain transcription regulatory proteins
   with their respective cognate DNA sites is also redox regulated.

6. Changes in the concentration of intracellular calcium ion control a wide variety of cellular functions including transcription and gene expression. Ca^{2+} driven protein phosphorylation and proteolytic processing of proteins are two major intracellular events that are implicated in signal transduction from the cell surface to the nucleus. Intracellular calcium homeostasis is regulated by the redox state of cellular thiols and it is evident that cell calcium may play a critical role in the activation of the redox sensitive transcription factor NF-κB.

7. Among the several thiol agents tested for their efficacy to modulate cellular redox status, N-acetyl-L-cysteine and α-lipoic acid hold most promise for human use. A strong therapeutic potential of strategies that would modulate the cellular thioredoxin system has been also evident.

8   ABBREVIATIONS

Ah:	aryl hydrocarbon
AhRE:	aromatic hydrocarbon responsive element
AP-1:	activator protein-1
ARNT:	Ah receptor nuclear translocator
BMK1:	big MAP kinase 1
CDK:	cyclin-dependent kinases
CYP1A1:	cytochrome P_1-450 gene
CYP1A2:	cytochrome P_3-450 gene
Egr-1:	early growth response-1
ER:	endoplasmic reticulum
ERK:	extracellular signal-regulated protein kinases
ErTRX:	exogenous recombinant human thioredoxin
GABP:	GA-binding protein
GSH:	reduced glutathione
GSNO:	nitrosoglutathione
GSSG:	glutathione disulfide
JNK:	c-Jun N-terminal kinases
MAP:	mitogen-activated protein
M Ø:	human macrophages
NAC:	N-acetyl-L-cysteine
NF:	nuclear factor
PDTC:	pyrrolidine dithiocarbamate
PKC:	protein kinase C
PMA:	phorbol 12-myristate 13-acetate
redox:	oxidative-reductive
ROS:	reactive oxygen species
-SH:	sulfhydryl
sIg:	surface immunoglobulin
STAT:	signal transducers and activators of transcription

TCR: T cell receptor
UVB: ultraviolet B

9   REFERENCES

1. Packer L. In: Methods in Enzymology, vol 251, 252. San Diego: Academic Press, 1995.
2. Sen CK, Packer L. Faseb J 1996;10:709—720.
3. Muller JM, Rupec RA, Baeuerle PA. Methods 1997;11:301—312.
4. Baeuml H, Behrends U, Peter RU, Mueller S, Kammerbauer C, Caughman SW, Degitz K. Free Radic Res 1997;27:127—142.
5. Grether-Beck S et al. Proc Natl Acad Sci USA 1996;93:14586—14591.
6. Ward, PA. Environ Health Perspect 1994;102(Suppl 10):13—16.
7. Sellak H, Franzini E, Hakim J, Pasquier C. Blood 1994;83:2669—2677.
8. Papa S, Skulachev VP. Mol Cell Biochem 1997;174:305—319.
9. Stadtman ER, Berlett, BS. Chem Res Toxicol 1997;10:485—494.
10. Richter C. Biosci Rep 1997;17:53—66.
11. Tabatabaie T, Potts JD, Floyd RA. Arch Biochem Biophys 1996;336:290—296.
12. Prehn JH, Jordan J, Ghadge GD, Preis E, Galindo MF, Roos RP, Krieglstein J, Miller RJ. J Neurochem 1997;68:1679—1685.
13. Li PF, Dietz R, von Harsdorf, R. FEBS Lett 1997;404:249—252.
14. Nakamura H, Nakamura K, Yodoi J. Annu Rev Immunol 1997;15:351—369.
15. Droge W, Schulze-Osthoff K, Mihm S, Galter D, Schenk H, Eck HP, Roth S, Gmunder, H. FASEB J 1994;8:1131—1138.
16. Arscott LD, Gromer S, Schirmer RH, Becker K, Williams CH Jr. Proc Natl Acad Sci USA 1997;94:3621—3626.
17. Ren X, Bjornstedt M, Shen B, Ericson ML, Holmgren A. Biochemistry 1993;32:9701—9708.
18. Grippo JF, Holmgren A, Pratt, WB. J Biol Chem 1985;260:93—97.
19. Chae HZ, Rhee SG. Biofactors 1994;4:177—180.
20. Yim MB, Chae HZ, Rhee SG, Chock PB, Stadtman ER. J Biol Chem 1994;269:1621—1626.
21. Netto LES, Chae HZ, Kang SW, Rhee SG, Stadtman ER. J Biol Chem 1996;271:15315—15321.
22. Spector A, Yan GZ, Huang RR, McDermott MJ, Gascoyne PR, Pigiet V. J Biol Chem 1988;263: 4984—4990.
23. Schallreuter KU, , Wood JM. Biochem Biophys Res Commun 1986;136:630—637.
24. Tanaka T, Nishiyama Y, Okada K, Hirota K, Matsui M, Yodoi J, Hiai H, Toyokuni S. Lab Invest 1997;77:145—155.
25. Nakamura H et al. Immunol Lett 1994;42:75—80.
26. May JM, Mendiratta S, Hill KE, Burk RF. J Biol Chem 1997;272:22607—22610.
27. Packer L, Witt EH, Tritschler HJ. Free Radic Biol Med 1995;19:227—250.
28. Sen CK, Hanninen O. In: Sen CK, Packer L, Hanninen O (eds) Exercise and oxygen toxicity. Amsterdam: Elsevier Science Publishers BV, 1994:89—126.
29. Iwata S, Hori T, Sato N, Hirota K, Sasada T, Mitsui A, Hirakawa T, Yodoi J. J Immunol 1997; 158:3108—3117.
30. Gasdaska JR, Kirkpatrick DL, Montfort W, Kuperus M, Hill SR, Berggren M, Powis G. Biochem Pharmacol 1996;52:1741—1747.
31. Patel JM, Zhang J, Block ER. Am J Respir Cell Mol Biol 1996;15:410—419.
32. Nikitovic D, Ho, Holmgren A. J Biol Chem 1996;271:19180—19185.
33. Droge W, Gross A, Hack V, Kinscherf R, Schykowski M, Bockstette M, Mihm S, Galter D. Adv Pharmacol 1997;38:581—600.
34. Anderson ME. Adv Pharmacol 1997;38:65—78.
35. ML OB, Tew KD. Eur J Cancer 1996;32A:967—978.
36. Taylor CG, Nagy LE, Bray TM. Curr Top Cell Regul 1996;34:189—208.

37. Lomaestro BM, Malone M. Ann Pharmacother 1995;29:1263—1273.
38. Meister A. Methods Enzymol 1995;251:3—7.
39. Sen CK. Journal of Nutritional Biochemistry 1997;8:660—672.
40. Sen CK, Khanna S, Reznick AZ, Roy S, Packer L. Biochemical and Biophysical Research Communications 1997;237:645—649.
41. Carelli S, Ceriotti A, Cabibbo A, Fassina G, Ruvo M, Sitia R. Science 1997;277:1681—1684.
42. Schieven GL, Ledbetter JA. J Immunother 1993;14:221—225.
43. Schieven GL, Kirihara JM, Myers DE, Ledbetter JA, Uckun FM. Blood 1993;82:1212—1220.
44. Hayashi T, Ueno Y, Okamoto T. J Biol Chem 1993;268:11380—11388.
45. Nakamura K, Hori T, Sato N, Sugie K, Kawakami T, Yodoi J. Oncogene 1993;8:3133—3139.
46. Yan SR, Berton G. J Biol Chem 1996;271:23464—23471.
47. Pu M et al. Oncogene 1996;13:2615—2622.
48. Nakamura K, Hori T, Yodoi J. Mol Immunol 1996;33:855—865.
49. Valle A, Kinet JP. FEBS Lett 1995;357:41—44.
50. Zor U, Ferber E, Gergely P, Szucs K, Dombradi V, Goldman R. Biochem J 1993;295:879—888.
51. Goldman R, Ferber E, Meller R, Zor U. Biochem Biophys Acta 1994;1222:265—276.
52. Meier B, Radeke HH, Selle S, Younes M, Sies H, Resch K, Habermehl GG. Biochem J 1989; 263:539—545.
53. Schieven GL, Mittler RS, Nadler SG, Kirihara JM, Bolen JB, Kanner SB, Ledbetter JA. J Biol Chem 1994;269:20718—20726.
54. Pellegrini S, Dusanter-Fourt I. Eur J Biochem 1997;248:615—633.
55. Symes A, Gearan T, Eby J, Fink JS. J Biol Chem 1997;272:9648—9654.
56. Kohlhuber F et al. Mol Cell Biol 1997;17:695—706.
57. Ihle JN. Proc Soc Exp Biol Med 1994;206:268—272.
58. Ihle JN, Witthuhn BA, Quelle FW, Yamamoto K, Thierfelder WE, Kreider B, Silvennoinen O. Trends Biochem Sci 1994;19:222—227.
59. Taniguchi T. Science 1995;268:251—255.
60. Weiss A, Littman DR. Cell 1994;76:263—274.
61. Knebel A, Rahmsdorf HJ, Ullrich A, Herrlich P. Embo J 1996;15:5314—5325.
62. Hansson T, Nordlund P, Aqvist J. J Mol Biol 1997;265:118—127.
63. Zhang ZY, Wu L. Biochemistry 1997;36:1362—1369.
64. Hecht D, Zick Y. Biochem Biophys Res Commun 1992;188:773—779.
65. Hadari YR, Geiger B, Nadiv O, Sabanay I, Roberts CT Jr, LeRoith D, Zick Y. Mol Cell Endocrinol 1993;97:9—17.
66. Sullivan SG, Chiu DT, Errasfa M, Wang JM, Qi JS, Stern A. Free Radic Biol Med 1994;16:399—403.
67. Zipser Y, Piade A, Kosower NS. FEBS Lett 1997;406:126—130.
68. Konishi H, Tanaka M, Takemura Y, Matsuzaki H, Ono Y, Kikkawa U, Nishizuka Y. Proc Natl Acad Sci USA 1997;94:11233—11237.
69. Abe J, Kusuhara M, Ulevitch RJ, Berk BC, Lee JD. J Biol Chem 1996;271:16586—16590.
70. Abe J, Takahashi M, Ishida M, Lee JD, Berk BC. J Biol Chem 1997;272:20389—20394.
71. Pombo CM, Bonventre JV, Molnar A, Kyriakis J, Force T. Embo J 1996;15:4537—4546.
72. Angel P, Karin M. Biochim Biophys Acta 1991;1072:129—157.
73. Karin M. J Biol Chem 1995;270:16483—16486.
74. Lo YYC, Wong JMS, Cruz TF. J Biol Chem 1996;271:15703—15707.
75. Irani K et al. Science 1997;275:1649—1652.
76. Qiu X, Forman HJ, Schonthal AH, Cadenas E. J Biol Chem 1996;271:31915—31921.
77. Lander HM, Ogiste JS, Teng KK, Novogrodsky A. J Biol Chem 1995;270:21195—21198.
78. Goldstone SD, Hunt NH. Biochim Biophys Acta 1997;1355:353—360.
79. Wilmer WA, Tan LC, Dickerson JA, Danne M, Rovin BH. J Biol Chem 1997;272:10877—10881.
80. Bhunia AK, Han H, Snowden A, Chatterjee S. J Biol Chem 1997;272:15642—15649.
81. Burdon RH, Alliangana D, Gill V. Free Radic Res 1994;21:121—133.

82. Dugan LL, Creedon DJ, Johnson EM Jr, Holtzman DM. Proc Natl Acad Sci USA 1997;94: 4086—4091.
83. Lander HM, Jacovina AT, Davis RJ, Tauras JM. J Biol Chem 1996;271:19705—19709.
84. Lander HM, Hajjar DP, Hempstead BL, Mirza UA, Chait BT, Campbell S, Quilliam LA. J Biol Chem 1997;272:4323—4326.
85. Biguet C, Wakasugi N, Mishal Z, Holmgren A, Chouaib S, Tursz T, Wakasugi H. J Biol Chem 1994;269:28865—28870.
86. Gomez del Arco P, Martinez-Martinez S, Calvo V, Armesilla AL, Redondo JM. J Biol Chem 1996;271:26335—26340.
87. Yamauchi A, Bloom ET. Blood 1997;89:4092—4099.
88. Yodoi J, Taniguchi Y, Sasada T, Hirota K. In: Montagnier L, Olivier R, Pasquier C (eds) Oxidative Stress Cancer, AIDS and Neurodegenerative Diseases. New York: Marcel Dekker Inc, 1997;247—250.
89. Bressler P, Brown K, Timmer W, Bours V, Siebenlist U, Fauci AS. J Virol 1993;67:288—293.
90. Kumar S, Rabson AB, Gelinas C. Mol Cell Biol 1992;12:3094—3106.
91. Toledano MB, Ghosh D, Trinh F, Leonard WJ. Mol Cell Biol 1993;13:852—860.
92. Matthews JR, Wakasugi N, Virelizier JL, Yodoi J, Hay RT. Nucleic Acids Res 1992;20: 3821—3830.
93. Mitomo K, Nakayama K, Fujimoto K, Sun X, Seki S, Yamamoto K. Gene 1994;145:197—203.
94. Xanthoudakis S, Miao G, Wang F, Pan YC, Curran T. Embo J 1992;11:3323—3335.
95. Xanthoudakis S, Curran T. Adv Exp Med Biol 1996;387:69—75.
96. Abate C, Patel L, Rauscher FJd, Curran T. Science 1990;249:1157—1161.
97. Okuno H, Akahori A, Sato H, Xanthoudakis S, Curran T, Iba H. Oncogene 1993;8:695—701.
98. Akamatsu Y, Ohno T, Hirota K, Kagoshima H, Yodoi J, Shigesada K. J Biol Chem 1997;272: 14497—14500.
99. Kambe F, Nomura Y, Okamoto T, Seo H. Mol Endocrinol 1996;10:801—812.
100. Schmidt JV, Bradfield CA. Ann Rev Cell Dev Biol 1996;12:55—89.
101. Safe S, Krishnan V. Arch Toxicol Suppl 1995;17:99—115.
102. Nebert DW. Crit Rev Toxicol 1989;20:153—174.
103. Otto DM, Sen CK, Casley WL, Moon TW. Comp Biochem Physiol C Pharmacol Toxicol Endocrinol 1997;117:299—309.
104. Otto DM, Sen CK, Casley WL, Moon TW. Biochem Mol Biol Int 1996;38:1127—1133.
105. Rowlands JC, Gustafsson JA. Crit Rev Toxicol 1997;27:109—134.
106. Whitlock JP Jr, Okino ST, Dong L, Ko HP, Clarke-Katzenberg R, Ma Q, Li H. Faseb J 1996;10: 809—818.
107. Fujii-Kuriyama Y, Ema M, Mimura J, Sogawa K. Exp Clin Immunogenet 1994;11:65—74.
108. Ireland RC, Li SY, Dougherty JJ. Arch Biochem Biophys 1995;319:470—480.
109. Nakshatri H, Bhat-Nakshatri P, Currie RA. J Biol Chem 1996;271:28784—28791.
110. Knoepfel L, Steinkuhler C, Carri MT, Rotilio G. Biochem Biophys Res Commun 1994;201: 871—877.
111. Wu X, Bishopric NH, Discher DJ, Murphy BJ, Webster KA. Mol Cell Biol 1996;16:1035—1046.
112. Schafer D, Hamm-Kunzelmann B, Hermfisse U, Brand K. FEBS Lett 1996;391:35—38.
113. Huang RP, Adamson ED. DNA Cell Biol 1993;12:265—273.
114. Nose K, Ohba M. Biochem J 1996;316:381—383.
115. Rouault TA, Klausner RD. Trends Biochem Sci 1996;21:174—177.
116. Leibrecht I, Kessler D. J Biol Chem 1997;272:10442—10447.
117. Martin ME, Chinenov Y, Yu M, Schmidt TK, Yang XY. J Biol Chem 1996;271:25617—25623.
118. Donoso P, Rodriguez P, Marambio P. Arch Biochem Biophys 1997;341:295—299.
119. Aizenman E, Hartnett KA, Reynolds IJ. Neuron 1990;5:841—846.
120. Zable AC, Favero TG, Abramson JJ. J Biol Chem 1997;272:7069—7077.
121. Campbell DL, Stamler JS, Strauss HC. J Gen Physiol 1996;108:277—293.
122. Sen CK, Roy S, Packer L. FEBS Lett 1996;385:58—62.

123. Suzuki YJ, Forman HJ, Sevanian A. Free Radic Biol Med 1997;22:269—285.

124. Henschke PN, Elliott SJ. Biochem J 1995;312:485—489.

125. Dolmetsch RE, Lewis RS, Goodnow CC, Healy JI. Nature 1997;386:855—858.

126. Staal FJT, Roederer M, Herzenberg LA, Herzenberg LA. Proceedings of the National Academy of Science USA 1990;87:9943—9947.

127. Bielefeldt K, Whiteis CA, Sharma RV, Abboud FM, Conklin JL. Am J Physiol 1997;272: G1439—G1450.

128. Thanos D, Maniatis T. Cell 1995;80:529—532.

129. Watt F, Molloy PL. Nucleic Acids Res 1993;21:5092—5100.

130. Liu ZQ, Kunimatsu M, Yang JP, Ozaki Y, Sasaki M, Okamoto T. FEBS Lett 1996;385:109—113.

131. Pahl HL, Baeuerle PA. FEBS Lett 1996;392:129—136.

132. Kurose I et al. J Clin Invest 1997;99:867—878.

133. Lopez-Zabalza MJ, Martinez-Lausin S, Bengoechea-Alonso MT, Lopez-Moratalla N, Gonzalez A, Santiago E. Arch Biochem Biophys 1997;338:136—142.

134. Jabado N, Pallier A, Le Deist F, Bernard F, Fischer A, Hivroz C. J Immunol 1997;158:94—103.

135. Kanno T, Siebenlist U. J Immunol 1996;157:5277—5283.

136. Sen CK, Roy S, Han D, Packer L. Free Radical Biology and Medicine 1997;22:1241—1257.

137. Sen CK, Roy, S and Packer, L. In: Montagnier L, Olivier R, Pasquier C (eds) Oxidative Stress Cancer, AIDS and Neurodegenerative Diseases. New York: Marcel Dekker Inc, 1997;251—267.

138. Holmgren A. J Biol Chem 1979;254:9627—9632.

139. Holmgren A. J Biol Chem 1989;264:13963—13966.

140. Spector A, Huang RR, Yan GZ, Wang RR. Biochem Biophys Res Commun 1988;150:156—162.

141. Packer L, Roy S, Sen CK. Adv Pharmacol 1997;38:79—101.

142. Newman GW, Balcewicz-Sablinska MK, Guarnaccia JR, Remold HG, Silberstein DS. J Exp Med 1994;180:359—363.

143. Nakamura H et al. Int Immunol 1996;8:603—611.

144. Okamoto T, Sakurada S, Yang JP, Merin JP. Curr Top Cell Regul 1997;35:149—161.

145. Sasada T et al. J Clin Invest 1996;97:2268—2276.

146. Wang J, Kobayashi M, Sakurada K, Imamura M, Moriuchi T, Hosokawa M. Blood 1997;89: 2480—2487.

147. Yokomizo A et al. Cancer Res 1995;55:4293—4296.

148. Gallegos A et al. Cancer Res 1996;56:5765—5770.

149. Lippoldt A, Padilla CA, Gerst H, Andbjer B, Richter E, Holmgren A, Fuxe K. J Neurosci 1995; 15:6747—6756.

150. Ichimiya S, Davis JG, O'Rourke DM, Katsumata M, Greene MI. DNA Cell Biol 1997;16:311— 321.

©2000 Elsevier Science B.V. All rights reserved.
Handbook of Oxidants and Antioxidants in Exercise.
C.K. Sen, L. Packer and O. Hänninen, editors.

Part VI • Chapter 16

Regulation and deregulation of vascular smooth muscle cells by reactive oxygen species and by α-tocopherol

A. Azzi[1], D. Boscoboinik[1], N. K. Özer[2], R. Ricciarelli[1] and E. Aratri[1]

[1]*Institute of Biochemistry and Molecular Biology, University of Bern, Bühlstrasse 28, 3012 Bern. Tel.: +41-31-6514131. Fax. +41-31-6513737. E-mail: E. angelo.azzi@mci.unibe.ch* [2]*Department of Biochemistry, Faculty of Medicine, Marmara University, 81326 Haydarpasa,Istanbul, Turkey. Tel.: +90-216-414-4733. Fax: +90-216-418-1047. E-mail: nkozer@escortnet.com*

1   INTRODUCTION
    1.1   The role of VSMCs in pathological conditions
        1.1.1   Atherosclerosis
        1.1.2   Restenosis
        1.1.3   Hypertension
    1.2   VSMC proliferation
    1.3   VSMC differentiation and phenotypic modulation
2   EFFECT OF REACTIVE OXYGEN SPECIES IN VSMCs
    2.1   Effects of reactive oxygen species on cell proliferation
    2.2   Reactive oxygen species effects on inducible gene expression
    2.3   Reactive oxygen species sensitivity of protein kinase C
    2.4   Reactive oxygen species sensitivity of tyrosine kinases
    2.5   Reactive oxygen species and MAP kinases
    2.6   Reactive oxygen species sensitivity of phosphatases
    2.7   Bcl-2 expression
    2.8   Reactive oxygen species sensitive proteases
    2.9   Paracrine modulation by reactive oxygen species
3   THE EFFECT OF d-α-TOCOPHEROL ON VSMCs
    3.1   Effect of tocopherols on cell proliferation
    3.2   Effect of tocopherols on PKC activity
    3.3   Effect of d-α-tocopherol on inducible gene expression
4   SUMMARY AND PERSPECTIVES
5   ACKNOWLEDGEMENTS
6   ABBREVIATIONS
7   REFERENCES

1   INTRODUCTION

All the arterial vessels with exception of the capillaries are composed of three layers: intima, media, and adventitia. The intima is the innermost layer and is in direct contact with the flowing blood. The intimal layer composed of a monolayer of endothelial cells lining the whole vascular wall, a very thin basal lamina, and subendothelial layer, composed of collagen bundles, elastic fibrils, smooth muscle cell (SMC) and some fibroblasts. The tunica media is the middle layer of the vascular wall. It is made up of many layers of SMCs, a varied number of elastic sheets, bundles of collagen fibrils, and a net work of elastic fibrils. The SMCs are separated from intima and adventitia by the internal and the external elastic lamina respectively. The adventitia is the outermost layer of the vascular wall. Its thickness varies considerably, depending on the type and location of the vessel. This layer consists of fibroelastic tissue containing smaller blood vessels and nerves without SMCs [1,2].

Although composed of distinct layers the vessel wall is entirely derived from the mesoderm. Mesenchymal cells initially form a lining of endothelial cells around spaces filled with fluid. Subsequently, additional mesenchymal cells accumulate and start to differentiate into SMCs. During most of the fetal and early postnatal period, the SMCs have a fibroblasts-like appearance with an extensive rough endoplasmic reticulum, a prominent Golgi complex, and only a few myofilaments. Their main functions are to proliferate and secrete extracellular matrix components like collagen and elastin. At this stage β-actin is the main actin isoform and vimentin is the main intermediate filament protein. This phenotype is termed "synthetic". As the vessels mature, the synthetic organelles decrease in size and myofilaments occupy successively larger parts of the cytoplasm. This is associated with a decrease in the β-actin expression and an increased expression of SMC specific α-actin. Moreover, the content of the intermediate filament protein desmin and the fraction of cells that show a positive staining for both vimentin and desmin increase. This phenotype is termed "contractile" and they have a muscle-like appearance and contract in response to chemical and mechanical stimuli. The changes in structure and function of arterial SMCs during development can be referred to as a shift from a synthetic to a contractile phenotype. However, these cells are able to return to a synthetic phenotype, this appears to be an important early event in atherogenesis [3,4].

The SMC, the only cell type present in the media of mammalian arteries, is responsible for maintaining tension via contraction-relaxation, as well as arterial integrity by proliferation and synthesis of extracellular matrix. The size, elasticity, and integrity of large arteries is determined by the SMC of the tunica media and by the connective tissue matrix including collagen, elastin and proteoglycans, synthesized and deposited by SMCs. Proliferation of a SMC is an important pathological event in a number of vascular disease processes including atherosclerosis, the response to endothelial injury, vascular rejection, restenosis and hypertension.

At least three mechanisms have been proposed to explain smooth muscle growth control. Firstly, smooth muscle growth may be controlled by growth factors released from blood cells. Secondly, smooth muscle growth may be controlled by inhibitors derived from the vessel wall or controlled by growth stimulant produced by the cells of the vessel wall themselves. These classic mitogens such as platelet growth factor and epidermal growth factor also cause contraction of vessels [1,5,6]. It now appears that the active oxygen species (i.e., O_2^-, H_2O_2, and $OH\hat{c}dot$) exhibit this same duality. Active oxygen species have been shown to contract aortic strips. It has also been shown that active oxygen species stimulate several growth factor-like cellular responses and may, therefore, act as vascular smooth muscle growth factors [7].

1.1 The role of VSMCs in pathological conditions

The VSMC of the arterial media plays a predominant role in functional and structural alterations of the arterial wall in pathophysiological processes such as atherosclerosis, restenosis, arterial hypertension and also normal aging. The observed alterations are related to the three activities of the VSMC, namely contractility, protein secretion, proliferation and migration.

1.1.1 Atherosclerosis

Atherosclerosis remains the major cause of death in the world. Although the etiology of this arteriopathy is undefined, several pathogenic hypotheses have been considered: monoclonal cell proliferation, thrombogenesis, lipid infiltration and response to injury [5,6,8,9]. In the early stages of disease, SMCs migrate from the media to the intima of the arterial wall, where they proliferate and deposit extracellular matrix components, thereby forming a lesion that protrudes into the vessel lumen. The SMCs are in this new location under the influence of a variety of factors, not only blood components, but also substances released by endothelial cells, platelets adhering to exposed subendothelial tissue, as well as macrophages and lymphocytes invading the vessel wall [10,11]. In addition, the SMCs may produce and release substances that affect their own function (see section 1.1.2). When cells are in the contractile phenotype in a normal artery they respond to agents that induce either vasoconstriction or vasodilatation such as endothelin, catecholamines, angiotensin II, prostaglandin E, prostaglandin I2, neuropeptides and, leukotrienes [6,12]. In forming atherosclerotic lesions, SMCs appear to regain the phenotypic characteristics of SMCs in young and developing arteries. In the lesion, SMCs are capable of expressing genes for a number of growth regulatory molecules and cytokines. They can also respond to growth factors by expressing appropriate receptors, and they can synthesize an extracellular matrix [3] (synthetic state). In atherosclerosis, SMCs can respond, in an autocrine style, by secreting platelet derived growth factor, as well as other possible growth stimulants. Furthermore, at sites where cell injury and necrosis occur, damaged SMCs could release fibroblast growth factor and in so doing could also stimulate neighboring SMCs, the overlying endothelium or vascular channels within the lesion [1,12]. Their synthetic activity will determine the matrix content of the lesion, which in turn could interact at their surface and modify their capability to respond to various agonists. Thus, the SMC plays the principal role in the fibroproliferative component of this disease process.

Accumulation of lipoproteins, including low-density lipoproteins, very low-density proteins and lipoprotein a, are important initial events in atherogenesis. The intimal generation of reactive oxygen species results in the oxidative modification of lipoproteins (Fig. 1). Their accumulation, via the scavenger receptor by newly recruited blood monocytes, this leads to the formation of foam cells in the arterial subendothelial [13]. Hydrogen peroxide and a reactive oxygen species are reported to induce protooncogene expression and replicative DNA synthesis in rat aortic SMCs [7]. Recently it has been shown that hydrogen peroxide induces c-fos mRNA expression via phospholipase A2 dependent activation of PKC in SMCs [14]. Thus, reactive oxygen species appear to play a pivotal role in both early and later phases of atherogenesis. Furthermore, an emerging and convincing body of evidence indicates that experimental atherosclerosis and foam cell formation can be effectively retarded by antioxidants. An example can be the antiatherogenic effect of probucol and butylated hydroxytoluene in hyperlipidemic Watanabe rabbits, (defective in the low-density lipoprotein (LDL)-receptor) and in rabbits that become hypercholesterolemic by dietary supplementation [15—17]. Lipoprotein may also directly modulate smooth muscle functions [18] and in particular low-density lipoproteins stimulate SMC proliferation [19]. This event is correlated with an increase in PKC activity that is sensitive to α-tocopherol [19].

1.1.2 Restenosis

Restenosis is a major unresolved complication following percutaneous coronary revascularization, bypass grafting and endarterectomy procedures. Restenosis is

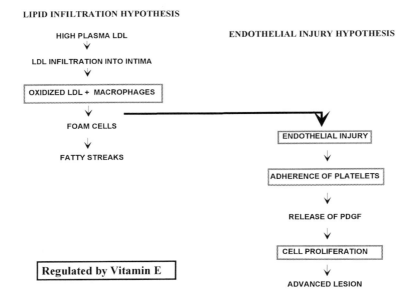

Fig. 1. Role of oxidants and α-tocopherol in the onset of atherosclerosis. The reactions that are sensitive to α-tocopherol are indicated with a frame.

associated with increase platelets adherence and aggregation, release of platelet granular components, migration and proliferation of medial SMCs into the intima [20]. The possibility of a change in VSMCs from a contractile (quiescent) phenotype to a synthetic or proliferating (activated) one [21] is also present. The transition of VSMCs to a proliferative state is preceded by the accumulation of platelets and leukocytes, which may release growth factors and cytokines at the site of injury [22]. (see section 1.1.3). The VSMCs may, therefore, play a dual role in vessel injury, both as a mediator of inflammatory response through chemoattractant release, and as an effector of the hyperplastic response through proliferation (intima hyperplasia) [23,24]. The basic fibroblast growth factor produces an antibody-sensitive smooth muscle proliferation in denuded carotid arteries [25]. In the percutaneous translumenal coronary angioplasty model, three stages of neointimal growth after arterial injury have been identified: an early thrombotic stage, blood coagulation, mechanical injury that first activates cytokine gene expression by macrophages and/or SMCs within the plaque. This cytokine expression would evoke secondary, self-sustaining, continuing autocrine and paracrine growth factor, along with cytokine expression by damaged cells, this includes leukocytes that could account for the lag between injury and restenosis [26].

1.1.3 Hypertension

Hypertension is another disease affecting the tunica media and its pathogenesis is still unclear. The tunica media of small muscular arteries regulates blood flow. The narrow lumen of these vessels produces an increased resistance, thereby reducing blood pressure to levels appropriate for metabolic exchange across the thin-walled capillaries. These vessels also serve to increase total peripheral resistance as reflected in systemic blood pressure. The disease represents a reversible narrowing of the lumen of resistance vessels resulting from contraction of smooth muscle mediated by neural or endogenous signals or increased sensitivity to vasoactive agents. The ultimate effect is an increased peripheral resistance and elevated blood pressure. This view of hypertension is complicated by the observation that even short periods of elevated pressure result in structural remodeling of the vessel wall, including an increase in smooth muscle mass and narrowing of the vessel lumen, to produce more permanent changes in vascular resistance [27]. Pathological change in the ratio of wall thickness to size of the lumen is central to elevation of blood pressure in hypertension. In arterial hypertension, VSMCs are functionally more contracted, structurally hypertrophic, and more collagen is secreted than under normal conditions. Hypertension may induce shear-related injury to the vessel. Endothelial injury (caused by hypertension) and vascular cell proliferation (induced by increased pressure and/or vasoactive substances) are effects that amplify the atherosclerotic process [28]. There are some data in literature on abnormalities in growth regulatory pathway in hypertension [6,29]. Morphometric studies have shown that SMC mass and connective tissue are both elevated in hypertensive arteries. Whether the increase in structural mass was due to hypertrophy or hyperplasia of the SMCs was, however, unclear. Somewhat surprisingly, it was found that the SMC of the adult, spontaneously hypertensive rat is polyploid, reflecting an increased cellular DNA content [30]. In hypertensive transgenic rats cellular mechanisms of proliferation was analyzed by the uptake of [^{3}H] thymidine in the presence and absence of phorbol-12, 13-dibutyrate, suggesting the involvement of a PKC-dependent pathway [31].

1.2 VSMC proliferation

Within the atherosclerotic lesions many cytokines and growth factors are formed but only a few play a dominant role in this process since their action is limited to the cells that express their specific surface receptors. The most important growth factors include both chains of platelet-derived growth factor (PDGF-A and PDGF-B), basic fibroblast growth factor (bFGF), insulin-like growth factor-I (IGF-I), epidermal growth factor (EGF), heparin-binding EGF-like growth factor (HB-EGF), macrophage-derived growth factor (MDGF) and transforming growth factor (TGF-α and TGF-β). The most relevant cytokines involved in atherosclerosis are tumor necrosis factor-α (TNF-α), interleukin-1 and interleukin-6 (IL-1 and IL-6) and interferon-γ (IFN-γ) [12]. Usually, growth factors and cytokines capable of stimulate SMC proliferation (PDGF, IGF, IL-1 and TNF-α) are undetectable in normal arteries but their expression is highly increased after injury or in the atherosclerotic lesions. On the contrary, bFGF is always present in high amounts in SMCs of the tunica media.

The most studied factor is PDGF [32] which induces directed migration and proliferation of SMCs, chemotaxis and chemokinesis [33]. PDGF is a competence factor and a potent mitogen for cells of mesenchymal origin (fibroblasts, glial cells and SMCs) and upon binding to its receptors stimulates rapid cellular responses. Paracrine and autocrine secretions have both been reported to be the sources of this factor, which is derived from clotted platelets. PDGF-like molecules are also released from endothelial cells, macrophages, or from the SMCs themselves. The importance of PDGF as a mediator in SMC hyperplasia is shown by the fact that its concentration increases in growing SMC in vitro [34], and that antibodies to PDGF inhibit neointimal SMC accumulation after angioplasty [24]. The response to PDGF stimulus includes a variety of intracellular signals. They involve activation of a tyrosine-specific protein kinase, phosphoinositide hydrolysis, activation of a phosphatidylinositol kinase, changes in intracellular pH and calcium, and increased expression of the c-fos and c-myc protooncogenes which encode proteins involved in the regulation of cell growth and differentiation. Human platelet PDGF is a 30 kD dimeric molecule composed of two disulfide-linked, partly homologous chains (A and B), that occurs as a homodimer (AA or BB) or a heterodimer (AB) [35]. SMCs appear to express only the A chain of PDGF and to synthesize PDGF-AA homodimers in a growth and differentiation-dependent manner, whereas endothelial cells and macrophages express mainly the B chain. The PDGF receptor was first identified as a 180- to 190-kD membrane glycoprotein and has an intrinsic tyrosine kinase activity [36]. Two types of receptors have been described, the α-type which preferentially binds A-chains and the β-type which binds B-chains. According to this model, preferential stimulation of either the α- or β-type receptor by the three different kinds of PDGF molecules could activate distinct signal transduction pathways [37]. The receptor can be found on VSMCs, fibroblasts and glial cells but it is not present in endothelial or on most hematopoietic cells. In cultured rat the VSMCs and the mitogenic responses to the three forms of PDGF are different, PDGF-BB being the most potent mitogen. The primary responses included the phosphorylation on tyrosine of phospholipase C-γ1 (PLC-γ1) and the PDGF receptor, which are key reactions in signal transduction associated to growth factor-induced cellular proliferation. PDGF-AB induced mitogenesis (measured as [³H] thymidine incorporation) but did not stimulate phosphorylation. PDGF-AA is a far weaker mitogen which does not elicit any transduction signal such as $[Ca^{2+}]_i$ elevation or Inostol 1,4,5-triosphosphate (IP₃) formation.

TGF-β) is a 25-kDa homodimer peptide that binds to specific cellular receptors in virtually all tissues, both normal and neoplastic [38]. As is the general case for the peptide growth factors, TGF-β is multifunctional and may exert proliferative effects, antiproliferative effects, or effects unrelated to proliferation [39,40]. TGF-β is synthesized by many cell types including smooth muscle, endothelial and macrophages and plays an important role in two process contributing to atherosclerosis, the SMC proliferation and the synthesis of connective tissue matrix collagen, proteoglycans and elastic fiber proteins [41]. TGF-β, usually present in a latent form, is activated by an acidic environment or by proteolytic enzymes, capable of releasing an active peptide [42]. A possible target for the actions of TGF-β is the phosphoinositide metabolism/PKC (PKC) pathway [43].

Many studies have shown the potential of PKC in regulating both normal and aberrant cell growth (reviewed in [44]). PKC became activated within the cell by translocation to the membrane where it binds to 1,2-diacylglycerol generated as a second messenger by phospholipase C [45]. In SMCs, TGF has diverse effects at the level of differentiation and growth [40,46,47]. These responses may vary depending on the cell type, whether the cells are from mesenchymal origin or ectodermal and the life cycle or cell density of that cell type [47]. In SMC from neural crest origin but not of mesenchymal origin, TGF signal transduction appears to be mediated by PKC and can potentiate PDGF-induced proliferation. However, TGF-β abolished PDGF-induced mitogenesis in mesenchymal VSMC [43]. DNA synthesis inhibition by TGF was also observed when SMCs from normal media or atheromatous intima were stimulated by fibroblast growth factor, SMC-derived growth factor or fetal calf serum [39]. TGF-β reversibly arrests SMCs at a point temporally located 1−2 h from S-phase, associated with this inhibitory effect is a decrease in the histone H1 kinase activity of p34^{cdc2} in the late G_1 phase [48]. TGF-β mRNA is rapidly induced following arterial injury and infusion of TGF-β in rats following aortic de-endothelialization enhanced neonitimal formation indicating the potential role of this factor in injury-induced atherogenesis [49]. Finally, it has been proposed that decreased TGF-β activity in vivo may contribute to the onset of vascular disease. In this context, compounds able to increase the levels of TGF may be beneficial in reducing SMC proliferation maintaining the vessel wall in a nonproliferating state. It has been found that heparin, heparan sulfate proteoglycan, tamoxifen and lipoprotein may keep the medial SMC in a quiescent state by releasing active TGF-β from inactive complexes with α_2 -macroglobulins or the extracellular matrix [50—52].

The cytokines IL-1 and TNF-α have been reported to have varying activities depending upon the type of cells which they act upon. IL-1 is able to induce in SMC the expression of PDGF-A chain and by the production of PDGF-AA this can exerts mitogenic effects on fibroblasts or SMCs. In a similar way, TNF-α can induce the formation of PDGF-B chain by arterial endothelial cells which in turn can affect surrounding cells in a paracrine manner [53].

Understanding the role of all these growth-regulatory molecules and their effects on the cells implicated in the atherosclerotic process will help to develop better strategies for diagnosis, treatment and prevention of the disease.

1.3 VSMCs differentiation and phenotypic modulation

SMCs are usually confined to the tunica media of the vessel wall where their contractile function serves to maintain vascular tone. SMCs exist both "in situ" and in culture as two different phenotypes: the contractile and the synthetic state. Contractile cells are differentiated, have a well developed contractile apparatus and their cytoplasm is packed with thin and thick myofilaments and dense bodies. On the contrary, synthetic cells are dedifferentiated, and undergo proliferation. Their main characteristics are a reduction in the volume fraction of myofilaments, an increase in the amounts of free ribosomes, mitochondria and rough endoplasmic reticulum and the loss of protein markers of contractility such as smooth muscle (SM) actin [3,54]. Synthetic cells are characteristic of the intimal lesions of atherosclerosis and of the vessels during embryonic development. The distinct phenotypes are only two points on a continuous spectrum of intermediate states of differentiation of SMC and the transition between the contractile to the synthetic state represents the phenotypic modulation [55]. This transition is correlated with changes in the levels of contractile and synthetic proteins.

During development or in pathological situations, biochemical and gene expression changes are correlated with the transition between phenotypes, and the expression of cytoskeletal and contractile proteins in skeletal muscle can serve as markers to characterize and describe the different stages of SMC differentiation [56,57]. The most studied proteins, actin and myosin, include specific isotypes which are characteristic of the different SMC states. The actin isoforms have been detected by isoelectrofocusing and include the α-SM specific actin which is the predominant form in normal arteries [58], the β-nonmuscle actin and the γ-isoactin which exists as both smooth muscle and nonmuscle isoforms [59—61]. Myosin is expressed in high amounts in contractile SMCs compared to the synthetic cells or fibroblasts.

In addition to the contractile proteins, two cytoplasmic structural proteins, vimentin and desmin, show changes with differentiation [60,62]. These proteins polymerize to form intermediate filaments characteristic of mesenchymal cells. Vimentin is found in many cell types whereas desmin is restricted to muscle cells (striated and smooth). VSMC express various ratios of desmin and vimentin that depend on both vessel type and biological species [63].

The process of SMC differentiation has been studied in cell culture models where changes similar to what occurs in vivo has been observed in cells undergoing proliferation. VSMC in vivo or freshly plated in vitro have a large volume fraction of myofilaments, they spontaneously contract or respond to vasoconstrictors, and synthesize small amounts of extracellular matrix. However, when growing in vitro, the cells undergo a spontaneous change in phenotype, they lose the ability to contract, the protein content changes, they respond to serum mitogens and increase their capability to divide and synthesize large amounts of extracellular matrix proteins [55]. Usually subcultured cells beyond passage 1 or 2 are in the irreversible synthetic state although some cells are able to express again the contractile phenotype when returning to quiescence [64]. Many studies have also shown that the induction of contractile proteins SM-specific is associated with growth arrest [61]. In particular, SM α-actin synthesis is rapidly induced after cell cycle withdrawal and its expression is repressed when postconfluent quiescent cultures are restimulated to initiate DNA synthesis by mitogenic agents.

An interesting observation by Blank et al. [65] was that PDGF was more effective than fetal calf serum in inhibiting α-actin synthesis. This suggests that potent mitogens such as PDGF may be involved in the control of SM cell differentiation, which correlates with the fact that PDGF expression is altered in pathological situations or during development [34].

2   EFFECT OF REACTIVE OXYGEN SPECIES IN VSMCs

2.1 Effects of reactive oxygen species on cell proliferation

VSMC proliferation is a significant pathological occurrence in a number of vascular diseases i.e., atherosclerosis, hypertension endothelial injury response and restenosis. The mechanisms at the basis of VSMC proliferation and the stimuli for its induction and maintenance are inadequately known. Recent reviews and articles deal with the initiation and the progression mechanisms leading to vascular muscular cell proliferation and their role in disease [12,66,67]. Understanding the molecular details of the altered signal transducing pathways in VSMCs may provide opportunities to develop new diagnostic, therapeutic and preventive tools for arteriosclerosis.

A number of observations suggest that cellular redox changes may be an important element in the control of cell growth and a role for oxidative stress in atherogenesis [68,69]. Reactive oxygen species have been reported in situations such as ischemia, thrombosis and angioplasty [70–74] that are associated with vascular smooth muscle proliferation and accelerated atherosclerosis. Consequently, the role of redox effects on the molecular events leading to SMC proliferation will be dealt with in the following parts of this chapter. Control of VSMC proliferation by reactive oxygen species has been less studied as in other cell types. The role of oxidants and antioxidants, proposed to be central in the pathogenesis of arteriosclerosis, gives these studies a special importance. Oxidants can stimulate proliferation in several cell types. Growth of melanoma cells is stimulated by ferricyanide [75], that of human skin fibroblasts [76] by active oxygen species with induction of c-fos and c-myc expression [77–79]. Oxidants also regulate nuclear factors and protein phosphorylation [14,80–88]. Probucol, a lipid-soluble antioxidant, administered to cholesterol-fed rabbits reduces the intima/media thickness ratio, inhibits neointimal macrophage accumulation in the balloon-catheterized carotid artery. These data suggest that reactive oxygen species may be involved in the intimal response to injury and that antioxidants may be therapeutically useful as inhibitors of restenosis [89]. Other results indicate that a high concentration of myocardial vitamin E can produce synergistic protective effects on recovery from ischemia during reperfusion [90].

In addition, α-tocopherol can partition the artery wall in critical cells such as SMCs, monocyte-macrophages, endothelial cells, and platelets, exerting beneficial effects. These effects can be illustrated by the inhibition of SMC proliferation, preservation of endothelial function, inhibition of monocyte-endothelial adhesion, inhibition of monocyte reactive oxygen species and cytokine release, and inhibition of platelet adhesion and aggregation [91]. A general scheme of signal transduction pathways and the effect of reactive oxygen species is shown in Fig. 2. Different reactive oxygen species exert distinct effects on VSMCs, with $O_2 \cdot^-$ – inducing proliferation and H_2O_2 causing apoptosis. Thus, reactive oxygen species might participate in atherosclerosis, restenosis, and hypertension in a dual manner by stimulating proliferation and triggering apoptosis of VSMCs [92].

Dicarbonyls regulate the expression of heparin-binding epidermal growth factor (HB-EGF) at the transcription level in rat aortic SMCs via production of intracellular peroxides. Since HB-EGF is known as a potent mitogen for SMCs and it is abundant in atherosclerotic plaques, the induction of HB-EGF, as well as the concomitant increment of intracellular peroxides, may trigger atherogenesis [93].

Elevated blood concentrations of lipoprotein a, constitute a major risk factor for atherosclerosis and stimulate the growth of human SMCs in culture [19,51,94]. Lipoproteins contain oxidized (possibly minimally oxidized) moieties [12] that may be responsible for the proliferative effects.

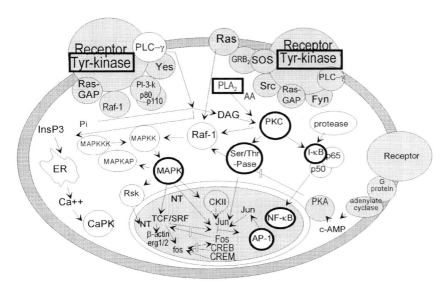

Fig. 2. Kinase cascade and possible sites of the interaction of oxygen radical species. The reactions that are sensitive to reactive oxygen species are circled with a heavy frame. Modified from Müller et al. **BBA** 1995;1155:151-179.

Carvedilol an antihypertension drug capable of attenuating oxygen free radical-initiated lipid peroxidation, inhibits mitogenesis in human cultured pulmonary artery VSMCs [95]. Carvedilol has been reported to reduce the neointimal growth following angioplasty by 84% and it was suggested that carvedilol may be effective in the treatment of atherosclerosis and vascular wall injury induced by angioplasty or coronary artery bypass [95].

2.2 Reactive oxygen species effects on inducible gene expression

Inducible gene expression in eukaryotes is mainly controlled by the activity of transcriptional activator proteins, such as nuclear factor κB (NF-κB) and activator protein-1 (AP-1). Oxidants and antioxidants affect these complexes in different ways and at different levels (Table 1). NF-κB is activated upon treatment of

Table 1. Redox changes at different levels affect the activation of AP-1 and NF-κB transcription factors.

	AP-1	NF-κB
Direct effects on the complex	[96]	[83,84,97,98]
Indirect effects on the signalling path leading to post-translational modifications	[99,100]	[101–103]
Transcriptional activation	[104]	?

cells with phorbol esters, lipopolysaccharides, IL-1 and TNF-α. Activation of NF-κB involves release of the inhibitory subunit nuclear factor κB inhibitor (I-κB) from a cytoplasmic complex with the DNA-binding subunits p65 and p50. Cell-free experiments have suggested that PKC and other kinases transfer phosphoryl groups onto I-κB causing release of I-κB and subsequent activation of NF-κB [101,105–109].

Although the intracellular pathways, leading to NF-κB activation are several and distinct, they may share a common intermediate step involving the synthesis of reactive oxygen intermediates [103]. Hydrogen peroxide and oxygen radicals are produced not only during inflammatory processes (reactive oxygen species), but also as an expression of regulatory processes (reactive oxygen intermediates). NF-κB can be in fact activated by an H_2O_2 treatment of cells from its inactive cytoplasmic form [102]. Moreover, treatment of cells with various protease inhibitors or an antioxidant completely prevented the inducible decay of I-κB, as well as the activation of NF-κB. NF-κB activation seems to rely on an inducible degradation of I-κB through a cytoplasmic, redox sensitive, chymotrypsin-like protease. In intact cells, phosphorylation of I-κB is apparently not sufficient for activation of NF-κB [101]. (Direct redox effects on NF-κB subunits have been also described [83,84,97,98].)

Fos and Jun form a dimeric complex (AP-1) [110–114] that controls basal and inducible transcription of several genes. AP-1 becomes activated through the phosphorylation cascade in which receptor-linked tyrosine kinases, PKC and the mitogen activated protein kinases (MAP-kinases) are involved.

The association of AP-1 with DNA sequences containing specific binding sites is sensitive to the reduction-oxidation status [96]. A single conserved cysteine residue, located in the DNA-binding domain has to be reduced either by reducing agents or by a nuclear redox factor (Ref-1), for AP-1 DNA-binding activity. Thus, direct redox regulation may limit the total level of functional fos-jun complexes in vivo and escaping from this control may lead to uncontrolled proliferation [96]. An antioxidant-responsive element [104] is also required for DNA binding of AP-1, this event being sensitive to the treatment with the antioxidants pyrrolidine dithiocarbamate and *N*-acetyl-L-cysteine. However, the latter may not be the same effect described by Curran's group [96] since a transcriptional induction of c-jun and c-fos genes appears to be at the basis of this antioxidant effect [104]. Hydrogen peroxide, on its own is only a weak inducer of AP-1, and suppresses phorbol ester activation of the factor. Similarly it has been shown that hydrogen peroxide can induce DNA synthesis in rat aortic SMCs [14]. Hydrogen peroxide and arachidonic acid could also induce c-jun mRNA in the aortic SMC in growth-arrested rat in a time-dependent manner. Phospholipase A_2 has been suggested to be the link between the former and the latter stimulus [99]. PKC plays a role in stimulating cell membrane associated phospholipase A_2 activity, and subsequent liberation of arachidonic acid from the exposure of rabbit pulmonary arterial SMCs to the oxidant hydrogen peroxide (H_2O_2) [100]. In macrophages, phorbol esters cause an increase in phosphorylation of the intracellular, high molecular weight phospholipase A_2. This increase in phosphorylation is accompanied by an increase in enzyme activity [115]. Phospholipase A_2 is, therefore, doubly regulated by Ca^{2+} (membrane interaction) and by phosphorylation (catalytic activity) and thus, PKC may be the primary target of oxidants, followed by further activation of other cellular events. The in vitro studies appear to reflect an in vivo situation since antioxidants protect against experimentally induced arterial lesions [116].

Neovascularization is a hallmark of neointimal formation in atherosclerotic plaques and restenotic lesions. Vascular endothelial growth factor promotes neovascular growth, whereas oxidative stress is a potent factor in vascular cell proliferation. H_2O elicits a dose- and time-dependent increase in vascular endothelial growth factor mRNA, protein expression and secretion. 4-Hydroxynonenal, an endogenous reactive oxygen species present in human atherosclerotic lesions, also increased vascular endothelial growth factor secretion in VSMCs. Regulators of vascular endothelial growth factor expression, such as reactive oxygen species, may enhance neovascularization of atherosclerotic and restenotic arteries [117].

Phorbol ester treatment of SMCs increases intracellular reactive oxygen and scavenger-receptor activity. Furthermore, direct treatment of SMCs with reactive oxygen species increases the scavenger-receptor activity. The increase in SMC scavenger-receptor expression this occurs at the level of gene transcription. Cytokines and growth factors that contribute to the generation of reactive oxygen species are present in atherosclerotic lesions. These factors may all contribute to the upregulation of SMC scavenger-receptor activity and, therefore, to the formation of smooth muscle foam cells [118].

Apoptosis of VSMC plays an important role in the genesis of atherosclerosis and restenosis. H_2O_2 and its derived form OH$\hat{c}dot$ might be related to apoptosis of VSMC in atherosclerosis and restenosis [119].

Reactive oxygen species increase the synthesis of IGF I and reduce the levels of the inhibitory IGF binding protein-4 in VSMCs. Furthermore, reactive oxygen species induce by DNA synthesis is inhibited by an anti-IGF I antiserum. These findings suggest that the autocrine IGF I system plays an important role in VSMC growth responses to reactive oxygen species [120].

2.3 Reactive oxygen species sensitivity of protein kinase C

As discussed in 2.2, a multiplicity of effects, sometimes of an opposite nature, on signal transduction, cell regulation and proliferation are caused by reactive oxygen species or by antioxidants. The use of comprehensive approaches (oxidative status or oxidative stress [121]) should now be assisted by analytical ones. This may lead to a more detailed understanding of the reactivity of different targets to specific oxidants and antioxidants. Protein kinase C, for example, can initially be activated by mild oxidative modification and subsequently inactivated by further oxidation. This dual activation-inactivation of PKC in response to H_2O_2 suggests an effective on/off signal mechanism able to influence cellular events

[122]. Periodate-induced modification of the regulatory domain of PKC causes activation of the kinase and loss of phorbol ester binding [123]. Thus, oxidant may be able to bypass normal transmembrane signalling systems to directly activate pathways involved in cellular regulation. PKC activity is increased several-fold in hepatocytes as a consequence of the production of quinone-generated active oxygen species. Thiol-reducing agents reverse quinone-mediated activation of PKC, suggesting a reduction-sensitive modification of its thiol/disulfide status [124]. An oxidation-induced persistent activation of PKC in hippocampal homogenates has also been reported [125]. Nitric oxide, an important cellular regulator, is involved in processes such as vasodilation, inhibition of platelet aggregation, and neurotransmission. Nitric oxide has been also shown to reversibly inactivate purified PKC and PKC in melanoma cells [126].

2.4 Reactive oxygen species sensitivity of tyrosine kinases

Receptor tyrosine kinases (such as EGF, PDGF etc, for a review see reference [127]) and nonreceptor tyrosine kinases (such as Src, Ras, etc, for a review see reference [128]) participate in normal cellular processes such as cell division, embryonic development and synaptic transmission [129]. They are also responsible, under certain circumstances, for pathological growth and development. The role of redox events as regulators of these central elements in the control of cell functions is poorly understood. However, information on different cell types begins to emerge, as reviewed below. No data are as yet available for SMCs.

Oxidants produced by redox cycling of naphthoquinones stimulate an adenosine- insensitive phosphatidylinositol kinase in rat liver membranes through tyrosine phosphorylation of the enzyme [130]. Exposure of human neutrophils to exogenous oxidants or endogenous production of superoxide induces marked tyrosine phosphorylation of several cellular proteins by effects of oxidation-sensitive tyrosine kinases and/or phosphatases [131]. Tyrosine-specific protein phosphorylation by rat liver plasma membranes and particulate fractions is markedly increased by quinones and inhibited by superoxide dismutase, catalase, and desferroxamine. A free radical-mediated mechanism is suggested for the quinone stimulation of protein phosphorylation [132]. A similarity was observed between the effects of redox cycling quinones and orthovanadate, a potent phosphotyrosyl phosphatase inhibitor, in the proliferation of 3T3-L1 cells cultured in serum-free media. Orthovanadate and 2,3-dimethoxy-1,4-naphthoquinone are alike in PI-3-kinase activation, c-fos proto-oncogene expression, and DNA synthesis, which are key events associated with cell growth. These data support the concept of an oxidant-mediated increase in tyrosine protein phosphorylation as an early event in the signal transduction cascade of growth factor receptors, leading to augmentation of cell proliferation [133,134]. p56lck is a Src-related protein-tyrosine kinase which has SH_2 and SH_3 domains and is involved in T cell signaling and oncogenic transformation. In T cells oxidative reagents such as hydrogen peroxide (H_2O_2) and diamide induce phosphorylation p56lck both at Tyr-394 (autophosphorylation site) and at Tyr-505 (negative regulatory site) [135]. Oxidative stress in T cells suppresses both CD3- and CD4-induced Ca^{2+} responses and correlates with a reduction in the level of phospholipase C-γ_1 tyrosine phosphorylation. Low concentrations of oxidant increase tyrosine kinase activity following cell stimulation. Signal transduction in T cells involves the activation of phospholipase C-γ_1 by tyrosine phosphorylation through an oxidation-sensitive intermediate between surface receptors and tyrosine kinases, perhaps including the interaction between CD4 and pp56lck [136]. Leukocyte tyrosine kinase is an unusual membrane protein lacking an extracellular domain, it resembles a receptor tyrosine kinase; it has a short, glycosylated, and cysteine-rich *N*-terminal domain. Yet, it appears to function with a ligand-independent mechanism. Its gene also produces a putative receptor tyrosine kinase for an unknown ligand [137]. Its in vivo catalytic activity is markedly enhanced by alkylating and thiol-oxidizing agents [86]. Hydrogen peroxide is an important reactive oxygen species implicated in lung vascular constriction and injury. Exposure to H_2O_2 causes smooth muscle contractions in isolated pulmonary arteries. Activation of tyrosine kinases mediates H_2O_2-induced contractions [138].

Oxygen-derived free radicals have also been shown to behave vasodilatory via enhancement of adenylyl cyclase activity. This activation occurs probably via tyrosine kinase-mediated effects on the catalytic subunit of adenylyl cyclase [139].

2.5 Reactive oxygen species and MAP kinases

Hydrogen peroxide induces phosphorylation of MAP-kinases. This event is markedly lower in the presence of protein tyrosine kinase inhibitors or in PKC down-regulated SMCs [140]. The expression of MAP kinase phosphatase-1 (MKP-1), a redox-sensitive protein tyrosine/threonine phosphatase (PTP), is transcriptionally and positively regulated by H_2O_2 and $O_2^- -$ [141]. H_2O_2 treatment stimulates extracellular signal-regulated protein kinase (ERK-$_1$) via successive activation of PKC, Raf-1, and mitogen-activated protein kinase (MEK1) [142].

2.6 Reactive oxygen species sensitivity of phosphatases

An SH-dependent protein phosphatase is inactivated during the early events of TNF/IL-1 signal transduction, hence inhibitors of protein phosphatases and H_2O_2 can mimic the early effects of TNF/IL-1 on cells [143]. A messenger RNA is highly inducible by oxidative stress and heat shock in human skin cells. The corresponding cDNA contains an open reading frame specifying a protein of M(r) 39.3 K with the structural features of a nonreceptor-type protein-tyrosine phosphatase and has significant amino-acid sequence similarity to a Tyr/Ser-protein phosphatase of vaccinia virus. The expressed and purified protein has intrinsic phosphatase activity [144].

Numerous reports have shown that cellular redox status plays an important role in signal transduction pathways that operate via tyrosine phosphorylation. H_2O_2 effects have been reported on three PTPs, PTP1, LAR (leukocyte antigen-related phosphatases), and VHR (vaccinia H1-related) and on three distinct serine/ threonine protein phosphatases (PP2Cα, calcineurin, and lambda phosphatase) were determined. Hydrogen peroxide had no apparent effect on serine/threonine protein phosphatase activity. In contrast, protein tyrosine phosphatases were rapidly inactivated with low μM concentrations of H_2O_2, but not with large alkyl hydroperoxides [145].

Reactive oxygen species lead to an increase in tyrosine phosphorylation, together with an increase in tyrosine phosphatase activity [146].

Calcineurin is the only protein phosphatase known to be under the control of Ca^{2+} and calmodulin. It is targeted by immunosuppressive drugs and has a critical role in T-cell activation. It is specifically inhibited by immunosuppressant immunophilin complexes and inactivated in vitro and in vivo by superoxide. Superoxide produces oxidative damage to the Fe-Zn active center of calcineurin. The redox-state of iron provides a mechanism to regulate calcineurin activity by desensitizing the enzyme and coupling Ca^{2+}-dependent protein dephosphorylation to the cellular redox state [147].

2.7 Bcl-2 expression

The protooncogene bcl-2 inhibits apoptotic cell death caused by a number of mechanisms involving reactive oxygen species [148]. Bcl-2 is localized to intracellular sites of oxygen free radical generation including the mitochondria, endoplasmic reticulum, and nuclear membranes. Bcl-2 protects cells from H_2O_2- and menadione-induced oxidative deaths. Bcl-2 has been suggested to regulate an antioxidant pathway at sites of free radical generation. [114,149,150]. The involvement of Bcl-2 in SMC proliferation control has not been studied yet. However, Bcl-2 may be a fundamental element, not only in preventing oxidant-induced cell death, but also in the regulation of oxidant induced cell proliferation.

2.8 Reactive oxygen species sensitive proteases

Inducible gene expression in eukaryotes is mainly controlled by the activity of transcriptional activator proteins, such as NF-κB. The activation of NF-κB is regulated by PKC and other kinases. Transfer of phosphoryl groups onto I-κB (inhibitory subunit of the complex) causes release of I-κB and subsequent activation of NF-κB. Treatment of cells with various protease inhibitors or an antioxidant prevents the I-κB decay and NF-κB activation. A chymotrypsin-like redox-sensitive protease or protease inhibitor may be responsible for the inducible degradation of I-κB [101]. Heparin, an inhibitor of VSMC proliferation and migration, affects a number of other cell functions. These effects include inhibition of growth factor binding, deposition of matrix proteins and gene expression. Various mechanisms have been proposed and, yet, how heparin works as an inhibitor remains unclear. It has been postulated [151] that heparin inhibits SMC growth and migration by suppressing the expression of matrix-degrading enzymes such as plasminogen activators and interstitial collagenase. The effect of protease inhibitors also confirms the role of proteases in the mechanism of SMC proliferation [152]. A subclass of thiol protease inhibitors (benzyloxycarbonyl-Leu-norleucinal and acetyl-Leu-Leu-norleucinal), that reversibly inhibit bovine aortic SMC proliferation in vitro, cause a block of platelet-derived growth factor-BB, as well as serum-inducible cell cycle progression at a point before the G_1-S boundary. Acetyl-Leu-Leu-norleucinal caused a 4-fold decrease in the transient elevation of fos and myc proto-oncogenes, as well as a decrease in the levels of both muscle and nonmuscle actin mRNA induced early after serum addition [152]. To what extent the activity of these proteases is redox sensitive has not yet been established. However, in liver cells evidence has been produced for enhanced expression of c-fos, c-jun, and the Ca^{2+}-activated neutral protease in response to oxidative cellular damage [153].

2.9 Paracrine modulation by reactive oxygen species

Effects of oxygen species may not only be direct on SMCs, but also indirect, on adjacent cells, such as endothelial cells or macrophages. As a result they may secrete growth factors responsible for the proliferation of SMCs. VSMCs proliferate in response to arterial injury. A common mechanism by which endothelial cells and inflammatory cells stimulate VSMCs growth could be the active oxygen species (i.e., O^{2-}, H_2O_2, and $\hat{c}dot OH$) generated during arterial injury [154]. Platelet-derived growth factor produced by endothelial cells, is a major stimulant for proliferation of VSMCs. Endothelial cells are apparently capable of sensing oxygen tension and discriminating and responding even to small differences in oxygen tension, resulting in dramatic upregulation of the platelet-derived growth factor gene [155]. Endothelial cells subjected to cell injury or to H_2O_2 are capable of producing platelet-derived growth factor, a mitogen for the stimulation of fibroblast and SMC proliferation [156].

3   THE EFFECT OF d-α-TOCOPHEROL ON VSMCs

3.1 Effect of tocopherols on cell proliferation

Tocopherols have been shown to modify the course of cell proliferation, in a positive or negative way depending on the preexisting situation. Lipid peroxidation occurs in small amounts when medial cells from guinea pig aorta are grown in tissue culture. Such an effect is strongly stimulated by polyunsaturated fatty acids and associated with inhibition of cell proliferation. d-α-Tocopherol when added to these cells in culture inhibits lipid peroxidation and enhances the extent of cell proliferation by overcoming the inhibitory effect of polyunsaturated fatty acid on the extent of cell proliferation [157—160]. Another indirect way for d-α-

Tocopherol to affect cell proliferation is through the protection of low-density lipoproteins from oxidative modification. d-α-Tocopherol has been shown to prevent LDL oxidation in vitro and retard the progression of atherosclerosis in animal models. In addition, supplementation of human subjects with antioxidants has been shown to increase the resistance of their low-density lipoproteins to oxidation and to protect against arteriosclerosis [161–165]. In other studies vitamin E both increased the cloning potential and the number of population increasing 2-fold for SMCs and the endothelial cell proliferation in culture [166,167]. From these and other studies it appears clear that in cells, possibly when their growth is inhibited by lipid peroxidation and antioxidants (and, therefore, also d-α-tocopherol) they may restimulate proliferation by removing the inhibitory lipid peroxide. d-α-Tocopherol has also a direct effect as cell growth inhibitor and this effect is not obviously mediated by its reduction-oxidation properties [19,89,168–170]. In fact, d-β-tocopherol (an equally potent antioxidant [171]) is not capable of inhibiting cell proliferation [89]. The inhibition by d-α-tocopherol of cell proliferation is cell type specific and depends on the mitogen responsible for stimulating growth.

d-α-Tocopherol (50 µM) inhibits cell growth approximately 50%. However, d-β-tocopherol, an analogue of d-α-tocopherol lacking a methyl group in position 7 of the chromanol ring, does not show any inhibition of cell proliferation. The amount of d-α- and d-β-tocopherol present in the cells as measured after 24 h incubation is not significantly different, indicating that the lack of inhibition is not due to a different uptake of d-β-tocopherol [89]. The effect of α-tocopherol depends on the type of mitogen utilized to stimulate cell proliferation. The inhibition of cell proliferation produced by 50 µM d-α-tocopherol is maximal when PDGF, endothelin or native LDL are used as growth stimulant. Other stimulants, such as lysophosphatidic acid, bombesin, and foetal calf serum (FCS) were less effective. When streptolysin-O makes the SMCs permeable a peptide substrate for PKC is introduced, d-α-tocopherol inhibits PKC activity, whereas β-tocopherol is much less effective [89]. Although the effect of d-α-tocopherol depends on the cell type (Table 2), all the SMC lines tested are inhibited by d-α-tocopherol, including two human primary cultures. The molecular basis of d-α-tocopherol specificity is not clear at the present moment. It can be based on a different signaling pathway used for proliferation in the various cell types (Table 3). It may be possible that d-α-tocopherol transport and metabolism is different, depending on the cell type. Finally, it may be conceivable that d-α-tocopherol binding proteins related to d-α-tocopherol inhibition are present in some cells and not in others [172].

3.2 Effect of tocopherols on PKC activity

It has been shown above that d-α-tocopherol causes inhibition of PKC activity, a signaling element that can regulate cell proliferation in some, but not all cells, depending on the type of mitogen employed to stimulate growth [45]. The time

Table 2. The growth inhibitory effect of d-α-tocopherol on different cell lines.

Tissue of origin	Sensitive	Insensitive
Rat aorta smooth muscle	A10/A7r5	
Human aorta smooth muscle	hAI	
Human tenon's fibroblasts	hTF	
Human skin fibroblasts	CCD-SK	
Mouse neuroblastoma	NB2A	
Human pigmented retinal epitelial cells	hPRE	
Human leukaemia	U937	
Human prostate tumor	DU-145,	
Mouse fibroblast	Balb/c-3T3	
Glioma	C6	
		HeLa
Chinese hamster lung		LR73
Chinese hamster ovary		CHO
Human osteosarcoma		Saos-2
Mouse macrophage		P388 Dl

of addition of d-α-tocopherol during the cell cycle appeared to determine the extent of PKC inhibition observed after several hours of incubation. The inhibitory effect disappearing if d-α-tocopherol is added in the late G_1-phase and PKC activity measured in the subsequent S-phase. Inhibition of activity is not caused by a decrease in the amount of PKC level.

The inhibition by d-α-tocopherol and the lack of inhibition by d-β-tocopherol of cell proliferation and PKC activity indicate that the mechanism involved is not related to the radical scavenging properties of these two molecules, which are essentially equal [171] (Table 4). On the basis of the analysis of several other tocopherols and similar compounds, a ligand -interaction mechanism has been proposed for the inhibition of cell proliferation by d-α-tocopherol. Although an

Table 3. Differential inhibition by d-α-tocopherol of A7r5 cells stimulated to proliferate with various mitogens.

Mitogenic stimulus	Inhibition by d-α-tocopherol, %
Lysophosphatidic acid (50 μM)	8 ± 1.5
Bombesin (20 nM)	26 ± 4.5
FCS (2%)	52 ± 2.0
PDGF-BB (20 ng/ml)	93 ± 3.0
Endothelin (80 nM)	94 ± 2.5
LDL (5 μg/ml)	99 ± 1.0

Quiescent cells were incubated in DMEM containing the indicated mitogens in the presence or absence of 50 μM d-α-tocopherol. [³H]Thymidine incorporation (in the case of lysophosphatidic acid, bombesin and endothelin) or cell number (in the case of the other mitogens) were determined. Results are expressed as percentage of the control incorporation for each mitogen measured in the absence of d-α-tocopherol and are the mean of triplicate determinations from a representative experiment.

Table 4. Comparison of d-α-and d-β-tocopherol antioxidant properties (from [171]).

Compound	Relative antioxidant potency	Stoichiometry factor
d-α-tocopherol	[1]	[2]
d-β-tocopherol	0.89	2.04

inhibition of PKC activity by d-α-tocopherol has been documented a detailed molecular mechanism of this inhibition is still elusive. PKC is inhibited at a cellular level d-α-tocopherol but not with the isolated enzyme, suggesting an indirect mechanism of action. The diminished phosphorylation of PKC specific substrates by d-α-tocopherol can be reconciled with the following hypothesis. d-α-Tocopherol prevents the activation of the enzyme by hindering its phosphorylation [173] (for a review see [45]), or it activates the phosphatase which dephosphorylates PKC [174,175]. It appears that the activation of a protein phosphatase (PP$_2$A) is related to the dephosphorylation and inactivation of PKC by α-tocopherol. The inhibition of SMCs proliferation by d-α-tocopherol at physiological concentrations may explain the notion that in vivo SMCs are quiescent and that they multiply only under stress condition [6,176]. Depletion of d-α-tocopherol may occur locally or generally as a consequence of oxidative stress [177–179] and such a condition would result in a cell growth stimulation. A dietary or oxidative diminution of d-α-tocopherol can thus, play a role in the onset and development of arteriosclerosis.

dl-α-tocopherol, added to a human erythroleukemia HEL and a megakaryoblastic leukemia, Meg-01, cell culture produces a reversible, dose-dependent inhibition of phorbol ester-induced adhesion. PKC appears to mediate shape change and adhesion, both of which are strongly inhibited by dl-α-tocopherol [180].

Platelet incorporation of α-tocopherol at levels attained with oral supplementation is associated with inhibition of platelet aggregation through a PKC-dependent mechanism. These observations may represent one potential mechanism for the observed beneficial effect of α-tocopherol in preventing the development of coronary artery disease [181].

Enrichment of vascular tissue with α-tocopherol protects the vascular endothelium from oxidized LDL-mediated dysfunction, at least in part, through the inhibition of PKC stimulation. These findings also suggest one potential mechanism for the observed beneficial effect of α-tocopherol in preventing the clinical expression of coronary artery disease that is distinct from the antioxidant protection of LDL [182].

Administration of vitamin E prevents hemodynamic changes in retina and renal glomeruli of diabetic rats. In addition, the inhibition of PKC β isoforms by a specific inhibitor (LY333531) can normalize the changes in gene expression of cytokines, caldesmon, and hemodynamics. These results provide supportive evidence that the activation of PKC, especially the β isoforms, is involved in the development of diabetic vascular complications, and that PKC β inhibitors can be used in the treatment of diabetic vascular complications [183].

In addition to decreasing LDL oxidation, α-tocopherol exerts intracellular effects on cells crucial in atherogenesis, such as monocytes. After α-tocopherol supplementation, there is a significant decrease in the release of reactive oxygen species, lipid oxidation, IL-1 β secretion, and monocyte-endothelial cell adhesion [184]. The inhibition of reactive oxygen species release and lipid oxidation is due to an inhibition of PKC activity by α-tocopherol. Thus, this study provides novel evidence for an intracellular effect of α-tocopherol in monocytes that is antiatherogenic [184]. α-Tocopherol, but not several tocopherol derivatives inhibit the superoxide generation of rat peritoneal neutrophils induced by phorbol 12-myristate 13-acetate. This phenomenon is associated with PKC inhibition [185].

3.3 Effect of d-α-tocopherol on inducible gene expression

Recent studies have examined the effects of a vitamin E analogue (2,2,5,7,8-Pentamethyl-6-hydroxychromane) on the tumor necrosis factor-α-induced NF-κB activation in Jurkat T cells causing complete inhibition of NF-κB activation [186]. AP-1 activation appears to be specifically caused by d-α-tocopherol and not by d-β-tocopherol (Träuble et al., unpublished). On the other hand, when the AP-1 complex was activated by phorbol esters, its DNA-binding was prevented by d-α-tocopherol but not by d-β-tocopherol, indicating a specific site of d-α-tocopherol interaction with the cell signaling pathway (Träuble et al., unpublished).

α-Tocopherol, as revealed by differential display mRNA analysis, increases the transcription of α-tropomyosin mRNA (isoform TMBr-2). As shown in Fig. 3, the protein expression increases, as well as in the α-tocopherol that was treated, synchronously growing SMCs reached a maximum after 4 h of restimulation. Tropomyosins are known for their role in muscular contraction, regulation of actin filament stability, intracellular granule movement, cell shape determination and cytokinesis. In light of these observations, it might be possible that the induction of this tropomyosin isoform is an early event induced by α-tocopherol, leading to cell proliferation inhibition (Aratri et al., unpublished).

PKC α-protein expression in human fibroblasts is increased approximately 8-fold from birth to 70 years of age. Collagenase (MMP-1) gene transcription and protein expression is also increased with age, in parallel to protein kinase C, as expected from the presence of a TRE element in collagenase gene promoter region. α-Tocopherol, which inhibits PKC activity, is able to diminish collagenase gene transcription without altering the level of its natural inhibitor, tissue inhibitor of metalloproteinase, TIMP-1. Tocopherol inhibition of PKC may be a natural way to protect against aging by bringing down the level of collagenase expression (Fig. 4; Ricciarelli et al., unpublished).

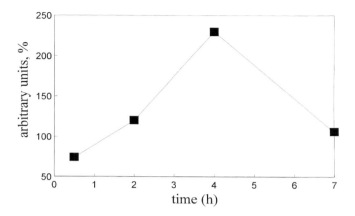

Fig. 3. Time course of tropomyosin protein expression in smooth muscle cells under the effect of α-to-copherol. Cells were harvested at the indicated time points after restimulation with fetal calf serum in the presence or absence of α-tocopherol. An antitropomyosin antiserum was used to detect the protein. Anti-actin antiserum was used to normalize protein levels.

4   SUMMARY AND PERSPECTIVES

1. Recent research at cellular level has shifted the accent from the phenomenolo-gical description of oxidant damage and antioxidant protection to the mecha-nisms of oxidant and antioxidant modification of molecular signaling.
2. The notion of sole radical damage of lipids, proteins and nucleic acids declines in favor of targeted reactive oxygen species.

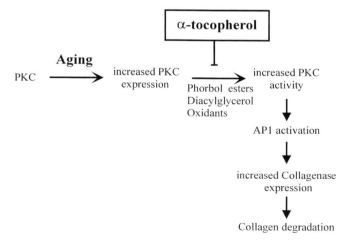

Fig. 4. α-Tocopherol prevents PKC mediated expression of collagenase in human fibroblast.

3. Reactive oxygen species have been found to have multiple interaction points in a cell with similar or opposite terminal effects.
4. Antioxidant molecules have additional nonantioxidant biological properties, which begin to emerge, as modulators of signal transduction enzymes and gene expression.

These new concepts are of great relevance for a better understanding of the molecular basis of disease and for their pharmacological implications. The field of the molecular interaction of antioxidants and oxidants with cell components is at the beginning of a prosperous future.

5   ACKNOWLEDGEMENTS

The present study has been supported by the Swiss Research Foundation, by F. Hoffman-La Roche, AG and by the Foundation for Nutrition Research in Switzerland.

6   ABBREVIATIONS

AP-1:	Activator protein-1
ERK:	Extracellular signal-regulated protein kinase
FCS:	Foetal calf serum
I-κB:	Nuclear factor κB inhibitor
IGF I:	Insulin like growth factor I
IL-1:	Interleukin-1
IP$_3$:	Inositol 1,4,5-trisphosphate
LAR:	Leukocyte antigen-related phosphate
LDL:	Low density lipoprotein
MAP-kinase:	Mitogen activated protein kinase
MEK:	Mitogen-activated protein kinase kinase
NF-κB:	Nuclear factor κB
PDGF:	Platelet derived growth factor
PKC:	Protein kinase C
PLC:	Phospholipase C
PP:	Protein phosphatase
PTP:	Protein tyrosine phosphatase
SMC:	Smooth muscle cell
TGF-β:	Transforming growth factor-β
TNF-α:	Tumor necrosis factor-α
VHR:	Vaccinia H1-related phosphatase
VSMC:	Vascular smooth muscle cell

7 REFERENCES

1. Schwartz SM, Heimark RL, Majesky MW. Physiol Rev 1990;70:1177–1209.
2. Campbell GR, Campbell JH. Exp Mol Pathol 1985;42:139–162.
3. Thyberg J, Hedin U, Sjolund M, Palmberg L, Bottger BA. Arteriosclerosis 1990;10:966–990.
4. Oertel WH, Kupsch A. Curr Opin Neurol Neurosurg 1993;6:323–332.
5. Badimon JJ, Fuster V, Badimon L. Circulation 1992;86:III86–III94.
6. Raines EW, Ross R. Br Heart J 1993;69:S30–S37.
7. Rao GN, Berk BC. Circ Rev 1992;70:593–599.
8. Fuster V, Badimon L, Badimon JJ, Chesebro JH. N Engl J Med 1992;326:242–250.
9. Bondjers G, Glukhova M, Hansson GK, Postnov YV, Reidy MA, Schwartz SM. Circulation 1991;84:V12–V16.
10. Ross R, Agius L. Diabetologia 1992;35(Suppl2):S34–S40.
11. Fuster V, Badimon JJ, Badimon L. Circulation 1992;86:III1–III11.
12. Ross R. Nature 1993;362:801–809.
13. Schwartz CJ, Valente AJ, Sprague EA. Am J Cardiol 1993;71:9B–14B.
14. Rao GN, Lassegue B, Griendling KK, Alexander RW, Berk BC. Nucl Acids Res 1993;21:1259–1263.
15. Kita T, Nagano Y, Yokode M, Ishii K, Kume N, Narumiya S, Kawai C. Am J Cardiol 1988;62:13B–19B.
16. Bjorkhem I, Henriksson Freyschuss A, Breuer O, Diczfalusy U, Berglund L, Henriksson P. Arteri400scl Thromb 1991;11:15–22.
17. Cushing SD, Berliner JA, Valente AJ, Territo MC, Navab M, Parhami F, Gerrity R, Schwartz CJ, Fogelman AM. Proc Natl Acad Sci USA 1990;87:5134–5138.
18. Witztum JL. Br Heart J 1993;69:S12–S18.
19. Özer NK, Palozza P, Boscoboinik D, Azzi A. FEBS Lett 1993;322:307–310.
20. Mercuro G, Cherchi A. Cardiologia 1991;36:291–297.
21. Simons M, Leclerc G, Safian RD, Isner JM, Weir L, Baim DS. N Engl J Med 1993;328:608–613.
22. Reidy MA. Arch Pathol Lab Med 1992;116:1276–1280.
23. Marmur JD, Poon M, Rossikhina M, Taubman MB. Circulation 1992;86:III53–III60.
24. Ferns GA, Raines EW, Sprugel KH, Motani AS, Reidy MA, Ross R. Science 1991;253:1129–1132.
25. Reidy MA, Fingerle J, Lindner V. Circulation 1992;86:III43–III46.
26. Libby P, Schwartz D, Brogi E, Tanaka H, Clinton SK. Circulation 1992;86:III47–III52.
27. Folkow B. Physiol Rev 1982;62:347–504.
28. Dzau VJ. J Cardiovasc Pharmacol 1990;15(Suppl 5):S59–S64.
29. Saltis J, Little P, Bobik A. Clin Exp Pharmacol Physiol 1991;18:319–322.
30. Owens GK, Schwartz SM. Circ Res 1982;51:280–289.
31. Peiro C, Rosa de Sagarra M, Redondo J, Sanchez Ferrer CF, Marin J. J Cardiovasc Pharmacol 1992;20(Suppl 12):S128–S131.
32. Williams HT, Fenna D, Macbeth RA. Surg Gynecol Obstet 1971;132:662–666.
33. Fingerle J, Johnson R, Clowes AW, Majesky MW, Reidy MA. Proc Natl Acad Sci USA 1989;86:8412–8416.
34. Walker LN, Bowen Pope DF, Ross R, Reidy MA. Proc Natl Acad Sci USA. 1986;83:7311–7315.
35. Hart CE, Bailey M, Curtis DA, Osborn S, Raines E, Ross R, Forstrom JW. Biochemistry 1990;29:166–172.
36. Heldin CH, Backstrom G, Ostman A, Hammacher A, Ronnstrand L, Rubin K, Nister M, Westermark B. EMBO J 1988;7:1387–1393.
37. Yarden Y, Escobedo JA, Kuang WJ, Yang Feng TL, Daniel TO, Tremble PM, Chen EY, Ando ME, Harkins RN, Francke U. Nature 1986;323:226–232.

38. Massague J, Cheifetz S, Boyd FT, Andres JL. Ann NY Acad Sci 1990;593:59–72.
39. Morisaki N, Kawano M, Koyama N, Koshikawa T, Umemiya K, Saito Y, Yoshida S. Atherosclerosis 1991;88:227–234.
40. Majack RA. J Cell Biol 1987;105:465–471.
41. Owens GK, Geisterfer AA, Yang YW, Komoriya A. J Cell Biol 1988;107:771–780.
42. Majack RA, Majesky MW, Goodman LV. J Cell Biol 1990;111:239–247.
43. Wrenn RW, Raeuber CL, Herman LE, Walton WJ, Rosenquist TH. In Vitro Cell Dev Biol 1993;29A:73–78.
44. Nishizuka Y. Nature 1984;308:693–698.
45. Azzi A, Boscoboinik D, Hensey C. Eur J Biochem 1992;208:547–557.
46. Assoian RK, Sporn MB. J Cell Biol 1986;102:1217–1223.
47. Goodman LV, Majack RA. J Biol Chem 1989;264:5241–5244.
48. Reddy KB, Howe PH. J Cell Physiol 1993;156:48–55.
49. Majesky MW, Lindner V, Twardzik DR, Schwartz SM, Reidy MA. J Clin Invest 1991;88:904–910.
50. Castellot JJ, Jr., Beeler DL, Rosenberg RD, Karnovsky MJ. J Cell Physiol 1984;120:315–320.
51. Grainger DJ, Kirschenlohr HL, Metcalfe JC, Weissberg PL, Wade DP, Lawn RM. Science 1993;260:1655–1658.
52. Grainger DJ, Weissberg PL, Metcalfe JC. Biochem J 1993;294:109–112.
53. Hajjar KA, Hajjar DP, Silverstein RL, Nachman RL. J Exp Med 1987;166:235–245.
54. Campbell GR, Campbell JH. Ann NY Acad Sci 1990;598:143–158.
55. Chamley Campbell J, Campbell GR, Ross R. Physiol Rev 1979;59:1–61.
56. Shanahan CM, Weissberg PL, Metcalfe JC. Circ Res 1993;73:193–204.
57. Glukhova MA, Kabakov AE, Frid MG, Ornatsky OI, Belkin AM, Mukhin DN, Orekhov AN, Koteliansky VE, Smirnov VN. Proc Natl Acad Sci USA 1988;85:9542–9546.
58. Clowes AW, Clowes MM, Kocher O, Ropraz P, Chaponnier C, Gabbiani G. J Cell Biol 1988;107:1939–1945.
59. Gabbiani G, Kocher O, Bloom WS, Vandekerckhove J, Weber K. J Clin Invest 1984;73:148–152.
60. Kocher O, Gabbiani G. Differentiation 1986;32:245–251.
61. Owens GK, Loeb A, Gordon D, Thompson MM. J Cell Biol 1986;102:343–352.
62. Lazarides E. Annu Rev Biochem 1982;51:219–250.
63. Kocher O, Skalli O, Bloom WS, Gabbiani G. Lab Invest 1984;50:645–652.
64. Thyberg J, Nilsson J, Palmberg L, Sjolund M. Cell Tissue Res 1985;239:69–74.
65. Blank RS, Thompson MM, Owens GK. J Cell Biol 1988;107:299–306.
66. Fleischer S, Fleischer B, Azzi A, Chance B. Biochim Biophys Acta 1971;225:194–200.
67. Azzi A, Rossi E, Azzone GF. Enzymo Biol Clin 1966;7:25–37.
68. Fridovich I. Science 1978;201:875–880.
69. Halliwell B. Br J Exp Pathol 1989;70:737–757.
70. Redl H, Gasser H, Schlag G, Marzi I. Br Med Bull 1993;49:556–565.
71. Ambrosio G, Zweier JL, Duilio C, Kuppusamy P, Santoro G, Elia PP, Tritto I, Cirillo P, Condorelli M, Chiariello M. J Biol Chem 1993;268:18532–18541.
72. Horton JW, Walker PB. J Appl Physiol 1993;74:1515–1520.
73. Granger DN, Kvietys PR, Perry MA. Can J Physiol Pharmacol 1993;71:67–75.
74. Kontos HA, Wei EP, Povlishock JT, Christman CW. Circ Res 1984;55:295–303.
75. Ellem KA, Kay GF. Biochem Biophys Res Commun 1983;112:183–190.
76. Murrell GA, Francis MJ, Bromley L. Biochem J 1990;265:659–665.
77. Shibanuma M, Kuroki T, Nose K. J Cell Physiol 1988;136:379–383.
78. Amstad P, Crawford D, Muehlematter D, Zbinden I, Larsson R, Cerutti P. Bull Cancer 1990;77:501–502.
79. Cerutti PA. Science 1985;227:375–381.
80. Malviya AN, Anglard P. FEBS Lett 1986;200:265–270.
81. Xanthoudakis S, Curran T. EMBO J 1992;11:653–665.

82. Abate C, Patel L, Rauscher FJ, Curran T. Science 1990;249:1157–1161.
83. Toledano MB, Ghosh D, Trinh F, Leonard WJ. Mol Cell Biol 1993;13:852–860.
84. Toledano MB, Leonard WJ. Proc Natl Acad Sci USA 1991;88:4328–4332.
85. Staal FJ, Roederer M, Herzenberg LA. Proc Natl Acad Sci USA 1990;87:9943–9947.
86. Bauskin AR, Alkalay I, Ben Neriah Y. Cell 1991;66:685–696.
87. Dartsch PC, Voisard R, Betz E. Res Exp Med 1990;190:77–87.
88. Dartsch PC, Voisard R, Bauriedel G, Hofling B, Betz E. Arteriosclerosis 1990;10:62–75.
89. Chatelain E, Boscoboinik DO, Bartoli GM, Kagan VE, Gey FK, Packer L, Azzi A. Biochim Biophys Acta 1993;1176:83–89.
90. Haramaki N, Packer L, Assadnazari H, Zimmer G. Biochem Biophys Res Commun 1993;196: 1101–1107.
91. Devaraj S, Jialal I. Curr Opin Lipid 1998;9:11–15.
92. Li PF, Dietz R, von Harsdorf R. Circulation 1997;96:3602–3609.
93. Che W, Asahi M, Takahashi M, Kaneto H, Okado A, Higashiyama S, Taniguchi N. J Biol Chem 1997;272:18453–18459.
94. Buhler FR, Tkachuk VA, Hahn AW, Resink TJ. J Hypertens 1991;9(Suppl):S28–S36.
95. Ohlstein EH, Douglas SA, Sung CP, Yue TL, Louden C, Arleth A, Poste G, Ruffolo RR, Jr., Feuerstein GZ. Proc Natl Acad Sci USA 1993;90:6189–6193.
96. Okuno H, Akahori A, Sato H, Xanthoudakis S, Curran T, Iba H. Oncogene 1993;8:695–701.
97. Schreck R, Zorbas H, Winnacker EL, Baeuerle PA. Nucleic Acids Res 1990;18:6497–6502.
98. Hayashi A, Suzuki T, Tajima S. J Biochem 1995;117:132–136.
99. Rao GN, Lassègue B, Griendling KK, Alexander RW. Oncogene 1993;8:2759–2764.
100. Chakraborti S, Michael JR. Mol Cell Biochem 1993;122:9–15.
101. Henkel T, Machleidt T, Alkalay I, Kronke M, Ben Neriah Y, Baeuerle P. Nature 1993;365: 182–185.
102. Schreck R, Albermann K, Baeuerle PA. Free Radic Res Commun 1992;17:221–237.
103. Schreck R, Rieber P, Baeuerle PA. EMBO J 1991;10:2247–2258.
104. Meyer M, Schreck R, Baeuerle PA. EMBO J 1993;12:2005–2015.
105. Baeuerle PA, Baltimore D. Genes Devel 1989;3:1689–1698.
106. Baeuerle PA, Baltimore D. Science 1988;242:540–546.
107. Baeuerle PA, Baltimore D. Cell 1988;53:211–217.
108. Baeuerle PA, Lenardo M, Pierce JW, Baltimore D. Cold Spring Harb Symp Quant Biol 1988;53(Part2):789–798.
109. Li S, Sedivy JM. Proc Natl Acad Sci USA 1993;90:9247–9251.
110. Lin A, Smeal T, Binetruy B, Deng T, Chambard JC, Karin M. Adv Second Messenger Phospho- protein Res 1993;28:255–260.
111. Angel P, Karin M. Biochim Biophys Acta 1991;1072:129–157.
112. Skroch P, Buchman C, Karin M. Prog Clin Biol Res 1993;380:113–128.
113. Chiu R, Imagawa M, Imbra RJ, Bockoven JR, Karin M. Nature 1987;329:648–651.
114. Jacobson MD, Burne JF, King MP, Miyashita T, Reed JC, Raff MC. Nature 1993;361:365–369.
115. Wijkander J, Sundler R. FEBS Lett 1992;311:299–301.
116. Ferns GA, Forster L, Stewart Lee A, Konneh M, Nourooz Zadeh J, Anggard EE. Proc Natl Acad Sci USA 1992;89:11312–11316.
117. Ruef J, Hu ZY, Yin LY, Wu Y, Hanson SR, Kelly AB, Harker LA, Rao GN, Runge MS, Patterson C. Circ Res 1997;81:24–33.
118. Mietus–Snyder M, Friera A, Glass CK, Pitas RE. Arterioscl Thromb Vasc Biol 1997;17: 969–978.
119. Li PF, Dietz R, von Harsdorf R. FEBS Lett 1997;404:249–252.
120. Delafontaine P, Ku L. Cardiovasc Res 1997;33:216–222.
121. Sies H. Eur J Biochem 1993;215:213–219.
122. Gopalakrishna R, Anderson WB. Proc Natl Acad Sci USA 1989;86:6758–6762.
123. Gopalakrishna R, Anderson WB. Arch Biochem Biophys 1991;285:382–387.

124. Kass GE, Duddy SK, Orrenius S. Biochem J 1989;260:499—507.
125. Palumbo EJ, Sweatt JD, Chen SJ, Klann E. Biochem Biophys Res Commun 1992;187: 1439—1445.
126. Gopalakrishna R, Chen ZH, Gundimeda U. J Biol Chem 1993;268:27180—27185.
127. Cadena DL, Gill GN. FASEB J 1992;6:2332—2337.
128. Toyoshima K, Yamanashi Y, Inoue K, Semba K, Yamamoto T, Akiyama T. Ciba Found Symp 1992;164:240—248.
129. Glenney JR, Jr. Biochim Biophys Acta 1992;1134:113—127.
130. Chen YX, Yang DC, Brown AB, Jeng Y, Tatoyan A, Chan TM. Arch Biochem Biophys 1990; 283:184—192.
131. Fialkow L, Chan CK, Grinstein S, Downey GP. J Biol Chem 1993;268:17131—17137.
132. Chan TM, Chen E, Tatoyan A, Shargill NS, Pleta M, Hochstein P. Biochem Biophys Res Commun 1986;139:439—445.
133. Chen Y, Chan TM. Arch Biochem Biophys 1993;305:9—16.
134. Zor U, Ferber E, Gergely P, Szucs K, Dombradi V, Goldman R. Biochem J 1993;295:879—888.
135. Nakamura K, Hori T, Sato N, Sugie K, Kawakami T, Yodoi J. Oncogene 1993;8:3133—3139.
136. Kanner SB, Kavanagh TJ, Grossmann A, Hu SL, Bolen JB, Rabinovitch PS, Ledbetter JA. Proc Natl Acad Sci USA 1992;89:300—304.
137. Toyoshima H, Kozutsumi H, Maru Y, Hagiwara K, Furuya A, Mioh H, Hanai N, Takaku F, Yazaki Y, Hirai H. Proc Natl Acad Sci USA 1993;90:5404—5408.
138. Jin N, Rhoades RA. Am J Physiol 1997;272:H2686—2692.
139. Tan CM, Xenoyannis S, Feldman RD. Circ Res 1995;77:710—717.
140. Cantoni O, Boscoboinik D, Fiorani M, Stauble B, Azzi A. FEBS Lett 1996;389:285—288.
141. Baas AS, Berk BC. Circ Res 1995;77:29—36.
142. Abe MK, Kartha S, Karpova AY, Li J, Liu PT, Kuo WL, Hershenson MB. Am J Respir Cell Mol Biol 1998;18:562—569.
143. Guy GR, Cairns J, Ng SB, Tan YH. J Biol Chem. 1993;268:2141—2148.
144. Keyse SM, Emslie EA. Nature 1992;359:644—647.
145. Denu JM, Tanner KG. Biochemistry 1998;37:5633—5642.
146. Lowe GM, Hulley CE, Rhodes ES, Young AJ, Bilton RF. Biochem Biophys Res Commun 1998;245:17—22.
147. Wang X, Culotta VC, Klee CB. Nature 1996;383:434—437.
148. Vaux DL. Proc Natl Acad Sci USA 1993;90:786—789.
149. Hockenbery DM, Oltvai ZN, Yin XM, Milliman CL, Korsmeyer SJ. Cell 1993;75:241—251.
150. Kane DJ, Sarafian TA, Anton R, Hahn H, Gralla EB, Valentine JS, Ord T, Bredesen DE. Science 1993;262:1274—1277.
151. Au YP, Kenagy RD, Clowes MM, Clowes AW. Haemostasis 1993; 23 Suppl1:177—182.
152. March KL, Wilensky RL, Roeske RW, Hathaway DR. Circ Res 1993;72:413—423.
153. Zawaski K, Grueble A, Kaplan D, Reddy S, Mortensen A, Novak RF. Biochem Biophys Res Commun 1994;197:585—590.
154. Rao GN, Baas AS, Glasgow WC, Eling TE, Runge MS, Alexander RW. J Biol Chem 1994;269: 32586—32591.
155. Kourembanas S, Hannan RL, Faller DV. J Clin Invest 1990;86:670—674.
156. Montisano DF, Mann T, Spragg RG. J Appl Physiol 1992;73:2255—2262.
157. Morisaki N, Yokote K, Saito Y. J Nutr Sci Vitaminol 1992; SpecNo:196—199.
158. Lindsey JA, Zhang HF, Kaseki H, Morisaki N, Sato T, Cornwell DG. Lipids 1985;20:151—157.
159. Morisaki N, Lindsey JA, Stitts JM, Zhang H, Cornwell DG. Lipids 1984;19:381—394.
160. Gavino VC, Miller JS, Ikharebha SO, Milo GE, Cornwell DG. J Lipid Res 1981;22:763—769.
161. Hennekens CH, Gaziano JM. Clin Cardiol 1993;16:10—13.
162. Jialal I, Fuller CJ. Clin Cardiol 1993;16:I6—I9.
163. Gey KF. Biochem Soc Trans 1990;18:1041—1045.
164. Rimm EB, Stampfer MJ, Ascherio A, Giovannucci E, Colditz GA, Willett WC. N Engl J Med

1993;328:1450—1456.

165. Stampfer MJ, Hennekens CH, Manson JE, Colditz GA, Rosner B, Willett WC. N Engl J Med 1993;328:1444—1449.

166. Kuzuya M, Naito M, Funaki C, Hayashi T, Yamada K, Asai K, Kuzuya F. Artery 1991;18: 115—124.

167. Morisaki N, Sprecher H, Milo GE, Cornwell DG. Lipids 1982;17:893—899.

168. Boscoboinik D, Chatelain E, Bartoli GM, Azzi A. Free radicals and aging. I Emerit and B Chance (eds) Birkhäuser Verlag. Basel-Boston-Berlin: 1992;164—177.

169. Boscoboinik D, Szewczyk A, Azzi A. Arch Biochem Biophys 1991;286:264—269.

170. Boscoboinik D, Szewczyk A, Hensey C, Azzi A. J Biol Chem 1991;266:6188—6194.

171. Pryor AW, Cornicelli JA, Devall LJ, Tait B, Trivedi BK, Witiak DT, Wu M. J Org Chem 1993;58:3521—3532.

172. Nalecz KA, Bolli R, Azzi A. Methods Enzymol 1986;126:45—64.

173. Pears C, Stabel S, Cazaubon S, Parker PJ. Biochem J 1992;283:515—518.

174. Clarke PR, Siddhanti SR, Cohen P, Blackshear PJ. FEBS Lett 1993;336:37—42.

175. Clément S, Tasinato A, Boscoboinik D, Azzi A. Eur J Biochem 1997;246:745—749.

176. Clowes AW, Schwartz SM. Circ Res 1985;56:139—145.

177. Traber MG, Rudel LL, Burton GW, Hughes L, Ingold KU, Kayden HJ. J Lipid Res 1990;31: 687—694.

178. Burton GW, Ingold KU. Ann NY Acad Sci 1989;570:7—22.

179. Sasaki H, Okabe E. Jpn J Pharmacol 1993;62:305—314.

180. Steiner M, Li W, Ciaramella JM, Anagnostou A, Sigounas G. J Cell Physiol 1997;172:351—360.

181. Freedman JE, Farhat JH, Loscalzo J, Keaney JF, Jr. Circulation 1996;94:2434—2440.

182. Keaney JF, Jr., Guo Y, Cunningham D, Shwaery GT, Xu AM, Vita JA. J Clin Invest 1996;98: 386—394.

183. Ishii H, Jirousek MR, Koya D, Takagi C, Xia P, Clermont A, Bursell SE, Kern TS, Ballas LM, Heath WF, Stramm LE, Feener EP, King GL. Science 1996;272:728—731.

184. Devaraj S, Li D, Jialal I. J Clin Invest 1996;98:756—763.

185. Kanno T, Utsumi T, Kobuchi H, Takehara Y, Akiyama J, Yoshioka T, Horton AA, Utsumi K. Free Radic Res 1995;22:431—440.

186. Suzuki YJ, Packer L. Biochem Biophys Res Commun 1993;193:277—283.

Part VII

Analytical methods

©2000 Elsevier Science B.V. All rights reserved.
Handbook of Oxidants and Antioxidants in Exercise.
C.K. Sen, L. Packer and O. Hänninen, editors.

Part VII • Chapter 17

Oxidative stress indices: analytical aspects and significance

Derick Han[1], Sonia Loukianoff[2] and Laura McLaughlin[3]

[1] *School of Pharmacy, University of Southern California, 1985 Zonal Avenue, Los Angeles, California 90033, USA. Tel.: +1-323-442-1420. E-mail: derickh@hsc.usc.edu*
[2] *Department of Molecular and Cell Biology, 251 LSA, University of California at Berkeley, California 94720-3202, USA. Tel.: +1-510-642-4549. Fax: +1-510-643-7935.*
[3] *School of Public Health, Harvard University, 651 Huntington Ave, Boston, Massachusetts, 02115, USA.*

1 INTRODUCTION
    1.1 Assessing oxidative stress
    1.2 General difficulties in oxidative stress determination
2 DETECTION OF REACTIVE OXYGEN SPECIES
    2.1 Electron paramagnetic resonance
    2.2 Detection of hydroxyl and superoxide radicals by spin traps
    2.3 Other methods to detect hydroxyl and superoxide radicals
    2.4 Hydrogen peroxide detection
3 MEASUREMENT OF ANTIOXIDANTS AS MARKERS OF OXIDATIVE STRESS
    3.1 Glutathione (GSH/GSSG)
    3.2 Vitamin E
    3.3 Ubiquinol/ubiquinone status
    3.4 Vitamin C and uric acid
    3.5 Total antioxidant assays
4 DETECTION OF OXIDATIVELY MODIFIED BIOMOLECULES
    4.1 DNA oxidation
    4.2 Lipid peroxidation products
    4.3 Protein oxidation
5 SUMMARY
6 PERSPECTIVES
7 ABBREVIATIONS
8 REFERENCES

1   INTRODUCTION

Oxidative stress has been defined as a shift in the normal pro-oxidant— antioxidant balance in favor of pro-oxidants [1,2]. Quantitation of oxidative stress has been a major challenge that has resulted in the development of a number of methodological approaches. While most methodological approaches have increased our understanding of oxidative stress in biological systems, some approaches have been inappropriately used and have provided misleading conclusions. The aim of this chapter is to review some of the key methodological approaches to evaluate oxidative stress. Some of the difficulties in quantitating oxidative stress, as well as controversies that have arisen over certain methods are discussed.

1.1 Assessment of oxidative stress

To assess oxidative stress in biological systems, typically, certain molecules are measured that are known to decrease or increase as a result of oxidative stress. Reliable markers of oxidative stress are generally: 1) chemically unique, 2) alter during times of oxidative stress, 3) are not affected by cellular processes (i.e., cell cycle, metabolism, etc.). Many molecules that fit these criteria have been identified and techniques to measure these "biomarkers" of oxidative stress will be the focus of this chapter.

During times of oxidative stress, pro-oxidants overwhelm the antioxidant defenses and damage cellular constituents. Thus, oxidative stress is generally characterized by the following parameters (Fig. 1):

1. An increase in the formation of reactive oxygen species (ROS).
2. A decrease in the levels of low molecular weight, water and/or lipid soluble antioxidants.
3. An increase in oxidative damage to cellular constituents: proteins, lipids and DNA.

Biomarkers used to assess oxidative stress fall into these three broad categories. For the measurement of ROS, exogenous biomarkers are used. A probe or trap is added to a biological system and if ROS are present, they will convert this probe or trap into a unique, oxidatively modified molecule. This newly formed, modified product can then be quantitated as a measure of ROS.

In the case of small molecular antioxidants, commonly measured biomarkers are antioxidants such as vitamin E, vitamin C, and glutathione. Since these chain-breaking antioxidants tend to decrease during times of oxidative stress, their measurement is frequently used to assess oxidative stress. However, the

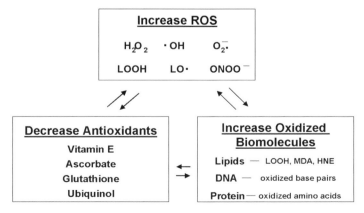

Fig. 1. General characteristics of oxidative stress.

loss of antioxidants in biological systems is not always a direct result of oxidative stress and should be accompanied by the measurement of other biomarkers.

In vitro studies have revealed that the oxidation of lipids, protein, and DNA provide a wide range of unique breakdown products that can be used as biomarkers of oxidative stress in in vivo studies. Measurement of these oxidative damage products provides a fingerprint of oxidative damage and provides the strongest evidence of oxidative stress in biological systems.

In addition, in oxidative stress assesment antioxidant treatment is often used in parallel with measurement of oxidative stress biomarkers. If antioxidant administration to a system can slow down or stop an event, this event is believed to involve oxidative stress. However, all antioxidants have some secondary effect, especially at the high levels that are sometimes used, and some caution should be used in the interpretation of these data. The combination of measuring parameters that characterize oxidative stress and the use of antioxidants are the most commonly used methods to assess oxidative stress in biological systems.

1.2 General difficulties in oxidative stress determination

Although there are many parameters to quantitate oxidative insult, the measurement of oxidative stress in biological systems has proven to be a difficult task. An examination of the literature reveals that different laboratories have published conflicting results on whether a biological process involves oxidative stress [3]. For example, some groups have reported that exercise causes lipid peroxidation, while others have reported no lipid peroxidation during exercise [4]. There is also a conflicting report on whether or not protein oxidation increases with age [5,6]. These inconsistencies may be related to technical difficulties that occur in measuring oxidative stress in biological systems. Some of these difficulties include the short lifetime of free radicals, the lack of specific and sensitive assays for oxidized biomolecules, and the tendency toward generating artifacts.

1.2.1 Short lifetime of free radicals

Because oxidative damage is mediated through free radicals, their measurement is important in understanding oxidative damage. However, free radicals are highly reactive, making their detection extremely difficult. Because oxygen-based free radicals have a very short lifetime and migration distance, their direct detection in biologiccal systems is virtually impossible. To overcome this problem, methods involving spin traps are commonly used. Spin traps react with free radicals to form a stable radical (with a relatively long lifetime) that can readily be detected. Spin traps have been useful in many cases, but there are limitations to their use, especially in vivo. Overcoming the difficulties in measuring free radicals in biological systems remains a significant challenge in this field.

1.2.2 Specificity and sensitivity

In vivo determination of oxidized biomolecules has been difficult to accomplish because of a lack of sensitive and selective assays. A high steady state level of oxidized biomolecules rarely occurs in vivo during times of oxidative stress. Oxidized protein, lipids, and DNA disrupt cell function and are rapidly removed by cellular repair systems. Cells contain GSH peroxidase that remove lipid peroxides, proteases that recognize and remove oxidized proteins, and DNA repair enzymes that remove oxidized DNA bases. In addition, while the oxidation of lipids, protein, and DNA generates unique products, these products still remain structurally similar to many other molecules that are also present in the cell and in much higher amounts. Assays with the specificity and sensitivity to detect a small number of oxidized molecules among many structurally similar compounds have been difficult to develop. False signals from interfering substances have been a common problem for many assays, the classic example being the thiobarbituric acid (TBA) assay. The TBA test is designed to measure malondialdehyde (MDA), a breakdown product of lipid peroxidation. This assay is based on the reaction of TBA with MDA to form a TBA-MDA adduct which can be measured spectrophotometrically. In simple in vitro systems, the TBA test has been a valuable tool for measuring lipid peroxidation. Unfortunately, when applied to biological systems, the assay cannot accurately quantitate MDA because many endogenous compounds can also conjugate with TBA to form a false signal. Nonspecificity has been a problem for many simple spectrophotometric assays. To overcome problems of sensitivity and selectivity, specialized equipment, such as gas chromatography-mass spectrometry (GC-MS) or high-performance liquid chromatography (HPLC) are generally needed.

1.2.3 Artifacts

One of the greatest problems in assessing oxidative stress is the generation of artifacts. The fact that we live in an atmosphere containing 20% oxygen creates a potential for the spontaneous oxidation of antioxidants, lipids, proteins, and DNA during sample processing. Oxidation of antioxidants and biomolecules will occur during extractions and sample processing, unless special precautions are taken. These precautions include the chelation of iron in solution, the bubbling of nitrogen or argon to deoxygenate solutions, and/or the addition of exogenous antioxidants to protect samples from atmospheric oxidation. Investigators have used different protocols to prevent oxidation of samples during sample processing, and some precautions prevent atmospheric oxidation more than others, creating a discrepancy in the measurement of antioxidants and oxidized biomolecules. The GSH/GSSG ratio in red blood cells has been reported to be as high as 500:1 and as low as 4:1 [7].

Assays requiring sample derivatization before detection are inherently problematic because of the reactive environment in which such a process must be conducted. For certain derivatization procedures, samples that normally would be kept at subzero temperatures, must be heated to higher temperatures at which oxidation will occur at a faster rate. Certain procedures for the derivatization of GSH [8] or DNA base pairs [9] have caused sample oxidation and yielded artificially high values. For such cases, it is recommended that the reduced and oxidized forms of a compound be separated before being derivatized. Thus, before oxidized guanine is derivatized for measurement by GC-MS, guanine should be removed by chromatography. This ensures that no guanine is present during the derivatization procedure, where it can oxidize and artificially inflate oxidized guanine values [9]. It is also recommended that GSH be neutralized prior to derivatizing GSSG for measurement [8].

1.2.4 *There is no one method that best assesses oxidative stress*

Although a general pattern for oxidative stress exists, a specific pattern of oxidative stress often varies from one biological system to another. There are numerous cellular sources of ROS and many different biomolecules with which ROS may react. This makes it difficult to predict a set outcome of oxidative damage. In certain cases, an increase in reactive oxygen species can occur without a significant decrease in certain antioxidants; or lipid peroxidation may occur without DNA oxidation. No one method best assesses oxidative stress; in most instances, many different methodologies must be implemented before an accurate assessment of oxidative stress can be made.

2 DETECTION OF REACTIVE OXYGEN SPECIES

Reactive oxygen species are primarily comprised of free radicals ($O_2^{\bullet -}$, $\cdot OH$, $NO\bullet$), peroxides (H_2O_2, LOOH), and strong oxidants such as peroxynitrite. Due to the short lifetime of most ROS, particularly free radicals, a reliable method has not yet been developed to directly detect ROS in biological systems. ROS are highly reactive and their detection relies on the use of exogenously added traps and probes that react with ROS to form unique products.

Spin traps, such as PBN and DMPO, are used to identify and quantitate a wide range of free radicals. Other agents, such as salicylic acid, are added to biological systems to capture hydroxyl radicals, which can then be detected by HPLC. To measure hydrogen peroxide, probes, like DCFH, are used in conjunction with flow cytometry or fluorescent microscopy. The disadvantage in using probes or traps is that they constitute an invasive detection scheme. Addition of these exogenous molecules to biological systems will, to some degree, perturb the system being measured. Many spin traps and probes are toxic and cannot be used in vivo. Until noninvasive methodologies are developed for the direct detection of ROS, probes and traps remain the most reliable methods available.

The primary focus of this chapter will be on superoxide, hydroxyl radical, and hydrogen peroxide detection methods. Nitric oxide, a very important free radical in signal transduction, will not be covered in this chapter, but the following book is recommended: [10].

2.1 Electron paramagnetic resonance

Electron paramagnetic resonance (EPR or also known as electron spin resonance, ESR) is the only method that can directly detect free radical species, such as the superoxide anion ($O_2^{\bullet-}$) and the hydroxyl free radical ($\cdot OH$). Detailed theory of EPR can be found in the literature [11]. EPR is a spectrophotometric technique that detects unpaired electrons. Electrons exist in two possible spin states, $+1/2$ and $-1/2$, and pair with electrons of the opposite spin, resulting in a net spin of zero. Unpaired electrons, which have charge and spin, act as tiny magnets that align themselves parallel or antiparallel to an external magnetic field. Unpaired electrons aligned parallel to the magnetic field exist in a lower energy state than do electrons aligned antiparallel to the field. When the appropriate amount of energy is applied in the form of electromagnetic radiation (generally in the microwave range), electrons move from the lower energy state (parallel to the magnetic field) to the higher energy state (antiparallel to the magnetic field). This resonance of electron spin states, or "flipping", depends on the frequency of energy used and the magnetic field. The magnetic field at which electron flipping occurs is called the "field of resonance". In EPR, the microwave frequency is generally kept constant, and the magnetic field is scanned. The energy absorbed during resonance can be used to quantitate free radical levels.

EPR cannot only be used to quantitate fre radicals but can also identify the free radical species generated. Each radical has a different hyperfine splitting pattern for a given set of EPR conditions (magnetic field strength and EM frequency) [12]. Atomic nuclei, like electrons, have spin and charge, and thus, behave like magnets. The nuclei affect the strength of the imposed magnetic field around the unpaired electron in a manner referred to as "shielding". Because nuclei can also align either parallel or antiparallel to the external magnetic field, unpaired electrons collectively experience two slightly different magnetic fields that result in the hyperfine splitting of the original spectra. Hyperfine splitting holds information about a compound's structure and can be used to verify the compound's identity. For example, tocopheroxyl radicals, ascorbyl radicals, and spin trap radicals all exhibit unique, hyperfine splitting patterns that can be readily identified by their EPR spectra.

Although EPR can directly detect free radicals, spin traps must be used for free radical measurements in biological systems. Generally, the steady state level of free radicals in biological systems is at or below the detection level of EPR. To directly detect oxygen-centered radicals by EPR without using spin traps, samples must be chilled to extremely low temperatures to slow down their rate of decay [13]. Because such techniques cannot be used with most biological samples, several different oxygen radical "traps" have been developed that can react with free radicals and give specific and stable products. Commonly used traps are nitrones, such as phenyl-tert-butylnitrone (PBN) and 5,5-dimethyl-1-pyrroline N-oxide (DMPO). When radicals are "trapped" by these compounds, the product formed also becomes a radical (although much more stable) and can be detected by EPR. A wide range of spin traps exist, varying in chemical structure and membrane permeability [12,14]. The use of spin traps with EPR remains the most useful method to measure free radicals in biological systems.

Detection of antioxidant radicals by EPR can be accomplished in biological systems without the use of spin traps. Tocopherol, ascorbate and other antioxidant radicals are relatively stable and can be measured by EPR at milder temperatures. EPR has been used to directly measure antioxidant radicals as markers of oxidative stress and to examine redox cycling of antioxidants. It was first shown by using EPR that the tocopheroxyl radical is recycled by ascorbate [15]. Ascorbyl radicals have been observed in skin after UV irradiation [18], have been associated with myocardial ischemia [19], and have been suggested to be an excellent marker of oxidative stress in biological systems [16,17].

2.2 Detection of hydroxyl and superoxide radicals by spin traps

Hydroxyl free radicals ($\cdot$OH) and superoxide anion ($O_2^{\bullet -}$) represent two of the most important radicals in free radical chemistry. Superoxide is believed to be the major radical generated during metabolism in aerobic organisms. $\bullet$OH is the most reactive oxygen species ($t_{1/2}$ of $\cdot$OH = 10^{-9} s, in cells) and is believed to be a key player in oxidative damage. Various spin traps have been employed for the measurement of superoxide and $\bullet$OH by EPR (Tables 1 and 2). Nitrone spins traps, such as PBN and DMPO, are commonly used. DEPMPO, an alkylated form of DMPO, has been shown to be an especially good trap for superoxide anion [20]. Figure 2 shows these spin trap structures and the structure formed after the trapping of a radical. The radical (i.e., superoxide) adds across the double bond of DMPO (or DEMPO), forming a nitroxide (N-O) spin adduct. Using these traps, $\bullet$OH can be detected in samples at room temperature with a fair amount of sensitivity [13]. The sensitivity can vary according to solvent condi-

Table 1. Hydroxyl free radical detection methods.

Method	Comments/references
EPR spin traps	PBN and DMPO are commonly used spin traps. EPR measures the steady state level of free radicals [13,14,21,23]
Salicylic acid	Hydroxyl free radicals attack salicylic acid to form oxidation products that can be measured by HPLC or GC-MS
HPLC methods	[27−29,248,249]
GC-MS method	[31]
Phenylalanine	Hydroxyl free radicals attack phenylalanine to form tyrosine oxidation products that can be measured by HPLC or GS-MS
HPLC	[27,250]
GS-MS	[32]

Table 2. Superoxide anion detection methods.

Method	Comments/references
EPR spin traps	PBN, DMPO, and DEPMPO are traps used in the measurement of super-oxide. EPR measures the steady state level of free radicals [13,14,20,21]
Luminol	Chemiluminescence probe. Should not be used to determine superoxide levels due to its ability to generate superoxide [36,39]
Lucigenin	Chemiluminescence probe. Use of lucigenin is controversial due to it's ability to undergo redox cycling and generate superoxide [39,40]
Aconitase activity	Aconitase Fe-S clusters are inactivated by superoxide. Measurement of aconitase activity is used to assess superoxide levels [44—47]
Hydroethindine	Fluorescent probe. Because the oxidation of HEt to Et is specific for super-oxide, the monitoring of Et fluorescence is used to estimate superoxide levels [41—43]

tions, in which a signal may be dampened in a protic solvent (water) vs. an apro-tic solvent (benzene).

The application of spin traps in biological systems can be difficult because: 1) spin traps like DMPO must be used in at high levels (high millimolar range) that can affect the system and 2) nitroxides can be reduced enzymatically or che-mically to hydroxylamine, a product that cannot be detected by EPR. Ascorbic acid, the mitochondrial electron transport chain, and cytochrome P-450 have all been shown to reduce nitroxide to hydroxylamine [21]. Reduction of nitroxides can decrease the sensitivity of detection and make quantification of radicals diffi-cult.

In vivo applications of EPR face additional difficulties. The toxicity of most spin traps has limited their use in vivo. Stable concentrations of nitroxide radicals are difficult to establish in vivo. The diffusion of spin traps from tissues and the breakdown of nitroxides by various biological components diminish nitroxide concentrations needed for in vivo detection. EPR techniques for biological sys-tems have been reviewed in numerous articles [13,14,21—23].

Despite some shortcomings, the use of EPR has remained an invaluable tool for free radical research. The ability of the EPR to monitor many different types of radicals in different biological samples makes it a versatile tool for research.

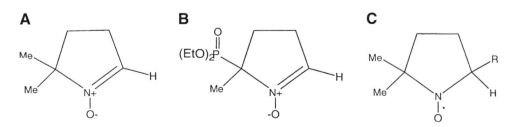

Fig. 2. Spin trap structures. **A:** DMPO. **B:** DEPMPO. **C:** DMPO in radical form where R represents the adduct formed upon "trapping" the radical.

With newer spin traps being developed and more intricate techniques such as EPR imaging, the use of EPR in free radical research will continue to grow.

2.3 Other methods to detect hydroxyl and superoxide radicals

2.3.1 Salicylate and phenylalanine traps to detect hydroxyl radicals

In addition to spin traps, •OH can be detected using exogenously added probes, such as salicylate or phenylalanine (Table 1). Both salicylate and phenylalanine are aromatic compounds that undergo addition reactions with HO• to give hydroxylation products.

1. salicylate   +   ·OH   →   (A)   2,3-dihydroxybenzoic acid (DHB)
                              (B)   2,5-DHB
                              (C)   catechol   + CO_2
                              (D)   salicylurate
                              (E)   others

2. phenylalanine   +   ·OH   →   *o*-, *m*-, and *p*-tyrosine   →   DOPA (not all reaction products are shown).

To measure HO• in biological systems, salicylate or phenylalanine are added, and high-performance liquid chromatography (HPLC) or gas chromatography-mass spectroscopy (GC-MS) is used to measure the hydroxylated molecules formed. These traps have an advantage over spin traps in that they are generally nontoxic and can be administered at lower doses than those for spin traps such as DMPO. These characteristics make phenylalanine and salicylate very suitable for in vivo studies of oxidative stress. By using these probes, it has been shown that HO• are generated during times of myocardial [24,25] and cerebral ischemia [26].

   The determination of DHBs by HPLC is accomplished with either amperometric or coulometric electrochemical detection [27—29]. 2,3-DHB and 2,5-DHB are two frequently measured hydroxylation products. It has been reported that 2,5-DHB may also be produced enzymatically via the cytochrome P-450 system. 2,5-DHB, therefore, may not be a specific marker of HO• and its measurement can give misleading results [30]. 2,3-DHB, on the other hand, is not generated by any known enzyme, and may be considered a specific marker for HO•. A GC-MS method also exists for the determination of DHB [31].

   The detection of the phenylalanine hydroxylation products, *o*-, *m*-, and *p*-tyrosine, can be done with either UV, fluorescence, or electrochemical detection in conjunction with HPLC [27], or by GC-MS [32].

2.3.2 Superoxide measurements

In addition to EPR, several other methods have been used to detect intracellular superoxide in biological systems (Table 2). Superoxide cannot cross the membrane and, therefore, intracellular detection of superoxide is usually achieved using membrane permeable probes. A few specialized cells, such as macrophages and neutrophils, generate superoxide at the outer plasma membrane during a respiratory burst. To detect superoxide production during respiratory bursts, methods that monitor cytochrome-c reduction and adrenochrome formation are used [33]. These assays, however, are sensitive to extracellular superoxide, and cannot be used for intracellular detection. The following section discusses methods for the determination of intracellular superoxide.

2.3.3 Superoxide probes

Two of the most widely used probes to measure intracellular superoxide are luminol and lucigenin. Lucigenin has been used to suggest that superoxide is involved in signal transduction [34,35]. It is assumed that after crossing the cell membrane, the probes chemiluminesce after reaction with superoxide. However, the chemistry involving the chemiluminescence of luminol and lucigenin is complicated [36]. Criticism has arisen over the fact that, in certain situations, both probes can undergo redox cycling and actually generate superoxide [36]. Lucigenin can be converted to its radical form by enzymes, such as xanthine oxidase and glucose oxidase, which can subsequently reduce oxygen to superoxide [37]. Vasquez-Vivar et al. also demonstrated that lucigenin stimulates superoxide production by nitric oxide synthase [38]. Based on these observations, Frivdovich has strongly warned against using lucigenin and luminol to measure superoxide. [39]. Li et al. argued that lucigenin, under certain conditions, is a valid probe to measure superoxide in enzymatic and cellular systems [40]. This group has demonstrated that, at low doses, lucigenin does not generate superoxide through redox cycling in biological systems. The level of lucigenin that can be used to measure superoxide and not undergo redox cycling must be determined for each new set of experimental conditions through other techniques, such as measuring oxygen consumption or by using DEPMPO as a spin trap. The use of lucigenin to measure superoxide in biological systems remains somewhat controversial.

Superoxide has been shown to oxidize hydroethidine (HEt) to ethidium (Et) [41,42]. The treatment of cells with HEt and the monitoring of Et fluorescence are frequently used to assess superoxide generation [41]. While the oxidation HEt to Et appears specific for superoxide, cellular alteration such as changes in the mitochondria membrane potential can affect Et fluorescence, and thus, caution must be used when using this probe in biological systems [43].

2.3.4 Aconitase activity to measure superoxide

According to Frivdovich, the measurement of aconitase activity in cells is one of the most specific methods available to monitor intracellular superoxide [39]. Aconitase is an enzyme that contains iron-sulfur clusters (4 Fe-4 S). Superoxide can inactivate Fe-S cluster enzymes, a process that is readily reversible. Decreases in aconitase activity that are chemically reversible are used to monitor superoxide production in cells. This method should be avoided in situations where GSH levels are depleted, since GSH has been shown to modulate aconitase activity [44]. Aconitase activity has been used to assess superoxide levels in bacteria and mammalian cells [45—47].

2.4 Hydrogen peroxide detection

Hydrogen peroxide, unlike superoxide, can readily transverse membranes. Intracellular levels of hydrogen peroxide or the efflux of hydrogen peroxide from a system can be monitored. Methods to measure hydrogen peroxide have been reviewed in the following references: [1,33,48] (Table 3).

2.4.1 Determination of intracellular levels of hydrogen peroxide

The determination of intracellular hydrogen peroxide is a difficult task. Due to interfering substances present within cells, only a few methods can be used to monitor intracellular hydrogen peroxide levels. Measurement of catalase intermediates and use of the probe, DCFH, are two commonly applied methods.

Table 3. Hydrogen peroxide detection methods.

Method	Comments/references
Intracellular hydrogen peroxide detection methods:	
Dichlorofluorescin	Fluorescent probe. Not specific for hydrogen peroxide; DCFH should be considered a general probe that measures oxidant levels [49,50,52,53,58]
Catalase intermediate	A generation of hydrogen peroxide will generate steady state concentration of a catalase-hydrogen peroxide intermediate (compound I). A dual wavelength spectrophotometer can be used to monitor the catalase-intermediate to assess the kinetics of hydrogen peroxide formation [48,62—64]
Measurement of hydrogen peroxide release or efflux:	
Horseradish peroxidase assay	Horseradish peroxidase will oxidize a wide range of hydrogen donor molecules in the presence of hydrogen peroxide; the resulting changes in hydrogen donor molecules are monitored. Commonly used hydrogen donors are scopoletin, DCFH, and Amplex Red [66,67,69]
Cytochrome c peroxidase	Cytochrome c peroxidase forms a stable complex with hydrogen peroxide that can be measured with a dual wavelength spectrophotometer [48,251]
GSSG reductase assay	The consumption of NADPH in the presence of GSH peroxidase peroxidase and GSSG reductase is monitored to estimate hydrogen peroxide levels [33,48]
Oxygen formation	The addition of catalase to samples containing hydrogen peroxide will lead to the formation of oxygen, which can be monitored using an oxygen electrode [33,48]
Luminol-hypochlorous assay	The oxidation of luminol by hypochlorous acid depends on hydrogen peroxide. Monitoring chemiluminescence of luminol in the presence of hypochlorous acid is a sensitive, nonenzymatic method to measure hydrogen peroxide release from cells [72]
Hydrogen peroxide electrode	A nonintrusive technique to measure hydrogen peroxide [252,253]

2.4.2 2',7'-dichlorofluorescin (DCFH)

DCFH is a nonfluorescent molecule that, upon oxidation, is converted to 2'7'-dichlorofluorescein (DCF), a fluorescent molecule [49,50]. Addition of DCFH to intavct cells and the monitoring of DCF fluorescence have been used by many invstigators as a method to measure intracellular hydrogen peroxide levels. It has been suggested using DCFH that processes such as signal transduction [54] and β-amyloid toxicity [55] involve hydrogen peroxide. DCFH has also been used to visualize oxidative stress in different biological systems [56,57].

There are, however, some serious questions about DCFH's use as a specific probe for hydrogen peroxide. Firstly, the chemistry by which DCFH oxidizes to DCF has not yet been completely characterized. Hydrogen peroxide has been shown to cause the slow oxidation of DCFH to DCF [52]. The addition of iron accelerates the oxidation of DCFH by hydrogen peroxide, suggesting that hydroxyl radicals may be involved in DCFH oxidation [58]. It has been demonstrated that DCFH itself is a substrate for many enzymes, including peroxidase [53] and oxidases such as xanthine oxidase and glucose oxidase [58]. Nitric oxide [59], lipid peroxides [50], and peroxynitrite [60] have also been shown to convert DCFH to DCF. Therefore, DCFH is rather nonspecific and should be used to monitor overall oxidant changes, rather than hydrogen peroxide levels specifically. To interpret DCF fluorescence as indicative of hydrogen peroxide levels gives misleading results. Until the chemistry of intracellular DCFH oxidation is characterized, it may be useful to consider DCFH as a probe that monitors the cell oxidation status.

In addition to DCFH, many other fluorescent probes have been used by researchers to measure ROS formation inside cells. C2938 [61], and dihydrorhodamine-123 [53] are some examples. As in the case with DCFH, the chemistry of these probes has not been completely elucidated. It is clear that these probes are monitoring a redox change in cells, but the exact nature of these changes is not completely understood. It is important to keep in mind that these probes are not specific for hydrogen peroxide.

The advantage of using DCFH and other fluorescent probes in cells is that they are relatively nontoxic, are membrane permeable, and are very easy to use. These factors have made DCFH and other probes popular to use in methods to measure oxidants in cells. Although one should always consider the aspect of nonspecificity when interpreting results from assays using DCFH and other probes, overall, they remain simple tools to monitor oxidative changes.

2.4.3 Monitoring of catalase intermediate

Generation of hydrogen peroxide will generate a steady state concentration of a catalase-hydrogen peroxide intermediate (compound I) [48]. A dual wavelength spectrophotometer can be used to measure the catalase-hydrogen peroxide intermediate. Because catalase is specific for hydrogen peroxide, monitoring of the catalase intermediate is a highly selective method to assess the steady state level of hydrogen peroxide. Measurement of this catalase intermediate has been used to measure hydrogen peroxide formation in bacteria, as well as in isolated organs [62—64]. While this method works well in cells that contain a high amount of catalase, it is difficult to use in cells with low levels of catalase, such as lymphocytes.

2.4.4 Determination of hydrogen peroxide release

Because the measurement of hydrogen peroxide release from cells into simple buffers presents an easier model than measuring hydrogen peroxide in the complex environment of the intracellular matrix, methods to measure hydrogen peroxide release are more commonly used. One of the few drawbacks to these methods is that endogenous catalase and GSH peroxidase only allow a fraction of cellular hydrogen peroxide to leave the cell, thereby underestimating actual hydrogen peroxide levels [48].

Nonspecific reactions can occur in even the simplest solutions, so it is important to perform proper controls to validate hydrogen peroxide measurements. The addition of excess catalase to a system is the easiest and most specific method to ensure the validity of these measurements. An excess of catalase will reduce hydrogen peroxide to water and oxygen. If the hydrogen peroxide signal is not quenched by the addition of catalase, the signal is not hydrogen peroxide. Such controls have been used to expose many plasma hydrogen peroxide measurements as erroneous [65].

2.4.5 Horseradish peroxidase assay

Horseradish peroxidase oxidizes a wide range of hydrogen donor molecules in the presence of hydrogen peroxide [48]. Resulting changes in hydrogen donor molecules in the presence of horseradish peroxidase can be monitored to quantitate hydrogen peroxide levels. The most commonly used hydrogen donor is scopoletin [66,67], a fluorescent molecule that, upon oxidation, loses its fluorescence. Other commonly used hydrogen donor molecules, including DCFH [68] and *N*-acetyl-3,7-dihydroxyphenoxazine (Amplex Red) [69], become fluorescent upon oxidation. Fluorescent monitoring of hydrogen donors has been used to quantitate hydrogen peroxide release from cells [70] and mitochondria [33,67,71].

Although horseradish peroxidase coupled to a hydrogen donor is frequently used, it has several inherent problems. Horseradish peroxidase accepts a wide range of hydrogen donors as substrates. Other hydrogen donors present in the sample can compete with the hydrogen donor being monitored, leading to an underestimation of hydrogen peroxide levels. This underestimation of hydrogen peroxide is difficult to overcome. Boveris et al. showed that commercial preparations of horseradish peroxidase contain some endogenous hydrogen donors [67] and that most measurements using this system underestimate hydrogen peroxide levels. There are also a large number of compounds, including glutathione, ascorbate, radical scavengers, and catalase that can potentially interfere with the assay [66]. Because of these interfering substances, this assay is usually performed in solutions in which hydrogen donors and other interfering substances are at a minimum. In complex systems, such as in cell culture, the high amount of competing hydrogen donors makes this assay impractical, but in simple systems, in which experimental conditions are carefully chosen, this assay is a valuable tool for the measurement of hydrogen peroxide.

2.4.6 GSSG reductase and GSH peroxidase

The use of GSSG reductase and GSH peroxidase allows for the specific measurement of hydrogen peroxide efflux. The following reactions are important:
1. H_2O_2 + 2GSH + $2H^+$ $\rightarrow$ $2H_2O$ + GSSG
   (catalyzed by GSH peroxidase)
2. GSSG + NADPH + H^+ $\rightarrow$ 2GSH + $NADP^+$
   (catalyzed by GSSG reductase)
NADPH is monitored spectrophotometrically to estimate hydrogen peroxide levels. The addition of cyanide is used to inactivate many, but not all, NADPH oxidases that may interfere with the assay [33,48].

2.4.7 Oxygen formation

Oxygen is generated when exogenous catalase is added to samples containing hydrogen peroxide. The formation of oxygen is a specific measure of hydrogen peroxide that can be monitored with an oxygen electrode [33,48].

2.4.8 Luminol-hypochlorous acid assay

The oxidation of luminol by hypochlorous acid is dependent on the concentration of hydrogen peroxide [72]. The chemiluminescence of luminol, in the presence of hypochlorous acid, is a sensitive, nonenzymatic method that measures hydrogen peroxide concentrations generated from cells. Mueller et al. monitored hydrogen peroxide changes from a respiratory burst with as few as 3,000 cells [72]. This method can be modified to measure catalase activity in intact cells [73,74].

3   MEASUREMENT OF ANTIOXIDANTS AS MARKERS OF OXIDATIVE STRESS

A decrease in small molecular weight antioxidants is a common occurrence after oxidative insult, and its measurement is frequently used as a marker of oxidative stress. Results can sometimes be misleading because a decrease in tissue antioxidant levels is an indirect measure of oxidative stress. Other factors, such as changes in cellular regulation and diet, can also affect the antioxidant levels. Tissue glutathione (GSH) levels are decreased during oxidative stress but may also be decreased due to the blockage of cystiene-cystine transport [75], medium and serum alterations [76,77], and changes in the cell cycle [78].

A better marker of oxidative stress is the measurement of the redox ratio (reduced/oxidized) of antioxidants. Ascorbate/dehydroascorbate, GSH/GSSG, and ubiquinol/ubiquinone ratios are often used as a measure of oxidative stress in biological systems. In most cases, decreases in antioxidant levels are used as supporting evidence for oxidative stress and not as the sole marker of oxidative insult.

Measurement of antioxidants is the least problematic parameter in assessing oxidative stress. Most antioxidants are found at relatively high concentrations in cells and in plasma, thereby, remaining within detection limits. Additionally, most antioxidants are redox active molecules that can be detected with HPLC-electrochemical detection, a highly sensitive method. The greatest difficulty in antioxidant measurements is the potential of auto-oxidation during sample preparation. In the following section, assays for GSH, ascorbate, vitamin E, and ubiquinol have been discussed, in addition to assays that measure total antioxidant status in biological fluids.

3.1 Glutathione (GSH/GSSG)

Glutathione (γ-glutamyl-L-cysteinylglycine), the major free thiol found in cells, participates in a number of cell functions, including amino acid transport, detoxification of exogenous compounds, and protection against oxygen radicals [79]. Many pathologies, including AIDS [80], Parkinson's disease [81], and cerebral ischemia [82], are associated with a decrease in intracellular GSH levels. GSH depletion generally precedes apoptosis, and its role in apoptosis is currently the focus of intense research [83,84]. Numerous methods exist, ranging from spectrophotometric assays to flow cytometric assays, that can measure GSH in biological systems (Table 4). The wide variety of methods has created a certain amount of discrepancies about the values of GSH and GSSG in biological fluids.

Intracellular GSH levels can be affected by nonoxidative processes, such as the inhibition of cysteine-cystine transport [75] and fluctuations with the cell cycle [85]. GSH-GSSG redox status is a more specific marker of oxidative stress than the measurement of GSH alone. It is generally accepted that the GSH/GSSG ratio is greater than 100:1 inside the cell [86]. Under oxidative conditions, this ratio can dramatically decrease. GSSG is either rapidly reduced by GSSG reductase to GSH or is transported out of the cell; this makes it difficult to see elevated levels of intracellular GSSG for extended periods, even under severe oxidative stress. GSSG efflux has been well-established in isolated, perfused liver when treated with oxidants such as diamide and *tert*-butylperoxide [87]. GSSG efflux out of tissues indicates that an oxidative insult has occurred. Glutathione can also crosslink with other thiols during oxidative stress. The measurement of GS-

Table 4. GSH/GSSG detection methods.

Method	Comments/references
Spectrophotometric assays:	
DTNB	DTNB reacts with all thiol groups. The measurement of nonprotein thiols provides an estimation of GSH levels [93]
GSSG reductase -DTNB assay	The rate of TNB color formation provides a quantitative value of the total glutathione level (GSH + GSSG) in the presence of GSSG reductase Individual GSH and GSSG values can be obtained if samples are run twice with the use of NEM or 2-VP [88,94,95]
Flow injection:	Combines the DTNB-GSSG reductase method with flow injection [254]
HPLC assays:	
UV detection	Samples must be derivatized with various chromaphores before detection by HPLC-UV. Derivatization will cause some GSH to oxidize to its disulfide form
	Compounds used in derivatization for UV detection:
	Iodoacetic acid/dinitrobenzene [99]
	4,4'-dithiodipyridine [255]
	DTNB [256]
Fluorometric detection	Samples must be derivatized with various fluorophores before detection. Derivatization will cause some GSH to oxidize to its disulfide form
	Compounds used in derivatization for fluorometric detection:
	N-chlorodansylamide [NCDA]/dansyl chloride [257,258]
	Monobromobimanes [259,260]
	o-phthalaldehyde [261,262]
Electrochemical detection	A sensitive method that does not require derivatization. Can suffer from problems such as electrode drift and changes in sensitivity due to corrosion of electrode surface
Glassy carbon	[102,103]
Gold-mercury	This electrode is more selective for thiols and disulfide[101]

thiol crosslinks can be determined with various spectrophotometric assays [88]. Protein-GSH crosslinking has been discussed in more detail in the protein oxidation section.

Methodologies used to determine GSSG remain somewhat controversial. As previously mentioned, GSSG values in cells had been reported to be as low as 0.2% and as high as 25% [7]. GSH oxidation to GSSG during sample processing is the main reason for this discrepancy in values.

3.1.1 Sample preparation

Samples for GSH analysis must be properly treated to prevent auto-oxidation after collection. Because the GSH/GSSG ratio is greater than 100:1, even a tiny amount of GSH oxidation can underestimate its redox state. GSH and thiols are reactive at neutral or basic pH. A high pH deprotonates the thiol group, making the sulfide an excellent nucleophile that can attack and crosslink other thiols. To prevent GSH oxidation to GSSG, samples should immediately be acidified after or during collection. Acids such as perchloric acid, *m*-phosphoric acid, 5-sulpho-salicylic acid, and picric acid are commonly used [89, 90]. For glutathione analysis, samples that are treated with acid and properly stored could remain stable for months at $-80°C$ [89].

3.1.2 Spectrophotometric assay

Ellman's reagent, (5,5′-dithiobis-(2-nitrobenzoic acid)) (DTNB), is one of the most commonly used reagents to measure thiols. The reaction of DTNB with thiols is shown in Fig. 3. The product of the reaction, 2-nitro-5-thiobenzoic acid (TNB), has an extremely high extinction coefficient ($\varepsilon = 13,600$ at 412 nm), and is used to quantitate thiol levels [92]. DTNB reacts with all thiols, including protein thiols and small molecular weight thiols, and so, protein and nonprotein constituents must first be separated before their respective thiol levels are measured [92,93]. GSH is the major low molecular weight thiol found in the cell. Thiol measurements of nonprotein fractions are often used as an indication of GSH levels in biological samples. This method, however, will always overestimate GSH levels.

For specific measurements of GSH, DTNB can be coupled with GSSG reductase and NADPH [94]. The probable reaction mechanism is as follows:

1. GSH + DTNB ⇌ GSTNB + TNB
2. GSH + GSTNB ⇌ GSSG + TNB
3. GSSG + NADPH + H$^+$ → 2GSH + NADP$^+$
   (catalyzed by GSSG reductase); or
4. GSTNB + NADPH + H$^+$ → GSH + TNB + NADP$^+$
   (catalyzed by GSSG reductase)

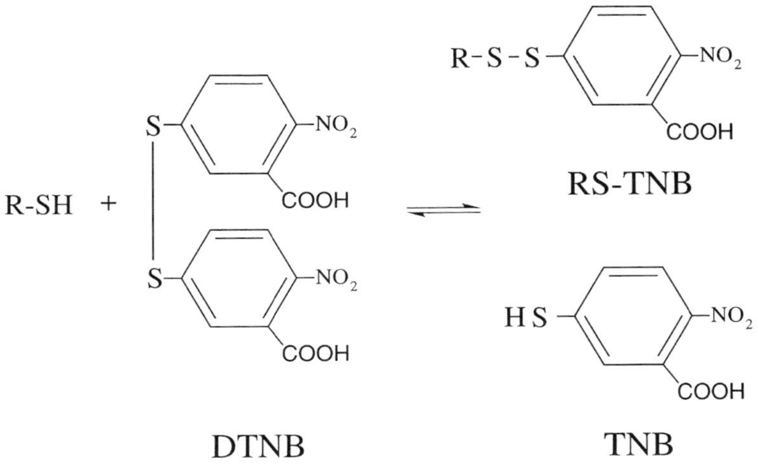

Fig. 3. Reaction of DTNB with thiols.

With the addition of excess GSSG reductase, the total amount of glutathione in the sample becomes a catalyst in the formation of TNB, using NADPH as the reducing equivalent. The rate of TNB color formation provides a quantitative value of the total glutathione (GSH + GSSG) in the sample (comparison with GSH standards is necessary) [94,95]. The high specificity of this quantitative technique is primarily due to the specificity of GSSG reductase for GSH.

Two sets of samples must be analyzed to obtain both GSH and GSSG levels. After total glutathione (GSH + GSSG) is determined, GSH is made chemically inert by the derivatization with either N-ethylmaleimide (NEM) [88] or 2-vinyl-pyridine (2-VP) [96,97], leaving only GSSG to be determined. GSH values are obtained by subtraction of GSSG from the total glutathione values. The sensitivity of the spectrophotometer assay is about 100 picomoles [95].

Some controversy remains about whether NEM or 2-VP is better to neutralize GSH. NEM reacts quickly with GSH [1–2 min], thereby making it less likely for GSH to auto-oxidize to GSSG during derivatization. Excess NEM will inhibit GSSG reductase and, therefore, must be removed by an ether extraction or by column separation, both of which are somewhat laborious procedures [88]. 2-VP does not interfere with GSSG reductase and does not need to be removed [96]. The derivatization of 2-VP takes a couple of hours, thus, providing a greater likelihood of GSH oxidation to GSSG [88]. This has lead some authors to suggest that 2-VP gives artificially high GSSG values and that NEM should be used instead [7,88].

3.1.3 HPLC Methods

3.1.3.1 UV-fluorescent methods. Sensitive measurements of GSH and GSSG can be achieved with the HPLC methods listed in Table 4. The UV and fluorescent HPLC methods shown here rely on the derivatization of GSH and GSSG with various chromophores and have a sensitivity range of 10–100 picomoles. A major problem with derivatization, besides a lengthy sample preparation, is the possibility of auto-oxidation. Most derivatization procedures require a high pH, where auto-oxidation of glutathione is bound to occur. Although it is practically impossible to derivatize a sample without some oxidation of GSH to GSSG, with the proper precautions, the amount of auto-oxidation can be limited. The commonly used method of Reed et al. has been reported to generate 0.7% oxidation of GSH to GSSG [98,99], although others have reported a higher value [8,100].

Some researchers suggest measuring GSSG separately [8,100] to avoid artificially high oxidation. In a method described by Asensi et al., GSH is neutralized by NEM, followed by the derivatization of GSSG [8,100]. This method ensures that the measured product is endogenous GSSG, and not GSSG generated during the derivatization process. Such a procedure limits auto-oxidization and is recommended for GSSG measurements.

3.1.3.2 Electrochemical detection. Electrochemical detection with HPLC has an advantage in that no derivatization is needed. Samples are acidified, the precipitated proteins are pelleted, and the supernatant is injected into the HPLC for analysis. Electrochemical detection is one of the most sensitive methods for GSH/GSSG detection (sensitivity limit = 10 picomoles), but it does suffer from such problems as drift and decreases in sensitivity due to the corrosion of the electrode surface.

There are primarily two types of electrochemical detectors that exist for GSH and GSSG measurements, gold-mercury and glassy carbon. The gold-mercury system is very selective for thiols due to a unique reaction between thiols and mercury that ultimately generates a current [101]. While this method is sensitive, there are several drawbacks due to the nature of the electrode. Not only does the gold-mercury electrode need to be routinely polished and recoated, this system also is associated with a high variability due to the coating process. The glassy carbon electrode, on the other hand, is extremely sensitive for both GSH and GSSG measurements, and requires less maintenance than the gold-mercury system. The disadvantage with the glassy carbon system is that it is not selective for thiols, thereby creating a greater possibility for interfering peaks. For GSSG detection, a voltage of 900 mV or greater [102,103] is usually required. In complex matrices, like plasma and culture medium, a high voltage causes a rapid corrosion of the electrode surface, leading to a decrease in sensitivity. In complex samples like these, sample purification steps are necessary to remove compounds that are attached to the surface of the electrode.

An additional advantage of HPLC is that other thiols (cystine, cysteine, *N*-acetylcysteine, S-methionine) can be measured simultaneously with GSH. Many methods for the simultaneous detection of free thiols exist in the literature. Other thiols, like lipoic acid and dihydrolipoic acid, can be measured by HPLC with minor modifications [104].

3.1.4 Flow cytometric analysis

A decrease in the T-cell glutathione content of AIDS patients was first demonstrated by flow cytometry. Monochlorobimane (MCB) [105] and monobromobimane (MBB) [106,107], two commonly used probes for thiol detection in flow cytometry, gain fluorescence upon conjugation with thiols. Because MCB and MBB react with all thiols, including protein thiols, they can only provide an estimate of cell thiol status and glutathione levels. MCB conjugation with GSH is dependent on GSH S-transferase activity [108,109], and results from these GSH measurements tend to reflect GSH S-transferase activity rather than actual GSH levels. For this reason, the use of MCB has been heavily criticized. Monobromobimane, on the other hand, is less dependent on GSH S-transferase for its conjugation with thiols and gives a better indication of GSH levels [106,107].

A significant drawback in using flow cytometry to measure GSH is that it is not quantitative, since MBB reacts with all thiols, including proteins thiols. However, this drawback can be adequately addressed by using appropriate chemical treatment procedures as described by Sen et al. [107]. Flow cytometry is advantageous in that the thiol heterogeneity of different cell populations can be seen. This technique has been used to demonstrate that GSH is not always homogenous throughout the whole cell population, but is, instead, heterogeneous, especially when treated with various agents [110]. Subsets of cells with drastically low GSH values have been detected in AIDS patients, showing its potential for GSH analysis in certain pathologies [80].

3.2 Vitamin E

Vitamin E is considered to be one of the major antioxidants involved in protecting cell membranes and lipoproteins against lipid peroxidation in vivo [111]. Several forms of vitamin E exist (α-, β-, γ-, δ-tocopherols and tocotrienols), with α- and γ-tocopherol being the most abundant forms found in mammalian cells. When vitamin E reacts with lipid peroxyl and alkoxyl radicals, it donates a hydrogen atom, thereby terminating the propagation of peroxidation while converting tocopherol to its radical form [111,112]:

$$\alpha-TH \quad + \quad LOO\cdot \quad \rightarrow \quad \alpha-T\cdot \quad + \quad LOOH$$

The tocopheroxyl radical formed has been demonstrated to be readily reduced back to α-tocopherol by ascorbate [15,113] or ubiquinol [114,115]. Because vitamin E is readily recycled by other antioxidants, it may be one of the last antioxidants to be depleted during times of oxidative stress. Many experiments have demonstrated that tocopherol depletion occurs only after ascorbate is consumed [113,116]. Vitamin E has been shown to be depleted after exposure to many different types of oxidative stresses, including exercise [117] and UV light [118,119].

Table 5. Vitamin E detection methods.

Method	Comments/references
HPLC:	
Electrochemical detection	The most sensitive HPLC method for tocopherol detection, but can suffer from problems, such as electrode drift [120,136,265,266]
Fluorometric detection	A sensitive and selective method that is fairly trouble-free [123,126,267]
UV detection	This method has limited sensitivity and is not applicable to all biological systems [124,268,269]
GC-MS	[125,270]

3.2.1 Measurement of α-tocopherol

Vitamin E is primarily determined by reverse-phase HPLC, with either UV, fluorescence, or electrochemical detection, or by GC-MS (Table 5). Several methods exist for the simultaneous detection of the vitamin E family. Since α- and γ-tocopherol are the major forms of vitamin E in cells, most methods focus on the detection of these tocopherols to assess oxidative stress.

Vitamin E, like most antioxidants, can undergo auto-oxidation during extracting and processing of samples. Consequently, some researchers add exogenous antioxidants, such as BHT or ascorbate, to prevent tocopherol loss during sample processing [120]. Apolar, organic solvents such as hexane or heptane are frequently used for the extraction of vitamin E from biological samples. To release tocopherol from tissues prior to extraction with hexane, sodium dodecyl sulfate (SDS) is frequently used [120,121]. For the release of vitamin E from tough tissue samples, saponification is effective [122,123]. Saponification involves the heating of tough tissues in a saturated KOH solution. Under such conditions, high levels of ascorbate must be added to the samples to prevent tocopherol oxidation during the heating process. Because α-tocopherol loss during extraction procedures can be a source of error, internal standards like tocopherol acetate [124,125] and tocol [122,126] can be used to increase reliability.

3.2.1.1 HPLC. While UV, fluorescence, and electrochemical detection (Table 5) have all been used with HPLC to determine tocopherols, there are differences between the detection methods. Detector sensitivity for vitamin E is as follows: electrochemical > fluorescence > UV. Electrochemical determination of vitamin E is one of the most frequently utilized methods of detection because of its high sensitivity. The drawback of this system is that, like all electrochemical detectors, they are subject to electrode drift and require some labor in maintenance. For samples that need extremely sensitive detection methods, electrochemical detection, despite these minor drawbacks, remains one of the best methods available. The fluorometric detector is advantageous over electrochemical detection in that there is little drift and less maintenance is required. Although fluorometric detection is less sensitive than electrochemical detection, for most biological samples the sensitivity of fluorescence detection suffices and represents a trouble-free method for tocopherol determination.

HPLC with UV detection can be problematic for two reasons. First, the extinction coefficient for tocopherol is not high ($\varepsilon = 3058$), and so this method lacks sensitivity. Secondly, the maximum absorption of tocopherol occurs at 294 nm, a wavelength at which many other biological compounds interfere. Even with HPLC separation, there is a higher likelihood that absorbing compounds will coelute with tocopherol, thereby decreasing the selectivity of the method. Thus, electrochemical or fluorescent detection is recommended over UV detection of biological samples for its sensitivity and selectivity. Despite these limitations, HPLC-UV, with the proper chromatographic conditions and amount of sample material, is applicable for the measurement of vitamin E in many systems. HPLC-UV in conjunction with an internal standard has been shown to be a reliable method for the measurement of vitamin E in plasma [125].

3.3 Ubiquinol/ubiquinone (coenzyme Q) status

Ubiquinone is a redox cycling, lipid soluble molecule that is an essential component of the mitochondrial respiratory chain. In addition to being present in mitochondrial membranes, ubiquinone is also found in the plasma membrane. Its reduced form, ubiquinol, is believed to be an important antioxidant in protecting both mitochondrial and plasma membranes [127]. Ubiquinols can prevent lipid peroxidation by directly acting as lipid peroxyl scavengers [114,127] and/or by regenerating vitamin E [115]. Like many antioxidants, the redox status of ubiquinone is often used as a marker of oxidative stress [128]. Ubiquinones have been shown to decrease with aging and in many pathologies, including myocardial disease [129] and HIV infection [130]. Ubiquinones exist in various chain lengths, with ubiquinone-9 being predominant in rats, while ubiquinone-10 is predominant in humans.

3.3.1 *Measurement of ubiquinone*

Being lipophilic molecules like vitamin E, ubiquinones/ubiquinols can be extracted by similar methods as described for vitamin E. Studies have shown that ubiquinol is less stable than vitamin E. Ubiquinol can rapidly oxidize to ubiquinone at room temperature [120]. To ensure the determination of an accurate redox status of coenzyme Q, antioxidants such as BHT should be added and samples should be processed on ice as quickly as possible [131].

There are three commonly used HPLC methods for the simultaneous detection of ubiquinone/ubiquinol: UV, a dual UV-electrochemical system, and a dual electrode electrochemical system (Table 6). Both ubiquinol and ubiquinone can be detected using UV detection at 210 nm [132,133] or, for greater specificity, 290 nm for ubiquinol and 275 nm for ubiquinone [131]. Although the use of

Table 6. Ubiquinol/ubiquinone detection methods.

Method	Comments/references
HPLC assays for simultaneous detection of ubiquinol/ubiquinone:	
UV detection	Limited sensitivity and selectivity [132,133].
Dual UV/electrochemical detection	UV detection is used for ubiquinone and electrochemical detection is used for ubiquinol [120,134].
Electrochemical dual electrode detection	Most sensitive HPLC method. Ubiquinone is converted to ubiquinol at the upstream electrode and is detected at the downstream electrode [128,135,136].

UV to determine ubiquinone/ubiquinol in tissue has been useful, this method is not extremely sensitive, particularly for ubiquinol detection at 290 nm.

Ubiquinol may also be detected by using electrochemical detection, a much more sensitive detection method. Because ubiquinone has a fairly strong extinction coefficient ($\varepsilon = 14,200$) at 275 nm, several researchers have coupled electrochemical and UV detectors for ubiquinol/ubiquinone detection [120,134]. Most biological samples fall within this method's sensitivity limits and so it is frequently used [117—119].

Perhaps the most sensitive way to simultaneously determine ubiquinone and ubiquinol is by a dual electrochemical system. In this system, the ubiquinone molecule is converted to ubiquinol by a high negative potential at the upstream electrode, and the newly converted ubiquinol molecule is detected at the downstream electrode [135,136]. Consequently, both molecules are detected at the downstream electrode as ubiquinol, but because HPLC separation of ubiquinone and ubiquinol occurs upstream of the electrode, the two compounds may be individually identified. Most of the methods described for ubiquinol/ubiquinone can also simultaneously detect vitamin E and β-carotene.

3.4 Vitamin C and uric acid

Ascorbic acid (vitamin C) has been described as the most effective antioxidant in protecting against oxidative stress in plasma [137]. Human plasma contains about 30—150 µM of ascorbic acid, a value that can alter during times of oxidative stress. Plasma levels of ascorbic acid have been shown to decrease with oxidative insults, such as cigarette smoke [138], iron overload [139], and in pathological conditions such as cystic fibrosis [140].

When ascorbate, an effective chain breaking antioxidant, encounters free radicals, the result is the formation of a stable semidehydroascorbate radical. Upon reaction with another semidehydroascorbate radical, dehydroascrobate is formed.

$$2 \text{ semidehydroascorbate} \quad \rightarrow \quad \text{ascorbate} \quad + \quad \text{dehydroascorbate}$$

The enzyme dehydroascorbate reductase uses GSH to reduce dehydroascorbate to ascorbate. The ascorbate/dehydroascorbate redox radio is commonly used as a marker of oxidative stress.

3.4.1 *Sample preparation*

Proper and immediate sample treatment is necessary due to the instability of ascorbate and dehydroascorbate. Ascorbate rapidly oxidizes to dehydroascorbate which rapidly oxidizes to L-2,3-diketogulonic acid. Since the latter step is considered irreversible, underestimation of ascorbate will occur unless samples are treated immediately. The addition of strong acids, such as *m*-phosphoric acid, can stop the breakdown of both ascorbate and dehydroascorbate [136,141].

Some researchers have suggested the use of a methanol/water/ethylenediamine-tetra-acetic acid (EDTA) mixture [142] or a combination of *m*-phosphoric acid/EDTA [142] to stabilize ascorbate in biological samples. To store samples for an extended period of time (months), the treatment of samples with *m*-phosphoric acid or dithiothreitol (DTT) at −80°C has been recommended [141,143].

3.4.2 HPLC

Ascorbate is primarily detected by reverse-phase HPLC with either UV or electrochemical (either amperometric or coulometric) detection (Table 7). Although ascorbate is a very polar molecule, the use of ion couplers allows for its separation via reverse-phase column chromatography. The UV determination of ascorbate at 254 nm has been used to measure ascorbic acid in animal tissue [144] and in urine [145]. This method is rather insensitive and cannot be used for many biological samples. Interference by other absorbing substances present in the sample, such as uric acid, hypoxanthine, or xanthine, make the use of UV determination impractical for most biological samples [146,147]. On the other hand, electrochemical detection for ascorbic acid is extremely sensitive and selective and is considered the method of choice for vitamin C detection. Electrochemical detection can be accomplished with either amperometric [136,148,149] or coulometric detectors [138,150]. Although electrochemical detection of ascorbate has some difficulties like electrode drift, we have found it to be the best quantitative method for measuring ascorbate. An advantage of the HPLC electrochemical detection system is the fact that uric acid, another important antioxidant found in plasma [151], can simultaneously be detected with ascorbate [136].

The detection of dehydroascorbate by HPLC is more troublesome and indirect

Table 7. Ascorbic acid detection methods.

Method	Comments/references
HPLC assays:	
UV detection	Little sensitivity and selectivity. Cannot be used with most biological systems [144,145]
Electrochemical detection	Sensitive method that can also measure uric acid. Two different designs of electrodes are used: amperometric and coulometric
Amperometric	[136,148,149]
Coulometric	[138,150]
Spectrophotometric assays:	
Colorimetric	Based on a reaction between ascorbate and 2,6-dichlorophenolindophenol. Some non-specific reactions can occur and cause artificially high values [154]
Ascorbate oxidase assay	Dehydroascorbic acid production is monitored. Ascorbic acid is determined as the difference between the initial dehydroascorbate value and dehydroascorbate value after ascorbate oxidase addition [146]

Table 8. Dehydroascorbate detection methods.

Method	Comments/references
HPLC:	
UV detection	Dehydroascorbate is derivatized with *o*-phenylenediamine for measurement [152,153]
Electrochemical detection	1) 2,3 dimercapto-1-propanol is used to reduce dehydroascorbate to ascorbate, which is then detected electrochemically. 2,3 dimercapto-1-propanol must be extracted out with ether before detection [142]
	2) DTT is used to reduce dehydroascorbate to ascorbate, which is then detected electrochemically. DTT does not need to be removed [138]
Spectrophotometric:	The kinetics of absorbance changes of dehydroascorbic acid in phosphate/methanol solutions are monitored [271]

(Table 8). Because dehydroascorbate cannot be directly detected electrochemically, two strategies have been used: 1) derivatization of dehydroascorbate with a strong chromaphore such as *o*-phenylenediamine [152,153] and detection by UV or fluorescence; or 2) reduction of dehydroascorbate to ascorbate using 2,3-dimercapto-1-propanol [142] or DTT [138] and detection of dehydroascorbate as ascorbate, electrochemically.

While both methods for dehydroascorbate detection have been used, the electrochemical method is better suited for biological samples. The derivatization of dehydroascorbate can cause the irreversible conversion of dehydroascorbate to 2,3-diketogulonic acid due to a lengthy derivatization process [138]. In order to use electrochemical detection, samples must be run twice. First, samples must be analyzed without DTT or 2,3-dimercapto-1-propanol treatment to obtain ascorbate values, and then measured again with such treatment to obtain the total ascorbate value. The dehydroascorbate value is obtained by subtracting the ascorbate value from the total ascorbate value. 2,3-dimercapto-1-propanol can interfere with ascorbate chromatography and must be extracted from the sample using an ether extraction method. The use of DTT is advantageous because it does not need to be extracted out, saving time and reducing sample variability [138].

3.4.3 *Spectrophotometry*

Spectrophotometric assays for ascorbic acid fall into two general categories: colorimetric and enzyme-linked assays (Table 7). The colorimetric assay is based on the reaction of ascorbate with 2,6-dichlorophenolindophenol [154]. Although the colorimetric assay is fairly sensitive, there is a chance of nonspecific reactions in biological systems. Baker et al. found a 12% higher value in spiked plasma due to nonspecific reactions, and so this assay should be limited to simple systems [150,153].

Greater specificity for ascorbate can be achieved if ascorbate oxidase is coupled with an assay for dehydroascorbate. Ascorbic acid oxidase catalyzes the following reaction:

$$\text{L} - \text{Ascorbate} \quad + \quad 1/2\text{O}_2 \quad \xrightarrow[\text{oxidase}]{\text{ascorbate}} \quad \text{dehydroascorbate} \quad + \quad \text{H}_2\text{O}$$

A spectrophotometric assay has been described in which ascorbic acid is monitored as the subsequent increase of dehydroascorbic acid that occurs upon the addition of ascorbate oxidase [146]. The ascorbate concentration is determined as the difference between the initial dehydroascorbate value and the enzyme generated dehydroascorbate value. The detection limit is less than 0.5 µM. This enzyme-linked method is specific for ascorbic acid due to the high specificity that ascorbate oxidase possesses for its natural substrate, ascorbic acid.

3.5 Total antioxidant status assays

An alternative to measuring individual antioxidants are assays that are designed to measure total antioxidant status in biological fluids (Table 9). In these assays, a free radical species is generated by a variety of chemical methods and is subsequently monitored. Different compounds, as well as biological samples, are then added and the ability of the added component to quench the radicals is used to assess its antioxidant capacity. Most researchers compare the free radical scavenging ability of a sample with the scavenging ability of trolox, a water soluble

Table 9. Assays for total antioxidant capacity.

Assay	Detection method	Principle/references
ABTS	Spectrophotometric	Myoglobin and peroxide generate an ABTS radical that can monitored spectrophotometrically. Ability of compounds to quench ABTS radicals are used to evaluate their antioxidant potential [156,158,272]
Phycoerythrin	Fluorescence	The ability of compounds to protect phycoerythrin from free radical damage is used to assess antioxidant capacity [273–276]
cis-Parinaric acid	Fluorescence	The ability of compounds to protect *cis*-parinaric acid in RBC membranes from free radical damage is used to assess antioxidant capacity [277]
TRAP	Oxygen electrode	The antioxidant capacity is determined by the ability of a compound to inhibit peroxide-dependent oxygen consumption [278]
Peroxidation potential	GC-MS	Free radicals are generated in plasma and the resulting peroxide is measured [279]
FRAP	Spectrophotometric	The ability of a compound to affect ferric to ferrous reduction is used to evaluate antioxidant capacity [280]
TOSCA	Gas chromatography	Ability of compounds to inhibit the conversion of KMBA to ethylene is used to evaluate antioxidant capacity [281]

form of vitamin E.

The strength of the total antioxidant assay lies in its ability to provide a quantitative value for general antioxidant levels in biological samples; such a process would be laborious if each individual antioxidant is measured separately. Conversely, a weakness of the assay is that it provides no indications of what antioxidants are being measured. Biological fluids contain molecules, such as protein thiols, urate, estrogen and bilirubin, that can exhibit antioxidant effects and could influence the outcome of this type of assay. Individual antioxidants need to be measured to better evaluate oxidative stress in many instances. Total antioxidant assays are also problematic in that they are not always as sensitive as most other assays developed to measure individual antioxidants. In addition, a study has shown that several of the commonly used assays do not correlate well when compared to each other [155]. Several pitfalls for some commonly used antioxidant assays exist and should be considered before their use [156–158].

4   DETECTION OF OXIDATIVELY MODIFIED BIOMOLECULES

ROS attack of lipids, protein, and DNA generates uniquely oxidized biomolecules that can be used as biomarkers, or fingerprints, to assess oxidative damage. Although the measurement of oxidized biomolecules is arguably the most important marker of oxidative stress, their measurement in biological systems, particularly in vivo, has been difficult. Oxidized biomolecules are found in extremely low amounts in cells, even during times of elevated oxidative stress.

Currently available methodologies can only give us a fractional representation of oxidative damage that occurs during times of oxidative stress. Dozens of oxidized biomolecules can be potentially generated from free radical attack to lipids, proteins and DNA. Unfortunately, most methods can measure only a few oxidatively modified molecules. Because no single method can cover all of the oxidative damage that occurs, a few key oxidatively modified biomarkers are used to estimate the overall severity of oxidative damage. This has been useful in assessing oxidative damage in many physiological and pathophysiological conditions, however, it provides only a limited understanding of the oxidative damage that has occurred. The reliance on only a few biomarkers to assess oxidative damage can often be misleading, since they may not always be representative of the total damage that has occurred.

Despite these limitations, there is a growing understanding of how oxidatively damaged biomolecules participate in pathological situations. Newer and more sensitive techniques are being developed to better understand oxidative damage in cells. Recently developed techniques such as the measurement of oxidized amino acids are providing better quantitative data about protein oxidation in different pathologies. The recent identification of oxidatively modified products, such as isoprostanes, have given us more noninvasive biomarkers to assess oxidative stress.

4.1 DNA oxidation

ROS can cause DNA strand breaks [159], DNA crosslinks, and base pair oxidation [160]. Methodologies that assess free radical damage to DNA have primarily focused on the measurement of oxidized DNA base pairs, particularly the oxidized base, 8-oxoguanine (8-oxoGua) or the oxidized nucleoside, 8-oxodGua. Unlike DNA strand breaks and crosslinks, oxidized base pairs represent specific biomarkers of ROS attack. 8-oxoGua has been the most widely used biomarker of DNA damage because of the observation that 8-oxoGua can mismatch (8-oxoGua matches with adenine instead of cytosine) during DNA replication [161]. The formation of 8-oxoGua and the consequent mismatching of base pairs have been suggested to be the major mechanism responsible for spontaneous mutations in cells [162]. 8-oxoGua formation has been shown to occur in cells during normal oxidative metabolism and to increase after oxidative insults, such as the addition of hydrogen peroxide [163]. Increased 8-oxoGua levels have also been found in pathological conditions such as Parkinson's disease [164] and smoking [165].

Methods to measure oxidized DNA base pairs are listed in Table 10. Measurements of 8-oxoGua formed by free radicals generated during oxidative metabolism have led to a wide discrepancy in values. Different methods have reported different values of 8-oxoGua formed each day in cells, as well as in tissues [166]. GC-MS has generally provided the highest values (ranging from 40 to 660 8-oxoGua or 8-oxodGua per 10^6 base pairs). HPLC measurement of 8-oxoGua have given intermediate values (ranging from 1.7 to 32 8-oxoGua or 8-oxodGua per 10^6 base pairs), while enzyme-based assays provide the lowest values (ranging from 0.08 to 0.24 8-oxoGua or 8-oxodGua per 10^6 base pairs) [166]. Artifacts

Table 10. 8-oxoGua/8-oxodGua detection methods.

Method	Comments/references
HPLC	A sensitive method that can measure 8-oxoGua and oxodGua. Traditional phenol extraction can cause artificially high oxidation values; newer and safer extraction procedures should be used [169,170,172]
GC-MS	A sensitive method that can measure many different oxidized base pairs. For measurement, samples must be derivatized, a process that will cause artificial oxidation. To avoid artifacts, oxidized base pairs must be separated from other nucleic acids before derivatization [9,167,168]

Enzymatic assays	Because formamidopyrimidine glycosylase [FPG] recognizes 8-oxoGua, incubation of DNA with FPG and endonucleases results in specific cleavage of DNA where 8-oxoGua is found. The resulting DNA breaks are measured using various techniques including alkaline unwinding, comet assay, and nick translation
	    Comet assay: [172,282]
	    Nick translation: [283]
	    Alkaline unwinding: [166]

Immunological methods	By using antibodies against 8-oxoGua, various immunological assays have been applied to measure 8-oxoGua [163,284]

generated during extraction and derivatization are responsible for most of the deviations in values among the different techniques [9].

4.1.1 GC-MS

GC-MS is very advantageous for the measurement of oxidized DNA due to its ability to analyze all oxidized DNA base pairs [167]. Oxidized DNA base pairs must be derivatized before detection by GC-MS. Recently, several papers have demonstrated that the high values of oxidized base pairs obtained by GC-MS were due, in part, to the oxidation of base pairs that occurs during the derivatization process [9]. To prevent oxidation, it has been suggested that nucleosides be separated from the oxidized nucleosides by column chromatography before derivatization [168]. This would ensure that only oxidized base pairs are present during derivatization, prevent artificially high results [9]. These recent improvements in GC-MS techniques have caused GC-MS measurements of cellular 8-oxoGua to approach those of HPLC.

4.1.2 HPLC

Floyd et al. first demonstrated that 8-oxoGua could be determined using HPLC-electrochemical detection [169]. Later, this method was adapted to simultaneously measure 8-oxoGua and 8-oxodGua [170]. HPLC values have generally yielded higher cellular 8-oxoGua values than those of enzymatic methodologies. The variation in values has been attributed to DNA extraction procedures. Phenol-chloroform, used to extract oxidized DNA, has been suggested to cause artificial oxidation [171]. Collins et al. used a milder extraction procedure to obtain 8-oxoGua values by HPLC, that were closer to the values derived using enzymatic assays [172]. Several DNA extraction procedures that lower artificially high values have been described in the following references: [171–174]. With the improved DNA extraction procedures, measurement of 8-oxoGua by HPLC remains a reliable and sensitive method.

4.1.3 Enzymatic methods

Because formamidopyridine glycosylase (FPG) recognizes 8-oxoGua, incubation of DNA with FPG and endonucleases results in specific cleavage of DNA at 8-oxo-Gua sites. The resulting DNA breaks are measured using various techniques, including alkaline unwinding, comet assay, and nick translation [166,172]. Enzymatic methods are advantageous in that they require less DNA than do HPLC and GC-MS methods, while still providing excellent sensitivity. Additionally, DNA is prepared for enzymatic analysis using a mild extraction, ensuring a lower probability for artificially high 8-oxoGua values [166]. Since enzymatic analysis requires less stringent extraction conditions than does either HPLC or GC-MS, it is believed that enzymatic assays have generally yielded the lowest 8-oxoGua values.

4.1.4 Measurement of 8-oxodGua in urine

The measurement of 8-oxodGua in urine represents a noninvasive method that can potentially be useful for clinical diagnosis. Increased urinary 8-oxodGua has been correlated with increased smoking [165], strenuous exercise [175], and in pathological conditions such as diabetes [176]. However, a great deal of controversy remains about whether urinary 8-oxodGua is an accurate marker of oxidative stress. One problem with measuring 8-oxodGua (the nucleoside), according to Lindahl, is that nucleosides are not a product of known excision repair pathways [162]. Bases, such as 8-oxoGua, are products of known excision repair pathways, but cannot be used to evaluate oxidative stress because these molecules can be influenced by diet as well as being a result of RNA breakdown [177]. Lindal has suggested that 8-oxodGua is the result of DNA breakdown from dead cells that become oxidized in the kidneys [162]. On the other hand, Shigenaga et al. reported that injection of radiolabeled guanosine in rats did not generate 8-oxodGua in urine, suggesting that the nucleosides do not oxidize in the kidneys [170]. It is clear that urinary 8-oxodGua increases in many diseases, but the question remains: is this increase due to an increase in oxidative stress, leading to 8-oxodGua formation and its excision, or is it merely due to an increase in cell death caused by the disease at hand? If the latter is true, then increasing urinary 8-oxodGua levels could be the result of DNA breakdown and oxidation that can occur after cell death. The source of 8-oxodGua in the urine still remains a matter of debate and its measurement as an accurate indicator of oxidative stress remains controversial.

4.2 Lipid peroxidation products

There is growing evidence that products generated during lipid peroxidation may play an important role in cellular pathologies [178]. Lipid hydroperoxides can alter membrane structures [179], and lipid peroxidation products, such as 4-hydroxynonenal (HNE) and malondialdehyde (MDA), have been shown to be mutagenic, cytotoxic, and to alter gene expression [178]. Lipid peroxidation of polyunsaturated fatty acids can generate lipid hydroperoxides and endoperoxides that can decompose into aldehydes, and into volatile hydrocarbons. A measurement of total lipid peroxidation is very difficult to quantitate because of the wide range of products that are generated. Lipid peroxidation products will vary, depending on the lipid composition, the species generating the lipid peroxidation, and the stage of the peroxidation process [180,181]. Certain oxidized biomolecules are found shortly after an oxidative insult, while other biomolecules form during later stages of oxidative stress. Consequently, using only one biomarker to evaluate lipid peroxidation as a whole can potentially be misleading [181].

The products of lipid peroxidation are displayed in Table 11. A wide range of biomarkers and techniques exist to measure lipid peroxidation, making it the most measured process involved in oxidative damage. While a few assays, such

Table 11. Lipid peroxidation product detection methods.

Compound	Comments/references
LOOH	LOOH are the initial products formed after the induction of lipid peroxidation. Because LOOH are rapidly cleared in cells, these hydroperoxides do not usually build up to high levels in the cell and are difficult to detect (Table 12)
Aldehydes (MDA, HNE)	These aldehydes are formed from the breakdown of lipid peroxides. Aldehydes can be found in their free form or bound to protein (Table 13)
Conjugated dienes	Both endoperoxides and LOOH possess a conjugated diene structure that have a characteristic absorbance at 234 nm. Conjugated diene measurements are not sensitive nor specific, thereby limiting their application in vivo
Spectrophotometric	The absorbance is measured at 234 nm after lipid extraction. Because of its nonspecificity, it has limited uses in biological samples [198]
Second derivative	An improvement of the spectrophotometric assay. Taking a derivative of the spectra provides greater resolution power [200,201]
HPLC-UV	HPLC separation provides greater selectivity. Lipid groups with conjugated dienes can be identified [199]
Volatile hydrocarbons	Volatile hydrocarbons, such as ethane and pentane, are generated during the breakdown of lipid peroxides. Generally, these are measured by gas-liquid chromatography with a flame ionization detector. This is a sensitive and noninvasive technique. However, it remains a difficult technique that is still in development for use as a clinical tool [217]
F2-Isoprostanes	F2-isoprostanes are prostaglandin-like compounds generated in vivo by non-cyclooxygenase dependent arachadonic acid peroxidation. F2-Isoprostanes have been found in biological fluids and plasma. Commonly measured in plasma or urine as a noninvasive technique [221]
GC-MS	[221,224]
Immunoassay	[225]
Fluorescent products	Aldehydes that form a Schiff base with protein are fluorescent. Measurement of fluorescence is not very specific in biological samples and should first be validated for the particular biological system being measured [219,220]
cis-Parinaric acid	PnA is a fluorescent polyunsaturated fatty acid not found endogenously. It is added to biological samples and its fluorescence is monitored. A decrease in PnA fluorescence suggests destruction of the fatty acid and is used as an indication of lipid peroxidation in the system
HPLC-detection	[227]
Fluorometry	[201,226]
Flow cytometry	[228]

as the TBA assay, have some inherent weaknesses, most techniques are highly specific and have been valuable tools to measure lipid oxidation in biological systems. In general, lipid hydroperoxides and their breakdown products are very unstable, and extra precaution must be taken during the processing and extraction procedures. Samples will either tend to increase in lipid peroxidation or decrease in lipid peroxidation, depending on the different processing procedures. Overviews on lipid peroxidation methodology can be found in the following reviews: [181−185].

4.2.1 *Lipid hydroperoxides (LOOH)*

LOOH are the major initial products formed after the induction of lipid peroxidation. LOOH are very unstable molecules that decompose to aldehydes or are rapidly broken down in cells through the action of GSH peroxidase. The measurement of LOOH generally reflects an early stage of lipid peroxidation. Because LOOH are rapidly cleared in cells, these hydroperoxides do not build up to high levels in the cell and are usually difficult to detect. The most frequently used methods to determine lipid hydroperoxides have been by HPLC, GC-MS, or enzymatic methods (Table 12).

4.2.1.1 HPLC. Chemiluminescence has been frequently used to measure LOOH [186]. Isoluminol [186] or luminol [187], in the presence of a heme molecule, react with LOOH and chemiluminesce. The chemiluminescence detection system is coupled with HPLC, downstream of the column. Here, HPLC provides two functions: 1) HPLC separates different LOOH species, allowing for specific identification by their different retention times; and 2) HPLC separates antioxidants and other compounds that would potentially interfere with the chemiluminescence detection system. Yamato et al. used HPLC-chemiluminescence, a commonly used system which utilizes microperoxidase, a heme fragment, and isoluminol to obtain chemiluminescence [187], while others have used cytochrome-c and luminol to generate chemiluminescence [188]. Although the HPLC-chemiluminescence detection system is fairly specific for LOOH, not all of the resulting peaks are indicative of LOOH. For example, ubiquinol has been shown to chemiluminesce when used with isoluminol [189]. One way to positively

Table 12. Lipid hydroperoxide detection methods.

Methods	Comments/references
HPLC	The chemiluminescence detection method is based on a reaction between isoluminol or luminol with LOOH. It is a specific and sensitive method when used with HPLC [187–189]
Iodometric	To quantitate lipid peroxide levels, iodine is added to the sample in excess, the I_2 that is formed is converted to I_3^- in the presence of excess iodide, and I_3^- is monitored. I_3^- contains a strong chromaphore and can easily be measured spectrophotometrically [196,197]
GC-MS (LOH)	LOOH is reduced to LOH (the hydroxyl derivative of LOOH), usually with sodium borohydride. The hydroxy-fatty acid is then derivatized, separated by gas chromatography and detected by mass spectrometry [190,191]
Enzymatic assays	
Cyclooxygenase	LOOH have been shown to activate cyclooxygenase, which can be measured by monitoring oxygen consumption [194,195]
GSH peroxidase	GSH peroxidase breaks down LOOH to their alcohol constituents by using the reducing power of GSH. LOOH in samples can be measured by the addition of GSH peroxidase and GSH and monitoring the GSSG formation [192,193]

identify LOOH from ubiquinol is to rerun samples with triphenylphosphate. LOOH are destroyed by triphenylphosphate, while ubiquinols are not. Although chemiluminescence is a sensitive method (picomole range), the postcolumn HPLC system is somewhat difficult to manage and suffers from high variability.

4.2.1.2 GC-MS. GC-MS is also a sensitive method to measure lipid hydroperoxides. LOOH is reduced to LOH (the corresponding hydroxyl derivative), usually with sodium borohydride. The hydroxy-fatty acid is then derivatized, separated by GC and detected by mass spectrometry [190,191].

4.2.1.3 Enzymatic methodologies. Selective assays for LOOH can be achieved by using enzymes that selectively react with LOOH. Two enzymatic systems use GSH peroxidase and cyclooxygenase. GSH peroxidase breaks down LOOH to their alcohol constituents by using the reducing power of GSH. LOOH in samples can be measured, after addition of GSH peroxidase and GSH, by monitoring the GSSG formation, using the DTNB-GSSG reductase assay previously described [192,193]. Similarly, cyclooxygenase activity of prostaglandin-H synthase has been used to selectively measure LOOH. LOOH has been shown to activate the cyclooxygenase and its activity can be measured by monitoring oxygen consumption [194,195]. Enzymatic methods are generally advantageous since they require a smaller sample size, however, these methods provide no information on which class of LOOH are being generated in a system.

4.2.1.4 Iodometric determination. There is a strict stoichiometric relationship between iodide ions in acidic solutions and peroxides.

$$ROOH \quad + \quad 2H^+ \quad + \quad 2I^- \quad \rightarrow \quad ROH \quad + \quad H_2O \quad + \quad I_2$$

To quantitate lipid peroxide levels, iodine is added to the sample in excess. The I_2 that is formed is converted to I_3^- in the presence of excess iodide, and I_3^- is monitored. I_3^- contains a strong chromaphore and can easily be measured spectrophotometrically [196,197]. Unfortunately, many other substances, such as oxygen, acetone, and ascorbate can interfere with the iodine assay. To avoid nonspecific reactions, lipids are sometimes extracted before the addition of the iodide solution.

4.2.2 Conjugated dienes

Both endoperoxides and LOOH possess a conjugated diene structure which absorbs UV at 234 nm. Consequently, conjugated dienes are frequently measured by spectrophotometry [198] or by HPLC-UV [199] as a biomarker of lipid peroxidation. Lipids are extracted using the standard Folch extraction method and the conjugated dienes are read at 234 nm. As many other molecules also absorb at 234 nm, a problem with spectrophotometric measurement of conjugated dienes is its lack of specificity and tendency to give artificially high values. In human fluids, molecules taken in from the diet and acquired from bacteria, such as octadeca-9(cis), 11(trans)-dienoic acid, have been shown to strongly absorb at 234 nm and interfere with conjugated diene values [181]. The use of second derivative spectroscopy has been shown to improve the conjugated diene assay [200,201]. HPLC with UV detection allows for the identification of lipids containing conjugated dienes. Such methods have been used to identify phospholipid peroxides and cholesterol ester peroxides formed during LDL oxidation [199]. Overall, measurement of conjugated dienes lacks the sensitivity needed to measure lipid peroxidation in more complex biological samples. Conjugated dienes represent a convenient and useful method to measure lipid peroxidation in simple in vitro systems, but are generally not selective and sensitive enough for analysis in most biological systems.

4.2.3 Aldehydes

The process of lipid peroxidation generates a wide variety of aldehydes, including malondialdehyde (MDA), 4-hydroxy-2-nonenal (HNE), 4-hydroxy-2-hexenal, 4-hydroxy-octenal, 2,4-heptadienal, pental, and hexanal [202]. MDA and HNE, the major species formed upon lipid peroxidation, are commonly studied aldehydes that have been shown to be cytotoxic and to exhibit mutagenic effects [178]. These aldehydes are relatively stable and can diffuse from their site of origin to different areas of the cell. Esterbauer has described aldehydes as "second toxic messengers" [178] because of their ability to diffuse and disrupt cell function. In the following section, methodologies for the determination of MDA and HNE are discussed (Table 13).

4.2.3.1 Malondialdehyde (MDA). MDA is a product of the oxidation of polyunsaturated fatty acids that contain more than two methylene-interrupted double bonds, such as arachadonic acid and docosahexaenoic acid [178]. In biological systems, MDA is either found in a free form or covalently bonded to protein in Schiff base linkages to lysine groups [203]. The liberation of bound MDA can be accomplished by heating MDA in hot acid or by alkaline digestion [204]. Many assays exist to measure MDA, including the TBA assay.

4.2.3.1.1 TBA assay. The most widely used method to detect MDA is the thiobarbituric acid (TBA) assay. The TBA assay is a colorimetric assay that is based on the conjugation between TBA and MDA. Samples are heated at a low pH to break the covalent bonds between MDA and proteins, as well as to catalyze MDA-TBA adduct formation. The MDA-TBA adduct has a high molar absorption at 532 nm ($\varepsilon = 153,000$), allowing for its measurement with conventional spectrophotometers [182,204,205].

Although the TBA assay has been an important tool for in vitro systems, its use in biological systems has been heavily criticized. A significant criticism with the

Table 13. Aldehyde detection methods.

Method	Comments/references
Malondialdehyde:	
Spectrophotometric	
TBA assay	MDA is conjugated with TBA and detected spectrophotometrically. This assay is nonspecific when applied to biological samples. If it is to be used, it should be validated by more specific methods, such as HPLC, for the biological system being measured [182,206]
HPLC	MDA can be detected using HPLC directly or after conjugation with TBA
TBA-MDA conjugate	As in the TBA assay, MDA is conjugated with TBA for measurement. The TBA-MDA conjugate may be separated using HPLC, and detected either by UV or fluorescent detection. HPLC helps to separate away interfering substances, providing for a specific assay [207,208,285,286]
MDA	Because MDA has a high extinction coefficient in the UV, it can be detected directly using HPLC-UV. This method detects free MDA only [206,209]
GC	Depending on which compound is used for derivatization, both free and protein bound MDA can be determined with great sensitivity [210]
Immunological methods	By using antibodies against MDA-protein or MDA-DNA adducts, various immunological techniques have been used to detect such adducts in pathological conditions [287−289]
4-Hydroxynonenal:	
HPLC	HNE can be detected by HPLC directly or as a derivatized product
UV detection	1) HNE has a high extinction coefficient and can be detected directly by HPLC-UV. This method measures only free HNE [215] 2) HNE is conjugated with DNPH and detected by HPLC-UV [206]
Fluorescence detection	HNE is derivatized with the fluorescent reagent 1,3-cyclohexanedione for measurement [214]
Electrochemical detection	HNE is derivatized with 2,4-dinitrophenylhydrazone and detected electrochemically. Electrochemical detection offers greater sensitivity [213]
GC-MS	A sensitive and selective method that can detect as low as 1 picomole of HNE [190,212]
Immunological methods	By using antibodies against HNE-protein adducts, various immunological techniques have been used to detect such adducts in pathological conditions [216,290−292]

TBA assay has been its nonspecificity which arises from two facts: 1) cells contain many endogenous pigments that absorb at 532 nm, leading to artificially high values; and 2) other aldehydes [204], amino acids, and sugars [181] can conjugate with TBA as well, also leading to artificially high values. Because of this nonspecificity, it is often considered an assay that measures thiobarbituric reactive substances (TBARS) more than just MDA alone.

Another significant problem with the TBA assay is that it is greatly influenced by the reaction conditions. TBA color formation is influenced by the heating time, acids used, and the temperature [205,206]. The addition of exogenous antioxidants also influences the outcome of the assay. If no exogenous antioxidants are added, the majority of the MDA being measured in the TBA assay is the result of the lipid peroxidation that has occurred during sample heating [182]. Some researchers add exogenous antioxidants like BHT, beforehand, to inhibit lipid peroxidation during sample heating. Due to the many different recipes for the TBA assay, MDA estimates are highly variable in the literature. MDA values in the plasma have been reported to be as high as 47 nmol/l and as low as 0 nmol/l [205]. The lack of standardization of the TBA assay has made comparison of TBA measurements almost impossible.

The TBA assay is a valuable tool for the following: 1) in measuring lipid peroxidation in simple in vitro systems; and 2) in determining the potential of a sample to undergo lipid peroxidation (no exogenous antioxidants should be added) [182]. The TBA assay is too nonspecific to be of any substantial value when measuring MDA in biological systems. Only if the TBA assay is first validated with another, more specific method (such as one using HPLC), can this assay be routinely used for a particular biological system [206].

4.2.3.1.2 HPLC. Coupling HPLC with the TBA assay allows for the separation of the MDA-TBA conjugates from other nonspecific TBA conjugates, thereby providing a more specific measurement of MDA [205,207,208]. TBA-MDA conjugates can be determined with UV or fluorescence detection, with the latter being the more sensitive and selective method. It is important to add BHT during the TBA-MDA conjugation process to prevent lipid peroxidation during heating. The HPLC-TBA system is a sensitive and selective method that has been used for the measurement of MDA in many clinical situations.

The high extinction coefficient ($\varepsilon = 31,500$ at 267 nm) of MDA allows for its measurement by HPLC-UV detection, without the conjugation of MDA [206,209]. Because, unlike in the TBA assay, there is no acid hydrolysis, this HPLC method measures only free MDA. Since the majority of MDA is believed to be bound to protein, this assay would greatly underestimate total MDA levels. In certain cases, such as in peroxidized mitochondria, MDA has been found to be predominantly in the free form [206].

4.2.3.1.3 Gas chromatography. Gas chromatography (GC) can be used to measure free or bound MDA in cells, depending on the material used to derivatize the MDA. Derivatization of MDA with compounds such as 2-hydroxypyrimidine can be used to detect total MDA, while methyl hydrazine can be used to determine free MDA [210]. GC can separate interfering substances and provide an accurate estimate for MDA levels in biological samples.

4.2.3.2 Hydroxynonenal (HNE). HNE is an aldehyde generated during the peroxidation of unsaturated fatty acids, such as linolenic acid and arachadonic acid [178]. HNE exhibits a wide range of deleterious effects in cells, including the alteration of gene expression [178], dissipation of the mitochondrial membrane potential [211], and inhibition of protein synthesis. HNE may be found in cells in its free or protein-bound form. When HNE binds to protein, it does so through the formation of a Schiff base or by binding protein sulfhydryl groups. Most methods designed to measure HNE can only detect the free form and Schiff base-bound molecules [212]. The HNE-sulfide linkages are difficult to reverse and thus, detection of total HNE values are difficult to obtain.

4.2.3.2.1 HPLC. HNE, as well as other aldehydes, can be detected by HPLC or TLC after conjugation with dinitrophenylhydrazine (DNPH) [206]. DNPH bound to an aldehyde exhibits a strong yellow color ($\varepsilon = 25,000-28,000$ at $360-380$ nm) that can easily be measured. The HNE-DNPH adduct can also be measured by HPLC-electrochemical detection with greater sensitivity [213]. Another agent, 1,3-cyclohexanedione, when conjugated to HNE, can be measured fluorometrically [214]. These methods can detect free and Schiff base-bound HNE.

HNE as a strong molar absorption (ε13,000 at 222 nm) in methanol and can be directly determined by HPLC-UV [215]. This HPLC method only detects free HNE, a minor form found in the cell.

4.2.3.2.2 GC-MS. Greater sensitivity and selectivity can be achieved with GC-MS detection. Generally HNE is derivatized with such compounds as *o*-(pentafluorobenzyl)hydroxylamine [190]. GC-MS can detect as low as $1-5$ picomole of HNE in biological samples [212].

4.2.3.2.3 Antibodies. Because the majority of HNE and MDA are bound to protein, antibodies have been developed that recognize HNE- and MDA-protein adducts. Such immunological techniques have been used to detect these adducts in pathological conditions such as cardiovascular disease [216].

4.2.4 *Volatile hydrocarbons*

Volatile hydrocarbons, such as ethane and pentane, are generated during the breakdown of lipid peroxides. It has been shown that hydrocarbons tend to increase after exercise and are elevated in many diseases. Measurement of volatile hydrocarbons is a highly sensitive, noninvasive technique with great clinical potential. The breath of subjects is collected and measured by gas-liquid chromatography with a flame ionization detector [217]. One problem with hydrocarbon measurements is that hydrocarbons can be generated from sources other than lipid peroxidation, such as intestinal bacteria. At present, the determination of hydrocarbons remains a difficult technique that is still in development for use as a clinical tool [217,218].

4.2.5 *Fluorescent products*

As previously mentioned, MDA can form Schiff bases with proteins. The bond formed ($-N=CHCH=CHNHR-$) is highly fluorescent. Other products of lipid peroxidation, such as lipofuscin (age pigment) and ceroid pigments also have a characteristically strong fluorescence [219]. Monitoring changes in fluorescent products have been frequently used to estimate lipid peroxidation [220]. While measurement of fluorescent products in simple systems is useful, in complex biological systems, the use of fluorescence to assess lipid peroxidation is nonspecific. Gutteridge and Halliwell pointed out that without detailed characterization it should never be assumed that fluorescent products are the end products of lipid peroxidation [181]. Therefore, this method should not be used in biological systems unless it is first validated for that particular system with a more specific assay.

4.2.6 *F2-Isoprostanes*

F2-isoprostanes are prostaglandin-like compounds generated in vivo by non-cyclooxygenase-dependent arachadonic acid peroxidation [221]. Four isoforms of isoprostanes are believed to be generated during arachadonic acid peroxidation. F2-isoprostanes have been shown to occur in all biological fluids and tissues measured and there is increasing evidence that they can alter cell function [222]. Increased isoprostane formation has been shown to occur in numerous diseases, including cardiovascular disease and diabetes mellitus [223]. The most widely used method to detect isoprostanes is by GC-MS [221,224]. Recently, an ELISA assay has been developed for the measurement of isoprostanes [225] and is commercially available. Urinary measurements of isoprostanes are used as a noninvasive measurement of oxidative stress.

4.2.7 *Cis-parinaric acid (PnA)*

PnA is a fluorescent polyunsaturated fatty acid that is frequently used to monitor lipid peroxidation in biological samples. PnA is not found endogenously and is added to biological samples, so that its fluorescence can be monitored. A decrease in PnA fluorescence suggests destruction of the fatty acid and is used as an indicator of lipid peroxidation. PnA can be measured by fluorometry [201,226], HPLC [227], or by flow cytometry. PnA has been used to monitor lipid peroxidation in many biological systems, including low density lipoprotein (LDL) [201] and cells [228]. The primary weakness of PnA is that it must be added exogenously, which can potentially disturb the system being measured. PnA must be added in moderation to cells, since it can affect membrane fluidity and can potentially affect lipid peroxidation rates. However, if used correctly, monitoring of PnA is a very sensitive and powerful method to determine lipid oxidation.

4.3 Protein oxidation

In vitro studies have shown that free radicals can damage the tertiary structure of

Table 14. Protein oxidation.

Method	Comments/references
Protein thiol/disulfide redox status	Most intracellular proteins are in the reduced thiol state, however, during times of oxidative stress, protein sulfhydryl groups can oxidize to their disulfide form. Protein redox status is monitored using various probes that label thiol groups or by EPR
	[93]
	[231]
DTNB	[232]
MBB	[233]
Iodoacetyl(^{125}I)3-iodotyrosine	
(^{3}H)acetyl-4-aminophenylarsine	[234,235]
oxide	Thiolation is the nonenzymatic linkage of GSH to protein
EPR	sulfhydryl groups that can occur during times of oxidative
S-Thiolation	stress. It is generally measured using radiolabelled cystine
	[236–238,293]
	Carbonyl groups are formed when amino acids (particularly histidine, arginine, lysine and proline) are attacked by ROS
Protein carbonyls	These groups are not a specific marker of oxidative damage because glycation also can form carbonyl structures.
	The carbonyl assay is based on the reaction between 2,4-di-nitrophenylhydrazine with protein carbonyls, whose product
Spectrophotometry	can be measured spectrophotometrically (usually at 370 nm). A controversial assay. Its specificity and reproducibility has been questioned [239,240,242].
HPLC	[240]
ELISA	[243]
Western blot	[244]
Oxidized amino acids	ROS attack to protein can oxidize a wide range of amino acids (Table 15)

proteins, cause protein fragmentation, oxidize thiol residues, and damage different amino acids [229]. Commonly used parameters to assess oxidative damage to protein include the measurement of thiol/disulfide redox status, S-thiolation, protein carbonyls, and oxidized amino acids (Table 14).

4.3.1 *Protein thiol/disulfide redox status*

Most intracellular proteins are found in the reduced thiol state. During oxidative stress, protein sulfhydryl groups can oxidize to their disulfide form. The formation of disulfides in intracellular proteins is considered consequence of oxidative stress [230]. The oxidation of protein thiols has been suggested to be important in the activity of key transcription factors such as NF-κ B and OxyR.

The thiol/disulfide protein redox status is difficult to directly determine and, in most cases, investigators only measure a decrease in protein thiol levels. Protein thiol status in biological samples can be measured with general thiol probes, such as DTNB [93] or MBB [231] as previously discussed in the GSH section. For the determination of thiol/disulfide redox status of specific proteins, several radiolabeled probes, such as *N*-iodoacetyl(^{125}I)-3-iodotyrosine [232] and (^3H) acetyl-4-aminophenylarsine oxide [233], have been developed. These labeled probes covalently bind to the free thiol groups of proteins, which are then analyzed. Several researchers have also applied EPR methods for the determination of cellular thiol status [234,235].

4.3.2 S-Thiolation

S-thiolation is the nonenzymatic linkage of GSH to protein and can occur in cells after treatment with peroxides and in monocytes undergoing respiratory burst. S-thiolation is generally believed to be mediated through GSSG formation. The protein-glutathione bond formed during oxidative stress can disrupt protein function and inactivate certain enzymes [230]. Radiolabeled cystine in cultured cells is a frequently used method that measures S-thiolation in biological systems [236,237]. Radiolabeled cystine is transported into the cells, reduced intracellularly to cysteine, and incorporated into GSH. The net result is radiolabeled GSH that will label protein if S-thiolation occurs. Protein synthesis inhibitors, such as cycloheximide, must also be added to the system to ensure that cysteine is not utilized for the synthesis of new proteins. S-thiolation is considered to be an early event in oxidative stress and has also been shown to be a reversible process [237, 238].

4.3.3 *Protein carbonyls*

Carbonyl groups (protein$-C=O$) are formed when amino acids (particularly histidine, arginine, lysine and proline) are attacked by ROS. A carbonyl assay, introduced by Levine et al. has frequently been used to measure carbonyl formation in proteins [239,240]. This assay is based on the reaction between 2,4-dinitrophenylhydrazine with protein carbonyls, whose product can be measured spectrophotometrically (usually at 370 nm). By using the carbonyl assay, researchers have demonstrated that protein carbonyls increase with age [5] and in pathological conditions such as Alzheimer's disease [241].

The carbonyl assay, like the TBA assay, has been widely used, but has also been heavily criticized for its lack of specificity and reproducibility. In essence, many of the problems that exist with the TBA assay also exist with the carbonyl assay. First, protein carbonyls themselves have been questioned as to whether or not they are a specific marker of oxidative stress. Carbonyls form not only as a consequence of oxidative stress, but also as a result of enzymatic and nonenzymatic protein glycosylation [240]. Carbonyl groups not related to oxidative stress are also found in nucleic acids and lipids and these other biomolecules must be extracted out, requiring difficult extraction procedures. DNA that is not completely extracted from samples can cause erroneously high carbonyl measurements

[6]. The carbonyl assay, like the TBA assay, is greatly influenced by reaction conditions. Carbonyl values can be influenced by the timing of the 2,4-dinitrophenyl-hydrazine addition to the reaction, as well as by how long the finished reaction sits before measurement [242]. Several investigators have introduced modifications of the carbonyl assay, making the comparison of results even more difficult [242].

Perhaps the most troubling aspect of the carbonyl assay is its irreproducibility that has been reported in the literature [6]. Studies that report increases in protein carbonyls with age and in motor neuron disease [242] have not been able to be reproduced [6]. Cao et al. has reported that the carbonyl assays are unreliable and attributes the irreproducibility to the inability to completely rid samples of interfering nucleic acids and to the interference of free DNPH [6]. The problems of reproducibility have led some researchers to seriously question the validity of the carbonyl assay [6].

To improve specificity of the carbonyl assay, ELISA [243], Western blot [244], and HPLC methods [240] have been developed. Unfortunately, even with such improvements, criticism still exists. One report has criticized the HPLC method for being nonspecific and unreliable [6]. The validity of these methods depends on whether or not carbonyls represent a good marker of protein oxidation. Because carbonyls are not a specific biomarker of oxidative stress, its use as a marker of oxidative protein damage remains somewhat controversial.

4.3.4 Oxidized amino acids

One of the best methods to assess oxidative stress in biological systems is the detection of oxidized amino acids. Table 15 shows some of the oxidized products of amino acids that form during protein oxidation. For a few amino acids, amino acid-peroxides can be formed during oxidative stress, and these peroxides are detected by similar methodologies that are used to detect lipid peroxides [245]. Before their analysis, proteins are broken down into their amino acid components

Table 15. Amino acid oxidation products.

Amino acid	Oxidized product	Method	References
Arginine	5-hydroxy-2-amino (HAVA)	GC-MS	[294,295]
Histidine	2-oxohistidine	HPLC mass spec.	[302,303]
Leucine	Hydroxyleucines, proline analogs	HPLC	[304]
Methionine	methione sulfoxide	HPLC	[246]
Phenylalanine	*o*-,*m*-,*p*-tyrosine	HPLC	[32,305,306]
Proline	5-hydroxy-2-amino (HAVA)	GC-MS	[294,295]
Tyrosine	Dityrosine	HPLC	[296,297]
	Nitrotyrosine	HPLC, GC-MS, antibodies	[32,298,299]
	Chlorotyrosine	GC-MS	[300]
	DOPA	HPLC, GC-MS	[245,301]
Valine	Valine hydroperoxides, hydroxides	HPLC	[307]

and are then detected for their oxidation products. Most of the oxidized amino acids are not produced by endogenous enzymes and represent specific markers of oxidative damage. For the most part, the various oxidized amino acids can be detected by HPLC and GC-MS.

Only in recent years have researchers vigorously searched for in vivo measurements of oxidized amino acid products. Analysis of certain oxidized amino acids has failed to show any increase with aging [32] while many pathologic conditions, such as arteriosclerosis and inflammatory lung disease [246] have been shown to be associated with increased oxidized amino acid levels. Generally, studies carried out to determine oxidized amino acids in pathophysiological conditions have been technically difficult because of the large number of amino acid oxidation products that can form [247]. Most methods allow for the determination of one or two oxidized amino acids and may only provide a limited view of the actual protein oxidation that has occurred. However, until better techniques are developed, measurement of oxidized amino acids represents one of the most specific markers of oxidative protein modification, and further use of this technique can provide us with a better understanding of protein oxidation in vivo.

5   SUMMARY

1. Oxidative stress is generally characterized by an increase in ROS, a decrease in antioxidants, and/or an increase in oxidized biomolecules (lipids, protein or DNA).
2. To assess oxidative stress, particular molecules from the above three categories that are known to decrease or increase during such stress are chosen for measurement. To be effective biomarkers of oxidative stress, these molecules must change only as a result of oxidative stress and cannot fluctuate with other cell processes.
3. Determination of oxidative stress in biological systems remains a difficult task. Some factors that contribute to its difficulty include the short lifetime of free radicals, the low levels of oxidized biomolecules, and the high probability for artificial oxidation during the extraction.
4. Given the short lifetime of ROS, especially of free radicals, their detection in biological systems is extremely difficult. Instead, ROS are detected indirectly by using spin traps or probes.
5. Antioxidants can be detected in vivo by a wide range of reliable methods. Precautions must be taken to avoid auto-oxidation of antioxidants during extraction procedures.
6. Oxidized lipids, proteins, and DNA are difficult to measure due to their low concentration inside cells. ROS attack lipids, proteins, and DNA and can create a wide range of products. Because no method exists to measure all of these breakdown products at once, an accurate assessment of total oxidative damage has been almost impossible to obtain. A few oxidized biomolecules are usually chosen as indicators of the severity of oxidative damage, and are

monitored as biomarkers of oxidative stress.

7. Many assays that determine oxidative stress in biological systems are non-specific. A classic example is the TBA assay used to measure lipid peroxidation. The use of these nonspecific assays should be avoided in vivo because their results can be misleading.

8. There is no one best method to assess oxidative stress. Because there are numerous potential cellular sources of ROS and many different biomolecules with which ROS may react, a set outcome of oxidative damage is difficult to predict. Several methods must be employed for an accurate assessment of oxidative stress.

6 PERSPECTIVES

While oxidative stress has been linked to physiological processes, such as signal transduction, and to pathophysiological conditions, such as Parkinson's, Alzheimer's and cancer, the extent of its involvement remains unclear. Whether oxidative stress is merely a byproduct of pathophysiological conditions or if it plays an active role in the progression of these pathologies has yet to be decided. Efforts to research this question have fallen short because of their reliance on nonspecific assays such as the TBA, carbonyl, and conjugated diene assays. While these assays are advantageous in that they are convenient and easy, their lack of specificity makes them a poor tool for the quantitative analysis of oxidative stress in vivo. Less use of these types of assays and utilization of newer developing methodologies, such as new visualization techniques that provide spatial and temporal understanding of ROS in cells, will furnish a more complete and precise understanding of oxidative stress. Still, it is clear that newer revolutionary techniques must be developed to better comprehend the role of oxidative stress in vivo. Until such methodologies are developed, the role of oxidative stress in physiological and pathological events will remain elusive.

7 ABBREVIATIONS

DCFH: 2',7'-dichlorofluorescin
DEPMPO: 5-diethoxyphophoryl-5-methyl-1-pyrroline-n-oxide
DHB: 2,3-dihydrobenzoic acid
DMPO: 5,5-dimethyl-1-pyrroline-N-oxide
DTNB: 5,5'-dithiobis-(2-nitrobenzoic acid)
DTT: dithiothreitol
EDTA: ethylenediaminetetraacetic acid
EPR: electron paramagnetic resonance
ESR: electron spin resonance
FPG: formamidopyrimidine glycosylase
GC: gas chromatography
GCMS: gas chromatography-mass spectroscopy

GSH: glutathione
GSSG: glutathione disulfide
H_2O_2:   hydrogen peroxide
HFR,·OH: hydroxyl free radical
HNE: 4-hydroxy-2-nonenal
HPLC: high performance liquid chromatography
LOH: lipid hydroxyl
LOOH: lipid hydroperoxides
LOOH: lipid peroxide
MBB: monobromobimane
MCB: monochlorobimane
MDA: malondialdehyde
NADPH: nicotinamide dinucleotide phosphate {reduced}
NEM: *N*-ethylmaliamide
$O_2^{\bullet-}$:   superoxide
OSS: oxidative stress status
PBN: phenyl-tert-butylnitrone
PnA: *cis*-parinaric acid
ROS: reactive oxygen species
SDS: sodium dodecyl sulfate
TBA: thiobarbituric acid
TBARS: thiobarbituric reactive substances
2-VP: 2-vinylpyridine
8-oxoGua: 8-oxoguanine
8-oxodGua: 8-oxodeoxyguanosine

8   REFERENCES

1. Halliwell B, Gutteridge JMC. Free radicals in biology and medicine. Oxford: Clarendon Press, 1985.
2. Sies H, Oxidative Stress. New York: Academic Press, 1985.
3. Smith CV. Free Radic Biol Med 1991;10:217–224.
4. Haramaki N, Packer L. Oxidative stress indices in exercise. In: Sen CK, Packer L, Hanninen O (eds) Exercise and oxygen toxicity. Elsevier: Amsterdam, 1994;77–87.
5. Stadtman ER. Science 1992;257:1220–1224.
6. Cao G, Cutler RG. Arch Biochem Biophys 1995;320:106–114.
7. Schofield D, Braganza JM. Clin Sci 1992;82:117–118.
8. Asensi M, Sastre J, Pallardo FV, Garcia de la Asuncion J, Estrela JM, Vina J. Anal Biochem 1994;217:323–328.
9. Ravanat JL, Turesky RJ, Gremaud E, Trudel LJ, Stadler RH. Chem Res Toxicol 1995;8:1039–1045.
10. Packer L. Nitric Oxide: Part A, Sources and Detection of NO, NO Synthase. Meth Enzymol 268. San Diego: Academic Press, 1996.
11. Weil JA, Bolton JR, Wertz JE. Electron paramagnetic resonance. Elementary theory and practical applications. New York: Wiley, 1994.
12. Buettner GR. Free Radic Biol Med 1987;3:259–303.
13. Mason RP, In vitro and in vivo detection of free radical metabolites with electron spin reso-

nance. In: Punchard NA, Kelly FJ (eds) Free Radicals: A Practical Approach. Oxford: Oxford University Press, 1996:11—24.

14. Buettner GR, Mason RP. Meth Enzymol 1990;186:127—133.
15. Packer JE, Slater TF, Willson RL. Nature 1979;278:737—738.
16. Buettner GR, Jurkiewicz BA. Free Radic Biol Med 1993;14:49—55.
17. Mori A, Wang X, Liu J. Meth Enzymol 1994;233:149—154.
18. Buettner GR, Motten AG, Hall RD, Chignell CF. Photochem Photobiol 1987;46:161—164.
19. Pietri S, Culcasi M, Stella L, Cozzone PJ. Eur J Biochem 1990;193:845—854.
20. Roubaud V, Sankarapandi S, Kuppusamy P, Tordo P, Zweier JL. Anal Biochem 1997;247: 404—411.
21. Rosen GM, Rauckman EJ. Meth Enzymol 1984;105:198—209.
22. Janzen EG. Spin trapping and new developments in EPR: Overview and advances. In: Davies KJA (ed) Oxidative Damage and Repair. Oxford: Pergamon, 1991.
23. Borg DC. Spin trapping and new developments in EPR; An Overvie. In: Davies KJA (ed) Oxidative Damage and Repair. Oxford: Pergamon, 1991.
24. Sun JZ, Kaur H, Halliwell B, Li XY, Bolli R. Circ Res 1993;73:534—549.
25. O'Neill CA, Fu LW, Halliwell B, Longhurst JC. Am J Physiol 1996;271:H660—667.
26. Piantadosi CA, Zhang J. Stroke 1996;27(discussion 332):327—331.
27. Kaur H, Halliwell B. Salicyclic acid and phenylalanine as probes to detect hydroxyl radicals. In: Punchard NA, Kelly FJ (eds) Free Radicals: A pratical approach. Oxford: Oxford University Press, 1996.
28. Floyd RA, Henderson R, Watson JJ, Wong PK. Free Radic Biol Med 1986;2:13—18.
29. Coudray C, Talla M, Martin S, Fatome M, Favier A. Anal Biochem 1995;227:101—111.
30. Halliwell B, Kaur H, Ingelman—Sundberg M. Free Radic Biol Med 1991;10:439—441.
31. Luo X, Lehotay DC. Clin Biochem 1997;30:41—46.
32. Leeuwenburgh C, Hansen P, Shaish A, Holloszy JO, Heinecke JW. Am J Physiol 1998;274: R453—461.
33. Forman HJ, Boveris A. Superoxide radical and hydrogen peroxide in mitochondria. In: Pryor WA (ed) Free Radicals in Biology. New York: Academic Press Inc, 1982;65—89
34. Clement MV, Stamenkovic I. Embo J 1996;15:216—225.
35. Irani K, Xia Y, Zweier JL, Sollott SJ, Der CJ, Fearon ER, Sundaresan M, Finkel T, Goldschmidt-Clermont PJ. Science 1997;275:1649—1652.
36. Faulkner K, Fridovich I. Free Radic Biol Med 1993;15:447—451.
37. Liochev SI, Fridovich I. Arch Biochem Biophys 1997;337:115—120.
38. Vasquez-Vivar J, Hogg N, Pritchard KA Jr, Martasek P, Kalyanaraman B. FEBS Lett 1997;403: 127—130.
39. Fridovich I. J Biol Chem 1997;272:18515—18517.
40. Li Y, Zhu H, Kuppusamy P, Roubaud V, Zweier JL, Trush MA. J Biol Chem 1998;273: 2015—2023.
41. Bindokas VP, Jordan J, Lee CC, Miller RJ. J Neurosci 1996;16:1324—1336.
42. Benov L, Sztejnberg L, Fridovich I. Free Radic Biol Med 1998;25:826—831.
43. Budd AL, Castilho RF, Nicholls DG. FEBS Lett 1997;415:21—24.
44. Gardner PR, Fridovich I. Arch Biochem Biophys 1993;301:98—102.
45. Gardner PR, Fridovich I. J Biol Chem 1992;267:8757—8763.
46. Gardner PR, Raineri I, Epstein LB, White CW. J Biol Chem 1995;270:13399—13405.
47. Gardner PR, White CW. Application of the aconitase method to the assay of superoxide in the mitochondria matrices of cultured cells: Effects of oxygen, redox—cycling agents, TNF—a, IL—1, LPS and inhibitors of respiration. In: Davies KJA, Ursini F (eds) The Oxygen Paradox. Padova: Cleup University Press, 1995.
48. Chance B, Sies H, Boveris A. Physiol Rev 1979;59:527—605.
49. Keston AS, Brandt RB. Anal Biochem 1965;11:1—5.
50. Cathcart R, Schwiers E, Ames BN. Anal Biochem 1983;134:111—116.

51. Han D, Sen CK, Roy S, Kobayashi MS, Tritschler HJ, Packer L. Am J Physiol 1997;273: R1771–1778.
52. LeBel CP, Ischiropoulos H, Bondy SC. Chem Res Toxicol 1992;5:227–231.
53. Royall JA, Ischiropoulos H. Arch Biochem Biophys 1993;302:348–355.
54. Sundaresan M, Yu ZX, Ferrans VJ, Irani K, Finkel T. Science 1995;270:296–299.
55. Behl C, Davis JB, Lesley R, Schubert D. Cell 1994;77:817–827.
56. Tsuchiya M, Suematsu M, Suzuki H. Meth Enzymol 1994;233:128–140.
57. Suematsu M, Schmid–Schonbein GW, Chavez–Chavez RH, Yee TT, Tamatani T, Miyasaka M, Delano FA, Zweifach BW. Am J Physiol 1993;264:H881–891.
58. Zhu H, Bannenberg GL, Moldeus P, Shertzer HG. Arch Toxicol 1994;68:582–587.
59. Rao KM, Padmanabhan J, Kilby DL, Cohen HJ, Currie MS, Weinberg JB. J Leukoc Biol 1992; 51:496–500.
60. Kooy NW, Royall JA, Ischiropoulos H. Free Radic Res 1997;27:245–254.
61. Quillet–Mary A, Jaffrezou JP, Mansat V, Bordier C, Naval J, Laurent G. J Biol Chem 1997;272: 21388–21395.
62. Sies H, Bucher T, Oshino N, Chance B. Arch Biochem Biophys 1973;154:106–116.
63. Oshino N, Chance B, Sies H, Bucher T. Arch Biochem Biophys 1973;154:117–131.
64. Oshino N, Jamieson D, Sugano T, Chance B. Biochem J 1975;146:67–77.
65. Nahum A, Wood LD, Sznajder JI. Free Radic Biol Med 1989;6:479–484.
66. Corbett JT. J Biochem Biophys Methods 1989;18:297–307.
67. Boveris A, Martino E, Stoppani AO. Anal Biochem 1977;80:145–158.
68. Hinkle PC, Butow RA, Racker E, Chance B. J Biol Chem 1967;242:5169–5173.
69. Zhou M, Diwu Z, Panchuk-Voloshina N, Haugland RP. Anal Biochem 1997;253:162–168.
70. Root RK, Metcalf J, Oshino N, Chance B. J Clin Invest 1975;55:945–955.
71. Loschen G, Azzi A, Flohe L. FEBS Lett 1973;33:84–87.
72. Mueller S, Arnhold J. J Biolumin Chemilumin 1995;10:229–237.
73. Mueller S, Riedel HD, Stremmel W. Blood 1997;90:4973–4978.
74. Mueller S, Riedel HD, Stremmel W. Anal Biochem 1997;245:55–60.
75. Bannai S, Tateishi N. J Membr Biol 1986;89:1–8.
76. Kang YJ, Enger MD. J Cell Physiol 1991;148:197–201.
77. Post GB, Keller DA, Connor KA, Menzel DB. Biochem Biophys Res Commun 1983;114: 737–742.
78. Shaw JP, Chou IN. J Cell Physiol 1986;129:193–198.
79. Meister A. Nutr Rev 1984;42:397–410.
80. Roederer M, Staal FJ, Osada H, Herzenberg LA. Int Immunol 1991;3:933–937.
81. Adams JD Jr, Odunze IN. Free Radic Biol Med 1991;10:161–169.
82. Panigrahi M, Sadguna Y, Shivakumar BR, Kolluri SV, Roy S, Packer L, Ravindranath V. Brain Res 1996;717:184–188.
83. Macho A, Hirsch T, Marzo I, Marchetti P, Dallaporta B, Susin SA, Zamzami N, Kroemer G. J Immunol 1997;158:4612–4619.
84. van den Dobbelsteen DJ, Nobel CSI, Schlegel J, Cotgreave IA, Orrenius S, Slater AF. J Biol Chem 1996;271:15420–15427.
85. Lee FY, Siemann DW, Allalunis-Turner MJ, Keng PC. Cancer Res 1988;48:3661–3665.
86. Kosower NS, Kosower EM. Int Rev Cytol 1978;54:109–160.
87. Sies H, Akerboom TP. Meth Enzymol 1984;105:445–451.
88. Akerboom TP, Sies H. Meth Enzymol 1981;77:373–382.
89. Roberts JC, Francetic DJ. Anal Biochem 1993;211:183–187.
90. Anderson ME. Glutathione. In: Punchard NA, Kelly FJ (eds) Free Radicals: A Practical Approach. Oxford: Oxford University Press, 1996.
91. Mills BJ, Richie JP Jr, Lang CA. Anal Biochem 1994;222:95–101.
92. Sedlak J, Lindsay RH. Anal Biochem 1968;25:192–205.
93. Boyne AF, Ellman GL. Anal Biochem 1972;46:639–653.

94. Tietze F. Anal Biochem 1969;27:502—522.
95. Eyer P, Podhradsky D. Anal Biochem 1986;153:57—66.
96. Griffith OW. Anal Biochem 1980;106:207—212.
97. Robertson JD, Maughan RJ, Duthie GG, Morrice PC. Clin Sci (Colch) 1991;80:611—618.
98. Reed DJ, Babson JR, Beatty PW, Brodie AE, Ellis WW, Potter DW. Anal Biochem 1980;106: 55—62.
99. Fariss MW, Reed DJ. Meth Enzymol 1987;143:101—109.
100. Asensi M, Sastre J, Pallardo FV, Estrela JM, Vina J. Meth Enzymol 1994;234:367—371.
101. Allison LA, Shoup RE. Anal Chem 1983;55:12—16.
102. Harvey PR, Ilson RG, Strasberg SM. Clin Chim Acta 1989;180:203—212.
103. Krien PM, Margou V, Kermici M. J Chromatogr 1992;576:255—261.
104. Han D, Handelman GJ, Packer L. Meth Enzymol 1995;251:315—25.
105. Rice GC, Bump EA, Shrieve DC, Lee W, Kovacs M. Cancer Res 1986;46:6105—6110.
106. Hedley DW, Chow S. Cytometry 1994;15:349—358.
107. Sen CK, Roy S, Han D, Packer L. Free Radic Biol Med 1997;22:1241—1257.
108. Ublacker GA, Johnson JA, Siegel FL, Mulcahy RT. Cancer Res 1991;51:1783—1788.
109. Cook JA, Iype SN, Mitchell JB. Cancer Res 1991;51:1606—1612.
110. Han D, Handelman G, Marcocci L, Sen CK, Roy S, Kobuchi H, Tritschler HJ, Flohe L, Packer L. Biofactors 1997;6:321—338.
111. Kamal—Eldin A, Appelqvist LA. Lipids 1996;31:671—701.
112. Cadenas E. Annu Rev Biochem 1989;58:79—110.
113. McCay PB. Annu Rev Nutr 1985;5:323—340.
114. Kagan VE, Serbinova EA, Koynova GM, Kitanova SA, Tyurin VA, Stoytchev TS, Quinn PJ, Packer L. Free Radic Biol Med 1990;9:117—126.
115. Kagan V, Serbinova E, Packer L. Biochem Biophys Res Commun 1990;169:851—857.
116. Niki E, Saito T, Kawakami A, Kamiya Y. J Biol Chem 1984;259:4177—4182.
117. Gohil K, Rothfuss L, Lang J, Packer L. J Appl Physiol 1987;63:1638—1641.
118. Shindo Y, Witt E, Han D, Epstein W, Packer L. J Invest Dermatol 1994;102:122—124.
119. Shindo Y, Witt E, Han D, Packer L. J Invest Dermatol 1994;102:470—475.
120. Lang JK, Gohil K, Packer L. Anal Biochem 1986;157:106—116.
121. Mitton KP, Trevithick JR. Meth Enzymol 1994;233:523—539.
122. Handelman GJ, Epstein WL, Machlin LJ, van Kuijk FJ, Dratz EA. Lipids 1988;23:598—604.
123. Schuep W, Rettenmaier R. Meth Enzymol 1994;234:294—302.
124. Talwar D, Ha TK, Cooney J, Brownlee C, O'Reilly DS. Clin Chim Acta 1998;270:85—100.
125. Kock R, Seitz S, Delvoux B, Greiling H. Eur J Clin Chem Clin Biochem 1997;35:371—378.
126. Handelman GJ, Machlin LJ, Fitch K, Weiter JJ, Dratz EA. J Nutr 1985;115:807—813.
127. Beyer RE. Free Radic Biol Med 1990;8:545—565.
128. Yamamoto Y, Yamashita S. Mol Aspects Med 1997;18:S79—84.
129. Mortensen SA, Vadhanavikit S, Muratsu K, Folkers K. Int J Tissue React 1990;12:155—162.
130. Folkers K, Langsjoen P, Nara Y, Muratsu K, Komorowski J, Richardson PC, Smith TH. Biochem Biophys Res Commun 1988;153:88—96.
131. Okamoto T, Fukui K, Nakamoto M, Kishi T, Okishio T, Yamagami T, Kanamori N, Kishi H, Hiraoka E. J Chromatogr 1985;342:35—46.
132. Elmberger PG, Egens I, Dallner G. Biomed Chromatogr 1989;3:20—28.
133. Aberg F, Appelkvist EL, Dallner G, Ernster L. Arch Biochem Biophys 1992;295:230—234.
134. Ikenoya S, Takada M, Yuzuriha T, Abe K, Katayama K. Chem Pharm Bull (Tokyo) 1981;29: 158—164.
135. Edlund PO. J Chromatogr 1988;425:87—97.
136. Motchnik PA, Frei B, Ames BN. Meth Enzymol 1994;234:269—279.
137. Frei B, Stocker R, England L, Ames BN. Adv Exp Med Biol 1990;264:155—163.
138. Lykkesfeldt J, Loft S, Nielsen JB, Poulsen HE. Am J Clin Nutr 1997;65:959—963.
139. Dabbagh AJ, Mannion T, Lynch SM, Frei B. Biochem J 1994;300:799—803.

140. Brown RK, Wyatt H, Price JF, Kelly FJ. Eur Respir J 1996;9:334—339.
141. Margolis SA, Paule RC, Ziegler RG. Clin Chem 1990;36:1750—1755.
142. Dhariwal KR, Hartzell WO, Levine M. Am J Clin Nutr 1991;54:712—716.
143. Margolis SA, Duewer DL. Clin Chem 1996;42:1257—1262.
144. Otsuka M, Kurata T, Suzuki E, Arakawa N, Inagaki C. J Nutr Sci Vitaminol 1981;27:9—15.
145. Hatch LL, Sevanian A. Anal Biochem 1984;138:324—328.
146. Moeslinger T, Brunner M, Volf I, Spieckermann PG. Clin Chem 1995;41:1177—1181.
147. Schofield D, Guyan PM, Braganza JM. Biochem Soc Trans 1990;18:1179—1180.
148. Behrens WA, Madere R. Anal Biochem 1987;165:102—107.
149. Kutnink MA, Hawkes WC, Schaus EE, Omaye ST. Anal Biochem 1987;166:424—430.
150. Washko PW, Hartzell WO, Levine M. Anal Biochem 1989;181:276—282.
151. Ames BN, Cathcart R, Schwiers E, Hochstein P. Proc Natl Acad Sci USA 1981;78:6858—6862.
152. Speek AJ, Schrijver J, Schreurs WH. J Chromatogr 1984;305:53—60.
153. Baker JK, Kapeghian J, Verlangieri A. J of Liquid Chromat 1983;6:1319—1332.
154. Omaye ST, Turnbull JD, Sauberlich HE. Meth Enzymol 1979;62:3—11.
155. Cao G, Prior RL. Clin Chem 1998;44:1309—1315.
156. Strube M, Haenen GR, Van Den Berg H, Bast A. Free Radic Res 1997;26:515—521.
157. Ghiselli A, Serafini M, Ferro-Luzzi A. Free Radic Biol Med 1994;16:135—137.
158. Rice-Evans C, Miller NJ. Meth Enzymol 1994;234:279—293.
159. Birnboim HC. Science 1982;215:1247—1249.
160. Breen AP, Murphy JA. Free Radic Biol Med 1995;18:1033—1077.
161. Shibutani S, Takeshita M, Grollman AP. Nature 1991;349:431—434.
162. Lindahl T. Nature 1993;362:709—715.
163. Musarrat J, Wani AA. Carcinogenesis 1994;15:2037—2043.
164. Alam ZI, Jenner A, Daniel SE, Lees AJ, Cairns N, Marsden CD, Jenner P, Halliwell B. J Neurochem 1997;69:1196—1203.
165. Loft S, Vistisen K, Ewertz M, Tjonneland A, Overvad K, Poulsen HE. Carcinogenesis 1992;13:2241—2247.
166. Collins A, Cadet J, Epe B, Gedik C. Carcinogenesis 1997;18:1833—1836.
167. Halliwell B, Dizdaroglu M. Free Radic Res Commun 1992;16:75—87.
168. Douki T, Delatour T, Bianchini F, Cadet J. Carcinogenesis 1996;17:347—353.
169. Floyd RA, Watson JJ, Wong PK, Altmiller DH, Rickard RC. Free Radic Res Commun 1986;1:163—172.
170. Shigenaga MK, Gimeno CJ, Ames BN. Proc Natl Acad Sci USA 1989;86:9697—9701.
171. Finnegan MT, Herbert KE, Evans MD, Griffiths HR, Lunec J. Free Radic Biol Med 1996;20:93—98.
172. Collins AR, Dusinska M, Gedik CM, Stetina R. Environ Health Perspect 104 Suppl 1996;3:465—469.
173. Adachi S, Zeisig M, Moller L. Carcinogenesis 1995;16:253—258.
174. Nakae D, Mizumoto Y, Kobayashi E, Noguchi O, Konishi Y. Cancer Lett 1995;97:233—239.
175. Okamura K, Doi T, Hamada K, Sakurai M, Yoshioka Y, Mitsuzono R, Migita T, Sumida S, Sugawa—Katayama Y. Free Radic Res 1997;26:507—514.
176. Leinonen J, Lehtimaki T, Toyokuni S, Okada K, Tanaka T, Hiai H, Ochi H, Laippala P, Rantalaiho V, Wirta O, Pasternack A, Alho H. FEBS Lett 1997;417:150—152.
177. Park EM, Shigenaga MK, Degan P, Korn TS, Kitzler JW, Wehr CM, Kolachana P, Ames BN. Proc Natl Acad Sci USA 1992;89:3375—3379.
178. Esterbauer H, Schaur RJ, Zollner H. Free Radic Biol Med 1991;11:81—128.
179. van Ginkel G, Sevanian A. Meth Enzymol 1994;233:273—288.
180. Kim RS, LaBella FS. J Lipid Res 1987;28:1110—1117.
181. Gutteridge JMC, Halliwell B. TIBS 1990;15:129—135.
182. Gutteridge JM. Free Radic Res Commun 1986;1:173—184.
183. Slater TF. Meth Enzymol 1984;105:283—293.

184. Smith CV, Anderson RE. Free Radic Biol Med 1987;3:341–344.
185. Dillard CJ, Tappel AL. Free Radic Biol Med 1989;7:193–196.
186. Iwaoka T, Tabata F, Takahashi T. Free Radic Biol Med 1987;3:329–333.
187. Yamamoto Y, Brodsky MH, Baker JC, Ames BN. Anal Biochem 1987;160:7–13.
188. Miyazawa T, Fujimoto K, Suzuki T, Yasuda K. Meth Enzymol 1994;233:324–332.
189. Frei B, Yamamoto Y, Niclas D, Ames BN. Anal Biochem 1988;175:120–130.
190. va Kuijk FJGM, Thomas DW, Stephens RJ, Dratz EA. Meth Enzymol 1990;186:388–398.
191. Thomas DW, van Kuijk FJ, Dratz EA, Stephens RJ. Anal Biochem 1991;198:104–111.
192. O'Gara CY, Maddipati KR, Marnett LJ. Chem Res Toxicol 1989;2:295–300.
193. Allen KGD, Huang CJ, Morin CL. Anal Biochem 1990;186:108–111.
194. Pendleton RB, Lands WE. Free Radic Biol Med 1987;3:337–339.
195. Marshall PJ, Warso MA, Lands WEM. Anal Biochem 1985;145:192–199.
196. Jessup W, Dean RT, Gebicki JM. Meth Enzymol 1994;233:289–303.
197. Cramer GL, Miller JF Jr, Pendleton RB, Lands WE. Anal Biochem 1991;193:204–211.
198. Casini AF, Farber JL. Am J Pathol 1981;105:138–148.
199. Handelman GJ, Frankel EN, Fenz R, German JB. Biochem Mol Biol Int 1993;31:777–788.
200. Corongiu FP, Banni S. Meth Enzymol 1994;233:303–310.
201. Laranjinha JAN, Almeida LM, Madeira VMC. Arch Biochem Biophys 1992;297:147–154.
202. Esterbauer H, Jurgens G, Quehenberger O, Koller E. J Lipid Res 1987;28:495–509.
203. Piche LA, Cole PD, Hadley M, van den Bergh R, Draper HH. Carcinogenesis 1988;9:473–477.
204. Draper HH, Hadley M. Meth Enzymol 1990;186:421–431.
205. Esterbauer H. Path Biol 1995;44:25–28.
206. Esterbauer H, Cheeseman KH. Meth Enzymol 1990;186:407–421.
207. Bird RP, Hung SS, Hadley M, Draper HH. Anal Biochem 1983;128:240–244.
208. Wong SH, Knight JA, Hopfer SM, Zaharia O, Leach CN Jr, Sunderman FW Jr. Clin Chem 1987;33:214–220.
209. Esterbauer H, Lang J, Zadravec S, Slater TF. Meth Enzymol 1984;105:319–328.
210. Dennis KJ, Shibamoto T. Free Radic Biol Med 1989;7:187–192.
211. Kristal BS, Park BK, Yu BP. J Biol Chem 1996;271:6033–6038.
212. Kinter M, Quantitative analysis of 4-hydroxy-2-nonenal. In: NA Punchard NA, Kelly FJ (eds) Free Radicals: A Practical Approach. Oxford: Oxford University Press, 1996.
213. Goldring C, Casini AF, Maellaro E, Del Bello B, Comporti M. Lipids 1993;28:141–145.
214. Yoshino K, Matsuura T, Sano M, Saito S, Tomita I. Chem Pharm Bull (Tokyo) 1986;34: 1694–1700.
215. Lang J, Celotto C, Esterbauer H. Anal Biochem 1985;150:369–378.
216. Uchida K, Itakura K, Kawakishi S, Hiai H, Toyokuni S, Stadtman ER. Arch Biochem Biophys 1995;324:241–248.
217. Kneepkens CM, Lepage G, Roy CC. Free Radic Biol Med 1994;17:127–160.
218. Jeejeebhoy KN. Free Radic Biol Med 1991;10:191–193.
219. Shimasaki H. Meth Enzymol 1994;233:338–346.
220. Iwata A, Kikugawa K. Chem Pharm Bull (Tokyo) 1987;35:5020–5023.
221. Morrow JD, Roberts II LJ. Free Radic Biol Med 1991;10:195–200.
222. Morrow JD, Roberts LJ. Biochem Pharmacol 1996;51(2):1–9.
223. Patrono C, FitzGerald GA. Arterioscler Thromb Vasc Biol 1997;17:2309–2315.
224. Morrow JD, Roberts LJ II. Meth Enzymol 1994;233:163–174.
225. Wang Z, Ciabattoni G, Creminon C, Lawson J, Fitzgerald GA, Patrono C, Maclouf J. J Pharmacol Exp Ther 1995;275:94–100.
226. Kuypers FA, van den Berg JJ, Schalkwijk C, Roelofsen B, Op den Kamp JA. Biochim Biophys Acta 1987;921:266–274.
227. Ritov VB, Banni S, Yalowich JC, Day BW, Claycamp HG, Corongiu FP, Kagan VE. Biochim Biophys Acta 1996;1283:127–140.
228. Hedley D, Chow S. Cytometry 1992;13:686–692.

229. Pacifici RE, Davies KJ. Meth Enzymol 1990;186:485—502.
230. Thomas JA, Poland B, Honzatko R. Arch Biochem Biophys 1995;319:1—9.
231. O'Keefe DO. Anal Biochem 1994;222:86—94.
232. Gitler C, Mogyoros M, Kalef E. Meth Enzymol 1994;233:403—415.
233. Frost SC, Schwalbe MS. Biochem J 1990;269:589.
234. Weiner LM. Meth Enzymol 1995;251:87—105.
235. Khramtsov VV, Yelinova VI, Weiner LM, Berezina TA, Martin VV, Volodarsky LB. Anal Biochem 1989;182:58—63.
236. Ravichandran V, Seres T, Moriguchi T, Thomas JA, Johnston RB Jr. J Biol Chem 1994;269: 25010—25015.
237. Schuppe-Koistinen I, Gerdes R, Moldeus P, Cotgreave IA. Arch Biochem Biophys 1994;315: 226—234.
238. Seres T, Ravichandran V, Moriguchi T, Rokutan K, Thomas JA, Johnston RB Jr. J Immunol 1996;156:1973—1980.
239. Lenz AG, Costabel U, Shaltiel S, Levine RL. Anal Biochem 1989;177:419—425.
240. Levine RL, Garland D, Oliver CN, Amici A, Climent I, Lenz AG, Ahn BW, Shaltiel S, Stadtman ER. Meth Enzymol 1990;186:464—478.
241. Smith MA, Perry G, Richey PL, Sayre L, Merson VE, Beal MF, Kowall N. Nature 1996;382: 120—121.
242. Lyras L, Evans PJ, Shaw PJ, Ince PG, Halliwell B. Free Radic Res 1996;24:397—406.
243. Buss H, Chan TP, Sluis KB, Domigan NM, Winterbourn CC. Free Radic Biol Med 1997;23: 361—366.
244. Shacter E, Williams JA, Lim M, Levine RL. Free Radic Biol Med 1994;17:429—437.
245. Dean RT, Fu S, Gieseg S, Armstrong SG. Protein hydroperoxides, protein hydroxides, protein-bound DOPA. In: Punchard NA, Kelly FJ (eds) Free Radicals: A Practical Approach. Oxford: Oxford University Press, 1996.
246. Maier KL, Lenz AG, Beck—Speier I, Costabel U. Meth Enzymol 1995;251:455—461.
247. Dean RT, Fu S, Stocker R, Davies MJ. Biochem J 1997;324:1—18.
248. McCabe DR, Maher TJ, Acworth IN. J Chromatogr B Biomed Sci Appl 1997;691:23—32.
249. Grootveld M, Halliwell B. Biochem J 1986;237:499—504.
250. Ishimitsu S, Fujimoto S, Ohara A. J Chromatogr 1989;489:377—383.
251. Boveris A, Oshino N, Chance B. Biochem J 1972;128:617—630.
252. Test ST, Weiss SJ. J Biol Chem 1984;259:399—405.
253. Kettle AJ, Carr AC, Winterbourn CC. Free Radic Biol Med 1994;17:161—164.
254. Redegeld FA, van Opstal MA, Houdkamp E, van Bennekom WP. Anal Biochem 1988;174: 489—495.
255. Andersson A, Isaksson A, Brattstrom L, Hultberg B. Clin Chem 1993;39:1590—1597.
256. Reeve J, Kuhlenkamp J, Kaplowitz N. J Chromatogr 1980;194:424.
257. Murayama K, Kinoshita T. Anal Lett 1981;14:1221.
258. Martin J, White IN. J Chromatogr 1991;568:219—225.
259. Fahey RC, Newton GL, Dorian R, Kosower EM. Anal Biochem 1981;111:357—365.
260. Newton GL, Dorian R, Fahey RC. Anal Biochem 1981;114:383—387.
261. Nakamura H, Tamura Z. Anal Chem 1982;54:1951—1955.
262. Keller DA, Menzel DB. Anal Biochem 1985;151:418—423.
263. Demaster EG, Shirota FN, Redfern B, Goon DJ, Nagasawa HT. J Chromatogr 1984;308: 83—91.
264. Richi JP Jr, Lang CA. Anal Biochem 1987;163:9—15.
265. Podda M, Weber C, Traber MG, Packer L. J Lipid Res 1996;37:893—901.
266. Ikenoya S, Abe K, Tsuda T, Yamano Y, Hiroshima O, Ohmae M, Kawabe K. Chem Pharm Bull (Tokyo) 1979;27:1237—1244.
267. Jansson L, Nilsson B, Lindgren R. J Chromatogr 1980;181:242—247.
268. McMurray CH, Blanchflower WJ. J Chromatogr 1979;178:525—531.

269. Mulholland M, Dolphin RJ. J Chromatogr 1985;350:285—291.
270. Thomas DW, Parkhurst RM, Negi DS, Lunan KD, Wen AC, Brandt AE, Stephens RJ. J Chromatogr 1981;225:433—439.
271. Moeslinger T, Brunner M, Spieckermann PG. Anal Biochem 1994;221:290—296.
272. Miller NJ, Rice—Evans C, Davies MJ, Gopinathan V, Milner A. Clin Sci (Colch) 1993;84: 407—412.
273. DeLange RJ, Glazer AN. Anal Biochem 1989;177:300—306.
274. Glazer AN. Meth Enzymol 1990;186:161—168.
275. Cao G, Alessio HM, Cutler RG. Free Radic Biol Med 1993;14:303—311.
276. Ghiselli A, Serafini M, Maiani G, Azzini E, Ferro—Luzzi A. Free Radic Biol Med 1995;18: 29—36.
277. McKenna R, Kezdy FJ, Epps DE. Anal Biochem 1991;196:443—450.
278. Wayner DD, Burton GW, Ingold KU, Locke S. FEBS Lett 1985;187:33—37.
279. Arshad MA, Bhadra S, Cohen RM, Subbiah MT. Clin Chem 1991;37:1756—1758.
280. Benzie IFF, Strain JJ. Anal Biochem 1996;239:70—76.
281. Winston GW, Regoli F, Dugas AJ Jr, Fong JH, Blanchard KA. Free Radic Biol Med 1998;24: 480—493.
282. Collins AR, Dobson VL, Dusinska M, Kennedy G, Stetina R. Mutat Res 1997;375:183—193.
283. Czene S, Harms—Ringdahl M. Mutat Res 1995;336:235—242.
284. Toyokuni S, Tanaka T, Hattori Y, Nishiyama Y, Yoshida A, Uchida K, Hiai H, Ochi H, Osawa T. Lab Invest 1997;76:365—374.
285. Draper HH, Squires EJ, Mahmoodi H, Wu J, Agarwal S, Hadley M. Free Radic Biol Med 1993; 15:353—363.
286. Chirico S. Meth Enzymol 1994;233:314—318.
287. Uchida K, Sakai K, Itakura K, Osawa T, Toyokuni S. Arch Biochem Biophys 1997;346:45—52.
288. Sevilla CL, Mahle NH, Eliezer N, Uzieblo A, O'Hara SM, Nokubo M, Miller R, Rouzer CA, Marnett LJ. Chem Res Toxicol 1997;10:172—180.
289. Hartley DP, Kroll DJ, Petersen DR. Chem Res Toxicol 1997;10:895—905.
290. Waeg G, Dimsity G, Esterbauer H. Free Radic Res 1996;25:149—159.
291. Uchida K, Szweda LI, Chae HZ, Stadtman ER. Proc Natl Acad Sci USA 1993;90:8742—8746.
292. Uchida K, Stadtman ER. Meth Enzymol 1994;233:371—380.
293. Thomas JA, Chai Y, Jung C. Meth Enzymol 1994;233:385—395.
294. Ayala A, Cutler RG. Free Radic Biol Med 1996;21:65—80.
295. Ayala A, Cutler RG. Free Radic Biol Med 1996;21:551—558.
296. Giulivi C, Davies KJ. Meth Enzymol 1994;233:363—371.
297. Giulivi C, Davies KJ. J Biol Chem 1993;268:8752—8759.
298. va der Vliet A, Eiserich JP, Kaur H, Cross CE, Halliwell B. Meth Enzymol 1996;269:175—184.
299. Halliwell B. FEBS Lett 1997;411:157—160.
300. Hazen SL, Crowley JR, Mueller DM, Heinecke JW. Free Radic Biol Med 1997;23:909—916.
301. Gieseg SP, Simpson JA, Charlton TS, Duncan MW, Dean RT. Biochemistry 1993;32: 4780—4786.
302. Lewisch SA, Levine RL. Anal Biochem 1995;231:440—446.
303. Uchida K, Kawakishi S. FEBS Lett 1993;332:208—210.
304. Fu SL, Dean RT. Biochem J 1997;324:41—48.
305. Ishimitsu S, Fujimoto S, Ohara A. Chem Pharm Bull (Tokyo) 1990;38:1417—1418.
306. Nair UJ, Nair J, Friesen MD, Bartsch H, Ohshima H. Carcinogenesis 1995;16:1195—1198.
307. Fu S, Hick LA, Sheil MM, Dean RT. Free Radic Biol Med 1995;19:281—289.

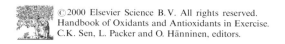
©2000 Elsevier Science B.V. All rights reserved.
Handbook of Oxidants and Antioxidants in Exercise.
C.K. Sen, L. Packer and O. Hänninen, editors.

485

Part VII • Chapter 18

Noninvasive measures of muscle metabolism

Takafumi Hamaoka[1], Kevin K. McCully[2], Toshihito Katsumura[1], Teruichi Shimomitsu[1] and Britton Chance[3]

[1]*Department of Preventive Medicine and Public Health, Tokyo Medical University, 6—1—1, Shinjuku, Shinjuku-ku, Tokyo 160-8402, Japan. Tel.: +81 3 5379 4339. E-mail: KYP02504@nifty.ne.jp*
[2]*Department of Exercise Science, University of Georgia, Athens, GA, USA.*
[3]*Department of Biochemistry and Biophysics, University of Pennsylvania, Philadelphia, USA.*

1   INTRODUCTION
     1.1   Control of oxidative energy metabolism
     1.2   Methods for evaluating energy metabolism
2   MAGNETIC RESONANCE SPECTROSCOPY
     2.1   Background
     2.2   Magnetic resonance equipment
     2.3   Oxidative metabolism
            2.3.1   Steady-state metabolism
            2.3.2   Recovery
3   NEAR INFRARED SPECTROSCOPY
     3.1   Background
     3.2   Principle of near infrared continuous wave spectroscopy
     3.3   Muscle oxygenation Measurements
            3.3.1   Ischemia
            3.3.2   Exercise
            3.3.3   Recovery
     3.4   Oxidative rate measurements
     3.5   Quantification
4   APPLICATION OF THE METHODS
     4.1   Athletes
            4.1.1   Magnetic resonance spectroscopy
            4.1.2   Near infrared spectroscopy
     4.2   Training and rehabilitation
            4.2.1   Magnetic resonance spectroscopy
            4.2.2   Near infrared spectroscopy
     4.3   Aging
     4.4   Disease
            4.4.1   Magnetic resonance spectroscopy
            4.4.2   Near infrared spectroscopy
5   SUMMARY
6   PERSPECTIVES
7   ACKNOWLEDGEMENTS
8   ABBREVIATIONS
9   REFERENCES

1   INTRODUCTION

This chapter reviews the various methods utilized for the evaluation of human skeletal muscle metabolism, focusing primarily on noninvasive approaches. Traditional methods using analytical biochemistry are based on obtaining biopsy specimens. Analytical biochemical approaches have provided information on muscle phosphorus compounds [1], $NAD^+/NADH$ (nicotinamide adenine dinucleotide/ reduced NAD) [2], and other important biochemical metabolites. Myoglobin O_2 saturation and NADH redox state can be detected using freeze clamped tissue [3]. The strength of the biopsy approach is that a wide array of metabolites can be measured to study specific metabolic pathways. The disadvantage of biopsy specimens is that, in addition to the invasive nature of sampling method, values for metabolites include both bound and free forms and thus, do not provide biologically active concentrations. Thus, there is a strong need for noninvasive approaches to measuring metabolites.

Magnetic resonance spectroscopy (MRS) [4—6] has been developed to measure free (active) forms of phosphate compounds and has developed as the "gold standard" for noninvasive evaluation of skeletal muscle bioenergetics since the late 1970s. The optical methods, using easy forms of the apparatus (near infrared spectroscopy, NIRS) [7—11], can be used to evaluate the kinetics of O_2 demand and O_2 supply in relation to muscle bioenergetics in human muscle in a more simple and portable way than MRS measurements. Later models of NIRS quantitatively measure the concentrations and O_2 saturations.

This chapter will primarily focus on MRS and NIRS approaches to evaluate skeletal muscle O_2 sufficiency and energy metabolism.

1.1 Control of oxidative energy metabolism

Skeletal muscle has some relatively unique metabolic characteristics, which include rapid changes in oxygen delivery that can reach 10-fold changes and metabolic rates that can change > 100-fold. The metabolic control of skeletal muscle has been of great interest to the historic biochemists such as Meyerhof, Krebs, etc., for many years. Studies to understand the metabolic control of mitochondrial function have been performed in earnest since the 1950s [12,13]. The net oxidative energy pathway in muscle tissues can be described by the following equation:

$$3ADP + 3Pi + NADH + H^+ + 1/2\ O_2 = 3ATP + NAD^+ + H_2O$$

The kinetic control model describes metabolic rate as a function of regulatory substrate concentrations using the Michaelis-Menten equation [6]:

$$V/Vm = 1/(1 + k1/ADP + k2/Pi + k3/O_2 + k4/NADH)$$

where V is the observed velocity, Vm is the maximal velocity, k1—4 represent affinity constants for the various substrates, Pi is the inorganic phosphate, PCr is the phosphocreatine, NADH is reduced nicotinamide adenine dinucleotide, and NAD is nicotinamide adenine dinucleotide.

Given the in vivo mitochondrial concentrations of ADP, inorganic phosphate, O_2, and reduced nicotinamide adenine dinucleotide are 20, 1000, 1, and 100 µM, respectively; and the Km (half maximum velocity) in vitro values for ADP, inorganic phosphate, O_2, and reduced nicotinamide adenine dinucleotide are 20, 300, 0.1, and ~ 10 µM, respectively, the primary candidate for metabolic control is ADP. It has been proposed that the rate of mitochondrial respiration can be determined by the rate of adenine nucleotide translocation and, therefore, the [ATP]/[ADP] ratio regulates the respiratory rate under physiological conditions [14]. Chance et al. illustrate the reversibility of electron transport in isolated mitochondria under anaerobic conditions. Holian et al. [15] demonstrated respiratory inhibition in isolated mitochondria. In addition, Holian et al. generalized metabolic control to include ATP as a controller, as well as ADP and inorganic phosphate. However, ATP is maintained constantly by the creatine kinase equilibrium in muscle and this is not effective in regulating respiration. Meyer et al. [16] used the thermodynamic model to verify that the relationship between the phosphocreatine level and the mitochondrial respiration rate is linear.

1.2 Methods for evaluating energy metabolism

Both invasive and noninvasive methods have been developed and applied for the evaluation of muscle energy metabolism. Methods for evaluating energy metabolism are classified into peripheral and cardiorespiratory measurements. Peripheral measurements can be used to obtain intravascular and intramuscular information. Invasive measurements include determining arterial-venous differences [17−19], washout of injected [133]xenon [20], and intramuscular measurements using tissue O_2 microelectrodes [21], myoglobin O_2 saturation by spectrophotometric analysis [3], and NADH analysis from exposed muscle surfaces [2]. Noninvasive methods include plethysmography [22] and the Doppler method [23] to measure arterial blood flow; MRS to measure phosphorus metabolites [4−6], and NIRS to measure oxygen dynamics [7−11,24]. Cardiorespiratory information can be obtained by cardiac output measurements [18] and by expiratory gas analysis [25]. The noninvasive methodology for muscle metabolism evaluation and their characteristics are summarized in Fig. 1.

2   MAGNETIC RESONANCE SPECTROSCOPY

2.1 Background

Nuclear magnetic resonance has become a very popular tool in the fields of both physiology and medicine since 1980, when it was first used on human subjects [26]. While nuclear magnetic resonance imaging (MRI) has shown its extraordinary capabilities in terms of imaging anatomical structures, spectroscopy (MRS) provides a wealth of biochemical information (Fig. 2). [31]Phosphorus magnetic resonance spectroscopy spectra contain five major peaks corresponding to con-

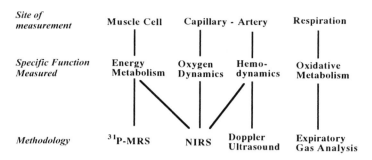

Fig. 1. Noninvasive methodology of muscle metabolism evaluation.

centrations of inorganic phosphate (Pi), phosphocreatine (PCr), and the three phosphates of ATP [27]. Other compounds are normally present in lower amounts such as phosphomonoesters (PME) and phosphodiesters (PDE) [28]. Free ADP concentrations are too low to be directly measured, but can be calculated via the creatine kinase equilibrium reaction. In addition, [31]phosphorus magnetic resonance spectroscopy allows the measurement of intracellular pH, based on a shift in the frequency of the inorganic phosphate peak, itself due to different concentrations of the mono- and diprotonated forms of inorganic phosphate (pK of 6.75 in muscle). Exchange between the two forms of inorganic phosphate is very fast,

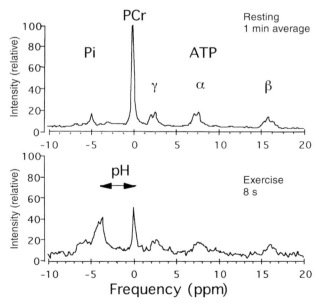

Fig. 2. Typical [31]phosphorus magnetic resonance spectroscopy (^{31}P-MRS) spectra at rest (top) and after strenuous exercise (bottom). Both spectra have 5-Hz line broadening and are presented in arbitrary units of intensity on the Y-axis.

so that only one peak with a weighted average frequency is seen in any given compartment. Nuclear magnetic resonance has become a very broad topic, with both magnetic resonance imaging and magnetic resonance spectroscopy measurements being made in a wide range of tissues using a wide range of techniques and nuclei. The most obvious advantage of magnetic resonance spectroscopy over other biochemical methods is its noninvasive character. Clinical magnetic resonance imaging measurements, with reasonable precautions, are considered to be a minimal or low risk procedure [29]. Magnetic resonance spectroscopy studies usually require shorter and weaker radio-frequency pulses.

In principle, all nuclei that have a nuclear spin can be studied by nuclear magnetic resonance. Other nuclei that have been commonly used to date are ^{1}proton (^{1}H), ^{2}deuterium (^{2}H), ^{7}lithium (^{7}Li), ^{13}carbon (^{13}C), ^{14}nitrogen (^{14}N), ^{19}fluorine (^{19}F), and ^{23}sodium (^{23}Na) [3,30–34]. The popularity of ^{31}phosphorus derives in part from the intimate relationship between phosphorylated metabolites and the function of muscle as a chemo-mechanical energy transducer. ^{31}Phosphorus is also the only naturally occurring isotope of phosphorus, so no isotopic enrichment is necessary. In addition, ^{31}phosphorus is one of the most sensitive nuclei, even though it is only $1/15$ as sensitive as ^{1}proton. As a result, ^{31}phosphorus signals are now relatively easy to detect. Nevertheless, they usually require some signal averaging to produce adequate signals to noise ratios, (signal-to-noise ratio increases with the square root of the number of signals used). It should be pointed out that at practical pulse repetition rates the ^{31}phosphorus signals have not completely relaxed, resulting in some loss of signal intensity, commonly referred to as 'saturation'. With pulse repetition times of 4 s, the amplitude of the inorganic phosphate and phosphocreatine signals are only 60% of the fully relaxed signals. Some studies have used pulse repetition times of 1 s or less, resulting in much greater amounts of saturation. Fortunately, the relative amounts of saturation for the inorganic phosphate and phosphocreatine peaks are similar (within 10%), and don not appear to change significantly with exercise intensity. Thus, ^{31}phosphorus data can be collected at relatively high repetition rates, and during different metabolic conditions with little effect on the inorganic phosphate/phosphocreatine ratio. The total time required to collect an adequate signal varies with magnet strength, the size of the collecting coil, and the sample volume. ^{31}Phosphorus signal collection times vary from as low as every 4 s from large muscles [26] to several minutes for localized signals from small muscle areas.

A second problem associated with in vivo magnetic resonance spectroscopy is accurate localization of the region of interest. Most magnetic resonance spectroscopy studies make use of a surface coil to achieve some form of localization. The 'sensitive volume' of a surface coil is typically a hemisphere with a radius approximately equal to the radius of the coil. More sophisticated localization techniques have been developed, from single volume localization methods [35] to multiple volume localization methods such as chemical shift imaging (CSI)[36,37] and Hadamard spectroscopic imaging (HSI)[38]. Multiple volume localization is particularly useful in studying muscle diseases which effect specific

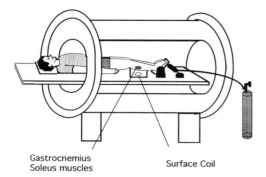

Gastrocnemius
Soleus muscles

Surface Coil

Fig. 3. Large bore magnet with subject arranged to exercise the calf muscles. A surface coil is mounted in the table which supports the subject. Resistance to exercise is provided by an air cylinder ergometer. Support straps used to hold the subject in place are not shown.

muscles, such as Becker and Duchenne dystrophies, since it can measure metabolite content in several muscles simultaneously. But the time required for a PCr image is quite long.

2.2 Magnetic resonance equipment

In human studies, first magnets could accommodate the foot. Thereafter, the magnets used have been in two basic sizes: 30- and 100-cm bore magnets (the actual 'clear' bore size is somewhat smaller). The magnetic fields have varied from 1.5 to 2.0 Tesla, although 4.7 Tesla magnets are available. In general, the stronger the magnetic field, the better the signal-to-noise ratios. The size of the magnets and the strength of the signals have served to limit the number of muscles that have been studied. The smaller magnets are pretty much limited to studies of forearm and calf muscles. Even in the larger magnets, most studied have been of the plantar flexor muscles in the lower leg (Fig. 3). However, it is possible to study almost any superficial muscle. Smaller magnets with higher field strengths have been used in animal studies.

2.3 Oxidative metabolism

2.3.1 Steady state measurements

Early magnetic resonance spectroscopy studies measured inorganic phosphate, phosphocreatine, ATP, and pH values during steady state exercise. In steady state, levels of ATP are normally quite constant in skeletal muscle, being around 8.3 mM [39] and phosphocreatine decreases with an increase in exercise intensity (Fig. 4).

Chance et al. [6] pioneered the use of the ratio of inorganic phosphate to phosphocreatine as an indicator of ADP levels. These studies showed that the primary

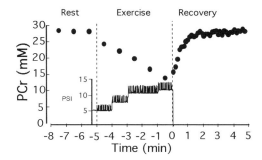

Fig. 4. Phosphocreatine (PCr) kinetics during steady-state exercise at different intensitys and during recovery.

control of oxidative metabolism during steady state exercise was ADP. Fitting the inorganic phosphate to phosphocreatine ratios and work levels to a Michaelis-Menten type equation yields a maximal velocity (Vmax) of the reaction, which was considered a measurement of oxidative capacity. This relationship has been described as the 'transfer function', indicating the relationship between the trans-duction of chemical energy into physical work. While the hyperbolic relationship between external work and inorganic phosphate to phosphocreatine ratio allow the qualitative determination of the Vmax of tissue respiration, the use of recipro-cal plots (EADIE, Hanes, etc.) provides a more accurate determination of maxi-mal velocity of the reaction. A number of studies have used steady state measure-ments of inorganic phosphate to phosphocreatine ratios to demonstrate differences between athletes, sedentary normal subjects, and patients with various diseases [6,9,40]. An example of one such study is shown in Fig. 5.

It is important to know that the use of inorganic phosphate to phosphocreatine ratios to approximate ADP levels assumes that there is no change in muscle pH (values around 7.0), as H^+ is part of the creatine kinase equation. Oxygen delivery

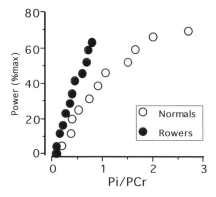

Fig. 5. Power output as a function of inorganic phosphate to phosphocreatine ratio.

is usually slightly lower than O_2 uptake, hemoglobin is desaturated significantly and O_2 delivery, as well as ADP, may regulate work. Finally, in skeletal muscle where blood flow is limited, such as in calf muscles distal to arterial stenosis, ADP is about its Km and the oxygen levels will be the major controlling variable.

2.3.2 Recovery

The rate of oxidative metabolism has also been measured under nonsteady state conditions, such as the rate of phosphocreatine resynthesis after submaximal exercise [41] (Fig. 6). Phosphocreatine recovery closely reflects oxygen consumption and the rate constant of phosphocreatine resynthesis is equivalent to the 'Vmax' calculated from the steady state measurements [42,43]. Submaximal exercise is used because decreases in muscle pH with higher levels of exercise slow the rate of phosphocreatine recovery due to mitochondrial inhibition. Time constants of phosphocreatine recovery (1/rate constant) vary from 18 s for endurance athletes to 30 s for young nonathletic controls [40]. McCully et al. [44] demonstrated that phosphocreatine recovery rate significantly correlated with mitochondrial oxidative enzymes measured with biopsy specimen (Fig. 7). Patients with various diseases can have slower rates of recovery, with peripheral vascular disease patients having recovery time constants of 200–250 s [40]. The main advantage of the recovery test for measuring oxidative metabolism is that the measurements are relatively independent of exercise intensity (Table 1), as long as muscle pH does not drop too much below 7.0. This means that the recovery test does not require accurate measurements of the amount of work being performed. This is an advantage in studies of human subjects because it is often difficult to accurately measure the work performed by the specific muscle being measured by magnetic resonance spectroscopy. The disadvantage of the recovery test is that it requires good time resolutions, with data points every 4–10 s for normal subjects. The advantage of the steady state measurements of muscle me-

$$PCr(t) = PCr_0 + \Delta PCr(1 - e^{-kt})$$
$$V_{max} = PCr_{end} * k$$

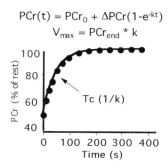

Fig. 6. The rate of oxidative metabolism calculated from phosphocreatine (PCr) resynthesis rate. This measurement assumes that muscle pH is at or near 7.0. PCr(t), PCr at a given time after exercise; PCr0, PCr at the end of exercise; ΔPCr, change in PCr from the cessation of exercise to the peak recovery; 1/k, time constant (Tc).

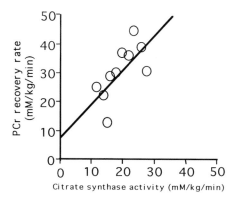

Fig. 7. Significant correlation between PCr recovery rate and mitochondrial oxidative enzyme activity.

Table 1. The effect of exercise intensity on recovery parameters in five young subjects.

Measurement	Light (target 75% PCr)	Medium (target 50% PCr)	Hard (target 25% PCr)
End Exercise PCr (%)	77.0	59.0	50.0
SD	6.7	4.3	9.0
Pi/PCr	0.42	0.86	1.2
SD	0.10	0.29	0.53
pH	7.05	6.78	6.74
SD	0.04	0.15	0.12
Initial PCr rate(mM/s)	14.1	17.3	25.9
SD	9.2	7.0	10.4
PCr T1/2 (s)	23.6	25.5	25.2
SD	6.5	5.1	3.8

MRS measurements were made in the calf muscles following plantar flexion exercise. Note that while end exercise PCr, Pi/PCr, and initial PCr resynthesis rates vary with exercise intensity, PCrT1/2 does not. This is due to the exponential nature of PCr recovery and relatively small changes in pH.

tabolism is that relatively long time periods (3—6 min) can be used to collect data at each work level, providing that fatigue does not occur.

3   NEAR INFRARED SPECTROSCOPY

3.1   *Background*

The optical technique has been used for noninvasive monitoring of changes in tissue oxygen levels since the 1930s [45,46] by using visible region light and by near infrared [47]. Such measurements rely on oxygen dependent absorption changes that occur in the heme and copper containing compounds of tissue. As a result of the great amount of visible light absorption by these chromophores, tissue exposure (removal of skin and subcutaneous fat) was necessary for the measurements. In order to solve this disadvantage, in 1977, Jobsis [7] applied a near infrared light (NIR) to tissue oxygenation monitoring, which shows adequate penetration into biological tissue. In 1980, Yoshiya et al. [48] developed a clinically popular, fingertip pulse oximeter. Also during the 1980s, many researchers [49–58] further developed the near infrared spectrometer (NIRS) for the evaluation of both brain and muscle oxygenation. The most common, commercially available NIRS device uses the continuous wave (NIR_{CWS}). NIR_{CWS} can only provide the relative values of tissue oxygenation, but it is simple and portable enough for widespread use. Chance et al. [56] developed a near infrared time-resolved spectroscopy (NIR_{TRS}) and compared the muscle deoxygenation, measured using $NIR_{CWS,}$ to that obtained by using NIR_{TRS}. The NIR_{TRS} provides data on quantitative hemoglobin/myoglobin changes in the skeletal muscle. However, methods of obtaining this type of data are complicated. The simpler phase modulation devices are more popular and afford quantification data. Since kinds of parameters are often suitable, we will concentrate on NIR_{CWS} measurements in this chapter.

3.2 Principle of NIR_{CWS}

Near infrared ranges from a wavelength of 700 to 3000 nm; this range shows much better penetration into biological tissue than visible light. In general, the 700 to 900 nm wavelength range is often used for the evaluation of the tissue oxygenation level, because a significant increase in water absorption occurs at wavelengths longer than 950 nm. The absorbing compounds of near infrared region (700–900 nm) are skin melanin, intravascular hemoglobin (Hb), intramuscular myoglobin (Mb), and cytochromes (Cyt) in the mitochondrial membrane. A similar absorption spectrum of hemoglobin and myoglobin makes it difficult to distinguish between two species by optical properties alone, however, [1]proton nuclear magnetic resonance using the water suppression method has successfully differentiated myoglobin from hemoglobin [59]. Figure 8 shows the spectrum of hemoglobin in the deoxygenated and oxygenated states. For example, as hemoglobin is oxygenated, the absorbance at 760 nm decreases, while the absorbance at 850 nm increases, providing a different signal.

The actual path of the light in tissue has been evaluated both by pulse measurements [60] and by Monte Carlo simulation [61]. The light from the probe permeates the skin and enters muscle tissue. It is then either absorbed, or scattered within tissue. Part of the scattered light subsequently returns back through the skin to the detectors. The pattern of the light path detected from input to output follows a banana shaped figure in which the penetration depth into the tissue is approximately equal to half the distance between the light and the detector [10].

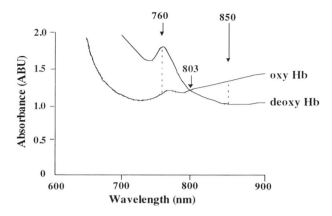

Fig. 8. Changes in optical density in accordance to a wavelength. The optical density (absorption) increases at 760 nm when the oxy-hemoglobin (Hb) is deoxygenated. When blood volume increases, the line shifts to the upper (increase in absorbance).

If optode separation was set to be 3 cm, penetration depth would be 1—2 cm and the measured volume would be approximately 4 cm^3 [56]. Because it tracks hemoglobin, myoglobin, and cytochrome, near infrared spectroscopy is sensitive to changes in muscle oxygenation, both at the level of the capillaries and venules, and at the intracellular sites of oxygen storage and oxygen uptake (myoglobin, mitochondria) [62].

To calculate the changes in oxy-hemoglobin/myoglobin, deoxy-hemoglobin/ myoglobin, or total-hemoglobin/myoglobin, the equation of a 2-, or multiple-wavelength method can be applied according to the following Beer-Lambert law [54]:

$$OD = -\log e(I/I_0) = \varepsilon L[C]$$

where ε is the extinction coefficient (/cm/mM); L is the photomigration path length; [C] is the concentration of absorber (mM); I is the detected light intensity; I_0 is the incident light intensity and OD is the optical density.

Several researchers have demonstrated and justified their own equations by in vitro and in vivo experiments. Chance et al. [10] adopted an "in vitro yeast and blood model" for the evaluation of the near infrared apparatus. The model system includes intralipid as a scatterer (0.5—1.0%) and blood at concentrations of 10—200 µM of hemoglobin. O_2 bubbling causes reoxygenation and the cessation of bubbling causes deoxygenation of the hemoglobin due to yeast respiration. The addition of blood simulates to the increased in vivo blood volume. Chance et al. found that the subtracted signals at 760 and 850 nm showed a linear relationship to hemoglobin deoxygenation. Wilson et al. [58] demonstrated a linear relationship between near infrared spectroscopy measurements and venous hemoglobin saturation in an animal model.

3.3 Muscle oxygenation measurements

3.3.1 *Ischemia*

In 1988, Hampson et al. [8], using NIR_{CWS}, demonstrated the changes in skeletal muscle O_2 store or O_2 content kinetics during 10 min ischemia in the human forearm. At the onset of arterial occlusion, muscle O_2 store began to decrease. Approximately 6 min after the onset of the arterial occlusion, muscle O_2 store was completely depleted (functional anoxia). During 10 min ischemia, Hampson et al. simultaneously monitored skin deoxygenation changes. The time course of skin deoxygenation changes during ischemia correlated poorly with the changes in the skeletal muscle. In their study, inflation of the pressure cuff to 170 mmHg and over, caused skin oxygenation to rapidly fall to 0 in 2—3 min, while muscle oxygenation fell in 6 min. Thigh muscle deoxygenation was studied [63] during 20 min arterial occlusion. A progressive decline in O_2 saturation was reported throughout ischemia. The half time of tissue deoxygenation during arterial occlusion was 2.3 ± 0.2 min (mean $\pm$ SE). Forearm oxygenation changes were studied during a 15 min ischemia (Fig. 9) [64]. The half time of tissue deoxygenation (2.33 ± 0.17 min (mean $\pm$ standard deviation)) during arterial occlusion was identical to the result of Sahlin [63], even though the limbs that were measured were different. The rate of muscle deoxygenation per min was $23.0 \pm 1.2\%$ of the resting O_2 storage amount. This rate was calculated from the linear portion of the O_2 decline, which indicates the basal oxidative rate. Interindividual variation of the decline rate was considerably smaller (coefficient of variation = 6.0%, n = 15). PCr breakdown began to occur around 4—5 min after the initiation of arterial occlusion and showed a linear decline (Fig. 9). Tissue deoxygenation during cuff ischemia was monitored [56] by NIR_{TRS} and NIR_{CWS}. The two measurements were then compared. It was concluded that the correlation between the data obtained by NIR_{TRS} and NIR_{CWS} was reasonable, but there was a greater response of the NIR_{CWS} measurement to hyperemia upon reflow. Ferrari et al. [65] demonstrated that by using time-resolved spectroscopy, scattering and absorption coefficients did not change during 10 min of forearm ischemia at 800 nm (isosbestic point). In contrast, absorption and scattering changes were observed at 760 nm of approximately 10% during ischemia. These studies showed that the muscle oxygenation gradually decreased, and almost completely depleted, in 6 min during ischemia.

3.3.2 *Exercise*

Chance et al. [10] studied the effects of exercise stress on skeletal muscle in elite rowers. They reported a progressive deoxygenation in the vastus lateralis muscle during exercise and an abrupt increase in reoxygenation upon the cessation of exercise. Hamaoka et al. [11] introduced a new method for the evaluation of muscle aerobic capacity by comparing ultra endurance to normal control athletes by

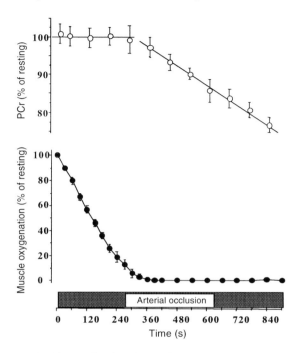

Fig. 9. Changes in phosphocreatine and oxygenation in human forearm during 15 min of arterial occlusion measured by near infrared spectroscopy and ^{31}P-magnetic resonance spectroscopy. No significant changes were found in pH and ATP throughout arterial occlusion.

using NIR_{CWS}. They used a bicycle ergometer for an exercise test in order to investigate the deoxygenation change during exercise and the reoxygenation change after 2 min of exercise at 50% of pulmonary maximal oxygen uptake.

Figure 10 shows the kinetics of the muscle oxygenation change during exercise and recovery. On the initiation of exercise, some oxygenation occurred due to a quicker response of oxygen supply to exercise than oxygen consumption or due to the "muscle pump effect" which squeeze out the deoxygenated blood. The appearance of deoxygenation indicated that homeostatic adjustments were insufficient to maintain a constant capillary oxygen concentration. After exercise was terminated, muscle oxygenation gradually recovered and surpassed the resting level, as oxygen consumption gradually decreased.

3.3.3 Recovery

Because NIR_{CWS} provides only the relative values of tissue oxygenation, some calibration is needed to compare the data between each individual. An arterial occlusion is one of the least invasive methods of determining physiological zero oxygenation or O_2 depleted level. However, this calibration is uncomfortable or even painful to the subjects. Thus, Chance et al. [10] proposed a "recovery time"

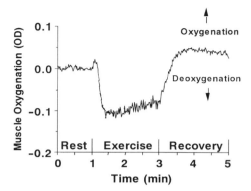

Fig. 10. Typical kinetics of muscle oxygenation during rest, exercise and recovery. The change is expressed as an arbitrary unit.

for hemoglobin/myoglobin desaturation in the capillary bed of exercising muscle. Recovery time reflects the balance of oxygen delivery and oxygen demand in localized muscles. Recovery time measurements are based on intensive studies of the recovery times of PCr, or on the ratio of PCr and Pi. Chance et al. [10] compared recovery times in submaximal and maximal work, with plasma lactate. They [10] also compared male elite rowers to female elite rowers and made suggestions for the direction of improved performance. They reported a prolonged recovery time, which suggested an increased energy deficit when the exercise intensity increased. Chance et al. also demonstrated a significant correlation between blood lactate and the recovery time of muscle reoxygenation after exercise.

The reproducibility of the recovery time for muscle oxygenation was investigated following bicycle exercise in normal controls [11]. The reproducibility of recovery time was good. The number of tests that 10 normal subjects performed varied from 3 to 10 times. The value of the recovery time ranged from 13.2 to 17.9 s (coefficient of variation $< 10\%$).

3.4 Oxidative rate measurements

Near infrared has been applied to monitor tissue oxygen availability. The near infrared spectroscopy technique, however, has difficulty in evaluating muscle energy metabolism because the value measured by near infrared spectroscopy does not reflect muscle oxygen consumption, but rather, it reflects the balance of muscle oxygen delivery in relation to muscle oxygen consumption. Because the absolute concentration changes of hemoglobin/myoglobin cannot be determined due to unquantifiable biophysical quantities (i.e., the optical path length in accordance with Beer-Lambert law) when NIR_{CWS} is used.

With the limitations mentioned above, skeletal muscle metabolism has been evaluated by measuring post-exercise recovery times for deoxygenated hemoglobin/myoglobin following exercise by near infrared spectroscopy [9–11]. However, the recovery time cannot be used for measuring energy metabolism during exercise.

Oxygen consumption was measured [66] in the calf by calculating the rate of conversion of oxyhemoglobin (HbO_2) to deoxyhemoglobin during a period of tourniquet-induced ischemia by NIR_{CWS}. Since NIR_{CWS} does not give absolute HbO_2 concentration because of an undetermined optical path length, Cheatle et al. [66] used 5.4 as the differential path-length factor, taken from their prior research on human forearms. The rate of HbO_2 decrease was converted into the rate of oxygen consumption in ml/100 g tissue/min utilizing an appropriate assumption. The resting oxygen consumption showed broad variability ranging from 4.46 to 24.55 µM/100 g. It seems that the path length variability in each subject caused this variability.

Changes in hemoglobin saturation and oxygen consumption (VO_2) were studied using NIR_{TRS} in the human forearm muscle at rest and subjected to a maximum increase in energy demand [67]. This study showed that the resting oxygen consumption was 4.96 ± 0.76 µM/100 g tissue/min, while oxygen consumption during isometric maximal voluntary contraction (MVC) was 65.04 ± 1.91 µM/100 g tissue/min. This study showed a smaller variability in oxygen consumption in the resting condition than that reported by Cheatle et al. [66]. De Blasi et al. [68] also applied this evaluation method to the study of the human forearm in untrained volunteers at rest and when a maximal increase of metabolic demand was achieved with and without blood flow limitation. De Blasi et al. concluded that the oxygen consumption during maximal voluntary contraction was very similar, both in the presence and absence of a limitation in blood flow in most of the subjects tested. These results suggest that muscle oxygen consumption might be accurately evaluated dynamically without cuff occlusion during maximal voluntary contractions, if the differential path length factor (DPF) is assumed to be constant.

Physiological calibration for the measurement of NIR_{CWS} was proposed [64] to eliminate the path length differences in each subject. This study investigated saturation changes and oxygen consumption of the human forearm muscle at rest and during isotonic (intermittent) muscle contractions. This study demonstrated that the variation of the resting oxygen consumption, which indicates muscle basal metabolic rate, was small in young, normal subjects. This was based on the evidence that the O_2 decline rate relative to the resting O_2 content during cuff ischemia was 23.0 ± 1.2%/min. In this text, oxygen consumption during exercise is expressed relative to the decline rate of resting O_2 content during arterial occlusion (Fig. 11).

3.5 Quantification

In a nonscattering medium like water, the path length can be defined as the distance between the input and output of the light. However, as biological tissue is a high scattering medium, photons randomly travel in tissue and are subsequently captured by the detector. The path length is unpredictable by NIR_{CWS}.

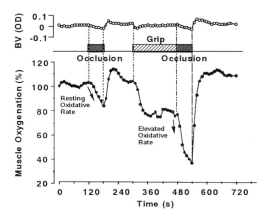

Fig. 11. The muscle oxygenation and blood volume (BV) kinetics in an arterial occlusion during rest and at 3 min exercise. Oxygen consumption at 3 min exercise was 8.3 times higher than that of the resting value. Muscle oxygenation level at rest was defined as 100%, while that at the minimum value during arterial occlusion was defined as 0%.

A DPF [53] was proposed to solve the limitation of undetermined path length measured by NIR_{CWS}. The average of the path lengths across the rat head is approximately 4.3 times the interoptode spacing. This average agrees with the data measured in the forearm and leg by Chance et al. [56] and in the forearm by Ferrari et al. [69]. Accordingly, quantitative evaluation is possible by multiplying the differential path-length factor for constant oxy-hemoglobin/hemoglobin values. However, some individual variation (a differential path-length factor of approximately 4–5 in 3 cm interoptode spacing), still exists when measured from the skin's surface, partly due to differences in the thickness of the subcutaneous adipose layer. In addition, it is reported that differential path-length factors were altered by the ischemic condition [69,70]. Further investigation is needed in order to clarify the differential path length factor variation and to determine a satisfactory technique for the evaluation of tissue oxygenation in a quantitative manner by NIR_{CWS}.

Sevick et al. [71] described the theoretical and experimental basis on tissue oxygenation by using time-resolved and frequency-resolved optical spectra. Sevick et al. reviewed the theory of light transport in a dense scattering medium and developed algorithms for the quantitation of hemoglobin saturation from the photon distribution as monitored by NIR_{TRS} and frequency-resolved spectroscopy (NIR_{PMS}). In order to calculate the path length, the amount of time the photons travel between the interoptode spacing had to be measured because the velocity of light is determinable. To determine the amount of time photons spend between the interoptode spacing, a dye laser was synchronously pumped to generate some 10-ps pulses of light. The detector quickly responded, capturing the photons that migrated from the tissue for 500 ps with approximately a 10-ps resolution. Thus, the distribution of light intensity as a function of time can be monitored by time resolved spectroscopy. It can also determine the optical properties in tissue and quantitative tissue oxygenation. Changes in muscle oxygenation and optical properties were studied by NIR_{TRS}, both in ischemic muscle [56,72] and in contracting muscle [72,73].

4   APPLICATION OF THE METHODS

4.1 Athletes

4.1.1   *Magnetic resonance spectroscopy*

The recovery rate of PCr after exercise has been used to evaluate oxidative capacity. McCully et al. [74] demonstrated that 6 young, normal humans showed the phosphocreatine recovery measurements to be reproducible, (standard error of 5% for each subject), and to be independent of the work level at submaximal exercise intensities. They also found a strong correlation between citrate synthase activity from muscle biopsies and phosphocreatine recovery rates measured in young and old healthy subjects, ($r^2 = 0.53$, $p = 0.002$, $n = 10$) (see Fig. 7) [44]. McCully et al. have found that the phosphocreatine recovery time constant is faster in endurance track athletes (18 ± 0.9 s) than in middle distance runners (30 ± 4.8 s) and sprinters (40 ± 3.3 s). Figure 12 summarizes phosphocreatine recovery rates in subjects with varied muscle functions.

4.2.2   *Near infrared spectroscopy*

Ultra endurance athletes and normal controls were compared using near infrared spectroscopy [11]. Hamaoka et al. utilized a bicycle ergometer for exercise testing to investigate deoxygenation and reoxygenation changes after 2 min of exercise at 50% of the maximal oxygen consumption. Hamaoka et al. demonstrated a significantly increased muscle aerobic function by 34% in triathletes, compared to that in the normal controls; 9.1 ± 2.0 s for triathletes vs. 14.7 ± 3.2 s for controls (Fig. 13). The magnitude of differences in muscle aerobic function between triathletes and controls were comparable to that of the maximal oxygen consumption differences between the two groups.

4.2 Training and rehabilitation

4.2.1   *Magnetic resonance spectroscopy*

A short 14-day training program consisting of 1 h per day of plantar flexion resulted in a significant improvement in the phosphocreatine time constant in four control subjects (pretraining = 25.4 ± 1.8 s, posttraining = 21.2 ± 1.7 s, and 1.5 months posttraining = 28.2 ± 2.1 s) [9] (Fig. 14).

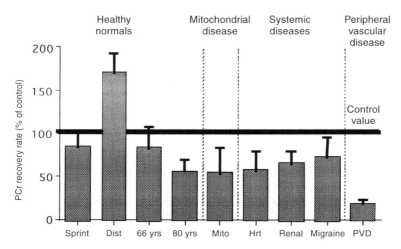

Fig. 12. PCr recovery rates in subjects with varied muscle functions. PCr, phosphocreatine; Sprint, sprinter; Dist, distance runner; Mito, mitochondria disease; Hrt, heart failure; Renal, renal disfunction; PVD, peripheral vascular disease.

4.2.2 Near infrared spectroscopy

Nishio et al. [75] illustrated the O_2 kinetics of atrophied forearm muscles after a 3-week immobilization due to bone fractures. Figure 15 demonstrated differences in O_2 kinetics in the atrophied and control muscle, especially in the recovery of O_2 content following muscle contraction. The half time of recovery (Tr) for control was around 15 s and the recovery time for the atrophied muscle was around 90 s. The Tr was shorter after training (rehabilitation), reaching the normal value in 3–4 weeks.

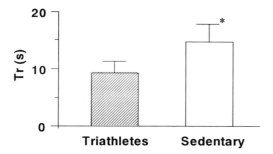

Fig. 13. Recovery time (Tr) for muscle oxygenation following exercise in triathletes and sedentary subjects. Tr for Triathletes is 9.1 ± 2.0 s (mean ± SD: n = 15) for 150 watts, and sedentary subjects 14.7 ± 3.2 s for 100 Watts (n = 10). *p < 0.01 compared to triathletes.

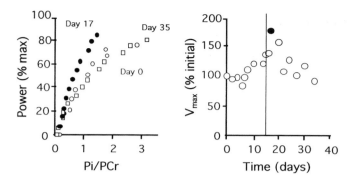

Fig. 14. Improved Pi/ PCr ratio by exercise training in normal subjects. V_{max}, maximal power relative to the initial value.

4.3 Aging

Organic functions gradually decline in elderly people [76—78]. Muscle endurance and mitochondrial function have also been shown to decrease with increasing age [79—81]. There was a significant age-related slowing of the phosphocreatine time constant in healthy subjects aged 25, 66, and 80 years of age (see Fig. 12).

4.4 Disease

4.4.1 Magnetic resonance spectroscopy

ATP concentration in muscles is usually constant in a physiological condition. An exception to this may be patients with phosphofructokinase (PFK) deficiency

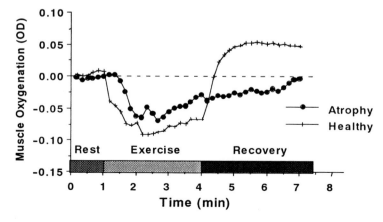

Fig. 15. Comparison of muscle oxygenation kinetics in the atrophied and intact forearm during grip contractions and recovery.

who may have abnormally low ATP levels ($\sim 70\%$ of normal) [82]. In a particular patient in whom cytochrome bc1 complex was shown to be deficient by biopsy, NMR was used to determine the very low value of PCr/Pi in the resting muscle to be near 1 [83]. This patient showed very low exercise endurance. A biochemical bypass was proposed using vitamin K3 as a biochemical bridge and ascorbate as a general reductant of the vitamin K3. The patient immediately responded with a rise in PCr/Pi to approximately 3 in the resting state and showed an increase in exercise capability, not previously observed. The patient has been functional since that day. This is the first instance of a diagnosis and a therapy, based upon magnetic resonance spectroscopy.

4.4.2 Near infrared spectroscopy

A number of studies on older healthy subjects and patients with mild peripheral vascular disease (PVD) have been presented using near infrared spectroscopy. Measurements of the rate of recovery in near infrared spectroscopy measurements of oxygen saturation following exercise were found to be similar in both young and old, healthy subjects [84]. However, subjects complaining of poor calf circulation (mean age = 72 years, n = 15) had recovery rates that were up to 5 times slower than healthy subjects (Fig. 16). A good correlation was found between measurements of Doppler pressure waveforms and ankle arm systolic pressures (AAI) and the near infrared spectroscopy recovery time constant [84].

Cheatle et al. [66] demonstrated a significant difference in the resting oxygen consumption between patients with peripheral vascular disease and normal subjects by using arterial occlusion to calculate the O_2 decline rate.

Komiyama et al. [85] successfully classified patients with a varied severity of peripheral vascular disease by using patterns of O_2 kinetics during exercise and recovery from exercise-induced desaturation of the calf muscle (Fig. 17).

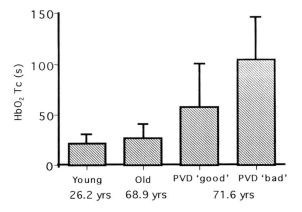

Fig. 16. Oxy-hemoglobin (HbO2) recovery rates (Tc) measured by near infrared spectroscopy in healthy subjects and patients with peripheral vascular disease (PVD).

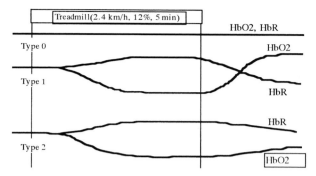

Fig. 17. Patterns of serial O_2 kinetics during exercise and recovery in the calf muscle. HbO_2, oxygenated hemoglobin; HbR, deoxygenated hemoglobin.

Komiyama et al. concluded that near infrared spectroscopy can be used to accurately assess the severity of patients with intermittent claudication.

The O_2 kinetics in the working skeletal muscle of patients with heart failure was investigated [58]. Arterial occlusion was used at the end of the exercise to determine the level of O_2 depletion. Wilson et al. concluded that patients with heart failure exhibited high deoxygenation compared to the normal control partly due to the pump failure of the heart, resulting in skeletal muscle hypoperfusion.

In the case of disease in the bioenergetic system, the uptake of oxygen by mitochondria diminishes considerably and the physiological increase of oxygen delivery (vasodilatation), stimulated by autonomic nerve activity and/or myogenic activity, provides a luxury perfusion of the limbs [86]. In Fig. 18, a documented cytochrome c oxidase deficiency, the deflection of the traces is in the opposite direction of the normal deflection, (i.e., an upward deflection on the starting exercise indicates a luxury perfusion). On cessation of exercise, instead of recovery from oxygen debt, there is recovery from O_2 surfeit (refer to the normal response shown in Fig. 10). This paradoxical response of the muscle oxygenation has been used as a diagnosis in many cases of suspected mitochondrial disease. However, Gellerich et al. has shown that this paradoxical response can be observed in normal subjects in the initial phase of muscle activity, but is soon replaced by the deoxygenation characteristic when approaching to the Vmax in a ramp study.

5 SUMMARY

1. Muscle energy metabolism can be quantitatively measured with analytical biochemistry by obtaining a biopsy specimen. However, obtaining a biopsy specimen requires an invasive procedure. In addition, information from biopsy specimens include information on the less biochemically active forms, that are not readily available for the biochemical process (i.e., oxidative phosphorylation).
2. Magnetic resonance spectroscopy (MRS) can detect free (active) forms of

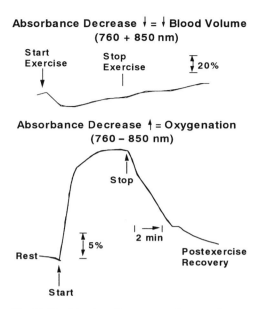

Fig. 18. The kinetics of gastrocnemius muscle oxygenation during treadmill exercise at 2 mile/h in patient with cytochrome oxidase deficient.

phosphate compounds and provides the gold standard for noninvasive evaluation of skeletal muscle bioenergetics, both during exercise by the inorganic phosphate to phosphocreatine ratio and in recovery from exercise by the phosphocreatine recovery rate. MRS has afforded diagnosis and therapy in the case of a mitochondrial genetic deficiency. This is the first example of a successful diagnosis and therapy carried out with MRS technology.

3. Optical methods can be used to evaluate the kinetics of O_2 demand and O_2 supply in relation to muscle bioenergetics in working human muscles in a more simple, portable, and affordable way than magnetic resonance spectroscopy measurements. Muscle O_2 consumption can be measured by the rate of O_2 decline during arterial occlusion. Time resolved spectroscopy has a great possibility for the quantitative assessment of muscle O_2 kinetics, while continuous wave spectroscopy can be developed as an easier and more practical tool when calibrated by the time-resolved spectroscopy method.

4. Simultaneous monitoring of muscle bioenergetics by magnetic resonance spectroscopy and O_2 kinetics by near infrared spectroscopy can provide a noninvasive and comprehensive evaluation of muscle energy metabolism.

6   PERSPECTIVES

This chapter reviewed the noninvasive methods available for the study of muscle metabolism, in particular MRS and NIRS. These methods are of use for the study of human subjects in varied physiological and pathological conditions. Optical methods are more suitable for both clinical and practical use than MRS measurements.

Medical engineering developments in the 21st century will make it possible to monitor specific metabolic changes occurring in the human body in a less invasive manner.

7 ACKNOWLEDGEMENTS

The authors acknowledge the help of colleagues in the Department of Preventive Medicine and Public Health, Tokyo Medical University. This work was supported in part by a Grant for the Encouragement of Young Scientists from the Ministry of Education, Science, Sports and Culture in Japan (# 09780087).

8 ABBREVIATIONS

ADP:	adenosine diphosphate
Cyt:	cytochromes
DPF:	differential path length factor
Hb:	hemoglobin
Km:	half maximum velocity
L:	light path length
Mb:	myoglobin
MRI:	nuclear magnetic resonance imaging
MRS:	magnetic resonance spectroscopy
MVC:	maximal voluntary contraction
NAD^+:	nicotinamide adenine dinucleotide
NADH:	reduced NAD
NIR_{CWS}:	near infrared continuous wave spectroscopy
NIR_{PMS}:	near infrared frequency-resolved spectroscopy
NIR_{TRS}:	near infrared time-resolved spectroscopy
NIRS:	near infrared spectroscopy
OD:	optical density
PCr:	phosphocreatine
PDE:	phosphodiesters
Pi:	inorganic phosphate
PME:	phosphomonoesters
PVD:	peripheral vascular disease
VO_2:	oxygen consumption

9 REFERENCES

1. Hill, DK. J Physiol (Lond) 1962;162:31–50.
2. Guezennec CY, Lienhard F, Louisy F, Renault G et al. Eur J Appl Physiol 1991;63:36–42.

3. Gayeski TEJ, Honig CR. Adv Exp Med Biol 1983;159:613—621.
4. Gadian DG, Hoult DI, Radda GK, Seeley PJ et al. Proc Natl Acad Sci 1976;73:446—448.
5. Chance B, Eleff S, Leigh JS. Proc Natl Acad Sci 1980;77:7430—7434.
6. Chance B, Leigh JS, Kent J, McCully K et al. Proc Natl Acad Sci 1986;83:9458—9462.
7. Jobsis FF. Science 1977;198:1264—1267.
8. Hampson NB, Piantadosi CA. J Appl Physiol 1988;64(6):2449—2457.
9. McCully KK, Kakihira H, Vandenborne K, Kent-Braun J. J Biomech 1991;24(1):153—161.
10. Chance B, Dait MT, Zhang C, Hamaoka T et al. Am J Physiol 1992;262(31):C766—775.
11. Hamaoka T, Albani C, Chance B, Iwane H. Med Sport Sci 1992;37:421—429.
12. Chance B, Williams GR. J Biol Chem 1955;217:409—427.
13. Chance B, Hollunger G. J Biol Chem 1961;236:1562—1568.
14. Kushmerick MJ. Energetics of muscle contraction. In: Peachey LD, Adrian RH, Gieger SR (eds) Handbook of Physiology. New York: Oxford 1983:189—236.
15. Holian A, Owen CS, Wilson DF. Arch Biochem Biophys 1977;181:164—171.
16. Meyer RA. Am J Physiol 1988;254(23):C548—553.
17. Jorfeldt L, Wahren J. Clin Sci 1971;41:459—473.
18. Pavek K. Circ Res 1964;15:311.
19. Wahren J. Acta Physiol Scand 1966;67(Suppl 269).
20. Cerretelli P, Marconi C, Pendergast D, Meyer M et al. J Appl Physiol 1984;56:24—30.
21. Clark LC, Jr. Trans Am Soc Art Intern Organs 1956;2:41.
22. Whitney RJ. J Physiol 1953;121:1—27.
23. Jager KA et al. J Ultrasound Med 1985;11(3):515—521.
24. De Blasi RA, Cope M, Ferrari M. Adv Exp Med Biol 1992:771—777.
25. Åstrand I. Acta Physiol Scand 1960;49(Suppl 169).
26. Chance B, Eleff S, Leigh JS et al. Proc Natl Acad Sci USA 1981;78:6714—6718.
27. Dawson MJ. Biosci Rep 1982;2:727—733.
28. Bertocci L, Haller R, Lewis S et al. J Appl Physiol 1991;70:1201—1207.
29. Kanal E, Shellock F. Magn Reson 1993;3(3):30—40.
30. Blum H, Schnall M, Chance B, Buzby G. Am J Physiol 1988;255:C377—C384.
31. Hetherington H, Hamm J, Pan J, Rothman D et al. J Magn Res 1989;82:86—96.
32. Renshaw P, Wicklund S. Biol Psych 1988;23:465—475.
33. Taylor R, Price T, Rothman D, Shulman R et al. Magn Reson Med 1992;27:13—20.
34. Noyszewski EA, Wang Z, McCully KK, Leigh JS. Biophys Mtg 1990.
35. Haselgrove J, Subramanian V, Leigh J, Gyulai L et al. Science (Wash DC) 1983;220:1170—1173.
36. Bailes D, Bryant D, Bydder G, Case H et al. J Magn Reson 1987;74:158—170.
37. Jeneson JA, Nelson SJ, Vigneron DB, Taylor JS et al. Am J Physiol 1992; 263:C357—364,
38. Goelman G, Walter G, Leigh JJ. Magn Reson Med 1992;25:349—354.
39. Taylor D, Styles P, Matthews P et al. Magn Reson Med 1986;3:44—54.
40. McCully KK, Vandenborne K, De Meirleir K, Posner J et al. Can J Physiol Pharmacol 1992;70: 1353—1359.
41. Barbiroli B, Montagna P, Cortelli P et al. Cephalalgia 1990;10:264—272.
42. Mahler M. J Gen Physiol 1985;86:135—165.
43. Meyer RA. Am J Physiol 1988;254:C548—C553.
44. McCully K, Fielding R, Evans W, Leigh J et al. J Appl Physiol 1993;75(2):813—819.
45. Millikan GA. Proc R Soc Lond B 1937;G23(123):218—241.
46. Matthes K, F Gross. Arch Exp Pathol Pharmakol 1939;191:381—390.
47. Kramer K. Z Biol 1934;95:126.
48. Yoshiya I, Shimada Y, Tanaka K. Med Biol Eng Comp 1980;18:27—32.
49. Ferrari M, Giannini I, Sideri G, Zanette E. Adv Exp Med Biol 1985;191:873—882.
50. Ferrari M, Wilson DA, Hanley DF, Hartmann JF et al. Am J Physiol 1989;256(25):H1493—H1499.
51. Piantadosi CA, Hemstreet TM, Jobsis-Vandervliet FF. Crit Care Med 1986;14(8):698—706.

52. Delpy DT, Cope MC, Cady EB, Wyatt JS. Scand J Clin Lab Invest 1987;(suppl 188):9—17.
53. Delpy DT, Cope M, Zee P, Arridge S et al. Phys Med Biol 1988;33(12):1433—1442.
54. Seiyama A, Hazeki O, Tamura M. Adv Exp Med Biol 1987;215:291—295.
55. Tamura M, Hazeki O, Nioka S, Chance B et al. Adv Exp Med Biol 1988;222:359—363.
56. Chance B, Nioka S, Kent J, McCully KK et al. Anal Biochem 1988;174:698—707.
57. Chance B. Adv Exp Med Biol 1989;248:21—31.
58. Wilson J, Mancini D, McCully KK, Ferraro N et al. Circulation 1989;80:1668—1674.
59. Wang Z, Wang DJ, Noyszewski E, Bogdan A et al. Magn Reson Med 1992;27:362—367.
60. Chance B, Maris M, Sorge J, Zhang MZ. Proc Soc Photo Optical Instrum Eng 1990;1204:481—491.
61. Patterson MS, Chance B, Wilson BC. J Appl Optics 1989;28:2331—2336.
62. Jobsis FF. Am Rev Respir Dis 1974;110:58—63.
63. Sahlin K. Int J Sport Med 1992;13:S157—S160
64. Hamaoka T, Iwane H, Shimomitsu T, Katsumura T et al. J Appl Physiol 1996;81(3):1410—1417.
65. Ferrari M, De Blasi R, Bruscaglioni P, Barilli M et al. Proc Soc Photo Optical Instrum Eng 1991;1431:276—283.
66. Cheatle TR, Potter LA, Cope M, Delpy DT. Br J Surg 1991;78:405—408.
67. De Blasi R, Cope M, Elwell C, Safoue F et al. Eur J Appl Physiol 1993;67:20—25.
68. De Blasi R, Ferrari M, Natali A, Conti G et al. J Appl Physiol 1994;76(3):1388—1393.
69. Ferrari M, Wei Q, Carraresi L, De Blasi R et al. J Photochem Photobiol B Biol 1992;16:141—153.
70. Van der Zee P, Cope M, Arridge SR, Essenpreis M et al. Adv Exp Med Biol 1992;316:143—153.
71. Sevick EM, Chance B, Leigh J, Nioka S et al. Anal Biochem 1991;195:330—351.
72. Hamaoka T, Iwane H, Shimomitsu T, Katsumura T et al. Annu Congr Frontiers in Sport Sci, Nice, France 1996;280—281.
73. De Blasi RA, Fantini S, Franceschini MA, Ferrari M et al. Med Biol Eng Comp 1995;33:228—230.
74. McCully K, C Strear, M Prammer, J Leigh, Jr. FASEB J 1990;4:A1212.
75. Nishio S, Iwane H, Hamaoka T, Shimomitsu T et al. Med Sci Sports Exerc 1994;26(5):S98.
76. Manton K, Soldo B. Milbank Memorial Fund Quarterly: Health and Society 1985;63:206—285.
77. Shephard R. Physical Activity and Aging. Chicago: Year Book Medical Publishers, 1978.
78. Williams M. J Am Geriatr Soc 1987;35:761—766.
79. Coggan A, Spina R, D King, M Rogers et al. J Gerontol 1992;47:71—76.
80. McCully KK, Forcia M, Hack L, Donlon E et al. Can J Physiol Pharmacol 1991;69:576—580.
81. Meredith C, Frontera W, Fisher E, Hughes V et al. J Appl Physiol 1989;66:2844—2849.
82. Argov Z, Bank W, Maris J, Leigh J et al. Ann Neurol 1987;22(1):46—51.
83. Eleff S, Kennaway NG, Buist NRM, Darley—Usmar VM et al. Proc Natl Acad Sci USA 1984;81:3529—3533.
84. McCully KK, Halber C, Posner J. J Geron Biol Sci 1994;49(3):128—134.
85. Komiyama T, Shigematsu H, Yasuhara H, Muto T. Eur J Vasc Surg 1994;8:294—296.
86. Bank W, Chance B. Ann Neurol 1994;36(6):830—837.

Part VIII

Environmental factors

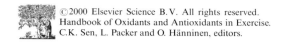

©2000 Elsevier Science B.V. All rights reserved.
Handbook of Oxidants and Antioxidants in Exercise.
C.K. Sen, L. Packer and O. Hänninen, editors.

513

Part VIII ● Chapter 19

Air pollution and oxidative stress

Dianne M. Meacher and Daniel B. Menzel

Department of Community and Environmental Medicine, 100 Faculty Research Facility, University of California at Irvine, Irvine, California 92697-1825, USA. E-mail: menzel@uci.edu

1   INTRODUCTION
2   ATMOSPHERIC OZONE AND NITROGEN DIOXIDE
3   DOSIMETRY MODELING OF OZONE AND NITROGEN DIOXIDE
    3.1   Ozone
    3.2   Nitrogen dioxide
4   LABORATORY HUMAN EXPOSURE WITH EXERCISE STUDIES
    4.1   Pulmonary function effects of acute ozone exposure
        4.1.1   Concentration-response relationship
        4.1.2   Reduction of exercise performance
        4.1.3   Recovery of pulmonary function following acute ozone exposure
        4.1.4   Mechanisms of pulmonary function effects of ozone
    4.2   Pulmonary inflammation following acute ozone exposure
    4.3   Airway responsiveness to ozone exposure
    4.4   Pulmonary function effects of prolonged ozone exposure
    4.5   Pulmonary function effects of mixtures of ozone and other air pollutants
    4.6   Pulmonary effects of nitrogen dioxide exposure
        4.6.1   Pulmonary function effects and airway responsiveness
        4.6.2   Inflammatory response and epithelial cell permeability
    4.7   Effects of urban air polluted with ozone and nitrogen dioxide
5   OUTDOOR STUDIES OF HUMAN AMBIENT AIR EXPOSURES
6   INFLAMMATORY RESPONSE TO OZONE
    6.1   In vitro studies
    6.2   Experimental in vivo studies
7   EXTRAPULMONARY EFFECTS OF OZONE AND NITROGEN DIOXIDE
    7.1   Ozone
    7.2   Nitrogen dioxide
8   MECHANISMS OF TOXICITY
    8.1   Ozone
        8.1.1   Lipid peroxidation
        8.1.2   Protein oxidation
    8.2   Nitrogen dioxide
9   BIOCHEMICAL EFFECTS
    9.1   Antioxidant enzyme activities
        9.1.1   Ozone
        9.1.2   Nitrogen dioxide
    9.2   Antioxidants
        9.2.1   Ozone
        9.2.2   Nitrogen dioxide
10 SUMMARY
11 PERSPECTIVES
12 ACKNOWLEDGEMENT
13 ABBREVIATION
14 REFERENCES

1   INTRODUCTION

The health effects of ozone and nitrogen dioxide, the major oxidant air pollutants, remain controversial after many years of study. There is little doubt that this is a complex subject compared to others in toxicology. This section is intended as a preface to the detailed data that will be presented in this chapter. The chapter is oriented to the topic of this volume so that some subjects regarding the toxicology of oxidant air pollutants have been deleted. We begin with the role of lung structure on toxicity and discuss features of the lung lining fluid. We propose that the toxicity of ozone and nitrogen dioxide can be explained from the direct chemical reaction of the oxidants with cellular constituents. Similarly, the protective effects of antioxidants can be ascribed to the lessening of oxidation in cells. We will also discuss the time course of ozone and nitrogen dioxide effects.

Mathematical models pioneered by Miller et al. [1] are the first steps toward a predictive theory of the human toxicity of ozone and nitrogen dioxide. According to mathematical models [1,2], the major driving force affecting ozone and nitrogen dioxide toxicity is deposition of the gases in the lung. The relative deposition of ozone and nitrogen dioxide in the three major regions of the respiratory tract of humans is shown schematically in Figs. 1 and 2. Although ozone and nitrogen dioxide are deposited throughout the lungs, the absorption of the gases into the lungs is uneven among the regions. The nasopharyngeal region plays an important protective role. In humans using nasal breathing, the nasopharyngeal cavity removes a major fraction of ozone (about 50%) from the inhaled air. An even larger fraction of inhaled nitrogen dioxide is removed in the nasopharyngeal region because of the relatively greater water solubility of nitrogen dioxide compared to ozone. During moderate and heavy exercise, an obligatory switch to a combination of mouth and nasal breathing occurs in humans. The removal of ozone and nitrogen dioxide by the nasopharyngeal region decreases during exercise because of the lower efficiency of the oral cavity compared to the nasopharyngeal region in removing both gases.

The regional uptake of ozone and nitrogen dioxide is controlled by the rates of reaction of the gases with the lung lining fluid. Even though the entire human lung is lined with fluid, the lung lining fluid is different in the alveolar region than it is in the conducting airways. Mucus, a glycoprotein mixture, covers the airways whereas lung surfactant, a protein-phospholipid complex composed mostly of phosphatidylcholine, covers the alveolar surface.

Figure 3 is a cartoon illustrating some of the features of the respiratory bronchiole and alveolus. One complicating aspect of understanding the effects of air pollutants on the lung is the cellular diversity present in the lung. Due to its specialized functions of oxygen transport and carbon dioxide excretion, the lung has evolved into some 40 or more different cell types arranged anatomically to facilitate gas exchange in the alveoli. A few of these cell types are depicted in Fig. 3.

The lung surfactant imparts ease of inflation and deflation to the alveoli so that all of the alveoli are inflated and collapsed at the same pace. Whereas most of

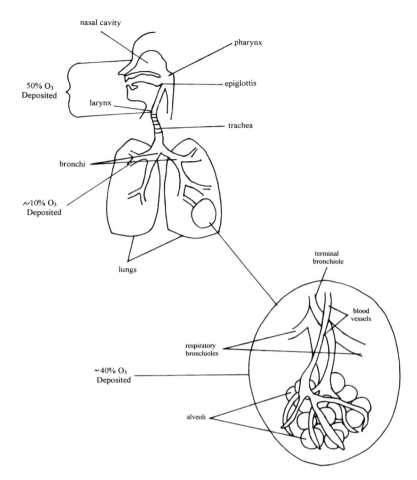

Fig. 1. A schematic representation of the deposition of ozone in the human respiratory tract. Ozone is poorly soluble in water so that removal in the nasopharyngeal region is less for ozone than for nitrogen dioxide. The deposition of ozone is mostly in the transitional zone of the lung, but all of the regions of the lung are damaged by ozone. In experimental animals, the most sensitive cells are the ciliated cells of the airways and type 1 cells of the alveoli. See Fig. 3 for detail on the transitional zone.

the fatty acid residues of the phospholipids in the lung surfactant are saturated palmitic acid residues, up to 30% are unsaturated. The polyunsaturated fatty acids in the lung lining fluid are rapidly oxidized by ozone and nitrogen dioxide, decreasing the surface-tension-lowering ability of the lung surfactant.

One hypothesis as to why ozone produces its greatest effects in the transitional or centriacinar zone is that ozone is more soluble in the lipid surfactant lining the alveoli than in the mucus lining the airways. The transitional zone includes the terminal bronchioles, respiratory bronchioles, and the immediately adjacent alveoli. As the lung surfactant contains mostly saturated fatty acids, it does not

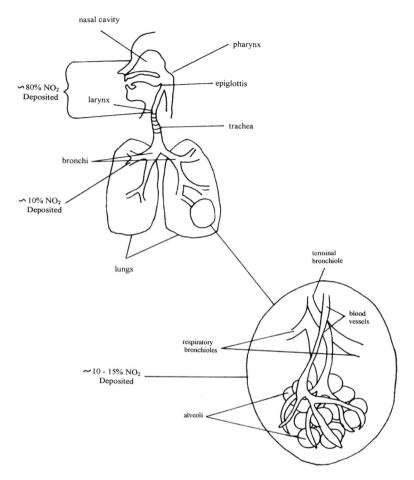

Fig. 2. A schematic representation of the deposition of nitrogen dioxide in the human respiratory tract. The nasopharyngeal region removes the majority of the inhaled nitrogen dioxide. The lower conducting airways and the pulmonary region also are sites of deposition. Nitrogen dioxide damage results mostly in the denuding of the ciliated regions of the transitional zone, but some damage to type 1 alveolar cells also occurs. See Fig. 3 for detailed structure of the transitional zone.

deplete the inhaled air of ozone or nitrogen dioxide before the gases can reach the cells lining the alveoli. The thin type 1 cells are low in mitochondria and protective antioxidants and thus are major targets for ozone and nitrogen dioxide toxicity. Type 2 cells, on the other hand, are secretory cells producing the lung surfactant. These cells are more metabolically capable than are the type 1 cells. Furthermore, in the transitional zone, bare patches or low coverage by mucus and lung surfactant result in greater ozone deposition in this region than in other regions of the lung. Ozone does injure the upper airways, but the most striking and critical long-term effect is in the transitional zone.

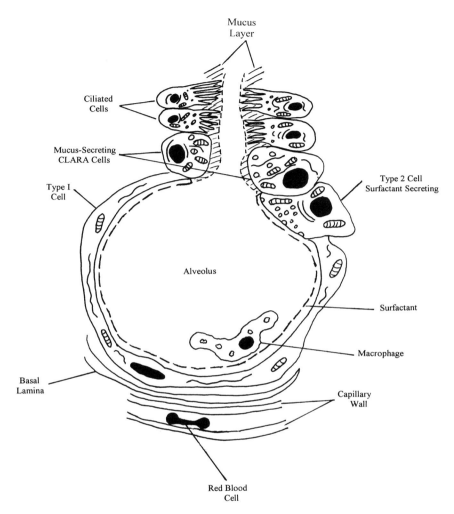

Fig. 3. A cross-section of the transitional zone of the lung. The key feature leading to the sensitivity of this region to ozone is the discontinuation of the aqueous mucus layer and the beginning of the surfactant layer. The main component of an alveolus is a single type 1 cell that lies in close proximity to capillaries. Type 2 cells secrete phospholipid constituents of the lung surfactant. When type 1 cells die, type 2 cells differentiate into type 1 cells. The bronchiole is lined with ciliated cells and mucussecreting cells like the Clara cell. Clara cells contain most of the drug-metabolizing activity of the lung. Ozone and nitrogen dioxide exposure injures the Clara cells and decreases the drug metabolizing capacity of the lung. This simplified drawing also illustrates that multiple cell types (some 40 or more in total) make up the lung. All are affected by air pollution to differing extents due their physiology and position within the lung.

Moreover, although ozone may not survive transit through the type 1 cell, some products of ozonation can diffuse from the type 1 cell into the blood (Fig. 3). To increase oxygen transport, the lung has evolved to have a very small separation between the alveolar lumen and the capillaries. Products such as ozonides and aldehydes can diffuse across this junction into the blood. The small space between the alveolar lumen and the capillaries explains why both ozone and nitrogen dioxide can affect distal tissues even though the original reaction products, such as the initial ozonide or lipid peroxyl radical, are too short-lived to exit into the blood.

As described in section 4, the contents of the fluid lining can be sampled using the procedure called bronchoalveolar lavage by introducing and withdrawing saline into one lobe of the lung. The lavage fluid contains cells, mucus, proteins, and small molecular weight compounds. The cell type most often found in the lavage fluid in a normal subject is the alveolar macrophage (Fig. 3). The alveolar macrophage is the first line of defense against microorganisms in the alveoli. The macrophages help kill and remove microorganisms from the lung by engulfing them and moving them to the mucus lining layer. The macrophages themselves can be killed by exposure to inhaled nitrogen dioxide and ozone. Exposure to these oxidants causes increased susceptibility of experimental animals to infection because the killing of macrophages by ozone and nitrogen dioxide allows microorganisms to multiply in the lung.

Injury to the cells lining the airways by air pollution attracts alveolar macrophages to the middle and upper airways from their normal domain in the alveoli. The digestion of dead or moribund cells by macrophages followed by the release of cytokines, eicosanoids, and other factors appears to attract inflammatory cells, which are found in lavage fluid during inflammation. Attraction of inflammatory cells to the lung requires time for the circulation of cytokines and expansion of inflammatory cell populations.

Interestingly, analysis of lung lavage fluid also yields ascorbic acid (vitamin C), glutathione, and vitamin E. The mechanisms by which these antioxidants are secreted into the lumen of the airways are unclear. During controlled human exposures to ozone and nitrogen dioxide, levels of some of these antioxidants decline possibly due to their destruction by reaction with inhaled ozone or nitrogen dioxide. Depletion or inhibition of transport of antioxidants into the airways could increase lung damage. There is little doubt that the lung lining fluid is the first protective barrier between an inhaled chemical or microorganism and the lung proper.

The site of the toxic reaction (i.e., the target of the toxic agent) is as important as the extent of the toxic reaction. The kinetics and mechanisms of reaction of inhaled agents teach us much about the parts of the lung that are affected. Regional effects clearly are important because they define the extent of a physiological decrement. Antigens act mostly in the upper airways, whereas ozone and nitrogen dioxide act mostly in the transitional zone of the lung. Antigenic effects are mostly in the bronchi. Chronic ozone or nitrogen dioxide exposure of animals leads to the loss of structure and function in the centriacinar region.

One of the challenges of extrapolating to humans the animal toxicity data from ozone and nitrogen dioxide exposures is the tremendous time scale over which toxic effects occur in humans compared to experimental animals. Experimental animals can be exposed to a constant ozone or nitrogen dioxide concentration over most of their lifetimes. In ambient air, humans are exposed to episodes of air pollution consisting of mixtures of ozone, nitrogen dioxide, polyaromatic hydrocarbons, inorganic particles, and much more. The concentration of ozone, for example, varies over the course of the day (Fig. 4). Chemical reactions leading to the ozonation of unsaturated fatty acids or the oxidation of unsaturated fatty acids by nitrogen dioxide have lifetimes of $10^{-3}-10^{-2}$ s whereas the health effects are seen clinically at 50–60 years or $10^{7}-10^{8}$ s of exposure. Few other toxicants exhibit this time scale in toxicity. Consequently, antioxidant prevention of lung disease caused by oxidant air pollutants cannot be expected to be evident after a few months or years. Long-term studies in humans are needed.

In Fig. 5, a hypothetical air pollution episode extending over 4 days is shown using the single-day ozone profile from Bakersfield, California (Fig. 4). The profile shown for Bakersfield is a very simple diurnal ozone pattern. Localities downwind from large metropolitan areas can have additional ozone peaks before dawn or at night because of so-called dark reactions contributing to ozone formation. Nitrogen dioxide concentrations follow more or less the same pattern as those of ozone except that nitrogen dioxide concentrations are greater at night than the ozone concentrations. The reason for this difference is that nitrogen dioxide is a reactant and hence a driving force in the formation of ozone by photochemical reactions. In the absence of light, nitrogen dioxide is not depleted by the reactions forming ozone.

In the summer, 3- to 4-day cycles of air pollution can occur across the USA and Europe with longer cycles of relatively clean air. These episodes of air pollution occur because of inversion layers or stagnant air over metropolitan air sheds.

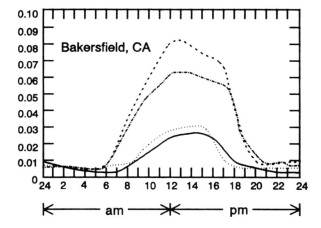

Fig. 4. Typical diurnal cycle of ozone in polluted air. Solid line represents 1st Quarter; alternating dashed and dotted line represents 2nd Quarter; dashed line represents 3rd Quarter; dotted line represents 4th Quarter. Taken from [8].

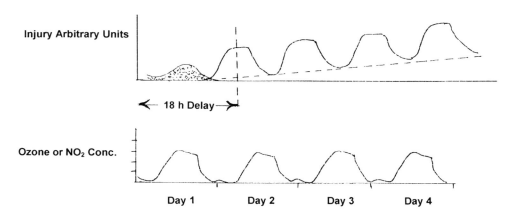

Fig. 5. Hypothetical lung injury from an air pollution episode. The lower chart shows a hypothetical 4-day exposure episode using the time course of ozone levels in Bakersfield, California (See Fig. 4). The upper chart represents the injury to the lung from the exposure. The stippled area represents the time course of chemical reactions that occur rapidly upon ozone or nitrogen dioxide exposure. The chemical reactions occur again with each ozone exposure. Reactive intermediates are formed each day during inhalation of polluted air. The health effects are not observable until about 18 h later. The "injury" curve is displaced from the ozone curve by about 18 h. When injury exceeds the ability to repair, repeated exposures will result in an accumulation of damage as shown by the dashed line. About 20 years of repeated exposure to ozone and nitrogen dioxide at the current standard are needed before conventional histopathologic changes can be observed.

In our schematic in Fig. 5, a 4-day period is shown with no accumulation of ozone or nitrogen dioxide from one day to the next. Under some meteorological conditions, ozone and nitrogen dioxide may accumulate by carry-over from prior days or from nitrogen dioxide and ozone formed upwind that drift over a metropolitan area. Nonetheless, an ozone and nitrogen dioxide maximum occurs at about noon.

Most in vitro studies indicate that the velocity of the oxidation of unsaturated fatty acids in cell membranes at low concentrations of ozone or nitrogen dioxide are likely to occur on the human lung surface is nearly first-order [3]. The formation of products from either ozone or nitrogen dioxide would be expected to rise as the exposure increases during the course of the day. The products of ozone and nitrogen dioxide reactions are also likely to decline in a first-order rate as do most other reactive intermediates formed in cells. The rates of formation and removal of reactive intermediates will result in a bell-shaped curve of concentration of reactive products vs. time as indicated in Fig. 5 by the stippled area. These reactive products will decline over time on their own. Probably, the antioxidants, particularly vitamin C in the lung lining fluid, will destroy them.

More reactive products are formed in the lung on inhalation with each successive day of air pollution. When more products are formed than can be removed, toxicity occurs. The toxic effect produced is shown in arbitrary units of injury on the upper graph of Fig. 5. Repair of injury, including elimination of oxidized cell constituents, probably also follows a general first-order process. In humans, about 18 h elapses between a single exposure to ozone or nitrogen dioxide and the maximum toxic effect in the lung. The time course of injury will follow the time course of ozone or nitrogen dioxide concentration in the inhaled air, but with some delay to account for absorption, the kinetics of reactions between ozone or nitrogen dioxide and cell components, and repair. We set the delay at 18 h to account for the observed time course of biomarkers of toxicity. Thus, the injury curve will rise and fall in the same manner as the ozone or nitrogen dioxide concentration rises and falls during the course of the day, however, the injury will be displaced in time by about 18 h. Breath-by-breath injury probably occurs but is obscured by the complexity of the process. Exercise, vs. rest, while breathing polluted air clearly increases lung deposition of pollutants in humans and may enhance the toxic effects of the diurnal ozone and nitrogen dioxide cycles. Thus, exercise at peak air pollution levels is inadvisable.

The model we have constructed for this review assumes that repair occurs throughout an exposure period. Toxic injury occurs because the rate of repair is slower than the rate of toxic injury. If the rate of the repair process is slower than the rate of formation of the toxic injury, some toxicity will be evident at a time when the air pollution rises again on the next day. In the model, the toxic injury to the lung gradually accumulates as is evident by the rising baseline of the toxic injury with the time curve (shown by the dashed line in Fig. 5). As the episodes of air pollution occur again and again over the years, some forms of toxic injury are not repaired causing permanent damage to the accumulate. Consequently, preventing human exposures to peak air pollution levels is a useful strategy for protection of the public health.

Because oxidizing air pollutants produce inflammation in the lung, repeated bouts of inflammation could result from air pollution episodes. The alarming rise in the prevalence and severity of asthma give added importance to the hypothesis that repeated bouts of air pollution cause inflammation leading to the initiation or exacerbation of bronchitis and asthma [4]. Viral lower respiratory tract infections are risk factors for both asthma and bronchitis.

The lungs of young people living in areas with high air pollution, such as Los Angeles, and dying violent deaths show histopathologic abnormalities at about age 20 years. This data, together with the data on the transient effects on lung function in normal and asthmatic subjects of ozone levels at or near the 0.12 ppm averaged over 1 h in the USA EPA National Ambient Air Quality Standard, prompted EPA to determine that the standard did not provide an adequate margin of safety. The ozone standard was revised to a lower level and the averaging time was chosen to eliminate exposures to short-time, but recurring, peaks of ozone. By changing the averaging time for ozone, EPA expects to reduce human exposures to ozone significantly.

In short-term studies of the protective effects of antioxidants on ozone or nitrogen dioxide toxicity, it has been difficult to demonstrate unequivocally that antioxidants are protective in humans. As an indirect measure of the susceptibility of human red cells to oxidative changes following fatty acid ozonide exposures mimicking ozone inhalation, vitamin E was protective at 300 to 600 IU/day in a small group of volunteers [5]. Even in cell membranes bearing the maximum vitamin E concentration, the vitamin E does not reduce the ozone or nitrogen dioxide reaction with fatty acids although it does terminate propagation of the chain reaction of peroxidation. That is, some, albeit reduced, injury is occurring in the protected individual.

On the other hand, near life-time studies in vitamin E deficient and vitamin E supplemented mice show that lung injury to the point of mortality is some 15- to 20-fold greater in the vitamin E deficient mice than in the vitamin E supplemented mice [6]. For the establishment of the essentiality of nutrients, data from experimental animal studies have been used as the best available data. In a similar manner, experimental animal studies show some of the best available data on the effects of long-term ozone and nitrogen dioxide exposure and of vitamin C and E protection.

Whereas vitamins E and C protect animals from ozone or nitrogen dioxide exposure effects, the rates and chemistry of the reaction of ozone and nitrogen dioxide with cellular constituents indicate that high levels of the antioxidants are needed to provide protection. Unfortunately, vitamin E and C supplementation at the levels likely to be effective for protection against damage from polluted air are not attainable by consumption of foods [7]. Thus, supplementation of adults with 1,000 IU of vitamin E and 1,000 mg vitamin C per day may be required before such protection is likely. Even in the presence of high levels of antioxidants, both ozone and nitrogen dioxide will react with cellular constituents to some small, but perhaps significant, effect [4]. Short-term effects of air pollution on pulmonary function and protection by vitamins C and E are difficult to demonstrate because of variations in pulmonary function among individuals are large compared to the air pollutant effects. Clearly, the preferable solution to the ozone and nitrogen dioxide problem is to reduce exposure to these air pollutants.

Controlled human studies have demonstrated that exposure to oxidant air pollution, and particularly to ozone, can lead to pain on inspiration, reversible pulmonary function decrements, hyperresponsiveness to bronchoconstrictor agents, airway inflammation, and exercise performance reduction. Although knowledge of the mechanisms responsible for the effects of air pollutants is incomplete, exercise appears to increase the risk of air pollutant-related consequences.

2   ATMOSPHERIC OZONE AND NITROGEN DIOXIDE

The principal oxidants in photochemical smog are ozone and nitrogen dioxide. The gases are potent respiratory tract oxidants and are of major public health concern. Typically, ozone is in higher concentration in ambient air than in nitrogen dioxide. Ozone is also a more powerful oxidant than is nitrogen dioxide. Incomplete combustion of fossil fuels by both stationary sources (e.g., electric power plants) and mobile sources (e.g., cars and trucks) provides the precursors of ozone and nitrogen dioxide formation in the atmosphere. Motor vehicles are the primary mobile sources of the precursors, and electric utilities followed by industries are the main stationary sources. In many cities around the world, automobile traffic gives rise to most of the oxidant air pollution.

Ozone and nitrogen dioxide are formed in the atmosphere through a series of reactions that involve nitric oxide, volatile organic compounds, and sunlight. Meteorological conditions such as strong ultraviolet radiation intensity, high temperature, and stagnated air can increase the production of photochemical smog. Ambient ozone levels in urban areas peak in the early afternoon (Fig. 4), whereas ambient nitrogen dioxide levels usually are highest in the late afternoon and evening hours [8,9]. An additional peak of nitrogen dioxide can occur in midmorning in cities with outdoor nitrogen dioxide levels greater than 0.2 ppm. Ozone levels are highest in the late spring or in summer in urban areas. In contrast, the maximum levels of nitrogen dioxide in outdoor urban air occur in the fall and winter months (Fig. 6). The time of day and site of exercising in an urban area are important in order to minimize exposure to oxidant air pollutants.

Ambient levels of ozone (Fig. 7) and nitrogen dioxide have been declining in the USA because of reductions in precursor emissions. Nevertheless, many urban areas in the USA do not meet the 1979 USA National Ambient Air Quality Standard for ozone of 0.12 ppm (averaged over 1 h), which is to be exceeded only once per year [8]. Reductions in the use of fossil fuels will be necessary to decrease further emissions of photochemical smog precursors. The USA National Ambient Air Quality Standard that was announced in July, 1997, establishes an 8-h standard of 0.08 ppm ozone in order to protect the public against exposures longer than 1 h. Photochemical smog is not a phenomenon restricted to urban areas in the USA and occurs in highly populated cities around the globe. In Mexico City, ozone levels are high and typically range from 0.15 to 0.25 ppm [10].

The USA National Ambient Air Quality Standard for nitrogen dioxide is an annual arithmetic mean of 0.053 ppm. In much of the USA, annual average out-

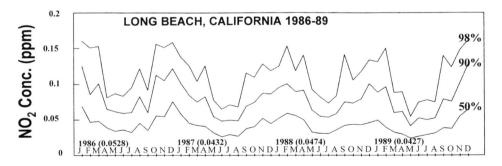

Fig. 6. Monthly 50th, 90th, and 98th percentiles of 1-h nitrogen dioxide concentrations at Long Beach, California, 1986 to 1989. The episodic and cyclic nature of NO_2 concentrations occurs in many other locations as well. Taken from [9].

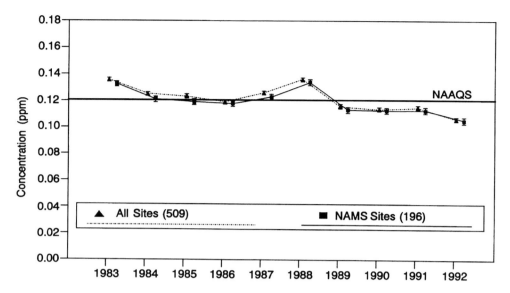

Fig. 7. The composite averages of the second highest maximum 1-hr ozone concentration with 95% confidence intervals at National Air Monitoring Stations (NAMS) and at all USA sites, 1983 to 1992, in relation to the USA National Ambient Air Quality Standard (NAAQS). Taken from [8].

door levels of nitrogen dioxide range from 0.015 to 0.035 ppm. Nonetheless, average hourly concentrations of nitrogen dioxide range from 0.02 to 0.20 ppm in moderately polluted urban areas and from 0.2 to 0.5 ppm in those that are heavily polluted [9].

Outdoor levels of ozone are almost always higher than the indoor levels because outdoor air is by far the primary source of indoor ozone. On the other hand, nitrogen dioxide is produced indoors, as well as outdoors, so that indoor levels of nitrogen dioxide can exceed those outdoors when gas appliances are used. Nitrogen dioxide levels can reach 0.6 ppm during cooking on a gas range [11].

3   DOSIMETRY MODELING OF OZONE AND NITROGEN DIOXIDE

Dosimetry is the process of measuring the amount of a substance that is absorbed at a target site. Absorption of air pollutants from the upper respiratory tract (nasopharyngeal region) and lower respiratory tract (tracheobronchial and pulmonary regions), as well as from the total respiratory tract, have been measured in experimental studies. Nevertheless, it has not been possible to determine absorption from smaller regions of the lung directly. Therefore, mathematical dosimetry models are especially useful for predicting the dose to particular areas of the lung.

3.1 Ozone

Because ozone is nearly insoluble in water, the gas penetrates into the pulmonary (gas-exchange) region of the lung even during restful breathing. Miller et al. [1] and Overton et al. [2] modeled the effects of exercise on the regional uptake of ozone in the lung. Simulations with human morphometric airway data predict little effect of exercise on tracheobronchial uptake but a marked effect on pulmonary uptake [1].

Dosimetry models predict that with exercise the dose of ozone delivered to the tracheobronchial region is slightly increased while the ozone dose to the pulmonary region is markedly increased. The model of Miller et al. [1] predicts that heavy exercise will cause the total mass uptake of ozone to increase 10-fold. According to Miller [12], human clinical studies consistently have shown that exposures with exercise to levels below 0.2 ppm ozone affect minute ventilation only slightly because a decrease in tidal volume occurs along with an increase in breathing frequency. Minute ventilation is the volume of gas exchanged in the lung per min.

Ozone is transported in the upper respiratory tract primarily by convection, or bulk movement, whereas the gas is transported in the pulmonary region of the lung mainly by diffusion. During heavy exercise, however, convection can contribute to gas transport in the pulmonary region [12].

Surprisingly, Gerrity et al. [13] found a small (approximately 10%) decrease in uptake of ozone in the upper respiratory tract during nasal breathing by healthy young male volunteers compared with oral or oronasal breathing. Total respiratory uptake of ozone was reported by Wiester et al. [14] to be slightly greater during oral rather than nasal breathing, however. This latter group of investigators also determined that the total respiratory uptake of ozone was about 75% in adult males during breathing at rest. The percentage of uptake varied substantially among subjects whereas intrasubject variability was moderate. In another human study, Kabel et al. [15] determined that 80% of the inhaled ozone was absorbed in the upper airways during nasal breathing compared with 50% during oral breathing. The point at which 90% of the inhaled ozone was absorbed was more distal with oral breathing. This finding implies that during exercise a switch from nasal to oral breathing can increase the risk of injury to the lower respiratory tract because of a greater dose.

Delivered dose of ozone, as determined mainly by minute ventilation, is suggested to account for part of the intersubject variability of pulmonary function response to ozone [16]. Subjects were exposed to 0.4 ppm ozone for 1 h during moderate intensity exercise and uptake efficiencies in the upper and lower respiratory tracts were measured. A significant relationship was found between either initial minute ventilation or average minute ventilation and forced expiratory volume in 1 s (FEV_1). FEV_1 is the volume of gas that can be exhaled in 1 s following a full inspiration. In other words, ozone decreased the flow from the lung at maximum effort. Probably, this is due to a smaller effective airway diameter.

3.2 Nitrogen dioxide

The dosimetry models for nitrogen dioxide evolved from the models developed for ozone. The uptake of nitrogen dioxide and ozone in the respiratory tract are similar because both of the gases are highly reactive and poorly soluble in water. Like ozone, nitrogen dioxide is absorbed throughout the respiratory tract and maximally in the centriacinar region (the junction between the conduction airways and the pulmonary region). Because nitrogen dioxide is more water soluble than ozone, deposition of nitrogen dioxide in the airways is predicted to be somewhat greater than that of ozone.

Total respiratory tract uptake of nitrogen dioxide has been measured experimentally in asthmatic and nonasthmatic humans. Healthy subjects exposed to 0.3—7.2 ppm nitrogen dioxide in a nitric oxide/nitrogen dioxide mixture absorbed 81—90% of the nitrogen dioxide while at rest [17]. Average uptake of nitrogen dioxide by adult asthmatic subjects exposed to 0.3 ppm nitrogen dioxide while at rest was 72% [18]. During exercise, uptake by both groups was similar, 81—90% for the healthy subjects and 88% for the asthmatic subjects.

Uptake of nitrogen dioxide by the upper and lower respiratory tract was determined in subjects exposed to 2 ppm nitrogen dioxide [19]. Nasal uptake, which was 44% at rest, diminished to 15% during heavy exercise. The total respiratory uptake was calculated to be 80% at rest and 91% during heavy exercise. The increased ventilation during exercise leads to a decreased percentage of nitrogen dioxide absorbed in the upper respiratory tract. The results indicate both a greatly increased uptake of nitrogen dioxide by the lower respiratory tract during exercise, as well as an increase in total respiratory tract uptake. Despite the greater uptake, nitrogen dioxide is less toxic than ozone because it reacts more slowly with cell constituents than does ozone.

4   LABORATORY HUMAN EXPOSURE WITH EXERCISE STUDIES

In controlled human studies of air pollutants, human volunteers are exposed to a fixed concentration of a gas under carefully controlled conditions. Methods commonly used to assess effects of air pollutants in human exposure studies include pulmonary function tests, bronchoalveolar lavage, and airway inhalation challenge tests. Pulmonary function tests involve noninvasive methods such as spirometric measures of lung volumes, measures of lung resistance, and measures of breathing patterns. Dynamic spirometry tests such as FEV_1 and plethysmographic tests such as specific airway resistance measurements provide information about large airway functions primarily. The coefficients of variation for these two specific tests are fairly low, about 3% for FEV_1 and about 10—20% for specific airway resistance measurements [11]. Because lung volume affects airway resistance, specific airway resistance measurements are calculated from resistance times volume.

Bronchoalveolar lavage is performed using a fiberoptic bronchoscope that is inserted into an airway and secured in a subsegmental bronchus [20]. Then, sterile buffered saline is used to remove cells and fluids lining the respiratory tract distal to the bronchoscope. Valuable information about the types of immune system cells in the segment, as well as the amount of protein and various other molecules, can be obtained using this procedure.

Airway inhalation challenge tests are used to examine the degree of responsiveness of the airways [21]. Responses include cough, bronchoconstriction, and increased mucus production. Commonly, the challenge is an inhaled agent such as methacholine, histamine, or carbachol that causes constriction of airways. Following each dose of a chemical provocation, airway resistance measurements or spirometry are performed. A target effect level, such as a 100% increase in airway resistance, is calculated from the concentration-effect curve.

4.1 Pulmonary function effects of acute ozone exposure

4.1.1 Concentration-response relationship

Studies conducted in the 1970s [22,23] demonstrated that, at a given ozone concentration, minute ventilation elevated by exercise exacerbated the pulmonary response to ozone and reduced the threshold for the response, as well. In these early studies, very low levels of exercise were used.

Later studies examined the effects of both multiple exposure concentrations and multiple intensities of either intermittent or continuous exercise [24,25]. The studies demonstrated that significant decrements in pulmonary responses result from exposure to 0.3 ppm ozone during moderate exercise. In addition, multiple regression analysis revealed that ozone concentration was primarily responsible for the pulmonary function variance [24].

A review of published data from pulmonary function studies that exposed normal subjects to ozone for 2 h during intermittent exercise confirmed that ozone concentration has a greater effect on pulmonary function than minute ventilation does[26]. In addition, the relationship between ozone concentration and alterations in pulmonary function was found to be nonlinear, and a threshold for pulmonary function effects caused by ozone could not be defined.

More recently, a number of investigators have shown that significant reductions in pulmonary function occur upon exposure of healthy subjects to ozone concentrations $\leqslant 0.2$ ppm during heavy exercise [27—30]. In order to cause a significant decline in pulmonary function in these studies, a minimum level of 0.1 to 0.18 ppm ozone for 1—3 h during moderate to heavy intermittent or continuous exercise was necessary.

In this chapter, the categories of ventilation levels will be described as follows: light exercise (~ 15 l/min), moderate exercise (20—40 l/min), and heavy exercise ($\geqslant 55$ l/min). In addition, the word significant will be used to describe a statistical significance at $p < 0.05$.

McKittrick and Adams [31] studied the effect of the exercise paradigm (intermittent or continuous exercise) on pulmonary function response when the ozone dose was held constant. Their results suggest that the exercise paradigm during exposures of 2 h or less has no effect on pulmonary function responses when the effective dose of ozone is equivalent at a given ozone concentration. The effective dose is a product of ozone concentration, ventilation, and exposure duration.

The dose-response relationship found by McKittrick and Adams [31] is interesting from a mechanistic view. By dimensional analysis,

$$\text{Ozone effective dose (g)} = \text{Ozone concentration (g/l)} \times \text{Ventilation (l/min)} \times \text{Exposure duration (min)}$$

If the reaction rate of ozone with lung constituents was the rate-limiting factor determining the toxicity in these experiments, the dose would not be the amount of ozone alone but a more complex function of the ozone concentration at the target site. That is, the transfer of ozone to the underlying tissues follows Henry's law and the kinetics of chemical reaction with mass transfer [1]. The ozone dose would depend on the location in the lung where ozone absorption is maximal.

Two factors may explain the differences found for exercise effects on ozone toxicity: 1) the endpoints used may be insensitive to ozone dose; and 2) the ozone reaction may be essentially instantaneous compared to the duration of subsequent biological measurements. It is our view that the latter is more likely. One should keep this possibility in mind when comparing clinical outcomes with the theory of how ozone produces its pulmonary toxicity. The matter is not trivial because the National Ambient Air Quality Standard for ozone has an averaging time-component. Generally, the component is chosen to provide the greatest protection of the population. The current averaging time of 8 h is aimed at reducing short-term exposures. Meteorology and air chemistry also influence the averaging time chosen. Nonetheless, further studies are needed to clarify the temporal relationships of ozone toxicity, especially during exercise.

Limited data suggests that healthy persons over 50 years of age show less of a pulmonary function response to ozone exposure than young adults do, especially those less than 25 years of age [32]. Whether a difference exists in sensitivity to ozone between men and women is yet to be determined.

A newly developed analyzer has been described that is expected to allow more accurate measurement of low doses of ozone (< 0.2 ppm) inhaled by human subjects during exercise [33]. The instrument can monitor ozone levels dynamically at the airway opening (nose or mouth). Such an instrument will be useful to confirm any interindividual differences in ozone sensitivity.

4.1.2 Reduction of exercise performance

As early as the 1960s, Wayne et al. [34] concluded from an epidemiologic study of high school cross-country runners that exercise performance is compromised by inhalation of oxidant air pollutants. Since that time, a number of controlled human studies have been conducted to examine the effects on exercise performance of acute (single 1- to 3-h) exposure to air pollutants and especially to ozone, the major oxidant in urban air pollution. Even though controlled human studies generally have a small sample size, they are valuable because they quantify concentration-response data.

The endpoints of controlled human studies of the effects of short-term exposure to ozone on exercise performance include maximal oxygen uptake and endurance (i.e., the ability to finish strenuous exercise tests). Of the three studies in the late 1970s that evaluated the effects of acute ozone exposure on maximal oxygen uptake [35—37], only one reported a significant reduction in maximal oxygen uptake [35].

More recently, controlled human studies of the effects of acute exposure to ozone on highly trained athletes [30] and trained nonathletes [38] have found significant reductions in maximal oxygen uptake as well as in other maximal exercise endpoints. The decreases in pulmonary function and symptoms of respiratory discomfort that occurred during the studies may have been responsible for the reductions in maximal oxygen uptake [38]. Symptoms of ozone exposure include coughing, pain on deep inspiration, shortness of breath, throat irritation, and wheezing.

Several controlled human studies of the effect of acute ozone exposures on endurance have shown that the ability of well-trained athletes to complete an exercise regimen is diminished [27—29,39]. In addition, subjective symptoms of respiratory discomfort are elevated in the subjects by the protocols.

The mechanisms responsible for the effects of ozone exposure on maximal oxygen uptake and endurance are unclear. Although symptoms of respiratory discomfort have been suggested to be the cause, evidence for such a conclusion is lacking. A reflex inhibition of α-motor neural activity during inspiration caused by ozone stimulation of neural receptors in the airways has been proposed [32]. Ozone reaction products could also reduce the airway caliber or thicken (via inflammation) the distance for diffusion of oxygen to the blood.

4.1.3 Recovery of pulmonary function following acute ozone exposure

Studies of repeated daily short-term ozone exposures to $\geqslant 0.2$ ppm ozone have shown that ozone exposure during moderate-heavy exercise can cause enhanced pulmonary responses on the second day [32]. Within 3 to 5 days, an attenuation of spirometric responses is typically observed irrespective of the dose rate of ozone exposure. The attenuated response can last for up to two weeks. These observations support the accumulated-damage hypothesis given in the introduction.

The relationship of pulmonary function responses and biomarkers of response in blood were measured in healthy subjects exposed to a pyramid-shaped profile of ambient ozone concentrations over three consecutive days (130 min/day) during light intermittent exercise [40]. The concentrations ranged from 0.25 ppm to 0.45 ppm ozone. Progressive decrements in forced vital capacity and FEV_1 began to diminish on the third day of exposure. These changes were accompanied by a significant decrease in serum α-tocopherol (vitamin E), as a measure of oxidative stress, and a significant increase in blastogenic activity of T lymphocytes, as a measure of immune function. Full recovery of pulmonary function had not occurred by 20 h after the third day of ozone exposure. The investigators speculate that, following intermittent ozone exposure, activated T lymphocytes may marginate and start the resolution of ozone-induced inflammation.

4.1.4 Mechanisms of pulmonary function effects of ozone

Although the mechanisms that lead to the pulmonary function responses induced by ozone exposure are not completely understood, the following three components of the chain-of-events are likely. The three components are:
1) reactions of ozone with constituents of the airway lining fluid and with epithelial cell membranes;
2) local tissue responses including injury and inflammation; and
3) stimulation of neural afferents (bronchial C fibers), which results in reflex responses and symptoms [32].

Hazbun et al. [41] tested the hypothesis that ozone acts via an oxidative reaction to reduce the activity of neutral endopeptidase in the airways. A reduction in neutral endopeptidase activity would lead to elevated levels of neuropeptides such as substance P. The investigators exposed healthy male and female subjects for 1 h to 0.25 ppm ozone during heavy exercise. Decrements in FEV_1 occurred. The airway lavage collected immediately after ozone exposure contained significantly higher levels of substance P and 8-epi-prostaglandin F_2 (a marker of oxidative free-radical reaction) than did that collected after filtered air exposure. These results agree with the findings in dogs that vagally mediated rapid breathing and bronchoconstriction induced by acute exposure to ozone are caused by stimulation of bronchial C fibers [42]. Substance P is released from the afferent endings of stimulated bronchial C fibers.

Pulmonary afferent C fibers are stimulated by prostaglandins [43,44]. A number of studies have implicated products of cyclooxygenase metabolism in the mediation of ozone-induced pulmonary function changes. In human subjects exposed to 0.4 ppm ozone for 2 h during heavy exercise, prostaglandin E_2 levels in bronchoalveolar lavage were increased at 1 h [45] and 18 h [46]. Furthermore, Schelegle et al. [47] showed that pulmonary function decrements in humans following inhalation of ozone for 1-h during heavy exercise are lessened markedly by pretreatment with the anti-inflammatory drug indomethacin, a cyclooxygenase inhibitor. A similar study by Ying et al. [48] also found that indomethacin attenuated the decline in pulmonary function induced by ozone.

Recently, Hazucha et al. [49] conducted a study in which ibuprofen (another inhibitor of cyclooxygenase activity) was given before and halfway-through exposure of subjects to 0.4 ppm ozone for 2 h with intermittent exercise. FEV_1 decrement was significantly lessened by the ibuprofen treatment although modest increases in specific airway resistance were not. Bronchoalveolar lavage collected immediately postexposure to ozone contained significantly lower levels of cyclooxygenase products prostaglandin E_2 and thromboxane B_2 after subjects were pretreated with ibuprofen. This latter result supports the hypothesis that arachidonic acid metabolites are involved in inhibiting inspiration, perhaps by stimulating nociceptive respiratory tract afferents. Of the proteins analyzed in the bronchoalveolar lavage, interleukin-6 was the only one that was significantly decreased by the treatment. Interleukin-6 has pro-inflammatory activities. No change was seen in neutrophil levels in the lavage, nor was a relationship between postexposure changes in constituents of bronchoalveolar lavage fluid and pulmonary function decrements observed.

At first glance, one might think the results of Hazucha et al. [49] to be at opposition to the general hypothesis that the oxidant air pollutants initiate lipid peroxidation. If so, there would be no need for cyclooxygenation to be initiated in order to form endoperoxides and then prostaglandins. Ozone can initiate peroxidation of arachidonic acid leading to cyclic peroxides (endoperoxides), but the measurable inflammatory effects in volunteers exposed to ozone are probably mediated by ozone-induced activation of cyclooxygenase as part of the inflammatory process. Thus, it is not surprising to see that cyclooxygenase inhibitors blunt the pulmonary function decrements caused by the inflammatory process. Despite blockade of cyclooxygenase, some airway effects remain that may be due to direct inflammatory hormone-like products of ozonation [50].

Although ozone itself is not a free radical, highly reactive hydroxyl radicals are generated during the decomposition of ozone in aqueous media [51]. In addition, singlet oxygen is produced in vitro when ozone reacts with various biological molecules [52]. Singlet oxygen reacts with protein in preference to lipids and DNA [53]. Hydroxyl radical production following ozone exposure has been found to correlate with decreases in lung function [54]. To ascertain whether hydroxyl radical formation occurs during ambient exposure to ozone, the investigators measured the concentration of *ortho*-tyrosine in nasal lavage fluid from healthy children following exposure to ozone levels that were "low" (about 0.070 ppm) and "high" (about 0.090 ppm). Hydroxyl radical reacts with endogenous phenylalanine to form *ortho*-tyrosine. Significantly higher levels of *ortho*-tyrosine, as a percentage of tyrosine, were measured following exposure to "high" compared with "low" concentrations of ozone. In addition, *ortho*-tyrosine levels varied inversely with forced vital capacity. No relationship was found between *ortho*-tyrosine levels and inflammation as determined by numbers of neutrophils, however. *ortho*-Tyrosine may be a marker of direct ozone oxidation.

4.2 Pulmonary inflammation following acute ozone exposure

An inflammatory response is of concern because of the presence of cells and factors in inflammatory exudate that can damage tissue. Neutrophils and macrophages can secrete substances capable of injuring lung tissue and compromising host defense mechanisms. The first evidence that ozone causes pulmonary inflammation was provided by Seltzer et al. [55] who performed bronchoalveolar lavage on subjects following exposure to 0.4 or 0.6 ppm ozone for 2 h during exercise. Later, a study by Koren et al. [46] confirmed the findings that exposure of humans to moderate levels of ozone during intermittent exercise results in enhanced levels of neutrophils and proinflammatory substances including prostaglandin E_2 in bronchoalveolar lavage fluid. The presence of neutrophils in the lung is recognized as a marker of acute inflammation.

Studies by Devlin et al. [56] indicate that inflammatory responses can occur in humans exposed to low levels of ozone (0.08 ppm) for 6.6 h while exercising moderately. The substantial range in response observed may indicate that some individuals are more susceptible to ozone damage than others are. Increases in inflammatory mediators in 18-h bronchoalveolar lavage fluid did not correlate with decrements in pulmonary function. Balmes et al. [57], too, found no correlation between the magnitude of decrements in pulmonary function and levels of inflammation in 18-h bronchoalveolar lavage fluid when healthy subjects were exposed to 0.2 ppm ozone for 4 h during exercise.

The lack of a correlation between pulmonary function decrements and inflammatory response may indicate that different mechanisms are responsible for the two responses. On the other hand, Schelegle et al. [58] showed that the time course of ozone-induced neutrophilia (increase in neutrophils) and decrements in FEV_1 differs. Furthermore, the investigators have demonstrated that the time course of ozone-induced neutrophilia in bronchoalveolar lavage of subjects undergoing heavy exercise differs in the proximal and distal respiratory tract. Comparing measurements taken at 1, 6, and 24 h, FEV_1 decreased only at 1 h following ozone exposure. In contrast, the greatest increase in neutrophils occurred at 6 h in the in bronchoalveolar lavage of the proximal airways and at 24 h in bronchoalveolar lavage of the distal airways and alveolar region.

Koren et al. [45] studied the time course of the inflammatory response following exposure of healthy subjects to 0.4 ppm ozone for 2 h during heavy exercise. Cellular and biochemical changes were detectable in bronchoalveolar lavage performed 1 h postexposure indicating that inflammatory response following ozone exposure develops quite rapidly. Levels of neutrophils, interleukin-6, and prostaglandin E_2 were higher at 1 h following ozone exposure than at 18 h. Other markers of inflammation including fibronectin, which has been related with fibrotic processes, and plasminogen activator, which in turn have been related with fibrinolytic processes, these were measured at higher levels at 18 h then at 1 h. These later changes could play a role in the long-term development of pulmonary fibrosis. Levels of tissue factor and protein were also elevated following ozone exposure, but the levels were similar at both time points. Tissue factor plays a role in fibrin formation, and an increase in protein in bronchoalveolar lavage indicates increased airway permeability. Similar results were reported by the same laboratories for another study in which subjects were exposed to 0.4 ppm ozone for 2 h while undergoing heavy exercise [59]. Therefore, maximal levels of the different inflammatory mediators in bronchoalveolar lavage fluid appear to vary temporally following ozone exposure.

Evidence of inflammation in airways 18 h after exposure of healthy athletes to 0.2 ppm ozone for 4 h during moderate exercise has also been found [60]. Significant increases in lactate dehydrogenase and the total number of cells were observed in lavage of mainstem bronchi, which was performed rather than bronchoalveolar lavage following the ozone exposure. Bronchoalveolar lavage is primarily a measure of conditions in the distal lung. Bronchial biopsies revealed that ozone exposure elevated the numbers of neutrophils present.

Concern exists that there may be subpopulations of individuals who are particularly susceptible to adverse health effects from ozone. Ozone may induce a greater inflammatory response in asthmatic subjects compared with normal subjects. Following exposure to 0.12 ppm or 0.24 ppm ozone for 90 min during intermittent moderate exercise, leukocytes and epithelial cells were significantly increased in nasal lavage of asthmatic subjects but not nonasthmatic subjects [61]. Although there were no significant differences in pulmonary function responses between asthmatic and normal subjects exposed to 0.2 ppm ozone for 4 h during exercise, the asthmatic subjects showed significantly greater increases in a number of inflammatory endpoints in bronchoalveolar lavage than the normal subjects did[62]. Hence, asthmatics may be at increased risk of pulmonary injury from ozone exposure.

By measuring clearance of radiolabeled technetium diethylene triamine pentacetic acid (^{99m}Tc-DTPA), Kehrl et al. [63] demonstrated increased epithelial cell permeability in subjects exposed to 0.4 ppm ozone while exercising heavily. Inflammatory cells and their products are thought to be involved in permeability changes in airways after ozone exposure [64].

Whether repeated periods in humans of ozone-induced acute inflammation progress into chronic pulmonary disease is unknown. Like pulmonary responses, attenuation of airway inflammation in humans seems to take place with repeated daily exposure to ozone [32]. Nevertheless, the extent of airway inflammation attenuation may be less complete and more gradual than the recovery of normal pulmonary responses. Some indicators of inflammation such as lactate dehydrogenase and elastase appear not to attenuate during repeated ozone exposure. Animal studies by Tepper et al. [65] showed that whereas decrements in pulmonary function attenuate with repeated exposure to ozone, inflammation and damage to epithelial cells advance and some biochemical markers remain elevated.

4.3 Airway responsiveness to ozone exposure

In several previously cited studies, healthy subjects exposed to 0.12 ppm ozone for short periods during exercise demonstrated increased airway responsiveness to the bronchoconstrictors methacholine or histamine [30,66]. Although acute increases in airway responsiveness are well documented following exposure to ozone, whether ozone causes prolonged increases in airway responsiveness, induces asthma, or increases susceptibility to asthma, is uncertain [32].

Methacholine responsiveness in healthy subjects exposed to 0.2 ppm ozone for 4 h with moderate exercise was not associated with a decreases in FEV_1 [67]. Therefore, in the absence of respiratory symptoms, an individual may not be aware of even large pulmonary function decrements and may remain in an injurious environment unknowingly.

Both healthy and mild-asthmatic subjects exposed to 0.4 ppm ozone for 2 h with intermittent exercise responded with an increase in the maximal degree of airway narrowing to methacholine 12 h after exposure [68]. The authors suggested that this temporal relationship between exposure and bronchoconstriction may explain the increase in hospital admissions for respiratory diseases 1 day after an ozone episode.

The mechanism of ozone-induced increases in airway responsiveness has not been elucidated. Nevertheless, soluble mediators of inflammation such as cytokines and arachidonic acid metabolites may play a role [32]. That is, both the initial peroxidation products and later inflammatory agents combine to enhance the airway permeability. The increased permeability of the airways following ozone exposure would increase the diffusion of vasoactive agonists to the site of action.

4.4 Pulmonary function effects of prolonged ozone exposure

A number of controlled human studies in which subjects were exposed to 0.08–0.12 ppm ozone for 6.6 h with moderate exercise found that FEV_1 was decreased compared to exposure to clean air [66,69,70]. Similar to the findings with acute ozone exposures, interindividual variation in response to prolonged exposures to ozone was considerable.

Studies with prolonged ozone exposure protocols ($\geqslant 4$ h) which result in modest changes in pulmonary function show evidence of a response plateau [66,71]. Responsiveness of subjects to exposure to varying levels of ozone suggests that the response plateau depends on ozone concentration, dose rate, and cumulative dose [71]. Based on results of this latter study, as well as those from numerous others, ozone concentration during prolonged exposures has a greater effect on pulmonary function than does exposure duration or volume of air inhaled [32].

In a study that examined pulmonary responses of asthmatic and nonasthmatic subjects to ozone, subjects were exposed to 0.16 ppm ozone for 7.6 h with intermittent light exercise [72]. Whereas decrements in FEV_1 were significantly greater for asthmatics than for nonasthmatics, no difference was observed for decrements in forced vital capacity between the two groups. The investigators concluded that bronchoconstriction was responsible for part of the ozone-induced pulmonary decrements.

Attenuation of pulmonary responses with repeated prolonged exposure to 0.12 ppm ozone during moderate exercise were examined by Folinsbee et al. [69]. Pulmonary function decrements were observed on the first day of exposure. The decrements were lessened on the second day and were absent compared with the control values on the last 3 days of ozone exposure.

4.5 Pulmonary function effects of mixtures of ozone and other air pollutants

Although humans are exposed to mixtures of pollutants in ambient air, most controlled human studies have examined the effects of single air pollutants. In general, studies of mixtures of air pollutants have found no significant differences between exposure to ozone alone and exposure to the mixtures.

Nevertheless, a few human studies of pulmonary function responses to mixtures of ozone and sulfur dioxide have demonstrated greater effects of the mixture than of either pollutant alone. In their study of allergic asthmatic adolescents, Koenig et al. [73] found that when the subjects were exposed sequentially to ozone and sulfur dioxide during intermittent exercise, significant changes in FEV_1 and total respiratory resistance occurred. No significant changes in pulmonary function occurred with sequential exposures to air and sulfur dioxide or to ozone and ozone. The response of asthmatic adolescents to sulfur dioxide may, therefore, be potentiated by exposure to ozone.

Linn et al. [74] studied the effects of ozone and aerosols of sulfuric acid on the pulmonary function of normal, atopic, and asthmatic subjects undergoing exercise. Both the exposure to ozone alone and ozone mixed with sulfuric acid aerosol caused significant decrements in FEV_1 and bronchial reactivity to methacholine. The investigators concluded that the pulmonary effects in their study population were caused predominantly by ozone. Nonetheless, because a few of the subjects demonstrated significantly greater effects from exposure to the mixture compared with ozone alone, a subpopulation of individuals sensitive to ozone plus sulfuric acid may exist.

Aris et al. [60] studied the exposure of human subjects during exercise to nitric acid gas followed by ozone (an exposure pattern typical in some coastal California regions). Nitric acid, the main acid air pollutant in the western USA, is capable of damaging the respiratory tract. Smaller reductions in pulmonary function were observed with air and ozone than with nitric acid and ozone. In other words, the nitric acid seemed to antagonize the effect of ozone. In a later study of simultaneous exposure of exercising human subjects to ozone and nitric acid gas, no significant differences in pulmonary function or cellular or biochemical components in bronchoalveolar lavage, proximal airway lavage, or bronchial biopsy specimens were observed in comparison with exposure to ozone plus air [75].

Low levels (< 0.6 ppm) of nitrogen dioxide do not seem to enhance pulmonary function responses to ozone. Moreover, synergism between nitrogen dioxide and other air pollutants has not been demonstrated. Exposure of healthy young adults during heavy exercise to filtered air, 0.60 ppm nitrogen dioxide, 0.30 ppm ozone, or 0.60 ppm nitrogen dioxide plus 0.30 ppm ozone revealed no significant effect on pulmonary function or symptoms of nitrogen dioxide either alone or in combination with ozone [76]. Nonetheless, results of a study of sequential exposures with intermittent exercise showed that exposure to nitrogen dioxide (0.6 ppm) followed by ozone (0.3 ppm) potentiated airway responsiveness to methacholine

[77]. In addition, small but significant differences in some pulmonary function measures were observed.

Young asthmatic subjects were exposed in a chamber to respirable acid aerosol (available hydrogen ions equivalent to 127 ug/m^3 sulfuric acid), 0.3 ppm nitrogen dioxide, and 0.2 ppm ozone in effort to simulate summertime air pollution [78]. The subjects were exposed on separate occasions to nitrogen dioxide and ozone without the acid and to clean air. Each exposure lasted 90 min and included intermittent exercise. No significant differences in group mean lung function were measured among the three exposures.

A number of studies of mixtures of ozone and the air pollutant peroxyacetyl nitrate have been conducted. Peroxyacetyl nitrate forms in the troposphere from organic peroxyl radicals and nitrogen dioxide. In general, results of these studies have shown that at common ambient levels of ozone and peroxyacetyl nitrate, no additional effects of peroxyacetyl nitrate are evident [32].

4.6 Pulmonary effects of nitrogen dioxide exposure

4.6.1 Pulmonary function effects and airway responsiveness

Avol et al. [79,80] detected attributable no effects in children and adolescents due to nitrogen dioxide exposure for 1 h during exercise as a constituent of ambient oxidant air pollution containing 0.04—0.05 ppm nitrogen dioxide. Moreover, exercise studies of the effects of nitrogen dioxide exposure for ≤4 h on normal subjects consistently show no pulmonary function changes at levels between 0.3—0.6 ppm [76,81—83].

Nevertheless, a small but significant decrease in values for FEV$_1$ was reported after young healthy subjects were exposed, while exercising maximally for 8 min, to city air, compared with an air-conditioned room [84]. The mean concentration of nitrogen dioxide in the city air was about 10-fold higher than that in the room air (0.038 vs. 0.004 ppm).

A change in airway responsiveness may be one of the most sensitive markers of a response to nitrogen dioxide exposure. Exposure of normal subjects to 1.5 ppm nitrogen dioxide for 3 h during intermittent moderate exercise increased airway reactivity [82]. Exposure of the subjects for 3 h during intermittent moderate exercise to a continuous supply of 0.6 ppm nitrogen dioxide or to 0.05 ppm nitrogen dioxide with three 15-min periods of 2.0 ppm nitrogen dioxide caused no effect, however.

Because individuals with asthma may be sensitive to nitrogen dioxide, numerous studies of the effects of nitrogen dioxide exposure on asthmatics have been conducted. In general, pulmonary function responses in asthmatics to ambient levels of nitrogen dioxide have been shown to be small relative to those following sulfur dioxide exposure. Asthmatic subjects exposed to 0.2 ppm nitrogen dioxide for 2 h with light intermittent exercise showed no significant effect on pulmonary function and only a small significant effect on symptoms [85]. Effects on bronchial reactivity were equivocal.

Exposure of asthmatic subjects to ambient air containing 0.01—0.26 ppm nitrogen dioxide (mean = 0.09 ppm) for 3 h during intermittent exercise had no significant effect of pulmonary function, symptoms, or bronchial reactivity to cold air [86]. Furthermore, no significant changes in pulmonary function responses or bronchial responsiveness were observed in subjects with moderate asthma that were exposed to 0.3 ppm nitrogen dioxide for 4 h during intermittent exercise [83].

Increased airway resistance in healthy subjects after exposure to high levels of nitrogen dioxide (5 ppm) for 2 h during intermittent light exercise have been reported [87]. No effects on airway resistance or symptoms of exposure of healthy and asthmatic subjects to 4 ppm nitrogen dioxide for 75 min during moderate or moderate-heavy exercise were observed, [88].

Importantly, a concentration-response relationship in asthmatic subjects has not been demonstrated for nitrogen dioxide and pulmonary function during exercise. A few exercise studies have indicated that modest changes in pulmonary function may occur when asthmatic subjects are exposed to 0.3 ppm nitrogen dioxide [18,86,89,90]. On the other hand, exercise studies that used a range of concentrations showed no concentration-related effect [89,90].

Nitrogen dioxide is thought to act principally on the small airways. Therefore, the lack of an effect of nitrogen dioxide exposure on the standard spirometric and airway resistance measurements that measure large airway function primarily does not prove conclusively that nitrogen dioxide has no effect on pulmonary functions.

4.6.2 *Inflammatory response and epithelial cell permeability*

Nitrogen dioxide exposure has not been shown to cause an increase in inflammatory cells in bronchoalveolar lavage fluid from exercising subjects. Frampton et al. [91] exposed normal subjects to nitrogen dioxide during intermittent moderate exercise for 3 h using three protocols in which bronchoalveolar lavage was performed 3.5-h postexposure:
1) continuous 0.6 ppm,
2) background 0.05 ppm with three 15-min periods of 2.0 ppm, and
3) continuous 1.5 ppm.
In a fourth protocol bronchoalveolar lavage was performed 18 h after continuous 0.6 ppm exposure for 3 h. No influx of inflammatory cells occurred, nor did epithelial cell permeability increase, following any of the protocols.

4.7 Effects of urban air polluted with ozone and nitrogen dioxide

Exposure to the complex mixture of air pollutants in ambient urban air may have different health consequences than exposure to one or a mixture of only a few air pollutants generated in a laboratory. Field studies using mobile exposure chambers can compare the acute effects of exposures to ambient air, filtered air, or air containing specific laboratory-generated air pollutants. A number of mobile laboratory studies of photochemical oxidants have been conducted at Rancho Los Amigos Medical Center in Duarte, California, a suburb of Los Angeles. These studies show that the exercise level, as well as the ozone concentration, has respiratory effects on residents in this metropolitan area [32]. For example, exposure for 1 h to ambient air with a mean ozone concentration of 0.144 ppm caused pulmonary function decrements in healthy adolescents exercising moderately [80]. Decrements in pulmonary function plus increases in respiratory symptoms were observed in heavily exercising athletes exposed for 1 h to ambient air with a mean ozone concentration of 0.153 ppm [28] and in healthy and asthmatic subjects exposed for 2 h to ambient air with a mean ozone concentration of 0.174 ppm with light intermittent exercise [92].

In a study that compared exposures of exercising athletes to ambient air (mean ozone concentration of 0.15 ppm) or purified air containing laboratory-generated ozone (0.16 ppm), no significant differences in pulmonary function or respiratory symptoms were observed [28]. The results indicate that pollutants other than ozone in ambient air on a summer day in the Los Angeles area contribute minimally to the respiratory effects.

Exposure of adults with moderate to severe asthma to ambient air containing a mean of 0.086 ppm nitrogen dioxide for 2 h with intermittent exercise caused no significant changes in lung function, symptoms, or bronchial reactivity compared with clean air [89]. The investigators concluded that, at least in the Los Angeles area, adults with moderate to severe asthma are not sensitive to ambient concentrations of nitrogen dioxide.

In a recent laboratory chamber exposure study of children, ambient acid summer haze was simulated by a mixture of 0.10 ppm ozone, 0.10 ppm sulfur dioxide, and 100 $\mu g/m^3$ 0.6 μm sulfuric acid aerosol [93]. The children were exposed for 4 h during intermittent exercise. No significant changes in spirometry or symptoms were observed in the group, which included healthy children as well as those with allergy or mild asthma.

5   OUTDOOR STUDIES OF HUMAN AMBIENT AIR EXPOSURES

In the field studies discussed in this section, the acute effects of photochemical oxidant air pollution on pulmonary function were assessed in subjects exercising outdoors. Pulmonary function was measured before and after a series of exercise regimens during which the subjects were exposed to ambient air pollution. Although the design of these studies is similar to that of the mobile laboratory studies described previously, the duration and intensity of the exercise is not controlled strictly and the minute ventilation attained frequently is not measured in the outdoor studies. On the other hand, the collection of repeated measurements on the same subject is simplified in outdoor studies [32].

The ranges of ozone exposure levels in five outdoor exercise studies [94—98] were similar, in general, and ranged from 0.004 to 0.135 ppm. In the three studies that involved adults, the exercise was moderate to heavy, and decrements in FEV_1 were negatively associated with ozone concentration. In contrast, two studies of children yielded no relationship between ozone concentration and decrements in FEV_1 perhaps because of the low intensity of the exercise or recent ozone exposures prior to the event.

A field study was conducted recently to determine whether, as in controlled laboratory studies of acute exposures to ozone, biomarkers of inflammation are detectable in humans exposed outdoors to polluted air containing ozone [99]. Bronchoalveolar lavage fluids were collected from recreational joggers during summer and winter. Significantly elevated levels of soluble factors such as lactate dehydrogenase (a marker of epithelial cell damage) and prostaglandin E_2 were measured in bronchoalveolar lavage fluids in summer compared with winter. In contrast, a significantly greater release of reactive oxygen species by stimulated bronchoalveolar lavage cells was observed in winter compared with summer. These findings may indicate the presence of continual pulmonary inflammation in recreational joggers exposed to ozone-polluted air.

6   INFLAMMATORY RESPONSE TO OZONE

6.1 In vitro studies

In vitro studies of epithelial cells or epithelial cell lines have provided insight into potential mechanisms by which ozone induces an inflammatory response. Ozone stimulates the release of arachidonic acid metabolites from the human bronchial cell line BEAS-S6 [100]. Eicosanoids from both the cyclooxygenase pathway (e.g., thromboxane B_2 and prostaglandin E_2) and the lipoxygenase pathway (e.g., leukotrienes C_4, D_4, and E_4) were elaborated from the cells after ozone exposure. These results indicate that eicosanoids also may be released from airway epithelial cells in humans exposed to ozone.

Human bronchial epithelial cells, as explant cultures, exposed to ambient concentrations of ozone (0.10−0.100 ppm) released the inflammatory cytokines interleukin-8, granulocyte/macrophage colony-stimulating factor, and tumor necrosis factor-α . The release of the proinflammatory mediators was inhibited by the anti-inflammatory drug nedocromil as well as by 0.4−0.6 mM glutathione, a normal component of cells. Therefore, airway inflammation may be produced when humans are exposed to ambient levels of ozone via the liberation of these inflammatory mediators from airway epithelial cells.

Prostaglandin E_2, lesser amounts of prostaglandin F_2, and 15-hydroxyeicosatetraenoic acid were released from primary cultured human tracheal epithelial cells exposed to 0.1−0.5 ppm ozone [102]. Prostaglandin E_2 release increased transiently and then decreased for an extended period of time. Ozone exposure caused a reduction in cyclooxygenase activity but no effect on 15-hydroxyeicosatetraenoic acid production. The authors suggested that, because prostaglandin

E$_2$ is a bronchodilator and has anti-inflammatory properties, an extended decrease in the level of the eicosanoid following ozone exposure may play a role in ozone-induced airway dysfunction.

In human nasal mucosa treated in vitro with 0.1 ppm ozone for 24 h, significantly greater levels of prostaglandin F$_{2\alpha}$ thromboxane B$_2$, and leukotriene B$_4$ were elaborated compared to control [103]. The results suggested that, in nasal mucosa, ozone acts as an oxidant to stimulate arachidonic metabolism, which leads an to increases in products from both the cyclooxygenase and the lipoxygenase pathways.

6.2 Experimental in vivo studies

Expression of macrophage inflammatory protein-2 mRNA is induced in rat lung following ozone exposure [104]. Because to the glucocorticoid dexamethasone blocked macrophage inflammatory protein-2 in mRNA induction by ozone, as well as the influx of neutrophils into the airways, macrophage inflammatory protein-2 may trigger ozone-induced neutrophilic inflammation of airways.

Ozone exposure may alter the function of surfactant protein A, which has been shown to stimulate macrophage chemotaxis [105]. Surfactant from bronchoalveolar lavage fluid of guinea pigs exposed to 0.8 ppm ozone for 6 h enhanced the respiratory burst of stimulated macrophages, which was blocked by antibodies against surfactant protein A. An increase in the chemotactic activity of surfactant protein A may contribute to the influx of monocytic cells in lavage fluid that occurs following ozone exposure.

7   EXTRAPULMONARY EFFECTS OF OZONE AND NITROGEN DIOXIDE

7.1 Ozone

Hematologic effects in laboratory animals and humans exposed to ozone provide evidence that ozone or its reaction products reach the bloodstream. Erythrocytes from mice exposed to 1 ppm ozone for 4 h exhibited reduced ability to deform, a characteristic needed for their passage through capillaries [106]. Vitamin E supplementation failed to protect against the rigidity, but appeared to protect somewhat against the ozone-induced increase in hematocrit, which is an indirect evaluation of erythrocyte deformability. Although the mechanism of action of ozone on erythrocyte deformability is unknown, the rigidity could result from the cross-linking of membrane components or oxidation of intracellular proteins.

Heinz bodies are formed in erythrocytes of mice exposed to 0.85 ppm ozone for 48 h and in mouse and human erythrocytes exposed to fatty acid ozonides in vitro [107]. Heinz bodies are aggregations of denatured hemoglobin bound to the interior of the erythrocyte cell membrane. Oral supplementation of humans with vitamin E prevented Heinz body formation in erythrocytes treated in vitro with methyl oleate ozonide [5], which suggests that vitamin E protects against oxidative damage by ozone-generated products.

Ozone exposure also has been shown to have an effect on the liver. Exposure of rats to $1-2$ ppm ozone for 3 h stimulated nitric oxide production and protein synthesis in hepatocytes [108]. Liver, as well as lung tissue in ozone-treated rats contained increased levels of tumor necrosis factor-α, which, along with interleukin-1, was induced in alveolar macrophages. The investigators proposed that inflammatory cytokines from activated pulmonary macrophages may mediate extrapulmonary effects of ozone.

7.2 Nitrogen dioxide

Apparently, like ozone, nitrogen dioxide and/or its reaction products are absorbed into the blood via the lungs. Animal experiments have shown that exposure to nitrogen dioxide causes changes in blood components and various organs [11]. Nevertheless, the data do not indicate that a particular extrapulmonary effect predominates.

Nitrogen dioxide, as well as ozone, has effects on hepatic drug metabolism in experimental animals. Pentobarbital sleeping time was prolonged by ambient concentrations of ozone in female mice, rats, and hamsters [109] and ambient concentrations of nitrogen dioxide in mice [110]. Phenobarbital is metabolized in the liver by cytochrome P450 enzymes. The mechanism of action for the effect of the gases on pentobarbital metabolism remains unknown.

8   MECHANISMS OF TOXICITY

Ozone and nitrogen dioxide generate free radicals in biological systems both in vitro and in vivo [111$-$113]. These oxidants cause the peroxidation of membrane lipids, a process that is initiated by free radicals. That the lipid-soluble molecule vitamin E breaks the chain reaction of lipid peroxidation is further evidence that ozone and nitrogen dioxide produce free radicals. Vitamin E interrupts lipid peroxidation by scavenging peroxyl radicals.

8.1 Ozone

8.1.1 Lipid peroxidation

One hypothesis regarding a mechanism for the biochemical effects of ozone is that lipid peroxidation is responsible for the toxicity of ozone. The reaction of ozone with unsaturated fatty acids is described by the Criegee ozonation hypothesis. The initial ozonide in the pathway of formation of the Criegee ozonide is a 1,2,3-trioxolane (Fig. 8). Pryor [3] suggests that the a diradical intermediate is produced from the trioxolane by O-O bond scission. The diradical can decompose into an aldehyde and a carbonyl oxide.

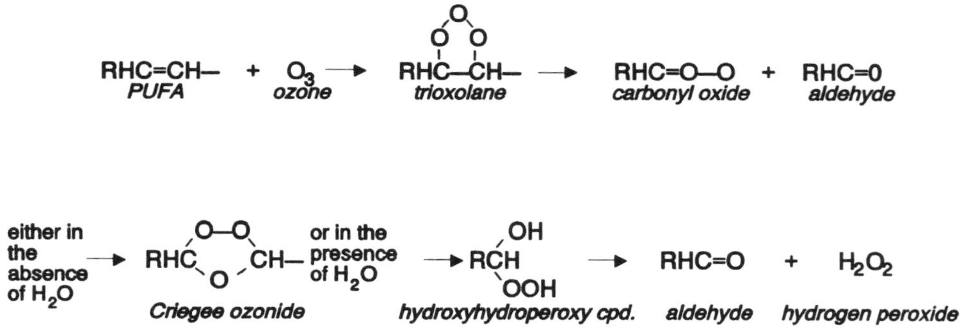

$$RHC=CH- \quad + \quad O_3 \quad \longrightarrow \quad RHC-CH- \quad \longrightarrow \quad RHC=O-O \quad + \quad RHC=O$$

PUFA   ozone   trioxolane   carbonyl oxide   aldehyde

either in
the
absence $\longrightarrow \quad RHC \quad CH-$ or in the presence of H_2O $\longrightarrow RCH \quad \longrightarrow \quad RHC=O \quad + \quad H_2O_2$
of H_2O

Criegee ozonide   hydroxyhydroperoxy cpd.   aldehyde   hydrogen peroxide

Fig. 8. Classic ozone addition to carbon-carbon double bonds of polyunsaturated fatty acids (PUFA) as residues of membrane phospholipids or in the lung lining fluid to form a 1,2,3-trioxolane. This initial ozonide via OO scission generates a diradical that decomposes by β-scission to form a carbonyl oxide and an aldehyde. In the relatively anhydrous environment of cell membranes, the initial ozonide rearranges to form the Criegee ozonide, which can decompose to a hydroperoxide and an aldehyde. The hydroperoxide can initiate lipid peroxidation. In an aqueous environment, the carbonyl oxide can form a hydroxyhydroperoxide, which breaks down to an aldehyde and hydrogen peroxide.

Pryor [3] also postulates a second mechanism of radical production in which ozone reacts with electron donors such as glutathione or its anion to generate the thiyl radical and the ozone radical anion. The ozone radical anion reacts with a proton to form the hydroxyl radical and molecular oxygen. Ozone also reacts with the unsaturated compounds cholesterol and tryptophan and with phenolic electron donors.

Pryor [3] predicts that the radicals are generated via the two mechanisms in only about 10% of the reactions of ozone with lung constituents. Usually, the 1,2,3-trioxolane decomposes into a carbonyl oxide and a carbonyl compound directly or via a diradical intermediate. When ozone reacts with unsaturated fatty acids in a cell membrane (a lipophilic environment), the carbonyl oxide and the carbonyl compound recombines to form a Criegee ozonide (Fig. 8).

In an aqueous medium such as the lung lining fluid, water reacts with the carbonyl compound generated from the decomposition of the 1,2,3-trioxolane to form a hydroxyhydroperoxide (Fig. 8). Hydrolysis of the hydroxyhydroperoxide produces hydrogen peroxide and aldehydes, including hexanal, heptanal, and nonanal [3]. Aldehydes also can be formed from Criegee ozonides. Marker molecules from the ozonation of unsaturated lipids have been detected in bronchoalveolar lavage fluid from rats and humans [3].

A gas chromatography-mass spectrometric method has been developed to detect and quantify aldehydes (as their 2,4-dinitrophenylhydrazones) that are biomarkers of lipid peroxidation [114]. Aldehydes such as 4-hydroxyalkenals, the most toxic aldehydes generated during lipid peroxidation, are detected. Using their method, the authors quantified 4-hydroxynonenal released into the medium from alveolar macrophages treated with 20 ppm nitrogen dioxide for 1 h and measured an equivalent of 1.3 ng of 4-hydroxynonenal per million cells. These high concentrations of nitrogen dioxide may produce aldehydes by mechanisms that do not occur in ambient air concentrations. Further studies are needed.

Criegee ozonides are toxic compounds that can initiate peroxidation of poly-unsaturated fatty acids and cell membranes in vitro (Menzel, unreported results). The peroxidation can be prevented by vitamin E (Menzel, unreported results), which indicates that peroxyl radicals are produced when Criegee ozonides react with unsaturated lipids.

The rates of reaction of vitamin E and polyunsaturated fatty acids with ozone are similar [3]. Yet, ozone is expected to react more often with unsaturated fatty acids than with vitamin E in the lung lining fluid and in cell membranes because of the much greater abundance of unsaturated fatty acids compared with vitamin E in both locations. Vitamin C and thiols such as glutathione, which react with ozone at a faster rate that unsaturated fatty acids do, can scavenge ozone in the lung lining fluid and prevent it from reaching cellular targets [3].

Strenuous exercise results in a temporary elevation of plasma vitamin E levels [115]. Following exposure to 0.5 ppm ozone for 5 days, the vitamin E content of lungs of vitamin E-supplemented rats increased significantly whereas the vitamin E content of the lungs of the vitamin E-deficient rats tended to decrease [116]. The investigators concluded that ozone exposure, an additional source of oxida-tive stress, might cause a mobilization of vitamin E to the lung from other parts of the body.

Due to its extreme reactivity, all of the ozone that is inhaled into the lungs is thought to combine with either constituents of the lung lining fluid or, when the fluid is absent or sparse, with the first layer of cells with which it comes in contact [117]. Ozone may interact directly with cells lining the distal conducting airways where the lung lining fluid may be scanty and with cells in the pulmonary region, which have no lung lining fluid layer [12]. Instead of lining fluid, the pulmonary region of the lung is covered with a surfactant layer, which has a few substances with which ozone reacts [12].

Ozonation byproducts that are more stable than ozone are proposed to account for the majority of the ozone-induced damage that occurs in the upper airways where the lung lining fluid is thicker [118]. The effects of ozone that occur beyond the first layer of lung cells, as well as those that are extrapulmonary, also are pro-posed to result from lipid ozonation products. Free radicals are not expected to relay the effects of ozone because they are too unstable to travel far within a tissue and, in addition, are in very low concentrations [3].

Criegee ozonides produced from the reaction of ozone with unsaturated fatty acids in membrane lipids are possible mediators of ozone toxicity. The half-life of Criegee ozonides is long (about 4—6 weeks) under physiological conditions [119]. Criegee ozonides or their decomposition products can initiate lipid peroxi-dation in vitro [120].

Other likely mediators of the toxic effects of ozone inhalation are the lipid per-oxidation products 4-hydroxynonenals, which can be found in both the cytosol and membranes [121]. Like Criegee ozonides, aldehydes have longer half-lives than do free radicals, which enables them to reach more distant targets. The most cytotoxic aldehyde produced from lipid peroxidation is 4-hydroxynonenal, which is generated from linoleic acid and arachidonic acid [122]. 4-Hydroxynonenal reacts easily and forms stable products with thiol groups on proteins and molecules such as glutathione [122]. Other amino acid groups on proteins also react with 4-hydroxynonenal.

Ozone has been shown to induce the production of 4-hydroxynonenal in vivo. Exposure of human subjects to 0.25 ppm ozone caused an increase in 4-hydroxynonenal protein adducts in lavage fluid and alveolar macrophages as determined by Western blot [123]. Lung lavage cells from mice exposed to 0.25 ppm ozone for 3 h also contained specific 4-hydroxynonenal-protein adducts [124]. Increased 4-hydroxynonenal adducts on two cellular proteins of approximately 32 kDa and 86–90 kDa were detected. The 32 kDa protein may be the stress protein heme oxygenase-1; the higher molecular weight protein may be another stress protein. Heme oxygenase 1 may be induced by oxidative stress and protect against it as well [125].

Oxidative stress has been suggested as a mediator of apoptosis (programmed cell death) [126]. Apoptosis in alveolar macrophages was detected after in vivo exposure of mice to 2.0 ppm ozone for 3 h [124]. In vitro, 4-hydroxynonenal was shown to induce apoptosis in murine alveolar macrophages [127]. Formation of the lipid peroxidation product 4-hydroxynonenal following ozone exposure may, therefore, play a role in the lung cell damage that results. Nevertheless, effects resulting from these extremely high ozone exposures may not be representative of effects in the lung during ambient exposures. More work is needed here.

Because biologically relevant concentrations of 4-hydroxynonenal ($<0.1\ \mu M$) stimulate chemotaxis of neutrophils in vitro [122], this lipid peroxidation product may contribute to the inflammatory process that results from ozone exposure by inducing the influx of neutrophils into the lung. 4-Hydroxynonenal has been shown to be produced by and to attract neutrophils in vitro [128]. To be convincing, it will need to be shown that such concentrations of the 4-hydroxynonenal are produced at ozone levels that are likely to occur at the lung surface during inhalation of ambient concentrations.

8.1.2 *Protein Oxidation*

Another hypothesis for the biological effects of ozone is that they result from its reaction with proteins. Using human erythrocytes as a membrane model, Freeman and Mudd [129] suggested that ozone reacts with proteins in preference to lipids in cell membranes, that it crosses the cell membrane to oxidize glutathione, and that it has no effect on hemoglobin. This last suggestion is contrary to the finding that synthetic fatty acid ozonides cause the formation of Heinz bodies in human erythrocytes [107]. In a study in which human erythrocyte ghosts were exposed to ozone, protein was found to be more susceptible to oxidation than lipid and only amino acids external to the membrane were oxidized [130].

Pryor and Uppu [131] found that tryptophan residues of proteins solubilized in reverse micelles were oxidized by ozone. Evidence suggests that the oxidation product was a Criegee ozonide. Results of experiments with human erythrocyte membranes showed that, in the presence of limiting amounts of ozone, ozonation of proteins and unsaturated lipids occurs concurrently and competitively [119]. Limiting amounts of ozone occur in environmental exposures, as well; that is, the number of molecules of ozone inhaled is much smaller than the number of molecules in the lung lining fluid with which ozone can react [132].

8.2 Nitrogen dioxide

As for ozone, the toxic effects of nitrogen dioxide inhalation are proposed to result from lipid peroxidation. Nitrogen dioxide causes lipid peroxidation when lipid bilayers are used as a model membrane system [133]. Vitamin E incorporated into the lipid bilayers protects unsaturated fatty acids against initiation of peroxidation by nitrogen dioxide [134]. Vitamin E provides greater protection against damage from nitrogen dioxide than against ozone [113,135]. More than likely, the reason for the difference in the protection is that ozonation products decompose into cytotoxic compounds not generated by nitrogen dioxide.

As a free radical, nitrogen dioxide is thought to attack unsaturated membrane lipids to produce carbon-centered free radicals, which begin the chain reaction of lipid peroxidation (Fig. 9). The mechanism of action of low concentrations of nitrogen dioxide with fatty acids that have doubly allylic hydrogen atoms is postulated to be hydrogen abstraction rather than addition to a double bond [136].

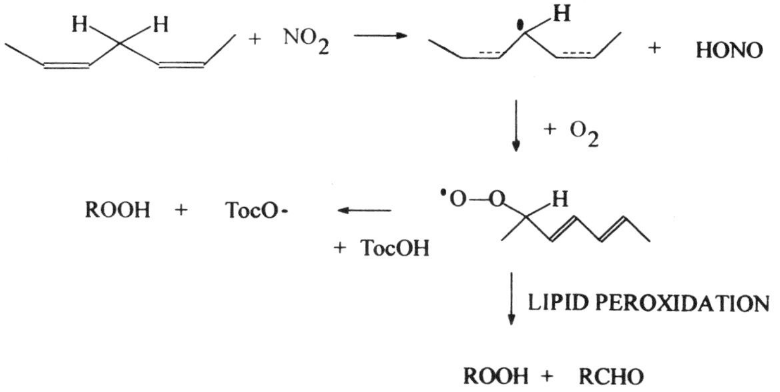

Fig. 9. Reaction of nitrogen dioxide with unsaturated fatty acids in cell membranes. Nitrogen dioxide, a radical, abstracts a methylenic hydrogen from unsaturated fatty acids and produces a carbon-centered free radical plus nitrous acid. The carbon free radical reacts with oxygen to form a peroxyl radical, which can initiate a chain reaction of lipid peroxidation. Vitamin E as α-tocopherol (TocOH) terminates lipid peroxidation by forming the relatively stable TocO radical, which can be reduced by vitamin C.

Another mechanism for the initiation of lipid peroxidation by inhaled nitrogen dioxide is via reactions with constituents of the lung lining fluid [137]. Free radicals generated from glutathione and vitamin C are proposed to initiate lipid peroxidation, which leads to cell damage.

Aldehydes may play a role in the toxicity of nitrogen dioxide as well as ozone. Nitrogen dioxide at noncytotoxic concentrations has been shown to cause the release of 4-hydroxynonenal along with other aldehydes from rat alveolar macrophages [138].

9.0 BIOCHEMICAL EFFECTS

9.1 Antioxidant enzyme activities

9.1.1   Ozone

Short-term exposure of rats to ozone has been shown to lead to an increase in the activities of the antioxidant enzymes copper-zinc superoxide dismutase, manganese superoxide dismutase, catalase, and glutathione peroxidase in the lung [139]. Manganese superoxide dismutase is induced in lung cells by various oxidants that cause inflammation and pulmonary fibrosis [140]. The glutathione antioxidant system composed of glutathione, glutathione peroxidase, and glutathione reductase is simulated in bronchoalveolar lavage cells of rats exposed to ozone acutely [141].

Site-specific changes in antioxidant enzyme activities in the lung were reported after long-term exposure of rats to ozone [142]. In the distal bronchioles, the activities of glutathione *S*-transferase, glutathione peroxidase, and superoxide dismutase increased significantly. Changes in the activities of the enzymes occurred in the distal trachea and major and minor daughter bronchi but not in other lung subcompartments.

9.1.2 Nitrogen dioxide

Temporal changes in lipid peroxidation and activities of antioxidant enzymes were studied in rat lungs following acute, subacute, and chronic exposures to a range of concentrations of nitrogen dioxide [143]. The activities of antioxidant enzymes initially increased and then slowly decreased. Lipid peroxides increased initially and then returned to control level before increasing again gradually. Lipid peroxidation as measured by ethane exhalation increased significantly in a dose-response manner throughout the long-term exposure. These results indicate that the protective effects of antioxidant enzymes against lipid peroxidation after acute exposure to nitrogen dioxide may be lacking during chronic exposure.

9.2 Antioxidants

9.2.1 Ozone

The depletion of the antioxidants ascorbic acid, uric acid, and glutathione was determined from human bronchoalveolar lavage fluid exposed to 0.05—1 ppm ozone [144]. Ozone depleted both vitamin C and uric acid from the fluid in a time- and concentration-dependent manner. Nevertheless, the rate of depletion showed substantial intersubject variability. For individuals, significant correlations were found between the rates of depletion of vitamin C and uric acid and the initial antioxidant concentrations. The rate of consumption of glutathione did not vary with ozone concentration. The investigators concluded that in human bronchoalveolar lavage fluid, the order of reactivity with ozone is vitamin C > uric acid > > glutathione.

When human plasma was used as a model for lung lining fluid, ozone at 2 ppm and 16 ppm also was found to react principally with vitamin C and uric acid [145]. Reactive absorption was surmised to be a mechanism of interaction. Neither glutathione nor dihydrolipoic acid blocked the oxidative damage to proteins and lipids that occurred after extended ozone treatment. Rates of consumption of vitamin C and uric acid also were unaffected by the thiol additions. The investigators concluded that the thiols increased the reactive absorption of ozone and that thiol supplementation may, therefore, protect the lower respiratory tract from injury by ozone.

9.2.2 Nitrogen Dioxide

Levels of lipid peroxidation products (mainly conjugated dienes) in alveolar lining fluid of human subjects exposed to 4 ppm nitrogen dioxide for 3 h were diminished considerably by supplementation with vitamins C and E for 4 weeks prior to exposure [146]. Vitamin C and E supplementation also prevented a reduction in the activity of α-1 protease inhibitor in the alveolar lining fluid by nitrogen dioxide exposure. α-1 Protease inhibitor protects the lung against proteolytic damage by blocking the activity of elastase, which is produced especially by neutrophils [19].

β-Carotene rapidly scavenges the free radicals nitrogen dioxide, thiyl radicals, and sulfonyl radicals [147]. The antioxidant reacts with the nitrogen dioxide by electron abstraction to form a radical cation whereas the reaction of β-carotene with the glutathione thiyl radical is a radical addition to form an adduct radical. Sulfonyl radicals react with β-carotene by both mechanisms. Both types of reaction products are stable and gradually decay to nonradical compounds. Further studies are needed to demonstrate these reactions in vivo.

10 SUMMARY

1. Ozone and nitrogen dioxide are the major oxidant air pollutants in smog.
2. Inhaled ozone and nitrogen dioxide cause toxicity primarily in the region of the lung where gas exchange takes place.
3. Exercise increases the deposition of ozone and nitrogen dioxide in the pulmonary region of the lung.
4. Acute exposure to ozone concentrations of 0.3 ppm during moderate exercise and of $\leqslant 0.2$ ppm during heavy exercise significantly reduces pulmonary function.
5. Exercise performance as determined by maximal oxygen uptake and endurance is reduced by acute ozone exposure.
6. Recovery of pulmonary function following acute ozone exposure typically occurs within 3—5 days.
7. Ozone effects on pulmonary function probably result from the reaction of ozone with the lung lining fluid and lung cells causing injury, inflammation, and the stimulation of neural pathways.
8. Increased airway responsiveness to bronchoconstrictors occurs following acute ozone exposure.
9. During moderate exercise, prolonged exposure to 0.08 ppm ozone causes pulmonary inflammation and to $\leqslant 0.12$ ppm ozone causes pulmonary function decrements.
10. Pulmonary function effects of mixtures of air pollutants in ambient air appear to be caused primarily by ozone.
11. The inflammatory response to ozone may be mediated by inflammatory cytokines and eicosanoids released from lung epithelial cells and macrophages.
12. Ozone and nitrogen dioxide inhalation can cause extrapulmonary effects.
13. Ozone and nitrogen dioxide cause peroxidation of unsaturated fatty acids in cell membranes; ozone also oxidizes cell membrane proteins.
14. Aldehydes and Criegee ozonides produced by the reaction of ozone with membrane lipids are possible mediators of ozone toxicity.
15. In experimental animals, exposure to ozone or nitrogen dioxide increases antioxidant enzyme activities in the lung.
16. Vitamin C in the lung lining fluid and vitamin E in cell membranes help protect against damage from inhaled ozone and nitrogen dioxide.

11 PERSPECTIVES

Ironically, the adverse health effects of air pollution on an individual are increased, not decreased, if the individual exercises while breathing polluted air. The chemical nature of the oxidant air pollutants is such that exercise increases the dose of nitrogen dioxide or ozone reaching the most distal portions of the lung. Outdoor exercise when ambient air pollutant levels are high (around noon to 1.00 pm) is to be avoided.

Despite considerable progress in reducing the amount of air pollution generated by each car in the USA, air pollution from mobile sources has increased or remained about the same due to the greater use of cars and other motor vehicles. Air pollution in developing or underdeveloped countries remains high and is increasing. In the future, major declines in ambient levels of nitrogen oxides and ozone are not likely unless there is an overall reduction in the transportation fleet or a change in the energy source driving the fleet. Electric cars are only marginally commercial, and it is unlikely that the ambitious goals set by the US EPA for replacement of internal combustion cars with electric cars will be met by the year 2010. Thus, health effects research on air pollution and particularly on nitrogen dioxide and ozone will be needed for the foreseeable future.

The national importance of air pollution also remains high because almost everyone is exposed to air pollution at levels likely to cause some kind of health effects. The episodic nature of air pollution moderates the health effects because periods of low air pollution exposure exist between periods of high air pollution exposure. An unknown is whether damage from air pollution over the short term is permanent or is fully repaired.

In this discussion, we have outlined the overall research on the short-term health effects in humans of ozone and nitrogen dioxide. Chronic health effects found in experimental animals clearly show that both oxidant air pollutants are major health hazards. The full impact of the oxidant air pollutants on human health is not known, but may be significant.

Obviously, reducing exposures to nitrogen dioxide and/or ozone is still the best public health policy. Recognizing that there are limits for reduction of oxidant air pollutants with present and foreseeable technology, research emphasis should be on quantifying the projected health effects at very low levels of the oxidants. Major studies of the long-term dose-response relationships of ozone and nitrogen dioxide in animals are needed so that oxidant air pollution levels can be extrapolated to below present ambient concentrations. If some biologically plausible estimate can be made of the improvement in public health by further reductions in oxidant air pollution, a value can be placed on the technology needed to move to another generation in mobile emissions technology.

To achieve such estimates, two types of research are needed. First, a much clearer understanding of the mechanisms of action of nitrogen dioxide and ozone is needed so that better experiments can be designed to gather the necessary data. Experiments are needed that are quantitative (not descriptive), that test a clear hypothesis, and that can be used in mathematical models on the health effects of the oxidant gases. The dosimetry model of ozone and nitrogen dioxide pioneered by Miller and his colleagues needs to be extended to an effects model. Secondly, better measures of interventions with antioxidants in the prevention of lung disease from oxidant air pollution are needed. It may be that the future of prevention of air pollution health effects falls to physiological or pharmacological interventions, rather than further reduction in sources of air pollution. Any therapeutic or preventive agent that can reduce the adverse health effects of air pollution will be useful immediately.

The public health costs of air pollution are enormous. The costs of emissions controls are equally enormous. Therefore, advances in this field have both national and international consequences. Because air pollution is a global problem, there is no population on earth that will not benefit from advances in preventing the adverse health effects of air pollution. There are about 14.6 million asthmatic and 14 million bronchitis patients in the USA [148]. Even if only 10% of the 28 million persons have a chronic respiratory disease due to air pollution, the prevention or cure of 2—3 million cases that might be due to oxidant air pollution would be a major public health achievement.

Despite much research, it is essential that the health effects of ozone and nitrogen dioxide at very low levels (e.g., less than the USA National Ambient Standards of 0.08 ppm for ozone and 0.053 ppm for nitrogen dioxide) be studied. We reviewed more than enough evidence to show that ozone and nitrogen dioxide are very toxic chemicals. Further, we purposely emphasized experiments at low levels (e.g., less than 0.5 ppm) because it is clear that different mechanisms underlie the chronic effects of ozone and nitrogen dioxide at ambient levels than at artificial levels of above 1 ppm. The evolving and exquisitely sensitive tools of molecular biology are needed here to quantify potential mechanisms of action. It is still unclear if ambient ozone and nitrogen dioxide cause permanent anatomical and functional alterations in the lung at levels that are likely to be present in the urban air through the next century. Because billions of people are exposed on every continent to oxidant air pollution, fully understanding why asthmatics and bronchitics appear to be more sensitive to ozone and nitrogen dioxide is one of the great public health challenges of our time.

12 ACKNOWLEDGEMENTS

We dedicate this paper to the memory of Mrs Lana Miller, wife of Dr Frederick J. Miller. As one of the long-suffering wives of the ozone research group of Dr David Coffin, Dr Donald E. Gardner, Dr Judith Graham, Dr Frederick J. Miller, and Dr Daniel B. Menzel, Lana encouraged and supported our endless debates over ozone on junkets throughout the world. Dr Daniel B. Menzel is also grateful to this discussion group for their ideas of the quantitative nature of ozone toxicity, to Dr John Overton for his insights into extrapolation modeling, to Prof William Pryor for his studies of the Criegee mechanism, to Prof Brian Mudd for his grasp of the effects of ozone on membrane proteins, to Dr Gary Hatch for his work on antioxidants in human lung lavage fluid, and to Prof Al Tappel for his comments on enzymatic antioxidants. We are also grateful to Dr Lester D. Grant of EPA and his staff for the use of the figures in this chapter, which are in the public domain. Mr John Bachman of EPA also provided critical views of the public health problem of air pollution. Prof Depak Bhalla shared data with us before publication and provided his views of the effects of ozone and nitrogen dioxide on the permeability of the lung. Prof Ronald E. Rasmussen provided invaluable help on the content, perspective, and biological aspects of the chapter. We thank Dr Peter Rombout for his insights into the global air pollution problem.

13 ABBREVIATION

FEV_1:   forced expiratory volume in 1 s

14 REFERENCES

1. Miller FJ, Overton JH, Jaskot RH, Menzel DB. Toxicol Appl Pharmacol 1985;79:11–27.
2. Overton JH, Graham RC, Miller FJ. Toxicol Appl Pharmacol 1987;88:418–432.
3. Pryor WA. Free Radic Biol Med 1994;17:451–465.
4. Menzel DB. Toxicol Ind Health 1993;9:323–336.
5. Menzel DB, Slaughter RJ, Bryant AM, Jauregui HO. Arch Env Health 1975;30:234–236.
6. Donovan DH, Williams SJ, Charles JM, Menzel DB. Toxicol Lett 1977;1:135–139.
7. Menzel DB. Ann NY Acad Sci 1992;669:141–155.
8. US Environmental Protection Agency. Air quality criteria for ozone and related photochemical oxidants, vol. 1. Research Triangle Park: US Environmental Protection Agency, 1996.
9. US Environmental Protection Agency. Air quality criteria for oxides of nitrogen, vol. 1. Research Triangle Park: US Environmental Protection Agency, 1993.
10. Medina-Navarro R, Lifshitz A, Wacher N, Hicks JJ. Arch Med Res 1997;28:205–208.
11. US Environmental Protection Agency. Air quality criteria for oxides of nitrogen, vol 3. Research Triangle Park: US Environmental Protection Agency, 1993.
12. Miller FJ. Toxicol Lett 1995;82–83:277–285.
13. Gerrity TR, Weaver RA, Berntsen J, House DE et al. J Appl Physiol 1988;65:393–400.
14. Wiester MJ, Stevens MA, Menache MG, McKee JL et al. Fund Appl Toxicol 1996;29:102–109.
15. Kabel JR, Ben-Jebria A, Ultman JS. J Appl Physiol 1994;77:2584–2592.
16. Gerrity TR, McDonnell WF, House DE. Toxicol Appl Pharmacol 1994;124:275-283.
17. Wagner HM. Staub Reinhalt Luft 1970;30:380–381.
18. Bauer MA, Utell MJ, Morrow PE, Speers DM et al. Am Rev Respir Dis 1986;134:1203–1208.
19. Mohsenin V. Toxicology 1994;89:301–312.
20. Reynolds HY. Am Rev Respir Dis 1987;135:250–263.
21. Chai H, Farr RS, Froehlich LA, Mathison DA et al. J Allergy Clin Immunol 1975;56:323–327.
22. Bates DV, Bell GM, Burnham CD, Hazucha M et al. J Appl Physiol 1972;32:176–181.
23. Hazucha M, Silverman F, Parent C, Field S et al. Arch Env Health 1973;27:183–188.
24. Adams WC, Savin WM, Christo AE. J Appl Physiol 1981;51:415–422.
25. Folinsbee LJ, Drinkwater BL, Bedi JF et al. Folinsbee LJ, Wagner JA, Borgia JF. Drinkwater BL, Gliner JA, Bedi JF (eds) Environmental stress: individual human adaptations. New York: Academic Press, 1978;125–145.
26. Hazucha MJ. J Appl Physiol 1987;62:1671–1680.
27. Adams WC, Schelegle ES. J Appl Physiol 1983;55:805–812.
28. Avol EL, Linn WS, Venet TG, Shamoo DA et al. J Air Pollut Control Assoc 1984;34:804–809.
29. Folinsbee LJ, Bedi JF, Horvath SM. J Appl Physiol 1984;57:984–988.
30. Gong HJ, Bradley PW, Simmons MS, Tashkin DP. Am Rev Respir Dis 1986;134:726–733.
31. McKittrick T, Adams WC. Arch Env Health 1995;50:153–158.
32. US Environmental Protection Agency. Air quality criteria for ozone and related photochemical oxidants, vol. 3. Research Triangle Park: US Environmental Protection Agency, 1996.
33. Ultman JS, Ben-Jebria A, MacDougall CS et al. Improvement of a respiratory ozone analyzer. Report No. 79. Cambridge: Health Effects Institute, 1997;1–22.

34. Wayne WS, Wehrle PF, Carroll RE. JAMA 1967;199:901—904.
35. Folinsbee LJ, Silverman F, Shepard RJ. J Appl Physiol 1977;42:531—536.
36. Horvath SM, Gliner JA, Matsen-Twisdale JA. Aviat Space Env Med 1979;50:901—905.
37. Savin WM, Adams WC. J Appl Physiol 1979;46:309—314.
38. Foxcroft WJ, Adams WC. J Appl Physiol 1986;61:960—966.
39. Schelegle ES, Adams WC. Med Sci Sports Exerc 1986;18:408—414.
40. Foster WM, Wills-Karp M, Tankersley CG, Chen X et al. J Appl Physiol 1996;81:794—800.
41. Hazbun ME, Hamilton R, Holian A, Eschenbacher WL. Am J Respir Cell Mol Biol 1993;9: 568—572.
42. Coleridge JC, Coleridge HM, Schelegle ES, Green JF. J Appl Physiol 1993;74:2345—2352.
43. Coleridge HM, Coleridge JC, Baker DG, Ginzel KH et al. Adv Exp Med Biol 1978;99: 291—305.
44. Coleridge HM, Coleridge JC, Ginzel KH, Baker DG et al. Nature 1976;264:451—453.
45. Koren HS, Devlin RB, Becker S, Perez R et al. Toxicol Pathol 1991;19:406—411.
46. Koren HS, Devlin RB, Graham DE, Mann R et al. Am Rev Respir Dis 1989;139:407—415.
47. Schelegle ES, Adams WC, Siefkin AD. Am Rev Respir Dis 1987;136:1350—1354.
48. Ying RL, Gross KB, Terzo TS, Eschenbacher WL. Am Rev Respir Dis 1990;142:817—821.
49. Hazucha MJ, Madden M, Pape G, Becker S et al. Eur J Appl Physiol 1996;73:17—27.
50. Roycroft JH, Gunter WB, Menzel DB. Toxicol Lett 1977;1:75—82.
51. Glaze WH. Envrion Health Perspect 1986;69:151—157.
52. Kanofsky JR, Sima P. J Biol Chem 1991;266:9039—9042.
53. Moller P, Wallin H, Knudsen LE. Chem Biol Interact 1996;102:17—36.
54. Frischer T, Pullwitt A, Kuhr J, Meinert R et al. Free Radic Biol Med 1997;22:201—207.
55. Seltzer J, Bigby BG, Stulbarg M, Holtzman MJ et al. J Appl Physiol 1986;60:1321—1326.
56. Devlin RB, McDonnell WF, Mann R, Becker S et al. Am J Respir Cell Mol Biol 1991;4:72—81.
57. Balmes JR, Chen LL, Scannell C, Tager I et al. Am J Respir Crit Care Med 1996;153:904—909.
58. Schelegle ES, Siefkin AD, McDonald RJ. Am Rev Respir Dis 1991;143:1353—1358.
59. Devlin RB, McDonnell WF, Becker S, Madden MC et al. Toxicol Appl Pharmacol 1996;138: 176—185.
60. Aris R, Christian D, Tager I, Ngo L et al. Am Rev Respir Dis 1993;148:965—973.
61. McBride DE, Koenig JQ, Luchtel DL, Williams PV et al. Am J Respir Crit Care Med 1994;149: 1192—1197.
62. Scannell C, Chen L, Aris RM, Tager I et al. Am J Respir Crit Care Med 1996;154:24—29.
63. Kehrl HR, Vincent LM, Kowalsky RJ, Horstman DH et al. Am Rev Respir Dis 1987;135: 1124—1128.
64. Bhalla DK, Daniels DS, Luu NT. Am J Respir Cell Mol Biol 1992;7:73—80.
65. Tepper JS, Costa DL, Lehmann JR, Weber MF et al. Am Rev Respir Dis 1989;140:493—501.
66. Horstman DH, Folinsbee LJ, Ives PJ, Abdul-Salaam S et al. Am Rev Respir Dis 1990;142: 1158—1163.
67. Aris RM, Tager I, Christian D, Kelly T et al. Chest 1995;107:621—628.
68. Hiltermann TJ, Stolk J, Hiemstra PS, Fokkens PH et al. Clin Sci (Colch) 1995;89:619—624.
69. Folinsbee LJ, Horstman DH, Kehrl HR, Harder S et al. Am J Respir Crit Care Med 1994;149: 98—105.
70. McDonnell WF, Kehrl HR, Abdul-Salaam S, Ives PJ et al. Arch Env Health 1991;46:145—150.
71. Hazucha MJ, Folinsbee LJ, Seal EJ. Am Rev Respir Dis 1992;146:1487—1493.
72. Horstman DH, Ball BA, Brown J, Gerrity T et al. Toxicol Ind Health 1995;11:369—385.
73. Koenig JQ, Covert DS, Hanley QS, van Belle G et al. Am Rev Respir Dis 1990;141:377—380.
74. Linn WS, Shamoo DA, Anderson KR, Peng RC et al. Am J Respir Crit Care Med 1994;150: 431—440.
75. Aris RM, Christian D, Hearne PQ, Kerr K et al. Am Rev Respir Dis 1993;148:1363—1372.
76. Adams WC, Brookes KA, Schelegle ES. J Appl Physiol 1987;62:1698—1704.
77. Hazucha MJ, Folinsbee LJ, Seal E, Bromberg PA. Am J Respir Crit Care Med 1994;150:

642−647.
78. Linn WS, Anderson KR, Shamoo DA, Edwards SA et al. Am J Respir Crit Care Med 1995;152: 885−891.
79. Avol EL, Linn WS, Shamoo DA, Spier CE et al. JAPCA 1987;37:158−162.
80. Avol EL, Linn WS, Shamoo DA, Valencia LM et al. Am Rev Respir Dis 1985;132:619−622.
81. Drechsler-Parks DM. Res Rep Health Eff Inst 1987;1−37.
82. Frampton MW, Morrow PE, Cox C, Gibb FR et al. Am Rev Respir Dis 1991;143:522−27.
83. Morrow PE, Utell MJ. Res Rep Health Eff Inst 1989;1−45.
84. Kulstrunk M, Bohni B. Schweiz Med Wochenschr 1992;122:375−381.
85. Kleinman MT, Bailey RM, Linn WS, Anderson KR et al. J Toxicol Env Health 1983;12: 815−826.
86. Avol EL, Linn WS, Peng RC, Whynot JD et al. Toxicol Ind Health 1989;5:1025−1034.
87. von Nieding G, Wagner HM, Krekeler H, Lollgen H et al. Int Arch Occup Env Health 1979;43: 195−210.
88. Linn WS, Solomon JC, Trim SC, Spier CE et al. Arch Env Health 1985;40:234−239.
89. Avol EL, Linn WS, Peng RC, Valencia G et al. Am Ind Hyg Assoc J 1988;49:143−149.
90. Roger LJ, Horstman DH, McDonnell W, Kehrl H et al. Toxicol Ind Health 1990;6:155−171.
91. Frampton MW, Finkelstein JN, Roberts NJ, Smeglin AM et al. Am J Respir Cell Mol Biol 1989; 1:499−505.
92. Linn WS, Jones MP, Bachmayer EA, Spier CE et al. Am Rev Respir Dis 1980;121:243−252.
93. Linn WS, Gong HJ, Shamoo DA, Anderson KR et al. Arch Env Health 1997;52:179−187.
94. Braun-Fahrlander C, Kunzli N, Domenighetti G, Carell CF et al. Pediatr Pulmonol 1994;17: 169−177.
95. Brunekreef B, Hoek G, Breugelmans O, Leentvaar M. Am J Respir Crit Care Med 1994;150: 962−966.
96. Hoek G, Fischer P, Brunekreef B, Lebret E et al. Am Rev Respir Dis 1993;147:111−117.
97. Selwyn, B.J., Stock, T.H., Hardy, R.J et al. In: Lee SD (ed) Evaluation of the scientific basis for ozone/oxidants standards: proceedings of an APCA international specialty conference; November 1984; Houston. Pittsburgh: Air Polution Control Association; 1985:281−296.
98. Spektor DM, Lippmann M, Thurston GD, Lioy PJ et al. Am Rev Respir Dis 1988;138:821−828.
99. Kinney PL, Nilsen DM, Lippmann M, Brescia M et al. Am J Respir Crit Care Med 1996;154: 1430−1435.
100. McKinnon KP, Madden MC, Noah TL, Devlin RB. Toxicol Appl Pharmacol 1993;118: 215−223.
101. Rusznak C, Devalia JL, Sapsford RJ, Davies RJ. Eur Respir J 1996;9:2298−2305.
102. Alpert SE, Walenga RW. Am J Physiol 1995;269:L734−743.
103. Schierhorn K, Zhang M, Kacy M, Kunkel G. Int Arch Allergy Immunol 1997;113:312−315.
104. Haddad EB, Salmon M, Sun J, Liu S et al. FEBS Lett 1995;363:285−288.
105. Su WY, Gordon T. J Appl Physiol 1996;80:1560−1567.
106. Morgan DL, Dorsey AF, Menzel DB. Fund Appl Toxicol 1985;5:137−143.
107. Menzel DB, Slaughter RJ, Bryant AM, Jauregui HO. Arch Env Health 1975;30:296−301.
108. Laskin DL, Pendino KJ, Punjabi CJ, Rodriguez del Valle M et al. Enviorn Health Perspect 1994; 102(Suppl 10):61−64.
109. Graham JA, Menzel DB, Miller FJ, Illing JW et al. Toxicol Appl Pharmacol 1981;61:64−73.
110. Miller FJ, Graham JA, Illing JW, Gardner DE. Toxicol Lett 1980;6:267−274.
111. Menzel DB. J Occ Med 1976;18:342−345.
112. Menzel DB. Annu Rev Pharmacol 1970;10:379−394.
113. Roehm JN, Hadley JG, Menzel DB. Arch Env Health 1971;23:142−148.
114. Thomas MJ, Robison TW, Samuel M, Forman HJ. Free Radic Biol Med 1995;18:553−537.
115. Pincemail J, Deby C, Camus G, Pirnay F et al. Eur J Appl Physiol 1988;57:189−191.
116. Elsayed NM, Mustafa MG, Mead JF. Arch Biochem Biophys 1990;282:263−269.
117. Pryor WA. Free Radic Biol Med 1992;12:83−88.

118. Pryor WA, Squadrito GL, Friedman M. Free Radic Biol Med 1995;19:935—941.
119. Uppu RM, Cueto R, Squadrito GL, Pryor WA. Arch Biochem Biophys 1995;319:257—266.
120. Pryor WA, Wu M. Chem Res Toxicol 1992;5:505—511.
121. Danielson UH, Esterbauer H, Mannervik B. Biochem J 1987;247:707—713.
122. Esterbauer H, Schaur RJ, Zollner H. Free Radic Biol Med 1991;11:81—128.
123. Hamilton RF, Hazbun ME, Jumper CA, Eschenbacher WL et al. Am J Respir Cell Mol Biol 1996;15:275—282.
124. Kirichenko A, Li L, Morandi MT, Holian A. Toxicol Appl Pharmacol 1996;141:416—424.
125. Abraham NG, Drummond GS, Lutton JD, Kappas A. Cell Physiol Biochem 1996;6:129—168.
126. Buttke TM, Sandstrom PA. Immunol Today 1994;15:7—10.
127. Li L, Hamilton RF, Kirichenko A, Holian A. Toxicol Appl Pharmacol 1996;139:135—143.
128. Schaur RJ, Dussing G, Kink E, Schauenstein E et al. Free Radic Res 1994;20:365—373.
129. Freeman BA, Mudd JB. Arch Biochem Biophys 1981;208:212—220.
130. Banerjee SK, Mudd JB. Arch Biochem Biophys 1992;295:84—89.
131. Pryor WA, Uppu RM. J Biol Chem 1993;268:3120—3126.
132. Pryor WA, Bermudez E, Cueto R, Squadrito GL. Fund Appl Toxicol 1996;34:148—156.
133. Shoaf CR, Wolpert RL, Menzel DB. Inhal Toxicol 1989;1:301—314.
134. Shoaf CR, Wolpert RL, Menzel DB. Inhal Toxicol 1989;1:315—329.
135. Menzel DB, Roehm JN, Lee SD. J Agric Food Chem 1972;20:481—486.
136. Gallon AA, Pryor WA. Lipids 1994;29:171—176.
137. Postlethwait EM, Langford SD, Jacobson LM, Bidani A. Free Radic Biol Med 1995;19:553—563.
138. Robison TW, Forman HJ, Thomas MJ. Biochim Biophys Acta 1995;1256:334—340.
139. Rahman I, Clerch LB, Massaro D. Am J Physiol 1991;260:L412—418.
140. Quinlan T, Spivack S, Mossman BT. Env Health Perspect 1994;102(Suppl)2:79—87.
141. Boehme DS, Hotchkiss JA, Henderson RF. Exp Mol Pathol 1992;56:37—48.
142. Plopper CG, Duan X, Buckpitt AR, Pinkerton KE. Toxicol Appl Pharmacol 1994;127:124—131.
143. Sagai M, Ichinose T. Environ Health Perspect 1987;73:179—189.
144. Mudway IS, Housley D, Eccles R, Richards RJ et al. Free Radic Res 1996;25:499—513.
145. van der Vliet A, O'Neil CA, Eiserich JP, Cross CE. Arch Biochem Biophys 1995;321:43—50.
146. Mohsenin V. J Appl Physiol 1991;70:1456—1462.
147. Everett SA, Dennis MF, Patel KB, Maddix S et al. J Biol Chem 1996;271:3988—3994.
148. US Bureau of the Census. Statistical abstract of the United States, 1994. Washington, D.C., US Dept. of Commerce, 1995.

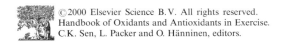

©2000 Elsevier Science B.V. All rights reserved.
Handbook of Oxidants and Antioxidants in Exercise.
C.K. Sen, L. Packer and O. Hänninen, editors.

555

Part VIII ● Chapter 20

Risk of oxidative stress at high altitude and possible benefit of antioxidant supplementation

I.M. Simon-Schnass

Nutrisan, Privat-Institute for Nutrition Research, Unterfeldstr. 5a, D-82377 Penzberg, Germany.

1   INTRODUCTION
2   PHYSICAL EXERCISE AT A HIGH ALTITUDE
    2.1   High altitude hypoxia
    2.2   Energy metabolism
    2.3   Evidence for increased oxidative stress at high altitudes
    2.4   Indirect studies on oxidative stress at a high altitude
3   INCREASED UV-RADIATION WITH INCREASING ALTITUDE
4   HIGH TEMPERATURE DIFFERENCES AT A HIGH ALTITUDE
5   DEHYDRATION
6   NUTRITIONAL DEFICITS
7   SUMMARY
8   ABBREVIATIONS
9   REFERENCES

1   INTRODUCTION

It is very likely that different readers may have very different expectations regarding this topic. The terms "exercise", as well as "high altitude" can be interpreted quite differently. This depends largely on the person's intention. It may be someone who wants to spend his holidays in a hotel in the mountains, or someone on a trekking tour in Europe or abroad. It might be an athlete participating in a training session at about 2,500 m or a high altitude mountaineer who will spend some weeks or months at an altitude of at least 4,000 m or higher. Or it might be someone living permanently at an altitude above 2,500 m who performs physical work or does some sport. Due to this, it is clear that motivation, training status and adaptation to altitude may be very different.

What are the main characteristics of high altitude with which people are confronted with? Initially one would think that high altitude concerns the decreased availability of oxygen with its influence on metabolism and thereby on physical and mental performance. However, there are other factors one must bear in mind too. The most important being increased UV-radiation, high temperature differences, sometimes increased psychological stress, dehydratation and malnutrition.

There is growing evidence that oxidative injury mediated by free radicals is an important factor in various pathologies including adverse metabolic reactions at high altitudes. All aerobic cells must adapt to develop and maintain a defence system against oxidative damage. The protection against these damaging free radicals is provided by cellular and extracellular antioxidants. Enzymes, as well as low molecular antioxidants, are components of this system. The "antioxidative strategy" of aerobic cells is targeted at inhibiting or blocking potentially toxic oxygen species, their derivatives at the various levels of formation or their reaction with biomolecules [1].

Typical "detoxification enzymes" are superoxide dismutase, the catalases and various peroxidases. If the organism is confronted with radicals, as is the case of physical activity, these enzymes are reactively synthesized to an elevated degree. Clearly, a certain time-lag between the occurrence of the noxae, (free radicals), and the higher enzymatic level as a protective measure cannot be avoided. If the stimulus for the increased enzyme formation does not occur any more, it drops back to its original level. This suggests that enzymatic protection against oxidation can only be effectively boosted by regular occurrence of free radicals. From this point of view, athletes who train irregularly, and/or at varying degrees of intensity, are relatively insufficiently protected against oxidative stress by enzymes [2]. On the other hand, populations with nutritional deficits may not be able to build up the defense system and may, therefore, be susceptible to oxidative stress, as could be shown in an Andean population [3].

On the other hand, the defence system comprises various antioxidants in addition to the antioxidative enzymes. Many substances that also occur physiologically represent antioxidants in vitro. Until now, practical relevance has only been found for vitamins E and C, β-carotene and some other carotenoids, as well as glutathione and, in certain cases, a-lipoic acid, uric acid, taurine, the amino acids cysteine and histidine, as well as several xenobiotics.

Vitamin E is a lipophilic radical inhibitor. Correspondingly, its action is mainly limited to the region of the lipophilic membrane and the lipoproteins in plasma. Because it is stored in the immediate vicinity of the substances in danger of oxidation, vitamin E can very effectively circumvent the peroxidation of fatty acids, as well as the oxidation of cholesterol and proteins. This is of great importance for membrane integrity. Even during vitamin E deficiency, no other antioxidant could yet be proven that acts to break the radical chain-reaction in the lipophilic area of the cell. This means that vitamin E cannot be replaced by any other substances at its functional site. In addition to the inhibition of lipid peroxidation in the lipophilic centers of biological membranes, vitamin E also appears to play a role in the repair of oxidated amino acids, which otherwise may build blocks of proteins. In this way, vitamin E could also be attributed to a special role in the repair of damaged amino acids in the integral membrane proteins [1]. Recent papers also suggest an important role of vitamin E in the intracellular signaling [4—6].

Vitamin C is known as an excellent water-soluble antioxidant with a strong reducing potential. It is capable of scavenging a wide variety of different oxidants. For example, it has been shown to scavenge superoxide anions, hydrogenperoxide, OH-radical, aqueous peroxyl radicals, as well as singlet oxygen effectively [7]. As an antioxidant, vitamin C undergoes a 2-electron oxidation to dehydroascorbic acid with intermediate formation of a relatively unreactive ascorbyl radical [8]. Dehydroascorbic acid is unstable and hydrolyses readily to diketogulonic acid. On the other hand, it also can be reduced back to ascorbic acid by glutathione in erythrocytes and other blood cells [9].

As a water soluble substance, vitamin C is predominantly found in plasma and the aqueous phase of the cell. In particular, vitamin C deactivates the extracellular oxidants generated by activated neutrophiles [10] and also quenches radicals diffused to the extracellular space. Moreover, vitamin C interacts with the membrane-bound vitamin E by reducing the tocopheryl radical back to tocopherol [11].

In addition to vitamin E, the β-carotene and some other carotenoids (also lipid-soluble) have been shown to be effective chain-breaking antioxidants. The peroxyl-trapping activity of β-carotene and possibly other carotenoids is dependent on the partial pressure of oxygen. It is less effective in the presence of air, but becomes a good peroxyl radical trap at low pO_2 which prevails in biological tissues [12]. At very low pO_2 (4 torr) it inhibited lipid peroxidation even better than vitamin E [13].

The antioxidative strategy of aerobic cells is aimed at reducing or blocking the potentially toxic effects of activated oxygen species, which are generated by various metabolic processes and which may cause oxidative stress. The question now is if there is oxidative stress during a (prolonged) stay at (high) altitude. In the following several possible sources of free radical generation are discussed.

2 PHYSICAL EXERCISE AT A HIGH ALTITUDE

2.1 High altitude hypoxia

Aerobic energy supply is necessary for all higher life forms. In accordance, an inadequate oxygen supply leads from unnoticed metabolic impairments up to a direct life threat. A drop in arterial oxygen pressure below a nominal level may be due to a number of factors, including a decreased oxygen partial pressure as occurs at high altitude.

Acute exposure to high altitude results in a fall in the amount of oxygen available to the body and thus, to a decreased arterial blood oxygen saturation. This leads to a reduction in maximal aerobic power of approximately 1% for every 100 m above 1,500 m [14]. However, as the body has compensation mechanisms to counteract the resulting hypoxia, acclimatization is possible. This includes an increase in hematocrit and hemoglobin to improve the transport capacity for oxygen (compensatory polycythemia), a shift in oxygen binding to hemoglobin, as well as an increase in capillary density, mitochondria, and tissue myoglobin [15,16]. Moreover, muscle glycogen is saved and mobilization and metabolism of free fatty acids improved as shown by a decrease in blood lactate and ammonia during submaximal exercise [17,18]. These changes are remarkably similar to those induced by endurance training and are aimed at reducing the oxygen demand of the body and optimizing the utilization of the available oxygen.

2.2 ENERGY METABOLISM

Physical performance can be looked at as stress and a regular training as an adaptation to stress. When the stimulus impairs homeostasis, catabolic processes are of major importance. Today, impairment of homeostasis is considered to be the cause of adaptive changes in the stressed system. The adaptation reactions cause homeostasis to be achieved at a higher level. This is where anabolic processes dominate.

Each movement is associated with the turnover of substrates, including oxygen and thus, with energy consumption. From a simplified point of view, blood circulation is no more than an aid to substrate delivery and removal.

Circulation increases during dynamic activity, as the increased consumption of substrates and the removal of end products would otherwise not be possible. However, muscular concentration also leads to vascular compression, which in turn may cause a regional and short-term reduction in circulation with limited hypoxia. This particularly applies to sports with concentrated power development. On the other hand, in sports with an emphasis on endurance and a less locally active force, the transport capacity of the blood and oxygen exchange into the cell become the limiting factors. In both cases, transient oxygen deficiency can occur, despite the high oxygen turnover [19].

Classical sports physiology has concerned itself intensively with the phenomena of availability, turnover and regeneration of substrates for obtaining energy. In addition to this, a fact that has as yet hardly been acknowledged, the effects on the structured components of the cell are of essential relevance. The cell membrane contains important switching points for transport processes, as well as for reactive processes. It is no coincidence that the compartmentalisation of the cell is a major feature of living structures. Indeed this is the basis from which the cell is able to function. Membranes participate in some form in the vast majority of metabolic processes. The main objective, even in the case of intense physical performance is always to maintain the integrity of the membrane structures, or at least that changes be reversible [20].

The major cause of membrane damage is the formation of free radicals, which can arise from various processes during metabolism. In the aerobic energy supply, most of the ATP is formed during endoxidation. This is when electrons of a substrate, (e.g., pyruvate or succinate), are transformed via a so-called redox chain into oxygen, the end product formed being water (reduction of the oxygen to water);

$$O_2 + 4H^+ + 4e \rightarrow 2H_2O \quad (water)$$

It is known that free radicals can arise in the case of incomplete oxygen reduction. If less than 4 electrons are made available, the following activated oxygen species are created:

$$O_2 + 1e \quad\quad\quad\quad \rightarrow \quad \cdot O_2^- \quad (superoxide\ radical)$$

$$O_2 + 2e + 2H^+ \quad\quad \rightarrow \quad H_2O_2 \quad (hydrogen\ peroxide)$$

$$O_2 + 3e + 3H^+ \quad\quad \rightarrow \quad HO^- + \cdot OH \quad (hydroxyl\ radical)$$

In the resting state, 250−300 ml of oxygen per min are usually taken up. Under physical exertion, oxygen uptake can increase to 4,700 ml per min, or even more, depending on training conditions. Around 3−10% of the metabolized oxygen is not completely reduced to water, but to these different radicals [20].

However, other metabolic processes also lead to the generation of free radicals. Physically strenuous activity induces certain inflammatory-like reactions which are associated with the increased formation of radicals, (e.g., leukocyte activation with phagocytosis, leukotriene synthesis). In addition, radicals from outside are taken up into the body, e.g., from UV-radiation, air pollution, cigarette smoke etc. This can also be of great relevance because the damaging reactive mechanisms of these radicals do not differ greatly from the reactions mentioned above [21].

One characteristic of free radicals is their high, if in part extremely high, reactive capability. Activated oxygen species react very readily with other substances and thus, form other radicals. Particular mention should be given to reactions with lipids, (formation of fatty acid radicals), and with proteins, particularly those which contain functional SH-groups (inactivation, formation of carbonyls). Destructive chain reactions which will be mentioned later, can be set off and lead to functional impairments and even complete destruction of the cell [21].

In case of extreme physical activity, (the term "extreme" being defined as of an individual nature), the following factors can lead to an increased discharge of free radicals. The oxygen turnover can be increased up to 20 times resting consumption. In accordance, the incomplete reduction of oxygen to water and the associated formation of free radicals can also increase. Hypoxic cells are particularly susceptible to oxidative stress. If there is not enough oxygen available to accept electrons, they will be transferred to other low molecular weight molecules which in turn induce radical chain reactions. When the pH drops, (metabolic acidosis during extreme physical exertion), O_2 can be converted into the highly toxic $\cdot OOH$ radical. $\cdot O2$ is derived from the respiratory chain, whereas the required hydrogen is supplied by the lactic acid which is formed. In the case of physiological pH, only around 1% of the $\cdot O2$ is converted to an $\cdot OOH$ radical. However, the percentage increases with increasing acidosis [20,22].

The imbalance between an increased formation of (oxygen) radicals and the antioxidative capacity of a cell, tissue or organism, is termed oxidative stress [23]. In recent reviews the evidence for oxidative stress and its potential cellular damage, as well as the role of antioxidants in the control of these processes, has been discussed [2,24−27]. Aerobic exercise may lead to the generation of radicals capable of damaging lipids, proteins, carbohydrates and DNA [28,29]. There is increasing evidence that vitamins E and C, together with other low molecular weight antioxidants and antioxidative enzymes, protect against the damage of reactive oxygen species generated during exercise [26,30].

2.3 Evidence for increased oxidative stress at high altitudes

One of the very few studies discussing the influence of an antioxidant (vitamin E) in a situation of oxidative stress at high altitude, (physical performance at varying altitudes), is that of Nagawa et al. of 1968 [31]. Twenty endurance-trained athletes participated in exercise tests carried out at sea level, and at 2700 m and 2900 m altitude. Two types of work load were used. A bicycle-ride to complete exhaustion at 1300 kpm/min at 75 rpm and an interval run in which 200 m dash (30 s) and jogging (60 s) were repeated 21 times. Among other parameters, oxygen intake, blood lactate and pyruvate were determined before and after exercise. In addition the athletes received 300 mg vitamin E/d or placebo.

In the bicycle ride, the maximum and the final values of oxygen intake and oxygen pulse were higher in the supplemented group. Although the performance of both groups was lowered at high altitude, the supplemented group showed better records in events longer than 5,000 m compared to the placebo group. Postexercise blood lactate was lower in the experimental group.

The authors conclude from these results that vitamin E might have an accelerating effect on endurance, due to its ability to increase activity of respiratory enzymes in mitochondria of muscle cells and thereby improving the utilization of oxygen in muscle during activity, especially a high altitude [31].

This hypothesis is supported by the results of a later study on the effect of vitamin E on physical performance a high altitude [32]. Twelve mountaineers were supplemented with 400 mg vitamin E/d (supplemented group) or a placebo (placebo group) during an expedition to K2 (8,611 m). Supplementation started before the departure. The base camp was established at about 5100 m. The anaerobic threshold was determined before departure and 3 times at base camp with an interval of 2 weeks. The anaerobic threshold is generally defined as the work load which leads to a lactic acid blood level of 4 mmol/l. Accumulation of lactic acid in serum was caused by performing graded exercise until exhaustion on a bicycle with 3-min load steps starting at 50 Watts and with increments of 50 Watts. Given the baseline performance at the anaerobic threshold at 100%, the other three terms are expressed in percent of baseline. These data are shown in Fig. 1.

There was no significant difference between the baseline values of the two groups. In the course of the experiment, the anaerobic threshold of the treatment group increased while in the placebo group it first increased, but to a smaller degree, and then decreased compared to the initial value. The difference between the changes of the anaerobic threshold of the treatment group and the placebo group became significant ($p < 0.01$) after 4 weeks, these are the terms 3 and 4.

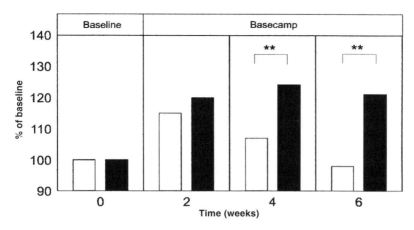

Fig. 1. Influence of vitamin E supplementation (400 IU/d) on performance at the anaerobic threshold shown as % of baseline. Open bar represents placebo group, closed bar supplemented group. Baseline determined before departure to altitude and after 2, 4 and 6 weeks at basecamp at 5,100 m (16,730 ft). Data are means (n = 12). **Significant difference at $p < 0.01$ compared with placebo.

The effect of altitude on the anaerobic threshold has been barely investigated. The results of the placebo group in the above described study, however, confirm the previous observation that a prolonged stay at a high altitude leads to a reduced physical performance, apparent as a decreased anaerobic threshold.

By its stabilizing effect on various components of the respiratory chain, vitamin E contributes to aerobic energy production [33—35]. A local vitamin E deficiency leads to disturbances of electron transport and thus, to reduced cell respiration [36—38]. This is especially apparent when the available oxygen is also limited, as occurs due to high demand, poor local supply or low partial pressure of oxygen. It can be expected that the impairment of metabolism is especially pronounced under conditions of increased physical load at high altitude. Investigations have shown that a prolonged stay at extreme altitudes leads to a loss of activity of succinate and lactate dehydrogenase [39]. The activity of both enzymes in skeletal muscle is also decreased by vitamin E deficiency [40—42]. This can be explained by their content of labile SH-groups, which have to be protected by the antioxidant.

The possible involvement of labile SH-groups suggests that free radical reaction have to be taken into consideration. There are very few studies performed which show that there is indeed an increased risk of free radical production during exercise at high altitude. In simulated altitude the plasma concentration of oxidized Glutathione (GSSG) increased significantly [43], which may be the result of an increased production of free radicals. Hoshikawa et al. [44] suggest that hypoxia causes oxidative stress in the lung tissue and that oxidative stress may have a role in the development of pulmonary hypertension, induced by chronic hypoxia. In their experiment it could be shown that a free radical scavenger (N-acetyl-L -

cystine) was able to prevent oxidative stress during chronic hypoxia in rats. Kou-delova and Mourek determined an increased lipid peroxidation in the cerebral cortex, the subcortical formations, the medulla oblongata and the cerebellum in rats exposed to a simulated altitude of 7,000 to 9,000 m (22,950 to 29,500 ft). Young animals were more vulnerable than older animals [45]. If this damage is caused by free radicals, oxidative stress may be connected to the increase in blood-brain barrier permeability observed at high altitude [46,47], which may contribute to the frequent occurrence of brain edema at high altitude.

Nakanishi et al. [48] measured the effects of hypobaric hypoxia on the antioxi-dant enzymes in rats. They found that under these conditions there was an increase in malondialdehyde (MDA), a product of lipid peroxidation, in plasma, heart, lung, liver and kidney of the rats, which supports the increased formation of free radicals. Reactively SOD increased in plasma, but decreased in liver and lungs. GSH-peroxidase increased in the heart and lungs but decreased in liver. Katalase decreased too in the liver and kidney. From these results the authors suppose that the liver is more vulnerable than other organs to oxidative stress at high altitude. These data are supported by the work of Costa et al. [49].

The exhalation of pentane can be considered to be a result of lipid peroxidation [50]. In animal, as well as in human studies, it could be related to the vitamin E status [35,51]. Various conditions, such as an increased energy turnover and/or hypoxia, favor lipid peroxidation [20,51]. Vitamin E is one of the most effective membrane-bound radical scavengers. In animals, exercise-induced lipid peroxi-dation could be prevented by vitamin E administration [21,52].

To test if there is indeed an increased oxidative stress leading to increased lipid peroxidation at high altitude, the amount of exhaled pentane was determined by gas-chromatography during the above described expedition to K2. Pentane was measured twice, the baseline value before departure and the second after two weeks at base camp. The results are shown in Fig. 2.

There was no significant difference between the initial pentane exhalation of the two groups, but after four weeks of supplementation and two weeks at high altitude, the exhaled pentane increased significantly ($p < 0.01$) in the placebo group. In the treatment group there was no noticeable change. It can be con-cluded from this study that high altitude climbing incurs a considerable risk of metabolically-induced cell damage. This can be counteracted by supplementation with antioxidants.

As mentioned above membranes are most susceptible to oxidative stress because of their high amount of polyunsaturated fatty acids. Erythrocytes are able to change their shape due to their membrane fluidity among others. The loss of this fluidity can be influenced by different factors such as acidosis, hyperthermia, immobilization (stasis) e.g., due to aggregation, membrane defects and cell aging [53]. As the important underlying phenomenon is considered to be an oxidative change of membrane lipids and proteins, it is suggested that they may be triggered by free radicals [50]. The filterability of the red blood cells is considered a measurement of their flexibility. This parameter was tested during

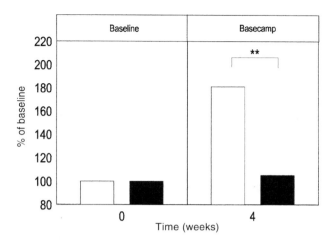

Fig. 2. Influence of vitamin E supplementation (400 IU/d) on pentane exhalation shown as % of baseline. Open bar represents placebo group, closed bar supplemented group. Baseline determined before departure to altitude and after 4 weeks at basecamp at 5,100 m (16,730 ft). Data are means (n = 12). **Significant difference at $p < 0.01$ compared with placebo.

two other expeditions at a high altitude.

During the first study, 12 mountaineers were supplemented with either 400 mg vitamin E/d (supplemented group) or a placebo (placebo group) during an expedition to Annapurna (8,091 m) [54]. Supplementation started before departure. The basecamp was established at 4,300 m. For standardization reasons the erythrocyte filterability is expressed as the quotient of an unfilterized to a filterized sample. Given the baseline filterability as 100%, the other two terms are expressed in percent of baseline. These data are given in Fig. 3.

It could be shown that red blood cell filterability deteriorates at a high altitude. The fact that no change in erythrocyte filterability was detected in the supplemented-group indicates that protection from oxidation was adequate there. The significant drop in filterability in the placebo group ($p < 0.05$) on the other hand, permits the conclusion that the oxidative stress led to depletion of vitamin E and/or other antioxidative substances.

In order to prove that the reason for this is indeed the effect of an increased free radical production, the test was repeated during an expedition to Solo Khumbu, close to Mt. Everest, comprising several different scientific projects. In this special unit 10 scientists were supplemented with either 400 mg vitamin E/d (supplemented group) or a placebo (placebo group). The tests were conducted in a permanently established laboratory at an altitude of 5,000 m. Unfortunately only data of 1 and 3 weeks after arrival at the laboratory are available because the organizers and some scientific heads could not be convinced to agree to the determination of low altitude values as well. Therefor in this case, the first term at altitude is the baseline value. The results are shown in Fig. 4. They are

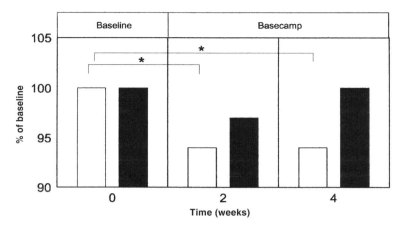

Fig. 3. Influence of vitamin E supplementation (400 IU/d) on erythrocyte filterability shown as % of baseline. Open bar represents placebo group, closed bar supplemented group. Baseline determined before departure to altitude and after 2 and 4 weeks at basecamp at 4,300 m (14,100 ft). Data are means (n = 12). *Significant difference at p < 0.05 compared with placebo.

very similar to the first experiment already described. The difference between the two groups after two weeks at altitude is again significant with p < 0.05 [55].

In addition, the susceptibility of the erythrocytes of the same blood sample against peroxidation was tested by measuring the amount of thiobarbituric acid reactive substances (TBARS). In contrast to the slight decrease in TBARS formation in the supplemented group, there is a tremendous increase in the placebo group. This clearly shows that there is indeed increased oxidative stress at a high altitude. As shown later, the average daily intake of vitamin E of this group was

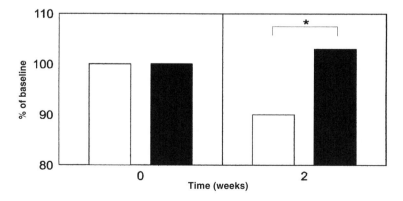

Fig. 4. Influence of vitamin E supplementation (400 IU/d) on erythrocyte filterability shown as % of baseline. Open bar represents placebo group, closed bar supplemented group. Baseline determined after arrival at altitude and after 2 weeks sojourn at 5,000 m (16,400 ft). Data are means (n = 12). *Significant difference at p < 0.05 compared with placebo.

16.8 mg. Obviously this amount was inadequate to meet with the demand at a high altitude. The data are given in Fig. 5.

There was also a negative correlation between the filterability of the erythrocytes and the amount of TBARS measured during this experiment (r = –0.9190 resp. r = –0.8218). This indicates that membranes which are more susceptible to oxidative stress in vitro (increased TBARS) are also more susceptible in vivo (decreased filterability) [55]. Together with the above given results of the pentane measurement, this shows that there is increased oxidative stress at a high altitude and that a supplementation with antioxidants can counteract with its negative consequences.

2.4 Indirect studies on oxidative stress at a high altitude

As shown, increased free radical production not only influences physical performance by deteriorating energy metabolism but also has a negative influence on membranes. This could be demonstrated by the experiments on red blood cells. This is of central importance, especially at a high altitude.

At high altitudes the body attempts to boost the blood's oxygen transport capacity by increasing erythropoiesis, resulting in a compensatory polycythemia. This has significant influence on capillary blood supply which is mainly determined by cardiac output, vascular resistance and the rheological properties of the blood or its constituents.

The special rheological properties of the blood arise from its two-phase composition of plasma and blood cells. The viscosity of the blood depends largely on the packed cell volume, plasma viscosity, the deformability of the erythrocytes and their tendency to aggregate [56,57].

Blood is a liquid without Newtonian properties. Instead its viscosity varies as a

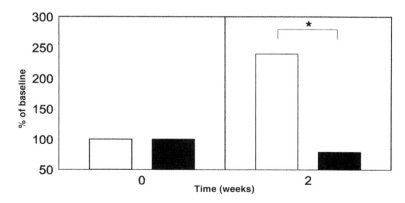

Fig. 5. Influence of vitamin E supplementation (400 IU/d) on thiobarbituric acid-reactive-substances (TBARS) shown as % of baseline. Open bar represents placebo group, closed bar supplemented group. Baseline determined after arrival at altitude and after 2 weeks sojourn at 5,000 m (16,400 ft). Data are means (n = 12). *Significant difference at p < 0.05 compared with placebo.

function of flow conditions. The very same blood can at one time be highly fluid and rapidly flowing, at another highly viscous with sluggish flow. In in vitro measurements an elevated hematocrit level is discernible immediately, whereas in vivo the situation is much more complex. Because of the special two-phase composition of blood, under otherwise normal conditions, a high hematocrit does not necessarily cause changes in flow characteristics in the terminal vessels, as the local hematocrit in the capillaries is much lower (with a high flow-rate) than in the larger blood vessels [58]. However, there are limits to even this mechanism. Thus, today it is also assumed that from hematocrit levels over 50—55%, the oxygen transport capacity falls again, even in pulmonary diseases [59,60]. Hematocrit levels of 60% and more are not a rare finding in high altitude climbers. In the event of a general or localized reduction in flow velocity, however, the capillary hematocrit level approaches the venous hematocrit, an aggregation occurs. In this case the hematocrit becomes highly important.

In case of a high hematocrit, one of the major factors determining if local oxygen supply is still improved or already decreased is the flexibility of the erythrocytes, which is highly dependent on membrane integrity. As discussed above, hypoxia leads to oxidative stress. There is increased formation of free radicals which triggers lipid peroxidation. As a result, membrane fluidity (measured by erythrocyte filterability) deteriorates. As vitamin E is directly incorporated into the membranes, it should counteract such processes there.

In addition to blood viscosity, the elasticity and integrity of the vascular wall plays an important role in capillary blood supply. Here too, oxidative changes are discussed as a pathogenetic factor [50]. The release of tissue hormones such as histamine, kinines and prostaglandins also play an important part in the damage of the vascular wall [58]. Endothelial lesions may lead to disturbances in microcirculation. These may be compounded by activation of the coagulation system, with resultant consumption coagulopathia. This can lead to the formation of microthrombi and, consequently, increased reactive fibrinolysis. This in turn then results in an increased tendency to hemorrhages [61].

The aforementioned disturbances are frequently found during a prolonged stay at a high altitude. Here, the pathological changes are mainly in the area of the pulmonary and cerebral capillaries, but also in those of the retina and the mucosa [62].

Both the radical-binding properties of vitamin E and its involvement in the metabolism of eicosanoids, (which may be related to each other), indicate that this vitamin has an effect on the phenomena described above [63—65].

In the aforementioned study, (expedition to Annapurna), the influence of a supplementation with 400 IE vitamin E/d on several of these rheological parameters was tested. Those included whole blood and plasma viscosity, white blood cells, platelets, antithrombin III and protein C. [54]. Here, only the data on white blood cells and two anti-aggregational substances are discussed.

The viscosity of blood is mainly determined by the amount of blood cells, their flexibility and the plasma viscosity. The results of our study and the experience of mountaineers [66] show that an adequate fluid intake not only maintains the hematocrit in a physiologically acceptable range, but can also prevent hemoconcentration and a related increase in plasma viscosity. As there was no correlation between hematocrit and plasma viscosity it can be assumed that the volunteers of our study did not experience any appreciable dehydration. The increase in whole blood viscosity was, therefore, mostly the result of the increase of blood cells and their membrane rigidity.

Because of their rigidity and spherical shape leukocytes (WBC) cannot pass through the terminal vessel as easily as erythrocytes. Even under physiological conditions there may be a reduction in flow velocity or even temporary stasis in the passage of leukocytes through the capillaries [67]. If the perfusion pressure falls, pronounced disturbances of microcirculation occur, mainly due to the white blood cells. Thus, there may also be, for example, occlusion of the arterioles and venules, e.g due to adhesions to the vascular walls [68,69]. Figure 6 shows the changes in total WBC, as well as the subgroup of granulocytes at high altitude with and without supplementation with vitamin E. Although there was an increase in total leucocytes in both groups it was much more pronounced in the placebo group (p < 0.05). A splitting into the different subgroups showed the most clear changes with respect to the granulocytes (p < 0.05).

After stimulation, e.g., by activation of complement, endotoxins, immune complexes, or leukotriene B4, there is a particularly substantial rise in the tendency of the leukocytes and, in particular, the granulacytes, to aggregate. This in turn leads not only to a further increased risk of occlusion, but also to increased

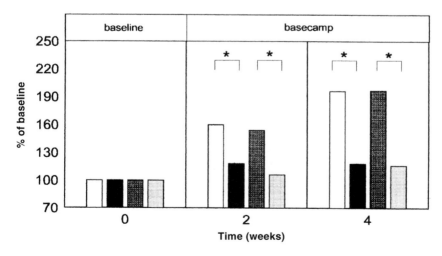

Fig. 6. Influence of vitamin E supplementation (400 IU/d) on granulocytes. Open bar represents placebo group, closed bar supplemented group and total white blood cells (WBC). Light grey bar represents placebo group, dark grey bar supplemented group, shown as % of baseline. Baseline determined before departure to altitude and after 2 and 4 weeks at basecamp at 4,300 m (14,100 ft). Data are means (n = 12). *Significant difference at p < 0.05 compared with placebo.

release of intracellular proteases [70].

On the basis of data in the literature it can be assumed that increased granulocyte stimulation occurs in such a situation. The proteases then released can split not only the endothelial cells and the proteins bound to the endothelial cells, but also proteins free in the plasma [71,72]. This could explain the significant drop in protein C, observed in the placebo group ($p < 0.05$) and of antithrombin III, which did not reach a significant level (see Fig. 7). Another possible cause seems to be a modulation of endothelial cell function in hemostasis. On the one hand, endotoxins (the presence of which was indicated by the rise of leukocytes), can reduce the concentration of available thrombomodulin so that there is only reduced protein C activation [73]. Blockade of the binding sites could then result in increased protein C clearance. On the other hand, increased formation of the inflammation mediator interleukin-1 may cause similar reactions [74]. A lot of these reactions produce or are influenced by free radicals. A supplementation with antioxidants seems to stabilize both leukocytes and the endothelial cells, and to protect against splitting of proteins.

Most interesting was also the marked increase in blood platelets in both groups (see Fig. 8). Whereas there was a 50% increase in the supplemented group it nearly doubled in the placebo group, but because of a very high variation within each group the differences did not reach statistic significance.

It should be emphasized that all the mentioned changes in the different tested parameters point clearly to impaired blood rheology at a high altitude. In this correlation, one should bear in mind that mountain sickness is often attributed

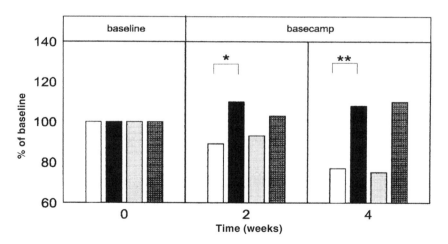

Fig. 7. Influence of vitamin E supplementation (400 IU/d) on the activity of Protein C, (open bar represents placebo group, closed bar supplemented group), and Antithromin III, (light grey bar represents placebo group, dark grey bar supplemented group) shown as % of baseline. Baseline determined before departure to altitude and 2 and 4 weeks at basecamp at 4,300 m (14,100 ft). Data are means (n = 12). *Significant difference at $p < 0.05$ compared with placebo. **Significant difference at $p < 0.01$ compared with placebo.

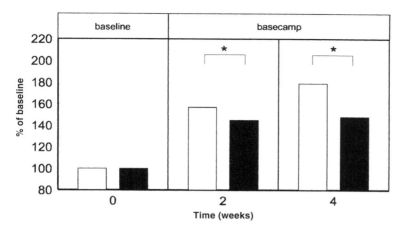

Fig. 8. Influence of vitamin E supplementation (400 IU/d) on the platelets shown as % of baseline. Open bar represents placebo group, closed bar supplemented group. Baseline determined before departure to altitude and 2 and 4 weeks at basecamp at 4,300 m (14,100 ft). Data are means (n = 12). *Significant difference at $p < 0.05$ compared with placebo.

to general microcirculation disturbances. This explains the tendency to frost bite but also to retinal hemorrhage, and to cerebral and pulmonary edema. As the supplementation with 400 IE vitamin E/d was able to prevent some of these changes and vitamin E is known to be an effective radical scavenger, free radical related reactions are most likely. Unfortunately there are still many more questions than answers, especially in this field of research.

3   INCREASED UV-RADIATION WITH INCREASING ALTITUDE

The skin is exposed to radiation of a wave length between about 300 nm to 3000 nm, including infrared, visible light and UV-radiation, made up by UV-A and UV-B. The proportion between the different kinds of radiation is not constant but is influenced by the sun's position, (depending on locus, season, and time of day), altitude, ozone content of the stratosphere, and extent of air pollution. Radiation intensity is proportional to the way the sunlight has to pass before it reaches the ground. The shorter the wave length, the higher the losses. Therefore, UV-B is much more susceptible to scattering than UV-A and visible light. This is also the reason why UV-B radiation increases excessively in clean air and high altitude. As shown in Table 1 for every 1,000 m of altitude the UV-B intensity increases by 15 to 20% whereas the UV-A intensity increases to a much lower degree [75].

The basis for a photochemical reaction in the skin is the interaction between a light quantum and biological material. That means that an electron is lifted to a higher orbit. In case of a stable electron condition the energy is absorbed. But there is a characteristic borderline, the so called ionization potential. If the

Table 1. Increase of UV radiation intensity at increasing altitude (sun at the zenith) [65].

Altitude	UV-B	UV-A
1,000 m (3,280 ft)	20%	17%
2,000 m (6,560 ft)	35%	27%
3,000 m (9,840 ft)	50%	34%
5,000 m (16,400 ft)	70%	44%

absorbed energy is higher than the binding energy of the electron, the electron is detached (ionized). Visible light and UV-radiation has a quantum energy of 40 to 150 kcal/mol. This is within the order of the intermolecular binding energy. This is the reason why singlet and triplet forms, as well as free radicals, can be produced 75). The increased UV-B radiation at high altitude may, therefore, be an important reason for increased oxidative stress at a high altitude.

Irradiation of the skin with UV-A and UV-B can induce the formation of lipid peroxidation products. In human skin surface lipids are peroxidized by UV-A radiation [76], whereas UV-B causes a remarkable decline in desaturation of fatty acids [77]. This increased lipid peroxidation could be proved by the elevated levels of TBARS in chronically sun-exposed human skin [78]. Lipid peroxides are cytotoxic and have a pro-inflammatory potency. Both are thought to play a role in UV-B-induced skin inflammation [79].

Various cellular compounds, such as carotenoids, vitamin E, vitamin C, and sulfhydryls are effective radical scavengers. Especially carotenoids may play a role in protection against UV-A damage. Carotenoids have been shown to inhibit UV-induced epidermal damage and tumor formation [80]. Vitamin E is increased in chronically sun-exposed skin, perhaps as an adaptive reaction of the body [81]. On the other hand, the vitamin E level is decreased immediately after UV-B irradiation. The total amount of vitamin C does not change, but there is no information about the ratio between ascorbic and dehydroascorbic acid [82].

Oral β-carotene administration significantly increased the minimal erythema dose of solar radiation in humans [83,84]. This may be caused by the photoprotective mechanism of β-carotene, a potent singlet oxygen scavenger at low oxygen partial pressure. A similar effect of vitamin E is likely [85].

Epidemiological investigations have shown a negative correlation between the incidence of age-dependent macula degeneration and the concentration of antioxidative vitamins and carotenoids in plasma [86—88]. UV-radiation is considered to be a causal factor within the development of the disease. In a situation characterized by high UV-load, for example high altitude, an insufficient supply with these substances should most probably be harmful.

As UV-radiation is increased tremendously at high altitudes (see Table 1) the prophylactic supplementation for people who want to go to the mountains is highly recommendable, although no specific investigations have been available until now. It seems noteworthy, however, that in nature this concept has already been realized. In plants, (pinus caribaea vars. bahamensis, pinus caribaea vars.

caribaea, pinus caribaea vars. hondurensis [89] and the snow algae Chlamydomonas nivalis), [90] and in animals, (the rodent Citellus pygmaeus), [91] the concentration of carotenoids increases with increasing altitude.

4   HIGH TEMPERATURE DIFFERENCES AT HIGH ALTITUDE

High temperature differences are typical at high altitudes. This includes not only considerable temperature differences between day and night but also depends upon the presence of sunshine or especially wind. For example, at an altitude of more than 4,000 m it is not rare to have a temperature in the afternoon sun of about 30 °C or more, and after sunset, temperatures dropped within 15 min to below O°C. To my knowledge, there have been no investigations on this, with respect to changes in metabolism caused by such a rapid change of air temperature. It might not be too speculative to suppose that.

Until now there has been no information concerning the production of free radicals increased in the heat. However, it has been suggested that work in the heat could create a hypoxic condition in the muscle due to the redistribution of blood from the muscle to the skin [92]. While no studies have examined the amount of lipid peroxidation in the heat, it is possible that the combination of hypoxia, dehydration, and other changes such as heat stress could exacerbate oxidative stress in the muscle. If this hypothesis could be confirmed, the use of antioxidants should be recommended [93].

Hypothermia on the other hand, may be an important reason for damage to the blood vessels and may induce a deterioration in the rheological properties of the blood. The degree varies, but is clearly temperature-dependent. Schmidt-Schönbein and Neumann [58] gave an excellent overview. Under hypothermic conditions erythrocytes tend to aggregate more easily and the aggregates are more resistant to hydrodynamic dispersion. This is consistent with the observation that together with a membrane stiffening, the deformation of aggregated red blood cells in stasis is enhanced in hypothermia. From the start it has been impossible to decide if the stiffening of the membranes are only a temperature phenomenon or the result of an increased lipid peroxidation. In any case, after stasis occurs, tissue hypoxia is most likely and thus, increased oxidative stress.

As far as things have been understood until now, blood rheology is dependent on a lot of factors. Clearly some very minute variables may have big effects in the end. The prophylactic use of antioxidants at a high altitude or in the cold may be one of these. Certainly they will not prevent frostbites in all conditions. However, it seems worthwhile to do more research on the possibility, to influence the metabolism in a way that makes blood cells and vessel intima more resistant to circumstances that initially disturb blood rheology, and thus prevent harmful events in some cases.

It is well known that temperature influences the hormonal status. Noradrenalin, for example, plays an important role in the nonshivering thermogenesis. It could be shown that incubation of mitochondria with noradrenalin caused a significant increase in hydrogen peroxide production and so to oxidative stress. The same author was able to demonstrated the same effect in animals exposed to cold temperatures [94].

One of the few experiments that indicate oxidative stress during exercise at cold temperatures is that of Panin et al. [95]. During the 6-week Soviet-Canadian transpolar ski trek, plasma and red blood cell levels of vitamin E and the fluorescent products of lipid peroxidation, as well as blood concentrations of MDA, were measured. Plasma MDA levels increased whereas tocopherol decreased. This was preceded by an increase in lipid peroxidation products both in plasma and red blood cells. Both make the increased production of free radicals in the cold very likely.

5   DEHYDRATION

Fluid demand is increased at high altitudes depending on temperature and humidity of the air. Working in a warm or even hot surroundings causes more or less intensive perspiring. As mentioned above, even at high altitudes temperatures may be considerably high. Working to a more or less intensive degree is obligatory when staying in the mountains. So fluid loss through perspiration is common. There is no doubt that these losses have to be substituted. In this case, the use of an electrolyte drink is useful.

With increasing altitude, fluid losses of the lungs as a consequence of the increasingly dry breathing air tend to dominate over perspiration. There is evidence that this fluid loss can increase until 6 and more liters per day at extremely high altitudes. As the melting of 1 liter of water from the snow takes about 1 h, under these conditions it is not surprising that high altitude climbers generally do not meet their fluid demand and return to base camp more or less dehydrated. In this case the fluid deficit can be compensated for by water only, in practice with tee.

As dehydration is one of the important risk factors for frost bites it is necessary to look for a proper fluid balance already before starting to climb. This can be easily controlled by checking hematocrit or urine osmolarity regularly.

To my knowledge there are no studies available, which have ever examined if dehydration is involved in increased free radical production. However, as energy production is impaired in such a condition, it is likely that partial hypoxia may occur and thus, oxidative stress. Clarkson mentions dehydration as a possible risk factor. As dehydration is such a big problem at high altitudes studies on this question are highly desirable [93].

6   NUTRITIONAL DEFICITS

Nutrient deficiency may already be a problem at low altitudes but it certainly is one at a high altitude. In the following, some data are shown, which were produced by calculating the nutrient intake during three different expeditions. The food supply of the first (to K2) was calculated carefully by a nutrition professional who took the limited possibilities during an expedition into consideration. The second was the scientific project in the Solo Khumbu for which the food supply was organized by experienced mountaineers. The third (to Kangchenjunga) was a "normal" climbing expedition organized by hobby mountaineers. In the first and the third case, data were obtained by weighing the food consumed and then calculating the average intake by dividing this amount per head and day at the basecamp. In the second case, nutrient intake was calculated from a 7-day-nutrition protocol. As there was not much chance for varying the meals individually, or during the time period, the data can be considered representative for the whole period of time [55]. In the following, data are limited to the intake of water and some vitamins and minerals.

From Fig. 9 it can be seen that nutrient deficiency may easily occur during high altitude climbing. This is especially true for the trace elements. The price and weight of food, as well as a fall in appetite, are often limiting factors, but this is not surprising. To my knowledge there are no existing investigations on nutrient intake during trekking and altitude training of athletes. As increased oxidative stress at high altitudes can be presumed, especially the antioxidative nutrients such as β-carotene, vitamin E, vitamin C, selenium and zinc, should be taken into consideration. The relatively high intake of vitamin C during the second expedition was due to a regular supply with fresh potatoes, cabbage, and apples. That depends largely on area and season and cannot be considered normal. In general, the food supply is limited, especially with respect to fresh food. Therefore, a supplementation is advisable.

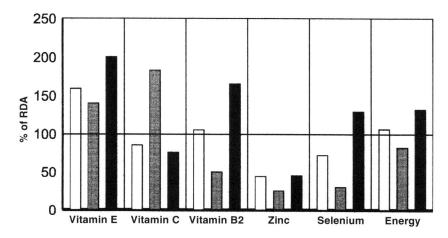

Fig. 9. Average daily intake of selected nutrients during three different expeditions to high altitudes shown as % of recommended dietary allowances (RDA). Open bar represents data from the expedition to K2, grey bar to Solo Khumbu, and closed bar to Kangchenjunga. Data are calculated from weighed foods or food records.

7   SUMMARY

1. There is considerable evidence that there is indeed increased oxidative stress at high altitudes.
2. The most important sources of free radicals are the respiratory chain itself, hypoxia, and increased UV-radiation. Whether high and low temperatures and dehydration lead to an increased formation of free radicals is not clear at the moment. Certainly there are some more causes for increased oxidative stress such as diseases and/or intake of medication. However, this should be discussed separately.
3. Several studies indicate that oxidative stress impairs physical performance, as well as blood flow. Both are of particular importance to people at high altitudes.
4. A nutritional survey showed that nutrient intake, especially of antioxidants, may not always meet with the increased demand at high altitudes. Deficiency of antioxidants clearly deteriorates metabolic functions at high altitudes.
5. Obviously the recommendations given for people living at lower altitudes are insufficient for this special situation.
6. As food supply is limited during a prolonged stay at high altitudes, e.g., during a trekking tour or an expedition, a supplementation with antioxidants is advisable.
7. To my knowledge the only studies available have shown a beneficial influence of vitamin E. However, the synergetic functions of other antioxidants, such as β-carotene and vitamin C, justify the recommendation of a supplementation.
8. Of course, not all of the aforementioned factors influence all groups of people to the same degree. It can be said however, that normally, their importance increases with altitude. There is no doubt that there is still a lot of research to be done in this area of biomedical importance.

8   ABBREVIATIONS

DNA:	desoxyribonuclein acid
GSH:	(reduced) glutathione
GSSG:	(oxidized) glutathione disulfide
MDA:	malondialdehyde
OH:	hydroxyl radical
pO_2:	oxygen partial pressure
SH:	sulfhydryl group
TBARS:	thiobarbituric acid reactive substances
UV:	ultra violet
WBC:	white blood cells

9   REFERENCES

1. Elstner EF. Die antioxidative Strategie. In: Der Sauerstoff. Mannheim: BI-Wissenschaftsverlag, 1990;267–342.
2. Alessio HM. In: Sen CK, Packer L, Hänninen O (eds) Exercise and Oxygen Toxicity. Amsterdam: Elsevier, 1994;269–295.
3. Agostoni A, Gerli GC, Beretta L, Palazzini G, Buso GP, Hu X, Moschini G. Clin Chim Acta 1983;133:153–157.
4. Azzi A, Boscoboinik D, Marilley D, Özer NK, Stäuble B, Tasinato A. Am J Clin Nutr 1995;62:1337S–1346S.
5. Azzi AM, Bartoli G, Boscoboinik D, Hensey C, Szewczyk A. In: Packer L, Fuchs J (eds) Vitamin E in Health and Disease. New York: Marcel Dekker, 1993;371–383.
6. Pool-Zobel BL, Bub A, Müller H, Wollowski I, Rechkemmer G. Carcinogenesis 1997;18:1847–1850.
7. Stocker R, Frei B. Oxidative Stress: In: Sies H (ed) Oxidants and Antioxidants. London: Academic Press, 1991;213–243.
8. Bielski BHJ, Richter HW. Ann NY Acad Sci 1975;258:231–237.
9. Hughes RE, Maton SC. Br J Haematol 1968;14:247–253.
10. Halliwell B, Wasil M, Grootveld M. FEBS Lett 1987;213:15–18.
11. Packer JE, Slater TF, Willson RL. Nature 1979;278:737–738.
12. Burton GW, Ingold KU. Science 1984;224:569–573.
13. Vile GF, Winterburn CC. FEBS Lett 1988;238:353–356.
14. Buskirk ER. In: Goddard RF (ed) The Effects of Altitude on Physical Performance. Chicago: Athetic Inst, 1966;65–72.
15. Eckhardt K, Boutellier U, Kurtz A, Schopen M, Koller E, Bauer C. J Appl Physiol 1989;66:1785–1788.
16. Hannon JP, Shields JL, Harris CW. J Appl Physiol 1969;26:540–547.
17. Young AJ, Evans WJ, Cymerman A, Pandolf KB, Knapik JJ, Maher JT. J Appl Physiol 1982;52:857–862.
18. Young PM, Rock PB, Fulco CS. J Appl Physiol 1987;63:738–764.
19. Berg A, Simon-Schnass I, Rokitzki L, Keul J. Dtsch Z Sportmed 1987;38:416–424.
20. Demopoulos HB, Santomier JP, Seligman ML, Pietronigro DD, Hogan P. In: Katch FI (ed) The 1984 Olympic Science Congress Proceedings. Champaign, Ill: Human Kinetiks, 1986;139–189.
21. Packer L. Med Biol Eng 1984;62:105–109.
22. Simon-Schnass I. In: Simopoulos AP, Pavlou KN (eds) Nutrition and Fitness for Athletes. World Review of Nutrition and Dietetics. Basel: Karger, 1993;144–153.
23. Sies H. In: Sies H (ed) Oxidative Stress. London: Academic Press, 1985;1–8.
24. Singh VN. J Nutr 1992; 122:760–765.
25. Witt EH, Reznick AZ, Viguie CA, Starke-Reed P, Packer L. J Nutr 1992;122:766–773.
26. Kagan VE, Spirichev VB, Serbinova EA, Witt EH, Erin AN, Packer L. In: Nutrition in Exercise and Sport. Boca Raton: CRC Press, 1994;185–213.
27. Goldfarb AH, Sen CK. In: Sen CK, Packer L, Hänninen O (eds) Exercise and Oxygen Toxicity. Amsterdam: Elsevier, 1994;163–189.
28. Jenkins RR, Krause K, Schofield LS. Med Sci Sport Exerc 1993;25:213–217.
29. Leaf DA, Kleinman MT, Hamilton M, Barstow TJ. Med Sci Sport Exerc 1997;29:1036–1039.
30. Jakeman P, Maxwell S. Eur J Appl Physiol 1993;67:426–430.
31. Nagawa T, Kita H, Aoki J, Maeshima T, Shiozawa K. Asian Med J 1968;11:619–633.
32. Simon-Schnass I, Pabst H. Int J Vit Nutr Res 1988;58:49–54.
33. Cormier M. Prog Food Nutr Sci 1977;2:347–356.
34. Schwarz K. Ann NY Acad Sci 1972;203:45–52.
35. Schwarz K. Vitam Horm 1962;20:463–484.

36. Carabello FB, Liu F, Eames O, Bird J. Fed Proc 1971;30:639.
37. Carabello FB. Can J Biochem 1974;52:679—688.
38. Fedelesova M, Sulaakhe PV, Yates JC, Dhalla NS. Can J Physiol Pharmacol 1971;49:909—918.
39. Cerretelli P, di Prampero PE. In: Rivolier J, Cerretelli P, Foray J (eds) High Altitude Deterioration. Basel: Karger, 1985;1—19.
40. Bertolotty E, Loidodice G, Quazza GF. Minerva Pediatrica 1965;17:873—877.
41. Chen LH, Lin CI. Nutr Rep Int 1980;21:387—395.
42. Tureen L, Simons R. Proc Soc Exp Biol Med 1968;129:384—390.
43. Chang SW, Stelzner TJ, Weil JV, Voelkel NF. Lung 1989;167:269—276.
44. Hoshikawa Y, Ono S, Tanita T, Sakuma T, Noda M, Tabata T, Ueda S, Ashino Y, Fujimura S. Jpn J Thorac Dis 1995;33:1168—1173.
45. Koudelova J, Mourek JK. Physiol Res 1992;41:207—212.
46. Chryssanthou C, Palaia T, Goldstein G, Stenger R. Aviat Space Env Med 1987;58:1082—1086.
47. Plateel M, Dehouck MP, Torpier G, Cecchelli R, Teissier E. J Neurochem 1995;65:2138—2145.
48. Nakanishi K, Tajima F, Nakamura A, Yagura S, Ookawara T, Yamashita H, Suzuki K, Taniguchi N, Ohno H. J Physiol 1995;489:869—876.
49. Costa LE, Llesuy S, Boveris A. Am J Physiol 1993;264:C1395—C1400.
50. Kappus H. In: Sies H (ed) Oxidative Stress. London: Academic Press, 1985;273—310.
51. Dillard CJ, Litov RE, Savin WM, Dumelin EE, Tappel AL. J Appl Physiol 1978;45:927—932.
52. Dillard CJ, Litov RE, Tappel AL. Lipids 1977;13:109—114.
53. Thews G, Mutschler E, Vaupel P. In: Anatomie, Physiologie und Pathophysiologie des Menschen. Stuttgart: Wissenschaftliche Verlagsgesellschaft mbH, 1982;180.
54. Simon-Schnass I, Korniszewski L. Int J Vit Nutr Res 1990;60:26—34.
55. Simon-Schnass I. In: Marriott BM, Carlson SJ (eds) Nutritional Needs in Cold and High-Altitude Environments. Washington, DC: National Academy Press, 1996;393—418.
56. Ernst E, Matrai A, Aschenbrenner E. J Sports Med 1985;25:207—210.
57. Ernst E, Matrai A. Clin Hemorheol (In press).
58. Schmid-Schönbein H, Neumann FJ. In: Rivolier J, Cerretelli P, Foray J (eds) High Altitude Deterioration. Basel: Karger, 1985;20—38.
59. Oelz O. In: Hypoxie. München-Deisenhofen: Dustrie Verlag, 1984;205—220.
60. Winslow RM. In: West JB, Lahiri S (eds) High Altitude and Man. Am Phys Soc 1984;163—172.
61. Hiller E, Riess H. In: Hämorrhagische Diathese und Thrombose. Stuttgart: Wissenschaftliche Verlagsgesellschaft mbH, 1988;93—107.
62. Volger E. In: Hypoxie. München-Deisenhofen: Dustrie Verlag, 1984;225—240.
63. Chow CK. Am J Clin Nutr 1979;32:1066—1081.
64. Leibovitz BE, Siegel BV. J Gerontol 1980;35:45—56.
65. Simon-Schnass I, Koeppe H-W. Z All Med 1983;59:1474—1476.
66. Oelz O. In: Brendel W, Zink RA (eds) High Altitude Physiology and Medicine. New York: Springer, 1982;298—300.
67. Asano M, Branemark PI, Castenholz A. Adv Microcirc 1973;5:1—31.
68. Bagge U, Blinxt A, Braide M. Clin Hemorheol 1986;6:365—372.
69. Lipowsky H, Usami S, Chien S. Microvasc Res 1980;19:297—319.
70. Harlan JM, Killen PD, Harken LA. J Clin Invest 1981;68:1394—1403.
71. Benjamini E, Leskowitz S. In: Immunologie. Stuttgart: Schwer Verlag, 1988;197—212.
72. Weis SJ, Regiani S. J Clin Invest 1984;73:1297—1303.
73. Moore KL, Andreollo SP, Esmon NL. J Clin Invest 1987;79:124—130.
74. Nawroth PP. Proc Natl Acad Sci 1986;83:3460—3464.
75. Kindl G, Raab W. In: Licht und Haut. Frankfurt am Main: Govi-Verlag, 1993;
76. Nazzaro-Porro M, Picardo M, Finotti E, Passi S. J Invest Dermatol 1986;89:320 (Abstract).
77. Horacek J, Cernikova-Brünn M. Arch Klin Exp Dermatol 1961;213:124—129.
78. Niwa Y, Kanoh T, Sakane T, Soh H, Kawai S, Miyachi Y. J Clin Biochem Nutr 1987;2:245—251.
79. Ohsawa K, Watanabe T, Matsukawa R, Yoshimura Y, Imaeda K. J Toxicol Sci 1984;9:151—159.

80. Mathews-Roth MM. Photochem Photobiol 1986;42:35—38.
81. De Simone C, Rusciani L, Vernier A. J Invest Dermatol 1987;89:317.
82. Fuchs J, Mehlhorn RJ, Packer L. J Invest Dermatol 1989;93:633—640.
83. Mathews-Roth MM, Pathak MA, Parrish J. J Invest Dermatol 1972;59:349—353.
84. Gollnick H, Hopfenmüller W, Hemmes C, Chun SC, Schmid C, Sundermeier K, Biesalski HK. Eur J Dermatol 1996;6:200—205.
85. Shindo Y, Witt EH, Packer L. J Invest Dermatol 1993;100:260—265.
86. Seddon JM, Ajani UA, Sperduto RD, Hiller R, Blair N, Burton TC, Farber MD, Gragoudas ES, Haller J, Miller DT, Yannuzzi LA, Willett W. J Am Med Assoc 1994;272:1413—1420.
87. Mares-Perlman JA, Brady WE, Klein BE, Stacewics-Sapuntzskis M, Palta M. Arch Ophth 1995;113:1518—1523.
88. Eye Disease Case-Controll Study Group. Arch Ophth 1993;111:104—109.
89. Venator CR, Howes CD, Telek L. Genetiks 1974;77:68.
90. Bidigare RR, Ondrusek ME, Kennicutt MC, Iturriaga R, Harvey HR, Hoham RW, Macko SA. J Phytol 1993;29:427—434.
91. Karnaukhov VN, Fedorov GG. Comp Biochem Physiol 1977;57:377—381.
92. Young AJ. In: Pandolf KE (ed) Exercise and Sport Sciences Reviews. Baltimore: Williams and Wilkins, 1990;65—117.
93. Clarkson PM. In: Marriott BM (ed) Nutritional Needs in Hot Environments. Washington, DC: National Academy Press, 1993;137—171.
94. Swaroop A, Patole MS, Puranam RS, Ramasarma T. Biochem J 1983;214:745—750.
95. Panin LE, Mayaskaya NM, Borodin AA. In: Shephard RJ, Rode A (eds) Observations on the Soviet-Canadian Transpolar Ski Trek. Basel: Karger, 1992;139—186.

©2000 Elsevier Science B.V. All rights reserved.
Handbook of Oxidants and Antioxidants in Exercise.
C.K. Sen, L. Packer and O. Hänninen, editors.

579

Part VIII • Chapter 21

Oxidants in skin pathophysiology

Stefan Weber

Department of Molecular and Cell Biology, University of California, Berkeley 251 LSA, Berkeley, California 94720-3200, USA

1 INTRODUCTION
    1.1   Aims
    1.2   Skin anatomy and physiology
    1.3   UV-light
    1.4   Ozone
2 ANTIOXIDANTS IN THE SKIN
3 FREE RADICALS IN THE SKIN
4 UV-INDUCED OXIDATIVE STRESS
    4.1   Photooxidative damage
    4.2   The sunburn reaction
    4.3   Skin cancer
    4.4   Photoaging
5 ANTIOXIDATIVE INTERVENTION
6 OZONE-INDUCED OXIDATIVE STRESS
    6.1   Possible reaction mechanisms
    6.2   Ozone-induced damage
7 SUMMARY
8 PERSPECTIVES
9 ABBREVIATIONS
10 REFERENCES

1 INTRODUCTION

1.1 Aims

During outdoor exercise the human body is exposed to environmental stressors. The skin, as the outermost part of the body, acts as a defense system against these stressors but is also the first target for oxidative damage due to this exposure.

UV light is certainly the most common and best studied environmental stressor to the skin. In recent years, progressive damage of the stratospheric ozone layer has led to increasing intensity of UV light at ground level. This problem is gaining more and more public awareness. Dangers involved in excessive UV exposure include accelerated aging of the skin and increased incidence of certain types of skin cancer. Increased UV irradiation in conjunction with the emission of carbon oxides and nitric oxides in industrialized countries leads to enhanced formation of photochemical smog including the production of ground level ozone.

Recently, several studies have indicated a possible role of ozone exposure in direct skin damage.

The aim of this chapter is to introduce the oxidative stressors, UV light and ozone, and to give an overview on their harmful effects to the skin. In addition, a possible role of antioxidative intervention in the modulation of oxidative skin damage is discussed.

1.2 Skin anatomy and physiology

The skin is the interface between the human body and the environment. It serves as a protective barrier against chemical, physical and biological stress and plays a vital part in prevention of transdermal water loss and in thermoregulation [1]. Moreover, it is an important organ of perception and immunity. Anatomically it consists of two main layers, the epidermis on the outside and the dermis underneath it (Fig. 1). The skin is placed on subcutaneous fat tissue. Each layer is subdivided and has its unique structure and function.

The epidermis is classified as a stratified cornifying squamous epithelium and is anchored on a basement membrane [2] (Fig. 2). The cell population consists predominantly of keratinocytes. The epidermis is regenerated continuously from the inside layer, the stratum basale. While ascending from the stratum basale, the keratinocytes undergo characteristic changes as they differentiate, forming

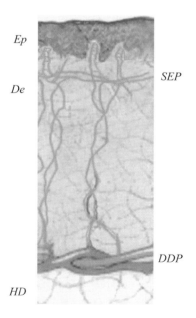

Fig. 1. Human skin: scheme of cross section; epidermis (Ep), dermis (De), hypodermis (HD), sub-epidermal vascular plexus (SEP), deep dermal plexus (DDP).

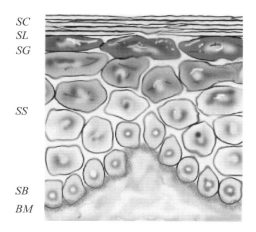

SC
SL
SG

SS

SB
BM

Fig. 2. Epidermis: scheme of cross section; stratum corneum (SC), stratum lucidum (SL), stratum granulosum (SG), stratum spinosum (SS), stratum basale (SB), basement membrane (BM).

morphologically distinct layers, the stratum spinosum, stratum granulosum, and the stratum lucidum. In the final step of differentiation, the cells lose their nuclei to form the stratum corneum (SC), which consists of enucleated corneocytes filled with core proteins in a wrapping of envelope proteins. A total of 15 to 20 layers of these cornified envelopes are embedded into lipid membrane bilayers acting as a physiological barrier against penetration from the outside and inside [3]. One such barrier function is the prevention of dehydration by limiting the transepidermal water loss. Also, it is a natural obstacle against penetration of exogenous chemicals, both toxic and therapeutic ones. Within 14 days the SC turns over, desquaming the outer layer.

Dendritic epidermal melanocytes are embedded in the basal layer. Depending on the skin type, they produce more or less of the tyrosine derivative melanin, a chromophore responsible for the skin's color. The melanin is packed in melanosomes, transported through the dendrites and transferred into keratinocytes. As the keratinocytes ascend, they are degraded into smaller particles in secondary lysosomes. UV irradiation stimulates the production of melanin as a protective mechanism [4].

The dermis is divided into a papillary and a reticular part. The upper, papillary part interdigitates with the epidermis, thus, enlarging the area of connection between the two layers. This provides the mechanical stability, as well as enhances the diffusion of nutrients into the epidermis. The papillary dermis carries blood vessels which form capillaries that reach out into the papillae in order to provide nutrients to the unperfused epidermis. Fibroblasts in the dermis are embedded in an extracellular matrix to produce collagen and elastin. This connective tissue accounts for the mechanical stability and elasticity of the skin [2].

Both the dermis and the epidermis participate in the immune system. Langerhans cells residing in the epidermis play an important role as antigen processing cells. In the perfused dermis, the whole range of humoral and cellular immune responses takes place.

There are also different types of skin appendages such as sweat glands and hair follicles. The skin is also a very important sensory organ for temperature, touch, vibration, and pain with specialized receptors. Lastly, there is a strong psychosomal bond between mind and skin. Many skin diseases are stress modulated, and since the skin is the most visual part of our body, the way our skin looks shapes the way we perceive ourselves.

1.3 UV light

Outdoor exercise exposes the skin of the human body to considerable amounts of UV light. The electromagnetic spectrum of solar light consists of an infrared (λ 760 nm — 10 μm), a visible (400—760 nm) and an ultraviolet (UV) (200—400 nm) portion. The UV spectrum is subdivided into UV-C,-B and -A (Fig. 3) depending on the wavelength [5]. Fortunately, earth's stratosphere filters out almost all of the high energy UV-C radiation and a considerable part of the UV-B portion. However, as explained in the next paragraph, the decaying ozone layer will most likely result in increased exposure to these types of UV radiation [6]. While the short-wave UV-C barely penetrates into the skin, UV-B enters the epidermis and UV-A can eventually reach the dermis and thus, the circulatory cells [7]. The lowest dose of UV-B radiation capable of causing an erythema (reddening) of the skin 24 h after exposure is called 1 minimal erythemal dose (MED). UV irradiation generates different reactive oxygen species (ROS) resulting in oxidative stress which has been implicated in skin aging and photocarcinogenesis.

1.4 Ozone

The damaging properties of smog have been documented for centuries. The first report on air pollution and its damaging effects on human health was filed during the reign of Richard III (1377 to 1399) in England [8]. Then, a connection between disease and air contamination in the surroundings of coal utilizing

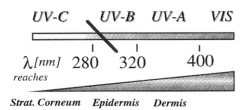

Fig. 3. UV-spectrum: electromagnetic spectrum in the UV and visible range. Wavelengths below 290 nm are mostly cut out by the atmosphere (black oblique bar).

industries was proposed. Today, ozone O_3 accounts for one of the major parts of air pollution [9]. While it is vital in the stratosphere for the survival of the current biosphere, it is unwanted and toxic at ground level.

Both contradicting features relate to the chemical properties of ozone: it is a fairly unstable and highly reactive gas. In the stratosphere, high energy UV radiation ($\lambda < 242$ nm) breaks dioxygen O_2 into atomic oxygen. This photochemical process absorbs the UV radiation, acting as an atmospheric filter for high energy UV radiation. The reaction of molecular oxygen with O_2 results in the formation of O_3. A dynamic equilibrium is reached, when ozone is destroyed again by reacting with atomic oxygen, hydroxyl radical or photochemical dissociation ($\lambda < 310$ nm) (Chapman reaction) [10] (Fig. 4). However, chlorofluorocarbons released from ground level can reach the stratosphere, where they act as strong catalysts in the destruction of ozone. Also, nitrogen oxides from supersonic flights have these effects [11]. This leads to the "ozone hole", an alarming decrease in ozone concentrations over the south pole [12].

In the troposphere (ground level), NO_2 from industry, home, and car emission can undergo photolysis by solar UV radiation ($\lambda < 370$ nm) forming NO and atomic oxygen. Atomic oxygen can then react with O_2 yielding ozone, as already pointed out in the Chapman cycle. NO usually destroys O_3 again, maintaining a cyclic balance [13]. Volatile organic compounds in smog like formaldehyde (HCHO) or nitrous acid (HONO) undergo photolysis and participate in the recycling of NO_2 from NO without destroying O_3, which leads to an accumulation of O_3. The concentration of tropospheric ozone is especially high in polluted

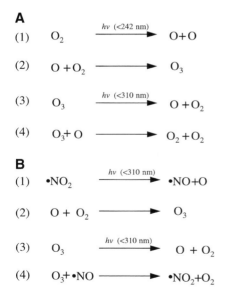

Fig. 4. Ozone chemistry in **A**: stratosphere, **B**: troposphere.

urban areas located in air basins with thermal inversion. For example, Los Angeles, located in the south coast air basin, suffered from high ozone concentrations in the past. Table 1 shows the development of O_3 levels in the south coast air basin [14]. Within the last three decades, tropospheric ozone levels have increased significantly. The increase in terrestrial UV-B irradiation is expected to further increase the ozone levels [15].

Ground level O_3 is known to exert harmful effects on the respiratory tract in fairly low doses: 0.12 ppm/h or 0.08 ppm in 8 h cause an average 10% drop in FEV_1, a parameter for respiratory function [9]. Especially in asthmatic patients but in healthy people as well, airway inflammation is triggered and a decrease in pulmonary function has been recorded. Countries like Germany even go so far as to issue special speed limits if O_3 levels exceed a safety limit of 0.12 ppm/ h [16].

2   ANTIOXIDANTS IN THE SKIN

All major intrinsic low molecular weight antioxidants have been found in human skin. Vitamin E and ubiquinol-10 are the main lipophilic antioxidants. Vitamin C, glutathione/ GSSG and uric acid are the main hydrophilic ones. Figure 5 shows their distribution in the different skin layers [17]. Interestingly, the epidermis is equipped with higher concentrations of antioxidants than the dermis. Recently, the concentration of vitamin E in the outermost part of the skin, the SC was found to increase with skin depth [18]. Different forms of vitamin E are present in the skin. In humans, α-tocopherol is predominant, while γ-tocopherol only accounts for a small percentage of the total vitamin E. This predominance of α-tocopherol is due to the action of α-tocopherol transfer protein (α-TTP) present in the liver [19]. Additional forms of vitamin E are not normally present in human skin. However, in hairless mice, tocotrienols account for almost 15% of vitamin E [20]. This phenomenon is probably caused by a tocotrienol rich diet.

Also, specialized antioxidant enzymes are found active in the skin: catalase, superoxide dismutase, glutathione peroxidase and reductase [21,22,17]. The same distribution pattern as for the low molecular weight antioxidants is observed, except in the case of glutathione peroxidase. Specifically, catalase activity in epidermis was reported to be 720% that in the dermis [17].

Table 1. South coast air basin: number of days exceeding health standard levels.

Year	Federal standard	$c(O_{3max})$
1955	no data	> 0.68
1979	169	0.45
1996	90	0.24

US federal safety standard: 0.12 ppm for 1 day a year; WHO safety standard: 0.75—0.1 ppm for 1 h (1 $\mu g/m^{-3} = 0.501 \times 10^{-3}$ ppm); (WHO 1995).

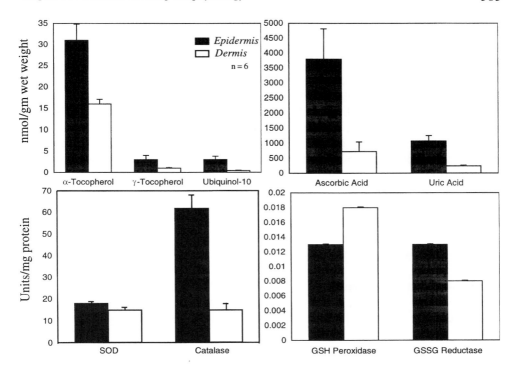

Fig. 5. Distribution of nonenzymatic and enzymatic antioxidants in epidermis and dermis of human skin (data from [17]).

3 FREE RADICALS IN THE SKIN

As in other living tissues, the skin cells themselves produce free radicals and reactive species as a byproduct of their regular energy metabolism, mainly from mitochondria. In inflammatory conditions, the oxidative stress is increased by cellular oxidative defense mechanisms such as the oxidative burst in neutrophils [23]. The direct detection of free radicals in the skin poses some problems due to their short half lives. However, spin trapping EPR techniques helped gain some insight into the free radical flux in skin. Lipid radicals [24] and the hydroxyl radical [25] were detected in skin cells during UV irradiation using several spin traps. Hydrogen peroxide was increased after UV irradiation as determined by dihydrorhodamine-123 [26]. UVA irradiation-induced the endogenous ascorbyl radical [27]. The vitamin E radical can be observed after topical enrichment of the skin with α-tocopherol [28].

How are free radicals produced by UV radiation? Depending on the wavelength, different mechanisms can be taken into consideration. The high energy UV-C irradiation is powerful enough to photolyse water directly (see [35]). The energy transfer is very rapid, which is the reason for its limited ability to penetrate deeply into the skin. UV-B acts partly through photodissociation of hydrogen peroxide (H_2O_2). Depending on their UV absorbance properties, some molecules can be directly photolysed, such as Vitamin E (A_{max} = 295 nm) [29] and DNA (A_{max} = 260 nm).

There is substantial evidence that UV-A radiation mainly acts via certain biomolecules absorbing in the UV-A range called, photosensitizers. Examples are porphyrins, flavins and the drug psoralen. Upon excitation, they are able to transfer energy in two different ways: in a type I photoreaction, the energy can be directly transferred to a target molecule, e.g., DNA leading to its oxidative modification. In a type II photoreaction, the energy transfer is directed to molecular oxygen in the ground state, leading to the formation of singlet oxygen and other reactive oxygen species. In a second step, they then can react with a target molecule [30].

4   UV-INDUCED OXIDATIVE STRESS

4.1 Photooxidative damage

Antioxidants

Extensive mouse studies were carried out to investigate dose response effects of acute UV radiation on epidermal and dermal antioxidants [22,31]. Vitamin C was the first to be depleted by a solar simulated spectrum. Doses from 2—10 MED caused the depletion of other antioxidants in the following order: ubiquinol-9, glutathione, and vitamin E in a dose-dependent manner. Recently, it was demonstrated that suberythmogenic doses of solar simulated UV radiation are capable of dramatically depleting vitamin E in the stratum corneum of human skin [18].

The lipophilic antioxidants vitamin E and ubiquinol decreased immediately after a single acute dose of UV radiation in the skin of hairless mice (10 MED) but were recovered within 24 h. The recovery period for the hydrophilic antioxidants (vitamin C and glutathione) was considerably longer, up to 120 h [32].

Antioxidants are known to interact with each other forming an antioxidant network [33]. There is considerable evidence of vitamin E recycling by ascorbate in skin [29]. Ultraviolet light induces the generation of vitamin E radicals, which can be recycled to vitamin E by vitamin C. The order of destruction and recovery of low molecular weight antioxidants suggests recycling mechanisms as well. However, the direct photodestruction of vitamin E could also lead to pro-oxidative effects by consumption of the networking antioxidants [28].

Lipids

UV irradiation of skin results in lipid peroxidation. Lipid hydroperoxides increase, as well as malondialdehyde, a product of lipid peroxidation [34,35].

Lipid peroxides are thought to be involved in the elevated prostaglandin E2 release after photooxidative insult.

Proteins

Proteins are a prime target for oxidative stress [36] modified by UV light. Collagen is a major structural protein in the dermis. It can be attacked and modified or degraded by reactive oxygen species [37,38]. In collagen, protein cross links induced by UV-A and near UV radiation were reported [39]. Macromolecular carbonyls (including those from proteins) were found to be increased in chronically exposed human stratum corneum [40]. Enzymes are also susceptible to UV. Acute UV exposure (solar simulated spectrum) inactivated catalase activity starting from 2 MED. 10 MED resulted in a dramatic loss in activity to only 12% of the original value in the epidermis [17]. This effect was reported to be due to direct photodestruction of the protein. Recently, it was demonstrated that singlet oxygen oxidizes catalase [41]. The effect on superoxide dismutase was also detectable but less pronounced [42]. Glutathione peroxidase and glutathione reductase were affected mildly. Generally, the changes in the epidermis were higher than in the dermis [17].

DNA

The study of oxidative DNA modification has been a focus of interest for many years, since DNA damage can lead to mutagenic and cancerogenic processes [43]. DNA absorbs in the UV-B range, which makes it rather susceptible to photochemical modification. Dimer formation in DNA after UV-B exposure has been shown to be ~ 5000 times greater than with long-wave UV-A [44]. UV-A was shown to induce pyridine dimers in DNA of human skin [45]. In conjunction with endogenous photosensitizers, UV-A can lead to base oxidation products such as 8-oxo-7,8-dihydroguanine [46]. Defective DNA repair enzymes, as in the autosomal recessive disease *Xeroderma pigmentosa*, result in skin cancer in sun exposed areas [47].

The skin is able to partly adapt to chronic photooxidative stress in several ways. Melanogenesis is activated to produce more of the chromophore melanin. Vitamin E levels in chronically exposed skin were found to be elevated [37]. One report indicated that chronic UV-B irradiation, but not UV-A, elevated superoxide dismutase activity in hairless mice [48].

4.2 The sunburn reaction

Acute UV-induced alterations have been well characterized clinically. The sunburn reaction includes erythema, heat, edema, pain and puritus followed by tanning and epidermal thickening [49]. The duration of the erythema depends on the wavelength: UV-C erythema fades 3 h after exposure, while the UV-B or -A

reaction may persist for days. Higher doses produce more pronounced and longer lasting reactions. The doses of radiation needed for UV-A-induced erythema
are about 100 times greater then those for UV-B. While UV-B erythema appears
2 to 4 h after irradiation and reaches a maximum after 24 to 48 h, the UV-A-
induced response exhibits a biphasic pattern. The initial erythema appears during exposure, fades away and then reaches a second peak several hours later
that may persist for more than 2 days. Histamine, kinins and lipid mediators
such as prostaglandin E2 are involved in the sunburn reaction [35].

4.3 Skin cancer

Within the last decades, the incidence of skin cancer has increased considerably.
Currently, it is the most common type of human cancer. The main types are
melanoma and nonmelanoma (NMSC). Annually ca. 1,200,000 cases of skin
cancer are reported in the US [50]. While the association of melanoma and UV
exposure is still controversial, the link between NMSC and UV irradiation is
well-established. Oxygen radicals have been shown to be involved in all three
stages of cancer development: tumor initiation, promotion and progression [51].
Both UV-B and -A induce reactive species and are currently considered to be
complete carcinogens [52]. The mutagenic potential of UV irradiation is one of
the main mechanisms by which skin cancer can evolve: genetic mutations occur
in tumor suppressor genes such as p53 and the patched gene, as well as in proto-
oncogenes/oncogenes like H-ras, K-ras and N-ras. Inactivation of tumor supres-
sors and activation of oncogenes lead to changes in the control of the cell cycle,
DNA repair and apoptosis, resulting in abnormal cell proliferation and clonal
expansion [5]. Chronic inflammation, caused by UV irradiation, may contribute
to tumor initiation and promote tumor invasion via degradation of connective
tissue [52]. Oxygen intermediates are involved in UV-induced damage of Langerhans cells, which may lead to a compromised immunosurveillance of mutated
cells in the epidermis [53].

4.4 Photoaging

Skin aging is a natural process. Intrinsic skin aging leads to subtle changes consisting primarily of laxity, fine wrinkling, and several benign neoplasms [54]. In
contrast to this type of aging, chronic UV exposure causes accelerated photoaging, termed dermatoheliosis. The skin appears wrinkly and coarse. The pig-
mentation is irregular. In addition to benign neoplasm, cancerous lesions are
found. The destruction of connective tissue is a hallmark of photoaging [54]. The
oxidative stress hypothesis claims that reactive species created by UV irradiation
are a main factor in the changes seen in skin aging by damaging crucial biomolecules [55]. There is evidence that the connective tissue, especially collagen, is
attacked by reactive species and slowly degraded [39]. UV irradiation causes a
chronic low level inflammation [56]. During this process, collagenases (metallo-

proteinases) are chronically elevated [57]. Tissue inhibitors of collagenases are excreted to limit the damage. A recent theory proposes that repair mechanisms (collagen synthesis) are incomplete and leave scars, leading to cumulative damage that finally results in a visible solar scar [58]. There is growing evidence that several signal transduction pathways are redox sensitive, among them transcription factors AP-1, AP-2 and NF-κB [59—61]. Proinflammatory (IL-1) and inflammatory (IL-8) cytokines, as well as collagenases are stimulated by UV light presumably via redox sensitive mechanisms [53,61,62]. A recent study also pointed out the importance of the ferric/ferrous ion in the UV mediated signal cascade [63].

5   ANTIOXIDATIVE INTERVENTION

Many antioxidants are being tested in the protection against photooxidative damage in the skin. The most commonly studied compounds are vitamin E and vitamin C. However, other antioxidants are also the subject of investigation. Polyphenols have shown anticarcinogenic properties in the mouse model [64].

This chapter will focus on vitamin E as an important example of some of the beneficiary effects of antioxidants. The majority of studies have been carried out in animal models, and only limited data exists for human studies. Topical application of vitamin E prevents depletion of endogenous vitamin E by UV irradiation (hairless mouse) [65]. Lipid peroxidation is inhibited after oral supplementation of vitamin E in mice [66] and also after topical application [67]. Several studies indicate that topically applied vitamin E inhibits UV-B-induced photodamage of DNA in a mouse model [68] and keratinocyte cultures (trolox) [69]. Protection against Langerhans cell depletion by UV light was observed after topical application of vitamin E in a mouse model [70].

α-Tocopherol and its sorbate ester were studied in a mouse model of skin aging. Both antioxidants were found to be effective, sorbate even more so, than α-tocopherol. [71]. Systemic administration of vitamin E in humans (in combination with vitamin C) increased the MED and reduced changes in skin blood flow after UV irradiation [72].

α-Tocopherol, the most commonly used form of vitamin E for external application, is quite unstable and light sensitive when used in topical formulations. The active hydroxyl group is, therefore, usually protected by esterification with acetate. This increases the stability but renders the compound redox inactive. When orally administered, vitamin E-acetate is hydrolyzed quantitatively in the gut [73]. There is some controversy to whether α-tocopherol acetate can be hydrolyzed in the skin. Chronic application of α-tocopherol acetate to hairless mice increases the level of free vitamin E significantly [74]. In the rat, slow bioconversion was observed which was enough to decrease the binding of 8-methoxypsoralen to macromolecules [75]. Recently, it was shown that UV-B increases the hydrolysis of α-tocopherol acetate to α-tocopherol in mouse skin by induction of nonspecific esterases [76] and could potentiate a 10- to 30-fold increase in free α-tocopherol. While one study suggested that bioconversion of α-tocopherol acetate does not occur in human skin, significant hydrolysis was demonstrated in recent studies using a human epidermis tissue culture model [77]. Yet several studies indicate that α-tocopherol acetate is not as effective as free vitamin E when applied topically. Inhibition of DNA mutation in mice was 5 to 10 times less effective [69]. Also in a mouse model, unlike free vitamin E, the acetate form seemed to be ineffective [71]. In summary, there is some considerable evidence that vitamin E is beneficial in limiting UV induced damage. However, further studies such as human trials and studies using the ester of vitamin E rather than the free form, are needed to better understand the actions of vitamin E supplementation in the skin.

6   OZONE-INDUCED OXIDATIVE STRESS

6.1 Possible reaction mechanisms

Ozone reacts readily with biomolecules. With its standard redox potential of +2.07 mV, it is [78] one of the most powerful oxidants known. It is not a biradical but resembles some characteristics of one, e.g., its ability to abstract hydrogen. Ozone is known to lead to the formation of free radicals and reactive intermediates and to the initiation of lipid peroxidation chain reactions. The oxidative loss of functional groups and the activities of biomolecules, including enzymes, has been reported. Also, alterations of membrane permeability and functions were observed, as well as the induction of inflammation [78].

Two main mechanisms were proposed [79] (Fig. 6) for the reaction of ozone with target molecules in the lung. In the first, an unsaturated hydrocarbon reacts with ozone, forming a peroxyl radical as an intermediate and finally hydrogen peroxide and two aldehydes. The second mechanism acts upon electron donors, such as glutathione and polyphenols. Hydrogen abstraction leads to the formation of a hydroxyl radical, dioxygen, and the radical of the electron donor.

A $RCH = CHR' + O_3 + H_2O \longrightarrow R\text{-}CHO + R'\text{-}CHO + H_2O_2$

B   (1) $X\!:\, +\ O_3 \longrightarrow X^\bullet + {}^\bullet O_3^-$

         (2) ${}^\bullet O_3^- + H^+ \longrightarrow HO^\bullet + O_2$

Fig. 6. Reaction mechanisms of ozone with target molecules in the lung [70]. **A**: with an olefin, and **B**: with and electron donor.

6.2 Ozone-induced damage

Keeping in mind the reactions of ozone with target molecules in the lung, it is easily conceivable that it also reacts with corresponding targets in the skin. Epidermal lipids are susceptible to peroxidation by UV. As to the stratum corneum lipids, the unsaturated lipids are limited to linoleic acid [80]. The presence of vitamin E in epidermis and in stratum corneum and the presence of glutathione in the epidermis is well-established. These and other molecules, depending on their accessibility, can be considered as possible direct or indirect targets.

So far, all data from ozone exposure of the skin has been generated in the hairless mouse model. Acute exposure of mice to 10 ppm for 2 h significantly depleted α-tocopherol and ascorbic acid in the upper epidermis of female SKH-1 hairless mice, while all deeper layers remained unaffected. Correspondingly, the formation of malondialdehyde (MDA), a product of lipid peroxidation, was increased dramatically in the upper epidermis and mildly in the lower epidermis/papillary dermis, while no changes were observed in the dermis [81].

The reactions in the stratum corneum can be analyzed separately by applying a tape stripping technique that is capable of sequentially removing the layers of the SC (Fig. 7). With this technique, lower doses of 5 and 1 ppm for 2 h were demonstrated to deplete α-tocopherol in a concentration-dependent manner. At 5 ppm, increased MDA formation was observed (Fig. 8). Chronic exposure with 6 times 1 ppm for 1 h each on 6 consecutive days depleted vitamin E and increased MDA formation in the stratum corneum [82].

It appears in these experiments that ozone reacts strongly with the outer limits of the skin, mainly the stratum corneum and the epidermis, while it most likeley

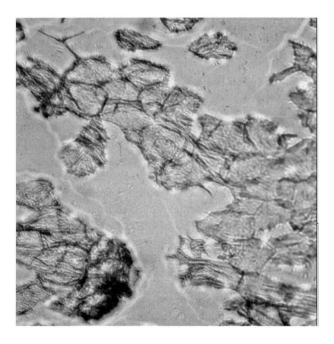

Fig. 7. Human corneocytes sticking to a transparent adhesive (micrograph magnification 40 × , DIC imaging).

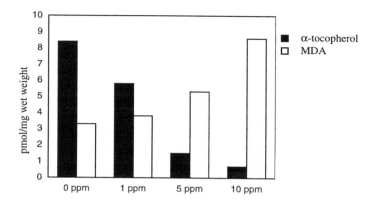

Fig. 8. Dose dependency of α-tocopherol depletion and MDA induction by ozone in murine stratum corneum ([82], reprinted by permission of Blackwell Science, Inc).

has no direct biochemical effect on deeper parts of the skin. However, it is conceivable that the structural integrity of the stratum corneum lipids could be compromised. Since the balance of the SC's lipid composition is vital for the body's barrier against transdermal water loss [83], a perturbation of the barrier could have possible health implications. A malfunctional barrier has been implicated in several dermal pathologies including atopic dermatitis and keloids. Barrier perturbation has been shown to evoke biological responses including increased gene transcription [84]. Repair mechanisms are stimulated with the formation of lamellar bodies aiming to replenish the SC lipids, but a proinflammatory response is also possible, since in the lung it has been shown to induce the nuclear factor NF-κB [85] which in turn stimulates the production of proinflammatory and inflammatory cytokines.

However, it is important to point out that the reported effects were observed only at doses exceeding the maximal ozone concentrations encountered currently. Therefore, it would be rather premature to consider current ozone levels to be an actual health risk to the skin. Still, the skin is not only exposed to ozone but to other components of photochemical smog as well, e.g., NO_2/NO and UV irradiation. NO_2 has been shown to exhibit synergistic effects with ozone in the lung, and UV irradiation could potentiate the ozone-induced damage to the skin.

7 SUMMARY

1. Outdoor exercise exposes the athlete to environmental stressors such as intense UV irradiation and ozone, a component of photochemical smog. As the stratospheric ozone layer continues to be depleted, both UV irradiation and ozone levels are likely to increase in the future.
2. The skin, as the outermost part of the body, is divided into the stratum corneum, epidermis, and dermis and is a primary target of environmental stres-

sors. The solar UV spectrum consists of a UV-B and a UV-A portion, which leads to the formation of radicals and reactive species via separate mechanisms.

3. The skin is protected from oxidative stress by a networking system of non-enzymatic (e.g., vitamin E, ubiquinone, vitamin C, glutathione) and enzymatic (e.g., superoxide dismutase, catalase, glutathione reductase and peroxidase) antioxidants.

4. UV irradiation depletes the antioxidant defenses in a dose-dependent manner. During phases of oxidative stress, biomolecules such as lipids, proteins and DNA are damaged.

5. This damage is believed to be causally involved in acute processes such as the sunburn reaction and in chronic pathologies like photoaging and photocancerogenesis.

6. Atmospheric ozone in high doses is found to deplete skin antioxidants and induce lipid damage. It is as yet unclear the consequences of this damage.

8   PERSPECTIVES

UV irradiation and ozone compromise the antioxidative defenses and cause oxidative stress and damage to biomolecules. UV irradiation is causally involved in photoaging and cancerogenesis. Extensive studies regarding ozone as a potential threat to human health have been carried out in the lung but are lacking in the skin. The outdoor athlete should try to minimize exposure to intense UV irradiation and photochemical smog. In any case, sufficient protection from sunlight by clothing and sunscreen are important to minimize the risk of photoaging and skin cancer. Future research is needed to elucidate the exact mechanism of how reactive species are involved in major skin pathologies. Thorough human studies should be directed toward the further characterization of the beneficiary effects of antioxidants to the skin.

9   ABBREVIATIONS

AP:	activator protein
IL:	interleukin
MDA:	malondialdehyde
MED:	minimal erythemal dose
NF-κB:	nuclear factor κB
NMSC:	nonmelanoma skin cancer
ROS:	reactive oxygen species
SC:	stratum corneum
TTP:	tocopherol transfer protein
UV:	ultraviolet

10 REFERENCES

1. Elias PM. Exp Dermatol 1996;5:191−201.
2. Quevedo WC, Holstein TJ. In: Norlund J (ed) The Pigmentary System. Oxford: Oxford University Press, 1998.
3. Odland GF. In: Goldsmith LA (ed) Physiology, Biochemistry, and Molecular Biology of the Skin. Oxford: Oxford University Press, 1991.
4. Jimbow K, Sugiyama S. In: Goldsmith LA (ed) Physiology, Biochemistry and Molecular Biology of the Skin. Oxford: Oxford University Press, 1991.
5. Soehnge H, Ouhtit A, Anathaswamy HN. Frontiers in Bioscience 1997;2:538−551.
6. World Meteorological Organization Global Ozone Research and Monitoring Project − Rep No 37 "Scientific Assesment of Ozone Depletion", 1994 Executive Summary.
7. Beissert S, Granstein RD. Crit Rev Biochem Molec Biol 1995;31:381−404.
8. Ayers SM, Evans RG, Buehler ME. Crit Rev Clin Lab Sci 1972;3:1−40.
9. Goldring J, Morris RD. Wisconsin Med J 1992;240−242.
10. Chapman S. Mem Roy Meteor Soc 1930;3:103−125.
11. Crutzen P. J Geophys Res 1971; 76:7311−7327.
12. Farman JB, Gardiner B, Shanklin J. Nature 1985;315:207−210.
13. Hagen−Smit AJ. Ind Eng Chem 1952;44:1342−1346.
14. South Coast Air Quality Management District: 1997 Annual Report (http://www.aqmd.gov).
15. WHO 1995. Update and revision of the air quality guidelines for Europe. EUR/ICP/EHAZ9405/Pb01.
16. German Government. "Ozongesetz", Bundesgesetzblatt 19 July 1995;part I:930.
17. Shindo Y, Witt E, Han D, Epstein W, Packer L. J Invest Dermatol 1994;102:122−124.
18. Thiele JJ, Traber MG, Packer L. J Invest Dermatol 1998;110:756−761.
19. Traber MG. Adv Pharmacol 1997;38:49−63.
20. Podda M, Weber C, Traber MG, Packer L. J Lipid Res 1996;37:893−901.
21. Fuchs J, Huflejt ME, Laurie M, Rothfuss AB, Wilson DS, Carcamo G, Packer L. J Invest Dermatol 1989;93:769−773.
22. Shindo Y, Witt E, Packer L. J Invest Dermatol 1993;100:260−265.
23. Smith JA. J Leukoc Biol 1994;56:672−686.
24. Ogura R, Sugiyama M, Nishi J, Haramaki N. J Invest Dermatol 1991;97:1044−1047.
25. Taira J, Mimura K, Yoneya T, Hagi A, Muramaki A, Makino K. J Biochem 1992;111:693−695.
26. Masaki H, Takamasa A, Sakurai H. Biochem Biophys Res Com 1995;206:474−479.
27. Buettner GR, Motten AG, Hall RD, Chignell CF. Photochem Photobiol 1987;46:161−164.
28. Kagan V, Witt E, Goldman R, Scita G, Packer L. Free Rad Res Comms 1991;16:51−64.
29. Kagan V, Witt E, Goldman R, Scita G, Packer L. Free Rad Res Comms 1992;16:51−64.
30. Foote CS. Photochem Photobiol 1991;54:659.
31. Fuchs J, Hufleit ME, Rothfuss LM, Wilson DS, Caramo G, Packer L. Photochem Photobiol 1989;50:739−744.
32. Shindo Y, Witt E, Han D, Tzeng B, Aziz T, Nguyen L, Packer L. Photodermatol Photoimmunol Photomed 1994;10:183−191.
33. Packer L. In: Rice−Evans CA, Burdon RH (eds) Free Radical Damage and its Control. Amsterdam: Elsevier Science, 1994.
34. Shindo Y, Witt E, Han D, Packer L. J Invest Dermatol 1994;102:470−475.
35. Fuchs J. Oxidative Injury in Dermatopathology. Berlin, New York: Springer, 1992.
36. Berlett BS, Stadtman ER. J Biol Chem 1997;33:20313−20316.
37. Monboisse JC, Braquet P, Randoux A, Borel JP. Biochem Pharmacol 1983;32:53−58.
38. Monboisse JC, Braquet P, Borel JP. Agents Action 1984;15:49−50.
39. Carbonare MD, Pathak MA. J Photochem Photobiol B, Biol 1992;14:105−124.
40. Thiele JJ, Traber MG, Re R, Espuno N, Yan LY, Cross CE, Packer L. FEBS Lett 1998;422:403−406.

41. Lledias F, Rangel P, Hansberg W. J Biol Chem 1998;273:10630—10637.
42. Miyachi Y, Imamura S, Niwa Y. J Invest Dermatol 1987;89:111—112.
43. Beckman KB, Ames BN. J Biol Chem 1997;32:19633—19636.
44. Freeman SE, Gange RW, Matzinger EA, Sutherland BM. J Invest Dermatol 1986;86:34—36.
45. Freeman SE, Gange RW, Sutherland JC, Matzinger EA, Sutherland BM. J Invest Dermatol 1987;88:430—433.
46. Cadet J, Berger M, Douki T, Morin B, Raoul S, Ravanat JL, Spinelli S. Biol Chem 1997;378:1275—1286.
47. Epstein JH, Fukuyama K, Read WB, Epstein WL. Science 1970;168:1477—1479.
48. Okada K, Takahashi Y, Ohnishi K, Ishikawa O, Miyachi Y. J Dermatol Sci 1994;8:183—186.
49. Shea CR, Parrish JA. In: Goldsmith LA (ed) Physiology, Biochemistry, and Molecular Biology of the Skin, vol 2. Oxford: Oxford University Press, 1991.
50. Miller DL, Weinstock MA. J Am Acad Dermatol 1994;30:774—778.
51. Cerruti PA. Lancet 1994;344:862—863.
52. Scharfetter—Kochanek K, Wlashek M, Brenneisen P, Schauen M, Blaudshun R, Wenk J. Biol Chem 1997;378:1247—1257.
53. Horio T, Okamoto H. J Invest Dermatol 1987;88:699—702.
54. Gilchrest BA. J Am Acad Dermatol 1989;3:610—613.
55. Packer L, Bertram J, Mori A (eds) Oxidative Stress and Aging. Basel: Birkenhauser Verlag, 1995.
56. Hruza LL, Pentland AP. J Invest Dermatol 1993;100:35S—41S.
57. Fisher GJ, Datta SC, Tlwar HS, Wang ZQ, Varani J, Kang S, Vorhees JJ. Nature 1996;379:335—339.
58. Fisher GJ, Wang ZQ, Datta SC, Varani J, Kang S, Vorhees JJ. N Engl J Med 1997;337:1419—1428.
59. Flohe L, Brigelius—Flohe R, Saliou C, Traber M, Packer L. Free Radical Biol Med 1996;22:1115—1126.
60. Sen CK, Packer L. Faseb J 1996;10:709—720.
61. Briviba K, Klotz LO, Sies H. Biol Chem 378:1259—1265.
62. Bender K, Blattner C, Knebel A, Iordanov M, Herrlich P, Rahmsdorf HJ. J Photochem Photobiol 1997;37:1—17.
63. Brenneisen P, Wenk J, Klotz LO, Wlashek M, Briviba K, Krieg T, Sies H, Sharffeter—Kochanek K. J Biol Chem 1998:5279—5287.
64. Mukthar H, Katiyar SK, Agarwal R. J Invest Dermatol 1994;102:3—7.
65. Weber C, Podda M, Rallis M, Thiele JJ, Traber MG, Packer L. Free Rad Biol Med 1997;22:761—769.
66. Packer L. Scientific American Sciene and Medicine 1994;1(1):54—63.
67. Lopez—Torres M, Thiele JJ, Shindo Y, Han D, Packer L. Br J Dermatol 1998;138:207—215.
68. McVean M, Liebler DC. Carcinogenesis 1997;18:1617—1622.
69. Stewart MS, Cameron GS, Pence BC. J Invest Dermatol 1996;106:1086—1089.
70. Yuen KS, Halliday GM. Photochem Photobiol 1997;65:587—592.
71. Jurkiewicz BA, Bisset DL, Buettner GR. J Invest Dermatol 1995;104:484—488.
72. Eberlein—Konig B, Placzek M, Przybilla B. J Am Acad Dermatol 1998;38:45—48.
73. Mathias PM, Harries JT, Peters TJ, Mueller DPR. J Lipid Res 1981;22:829—837.
74. Norkus EP, Bryce GF, Bhagavan HN. Photochem Photobiol 1993;57:613—615.
75. Beijersbergen van Henegouwen GMJ, Junginger HE, de Vries H. J Photochem Photobiol B: Biol 1995;29:45—51.
76. Kramer—Stickland K, Liebler DC. J Invest Dermatol 1998;111:302—307.
77. Nabi Z, Tavakkol A, Soliman N, Polefka TG. J Invest Dermatol 1998;110:679.
78. Mustafa MG. Free Rad Biol Med 1990;9:245—265.
79. Pryor WA. Free Rad Biol Med 1994;17:451—465.
80. Elias PM, Brown BE, Ziboh VA. J Invest Dermatol 1980;74:230—233.

81. Thiele JJ, Traber MG, Tsang K, Cross CE, Packer L. Free Rad Biol Med 1997;23:385—391.
82. Thiele JJ, Traber MG, Polefka TG, Cross CE, Packer L. J Invest Dermatol 1997;108:753—757.
83. Elias PM, Feingold KR. Semin Dermatol 1992;11:176—182.
84. Harris IR, Farrell AM, Grunfeld C, Holleran WM, Elias PM, Feingold KR. J Invest Dermatol 1997;109:783—787.
85. Haddad EB, Salmon M, Koto H, Barnes PJ, Adcock I, Chung KF. FEBS Lett 1996;379: 265—268.

Part IX

Organ functions

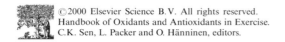
©2000 Elsevier Science B.V. All rights reserved.
Handbook of Oxidants and Antioxidants in Exercise.
C.K. Sen, L. Packer and O. Hänninen, editors.

Part IX • Chapter 22

Muscle fatigue: mechanisms and regulation

Michael B. Reid

Department of Medicine, Pulmonary Section, Baylor College of Medicine, One Baylor Plaza, Suite 520B, Houston, Texas 77030, USA. Tel.: +1-713-798-7224. E-mail: reid@bcm.tmc.edu

1   INTRODUCTION
    1.1   Early detection of free radicals in muscle
    1.2   Exercise and oxidative stress
    1.3   Nutritional supplements and exercise performance
    1.4   From phenomenology to mechanism
2   OXIDANT PRODUCTION BY SKELETAL MUSCLE
    2.1   Reactive oxygen species (ROS)
    2.2   Nitric oxide (NO) derivatives
3   REDOX MODULATION OF CONTRACTILE FUNCTION
    3.1   Basics of muscle contraction
    3.2   Contraction of unfatigued muscle
        3.2.1   Enhancement by ROS
        3.2.2   Inhibition by NO
    3.3   Muscle fatigue
        3.3.1   ROS as a cause of fatigue
        3.3.2   NO involvement
    3.4   ROS homeostasis in muscle
4   CELLULAR AND MOLECULAR MECHANISMS
    4.1   Effects on excitation-contraction coupling
        4.1.1   Sarcolemma
        4.1.2   Sarcoplasmic reticulum (SR)
            4.1.2.1   Calcium release channel
            4.1.2.2   Calcium-dependent ATPase
        4.1.3   Myofilaments
    4.2   Indirect mechanisms
        4.2.1   Mitochondrial dysfunction
        4.2.2   Loss of vascular control
        4.2.3   Altered motor control
5   SUMMARY
6   PERSPECTIVES
7   ACKNOWLEDGMENTS
8   ABBREVIATIONS
9   REFERENCES

1   INTRODUCTION

Over the past decade, the association of oxidative stress and exercise has become widely recognized in our society. Antioxidant intake is believed by many to affect athletic performance. Coaches, trainers, and sports nutritionists have introduced antioxidants to the training table. Feature articles in magazines and newspapers regularly report on the importance of antioxidants for professional and amateur athletes alike. In response, the antioxidant properties of food products are now advertised aggressively and over-the-counter sales of nutritional supplements is a major industry worldwide. But what is the scientific basis for this phenomenon? Where did the idea arise and how valid is it?

1.1 Early detection of free radicals in muscle

The story began with the advent of a new technology: electron spin resonance (ESR) spectroscopy. Prior to the advent of ESR, indirect evidence led bio-chemists to infer that free radicals existed as reaction intermediates but such short-lived molecular species could not be measured in biological systems. ESR provided a method to do so. ESR signals can be used to detect carbon-centered radicals in tissue samples, e.g., semiquinones. These signals generally are thought to reflect redox intermediates in the mitochondrial electron transport chain [1—8]. ESR was the method first used to establish the existence of free radicals in muscle and to demonstrate their physiologic relevance.

In 1954, Commoner and co-workers [1] used ESR techniques to detect free radicals in a variety of biological samples including freeze-dried rabbit muscle (Fig. 1). Seven years later, this same group [2] assessed the free-radical content of surviving tissues from guinea pig, rat, and mouse and reported that, "ESR signals are usually undetectable in samples of skeletal muscle from all three animals; occasionally, it is possible to detect a very weak signal". Not a very interesting finding. It was two decades before the topic of free radicals in skeletal muscle reappeared in the scientific literature.

The early 1980s produced several landmark papers which demonstrated that contractile activity increased free radical levels in muscle. Koren et al. [3] first studied isolated frog limb muscles that were stimulated to contract under isotonic conditions. During a 20-s tetanic contraction, free radical content increased from 7×10^7 centers/g under baseline conditions to approximately 17.5×10^7 centers/g. Longer contractions caused free radical content to return to baseline levels within 60 s; this was associated with a slow decline in the ability of the muscle to shorten. The authors attributed the transient rise in free radical content to a change in the metabolic state of muscle mitochondria. They subsequently bolstered this postulate by demonstrating that potassium cyanide disrupts the relationship between free radical concentration and muscle contraction [4].

One month later, Davies and co-workers [5] published a landmark report that dramatically increased scientific interest in this field. They measured a 2- to 3-fold increase in the free radical content of skeletal muscle of rats run to exhaustion. This was associated with decreased control of mitochondrial respiration, loss of integrity of the sarcoplasmic reticulum, and increased lipid peroxidation. These changes were exaggerated by vitamin E deficiency. Davies and colleagues reasoned that redox changes were a physiologic component of the exercise response and that increases in free radical content might influence muscle adap-

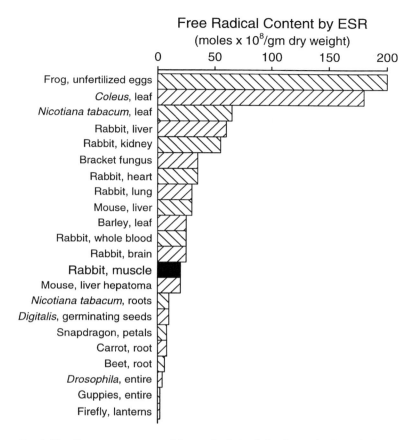

Free Radical Content by ESR
(moles x 10^8/gm dry weight)

Fig. 1. The first measurement of free radicals in skeletal muscle. Bars depict measurements by ESR spectroscopy from 500 mg samples of lyophilized, powdered tissue; biological signals from muscle (solid bar) and nonmuscle tissue (hatched bars) were compared with the absorption of 10^{-8} mol diphenyl picryl hydrazyl free radical under identical conditions; data replotted from Commoner, Townsend and Pike [1].

tation to exercise by stimulating mitochondrial biogenesis. The physiologic relevance of these events were further underscored by Jackson et al. [6] who demonstrated that free radicals were measurable in intact limb muscles and in human skeletal muscle and confirmed that excessive contractile activity increased free radical content. Almost a decade later, ESR techniques continue to be used in studies of skeletal muscle. Borzone et al. [7] recently demonstrated that the free radical content of the rat diaphragm is increased following a bout of inspiratory resistive loading. Under similar conditions, Hartell and co-workers [8] have shown that resistive breathing also increases free radical content in the systemic circulation.

1.2 Exercise and oxidative stress

The discovery that contractile activity stimulates free radical production in muscle caused a flurry of research activity. These investigations linked heavy exercise with oxidative stress, defined as a shift in the pro-oxidant/antioxidant balance toward oxidants [9]. Authoritative reviews by Sen [10] and Alessio [11] detail this association which is based on two parallel lines of evidence.

First, strenuous exercise increases biochemical markers of oxidative stress. The most common are by-products of lipid peroxidation. Free radical attack of biological membranes yields an array of lipid derivatives including malondialdehyde, thiobarbituric acid reactive substances, conjugated dienes, and pentane. These markers of lipid peroxidation are increased in experimental animals subjected to either muscle stimulation or whole-body exercise and in exercising humans. Glutathione oxidation is another widely used marker of oxidative stress. Reduced glutathione (GSH) is the primary antioxidant defense within eukaryotic cells. GSH is oxidized by free radicals and free radical derivatives to form glutathione disulfide (GSSG). Exercise drives this reaction, increasing GSSG levels in muscle and in the circulation and depleting total glutathione (GSH + GSSG) in skeletal muscle, heart, and liver. Protein oxidation is another index of oxidative stress that is elevated by exercise. Such reactions are likely to occur earlier than lipid peroxidation or GSH depletion and have obvious implications for muscle function. Surprisingly little is known about the extent of protein oxidation in working muscle or the relative susceptibility of regulatory proteins. Finally, exercise may cause oxidative modification of nucleic acids but this marker is not consistently altered by exercise.

Second, antioxidant depletion lowers exercise capacity and exaggerates exercise-induced muscle injury. The best documented example of this is vitamin E deficiency which leads to enhanced lipid peroxidation in muscle and other tissues, increased susceptibility to muscle injury, and a reduction in exercise performance. Disruption of the glutathione cycle has also been shown to cause decreased endurance in whole body exercise and in isolated muscle preparations. Unlike vitamin E deficiency, however, perturbation of GSH homeostasis does not consistently produce biochemical evidence of oxidative stress.

1.3 Nutritional supplements and exercise performance

If antioxidant deficiency compromises endurance performance, it logically follows that antioxidant supplementation might enhance performance. Much time and effort has been consumed in the attempt to demonstrate this principle. Supplements containing vitamin E, vitamin C, β-carotene, and other antioxidant nutrients — either alone or in combination — have been administered to experimental animals and to human volunteers for varying amounts of time. Results of these studies show that such interventions can reverse the effects of nutritional deficiencies. In the absence of malnutrition, antioxidant supplements also can decrease the biochemical markers of oxidative stress produced during exercise and can lessen exercise-induced muscle injury. However, dozens of carefully designed, rigorously conducted studies have failed to demonstrate improvements in either strength or endurance performance. Reviews of this literature by Gold-farb [12], Kanter [13], and Packer [14] have concluded that nutritional antioxidants generally are not effective as ergogenic aids.

1.4 From phenomenology to mechanism

At the beginning of this decade, the field began to change. New experimental approaches were used to address old questions and new, more mechanistic questions were raised. What is the nature of free radicals produced by skeletal muscle and what is their source? Is oxidative stress a cause of muscle fatigue or merely an effect? Do endogenous oxidants influence contractile function of unfatigued muscle? What are the molecular targets of free radical action?

Attempts to address these questions have revealed that free radical homeostasis is fundamental to skeletal muscle physiology. In the unfatigued state, skeletal muscle produces a wide array of free radicals and low molecular weight derivatives that are essential for normal contractile function. During strenuous exercise, redox active molecules accumulate within the working myocyte and depress cellular function, playing a causal role in muscle fatigue. Redox effects on contraction are mediated by regulatory proteins in the muscle fiber that react directly with free radicals and their derivatives. Such reactions reversibly alter protein function via covalent and allosteric modifications. The remainder of the chapter reviews this recent literature, detailing the research on which these concepts are based.

2   OXIDANT PRODUCTION BY SKELETAL MUSCLE

Rapid progress has been made over the last few years in our appreciation of the low molecular weight oxidants produced by skeletal muscle. These include reactive oxygen species and nitric oxide derivatives. These two classes of redox mediators are closely related chemically and are functionally interdependent in biological systems. For clarity, however, each is discussed separately in the sections that follow.

2.1 Reactive oxygen species (ROS)

Table 1 summarizes the evidence that skeletal muscle produces ROS in the absence of disease. Our laboratory used an intracellular fluorochrome probe to detect ROS in the cytosol of intact muscle fibers [15]. Both superoxide anions and hydrogen peroxide were detectable in unfatigued muscle fibers. Repetitive, electrically stimulated contractions caused oxidant levels in the cytosol to increase. A follow-up study [16] discovered that isolated muscle also releases

Table 1. Measurements of ROS production by skeletal muscle.

Muscle preparation	ROS detected	Localization in tissue	Detection assay	Reference
Rat diaphragm in vitro	O_2^-, H_2O_2	Muscle fiber cytosol	Intracellular fluorochrome[a]	Reid et al. [15]
Rat diaphragm in vitro	O_2^-	Extracellular space	Cytochrome c reduction	Reid et al. [16]
Rat diaphragm in vitro	·OH	Tissue homogenate	Salicylate hydroxylation	Diaz et al. [18]
Cat triceps surae in situ	·OH	Venous blood	Phenylalanine hydroxylation	O'Neill et al. [20]
Rat diaphragm in situ	O_2^-	Venous blood	Cytochrome c reduction	Kolbeck et al. [17]
Rat diaphragm in vivo	·OH	Tissue homogenate	Salicylate hydroxylation	Hasegawa et al. [19]

All studies documented an increase in ROS production during fatiguing exercise compared with resting muscle. [a]2′,7′-dichlorofluorescin diacetate.

superoxide anions into the extracellular space. Superoxide was released at a slow rate under passive conditions. During repetitive contractions, this signal increased 400% and was correlated with the fatigue characteristics of individual muscle preparations. Kolbeck et al. [17] have confirmed the physiologic relevance of superoxide release by working muscle. They measured minute-by-minute changes in superoxide levels of blood perfusing the canine diaphragm. Under passive conditions, no superoxide was detected in the vascular compartment. However, a bout of fatiguing stimulation induced superoxide production at the rate of 0.7 nmol/min. Superoxide release was elevated within the first minute, remained elevated throughout the fatigue protocol, and returned to baseline levels when muscle contraction ceased.

Superoxide anions and hydrogen peroxide appear to react via Fenton chemistry to produce hydroxyl radicals in skeletal muscle. Diaz and co-workers [18] first demonstrated that fatiguing muscle produces hydroxyl radicals. They studied muscle preparations isolated from rat diaphragm and found that the tissue content of hydroxyl radicals was increased by fatiguing stimulation. This signal was proportional to the accumulated tension-time product developed during fatigue. More recently, Hasegawa et al. [19] reported similar findings in studies of rat diaphragm in vivo. Fatiguing contractions increased the hydroxyl radical content of muscle and this increase correlated with force development. As observed for superoxide, hydroxyl radicals also appear to reach the vascular compartment in muscle. O'Neill et al. [20] showed that hydroxyl radicals are released into blood perfusing the cat hindlimb in proportion to the force of limb muscle contractions. Hydroxyl radical production was elevated in the absence of detectable fatigue and could be blocked by an iron chelator (deferoxamine) suggesting hydroxyl radicals are formed in the muscle via a Fenton-like reaction. It appears that nutritional status may influence the activity of this pathway. Rock et al. [21] have shown that hydroxyl radical signals from rat limb muscle homogenates are increased by chronic magnesium deficiency.

2.2 Nitric oxide (NO) derivatives

NO is a free radical synthesized enzymatically from L-citrulline by NO synthase (NOS). Two NOS isoforms are expressed constitutively by mammalian cells, the neuronal type NOS (nNOS) and the endothelial type (eNOS). Both isoforms are calcium-dependent. A third isoform, inducible NOS or iNOS, synthesizes NO at a rapid rate that is substrate limited and is not regulated by calcium. iNOS is not generally detectable in skeletal muscle under physiologic conditions [22] but has been reported in guinea pig muscle [23] and can be expressed by skeletal muscle in inflammatory disease [24,25]. NO is electrically neutral and freely diffusible in biological systems. NO reacts with molecular oxygen to yield an array of low molecular weight, redox-active derivatives. NO and its derivatives react with sulfhydryl groups and transition metal centers of regulatory proteins to influence cellular function.

The first suggestion that NO might be important in skeletal muscle was a report by Nakane et al. [26] that human skeletal muscle contains mRNA for nNOS. This isoform was named for the neural tissue in which it was originally discovered and nerve roots that pass through skeletal muscle tissue clearly express nNOS [27]. However, Kobzik et al. [28] demonstrated that skeletal muscle fibers also express nNOS which is localized to the sarcolemma of fast type fibers, a finding later confirmed by this same group [29] and by Grozdonovic et al. [30]. Brenman and co-workers [31,32] then determined that nNOS is concentrated in the subsarcolemmal region near the motor end-plate and is associated with the α1-syntrophin protein of the dystrophin complex. Several studies suggest that nNOS expression varies importantly among muscles and among mammalian species [22,30]. A second source of NO in skeletal muscle is the eNOS isoform. eNOS is evident in the endothelial cells of muscle capillaries but also is expressed by skeletal muscle fibers. Kobzik and co-workers [29] found that eNOS expression is not linked to myosin-based fiber type, a finding confirmed by Hussain and co-workers [22]. Rather, eNOS is associated with muscle mitochondria and acts to limit oxidative metabolism via direct effects of NO on electron transport [29]. Endurance training influences NOS expression in muscle. Balon and Nadler [33] have shown that both nNOS and eNOS isoforms are upregulated in rodent limb muscle after training.

It is clear that NO and its derivatives are normal components of the physiologic milieu in skeletal muscle. Isolated muscle preparations release NO derivatives into the extracellular space at a rate of approximately 1 pmol/mg/min during passive incubation [28,34]. Balon and Nadler [34] showed that repetitive muscle contraction accelerates NO synthesis by muscle. Thus, NO production is activity-dependent.

3   REDOX MODULATION OF CONTRACTILE FUNCTION

The contractile function of skeletal muscle appears to be strongly influenced by redox mechanisms. In unfatigued muscle, ROS and NO exert opposing effects; ROS increase force and NO derivatives depress force. Contractile function is determined by the balance between these two factors. During strenuous activity, increased ROS production can induce oxidative stress and loss of muscle function. The following sections describe basic concepts in muscle contraction and review our understanding of redox effects on muscle contraction, both in the unfatigued state and during fatigue.

3.1 Basics of muscle contraction

This section offers a brief overview of the cellular events that mediate skeletal muscle contraction (Fig. 2). Readers familiar with these aspects of muscle physiology may choose to skip this material. Those wishing a more detailed understanding may benefit from recent reviews that discuss motor control [35], excitation-contraction coupling [36,37], and muscle metabolism [38,39] in greater depth.

Unlike cardiac and smooth muscle, skeletal muscle is under direct control of the central nervous system. Action potentials originate in the motor cortex or premotor cortex of the brain. They propagate to the periphery via motor axons and stimulate acetylcholine release from the axon terminal. Each axon terminal

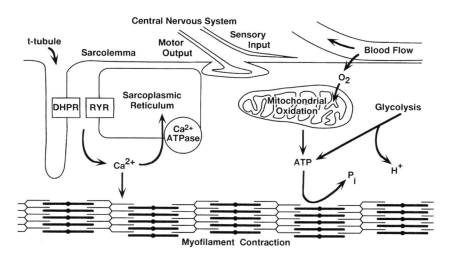

Fig. 2. Regulation of muscle contraction. Diagram depicts structures and processes described in section 3.1; DHPR, dihydropyridine-sensitive voltage sensor; RYR, ryanodine-sensitive SR calcium release channel; Ca^{2+} ATPase, SR calcium-dependent ATPase; Ca^{2+}, calcium; ATP, adenosine triphosphate; P_i, inorganic phosphate; H^+, hydrogen ion; O_2, molecular oxygen.

is localized to a specialized site on the muscle fiber membrane (sarcolemma) which contains acetylcholine receptors. Binding of acetylcholine to surface receptors triggers an action potential on the sarcolemma.

Sarcolemmal action potentials propagate along the surface of the muscle fiber and deep into the cell via membrane invaginations known as t-tubules. T-tubules are closely apposed to the sarcoplasmic reticulum (SR), an extensive, membrane-bound syncytium specialized for intracellular calcium storage. Action potential propagation along the t-tubule triggers calcium release from the SR. Voltage-dependent calcium release is thought to involve mechanical interaction of the dihydropyridine-sensitive voltage sensor, a membrane-spanning protein in the t-tubule, with the ryanodine-sensitive calcium release channel of the SR. Calcium is thereby released from SR stores. The ensuing rise in cytoplasmic calcium activates a calcium-sensitive regulatory protein in the myofilament lattice (troponin c) and stimulates muscle contraction.

Contraction reflects the transduction of chemical to mechanical energy by muscle myofilaments. Myosin cross-bridges interact with calcium-activated sites on the adjacent actin filaments. This reaction is ATP-dependent. Its mechanical product varies according to the constraints on the muscle and the intensity of activation. Under physiologic conditions, contraction results in force production by the muscle, active shortening, or both. Under laboratory conditions, muscle shortening is usually constrained and contraction intensity is measured as force output. The intensity of skeletal muscle contraction is proportional to the frequency of fiber stimulation and the number of muscle fibers that are activated. During volitional exercise, intact muscles are stimulated by the central nervous system using a complex activation pattern in which the frequency of fiber stimulation and the number of recruited fibers varies widely. In experimental systems, muscles are usually activated by electrical stimulation. The intensity of contraction is altered by varying stimulation frequency. The mechanical response to a single stimulus is a twitch. Repetitive stimulation evokes prolonged tetanic contractions that develop higher forces. The force of tetanic contraction can increase 3- to 10-fold beyond twitch force as stimulus frequency increases.

When muscle stimulation stops, contraction is rapidly terminated by reversal of the processes outlined above. Calcium release channels in the SR close and ATP-dependent calcium pumps (SR calcium ATPase) actively transport calcium back into the SR lumen. Subsequently, cytosolic calcium concentration returns to baseline levels and actin-myosin interaction is inhibited.

The events described above are energy-dependent. Glycolytic pathways respond rapidly to muscle activation and can meet metabolic needs for brief periods. However, endurance exercise depends critically on aerobic metabolism. Muscle mitochondria hydrolyze substrates and produce ATP via oxidative phosphorylation. The upper limit of muscle metabolism is, therefore, linked to mitochondrial content. However, oxidative phosphorylation requires continual delivery of molecular oxygen to the inner mitochondrial membrane. In perfused muscles, capillary blood flow delivers oxygen and substrate to the tissue. Blood flow also removes metabolic by-products that would otherwise accumulate in the tissue and inhibit muscle function. Adequate blood flow, therefore, is essential for optimal metabolism. Factors that restrict blood flow or that disrupt its distribution within the tissue can limit metabolism and thereby limit performance.

3.2 Contraction of unfatigued muscle

Under basal conditions, the contractile function of skeletal muscle is clearly sensitive to changes in redox status. Antioxidants appear to depress force whereas low level oxidant exposure can increase force production. Puppi et al. [40] demonstrated the general principle in early studies of unfatigued limb muscle from frogs. They observed that exposure to a reducing agent (ascorbate) decreased force whereas an oxidizing agent (threonine) increased force. As detailed below, subsequent research has established that ROS and NO exert similar effects on unfatigued muscle.

3.2.1 Enhancement by ROS

Endogenous ROS appear to be essential for normal force production by unfatigued muscle. This was first suggested by the pilot studies of Regnier and co-workers [41] in which ROS depletion appeared to diminish force production. Figure 3 shows data obtained using single fibers isolated from frog limb muscle. Fibers incubated with exogenous superoxide dismutase (SOD; dismutes superoxide anions) or catalase (dehydrates hydrogen peroxide) underwent marked

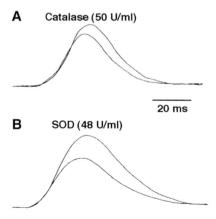

A   Catalase (50 U/ml)

20 ms

B   SOD (48 U/ml)

Fig. 3. ROS depletion inhibits twitch contraction in unfatigued muscle. Tracings depict the force of twitch contractions by intact skeletal muscle fibers from frog limb muscle; curarized fibers at optimal length were stimulated directly (supramaximal voltage, 0.2 ms pulse) at 22°C; data collected before and after treatment with catalase 50 U/ml (**A**) or superoxide dismutase (SOD; **B**); in each panel, force tracings affected by catalase or SOD falls below the corresponding control trace; reproduced from a preliminary report by Regnier and co-workers [41] with permission of the authors.

reductions in twitch force. We formally confirmed these observations in studies of fiber bundles isolated from rat diaphragm [42]. Incubation with either SOD or catalase decreased the forces developed during twitch and tetanic contractions. ROS depletion depressed the force-frequency relationship and shifted it rightward in a dose-dependent manner. This effect was quite dramatic. Maximal tetanic force could be depressed by 50% or more, yet force recovered almost completely after the anti-ROS enzyme was washed out. Most recently, Andrade et al. [43] evaluated the redox sensitivity of unfatigued muscle using intact single fibers from mouse limb muscle. The reducing agent dithiothreitol was found to depress force. This effect was reversed by hydrogen peroxide exposure which returned force to control levels. Other studies also have shown that force production by unfatigued rodent diaphragm is decreased by nonspecific antioxidants including *N*-acetylcysteine [44] and dimethyl sulfoxide [45,46]. These findings suggest that oxidant depletion has a stereotypical effect on intact muscle fibers in the unfatigued state. Force production is depressed by oxidant depletion and such decrements are acutely reversible. Endogenous ROS thus, appear to be essential for normal contractile function.

To a limited extent, increasing the ROS levels in unfatigued muscle can have the opposite effect: force production increases. We first observed this phenomenon in studies of rodent diaphragm [42]. Hydrogen peroxide exposure modestly increased twitch characteristics (peak force, time-to-peak force, half-relaxation time), opposing the effects of SOD and catalase. Similarly Oba et al. [47] found that the initial response of frog skeletal muscle fibers to exogenous hydrogen peroxide was a rise in twitch tension. More extensive measurements were made by Lawler and co-workers [48] using diaphragm strips from young rats. Unfatigued muscles were incubated with a xanthine oxidase/hypoxanthine system that generated superoxide anions. Twitch and submaximal tetanic forces were increased with no change in maximal tetanic force, indicating a leftward shift of the force-frequency curve. Interestingly, muscles from old animals did not respond to this ROS challenge. Andrade and co-workers [43] have systematically studied this response using intact single fibers from mouse limb muscle. Brief exposure of unfatigued fibers to hydrogen peroxide caused submaximal tetanic force to increase relative to baseline conditions, an effect reversed by the reducing agent dithiothreitol. Data from these studies suggest that unfatigued muscle maintains the intracellular environment in a relatively reduced state and that this reducing environment limits contractile function. Modest ROS supplementation, therefore, increases force production. (Note that excessive ROS stimulation is toxic to all eukaryotic cells and skeletal muscle myocytes are no exception. Hydrogen peroxide effects on unfatigued muscle are well documented. Toxicity increases in proportion to concentration [42] and the duration of exposure [43,47] and is characterized by rapid loss of force leading to muscle contracture [42,43,47].)

3.2.2 Inhibition by NO

NO opposes ROS effects on unfatigued muscle. Blockade of NO synthesis increases the force of submaximal contractions and shifts the force-frequency relationship leftward; NO donors have opposite effects, decreasing force [23,27,28]. During loaded shortening, endogenous NO appears to be required for optimal power output; NOS blockade reduces power output by decreasing the velocity of loaded shortening [49,50].

NO appears to depress force by two distinct mechanisms. First, cyclic guanosine monophosphate (cGMP) is a second messenger for NO in skeletal muscle. NO stimulates cGMP synthesis by soluble guanylyl cyclase [28,51,52]. The ensuing rise in cGMP depresses force [28,52]. However, cGMP signaling cannot fully account for the action of NO in unfatigued muscle. Thus, a second mechanism of action has been postulated [53] whereby NO may function as an antioxidant, opposing ROS effects on regulatory proteins in muscle. This postulate is based on the established antioxidant properties of NO in other tissues [54]. NO can function as an antioxidant either by nitrosylating reactive sulfhydryls and thereby limiting disulfide formation or by reacting directly with ROS to limit diffusion [55].

3.3 Muscle fatigue

For the purposes of this chapter, muscle fatigue can be defined as a loss of contractile capacity that is caused by exercise and is reversible with rest. In volitional exercise, fatigue is commonly assessed by measuring the amount of time that an exercise task can be maintained. In electrically stimulated muscle preparations, fatigue is reflected by a progressive loss of mechanical output, e.g., isometric force. There are two extremes of electrically stimulated fatigue, each representing a different mechanism. Fatigue caused by low-frequency stimulation resembles the physiologic fatigue that occurs during volitional exercise. Both are associated with phosphocreatine depletion, acidosis, and delayed recovery of function. In contrast, fatigue caused by intense high-frequency stimulation is caused by t-tubule conduction failure and is associated with rapid recovery. This phenomenon is termed "high-frequency fatigue" and generally is considered nonphysiologic. Both volitional exercise and muscle stimulation have been used to test the importance of oxidative stress in fatigue. The data summarized in Fig. 4 clearly demonstrate that pretreatment with antioxidant probes — either ROS-selective enzymes, pharmacologic agents, or vitamin E — can inhibit fatigue under a wide variety of experimental conditions. These findings establish a cause-effect relationship. Oxidative stress contributes to fatigue caused either by volitional exercise or by low-frequency electrical stimulation. As detailed below, ROS play a central role in the fatigue process whereas NO appears to influence fatigue indirectly.

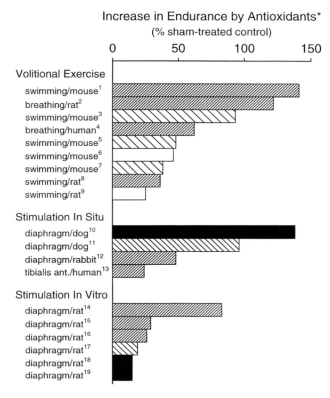

Fig. 4. Antioxidants inhibit muscle fatigue. Bars depict increase in endurance caused by pretreatment with ROS-specific enzymes (solid), thiol donors (fine hatching), vitamin E (open), or other nonspecific antioxidants (coarse hatching); data replotted from all published reports of positive antioxidant effects except Barclay and Hansel [57] and Moriura, et al. [66] that could not be expressed in the present units; footnotes depict antioxidants used: [1]reduced glutathione (GSH) 1000 mg/kg by intraperitoneal injection (ip) [65]; [2]N-acetylcysteine (NAC) 150 mg/kg by intravenous injection (iv) [62]; [3]5,5-dimethyl-1-pirrolyn-N-oxide 100 mM, 0.2 ml ip [65]; [4]NAC 150 mg/kg iv [61]; [5]α-4-pyridyil-1-oxide-N-tert-butyl-nitrone 100 mM, 0.2 ml ip [65]; [6]α-tocopherol 100 mg/kg/day × 3 days by intramuscular injection (im) [65]; [7]N-tert-butyl-α-phenyl-nitrone 100 mM, 0.2 mg ip [65]; [8]GSH 1000 mg/kg by oral administration (po) [60]; [9]vitamin E 500 mg/kg po [60]; [10]polyethylene glycol-adsorbed SOD 2,000 U/kg iv [56]; [11]dimethyl sulfoxide (DMSO) 50% solution 0.5 mg/kg iv [56]; [12] NAC 150 mg/kg iv [64]; [13]NAC 150 mg/kg iv [58]; [14]NAC 4 mg/ml incubation, indirect stimulation [63]; [15]NAC 10 mM incubation [44]; [16]NAC 4 mg/ml incubation, direct stimulation [63]; [17]DMSO 6.4 mM incubation [15]; [18]SOD 500 U/ml incubation [15]; [19]catalase 18,000 U/ml incubation [15].

3.3.1 ROS as a cause of fatigue

Endogenously produced ROS directly contribute to loss of mechanical function in muscle fatigue. This has been established by observations that SOD or catalase pretreatment can slow the fall in force during fatiguing exercise [15,56]. Figure 4 depicts the magnitude of fatigue-sparing effects that have been reported for

ROS-selective enzymes and other antioxidants; these include xanthine oxidase inhibitors [57], iron chelators [57], thiol donors [44,58−64], vitamin E [60,65], spin-traps [65], dimethyl sulfoxide [15,56,57], and other nonspecific antioxidants [66]. The efficacy of antioxidant interventions appears to be robust. Positive effects have been demonstrated in volitional exercise and in muscles activated electrically using preparations that range from isolated muscles to intact humans. The magnitude of antioxidant effects varies widely among studies but existing data suggest that oxidative stress may account for up to one-half of the mechanical losses that occur in acute fatigue.

Westerblad and colleagues [67] have suggested that the fatigue process involves a series of intracellular events that occur in sequence. To the extent this is true, ROS appear to preferentially influence the events that occur early in fatigue. This is evident in experiments that have tested antioxidant effects during repetitive electrical stimulation [15,44,56,58,64]. In these protocols, force fell rapidly during the first few minutes of stimulation; ROS scavengers and other antioxidants primarily acted to slow this early phase of fatigue. Force fell more slowly during the late phase of these protocols and the rate of force decline was less affected by antioxidants.

Antioxidants have only proven to be effective in volitional exercise or in stimulation protocols that utilize low-frequency, quasi-physiologic stimulus patterns. So-called "high-frequency" fatigue is a more artificial process that appears to be insensitive to antioxidant pretreatment [15,58]. Acute recovery from fatigue also appears to be unaffected by antioxidant pretreatment. Studies conducted in vitro [15,63] and in vivo [56,58,64] have monitored the increase in force that occurs immediately after fatiguing exercise. Antioxidants had no obvious effect on recovery of force.

Exogenous ROS have the opposite effect on exercising muscle. ROS exposure accelerates the loss of force that occurs during fatigue [48,57,68,69]. Thus, the effects of antioxidant pretreatment and ROS exposure are qualitatively different between unfatigued and fatiguing muscle. The most likely explanation for this apparent conundrum is that ROS production by intramuscular sources is accelerated during fatiguing exercise. Accumulation of endogenous ROS promotes oxidative stress and tends to compromise function. Antioxidants act to limit this shift and inhibit fatigue whereas exogenous ROS have an additive effect, promoting further loss of function.

Why do antioxidant enzymes and pharmacologic agents inhibit fatigue whereas nutritional supplements do not? The most likely explanation is that cellular uptake and tissue distribution of nutritional elements is regulated by the muscle. Perhaps muscle tissue does not incorporate nutrients at sufficiently high levels to be therapeutic. Alternatively, intracellular localization may be critical. Nutrients may not be concentrated near the cellular structure(s) that undergo oxidative modification during fatigue.

3.3.2 NO involvement

The direct effect of endogenous NO on fatiguing muscle have not been tested systematically. In theory, NO could either inhibit or promote fatigue based on its interactions with ROS. If antioxidant effects [54] predominate, NO would act to slow fatigue. Alternatively, high ROS levels favor NO conversion to peroxynitrite, a highly reactive radical that mediates nitrosative stress [70]. This pathway should accelerate fatigue. Pilot experiments by Abraham and co-workers [71] suggest that neither NO effect is prominent in excised muscle. As shown in Fig. 5, acute fatigue of isolated limb and respiratory muscles was not altered systematically

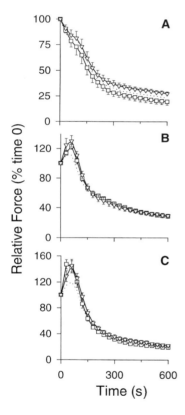

Fig. 5. NO effects on muscle fatigue in vitro. Mean forces ± SE developed by rat soleus (**A**), diaphragm (**B**) or extensor digitorum longus (EDL; **C**); muscles studied at optimal length and 37°C during direct submaximal-tetanic stimulation using supramaximal voltage, 0.2 ms pulses, 500 ms trains every 2 s at 15 Hz (soleus), 30 Hz (diaphragm), or 60 Hz (EDL); open squares depict data from muscles treated with an NO donor (sodium nitroprusside 1 mM; SNP); open triangles are data following NOS blockade ($N\omega$-nitro-L-arginine 10 mM; NLA); mean relationships for control data shown as dashed lines; for soleus, SNP and NLA curves each differ from Control at times 300–600 s ($p < 0.0001$); for diaphragm and EDL, SNP and NLA curves exceeded control at times 60–90 s. ($p < 0.01$). Data replotted from preliminary report of Abraham et al. [71] with permission of the authors.

by either NOS blockade or an NO donor. In a series of related studies, Murrant and co-workers [72—74] have tested the effects of NO donors on rodent limb muscle during infrequent, near maximal contractions in vitro. They found that exposure to a supplementary NO source slowed the progressive, irreversible loss of force that occurred under control conditions. Their observations suggest that exogenous NO may increase the stability of excised muscle.

There is evidence to suggest that NO influences fatigue of intact muscle via indirect effects on blood flow. Exercise hyperemia slows the development of muscle fatigue and is mediated in part by NO [75,76]. Recent experiments by Albertini et al. [77] indicate that NO homeostasis may be essential for this response. Systemic administration of a NOS inhibitor accelerated fatigue of working muscle by increasing local vascular resistance and compromising muscle blood flow. An NO donor increased fatigue by lowering perfusion pressure and thereby limiting flow. Thus, NO appears to be necessary for normal vascular regulation within working muscle. Loss of regulatory control predisposes the exercising muscle to fatigue.

3.4 ROS homeostasis in muscle

The ROS produced within muscle are buffered by an array of endogenous antioxidants that maintain ROS concentrations at low levels under baseline conditions. The balance between ROS production and intracellular buffering capacity can be perturbed in several ways. Increased production, exposure to exogenous sources, or an antioxidant deficiency will cause ROS levels to rise. Conversely, antioxidant supplementation or a decline in production will lower ROS levels. Data described in the preceding sections suggest that extreme shifts in either direction will compromise contractile function and that force production is optimal at some intermediate redox state. This suggests that cellular redox state may be regulated homeostatically and provides a context for oxidative involvement in muscle fatigue.

The diagram in Fig. 6 depicts a model that integrates the known effects of ROS on force production. Data from unfatigued muscles (section 3.2) suggest that endogenous ROS levels are less than optimal under basal conditions (A in Fig. 6). ROS depletion by exogenous antioxidants appears to depress force production by unfatigued muscle (B) whereas external ROS sources can increase intramuscular levels and optimize force (C). The effect of increasing ROS is biphasic, however. Excessive accumulation within the muscle appears to induce oxidative stress and decrease contractile function (D). Such shifts are evident in unfatigued muscles exposed to high levels of exogenous ROS. The right half of the model also describes fatiguing muscle (section 3.3) in which endogenous ROS production exceeds buffering capacity. This imbalance causes ROS to accumulate within the fatiguing muscle and contribute to the decline in force. Once a muscle has been driven rightward along the curve — either by ROS exposure or by accelerated production — exogenous antioxidants become beneficial. Antioxidants act to re-

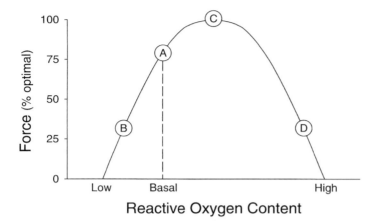

Fig. 6. Biphasic influence of reactive oxygen on skeletal muscle force production. Model integrates data from unfatigued and fatigued muscle. A, basal state of unfatigued muscle; B, fall in force production by unfatigued muscle following ROS depletion or antioxidant treatment; C, increase in force by unfatigued muscle following modest ROS exposure; D, fall in force following excessive ROS exposure. Adapted from previous depictions [42,43,53].

establish homeostasis by scavenging ROS, reversing oxidative modification of target proteins, or both. These effects drive the muscle leftward along the curve (e.g., from D toward point C) thereby increasing force production.

These concepts were originally developed to integrate the reported effects of ROS on unfatigued and fatigued muscle [42] and have been refined to incorporate new data as the field matures [53]. Recent studies by Andrade and co-workers [43] have tested aspects of this model experimentally and have validated its general principles. However, to understand the fatigue process it is essential that we progress beyond functional models to evaluate underlying mechanism(s). The following section reviews the intracellular processes that are sensitive to ROS and NO and the molecular events triggered by redox mechanisms.

4   CELLULAR AND MOLECULAR MECHANISMS

Authoritative reviews by Fitts [78] and Westerblad et al. [79] detail the prevailing view of intracellular events that mediate fatigue. Under physiological conditions, many aspects of muscle function remain within normal limits and are thought not to limit performance. Thus, neuromuscular activation, sarcolemmal depolarization, and ATP availability probably do not mediate fatigue directly. In contrast, calcium homeostasis and myofilament function are clearly compromised in fatiguing muscle and are the primary focus of mechanistic research in this field. Calcium handling by the sarcoplasmic reticulum (SR) becomes disrupted in the late phase of muscle fatigue, depressing the force of contraction and predisposing the muscle to incomplete relaxation between contractions. The myofilaments also lose function in fatigue, becoming less sensitive to calcium activation. Factors that decrease calcium sensitivity of the myofilaments include inorganic phosphate and hydrogen ions that accumulate in fatiguing muscle. Both metabolites act directly on myofilament proteins to inhibit cross-bridge interaction and decrease the force of contraction.

The relationship between these traditional mechanisms and the redox events that contribute to fatigue has not been established. A range of possible interactions exist as illustrated in Fig. 7. On the one hand, ROS and related oxidants act directly on regulatory proteins in the myocyte to inhibit muscle function. This is supported by observations that proteins critical to excitation-contraction coupling are sensitive to redox modulation. Alternatively, traditional mechanisms and redox effects may be interdependent. Oxidative stress may act at upstream sites to stimulate recognized pathways, e.g., by inhibiting mitochondrial metabolism or by compromising blood flow. Subsequent sections will address each of these possibilities individually, discussing the direct effects of ROS on excitation-contraction coupling (section 4.1) and possible indirect effects (section 4.2).

4.1 Effects on excitation-contraction coupling

At the most fundamental level, fatigue represents a failure of excitation-contraction coupling defined by Catterall [36] as, "... the process of coupling chemical and electrical signals at the cell surface to the intracellular release of calcium and ultimate contraction of muscle fibers". In fatiguing muscle, excitation-

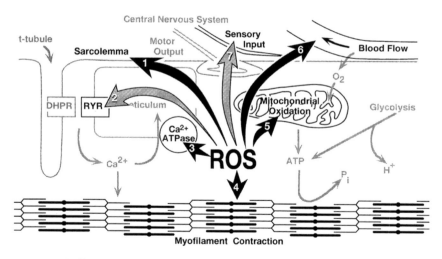

Fig. 7. ROS effects on muscle contraction. Diagram illustrates aspects of skeletal muscle contraction that ROS may inhibit (solid arrows) or exaggerate (shaded arrows): 1, sarcolemmal function; 2, calcium release from the SR; 3, calcium reuptake by the SR calcium ATPase; 4, myofilament contraction; 5, mitochondrial oxidation; 6, vascular control; 7, afferent feedback to the central nervous system. Abbreviations as in Fig. 2. See section 4 for details.

contraction coupling appears to be compromised by failure of sarcolemmal excitability, calcium homeostasis, or myofilament function. Proteins that regulate each of these processes can be disrupted by oxidative modification [79—81] suggesting multiple sites of oxidative action.

4.1.1 Sarcolemma

Electrical failure of the sarcolemma is thought to mediate "high-frequency fatigue". In this form of fatigue, the underlying mechanism is t-tubule depolarization [67]. Potassium accumulates in the t-tubules of during contraction, stabilizing the membrane and inhibiting action potential propagation into central regions of the myocyte. Accordingly, voltage-dependent calcium release is inhibited.

In theory, increased ROS production by contracting muscle could contribute to high-frequency fatigue by compromising potassium homeostasis. Experiments using skeletal muscle-derived L6 cells have demonstrated that sarcolemmal regulatory proteins are sensitive to oxidative modification [82]. Peroxide exposure activates the sodium-potassium pump, inhibits the sodium-potassium-chloride cotransporter, and inhibits passive influx of potassium into the cell. Such changes could contribute to high-frequency fatigue. Existing data do not support this mechanism, however, since antioxidant pretreatment does not appear to inhibit high-frequency fatigue [15,58].

Oxidative inhibition of the t-tubule voltage sensor could contribute to fatigue under more physiologic conditions. Several recent studies of isolated, skinned muscle fibers have demonstrated that oxidant exposure selectively compromises depolarization-induced force production without altering myofilament function [83,84]. Modest changes in SR function were noted — either calcium leak [84] or calcium-induced calcium release [83] — but these did not fully account for the loss of function. These observations suggest that the voltage sensor may have been inactivated by oxidant exposure. Voltage sensor inactivation acts to depress calcium transients in muscle and calcium transients are decreased by fatigue using low-frequency stimulation. The potential link between these two events has not yet been tested, however.

4.1.2 Sarcoplasmic reticulum (SR)

Calcium regulation by the SR is altered during exercise and this phenomenon contributes to fatigue [85—87]. SR function is strongly influenced by redox perturbations [47,79,83,88,89] due to critical regulatory proteins that are sensitive to oxidant effects [47,90,91]. These include both the calcium release channels and the calcium-dependent ATPase as detailed below.

4.1.2.1 Calcium release channel. Oxidant exposure stimulates isolated SR vesicles to release calcium. This phenomenon has been established using various chemical oxidants [92—95] including ROS [47,96] and is primarily attributed to oxidative modification of the calcium release channel [47,97,98]. Studies of isolated calcium release channels have confirmed that ROS promote channel opening. Single channel recordings have demonstrated that both the frequency and duration of spontaneous opening events are increased by ROS exposure [47,96,99]. ROS also enhance ryanodine binding to the channel [96] providing additional evidence for increased activity. Oxidative activation of the channel is acutely reversible by reducing agents [47,96,98] which fulfills a basic criterion for physiologic modulation via redox mechanisms.

Nitric oxide appears to have biphasic effects on the channel. At low concentrations, NO donors inhibit oxidative modification and thereby act to limit channel opening [99,100]. This suggests a cGMP-independent mechanism whereby NO may limit SR calcium release and depress force in unfatigued muscle. At higher concentrations, NO donors promote channel opening and stimulate disulfide formation [99,101]. These effects are indistinguishable from hydrogen peroxide effects in the same system [99] and suggest a mechanism whereby NO may compromise calcium homeostasis and contractile function when NO levels are elevated, e.g., by exercise or sepsis.

Recent research by Wu and co-workers [102] demonstrate that changes in function of the SR calcium release channel have a structural basis. The channel is a huge homotetrameric protein composed of four monomeric subunits; each has a molecular mass of 535 kD. Oxidation of the protein stimulates formation of intermolecular disulfide bonds between monomeric subunits, inducing dimerization. Intramolecular cross-links also are formed. These modifications correlate with increased channel opening and have been localized to specific regions of the protein. The cysteines that undergo oxidative cross-linking are located in the cytoplasmic domain between amino acids $\sim 2,100$ and 2,843 or between amino acids 2,844 and 4,685. The cysteines that are most sensitive to modification and, therefore, are most likely to participate in physiologic regulation are localized to the N-terminal domain between amino acids 426 and 1,396. These findings suggest that redox modulation of calcium channel activity is regulated by interactions between the N-terminal region and regions of the cytoplasmic domain.

4.1.2.2 Calcium-dependent ATPase. Acute fatigue slows the SR calcium-dependent ATPase, or calcium pump, both in excised rodent muscle [103] and in human limb muscle [104]. Slowing of pump activity may slow calcium reuptake or cause cytosolic calcium concentration to increase, changes that occurs in fatiguing muscle [105,106]. One mechanism that can slow the calcium pump is redox modification of protein thiols or tyrosine residues. In isolated cells and SR vesicle preparations, calcium pump activity is slowed by artificial oxidants [89,91,107,108] or by systems that generate ROS including hydrogen peroxide [109], singlet oxygen [110], and hydroxyl radicals [108,111,112]. The pump is also inhibited by peroxynitrite exposure which causes protein thiol oxidation [113] and nitrotyrosine formation [114]. Oxidative slowing of the SR pump during fatigue has not been tested systematically. However, the concept is supported by pilot data from Byrd and co-workers [115]. They observed that fatiguing exercise slows pump activity in equine limb muscle and that pump function is rapidly rescued by the reducing agent dithiothreitol.

Sensitivity to redox modulation appears to differ among calcium pump isoforms. The SERCA2b isoform from slow-type skeletal muscle is more sensitive to peroxynitrite modification than is the SERCA1a isoform from fast-type muscle [116]. SERCA2b is more sensitive to hydrogen peroxide than is SERCA3 [109]. As with most proteins, redox extremes damage the calcium pump. Prolonged exposure to high oxidant levels causes amino acid oxidation, protein fragmentation, and irreversible loss of enzymatic activity function [117]. Conversely, reductive stress also inhibits pump activity. This has been attributed to the reduction of vicinal thiols that must exist in an oxidized state for ATP hydrolysis [118].

The structural basis for redox sensitivity of the pump is likely to hinge on a small population of amino acids. Both oxidative and reductive stress are reported to influence phosphoenzyme formation by modifying a small number of critical thiol residues at the enzyme active site, perhaps as few as two per pump [91,112,118]. The precise location of these residues has not been determined but progress is being made. Recent studies indicate that oxidation primarily affects amino acids at six regions of the protein: 1) Glu121 to Lys128, 2) His190 to Lys218, 3) Asn330 to Lys352, 4) Gly432 to Lys436, 5) Glu551 to Arg604, and 6) Glu657 to Arg671 [114].

4.1.3 Myofilaments

Intact single fibers have been used to simultaneously measure force development and intracellular calcium transients during fatiguing exercise. These studies demonstrate that a significant component of fatigue is caused by loss of myofilament function, i.e., force is diminished at a given calcium concentration [67]. This finding indicates that fatigue reduces myofibrillar calcium sensitivity, slows cross-bridge kinetics, or both [119].

Myofilament function is directly inhibited by metabolites that accumulate in the exercising muscle including ROS [43] and NO derivatives [120]. Critical regulatory proteins in the myofilament lattice are sensitive to redox modification [80,81] and are putative sites of oxidative or nitrosative inhibition in fatigue. The sensitivity of constitutive proteins appears to vary. Some targets are more sensitive to redox changes than others. The proteins that appear to be least sensitive are actin and tropomyosin [121,122]. Myosin heavy chains possess thiol residues that are redox sensitive [123] and are commonly used for experimental manipulation of the protein [124]; however, thiol modification does not alter myosin function dramatically [125].

Calcium sensitivity of the myofilaments is primarily determined by troponin and by regulatory myosin light chains [119,126]. The primary amino acid sequences of these proteins show significant homology with calcium-binding proteins [127]. Both troponin and myosin light chains are potential targets for redox regulation. Studies of cardiac troponin C have shown that oxidation inhibits regulatory function: disulfide formation decreases calcium sensitivity of the protein [128]. Similar changes in skeletal muscle troponin during fatigue also would contribute to loss of force.

4.2 Indirect mechanisms

Oxidative stress may contribute to fatigue indirectly by altering processes other than excitation-contraction coupling. Most notable among these is muscle metabolism which closely influences endurance performance. Aerobic metabolism is critical for sustained exercise and factors that limit aerobic metabolism also promote fatigue. Thus, reductions in mitochondrial function or in vascular perfusion will tend to decrease aerobic capacity and thereby accelerate fatigue. Existing data suggest that these processes may be compromised by oxidative stress.

4.2.1 Mitochondrial dysfunction

As reviewed by Chance et al. [129], mitochondria are a major source of ROS production in mammalian cells. Superoxide anions are formed due to incomplete reduction of molecular oxygen at complexes I and III of the electron transport chain. As a result, 3 to 5% of mitochondrial oxygen consumption is shunted into production of superoxide anions. Increases in oxygen consumption generally produce a corresponding increase in ROS synthesis and the oxygen consumption of skeletal muscle can increase 10- to 20-fold during heavy exercise. Thus, mitochondrial ROS production is thought to be a major contributor to exercise-induced oxidative stress [10,11].

So, do ROS contribute to fatigue by stimulating mitochondrial autotoxicity? Might local ROS production lead to oxidative inhibition of mitochondrial proteins, thereby limiting aerobic metabolism and promoting fatigue? There are data to support this concept. Mitochondrial proteins are more susceptible to ROS-induced injury than other muscle proteins. For example, Haycock and co-workers [80] induced ROS injury of human skeletal muscle tissue using γ-radiation and screened a panel of structural and regulatory proteins for evidence of oxidative modification. The proteins most susceptible to oxidative injury were those of mitochondria including succinate dehydrogenase and cytochrome oxidase. Other studies have shown that oxidative stress inhibits mitochondrial function in skeletal muscle [38,130] and the hypothesis that exercise might cause oxidative injury to mitochondria is attractive. However, a cause-effect relationship has not been established between ROS effects on mitochondria and muscle fatigue. On the contrary, Brierley and colleagues [38] have suggested that physical activity may protect mitochondria against the oxidative insults associated with aging.

4.2.2 Loss of vascular control

Blood flow to working muscle determines the rate of oxygen delivery and governs the clearance of deleterious metabolites. Loss of vascular control disrupts these functions. Vascular dysfunction can accelerate fatigue by decreasing total blood flow to the muscle or, more subtly, by causing maldistribution of flow within the tissue.

As reviewed by Rubyani [131], ROS have complex vascular effects that could promote such disruption. ROS can function either as vasoconstrictors or vasodilators. Oxidative injury can damage smooth muscle, altering vascular tone directly, and can injure vascular endothelial cells that produce humoral mediators. ROS also react with vasoactive substances such as NO and catecholamines, thereby perturbing vascular control indirectly. The effects of ROS appear to depend on the specific molecular species involved, e.g., hydrogen peroxide effects differ from those of hydroxyl radicals, and the local concentration. As these actions predict, vascular control can be markedly compromised by excess ROS production.

Might this contribute to fatigue of intact muscle? Exercising muscle produces ROS at exaggerated rates (Table 1) that cause a marked rise in free radical content within the vascular compartment [8,17]. ROS scavengers increase the endurance of perfused muscle preparations (Fig. 4) but this is not accompanied by increases in arterial perfusion pressure [56,64] or total blood flow [56]. Thus, there is no evidence that endogenous ROS restrict overall delivery of blood to fatiguing muscle. The alternative possibility is that endogenous ROS may disrupt the distribution of blood flow without altering total perfusion. In principle, this would predispose exercising muscle to fatigue but the influence of ROS on flow distribution has not been tested.

4.2.3 Altered motor control

During volitional exercise, fatigue is most commonly reflected by "task failure" which is defined as an inability to sustain a desired level of exercise. Task failure is influenced by muscle fatigue (the peripheral process outlined in section 4) but does not directly reflect muscle failure. Instead, task failure often reflects loss of neural activation to the fatiguing muscles [35]. This can be caused by either of two neural mechanisms. Activation may be decreased unconsciously via inhibitory spinal reflexes that are stimulated by afferent nerve endings in the working muscle [132]. Alternatively, the subject may consciously decide to quit exercising because the task has become uncomfortable. This represents the most common cause of task failure under physiologic conditions.

Both neural mechanisms depend on an afferent signal from the exercising muscle that can be used by the central nervous system to monitor fatigue. The free nerve endings of group III and group IV afferents are sensitive to a variety of physiologic stimuli and may mediate either reflex or conscious adjustments to motor output. Recent data indicate that ROS activate skeletal muscle afferents without damaging the nerve endings [133]. Exercising muscle releases ROS into the extracellular space in proportion to fatigue [16,20]. This signal could stimulate the inhibitory motor reflexes that contribute to task failure; or fibers activated by ROS may influence the conscious perception of exercise-induced discomfort. Neither possibility has been tested experimentally.

5   SUMMARY

Early evidence that skeletal muscle generates free radicals has led to our current awareness of ROS and NO activity in muscle. It now is clear that muscle fibers continually produce both classes of free radical derivatives and that redox mechanisms strongly influence contractile function. In unfatigued muscle, low levels of endogenous ROS are essential for normal force production. The positive effects of ROS are opposed by endogenous NO which acts to depress force. The net effect of redox mechanisms on contraction is determined by the balance between these two influences. During fatiguing exercise, ROS production drastically increases in muscle and ROS play a causal role in fatigue. The physiologic importance of this pathway is underscored by evidence that antioxidant pretreatment can partially inhibit fatigue.

Mechanistic studies indicate that ROS accelerate fatigue by compromising regulatory processes within muscle fibers. The most fundamental is excitation-contraction coupling. Elevated ROS levels disrupt calcium regulation by the SR and calcium sensitivity of the myofilaments. The molecular mechanisms are best understood for the SR. Oxidation alters the structure of SR calcium release channels and stimulates channel opening via thiol modification. Oxidation of the SR calcium pump inhibits calcium reuptake which is attributed to disulfide bridge formation at the ATPase active site. ROS may also act upstream of excitation-contraction coupling. Mitochondria are a primary site of ROS production and mitochondrial proteins are especially sensitive to oxidative modification. Increases in mitochondrial ROS levels during exercise may cause oxidation of regulatory proteins thereby disrupting cellular metabolism.

At the tissue level, ROS may further accelerate fatigue via indirect effects. Oxidative stress compromises vascular control and could influence the distribution of blood flow within working muscle. ROS also stimulate sensory visceral neurons. The resulting afferent signals could conceivably depress motor drive to the muscle either by reflex mechanisms or by altering conscious perception.

6   PERSPECTIVES

Our understanding of oxidative stress in muscle fatigue is rapidly advancing. The challenge for the immediate future is 3-fold. First, the sources of ROS within muscle must be identified and the factors that regulate ROS production must be determined. It is possible that mitochondria are the primary source of ROS in exercising muscle but this has not been established experimentally. This is not an unresolved issue or a matter of controversy. There simply are no data to address the question. Systematic studies in this area are badly needed. Second, the cellular processes that are most sensitive to oxidative modification in exercising muscle must be identified. It makes little sense to aggressively investigate ROS effects on one particular process — myofilament contraction, calcium release, etc. — if some other aspect of endurance performance is more sensitive to ROS effects in vivo. Third, once the redox bottleneck has been established it will be necessary to determine molecular mechanism. What regulatory protein is primarily affected by oxidative stress and how do ROS alter the underlying chemistry of this target? These are the fundamental issues that must be resolved in order to understand the mechanism of ROS action in fatiguing muscle.

7 ACKNOWLEDGMENTS

I wish to thank Melanie Moody and Paulette Stone for assistance with graphics, Dr Michael Regnier for providing original tracings used in Fig. 3, and the National Institutes of Health for continued support of our research in this field (grant No. HL45721).

8 ABBREVIATIONS

Arg:	arginine
Asn:	asparagine
ATP:	adenosine triphosphate
Ca^{2+}:	calcium
Ca^{2+} ATPase:	
	SR Ca^{2+}-dependent ATPase
cGMP:	cyclic guanosine monophosphate
DHPR:	dihydropyridine-sensitive voltage sensor
DMSO:	dimethyl sulfoxide
EDL:	extensor digitorum longus
eNOS:	endothelial (type III) NO synthase
ESR:	electron spin resonance
Glu:	glutamine
Gly:	glycine
GSH:	reduced glutathione
GSSH:	glutathione disulfide
H^+:	hydrogen ion
His:	histidine
H_2O_2:	hydrogen peroxide
Hz:	Hertz
iNOS:	inducible (type II) NO synthase
ip:	intraperitoneal injection

iv: intravenous injection
Lys: lysine
NAC: *N*-acetylcysteine
NLA: *N*ω-nitro-L-argine
nNOS: neuronal (type I) NO synthase
NO: nitric oxide
O_2:   oxygen
O_2^-:   superoxide anion radical
·OH: hydroxyl radical
P_i: inorganic phosphate
po: oral administration
ROS: reactive oxygen species
RYR: ryanodine-sensitive SR Ca^{2+} release channel
SNP: sodium nitroprusside
SOD: superoxide dimutase
SR: sarcoplasmic reticulum

9   REFERENCES

1. Commoner B, Townsend J, Pike GE. Free radicals in biological materials. Nature 1954;174: 689—691.
2. Commoner B, Ternberg JL. Free radicals in surviving tissues. Proc Nat Acad Sci USA 1961;47: 1374—1384.
3. Koren A, Schara M, Sentjurc M. EPR measurements of free radicals during tetanic contraction of frog skeletal muscle. Period Biol 1980;82:399—401.
4. Koren A, Sauber C, Sentjurc M, Schara M. Free radicals in tetanic activity of isolated skeletal muscle. Comp Biochem Physiol 1983;74B:633—635.
5. Davies KJA, Quintanilha AT, Brooks GA, Packer L. Free radicals and tissue damage produced by exercise. Biochem Biophys Res Commun 1982;107(4):1198—1205.
6. Jackson MJ, Edwards RHT, Symons MCR. Electron spin-resonance studies of intact mammalian skeletal muscle. Biochem et Biophys Acta 1985;847:185—190.
7. Borzone G, Zhao B, Merola AJ, Berliner L, Clanton TL. Detection of free radicals by electron spin resonance in rat diaphragm after resistive loading. J Appl Physiol 1994;77(2):812—818.
8. Hartell MG, Borzone G, Clanton TL, Berliner LJ. Detection of free radicals in blood by electron spin resonance in a model of respiratory failure in the rat. Free Radic Biol Med 1994;17(5): 467—472.
9. Kehrer JP, Lund LG. Cellular reducing equivalents and oxidative stress. Free Radic Biol Med 1998;17(1):65—75.
10. Sen CK. Oxidants and antioxidants in exercise. J Appl Physiol 1995;79(3):675—686.
11. Alessio HM. Exercise-induced oxidative stress. Med Sci Sports Exerc 1993;25(2):218—224.
12. Goldfarb AH. Antioxidants: role of supplementation to prevent exercise-induced oxidative stress. Med Sci Sports Exerc 1993;25(2):232—236.
13. Kanter MM. Free radicals, exercise, and antioxidant supplementation. Int J Sport Nutr 1994;4 (3):205—220.
14. Packer L. Oxidants, antioxidant nutrients, and the athlete. J Sports Sci 1997;15(3):353—363.
15. Reid MB, Haack KE, Franchek KM, Valberg PA, Kobzik L, West MS. Reactive oxygen in skeletal muscle: I. Intracellular oxidant kinetics and fatigue in vitro. J Appl Physiol 1992;73(5): 1797—1804.

16. Reid MB, Shoji T, Moody MR, Entman ML. Reactive oxygen in skeletal muscle: II. Extracellular release of free radicals. J Appl Physiol 1992;73(5):1805—1809.
17. Kolbeck RC, She Z-W, Callahan LA, Nosek TM. Increased superoxide production during fatigue in the perfused rat diaphragm. Am J Resp Crit Care Med 1997;156:140—145.
18. Diaz PT, She Z-W, Davis WB, Clanton TL. Hydroxylation of salicylate by the in vitro diaphragm: evidence for hydroxyl radical production during fatigue. J Appl Physiol 1993;75(2):540—545.
19. Hasegawa A, Suzuki S, Matsumoto Y, Okubo T. In vivo fatiguing contraction of rat diaphragm produces hydroxyl radicals. Free Radic Biol Med 1997;22(1/2):349—354.
20. O'Neill CA, Stebbins CL, Bonigut S, Halliwell B, Longhurst JC. Production of hydroxyl radicals in contracting skeletal muscle of cats. J Appl Physiol 1996;81(3):1197—1206.
21. Rock E, Astier C, Lab C, Vignon X, Gueux E, Motta C, Rayssiguier Y. Dietary magnesium deficiency in rats enhances free radical production in skeletal muscle. J Nutr 1995;125:1205—1210.
22. Hussain SN, El-Dwairi Q, Abdul-Hussain MN, Sakkal D. Espression of nitric oxide synthase isoforms in normal ventilatory and limb muscles. J Appl Physiol 1997;83(2):348—353.
23. Gath I, Closs EI, Godtel-Armbust U, Schmitt S, Nakane M, Wessler I, Forstermann U. Inducible NO synthase II and neuronal NO synthase I are constitutively expressed in different structures of guinea pig skeletal muscle: implications for contractile function. FASEB J 1996;10:1614—1620.
24. Williams G, Brown T, Becker M, Prager M, Giroir BP. Cytokine-induced expression of nitric oxide synthase in C2C12 skeletal muscle myocytes. Am J Physiol 1994;267:R1020—1025.
25. Hussain SN, Giaid A, El Dawiri Q, Sakkal D, Hattori R, Guo Y. Expression of nitric oxide synthases and GTP cyclohydrolase I in the ventilatory and limb muscles during endotoxemia. Am J Resp Cell Molec Biol 1997;17(2):173—180.
26. Nakane M, Schmidt HH, Pollock JS, Forstermann U, Murad F. Cloned human brain nitric oxide synthase is highly expressed in skeletal muscle. FEBS Lett 1993;316(2):175—180.
27. Reid MB, Kobzik L, Bredt DS, Stamler JS. Nitric oxide modulates excitation-contraction coupling in the diaphragm. Comp Biochem Physiol 1998;119(1):211—218.
28. Kobzik L, Reid MB, Bredt DS, Stamler JS. Nitric oxide in skeletal muscle. Nature 1994;372:546—548.
29. Kobzik L, Stringer B, Balligand J-L, Reid MB, Stamler JS. Endothelial type nitric oxide synthase in skeletal muscle fibers: mitochondrial relationships. Biochem Biophys Res Commun 1995;211:375—381.
30. Grozdanovic Z, Nakos G, Dahrmann G, Mayer B, Gossrau R. Species-independent expression of nitric oxide synthase in the sarcolemma region of visceral and somatic striated muscle fibers. Cell Tis Res 1995;281:493—499.
31. Brenman JE, Chao DS, Xia H, Aldape K, Bredt DS. Nitric oxide synthase complexed with dystrophin and absent from skeletal muscle sarcolemma in Duchenne muscular dystrophy. Cell 1995;82(5):743—752.
32. Brenman JE, Chao DS, Gee SH, McGee AW, Craven SE, Santillano Dr, Wu Z, Huang F, Xia H, Peters MF et al. Interaction of nitric oxide synthase with the postsynaptic density protein PSD-95 and α1-syntrophin mediated by PDZ domains. Cell 1996;84(5):757—767.
33. Balon TW, Nadler JL. Evidence that nitric oxide increases glucose transport in skeletal muscle. J Appl Physiol 1997;82(1):359—363.
34. Balon TW, Nadler JL. Nitric oxide release is present from incubated skeletal muscle preparations. J Appl Physiol 1994;77(6):2519—2521.
35. Gandevia SG. Insights into motor performance and muscle fatigue based on transcranial stimulation of the human motor cortex. Clin Exp Pharmacol Physiol 1996;23(10—11):957—960.
36. Catterall WA. Excitation-contraction coupling in vertebrate skeletal muscle: a tale of two calcium channels. Cell 1991;64:871—874.
37. Melzer W, Herrmann-Frank A, Luttgau HC. The role of Ca^{2+} ions in excitation-contraction coupling of skeletal muscle fibres. Biochim Biophys Acta 1995;1241(1):59—116.
38. Brierley EJ, Johnson MA, James OF, Turnbull DM. Effects of physical activity and age on mito-

chondrial function. QJM 1996;89(4):251−258.

39. Voollestad NK, Verburg E. Muscular function, metabolism and electolyte shifts during prolonged repetitive exercise in humans. Acta Physiol Scand 1996;156(3):271−278.

40. Puppi A, Szekeres S, Dely M. Correlations between the tissue redox-state and potassium-contractures. Acta Physiol Hung 1990;75(3):253−259.

41. Regnier M, Lorenz RR, Sieck GC. Effects of oxygen radical scavengers on force production in single living frog skeletal muscle fibers. (Abstract) FASEB J 1992;6(5):A1819.

42. Reid MB, Khawli FA, Moody MR. Reactive oxygen in skeletal muscle: III. Contractility of unfatigued muscle. J Appl Physiol 1993;75(3):1081−1087.

43. Andrade FH, Reid MB, Allen DG,Westerblad H. Effect of hydrogen peroxide and dithiothreitol on contractile function of single skeletal muscle fibres from mouse. J Physiol (Lond) 1998;509: 565−575.

44. Khawli FA, Reid MB. *N*-acetylcysteine depresses contractility and inhibits fatigue of diaphragm in vitro. J Appl Physiol 1994;77(1):317−324.

45. Sams WM, Carroll NV, Crantz PL. Effect of dimethyl sulfoxide on isolated-innervated skeletal, smooth, and cardiac muscle. Proc Soc Exp Biol Med 1966;122:103−107.

46. Reid MB, Moody MR. Dimethyl sulfoxide depresses skeletal muscle contractility. J Appl Physiol 1994;76:2186−2190.

47. Oba T, Koshita M, Yamaguchi M. H2O2 modulates twitch tension and increases Po of Ca^{2+} release channel in frog skeletal muscle. Am J Physiol 1996;63:460−468.

48. Lawler JM, Cline CC, Hu Z, Coast JR. Effect of oxidant challenge on contractile function of the aging rat diaphragm. Am J Physiol 1997;272(2 Part 1):E201−207.

49. Morrison RJ, Miller III, Reid MB. Nitric oxide effects on shortening velocity and power production in the rat diaphragm. J Appl Physiol 1996;80(3):1065−1069.

50. Morrison RJ, Miller CC, Reid MB. Nitric oxide effects on force-velocity characteristics of the rat diaphragm. Comp Biochem Physiol 1998;119A(1):203−209.

51. Arnold WP, Mittal CK, Katsuki S, Murad F. Nitric oxide activates guanylate cyclase and increases guanosine 3':5'-cyclic monophosphate levels in various tissue preparations. Proc Natl Acad Sci 1977;74(8):3203−3207.

52. Abraham RZ, Kobzik L, Moody MR, Reid MB, Stamler JS. Cyclic GMP is a second messenger by which nitric oxide inhibits diaphragm contraction. Comp Biochem Physiol 1998;119A(1): 177−183.

53. Reid MB. Reactive oxygen and nitric oxide in skeletal muscle. New Physiol Sci 1996;11: 114−119.

54. Kanner J, Harel S, Granit R. Nitric oxide as an antioxidant. Arch Biochem Biophys 1991;289 (1):130−136.

55. Stamler JS. Redox signaling: nitrosylation and related target interactions of nitric oxide. Cell 1994;78:931−936.

56. Supinski G, Nethery D, Stofan D, Dimarco A. Effect of free radical scavengers on diaphragmatic fatigue. Am J Respir Crit Care Med 1997;155:622−629.

57. Barclay JK, Hansel M. Free radicals may contribute to oxidative skeletal muscle fatigue. Can J Physiol Pharmacol 1991;69:279−284.

58. Reid MB, Stokic DS, Koch SM, Khawli FA, Leis AA. *N*-acetylcysteine inhibits muscle fatigue in humans. J Clin Invest 1994;94:2468−2474.

59. Novelli GP, Falsini S, Bracciotti G. Exogenous glutathione increases endurance to muscle effort in mice. Pharmacol Res 1991;23:149−155.

60. Cazzulani P, Cassin M, Ceserani R. Increased endurance to physical exercise in mice given oral reduced glutathione (GSH). Med Sci Res 1991;19:543−544.

61. Travaline JM, Sudarshan S, Roy BG, Cordova F, Leyenson V, Criner GJ. Effect of *N*-acetylcysteine on human diaphragm strength and fatigue. Am J Respir Crit Care Med 1997;156: 1567−1571.

62. Supinski GS, Stofan D, Ciufo R, Dimarco A. *N*-acetylcysteine administration alters the

response to inspiratory loading in oxygen-supplemented rats. J Appl Physiol 1997;82(4): 1119–1125.

63. Diaz PT, Brownstein E, Clanton TL. Fatigue-sparing effects of acetylcysteine on the diaphragm are temperature-dependent. J Appl Physiol 1994;77(5):2434–2439.
64. Shindoh C, Dimarco A, Thomas A, Manubray P, Supinski G. Effect of *N*-acetylcysteine on diaphragm fatigue. J Appl Physiol 1990;68(5):2107–2113.
65. Novelli GP, Bracciotti G, Falsini S. Spin-trappers and vitamin E prolong endurance to muscle fatigue in mice. Free Radical Biol Med 1990;8(1):9–13.
66. Moriura T, Matsuda H, Kubo M. Pharmacological study on Agkistrodon blomhoffii blomhoffii BOIE. V Anti-fatigue effect of the 50% ethanol extract in acute weight-loaded forced swimming-treated rats. Biol Pharm Bull 1996;19(1):62–66.
67. Westerblad H, Lee JA, Lannergren J, Allen DG. Cellular mechanisms of fatigue in skeletal muscle. Am J Physiol 1991;261:C195–209.
68. Nashawati E, Dimarco A, Supinski G. Effects produced by infusion of a free radical-generating solution into the diaphragm. Am Rev Resp Dis 1993;147(1):60–65.
69. Lawler JM, Cline CC, Hu Z, Coast JR. Effect of oxidative stress and acidosis on diaphragm contractile function. Am J Physiol 1997;273(2 Part 2):R630–636.
70. Freeman B. Free radical chemistry of nitric oxide; looking at the dark side. Chest 1994;105(3): 79S–84S.
71. Abraham RZ, Miller III, Reid MB. The contractile response to nitric oxide (NO) varies among skeletal muscle. (Abstract) Endothelium 1995;3(Suppl):S108.
72. Murrant CL, Woodley NE, Barclay JK. Effect of nitroprusside and endothelium-derived products on slow-twitch skeletal muscle function in vitro. Can J Physiol Pharmacol 1994;72: 1089–1093.
73. Murrant CL, Barclay JK. Endothelial cell products alter mammalian skeletal muscle function in vitro. Can J Physiol Pharmacol 1995;73:736–741.
74. Murrant CL, Frisbee JC, Barclay JK. The effect of nitric oxide and endothelin on skeletal muscle contractility changes when stimulation is altered. Can J Physiol Pharmacol 1997;75(5): 414–422.
75. McAllister RM, Hirai T, Musch TI. Contribution of endothelium-derived nitric oxide (EDNO) to the skeletal muscle blood flow response to exercise. Med Sci Sports Exer 1995;27(8): 1145–1151.
76. Shen W, Zhang X, Zhao G, Wolin MS, Sessa W, Hintze TH. Nitric oxide production and NO synthase gene expression contribute to vascular regulation during exercise. Med Sci Sports Exer 1995;27(8):1125–1134.
77. Albertini M, Lafortuna C, Aguggini G. Effects of nitric oxide on diaphragmatic muscle endurance and strength in pigs. Exp Physiol 1997;82(1):99–106.
78. Fitts RH. Cellular mechanisms of muscle fatigue. Physiol Rev 1994;74(1):49–94.
79. Trimm JL, Salama G, Abramson JJ. Limited tryptic modification stimulates activation of Ca^{2+} release from isolated sarcoplasmic reticulum vesicles. J Biol Chem 1988;263(33):17443–17451.
80. Haycock JW, Jones P, Harris JB, Mantle D. Differential susceptibility of human skeletal muscle proteins to free radical induced oxidative damage: a histochemical, immunocytochemical and electron microscopic study in vitro. Acta Neuropathol 1996;92(4):331–340.
81. Nagasawa T, Hatayama T, Watanabe Y, Tanaka M, Niisato Y, Kitts DD. Free radical-mediated effects on skeletal muscle protein in rats treated with Fe-nitrilotriacetate. Biochem Biophys Res Commun 1997;231(1):37–41.
82. Sen CK, Kolosova I, Hanninen O, Orlov SN. Inward potassium transport systems in skeletal muscle-derived cells are highly sensitive to oxidant exposure. Free Radic Biol Med 1995;18(4): 795–800.
83. Brotto MAP, Nosek TM. Hydrogen peroxide disrupts calcium release from the sarcoplasmic reticulum of rat skeletal muscle fibers. J Appl Physiol 1996;81(2):731–737.
84. Posterino GS, Lamb GD. Effects of reducing agents and oxidants on excitation-contraction cou-

pling in skeletal muscle fibres of rat and toad. J Physiol (Lond) 1996;496:809–825.

85. Chin ER, Allen DG. The role of elevations in intracellular $[Ca^{2+}]$ in the development of low frequency fatigue in mouse single muscle fibres. J Physiol 1996;491:813–824.

86. Williams JH, Klug GA. Calcium exchange hypothesis of skeletal muscle fatigue: a brief review. Muscle Nerve 1995;18(4):421–434.

87. Stephenson DG, Lamb GD, Stephenson GM, Fryer MW. Mechanisms of excitation-contraction coupling relevant to skeletal muscle fatigue. Adv Exp Med Biol 1995;384:45–56.

88. Trimm JL, Salama G, Abramson JJ. Sulfhydryl oxidation induces rapid calcium release from sarcoplasmic reticulum vesicles. J Biol Chem 1986;261:16092–16098.

89. Scherer NM, Deamer DW. Oxidative stress impairs the function of sarcoplasmic reticulum by oxidation. Arch Biochem Biophys 1986;216:589–601.

90. Abramson JJ, Salama G. Sulfhydryl oxidation and Ca^{2+} release from sarcoplasmic reticulum. Mol Cell Biochem 1988;82(1–2):81–84.

91. Scherer NM, Deamer DW. Oxidation of thiols in the calcium-ATPase of sarcoplasmic reticulum microsomes. Biochim Biophys Acta 1986;862:309–317.

92. Xiong H, Buck E, Stuart J, Pessah IN, Salama G, Abramson JJ. Rose bengal activates the Ca^{2+} release channel from skeletal muscle sarcoplasmic reticulum. Arch Biochem Biophys 1992;292 (2):522–528.

93. Stuart J, Pessah IN, Favero TG, Abramson JJ. Photooxidation of skeletal muscle sarcoplasmic reticulum induces rapid calcium release. Arch Biochem Biophys 1992;292(2):512–521.

94. Abramson JJ, Buck E, Salama G, Casida JE, Pessah IN. Mechanism of anthraquinone-induced calcium release from skeletal muscle sarcoplasmic reticulum. J Biol Chem 1988;263(35): 18750–18758.

95. Abramson JJ, Cronin JR, Salama G. Oxidation induced by phethalocyanine dyes causes rapid calcium release from sarcoplasmic reticulum vesicles. Arch Biochem Biophys 1988;263(2): 245–255.

96. Favero TG, Zable AC, Abramson JJ. Hydrogen peroxide stimulates the Ca^{2+} release channel from skeletal muscle sarcoplasmic reticulum. J Biol Chem 1995;270(43):25557–25563.

97. Liu G, Abramson JJ, Zable AC, Pessah IN. Direct evidence for the existance and functional role of hyperreactive sulfhydryls on the ryanodine receptor-triadin complex selectively labeled by the coumarin maleimide 7-diethylamino-3-(4'-maleimidylphenyl)-4-methylcoumarin. Mol Pharmacol 1994;45(2):189–200.

98. Aghdasi B, Zhang J-Z, Wu Y, Reid MB, Hamilton SL. Multiple classes of sulfhydryls modulate the skeletal muscle Ca^{2+} release channel. J Biol Chem 1997;272(6):3739–3748.

99. Aghdasi B, Reid MB, Hamilton SL. Nitric oxide protects the skeletal muscle Ca^{2+} release channel from oxidation induced activation. J Biol Chem 1997;272(41):25462–25467.

100. Meszaros LG, Minarovic I, Zahradnikova A. Inhibition of the skeletal muscle ryanodine receptor calcium release channel by nitric oxide. FEBS Lett 1996;380(1–2):49–52.

101. Stoyanovsky DA, Murphy TD, Anno PR, Kim Y-M, Salama G. Nitric oxide activates skeletal and cardiac ryanodine receptors. Cell Calcium 1997;21(1):19–29.

102. Wu Y, Aghdasi B, Dou SJ, Zhang ZJ, Liu SQ, Hamilton SL. Functional interactions between cytoplasmic domains of the skeletal muscle Ca^{2+} release channel. J Biol Chem 1997;272(40): 25051–25061.

103. Ferrington DA, Reijneveld JC, Bar PR, Bigelow DJ. Activation of the sarcoplasmic reticulum Ca^{2+}-ATPase induced by exercise. Biochim Biophys Acta 1996;1279(2):203–213.

104. Booth J, McKenna MJ, Ruell PA, Gwinn TH, Davis GM, Thompson MW, Harmer AR, Hunter SK, Sutton JR. Impaired calcium pump function does not slow relaxation in human skeletal muscle after prolonged exercise. J Appl Physiol 1997;83(2):511–521.

105. Westerblad H, Duty S, Allen DG. Intracellular calcium concentration during low-frequency fatigue in isolated single fibers of mouse skeletal muscle. J Appl Physiol 1993;75(1):382–388.

106. Westerblad H, Allen DG. The contribution of $[Ca^{2+}]i$ to the slowing of relaxation in fatigued single fibres from mouse skeletal muscle. J Physiol 1993;468:729–740.

107. Ritov VB, Goldman R, Stoyanovsky DA, Menshikova EV, Kagan VE. Antioxidant paradoxes of phenolic compounds: peroxyl radical scavenger and lipid antioxidant, etoposide (VP-16), inhibits sarcoplasmic reticulum Ca^{2+}-ATPase via thiol oxidation by its phenoxyl radical. Arch Biochem Biophys 1995;321(1):140—152.
108. Morris TE, Sulakhe PV. Sarcoplasmic reticulum Ca^{2+}-pump dysfunction in rat cardiomyocytes briefly exposed to hydroxyl radicals. Free Radical Biol Med 1997;22(1—2):37—47.
109. Grover AK, Samson SE, Misquitta CM. Sarco(endo)plasmic reticulum Ca^{2+} pump isoform SERCA3 is more resistant than SERCA2b to peroxide. Am J Physiol 1997;273(2 Part 1): C420—425.
110. Ishibashi T, Lee CI, Okabe E. Skeletal sarcoplasmic reticulum dysfunction induced by reactive oxygen intermediates derived from photoactivated rose bengal. J Pharmacol Exp Therapeut 1996;277(1):350—358.
111. Lee C, Okabe E. Hydroxyl radical-mediated reduction of Ca^{2+}-ATPase activity of masseter muscle sarcoplasmic reticulum. Japanese J Pharmacol 1995;67(1):21—28.
112. Xu KY, Zweier JL, Becker LC. Hydroxyl radical inhibits sarcoplasmic reticulum Ca^{2+}-ATPase function by direct attack on the ATP binding site. Circ Res 1997;80(1):76—81.
113. Viner RI, Huhmer AF, Bigelow DJ, Schoneich C. The oxidative inactivation of sarcoplasmic reticulum Ca^{2+}-ATPase by peroxynitrite. Free Radical Res 1996;24(4):243—259.
114. Viner RI, Krainev AG, Williams TD, Schoneich C, Bigelow DJ. Identification of oxidation-sensitive peptides within the cytoplasmic domain of the sarcoplasmic reticulum Ca^{2+}-ATPase. Biochem 1997;36(25):7706—7716.
115. Byrd SK. Modification of sarcoplasmic Ca-ATPase sulfhydryls after exercise and protection by dithiothreitol. (Abstract) FASEB J 1993;7(4):A526.
116. Viner RI, Ferrington DA, Huhmer AFR, Bigelow DJ, Schoneich C. Accumulation of nitrotyrosine on the SERCA2a isoform of SR Ca-ATPase of rat skeletal muscle during aging: a peroxynitrite-mediated process? FEBS Lett 1996;379:286—290.
117. Castilho RF, Carvalho-Alves PC, Vercesi AE, Ferreira ST. Oxidative damage to sarcoplasmic reticulum Ca^{2+}-pump induced by Fe^{2+}/H_2O_2/ascorbate is not mediated by lipid peroxidation or thiol oxidation and leads to protein fragmentation. Mol Cell Biochem 1996;159(2):105—114.
118. Daiho T, Kanazawa T. Reduction of disulfide bonds in sarcoplasmic reticulum Ca^{2+}-ATPase by dithiothreitol causes inhibition of phosphoenzyme isomerization in catalytic cycle. This reduction requires binding of both purine nucleotide and Ca^{2+} to enzyme. J Biol Chem 1994;269 (15):11060—11064.
119. Brenner B. Effect of Ca^{2+} on cross-bridge turnover kinetics in skinned single rabbit psoas fibers: implications for regulation of muscle contraction. Proc Nat Acad Sci USA 1988;85:3265—3269.
120. Andrade FH, Reid MB, Allen DG, Westerblad H. Nitric oxide decreases myofibrillar Ca^{2+} sensitivity in single skeletal muscle fibres. J Physiol (Lond) 1998;577—586.
121. Williams DL Jr, Swenson CA. Disulfide bridges in tropomyosin. Eur J Biochem 1982;127: 495—499.
122. Liu DF, Wang D, Stracher A. The accessibility of the thiol groups on G- and F-actin of rabbit muscle. Biochem J 1990;266:453—459.
123. Bailey K, Perry SV. The role of sulfhydryl groups in the interaction of myosin and actin. 1947 "classical article". Biochim Biophys Acta 1989;1000:177—178.
124. Burghardt T-P, Ajtai K. Mapping global angular transitions of proteins in assemblies using multiple extrinsic reporter groups. Biochem 1992;31(1):200—206.
125. Crowder MS, Cooke R. The effect of myosin sulfhydryl modification on the mechanics of fiber contraction. J Muscle Res Cell Motility 1984;5:131—146.
126. Metzger JM, Moss RL. Myosin light chain 2 modulates calcium-sensitive cross-bridge transitions in vertebrate skeletal muscle. Biochem J 1992;63:460—468.
127. Collins JH. Homology of myosin DTNB light chains with alkali light chains, troponin C, and parvalbumin. Nature 1976;259:699—700.
128. Putkey JA, Dotson DG, Mouawad P. Formation of inter- and intramolecular bonds can activate

cardiac troponin C. J Biol Chem 1993;268:6827—6830.

129. Chance B, Sies H, Boveris A. Hydroperoxide metabolism in mammalian organs. Physiol Rev 1979;59(3):527—605.

130. Llesuy S, Evelson P, Gonzalez-Flecha B, Peralta J, Carreras MC, Poderoso JJ, Boveris A. Oxidative stress in muscle and liver of rats with septic syndrome. Free Radic Biol Med 1994;16(4): 445—451.

131. Rubyani GM. Vascular effects of oxygen-derived free radicals. Free Radic Biol Med 1988;4(2): 107—120.

132. Garland SJ, Kaufman MP. Role of muscle afferents in the inhibition of motorneurons during fatigue. Adv Exp Med Biol 1995;384:271—278.

133. Bonigut S, Stebbins CL, Longhurst JC. Reactive oxygen species modify reflex cardiovascular responses to static contraction. J Appl Physiol 1996;81(3):1207—1212.

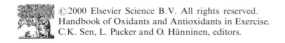
©2000 Elsevier Science B.V. All rights reserved.
Handbook of Oxidants and Antioxidants in Exercise.
C.K. Sen, L. Packer and O. Hänninen, editors.

Part IX • Chapter 23

Oxidative stress in muscular atrophy

Hisao Kondo

Cambridge Institute for Medical Research, University of Cambridge, Level 5 (room 5.36), Wellcome Trust/MRC Building, Hills Road, Cambridge CB2 2XY, UK. Fax: +44-1223-762640.
E-mail: hk228@cam.ac.uk

1   INTRODUCTION
2   OXIDATIVE STRESS IN SKELETAL MUSCLE ATROPHIED BY IMMOBILIZATION
3   MECHANISM OF OXIDATIVE STRESS IN ATROPHIED MUSCLE
    3.1   Antioxidant enzyme systems
    3.2   Cytochemical study of hydrogen peroxide
    3.3   Source of superoxide anions in the cytoplasm
    3.4   Iron movement
    3.5   Role of iron
    3.6   Production of nitric oxide
4   ROLE OF OXIDATIVE STRESS IN MUSCULAR ATROPHY
5   OXIDATIVE STRESS DURING RECOVERY FROM MUSCULAR ATROPHY
6   OXIDATIVE STRESS IN THE OTHER MUSCULAR DISEASES
    6.1   Muscular atrophy induced by denervation
    6.2   Duchenne muscular dystrophy
7   SUMMARY
8   ACKNOWLEDGEMENTS
9   ABBREVIATIONS
10 REFERENCES

1   INTRODUCTION

The production of free radicals in the mitochondria has been investigated a lot more compared with other organelles, and it is believed to play a major role in the oxidative stress of the cell. In the muscle, the increase of muscular activity enhances the oxygen consumption and increased oxygen consumption accelerates the production of free radicals in the mitochondria [1]. In view of this, it was believed without consideration of the production of free radicals in the cytoplasm that the oxidative stress in the muscle might parallel the muscular activity; that is, the oxidative stress might decrease in the muscular atrophy. This might be the reason why there were so few reports on the oxidative stress during disuse muscular atrophy, although numerous studies on oxidative stress during exercise have been carried out in this decade.

At first I will describe the enhanced oxidative stress in the course of the disuse muscular atrophy in section 2 and explain its mechanism from the view of cell biology in section 3. Its role in muscular atrophy will be discussed in section 4.

The recovery from the muscular atrophy is also accompanied by oxidative stress, which will finally be explained.

2 OXIDATIVE STRESS IN SKELETAL MUSCLE ATROPHIED BY IMMOBILIZATION

The skeletal muscle disuse atrophy has been an important problem in the field of rehabilitation and space biology. This atrophy was known from old times and many investigations on it have been performed for more than 100 years and reviews have been produced by others [2,3]. Many experimental models for disuse atrophy have been devised; in order to reduce muscular activity, immobilization, denervation, tetonomy, and tail suspension were adopted. In our experiment the immobilization model was used, because it causes muscular atrophy rapidly and reversibly, and produces exactly the same conditions for the muscles. Many biochemical changes have been investigated using this model also. Nick et al. [4] reported that atrophy produced by immobilization is the result of atrophy of the muscle cell without a decrease in muscle cell number. The infiltration of other cells such as phagocyte are rarely found in the early phase of atrophy [5]. Additionally, since the amount of mitochondria is maintained in the soleus muscle in disuse [6], the activities of the enzymes in mitochondria, such as Mn-containing superoxide dismutase, cannot be considered as reflecting the amount of mitochondria present, rather than indicating the amount of enzyme per mitochondria. Taking these into consideration, the muscular atrophy produced by immobilization is regarded as a good model to use to study cellular atrophy.

As a model animal, we used male Wistar rats (14- to 16-week-old) whose one ankle joints were immobilized in the fully extended position (i.e., with the soleus muscle in a shortened position) [7]. The periods of immobilization were 4, 8, and 12 days in order to investigate the metabolic change during the atrophy proceeds rapidly. After immobilization, soleus, a typical slow red muscles from immobilized and intact hindlimbs were collected (atrophied and contralateral control muscles, respectively). The degree of atrophy is shown in Fig. 1. In our model, the atrophy proceeded rapidly until the 8th day and slowly from the 8th to the 12th day (Fig. 1).

Thiobarbituric acid-reactive substance (TBARS), total glutathione (total GSH), and oxidized glutathione (GSSG) were measured to estimate the level of oxidative stress.

As shown in Fig. 2, TBARS level in atrophy did not change until 4th day and increased significantly from the 8th day; TBARS concentration on the 12th day was higher by 60% compared with that of control. The increase of TBARS level strongly suggests acceleration of lipid peroxidation (Fig. 2–4).

The levels of total GSH and GSSG and the ratio of GSSG-to-total GSH in a 12-day atrophy are shown in Fig. 3. In atrophy, total GSH concentration significantly decreased, and GSSG concentration significantly increased by 43% as compared with those in control. The activity of glutathione reductase (GSSGRx),

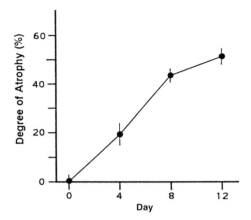

Fig. 1. Changes in the degree of atrophy as a function of the number of days after immobilization began. Each point is mean ± SE (n = 5).

which plays the main role in the conversion of GSSG into the reduced form of GSH, increased in atrophy (see Fig. 4). It is thought that the increase of oxidative reactions exceeded that of GSSGRx activity, which resulted in the increased level of GSSG in atrophy. Thus, the increases of GSSG and TBARS prove the enhanced oxidative stress in the skeletal muscle atrophied by immobilization.

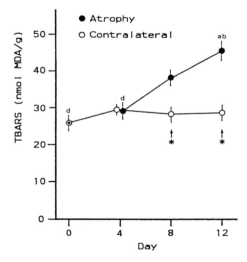

Fig. 2. Changes in thiobarbituric acid-reactive substance (TBARS) level in atrophied and contralateral muscles as a function of the number of days after immobilization began. Day 0 is the control. Each point is the mean ± SE (n = 5). a, b, c, and d indicate significant differences at $p < 0.05$ compared with 0, 4, 8, and 12 days, respectively. *Significant difference at $p < 0.05$ between atrophied and contralateral muscles.

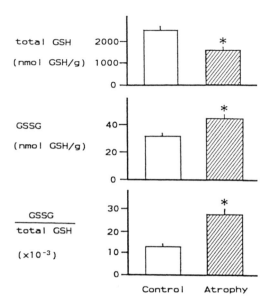

Fig. 3. Level of total glutathione (GSH), oxidized GSH (GSSG), and the ratio of GSSG to total GSH in a 12-day atrophied and contralateral (control) muscles. Data are means ± SE (n = 5). *Significant difference at $p < 0.05$ compared with the control.

Furthermore, the increased activity of GSSGRx on the 4th day suggests that the oxidative stress had already increased on the 4th day, although the TBARS level did not increase simultaneously.

On the other hand, Gilbert [8] has reported the possibilities of enzyme regulation by thiol-disulfide exchange and modulation of thiol/disulfide ratio in vivo

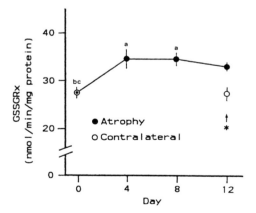

Fig. 4. Changes in glutathione reductase (GSSGRx) activities (ordinate) as a function of the number of days after immobilization began. Symbols explained in Fig. 2. Data have means ± SE (n = 6).

to serve as a "third messenger" in response to adenosine $3',5'$-cyclic mono-phosphate levels. The increased ratio of GSSG-to-total GSH in atrophy (Fig. 3) indicates one of the causes of the metabolic change in atrophied muscle.

3   MECHANISM OF OXIDATIVE STRESS IN ATROPHIED MUSCLE

In the previous section, oxidative stress is shown to increase in the skeletal muscle atrophied by immobilization, while it has also been reported to increase during the exhaustive exercise. Both the increased and decreased muscle activities cause elevated oxidative stress in skeletal muscle. The mechanism of oxidative stress during exercise will be explained in detail in the other chapters. In this section, I will describe the metabolism of active oxygen species and transition metals to clarify the mechanism of oxidative stress in muscular atrophy [9—11].

3.1 Antioxidant enzyme systems

Superoxide dismutase (SOD), acts as a converter of superoxide anion to hydrogen peroxide, this has two forms; namely, Cu,Zn-SOD in the cytoplasm and Mn-SOD in the mitochondria. As shown in Figs. 5 and 6, interestingly, the two forms of SOD showed entirely different responses in atrophy. The activity of Cu,Zn-SOD kept increasing throughout the 12 days; its activity on the 8th and 12th day were significantly higher than that of the control. The activity of Mn-SOD tended to increase from the 8th day, and its activity on the 12th day significantly decreased to 60% of the control value. Since it is generally known that SOD is induced by superoxide anions [12], the SOD level may be thought to reflect the generation of superoxide anions. It is also known that superoxide anions usually

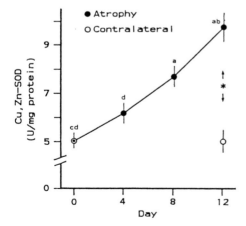

Fig. 5. Changes in Cu,Zn-containing superoxide dismutase (Cu,Zn-SOD) activities are as a function the of number of days after immobilization began. Data show means ± SE (n = 6). Symbols are explained in Fig. 2.

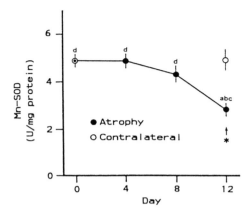

Fig. 6. Changes in Mn-containing Superoxide dismutase (Mn-SOD) activities as a function of the number of days after immobilization began. Data shows means ± SE (n = 6). Symbols are explained in Fig. 2.

cannot cross biological membranes [13]. Taking these aspects into consideration, the increased cytoplasmic form of SOD (Cu,Zn-SOD) and the decreased mitochondrial form of SOD (Mn-SOD) may reflect an increased production of superoxide anions in the cytoplasm and a decreased production in the mitochondria.

The elevated Cu,Zn-SOD level also indicates that the generation of hydrogen peroxide, the product of the reaction catalyzed by SOD, may be enhanced in the cytoplasm. It is generally known that Se-dependent glutathione peroxidase (Se-GSHPx) and catalase have the ability to degrade hydrogen peroxide [13]. The activities of Se-GSHPx did not change significantly throughout 12 days (Fig. 7). The GSH level is known to limit the function in vivo of Se-GSHPx [14] and, as shown in Fig. 3, its level decreased in the atrophied muscle. Accordingly,

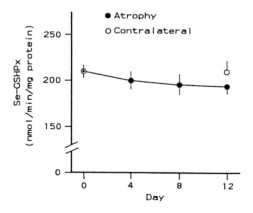

Fig. 7. Changes in Se-dependent glutathione peroxidase (Se-GSHPx) activities as a function of the number of days after immobilization began. Data shown as means ± SE (n = 6).

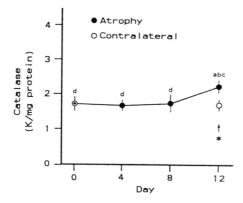

Fig. 8. Changes in catalase activities as a function of the number of days after immobilization began. Data show means ± SE (n = 6). Symbols are explained in Fig. 2.

although the activity of Se-GSHPx did not change, its function in vivo could be anticipated to decrease in the atrophied muscle. The catalase activity also did not increase until the 8th day and increased only slightly on the 12th day (Fig. 8). Although the activity of glutathione S-transferase (GST), which also shows some GSHPx activity, rose in atrophy [11], this enzyme is unable to utilize hydrogen peroxide as substrate [15]. Hence, the level of hydrogen peroxide may well be increased, especially in the cytoplasm.

3.2 Cytochemical study of hydrogen peroxide

Is the prediction in the above section actually brought about? To answer this question, we assessed the level of hydrogen peroxides in the atrophied muscular cell by a cytochemical study using an electron microscope [11].

The cytochemical study was carried out according to the method of Babbs et al. [16]. Briefly, samples are incubated in short-term organ culture in the presence of 3,3'-diaminobenzidine (DAB), and generated hydrogen peroxide is allowed to react with DAB through the catalysis of the endogenous peroxidase to produce oxidized DAB, which deposits as an osmiophilic polymer in the cell. The number of oxidized DAB deposits reflects the level of hydrogen peroxide in the cell, and, thereby, the deposits are scored using only the electron microscope to estimate the level of hydrogen peroxide generated in organ culture.

As shown in Fig. 9, the number of positive stains increased in atrophy. Since the activities of peroxidase in an 8-day atrophy were the same as those in the control (refer to section 3.1), the density of stains can be thought to reflect the level of hydrogen peroxide. Taking these into consideration, the present cytochemical study indicated the increased generation of hydrogen peroxide in the cytoplasm of the atrophied muscle cell in a short-term organ culture. Capillary density increases in the atrophied soleus muscle [17]. Due to oxygen delivery being lim-

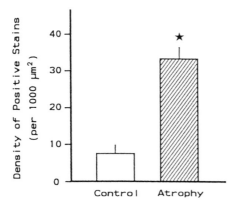

Fig. 9. Densities of positive stains revealed by electron-microscopic cytochemistry per 1,000 μm² in an 8-day atrophy and control. Data show means ± SE (n = 6). *Significant difference at p < 0.05 compared with the control.

ited by capillary density, oxygen delivery in vivo to the atrophied muscle cell should not be less than that in the control [2]. Thereby, this cytochemical study may suggest that the elevated level of hydrogen peroxide in vivo, in the cytoplasm of the atrophied muscle cell, reinforces the preceding prediction.

3.3 Source of superoxide anions in the cytoplasm

The next question is what is the source of superoxide anions in the cytoplasm of the atrophied muscle. Stripe and Corte reported [18] that the xanthine oxidase (XOD) is localized in the cytoplasm and exists in the following two forms: NAD-dependent XOD (type D) and superoxide-producing XOD (type O). As presented in Fig. 10, the XOD activities in atrophy were significantly higher than those in the control, and, especially, the activity of type O increased as much as 2.3-fold. The substrates of XOD, xanthine and hypoxanthine, increased in atrophy. However, urate, the product of the reaction catalyzed by XOD, increased in atrophy (Fig. 11). Therefore, superoxide-producing XOD might function more greatly in the atrophied muscle, which is thought to be the important source of superoxide anions in the cytoplasm (Fig. 10)

Booth and Giannetta reported [19] an increased calcium concentration in a whole tissue of atrophied gastrocnemius muscle. Since calcium is rich in extracellular space, this unfortunately means its intracellular level cannot be estimated by its concentration in the whole tissue. Therefore, to clarify the intracellular calcium level in the atrophied muscle cell, we performed an electron probe X-ray microanalysis [9]. Figure 12 shows the intracellular calcium concentration. The intracellular calcium level in atrophy was significantly higher than that in the control. On the other hand, the increased ratio of type O-to-total XOD in atrophy (Fig. 10) indicates an enhanced conversion to type O from type D of XOD.

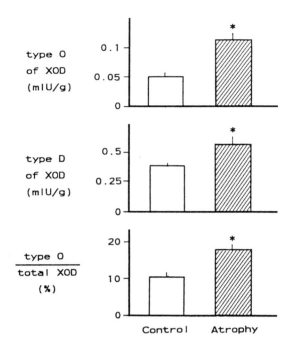

type O
of XOD
(mlU/g)

type D
of XOD
(mlU/g)

type O
―――――
total XOD
(%)

Control   Atrophy

Fig. 10. Activities of superoxide-producing xanthine oxidase (type O of XOD), NAD-dependent xanthine oxidase (type D of XOD) and ratio of type O to total XOD activity in a 12-day atrophied and contralateral (control) muscles. Data show mean ± SE (n = 6). *Significant difference at $p < 0.05$ compared with control.

It is generally known that the calcium-activated protease participates in the conversion [20]. Accordingly, the increased intracellular calcium in the atrophied muscle cell may cause the conversion via the activation of the protease (Fig. 12).

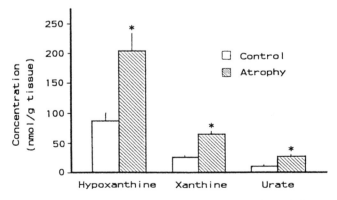

□ Control
▨ Atrophy

Concentration
(nmol/g tissue)

Hypoxanthine   Xanthine   Urate

Fig. 11. Levels of hypoxanthine, xanthine, and urate in a 12-day atrophied and contralateral (control) muscles. Data show mean ± SE (n = 6). *Significant difference at $p < 0.05$ compared with the control.

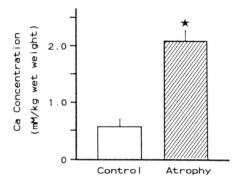

Fig. 12. Calcium level in sarcomere (A band) in an 8-day atrophied and contralateral (control) muscles. Data show mean ± SE (n = 15). *Significant difference at $p < 0.05$ compared with the control.

3.4 Iron movement

The generation of superoxide anions and hydrogen peroxides increased in the atrophied muscle cell, as described above. Although their reactivity is moderate, the very reactive radicals, hydroxyl radicals, are generated from them (so-called "Harber-Weiss reaction"). This reaction is generally very slow. If transition metal ions, such as iron and copper, exist in this reaction system, it will proceed alot faster [13]. Hence, it is necessary to investigate transition metals in the atrophied muscle in order to clarify the metabolism of active oxygen species. Moreover, the muscular atrophy induced by immobilization cause a rapid atrophy of the muscle cell [4]. Under the condition that the cell volume decreases rapidly and the cell structure changes dynamically, the distribution and balance of metals are expected to be disturbed [8,21].

Figure 13 shows the movements of metals in the course of atrophy. The concentration of iron, is known to play an important role in the generation of hydroxyl radicals, this kept increasing throughout the 12 days. To clarify this increased iron in whole tissues and the subcellular distribution of iron in atrophy was investigated (Fig. 14). The iron concentrations of microsomal and supernatant fractions increased in atrophy; particularly, the microsomal iron kept increasing throughout 12 days, and on the 12th day was about 3-fold higher than that of control.

This increase of microsomal iron suggested the possibility that iron-binding proteins appeared in the microsome of the atrophied muscle. Hence, we checked the iron-binding proteins in the Sarcoplasmic reticulum of the atrophied soleus muscle, and found the induction of iron-binding protein, 54 kDa in atrophy. This 54-kDa protein had already increased by the 4th day and the increased microsomal iron may be held by this protein.

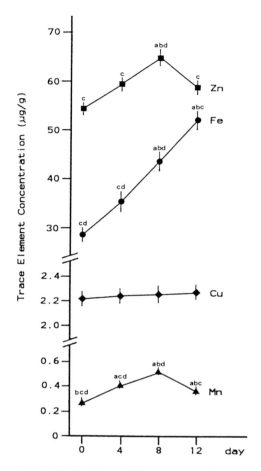

Fig. 13. Fe, Zn, Mn, and Cu movements in atrophied muscle as a function of the number of days after immobilization began. Data show mean ± SE (n = 5). Symbols are explained in Fig. 2.

3.5 Role of iron

Did the increased iron in the atrophied muscle play an important role in oxidative stress? To clarify the role of iron, we investigated the effect of deferoxamine (DFX) — an iron-chelating agent. DFX was administered at a rate of 0.21 mmol/day/kg body weight via an osmotic pumps that was implanted subcutaneously on the 4th day after immobilization started [22] (Table 1).

In DFX injection group (DFX group in Table 1), the increase of TBARS and GSSG were suppressed in the atrophied muscle. The increased TBARS level strongly suggests acceleration of lipid peroxidation. It also generally accepted that, under conditions of increased oxidative stress, the level of GSSG is normally increased [23]. Hence, DFX is thought to suppress oxidative stress. Iron-

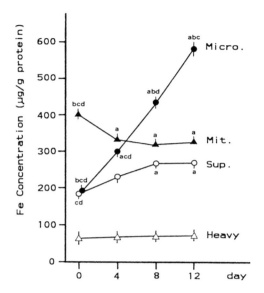

Fig. 14. Changes of iron concentration in subcellular fractions of atrophied muscle as a function of the number of days after immobilization began. Day 0 is the control. Each point is the mean ± SE (n = 5). Heavy: heavy fraction; Mit: mitochondrial fraction; Micro: microsomal fraction; Sup: supernatant fraction; Symbols are explained in Fig. 2.

Table 1. Effect of deferoxamine on muscle atrophy.

	Control		DFX		DFX + Fe	
	C	A	C	A	C	A
Muscle weight (mg)	158.2 ± 3.3^a	73.6 ± 2.6	144.4 ± 6.2^a	84.3 ± 4.3^c	156.9 ± 6.3^a	68.8 ± 2.4
Degree of atrophy (%)	53.5 ± 1.3	53.5 ± 1.3	$41.6 \pm 1.1^{b,c}$	41.6 ± 1.1	56.1 ± 0.7	56.1 ± 0.7
TBARS (nmol GSH/g)	24.6 ± 1.2^a	38.6 ± 1.5	25.3 ± 1.0	$27.7 \pm 1.5^{b,c}$	25.8 ± 1.6^a	38.5 ± 2.0
Total GSH (nmol GSH/g)	2928 ± 118^a	1805 ± 59	2867 ± 180^a	1883 ± 85	2753 ± 112^a	1869 ± 57
GSSG (nmol GSH/g)	51.6 ± 7.3^a	64.0 ± 4.7	57.6 ± 5.2^a	$33.0 \pm 3.5^{b,c}$	56.0 ± 11.5	59.0 ± 5.3
GSSG/total GSH (%)	1.75 ± 0.22^a	3.60 ± 0.33	2.04 ± 0.20	$1.95 \pm 0.26^{b,c}$	1.68 ± 0.41^a	3.21 ± 0.23

Values show means ± SE (n = 5). Control: doubled-distilled water injection group; DFX: deferoxamine injection group; DFX+Fe; iron-saturated deferoxamine injection group; C: contralateral muscle; A: 12-day atrophied muscle. [a]: significant difference at $p < 0.05$ compared with atrophied muscle by a paired t test; [b,c]significant differences at $p < 0.05$ compared with the Control and DFX+Fe group, respectivley by Bonferroni method.

saturated DFX did not have such an effect on oxidative stress (DFX+Fe group in Table 1). This indicates that DFX suppressed the oxidative stress by its iron-chelating action. In other words, this means that iron plays an important role in increasing oxidative stress in the atrophied muscle.

On the other hand, the level of TBARS increased only in the microsome in atrophy [9]. Free radicals that are harmful to the biological system are very reactive, and so the distance they can reach is very short. Taking these into consideration, the increased iron in the microsome is thought to participate in the generation of free radicals in atrophy. It is generally known that hydroxyl radicals, the most reactive of radicals, are generated from hydrogen peroxides and superoxide anions in the presence of iron [13]. In view of this simultaneous increase in microsomal iron and the increase in hydrogen peroxides and superoxide anions in the cytoplasm, it is to be expected that the generation of hydroxyl radicals may increase in the microsome of atrophied muscles.

Therefore, we measured the in vivo generation of hydroxyl radicals in atrophied muscle [24]. Salicylate was used as a trapping reagent for hydroxyl radicals. When small amounts of salicylate are added into a biological system, its phenolic ring can be attacked by hydroxyl radicals to yield dihydroxybenzoic acids (DHBs), which can then be determined using high-performance liquid chromatography. There was a significant increase in 2,3-DHB in the atrophied muscle. This result strongly suggested the enhanced generation in vivo of hydroxyl radicals in atrophied muscle.

Figure 15 presents schematically the possible mechanism of the oxidative stress in atrophy.

3.6 Production of nitric oxide

Endogenous nitric oxide (NO) has been reported to influence cell function [25]. Its function is "double-edged sword"; it works as a messenger and sometimes as a toxin. As a NOS, two types are known; constitutive NOS (cNOS) and inducible NOS (iNOS). The activity of cNOS is Ca-dependent, and that of iNOS is Ca-independent.

The activity of NOS was measured using the citrulline method, The cNOS activity significantly increased in the atrophied muscle as shown in Fig. 16, while that of iNOS did not changed. On the 8th day, the cNOS activity in the atrophied muscle increased up to 150% of the control. Considering, that the Ca level increased in the atrophy (Fig. 13), the increase of Ca-dependent NOS (cNOS) may be reasonable.

What function does the increased NO have in the muscular atrophy? Unfortunately, we don't have any clear answer. One interesting hypothesis is that the NO from atrophied muscle cell may stimulate the proliferation and differentiation of satellite cell. NO may work as a signal from the atrophied cell to the neighbor satellite cell (Fig. 16).

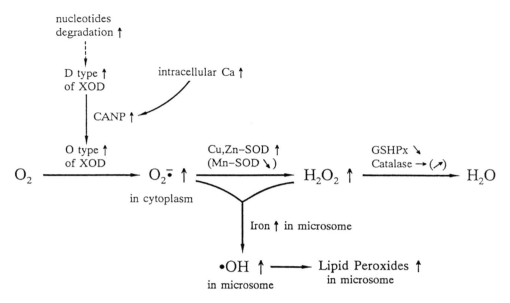

Fig. 15. Mechanism of oxidative stress in the skeletal muscle atrophied by immobilization. O_2: molecular oxygen; O_2^-: superoxide anion; H_2O_2: hydrogen peroxide; OH: hydroxyl radical; H_2O: water; D-type of XOD: NAD-dependent xanthine oxidase; O-type of XOD : superoxide-producing xanthine oxidase; CANP: calcium activated neutral protease; Cu,Zn-SOD: cytoplasmic form of superoxide dismutase; Mn-SOD: mitochondrial form of superoxide dismutase; GSHPx: Se-dependent glutathione peroxidase.

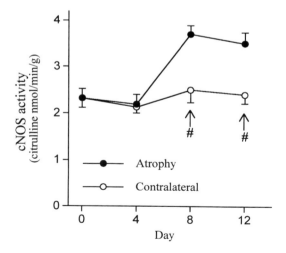

Fig. 16. Changes in constitutive nitric oxide synthase (cNOS) activities in atrophied and contralateral muscles as a function of the number of days after immobilization began. Day 0 is the control. Each point is the mean ± SE (n = 5). #Significant difference at $p < 0.05$ between atrophied and contralateral muscles.

4   ROLE OF OXIDATIVE STRESS IN MUSCULAR ATROPHY

Did the oxidative stress play a role in the progress of muscular atrophy or not? To answer this question, we have done an antioxidant-injection experiment. As antioxidant, vitamin E was injected intraperitoneally one time daily for 6 days before the immobilization period and every other day during the immobilization period in the form of DL-α-tocopherol at a dose of 30 mg/kg body weight [7] (Fig. 17).

In the vitamin E group the TBARS level in the atrophied muscle decreased significantly compared with that in the placebo group, which shows that vitamin E injected intraperitoneally served effectively as an antioxidant to lessen the oxidative stress in the atrophied muscle. In the vitamin E group, the muscle weight was significantly heavier, and the degree of atrophy significantly decreased 15% compared with those in the placebo group. The decrease of the degree of atrophy in the vitamin E group suggests that muscular atrophy proceeded mildly with lower oxidative stress. Thus, this indicates that oxidative stress accelerated the muscular atrophy.

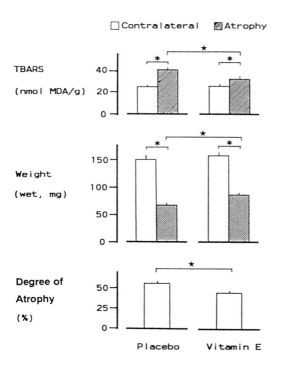

Fig. 17. Effect of vitamin E on a 12-day muscle atrophy. In vitamin E and Placebo groups, TBARS levels, muscle weights, and degree of atrophy in atrophied and contralateral muscles are shown. Data are means ± SE (n = 5). Ssignificant differences at p < 0.05 between atrophied and contralateral muscles. Star indicates significant difference at p < 0.05 between Vitamin E and Placebo groups.

As shown in Table 1, DFX diminished to the degree of atrophy by 22%. Considering that DFX suppressed the increase of oxidative stress in atrophied muscles, the effect of DFX on atrophy is thought to be mediated by the suppression of oxidative stress.

It is unclear how oxidative stress accelerated the muscular atrophy, but some possible mechanisms can be proposed:

1. The plasma membrane and sarcoplasmic reticulum are damaged by lipid peroxidation, allowing calcium to accumulate in the cell [26]. Ohta et al. [27] have reported that the inhibition of Ca^{2+}-ATPase by lipid peroxidation in vitro. Increased calcium has been reported to stimulate both phospholipid hydrolysis and nonlysosomal proteolysis [28,29]. We have shown an increase of calcium concentration in the sarcomere of atrophied muscle using electron probe X-ray microanalysis (refer to section 3.3). Although we cannot conclude whether this increase of intracellular calcium was a cause or a consequence of increased oxidative stress in the muscular atrophy, we suppose that its initial increase caused the oxidative stress which in turn accelerated its increase.

2. Free radical damage to proteins can make the proteins more susceptible to proteolysis [30]. The attack of free radicals can directly fragment proteins, followed by an increase of the enzymatic proteolysis of the fragments [31,32]. If the attacked proteins also have cross-linking and conformational changes, they are more susceptible to proteolysis [31].

3. The damage of lysosomal membrane by free radicals causes the leakage of lysosomal protease into the cytoplasm [33]. Actually, the activities of some lysosomal protease are reported to increase in muscular atrophy induced by immobilization [34].

It is also thought that the oxidative stress might have some effects on the physiological condition of the atrophied muscles. The possibility has also been explained that increased disulfide may also be one of the causes of metabolic changes. However, it remains uncertain which physiological and biochemical functions have changed in the atrophied muscle.

5   OXIDATIVE STRESS DURING RECOVERY FROM MUSCULAR ATROPHY

Oxygen consumption is expected to increase in the recovering muscle. Taking into account the catalytic action of the increased iron in the atrophied muscle, it is thought that the oxygen radicals may possibly increase during the recovery from muscle atrophy.

Some rats were exsanguinated after a 7-day immobilization (Atrophy group). The ankle joints of the other rats were remobilized after a 7-day immobilization and they were exsanguinated after a 5-day remobilization (Recovery group). The soleus muscles from both hindlimbs (atrophic and contralateral) were collected, and their levels of TBARS, total GSH, and GSSG were measured as a parameter of oxidative stress [35]. The levels of TBARS and GSSG increased significantly in atrophic muscles in the recovery group. These findings prove the enhanced level of oxidative stress during the recovery from muscle atrophy (Figs. 18 and 19).

To clarify the role of the oxidative stress during the recovery, the effect of vitamin E on the recovery from atrophy was examined (Fig. 20). Vitamin E was injected intraperitoneally in the form of *dl*-α-tocopherol at a dose of 30 mg/kg body weight one time daily during the remobilization period [35]. In the vitamin E group the TBARS level in atrophic muscle decreased significantly compared with that in the placebo group, and, hence, vitamin E injected intraperitoneally was thought to serve effectively as an antioxidant to lessen the oxidative stress. Moreover, since the degree of atrophy significantly decreased in the vitamin E group, it was suggested that recovery proceeded rapidly with lower oxidative stress. In other words, this indicates that oxidative stress slowed down the recovery from atrophy (Fig. 20).

6   OXIDATIVE STRESS IN OTHER MUSCULAR DISEASES.

So far, the oxidative stress in the muscular atrophy produced by immobilization has been discussed. The muscular atrophy is caused under various conditions in addition to muscular disuse. The deficiency of most nutrients is known to accompany muscular atrophy, as well as antioxidants such as vitamin E and selenium. Many diseases, containing neurogenic and muscular diseases, show the symptoms of muscular atrophy, as well. Among these muscular atrophies, we will choose two and discuss them in this section. One is the muscular atrophy by denervation, which has also been known as a model of disuse muscular atrophy. The other is Duchenne muscular atrophy.

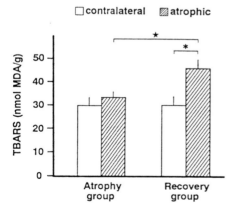

Fig. 18. Effect of a 5-day remobilization on TBARS level. Data show mean ± SE (n = 6). Star indicates significant difference at p < 0.05 between atrophy and recovery groups. *Significant difference at p < 0.05 between atrophic and contralateral muscles.

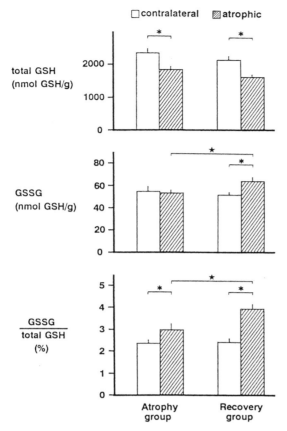

Fig. 19. Effect of a 5-day remobilization on levels of total GSH, GSSG, and ratio of GSSG to total GSH. Data show mean ± SE (n = 6). *Significant difference at p < 0.05 between atrophic and contralateral muscles.

6.1 Muscular atrophy induced by denervation.

Although denervation causes muscular atrophy and is used as a model of muscular disuse, its atrophy is reported to have various differences from the atrophy produced by immobilization [3]. Is there the oxidative stress in the muscular atrophy induced by denervation, too? There have been a few studies that can clearly answer this question. However, a few investigators reported on the activities of certain antioxidant enzyme.

Jenkins et al. [36] reported that denervation caused the activity of catalase to increase markedly in both red and white muscles; after only 2 days, denervation produced a rise of more than 200% in both soleus (red muscle; predominantly type I fiber) and extensor digitorum longus (EDL, white muscle; predominantly type II fiber). An increase in the catalase activity suggests that there is the possibility of the enhanced oxidative stress.

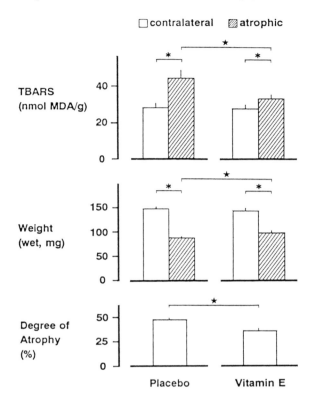

Fig. 20. Effect of vitamin E on the recovery from muscle atrophy. In vitamin E and Placebo groups, TBARS levels, muscle weights, and degree of atrophy in atrophied and contralateral muscles are shown. Data show means ± SE (n = 8). Significant differences at p < 0.05 between atrophic and contralateral muscles. Star mark, shows significant difference at p < 0.05 between vitamin E and placebo groups.

Asayama et al. [37] reported the activities of Mn-SOD, Cu,Zn-SOD, and GSHPx in the muscle atrophied by denervation. Although Cu,Zn-SOD concentrations showed no changes in the atrophied muscles, Mn-SOD concentrations decreased to 28% and 49% in the control in the soleus and EDL, respectively. The marked decrease of Mn-SOD might indicate the decreased production of free radicals in the mitochondria. The activities of GSHPx showed entirely different movements in soleus and EDL muscles; 2 weeks after denervation, its activity increased to 257% of the control in the EDL muscle and decreased to 22% of the control in the soleus muscle. It is very difficult to interpret those GSHPx activities in two muscles. The type I fiber shows the highest activity of GSHPx than the type II fiber, and the proportion of type II fiber is increased in the atrophic soleus muscle [2]. Considering these, Asayama et al. speculated that the decrease of its activity in the soleus to a level comparable to that of EDL may be influenced by the metabolic alternation related to the conversion of type

I to type II fibers.

The increased activities of some antioxidant enzymes is thought to suggest that oxidative stress may be enhanced in the skeletal muscle atrophied by denervation. Unfortunately, there has been no report to attempt to prove it. Personally, I think that when investigating this, the experimental period can be one of the most important factors. The stage that atrophy rapidly proceed is entirely different from the following stage. These two stages must be clearly distinguished in the investigation, otherwise some confusions might be caused.

6.2 Duchenne muscular dystrophy

On the other hand, there have been numerous studies on the oxidative stress in the Duchenne muscular dystrophy [38]. A lot of investigators have shown that the dystrophic human [39,40], mouse [41], and chicken [41,42] muscles contained higher levels of TBARS than normal. In the dystrophic chicken muscle, the level of GSSG increased even considering the elevated GSH [43]. The dystrophic chicken muscle showed a higher level of taurine — the fully oxidized metabolite of cysteine [44]. α-tocopherol (one of vitamin E family) is the major lipid-soluble antioxidant present in membranes and may be critical in the maintenance of sulf-hydryl group in cellular proteins. In the dystrophic chicken, the content of α-toco-pherol decreased even before secondary pathological symptoms of the disease become evident and the content of tocopheryl quinone (irreversible oxidation product of tocopherol) was increased, indicating that α-tocopherol was oxidized at a higher rate in the dystrophic muscle than in the relatively early phase [45]. The antioxidant enzymes increased or tended to be increased in the dystrophic muscles. In patients muscles, the SOD activity was unchanged [39,40] or slightly increased [43], while the activities of catalase [39,46], GSHPx [46], and GSSGRx [39] increased. In chicken, the dystrophic muscle showed higher activities of Cu,Zn-SOD [42,47], Mn-SOD [42,47], catalase [42,47], GSHPx [41,42,47], GST [46], and GSSGRx [41,42] than the normal. If the elevated activities of antioxi-dant enzymes is thought to be an adaptive response to oxidative stress, this may suggest why there is an increased oxidative stress. Considering these findings, it may be concluded that the Duchenne muscular dystrophy is accompanied by oxi-dative stress.

Is the oxidative stress related to the pathogenesis of muscular dystrophy? If so, antioxidant therapy may be effective in muscular dystrophy. Unfortunately, how-ever, many attempts at treatment of Duchenne muscular dystrophy had been rewarded only to demonstrate repeatedly its ineffectiveness [48]. Vitamin E [49,50], SOD [51], selenium [52], and allopurinol [53,54] were tested to treat the patients, but this was without success. It must be concluded that there is no strong evidence that the oxidative stress plays a causal role in the initiation of the Duchenne muscular dystrophy.

7   SUMMARY

1. Atrophied soleus muscles were collected from male Wistar rats (14- to 16-week-old), one ankle joint of which had been immobilized in the fully extended position. The degree of atrophy increased rapidly until the 8th day and slowly after that. TBARS and GSSG increased in the atrophied muscle, indicating the enhanced oxidative stress in atrophy.

2. In atrophy, Cu,Zn-containing superoxide dismutase (Cu,Zn-SOD) increased and Mn-containing superoxide dismutase decreased this might reflect the increased generation of superoxide anions in the cytoplasm rather than in the mitochondria. The source of superoxide anions in the cytoplasm may be the increased superoxide-producing XOD. Enhanced generation of superoxide anions and increased Cu,Zn-SOD activity in atrophy suggested an enhanced generation of hydrogen peroxide in the cytoplasm. Due to the unchanged activity of Se-dependent GSHPx and the unchanged or slightly increased activity of catalase, the ability to degrade hydrogen peroxide might not increase as much. Hence, hydrogen peroxide is expected to be increased in atrophy. The cytochemical study supported this expectation.

3. We also found an increased iron level, especially in the microsome, in the atrophied muscle and this proved its important role in oxidative stress by showing that the injection of DFX, iron-chelating agent, suppressed the enhanced oxidative stress in atrophy. The increased iron, which may be held by the 54-kDa protein, is thought to accelerate the Harber-Weiss reaction under increased superoxide anion and hydrogen peroxide in the cytoplasm. Consequently, the production of hydroxyl radicals, the most aggressive of radicals, might be elevated in the microsomes of the atrophied muscle. This is supported by our observation that only the microsomal fraction showed an increased in TBARS level in atrophy.

4. Vitamin E injection lessened the degree of atrophy, this suggests that muscular atrophy proceeded mildly with lower oxidative stress, i.e., the oxidative stress accelerates muscular atrophy.

5. Single angle joints of rats were immobilized for 7 days and remobilized for 5 days after the immobilization period. The levels of TBARS and GSSG increased in the recovering muscle, which strongly suggest that enhanced oxidative stress occurred during the recovery from disuse muscular atrophy. Vitamin E injection accelerated the recovery from atrophy, thus, showing that oxidative stress slowed it down.

6. In the skeletal muscle atrophied by denervation, the increased activities of some antioxidant enzymes suggests the possibility of enhanced oxidative stress and yet there is no report to prove it. In Duchenne muscular dystrophy, the increased oxidative stress has been generally accepted. However, there is no strong evidence that this is related to its pathogenesis.

8 ACKNOWLEDGEMENTS

This works were supported by the following funds; Inamori Foundation, Nakatomi Foundation, Uehara Foundation, Foundation for Pathological and Metabolic Research, Scientific Research Fund of the Ministry of Education, Science and Culture of the Government of Japan. I am grateful to Mrs Shoko Kondo for her kind assistance in the preparation of the manuscript. Special thanks go to Dr Chandan K. Sen for encouragement.

9 ABBREVIATIONS

TBARS: thiobarbituric acid-reactive substance
GSH: glutathione
GSSG: oxidized glutathione
GSSGRx: glutathione reductase
SOD: superoxide dismutase
GSHPx: glutathione peroxidase
GST: glutathione S-transferase
DAB: 3,3'-diaminobenzidine
XOD: xanthine oxidase
DFX: deferoxamine
DHB: dihydroxybenzoic acid
NO: nitric oxide
NOS: nitric oxide synthase

10 REFERENCES

1. Asayama K, Kato K. Free Radic Biol Med 1990;8:293−303.
2. Thomason DB, Booth FW. J Appl Physiol 1990;68:1−12.
3. Appell HJ. Sports Med 1990;10:42−58.
4. Nick DK, Beneke WM, Key RM, Timson B. J Anat 1989;163:1−5.
5. Cooper RR. J Bone Joint Surg (Am) 1972;54A:919−953.
6. Nemeth PM, Meyer D, Kark AP. J Neurochem 1980;35:1351−1360.
7. Kondo H, Miura M, Itokawa Y. Acta Physiol Scand 1991;142:527−528.
8. Gilbert HF. J Biol Chem 1982;257:12086−12091.
9. Kondo H, Miura M, Nakagaki I, Sasaki S, Itokawa Y. Am J Physiol 1992;262:E583−E590.
10. Kondo H, Miura M, Itokawa Y. Pflügers Arch 1993;422:404−406.
11. Kondo H, Nakagaki I, Sasaki S, Hori S, Itokawa Y. Am J Physiol 1993;265:E839−E844.
12. Hassan HM. Free Radic Biol Med 1988;5:377−385.
13. Halliwell B, Gutteridge JMC. Arch Biochem Biophys 1986;246:501−514.
14. Flohe L, Günzuler WA. Meth Enzymol 1984;105:114−121.
15. Habig WH, Pabst MJ, Jakoby WB. J Biol Chem 1974;249:7130−7139.
16. Babbs CF, Salaris SC, Turek JJ. Am J Physiol 1991;260:H123−H129.
17. Desplanches D, Mayet MH, Sempore B, Flandrois R. J Appl Physiol 1987;63:558−563.
18. Stripe F, Corte D. J Biol Chem 1969;244:3855−3863.
19. Booth FW, Giannetta CL. Calcif Tis Res 1973;13:327−330.
20. McCord JM. N Engl J Med 1985;312:159−163.

21. Kondo H, Kimura M, Itokawa Y. Proc Soc Exp Biol Med 1991;196:83—88.
22. Kondo H, Miura M, Kodama J, Ahmed SM, Itokawa Y. Pflügers Arch 1992;421:295—297.
23. Lew H, Pykes S, Quintanilha A. FEBS Lett 1985;185:262—266.
24. Kondo H, Nishino K, Itokawa Y. FEBS Lett 1994;349:169—172.
25. Nathan C, Xie Q. Cell 1994;78:915—918.
26. Mourelle M, Meza MA. J Appl Toxicol 1991;10:23—27.
27. Ohta A, Mohri T, Ohyashiki T. Biochem Biophys Acta 1989;984:151—157.
28. Nicotera P, Hartzell P, Baldi C, Svensson S, Bellomo G, Orrenius S. J Biol Chem 1986;261: 14628—14635.
29. Pascoe GA, Reed DJ. Free Radic Biol Med 1989;6:209—224.
30. Davis KJA, Goldberg AL. J Biol Chem 1987;262:8220—8226.
31. Davis KJA. J Biol Chem 1987;262:9895—9901.
32. Hunt JV, Simpson JA, Dean RT. Biochem J 1988;250:87—93.
33. Mak IT, Misra HP, Weglicki WB. J Biol Chem 1983;258:13733—13737.
34. Max SR, Maier RF, Vogelsang L. Arch Biochem Biophys 1971;146:227—232.
35. Kondo H, Kodama J, Kishibe T, Itokawa Y. FEBS Lett 1993;326:189—191.
36. Jenkins RR, Newsham D, Rushmore P, Tenjie J. Biochem Med 1982;27:195—199.
37. Asayama K, Dettbarn WD, Burr IM. J Neurochem 1986;46:604—609.
38. Murphy ME, Kehrer JP. Chem Biol Interact 1989;69:101—173.
39. Kar NC, Pearson CM. Clin Chim Acta 1979;94:277—280.
40. Mecheler F, Imre S, Dioszeghy P. J Neurol Sci 1984;63:279—283.
41. Omaye ST, Tappel AL. Life Sci 1974;15:137—145.
42. Mizuno Y. Exp Neurol 1984;84:58—73.
43. Murphy ME, Kehrer JP. Biochem J 1989;260:359—364.
44. Peterson DW, Lilyblade AL, Lyon J. Proc Soc Exp Biol Med 1963;113:798—802.
45. Murphy ME, Kehrer JP. Biochem Med Metab Biol 1989;41:234—245.
46. Burr IM, Asayama K, Fenichel GM. Muscle Nerve 1987;10:150—154.
47. Murphy ME, Kehrer JP. Biochem Biophys Res Commun 1986;134:550—556.
48. Jackson MJ, Edwards RH. Adv Exp Med Biol 1990;264:485—491.
49. Berneske GM, Burton ARC, Gould EN, Levy D. Neurology 1960;35:61—65.
50. Edwards RHT, Jones DA, Jackson MJ. Med Biol 1984;62:143—147.
51. Stern LZ, Ringel SP, Ziter FA, Menander-Huber KB, Ionasacu V, Pellegrio RJ, Snyder RD. Arch Neurol 1982;39:342—346.
52. Jackson MJ, Coakley J, Stokes M, Rdwards RHT, Oster O. Neurology 1989;39:655—659.
53. Mendell JR, Winchers DO. Muscle Nerve 1979;2:53—56.
54. Griffirhs RD, Cady EB, Edwards RHT, Wilkie DR. Muscle Nerve 1985; 8: 760—767.

©2000 Elsevier Science B.V. All rights reserved.
Handbook of Oxidants and Antioxidants in Exercise.
C.K. Sen, L. Packer and O. Hänninen, editors.

Part IX • Chapter 24

Protection against free radical injury in the heart and cardiac performance

D.K. Das and N. Maulik

Cardiovascular Division, Department of Surgery, The School of Medicine, University of Connecticut 263, Farmington Avenue, Farmington, CT 06030-1110, USA. Tel.: +1 860 679 3687. Fax: +1 860 679 4606. E-mail: ddas@neuron.uchc.edu

1   INTRODUCTION
2   HEART FAILURE
3   VALVULAR HEART DISEASE
         3.1   Cardiomyopathy
         3.2   Hypertrophy
4   DIABETES
5   ATHEROSCLEROSIS
6   ISCHEMIC HEART DISEASE
         6.1   Angina pectoris
         6.2   Ischemia/reperfusion injury
         6.3   ischemic preconditioning and myocardial adaptation to ischemia
         6.4   Apoptosis in reperfusion injury
         6.5   Nitric oxide: a double-edged sword
         6.6   Stunning
         6.7   Arrhythmias
7   AGING
8   STRESS
9   INTERVENTIONAL/INTRAOPERATIVE CORRECTIVE MANIPULATIONS
         9.1   Angioplasty
         9.2   Cardiac surgery
         9.3   Transplantation
10   SUMMARY
11   ABBREVIATIONS
12   REFERENCES

1   INTRODUCTION

The heart is an organ which is in continuous motion with the never ending task of pumping blood, as well as being in a constant state of mechanical and metabolic flux. It is not just a pump, but it can adapt itself by carefully regulating the rate and force of cardiac contractions by responding to the needs of the body during various performances, such as exercise and pathophysiological conditions.

When a heart fails to perform its tasks, it is deemed a failing heart. The biochemical basis of heart failure is in many ways different from that of myocardial infarction. The principle reason being that diverse diseases can lead to heart failure, whereas myocardial infarction is synonymous with ischemia of the heart. Diseases that can cause heart failure are numerous, some of which include ischemic heart disease, atherosclerosis, hypertrophy, cardiomyopathy, hypertension, arrhythmias, streneous exercise and diabetes, together with diseases originating in other organs. A large number of factors are likely to be responsible for the pathogenesis of the malfunction in cardiac performance. However, out of all these diseases, oxidative stress ought to be singled out. Indeed, reactive oxygen species have been implicated in all of the above mentioned coronary diseases. This review will focus on the role of oxygen free radicals in the dysfunction of cardiac performances associated with these heart diseases.

2   HEART FAILURE

Heart failure is a pathological state in which the heart is unable to pump sufficient blood to meet the metabolic needs of various tissues. Among other factors, free radicals have also been implicated in the pathogenesis of chronic heart failure. For example, there is evidence to suggest that increased production of prostaglandins in human heart failure patients is associated with the enhanced production of oxygen free radicals through arachidonic acid cascade [1]. This receives further support from the findings that circulating catecholamine formation increases in the failing heart, which, upon auto-oxidation may result in the generation of oxygen-derived free radicals [2]. The free radical generating activities of polymorphonuclear leukocytes (PMN) in dogs with heart failure were found to be greater in comparison to those in control dogs [3]. Adriamycin-induced heart failure is associated with the production of oxygen free radicals [4]. Recently, plasma of patients with heart failure was found to contain increased level of malonaldehyde, a presumptive marker for free radical production [5].

In congestive heart failure, myocardial dysfunctions occur primarily because of the impairment of cardiac contractility, either through the partial loss of muscle or by overload manifested by volume or pressure [6]. A decrease in the myocardial contractility functions and an increase in the left ventricular end-diastolic pressure in the failing dog hearts was attributed to an enhanced phagocytic activity of PMNs [7]. A study with human patients indicated a close correlation between the cardiac functions and free radical generation in congestive heart failure. For example, left ventricular ejection factor of these patients showed an inverse relationship with plasma MDA concentrations with an r value of -0.35 ($p < 0.05$) and a direct relationship with plasma thiol activities with an r value of 0.39 ($p < 0.01$) (Fig. 1). Furthermore, an angiotensin-converting enzyme (ACE), inhibitor captopril, was shown to improve myocardial functions of the patients [1], presumably by the free radical scavenging activities of captopril [8]. More recently, patients of congestive heart failure were found to have an elevated level of breath pentane, a marker for lipid peroxidation and free radical formation [9]. Again, captopril was able to reduce the breath pentane level, presumably through its free radical scavenging activities.

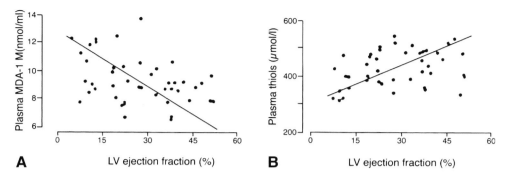

Fig. 1. Correlation curves for plasma concentration of malonaldehyde-like material (MDA-LM). Left ventricular (LV) ejection fraction (**A**) and plasma thiols and LV ejection fraction (**B**) in patients with congestive heart failure. (Data reproduced with permission from [5]).

3   VALVULAR HEART DISEASE

The contrasting effects of pressure and volume overload may lead to several forms of vascular heart disease. In aortic stenosis, the left ventricle undergoes concentric hypertrophy that enables it to overcome otherwise abnormally high wall tension, according to Laplace's law, and leads to pressure overload. In chronic aortic regurgitation, the primary effect is volume overload, but since the wall tension also rises, pressure hypertrophy is also developed to adjust the systolic wall tension to a normal level. Mitral stenosis, on the other hand, is not a manifestation of pressure or volume overload, but it is related to problems of a poorly filling left ventricle with a low cardiac output which is compensated by increased left atrial filling pressure. This leads to left atrial enlargement which can result in atrial fibrillation and increased pulmonary venous pressure. All valvular heart diseases can ultimately lead to heart failure. As discussed above, oxygen free radicals may play a role in the pathogenesis of congestive heart failure. It is also likely that the reactive oxygen species may be involved in the pathophysiology of valvular heart diseases that can lead to heart failure.

3.1 Cardiomyopathy

It should be clear from the above discussion that cardiomyopathy results from the myocardial adaptation to abnormal conditions. Many forms of cardiomyopathy exist in literature and, depending on the origin, include hypertrophic cardiomyopathy, ischemic cardiomyopathy, dilated cardiomyopathy, diabetic cardiomyopathy, metabolic cardiomyopathy and congestive cardiomyopathy. Many agents, such as alcohol, catecholamines, doxorubicin and adriamycin, can result in cardiomyopathy.

Reactive oxygen species have been implicated in the pathogenesis of cardiomyopathy. For example, antioxidant therapy was found to protect against catecholamine cardiomyopathies in an animal model [10,11]. Myocardial antioxidant defense mechanism is depressed in alcohol-induced congestive cardiomyopathy [12]. Oxygen-derived free radicals are increased in adriamycin cardiomyopathy [13]. Pretreatment of animals with α-tocopherol significantly reduced myocardial damage caused by doxorubicin or isoproterenol-induced cardiomyopathy [14]. A recent study also demonstrated the protective effect of α-tocopherol in Bio 14.6 hamsters treated during the early stage of cardiomyopathy [15]. In this study, the authors used morphometric analysis to assess the degree of protection by α-tocopherol. The total damaged area (%) in the treated group was significantly smaller than that in the control group (Fig. 2). Myocardium of 60-day-old Bio 14.6 hamsters have been found to be deficient in vitamin E and more susceptible to lipid peroxidation [16]. In another recent study, GSH peroxidase level of a 30-day-old Bio 14.6 cardiomyopathic Syrian hamster heart was found to be higher compared to that of an age-matched control [17]. The authors cited that increased antioxidant level was due to myocardial adaptation to oxidative stress. However, the concentrations of mitochondrial generation of free radicals were higher in the hearts of 40- and 90-day-old animals. A protective effect of α-tocopherol therapy was shown in these hamsters only during the early stage of cardiomyopathy. Another related study demonstrated reduction of catecholamine cardiomyopathy by allopurinol, a xanthine oxidase inhibitor [18]. Cardiomyopathy induced by magnesium deficiency was found to have increased the number and size of lesions, which were reduced by treatment with α-tocopherol [19].

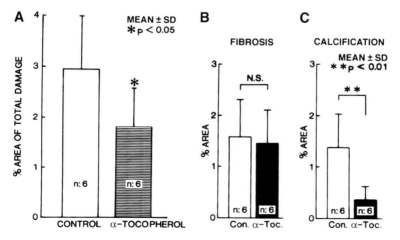

Fig. 2. Effect of α-tocopherol on the percentage area of total myocardial damage (**A**), area of fibrosis (**B**), and calcification (**C**) in Bio 14.6 cardiomyopathic hamsters. N.S: Not significant. (Data reproduced with permission from [15]).

3.2 Hypertrophy

Abnormal hemodynamic load originating from a change in demand may lead to an increase in heart to body weight ratio compared to that typical in a normal animal. Such an enlargement in heart size is referred to as hypertrophy. Hypertrophy can be manifested experimentally by applying either pressure, volume overload or by other means. For example, aortic stenosis, pulmonary artery stenosis, hypertension or renal ischemia can cause pressure overload [20]; aortic insufficiency or bradycardia can cause volume overload [21]; and hypoxia, exercise, or cardiomyopathy can also lead to overload [22]. Overload can be achieved by chemical factors such as catecholamines or carbon monoxide exposure [22,23].

Clinically, patients with hypertrophic cardiac disease are more sensitive to ischemia/ reperfusion injury compared to normal persons [24]. The fact that ischemia/reperfusion leads to the generation of reactive oxygen species in turn leads many investigators to wonder whether hypertrophic hearts are under oxidative stress. Hypertrophic cardiac tissue is even more sensitive to the toxic effects of adriamycin [25]. A recent study demonstrated that SOD content in a heart from a spontaneously hypertensive rat is approximately 50% lower compared to that in a genetically identical control animal [26]. In addition, xanthine oxidase content of these hypertrohic hearts was 75% higher compared to that in normal hearts. Xanthine oxidase being a well-known source of oxygen free radicals [27] would tend to support the observation that hypertrophic hearts are more susceptible to ischemia/ reperfusion injury. In this study, the authors found that the left ventricular functional recovery after ischemia was reduced in a spontaneously hypertensive heart, compared to that in otherwise genetically identical control Wister-Kyoto animals (Table 1). In hypertrophied rabbit cardiac muscle, unloaded shortening velocity (V_{max}) was found to be 36% lower compared to that in normal heart muscle [28].

4   DIABETES

Myocardial diseases and complications are more frequent in diabetes patients. The two degenerative diseases, cardiomyopathy and nephropathy, share a common etiology resulting from the altered metabolic fate from the lack of insulin.

Table 1. Left Ventricular Recovery After Ischemia and Antioxidant Enzymes in Control and Hypertensive Hearts. Results are expressed as Means ± SD of six animals/group for functional measurements and ten animals/group for SOD and XO activities (Data obtained from ref. 26).

	LVDP	LVEDP	LVdp/dt	SOD	XO
Control	62.4 ± 3.5	145 ± 34	62 ± 3.3	119 ± 68	1.4 ± 2
Hypertensive	42.8 ± 6.8*	361 ± 57*	39 ± 6.9*	67 ± 11.4*	2.2 ± 7*

*$p < 0.05$ compared to control.

Evidence present in the literature suggests that similar mechanisms, i.e., a role of oxygen free radicals, may be involved in the pathogenesis of these diseases even though different tissues are involved. Among many metabolic and biochemical factors that result in diabetic patients, development of oxidative stress plays a prominant role. It has long been known that diabetes can be experimentally induced by injecting alloxan, an oxidant that damages the β cell of the pancreas through the production of reactive oxygen species [29]. Free radical hypothesis receives further support from the observation that antioxidants can protect islet β cells from oxygen free radicals generated by cytokines [30,31]. Increased lipid peroxidation has been found to occur in diabetic patients, particularly in patients with vascular complications [32,33]. Diabetes can alter the free radical metabolism in blood, as well as in tissues [32–35].

Functional disturbances may occur in a diabetic heart. For example, the magnitude of post rest contraction (PRC) is significantly smaller in the diabetic than in the normal heart [36,37]. An example of a decrease in the developed contraction and prolongation of relaxation time of the contraction in a diabetic heart is shown in Fig. 3. Diabetes can lead to atherosclerosis, related to hypertriglyceridemia and altered lipoproteins that cause increased risk of myocardial infarction. Another heart disease, diabetic cardiomyopathy, that causes contractile dysfunctions, has already been discussed under cardiomyopathy.

Development of oxidative stress in the heart of the diabetic animals receives further support from the observation that diabetic hearts exibit increased resistance to lipid peroxidation [38] (Table 2). In this study, diabetic rat hearts contained significantly lower levels of thiobarbituric acid reactive substances than those present in normal animals. In addition, diabetic hearts contain higher levels of glutathione, as well as antioxidant enzymes such as catalase and glutathione reductase [35], suggesting that these hearts undergo adaptive modification due to oxidative stress. Another related study has demonstrated that diabetic rat hearts are more resistant to ischemia/reperfusion injury [39].

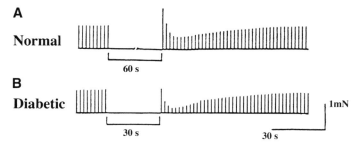

Fig. 3. Original examples of the maximum postrest contraction in the normal, (**A**), and the diabetic, (lower panel), heart. (Data reproduced with permission from [36]).

Table 2. In vivo TBARS, lipid hydroperoxides, and total GSH levels in the hearts of normal and diabetic rats (n = 4/group). All values are means ± SD. Each value is an average of four individual determinations. (Data reproduced with permission from [38].)

	Normal	Diabetic
TBARS (nmol/μmol lipid P)	3.78 ± 0.77	2.08 ± 0.51*
Lipid hydroperoxides (nmol/μmol lipid P)	29.3 ± 2.02	24.2 ± 1.03*
Glutathione (GSH) (μg/gm wet wt)	238 ± 9.56	305 ± 78.7*

*p < 0.05 compared to normal; TBARS: Thiobarbituric acid-reactive substances.

5   ATHEROSCLEROSIS

A growing body of evidence suggests the role of oxidatively modified low-density lipoprotein (LDL) in the pathogenesis of atherosclerosis [40]. LDL mainly consists of free and esterified cholesterol, triglycerides, phospholipids and free fatty acids. Upon oxidation these heterogeneous lipid populations are transformed into a more heterogeneous mixture, containing numerous newly formed lipid products in addition to the original lipid families. These complex lipid products potentiate a cascade of reactions, including the expression of several chemotactic factors and cytokines that lead to the formation of reactive oxygen species and the development of oxidative stress. Endothelial cell injury is one of the early events associated with atherosclerosis which may be potentiated by several factors including lipid peroxidation [41]. Blood level of lipid peroxidation product, malonaldehyde, is increased in hypercholesterolemic atherosclerosis [42]. Moreover, the supplementation of the diet with the antioxidant, vitamin E, reduced the aortic tissue malonaldehyde, simultaneously decreasing the amount of atherosclerotic plaques as shown in Fig. 4.

Increased levels of cholesterol oxides and oxidant-modified proteins have been reported in hypercholesterolemic hearts suggesting the increased presence of oxygen free radicals [43]. The efficacy of antilipolytic drug probucol in the reduction of intimal lesion formation in Watanabe hyperlipidemic rabbits have been attributed to its antioxidant properties [44].

The role of reactive oxygen species has been directly related to the pathogenesis of atherosclerosis from the findings that oxygen radicals can modify the low-density lipoproteins (LDL) [45]. Such oxidative modification of LDL presumably occurs by converting this lipoprotein to a modified form that is recognized by the macrophage scavenger receptors. Both endothelial and smooth muscle cells can oxidize LDL and are likely to serve as potential sources for oxidative modification [46]. Free radical hypothesis for the pathogenesis of atherosclerosis has received further support from the demonstration that not only are the malonaldehyde-lysine residues found in the hyperlipidemic rabbit atherosclerotic lesions [47], but also from the documentated evidence for the presence of several antioxidant enzymes in the atherosclerotic arteries [48]. In addition, the presence of autoantibodies to malonaldehydelysine has been recently well-documented in

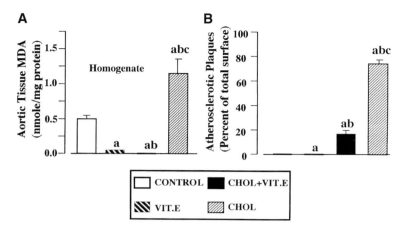

Fig. 4. Effects of four different types of diets on the development of atherosclerotic plaques in aorta (**B**) and aortic tissue malonaldehyde (**A**. The results are expressed as mean ± SEM. Chol: cholesterol. ap < 0.05, group I vs. groups II, III and IV. bp < 0.05, group II vs. groups III and IV. cp < 0.05, group III vs. group IV. Note that group I and II in the right(**B**) panel show some values for atherosclerotic plaques. This is just to show the location of groups I and II. There were no atherosclerotic plaques in these two groups (Data reproduced with permission from [42]).

the plasma of rabbit and man [49]. The same group have demonstrated a connection between the modification of LDL and lipid peroxidation [50]. More recently, a role of peroxynitrite radical, resulting from the reaction of superoxide and nitric oxide, has also been implicated in atherosclerosis [51].

6   ISCHEMIC HEART DISEASE

Ischemic heart disease remains a widespread cause of morbidity and mortality in the developed countries such as the USA. The term ischemia represents complete or partial reduction of coronary blood flow in conjunction with hypoxia, such that the supply of oxygen to the myocardium is inadequate for the oxygen demands of the tissue. Depending on the degree of ischemia, ischemic heart disease may be categorized in several forms. Angina pectoris, which means pin of the chest, is a complex clinical situation in which an acute attack of a chest pain is evoked by stress and is either relieved upon rest or occurs spontaneously through rest. In the advanced stage, angina pectoris may lead to myocardial infarction resulting in scared tissue and cell death. Thus, depending on the progression of ischemia, a mild or severe heart attack may result. A major percentage of the deaths that occur suddenly are apparently due to arrhythmias. Although diverse mechanisms exist behind the pathogenesis of ischemic heart disease, development of oxidative stress has been implicated as one of the potential mediators of this disease. These are discussed in the following sections.

6.1 Angina pectoris

Whether it is stable or unstable angina, during both conditions of angina there is a reduction in coronary blood flow to the myocardium. Transient vasoconstriction at the site of an epicardial stenosis during exercise may cause hypoperfusion in patients with stable angina [52]. Whereas thrombosis or aggregation of platelets at the site of an atherosclerotic plaque may be the reason for the reduced coronary flow in patients during unstable angina [53]. Since the relief occurs by the restoration of blood flow to the ischemic myocardium, it is likely that the reperfused myocardium would be subjected to oxidative stress. A recent study has demonstrated that lipid peroxides and conjugated dienes were elevated in patients with both stable and unstable angina [54]. In the case of a stable angina, the erythrocytes expressed a diminished activity of SOD and normal activities of catalase and glutathione peroxidase. Whereas in an unstable angina, enhanced activities of both SOD and catalase were observed. A significant increase was also noticed in the levels of ceruloplasmin and α-tocopherol during both types of angina, indicating that oxygen free radicals may play a role in the pathogenesis of angina pectoris.

6.2 Ischemia/reperfusion injury

Myocardial cellular injury associated with the reperfusion of ischemic myocardium has been attributed to many interrelated factors that include intracellular Ca^{2+} overloading, loss of sarcolemmal phospholipids and oxygen free radical generation [55]. The participation of free radicals has been demonstrated from the beneficial effects of antioxidants and antioxidant enzymes [56,57], as well as free radical scavengers [58]. In addition, the consequence of a free radical attack has been demonstrated by identifying the lipid peroxidative products in reoxygenated or reperfused myocardium [59]. The presence of free radicals has also been demonstrated in an ischemic reperfused heart [60].

There is general agreement that the amount of several antioxidants and antioxidant enzymes are significantly reduced after ischemia and reperfusion. For example, reduced amount of SOD, catalase and glutathione peroxidase enzymes, as well as α-tocopherol and ascorbic acid, have been found in the ischemic reperfused myocardium [59,61]. The loss of the key antioxidant enzymes and antioxidants reduces the overall antioxidant reserve of the heart and make the heart susceptible to ischemia/reperfusion injury. One of the major functions of antioxidants is to block the free radical formation. Thus, it is not difficult to comprehend that reduced antioxidative defense is not capable of providing complete protection against increased activities of the reactive oxygen species.

Evidence exists in the literature to support the idea that a large quantity of oxygen free radicals are generated in the postischemic heart upon reperfusion. They have been detected directly by HPLC, using an electrochemical detection technique [62], an ESR spectroscopy [63] and indirectly by the formation of malonaldehyde and conjugated dienes [64,65]. In a recent study, the presence of OH· was compared by two different methods [60]. Isolated buffer-perfused rat hearts were subjected to 30 min of normothermic global ischemia followed by 30 min of reperfusion. 5,5-Dimethyl-pyrroline-*N*-oxide (DMPO) was used as a spin-trap agent to detect OH· radicals. In additional HPLC studies, salicylic acid was infused into the heart for the detection of OH· radicals. In all studies, the effects of SOD and catalase on the OH· formation were examined. Irrespective of the methods used, OH· concentration was found to have increased drammatically between 60 and 90 s of reperfusion, peaked between 180 and 210 s, and then progressively decreased (Fig. 5). In all cases, SOD plus catalase were able to reduce the formation of OH· radicals. The results further demonstrated that OH· was produced only in the fibrillating hearts, but not in the nonfibrillating hearts.

Indirectly, numerous studies have demonstrated the increased formation of malonaldehyde in the ischemic reperfused myocardium [64—66]. Recently, a HPLC method has been described to monitor the malonaldehyde in hearts that utilized the 2,4-dinitrophenylhydrazine derivatization of the lipid metabolites [64]. The results of the study demonstrated the progressive increase of malonaldehyde and other lipid metabolites, supporting the previous reports concerning the increased formation of lipid peroxidation products during the reperfusion.

Although the development of oxidative stress in the ischemic reperfused myocardium has been confirmed, the literature is full of conflicting reports regarding the source(s) of these free radicals. These include polymorphonuclear leukocytes, mitochondrial, together with microsomal respiratory chains, arachidonic acid cascade, xanthine oxidase, catecholamine autooxidation, and oxygen-carrying proteins. All of which have been attributed to potential generators of oxygen free radicals [27,55,56,59,67,68] (Fig. 6). The precise role of free radicals in the mediation of ischemic reperfusion injury also remains unknown.

Irrespective of the source of free radicals, the role of the reactive oxygen species in the pathogenesis of ischemia/reperfusion injury cannot be excluded. For

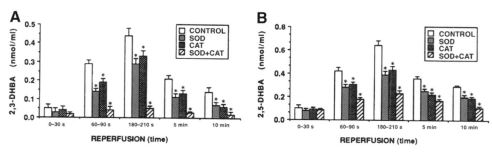

Fig. 5. (A) 2,3- and (B) 2,5-Dihydroxybenzoic acid concentrations in the effluents of reperfused hearts, subjected to 30 min normothermic global ischemia followed by reperfusion in the presence of 1 mmol/l of salicylic acid in the control, SOD, catalase, and SOD plus catalase-treated groups. The sampling time was: 0—30, 60—90, 180—210, 270—300, and 570—600 s, respectively, during reperfusion. Values are means ± SEM. Comparisons were made to the time-matched control values. *p < 0.05. (Data reproduced with permission from [60]).

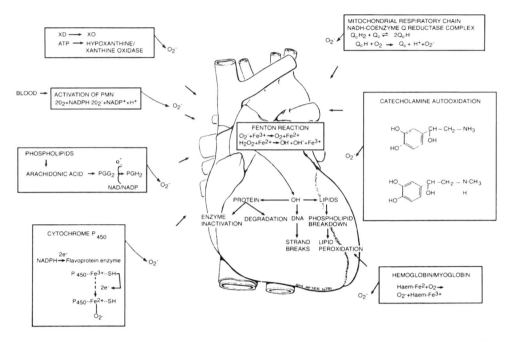

Fig. 6. Various mechanisms for the generation of oxygen-derived free radicals during reperfusion of ischemic myocardium. (Data reproduced with permission from [55].)

example, antioxidants and free radical scavengers can remove the oxygen radicals, simultaneously ameliorating the postischemic ventricular dysfunctions. A partial list of the beneficial effects of free radical scavengers and antioxidants on the postischemic ventricular functions and cellular injury in the ischemic reperfused heart [69—80] is shown in Table 3.

6.3 Ischemic preconditioning and myocardial adaptation to ischemia

Hearts subjected to stress, induced by cyclic episodes (usually four cycles) of short durations of ischemia (usually 5 min), each followed by another short duration of reperfusion (usually 10 min), renders the hearts resistence to subsequent lethal ischemic injury. This phenomenon has been termed as ischemic preconditioning or myocardial adaptation to ischemia [89,90]. Although significant controversy exists regarding the mechanism of ischemic adaptation, it is generally believed that adaptation occurs through the upregulation of an endogenous defence system of the heart [91]. Among several factors, antioxidants and antioxidant enzymes have been shown to play a significant role in myocardial adaptation [92]. A number of oxidative stress-inducible genes are induced by ischemic preconditioning suggesting a role of oxygen free radicals in ischemic preconditioning [93]. A recent study from our laboratory indicated free radicals as the initial signaling agent for myocardial ischemic adaptation [94].

Table 3. Beneficial effects of antioxidants in ischemia/reperfusion injury.

Antioxidant	Mode of action	Species	Beneficial effects	Refs
SOD	Dismutates O_2^-	DOG	Improves function	69
Catalase	Removes H_2O_2	DOG	Supresses T × B_2	70
SOD + Catalase	Scavengers O_2^- and H_2O_2	Dog Rat Pig	Reduces infarct Improves function Improves function, reduces CK release	70 71 72
Glutathione	Scavenges O_2^- and protects SH-group	Rat	Reduces membrane damage	73
α-Tocopherol	Breaks radical chain reactions	Rat	Improves contractile functions, reduces LDH release	74
		Rabbit	Preserves ATP, CP, reduces CK release	75
Trolox	Same as α-tocopherol	Dog	Reduces tissue necrosis	76
Ascorbic acid	Prevents oxy radical formation and regenerates α-tocopherol	Dog	Reduces tissue necrosis	76
Fatty acid binding protein (FABP)	Scavenges oxy radicals	Rat	Improves function, reduces CK release	77
ONO-3144	Scavenges OH	Pig	Improves function, reduces CK release	78
Allopurinol	XO-Inhibitor, removes OH	Pig	Improves function, reduces CK release	79
Deferoxamine	Chelates iron	Rat	Reduces fibrillation normalised contractility	80
		Dog	Reduces infarct	81
Fenozan	—	Rat	Improves function	82
Dimercapto-propanol	Protects -SH group	Rabbit	Reduces injury	83
Indapamine	Scavenges free radical interme-diates	Rat	Improves function, reduces LDH release	84

(Continued)

Table 3. (Continued).

Antioxidant	Mode of action	Species	Beneficial effects	Refs
IRFI-016	Scavenges free radicals	Rat	Reduces CK, attenuates ST segment rise	85
Phytic acid	Scavenges OH and chelates iron	Rat	Improves function, reduces CK release	86
Emoxipine	Enhances GSH-peroxidase and reductase	Human	Reduces injury	87
EGB 671	Scavenges O_2^- and OH	Rat	Reduces incidence of arrhythmias	88

6.4 Apoptosis in reperfusion injury

A growing body of evidence is rapidly accumulating to indicate that cardiomyocytes undergo apoptotic cell death during prolonged reperfusion. One of the inducers of apoptosis is oxidative stress which is also implicated in the pathogenesis of reperfusion injury. In a recent study, isolated rat hearts subjected to 90 min and 120 min of reperfusion, following 15 min of ischemia, were found to be associated with apoptotic cardiomyocytes [95]. Isolated hearts subjected to up to 60 min of ischemia without any reperfusion showed no evidence of apoptosis. These results corroborated with the findings of DNA fragmentation which showed increased ladders of DNA bands in the same reperfused hearts, representing integer multiples of the internucleosomal DNA length (about 180 bp), (Figs. 7 and 8). The presence of apoptotic cells and DNA fragmentation in the

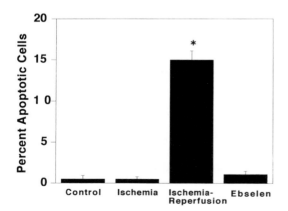

Fig. 7. Estimation of apoptotic cells. Apoptotic cells expressed as % of total number of cardiomyocytes in control, ischenic, reperfused, ebselen-treated and preconditioned(PC) group. *$p < 0.05$. (Data reproduced with permission from Free Radical Biology Medicine [24].)

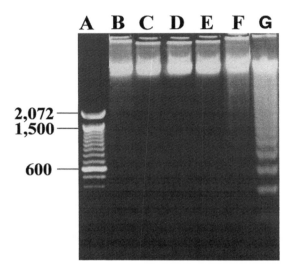

Fig. 8. Effects of ischemia/reperfusion, ebselen and preconditioning on DNA laddering. DNA isolated from cardiomyocytes were subjected to 1.8% agarose gel electrophoresis. 100 bp DNA ladder was used as molecular weight marker (A). Control (B); 30 min ischemia (C); Preconditioning + 15 min ischemia/2 h reperfusion (D); Ebselen + 15 min ischemia/2 h reperfusion (E); 15 min ischemia/90 min reperfusion (F); 15 min ischemia/2 h reperfusion (G).

myocardium were abolished by preperfusing the hearts in the presence of ebselen, a glutathione peroxidase mimic, which also removed the oxidative stress developed in the heart. Taken together, these results clearly demonstrate that oxidative stress developed in the ischemic reperfused myocardium induces apoptosis.

The role of apoptosis in reperfusion injury receives further support from a recent finding that myocardial adaptation to ischemia reduces apoptotic cell death and DNA fragmention [95,96]. Isolated rat hearts subjected to four cyclic episodes of 5 min ischemia, each followed by another 10 min of reperfusion, were found to be associated with a reduced number of apoptotic cardiomyocytes and DNA ladders compared to corresponding control hearts (Figs. 7 and 8).

6.5 Nitric oxide: a double-edged sword

By definition, NO is a free radical because one atom of nitrogen combines with one atom of oxygen to produce NO with an unpaired electron. Unlike highly detrimental reactive oxygen species, such as hydroxyl radical, $OH\cdot$ which attacks a large number of biomolecules, NO can only react with a small range of compounds. Compared to $OH\cdot$, it is virtually harmless. Nevertheless, NO can rapidly react at near diffusion-limited rate $(6.7 \times 10^9 \ M^{-1}s^{-1})$ with superoxide anion (O_2^-) to form highly reactive peroxynitrite radical $(ONOO^-)$ which is subsequently protonated to form $OH\cdot$ according to the following scheme:

$$NO \cdot + O_2^- \quad \longrightarrow ONOO^- \tag{1}$$
$$ONOO- + H^+ \quad \longrightarrow ONOOH \tag{2}$$
$$ONOOH \quad \longrightarrow OH \cdot + NO_2 \tag{3}$$

Although this scheme occurs in in vitro system, there is little evidence that such a system can occur in a physiological system. To the contrary, $ONOO^-$ radical should preferably react with -SH group and ascorbate that are present in most of the biological systems including the heart. In this regard, NO can be considered as an antioxidant. In addition, the affinity of NO towards O_2^- is greater than that of SOD for O_2^-. In fact, NO may compete with SOD for O_2^-, thereby removing O_2^- and preserving superoxide dismutase (SOD), further supporting its antioxidant role.

Several studies from this laboratory demonstrated that in ischemic reperfused myocardium, NO functions more as an antioxidant than as prooxidant [97–100]. The antioxidant activity of NO· may be realized through the reduction of reactive oxygen species produced by myoglobin (Mb) in the presence of H_2O_2 and organic hydroperoxide. In particular, our in vitro study has demonstrated that oxoferrylmyoglobin and related free radical species formed from metmyoglobin (metMb) and tertbutyl hydroperoxide (t-BuOOH) can be directly reduced by NO· to ferric metMb. As a result of this, NO· can protect against oxidative damage, produced by oxoferrylmyoglobin (oxoferryl Mb), as evident by the ability of NO· to inhibit oxoferrylMb radical-catalyzed oxidation of *cis*-parinaric acid. This effect of NO· is likely to contribute to protect against ischemia reperfusion injury of the heart where high concentrations of Mb and peroxidation products (viz., lipid hydroperoxides) set the stage for the enhancement of oxidative damage through the formation of oxoferryl-Mb.

Myoglobin (Mb) is the major heme-containing protein of cardiomyocytes that is involved in the intracellular transport and storage of molecular oxygen. Under conditions of oxidative stress in the heart, such as during ischemia and reperfusion, the potentially damaging role of Mb has been proposed to be associated with its ability to form a potent oxidant, oxoferrylMb, through the interactions with H_2O_2 or lipid peroxidation products (e.g., lipid hydroperoxides) [101]. In particular oxoferrylMb has been implicated to be one of the important pathogenetic mechanisms of ischemia/reperfusion-induced oxidative injury to the heart [102]. The results of our experiments demonstrate that NO· may counteract the damaging effect of oxoferryl-Mb. NO can act directly as a reductant to quench oxoferrylMb-derived free radical species and protect the heart against oxoferrylMb-induced peroxidations similar to ischemia reperfusion scenario.

The chemical reactions responsible for the biological activities of NO· appear to be its coordinate covalent binding to Fe and Cu in metalloproteins and its covalent modification of sulfhydryl groups in proteins. In biological systems such as during myocardial ischemia and reperfusion, NO· is likely to undergo numerous redox reactions, and simultaneously acts as either a weak oxidizing agent or a potent reducing agent. As discussed earlier, one of the most important reactions of NO· is its interaction with superoxide to form peroxynitrite (-OONO), which can decompose to yield highly reactive OH. radical. The reaction is considered to be responsible for the oxidative damage associated with NO. On the other hand, strong radical scavenging effects of NO· towards peroxyl radicals and OH· radicals, as well as towards oxoferryl-hemoproteins, as shown in the abovementioned study, strongly supports the notion that NO acts as an antioxidant rather than a prooxidant (Fig. 9). Indeed our results have demonstrated decreased oxidative stress by NO as evident in the reduced MDA formation.

6.6 Stunning

Considerable evidence suggests that myocardial stunning is a manifestation of reperfusion injury. By definition, stunning is a phenomenon associated with the reperfusion of myocardium after a brief, reversible ischemia. It is characterized by the prolonged depression of contractile functions in conjunction with a variety of ultrastructural, metabolic and electrophysiological disturbances [103]. Recent studies have demonstrated that myocardial stunning can be attenuated by antioxidants such as SOD, catalase, N-(2-mercaptopropionyl)-glycine (MPG), and dimethyl thiourea (DMTU) suggesting that oxygen-derived free radicals may play a role in the pathogenesis of stunning [104,105].

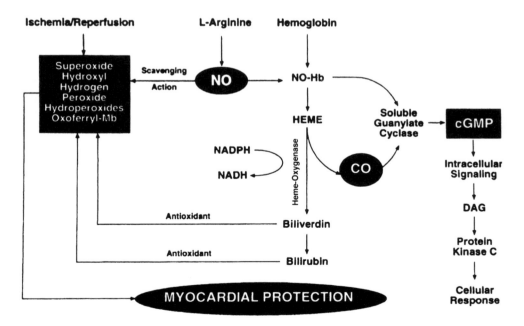

Fig. 9. Proposed mechanism of NO action in heart. (Reproduced with permission from Circulation 1996;94(2):398–406.)

More recently, SOD plus catalase were also shown to significantly attenuate the stunning in consious, unsedated dogs [106]. In this study, consious unsedated dogs undergoing a 15-min coronary occlusion were randomized to an intravenous infusion of either saline or SOD plus catalase. Despite the fact that plasma levels of SOD and catalase declined rapidly after reperfusion, postischemic wall thickening was significantly greater in treated, compared with saline-treated, control dogs throughout the first 6 h of reflow.

Generation of free radicals in the stunned myocardium has been demonstrated by using spin traps such as α-phenyl-*N*-tert-butyl nitrone (PBN) [107]. Conscious dogs undergoing a 15 min coronary occlusion were given PBN and the local coronary venous plasma was analyzed by electron paramagnetic resonance spectroscopy (ESR). In this study the authors observed a prolonged myocardial release of PBN radical adducts, which exhibited a burst in the initial minutes of reflow peaking at 3 min. Computer simulation revealed the presence of at least two PBN adducts, both consistent with the trapping of secondary carbon-centered radicals. A portion of the ESR signals was also due to α-tocopheroxyl radicals.

Among the large variety of oxygen-derived free radical species, OH· is believed to be the major reactive oxygen species that is responsible for the myocardial stunning. This receives further support from the observation that the presence of OH· has been demonstrated in stunned myocardium [108] and that antioxidant therapy inhibits OH· production, simultaneously enhancing the recovery of contractility. For example, SOD plus catalase have been shown to improve the regional coronary blood and left ventricular functions during stunning [109]. Phenylalanine, which reacts with OH· to form hydroxylated ortho, meta and paratyrosines also improved the stunning-mediated contractile dysfunctions simultaneously scavenging OH· [108].

6.7 Arrhythmias

Life-threatening ventricular arrhythmias such as ventricular tachycardia (VT) or ventricular fibrillation (VF) may occur during the reperfusion of ischemic myocardium [109]. Clinical autopsy data from victims of VF have shown that acute coronary thrombosis or acute myocardial infarction occurs only in a few cases. In these instances, the cause of VF has been attributed to the reperfusion after coronary artery spasm or transient thrombotic coronary occlusion [110]. Experimental studies suggest that myocardial salvage after reperfusion might be limited by deleterious biochemical events occurring concomitantly. The precise identity of the factor(s) responsible for reperfusion-induced injury and arrhythmias remains to be resolved, but it is likely that several simultaneous interacting triggers are involved that include the generation of oxygen free radicals. This has provoked much interest, because a close relationship has been established between free radical formation and the incidence of reperfusion-induced arrhythmias. Such a correlation has been evidenced from at least three distinct observations:
1. Reperfusion of the ischemic myocardium potentiates the incidence of arrhyth-

mias, and free radical scavengers protect the heart against reperfusion arrhythmias.

2. Exposure of either myocardium or single myocytes to free radical species produces many features similar to ischemia/ reperfusion injury, and instantly causes arrhythmias and electro physiological alterations.

3. Electrically fibrillating hearts can induce free radical formation even in the absence of myocardial ischemia.

In an early study of the effect of coronary occlusion on myocardial contraction in dogs, the authors serendipitously noted an event that was unrelated to their primary investigation, but is now generally heralded as the first description of reperfusion arrhythmias [111]. These investigators observed that in several experiments ventricular fibrillation occurred either before or just after the release of the clamp. Many subsequent studies have confirmed that arrhythmias are indeed associated with myocardial reperfusion, the severity of arrhythmias ranging from ventricular premature beats to ventricular fibrillation, both in experimental animals and human subjects [112]. The mechanism(s) of reperfusion-induced arrhythmias is controversial and unsettled, but the three most important hypotheses explaining the cellular events involved in reperfusion arrhythmias are intracellular calcium overloading, loss of sarcolemmal phospholipids and free radical generation. Numerous studies indicate that elimination of free radicals by free radical scavengers can ameliorate myocardial ischemia/reperfusion injury. For instance, scavengers of oxygen free radicals, superoxide dismutase (SOD) and catalase, deferoxamine, dimethyl thiourea, etc., can virtually eliminate free radicals, simultaneously salvaging the ischemic hearts from the reperfusion injury. Bernier and his co-workers studied the effects of six agents known to inhibit or scavenge the oxygen free radical formation in ischemic reperfused heart and found that all of these agents reduced the incidence of reperfusion-induced ventricular fibrillation [113]. Interestingly, many spin trapping agents, such as DMPO which removes free radicals by trapping, have also been found to reduce the incidence of reperfusion-induced arrhythmias.

In support of the free radical hypothesis, a number of electrophysiologic studies with free radical generating systems have shown that reactive oxygen species can induce changes in membrane action, potential characteristics that would be associated with an enhanced vulnerability to arrhythmias. Recently, Hearse and his colleagues have addressed the issue of the rapidity with which oxidant stress can cause electrophysiologic alterations [114]. They have achieved this by exploiting the photodynamic properties of rose bengal. When hearts were irradiated with green light, rose bengal was excited to a high energy state, which in the presence of molecular oxygen led to the generation of singlet oxygen and superoxide anion. Through the development of a perfusion chamber surrounded by a fiber optic cable, it was possible to photosensitize rose bengal in situ, and study the dose and light dependency of the electrocardiographic changes of bursts of oxidant stress under aerobic conditions. Their studies have demonstrated extremely rapid electrocardiographic changes which lead to severe arrhythmias. In another related study, Bernier et al. noted that the addition of a free radical generating system to the perfusion fluid markedly increased the incidence of reperfusion arrhythmias [113].

Several recent reports from our laboratory indicated that the generation of oxygen free radicals occur only in the fibrillating hearts and not in the nonfibrillating hearts [115]. Our conclusion was based on the direct measurement of the free radical generation using both ESR and HPLC methods. This observation led us to speculate that the formation of oxygen free radicals might be seen in the nonischemic electrically fibrillating heart. Consequently, we developed a model to examine this phenomenon. Figure 10 shows, under aerobic perfusion, the formation of oxygen free radicals was not observed (A), but after 1 min of pacing-induced VF a prominant ESR spectrum using 5,5-dimethyl-pyrroline-*N*-oxide (DMPO) as spin trap, was detected consisting of a 1:2:2:1 quartet (B). The maximum signal intensity was observed at 3 min of pacing-induced ventricular fibrillation (C), followed by a gradual decline over the next few minutes (D,E). This time course of free radical generation in electrically fibrillated hearts was similar to that found in fibrillating hearts upon reperfusion (Fig. 10B). A moderate elevation in end-diastolic pressure during the postfibrillating period might be a marker for the pacing-induced subendocardial ischemia although sig-

A   B

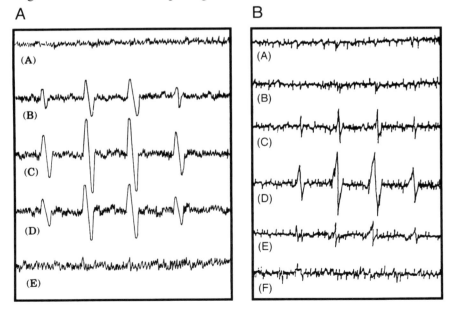

Fig. 10. Representative spectra of free radical formation in electrically fibrillated hearts (**A**). The heart was electrically fibrillated (20 Hz, 1200 beats/min) and oxygen radical formation was recorded using ESR spectroscopy before fibrillation (A), and after 1 min (B), 3 min (C), 5 min (D), and 10 min (E) of fibrillation, respectively. Representative spectra (**B**) of free radical formation in ischemic/reperfused hearts. Oxygen radical formation was measured using DMPO as a spin trap before ischemia (A), after 30 s (B), 1 min (C), 3 min (D), 5 min (E), and 10 min (F) of reperfusion in fibrillating hearts.

nificant changes were not observed in coronary flow rates either during the fibrillation or postfibrillating period. The results of our study suggest that this moderate elevation in end-diastolic pressure is not enough to produce oxygen free radicals at a detectable level in the effluents of hearts. Therefore, it seems reasonable to speculate that ventricular fibrillation is a necessary condition along with ischemia/reperfusion injury for free radical production. The discrimination between fibrillating and nonfibrillating hearts seems to be an absolute requirement in order to correlate the incidence of ventricular fibrillation and free radical generation in the postischemic hearts, and should be considered when making therapeutic interventions and risk assessments in this setting. The lack of this consideration might be responsible for the relatively high variability of the results obtained from different laboratories, and the controversy about the importance of free radicals in reperfusion injury and reperfusion arrhythmias.

7   AGING

The fact that oxygen free radicals are also implicated in the aging process, and that neonatal hearts are more susceptible to cellular injury compared to adult hearts, prompted many investigators to examine the antioxidant reserve of the neonates. For example, earlier studies demonstrated that in porcine myocardium, major antioxidant enzymes, SOD, catalase, GSH peroxidase and GSH reductase increase up to 8–10 days after birth [116,117]. SOD activity was found to be higher in a 3-month-old rat heart compared to that of an 18-month-old heart [118]. GSH level of an adult (12 month) rat heart was lower compared to that of a young (3 month) rat heart [119]. A unique age-specific myocardial lipid peroxidation expressed in terms of malonaldehyde formation occurred after incubation of neonatal and adult pig heart homogenates in the absence of any added factors [116]. Very little malonaldehyde release was noticed in the 0- to 2-day-old age group, while considerably higher activity was found in the 8- to 10-day old animals, the 2-month-old pig heart formed very little malonaldehyde. Myocardial injury from lipid peroxidation was highest in the 0- to 2-day-old age group, as evident in the release of oxidized glutathione, lactate dehydrogenase and creatine kinase. Release of glutathione, lactate dehydrogenase and creatine kinase decreased with age and was minimal in the adult group. Increasing evidence thus, suggest a link between the occurrence of cardiovascular diseases and the aging process with the development of oxidative stress [120].

Recently, the developmental profiles of myocardial antioxidant enzymes during neonatal growth was examined in rabbits of five different age groups; newborn, 7-, 14-, 35- and 45-day-old neonates [121]. The activities of five major antioxidant enzymes, superoxide dismutase (SOD), catalase, glutathione (GSH) peroxidase, GSH reductase, and glucose-6-phosphate dehydrogenase (G-6-P dehydrogenase), were enhanced during early neonatal growth of up to 14 days, and then with the exception of SOD and catalase, the enzyme activities declined to the baseline levels (Table 4).

Table 4. Activities of antioxidative enzymes as a function of neonatal age.

Antioxidative enzymes (n = 8) (units/mg protein)	Neonatal age (days)									
	0		7		14		35		49	
	LV	RV	LV	RV	LV	RV	LV	RV	LV	RV
G-6-P dehydrogenase	4.65	3.32	7.92*	3.54	20.20*	11.20	3.60	3.50	5.30	4.00
GSH reductase	18.8	19.6	24.4	26.0	99.6	92.0	42.0*	28.3	40.0	32.6
GSH peroxidase	85.4	106.0	113.0	153.0	232.0	215.0	132.0	83.9	109.0	101.0
Catalase	10.0	11.3	19.1	15.7	127.0*	88.4	98.0*	72.0	80.3*	63.2
SOD	13.7	11.7	17.4	15.7	27.2	31.4	30.1	30.7	20.7	24.9

*$p < 0.05$ compared to RV.

When these enzyme activities were compared between the left ventricle (LV) and the right ventricle (RV), similar developmental profiles were observed between LV and RV; except that catalase (for a 14- and 35-day old rabbit), GSH-peroxidase (for a 35-day-old rabbit), and glucose-6-P dehydrogenase (for a 7- and 14-day-old rabbit) activities were higher in LV compared to those in RV. The GSH content of the heart was also measured and did not vary between LV and RV, but increased up to 14 days after birth and then progressively dropped to the baseline values. These results indicate that newborn rabbit hearts are equipped with adequate antioxidant enzymes, which undergo significant developmental changes during the initial phase of neonatal growth.

The findings of this study are also clinically relevant. Recent studies demonstrated that adults are more susceptible to the ischemic injury than neonates. In another study, isolated neonatal pig hearts from two different age groups, 0—2 days old (newborn) and 7—9 days old (week-old), were subjected to 60 min of normothermic global ischemia followed by 60 min of reperfusion (122). Although myocardial ischemia reduced SOD, catalase and glutathione peroxidase activities in both age groups, SOD and catalase activities remained significantly lower in the newborn pig hearts during ischemia and reperfusion. Oxidized glutathione released from the neonatal pig hearts was at minimum levels before ischemia, but it increased 10-fold at the onset of reperfusion and was significantly higher in the newborn heart, indicating greater oxidative stress in born hearts compared with that in the week-old heart. Newborn hearts appear to be more susceptible to the ischemia/reperfusion injury as evident in the increased release of creatine kinase and decreased content of high energy phosphate compounds as compared to those in week old hearts. The decreased susceptibility of a week old heart to ischemia/reperfusion injury may be explained from the presence of increased levels of antioxidant enzymes in these hearts.

In summary, the evidence present in the literature indicate that glutathione redox cycle of heart undergoes significant alterations after birth. Although a large number of data is available regarding the fate of glutathione and antioxidant enzymes during adult and old ages, only a limited number of reports are available in the literature regarding the regulation of these antioxidants during early neonatal life. It appears that major antioxidant enzymes, as well as glutathione content are enhanced after birth, reaching the maximal level between the age of 14—21 days, and then drop gradually and progressively to baseline or below baseline levels which are maintained during further growth and development. It is tempting to speculate that after coming out of the womb where relatively hypoxic meliu is maintained, the newborns are likely to be subjected to oxidative stress. Such oxidative stress may be instrumental for the stimulation of glutathione and the enzymes of glutathione redox cycle because oxidative stress has been found to stimulate the antioxidants/antioxidant enzymes [123]. Such increased antioxidants may be necessary for the survival of the newborn hearts because of the exposure of the newborn hearts to increased amounts of potentially harmful toxic oxygen metabolites such as superoxide anions, hydroxyl radicals, etc.

8   STRESS

A variety of stressful conditions, such as exhaustive endurance exercise can lead to an increased metabolism and induce ischemic episodes in the heart, simultaneously developing oxidative stress. A recent study has demonstrated that daily exhaustive exercise of rats for a two month period increased the presence of reactive oxygen species in heart, and dietary supplementation of vitamin E reduced the amount of oxy radicals (124) supporting the previous finding that strenuous physical exercise leads to the development of oxidative stress (125, 126). Exhaustive exercise at submaximal workload in rats increased the free radical production as determined by ESR spectroscopy. In this study exercise also resulted in the decreased mitochondrial respiratory control and increased level of lipid peroxidation. However, prolonged exercise, possibly by way of adaptation, may stimulate the antioxidant reserve that combats free radical damage [127,128]. Another related study, on the other hand, showed that myocardial dysfunctions resulting from exercise were not modulated by treating the dogs with SOD plus catalase [129].

Several mechanisms may be considered for the development of oxidative stress in hearts during exercise. There is no doubt that exercise simulates ischemia in the heart because blood flow is directed towards the stressed muscle thus, reducing the blood supply to tissues that include the heart. After the exercise, the blood flow is resumed causing the simulation of the episode of ischemia/reperfusion. Secondly, the shearing forces resulting from strenuous exercise are likely to cause muscle damage thereby causing inflammatory response which may attract the PMNs at the site of injury. Thirdly, exercise can cause the release of catecholamines in blood which upon entry into the coronary circulation, may produce reactive oxygen species by autooxidation. Finally, the oxygen consumption in the exercising muscle can increase severalfold, which may enhance the production of oxygen radicals in the mitochondrial respiratory chain.

As mentioned earlier, antioxidants such as α-tocopherol can reduce the exercise-induced increase in free radical production [130]. In a study using human volunteers, exercise was found to enhance the amount of lipid peroxidation, as measured by exhaled pentane, which was suppressed by the daily supplementation of vitamin E to the volunteers [131]. Several related studies also demonstrated that exercise caused the development of oxidative stress that was reduced by antioxidants such as α-tocopherol [132–134]. Several studies from our laboratory have demonstrated that stress induced by diverse environmental factors such as heat shock, oxidative stress and ischemia/reperfusion can adapt the heart to withstand subsequent stress insults. Such adaptation occurs through the upregulation of the myocardial defense system which includes antioxidants, antioxidant enzymes in the first line of defence (Fig. 11). Our studies also demonstrated that a variety of oxidative stress inducible genes are induced in response to stress and may constitute members of the defense system against subsequent stress insult (91).

9 INTERVENTIONAL/INTRAOPERATIVE CORRECTIVE MANIPULATIONS

9.1 Angioplasty

Percutaneous transluminal coronary angioplasty (PTCA) is an alternative to coronary artery bypass surgery in certain patients. After removal of the obstruc-

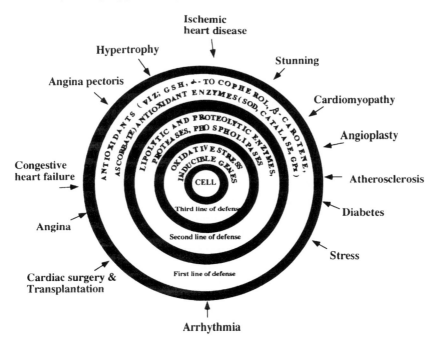

Fig. 11. Antioxidant defence against acute stress. (Reproduced with permission from J Molec Cell Cardiol 1995;27:181–193.)

tion in the infarct-related coronary artery, revascularization occurs, simulating the phenomenon of ischemia/reperfusion injury. A recent study has demonstrated that malonaldehyde and uric acid contents of vein-arterial plasma increased progressively up to 5 min following the PTCA [135], suggesting that the development of oxidative stress occurs in conjunction with angioplasty. In another related study, it was reported that treatment with SOD reduced the incidence of reperfusion arrhythmias following PTCA. Similar results were also reported by Yoshiharu et al. [136].

9.2 Cardiac surgery

Intraoperative myocardial preservation techniques have undergone substantial developmental changes during the past thirty years, resulting in a reduction of operative mortality and morbidity. While there has been significant improvement in intraoperative myocardial preservation techniques during the last decade, complications related to inadequate cardiac protection still exist, particularly in high-risk patients such as those undergoing repeat operations, emergent revascularization for acute myocardial infarcts, or failed percutaneous transluminal coronary angio-plasties (PTCA).

Cardiac surgery causes obligated ischemia to the heart, because the total cessation of coronary blood flow and a flaccid arrested heart, combined with a bloodless operative field is required for precise surgical repair. Therefore, it may be comprehensible that free radicals play a role in the pathogenesis of cellular injury associated with the revascularization of the arrested heart. The source of reactive oxygen species in cardiac surgery may be divided into two compartments: the blood borne and the cardiac-derived [137]. During open-heart surgical procedures, cardiopulmonary bypass per se result in the complement-mediated activation of PMNs [138] that become sequestered by the injured surface of the myocardium. This activation corresponds, among other events, to a production of oxygen free radicals. After it has become globally ischemic by the application of aortic cross-clamping, the myocardium itself is expected to become a source of free radicals at the time of its reoxygenation. Depletion of antioxidants has been reported after aortic cross-clamping associated with open heart surgery, with concomitant increase in plasma α-tocopherol, ascorbic acid and SH groups [61].

A large number of experimental studies have demonstrated the beneficial effects of free radical scavengerrs in reducing myocardial injury following cardioplegic arrest [58]. The effects of SOD and catalase as cardioplegic supplement were reported by Schlafer et al. [139]. The addition of exogenous SOD and catalase improved LV contractility after hypothermic cardioplegic arrest [58,140]. The role of supplementing SOD, catalase, deferoxamine and allopurinol separately was also examined in isolated heart preparations [141]. The benefical role of angiotensin-converting enzyme inhibitor, captopril, in conjunction with cardiac surgery have been attributed to its free radical scavenging properties [142] (Fig. 12). Antioxidants such as α-tocopherol have been shown to reduce lipid peroxidation during cardiopulmonary bypass in patients. Since the production of OH· is dependent on the catalization with a transition metal such as Fe^{3+}, chelation of iron as a modality to reduce the effects of reactive oxygen species has been well studied. For example, Ferreira et al. recently demonstrated the beneficial effects of supplementing cardioplegic solution with deferoxamine on reperfused human myocardium [143]. In this study, the authors demonstrated that although reperfusion of an arrested heart significantly increased the prevalence of grade 4 swelling (% of severely damaged mitochondria) in both control and

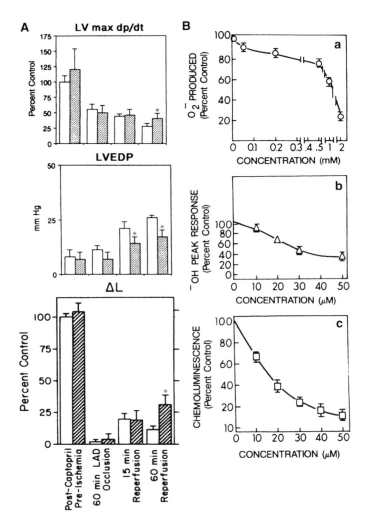

Fig. 12. Effects of captopril on the global (LVmax dp/dt and LVEDP) and regional (AL) functions during the reperfusion of arrested heart (**A**). The in vitro free radical scavenging function of captopril is shown in the right panel **B**. (The results are reproduced with permission from publisher [142].)

deferoxamine groups as compared with preischemic samples, deferoxamine significantly reduced the percentage of grade 4 damaged mitochondria (Table 5). Menasche et al. also showed that the addition of deferoxamine improved the LVmax dp/dt following 3 h of cardioplegic arrest in an isolated rat heart [137]. Illes et al. studied the effects of deferoxamine-blood cardioplegia on amelioration of postischemic stunning in dogs subject to short durations of LAD and circumflex occlusion followed by hypothermic cardioplegic arrest [144]. The regional stroke work was significantly improved by deferoxamine cardioplegia. Deferoxamine is approved for use in treating acute and chronic iron overload, and a great deal of clinical experience has demonstrated that it has minimal side effects thus, making it an attractive drug for potential therapy to reduce reperfusion injury in cardiac surgery.

9.3 Transplantation

An important aspect of a heart and lung transplantation is the sensitivity of these tissues to ischemia/reperfusion injury. Accordingly, much attention has been directed to protecting the tissues from the injury resulting from the reactive oxygen species. A recent study has demonstrated that allopurinol, a xanthine oxidase inhibitor and oxygen free radical scavenger, was able to better preserve a swine heart during transplantation [145]. In this study, the authors showed that the animals responding to allopurinol treatment with significantly reduced production of malonaldehyde following exposure of their red cells to tert-butyl hydroperoxide, demonstrated markedly superior respiratory functional status when compared with nonresponders. In another study, the same author demonstrated superior heart and lung functions through a combined treatment with allopurinol and deferoxamine. There is evidence that hypothermic perfusion of an isolated heart with an oxygenated solution may stimulate the production of reactive oxygen species [146]. These studies have demonstrated that a treatment with SOD plus catalase can provide significant myocardial protection when added to the cardioplegic solution.

Table 5. Grading of mitochondrial damage in control and deferoxamine treated hearts. (Data obtained from [143].)

	Mitochondrial grade (%)					No. of mitochondria checked
	0	1	2	3	4	
Control						
Preischemia	61 ± 7.7	16 ± 4.2	12 ± 3	6 ± 1	4.7 ± 1	205.7 ± 15
Reperfusion	38 ± 6	16 ± 2	15 ± 3	16 ± 4.3	14 ± 1.5	183.7 ± 14
Deferoxamine	60 ± 9.2	17 ± 2.5	16 ± 5.7	3 ± 1	4 ± 0.7	263.0 ± 39
Preischemia	53 ± 9	16 ± 4	18 ± 6.5	6 ± 2.3	7 ± 2	384.0 ± 62.8
Reperfusion						

10 SUMMARY

1. It should be clear from this review that free radicals and/or oxidative stress play a significant role in a large variety of cardiovascular diseases. Since the implication of oxygen free radicals in the pathogenesis of myocardial ischemia/reperfusion injury more than two decades ago, the role of these reactive oxygen species in many other cardiovascular diseases is becoming increasingly apparent. Under normal conditions there is a balance between the formation of prooxidants (oxygen free radicals) and the amount of antioxidants present. This steady-state condition is interrupted in pathophysiological conditions because of the excessive production of free radicals, or decrease in antioxidants or both.

2. Among the reactive oxygen species that are known to play a role in the cardiovascular diseases include; superoxide anion (O_2^-), hydroxyl radical (OH·), perhydroxy radical (HO_2·), alkoxy radical (RO·), peroxy radical (ROO·), singlet oxygen ($^1O_2$), as well as hydrogen peroxide (H_2O_2) and hydroperoxides (ROOH).

3. Nitric oxide which may have detrimental effects on mammalian cells, functions more as an antioxidant than as a prooxidant probably by virtue of its ability to remove oxygen free radicals that are being produced during the reperfusion of ischemic myocardium.

4. The antioxidant defense system consists of several antioxidants such as α-tocopherol, ascorbic acid, glutathione, β-carotene, flavanoids, uric acid and plasma proteins (viz., albumin, fatty acid binding protein, etc.,); and antioxidant enzymes such as SOD, catalase, GSH-peroxidase, GSH-reductase, etc. Myocardial cells are equipped with this antioxidant defense, which may also be termed as the antioxidant reserve of the heart. In addition, certain other enzymes such as oxidoreductases, hydrolases, GSH-transferases, etc., and NADPH supply are also the members of the antioxidant reserve.

5. Excessive production of reactive oxygen species and/ or reduction of antioxidant reserve have been implicated in the pathogenesis of cardiovascular diseases such as ischemic heart disease, arteriosclerosis, congestive heart failure, cardiomyopathy, hypertrophy, diabetes, arrhythmias, etc. Apart from the experimental studies mentioned in this review, epidemiological relationships also exist between oxidative stress and occurrance of cardiovascular diseases that include ischemic heart disease [147] and arteriosclerosis [148].

6. The regulation of antioxidant enzymes in the heart is under the genetic control. In both prokaryotic and eukaryotic systems, there is an upregulation of SOD and catalase mRNAs under oxidative stress; and this upregulation seems to be due to the adaptive modication of the enzyme activities. In a prokaryotic system, oxidative adaptation of S.typhimurium was associated with the induction of 30 new proteins, nine of which were under the positive control of the oxyR regulon for defenses against oxidative stress [149]. The oxyR is readily stimulated by oxidation. Recent studies indicate that adaptive modi-

fication of antioxidant enzymes can also occur in mammalian systems [123,150]. Recent studies from this laboratory identified several oxidative stress inducible genes in rat hearts [151]. In these studies, the adaptive stimulation of antioxidant enzymes has been found to be directly related to the protection of myocardial cells from the ischemia/reperfusion injury.

7. Prolonged reperfusion after even a brief period of ischemia causes apoptotic cardiomyocyte death associated with DNA laddering. Such apoptosis is under redox regulation because ebselen, a glutathione peroxide mimic, almost completely blocks apoptosis and DNA fragmentation.

8. Myocardial adaptation to ischemia, induced by cyclic episodes of brief periods of ischemia, each followed by another brief periods of reperfusion renders the heart tolerant to subsequent lethal ischemic reperfusion injury. Oxygen free radicals are believed to play a role in the ischemic adaptation of the heart. Like free radical scavengers, ischemic adaptation also reduces apoptotic cardiomyocyte death.

9. Although increased presence of reactive oxygen species or enhanced oxidative stress becomes obvious in the aforementioned cardiovascular diseases, in such cases, the increased oxidative stress may be secondary to the primary disease process. For example, inflammatory response during the disease process may cause the activation of phagocytes which in turn can produce, O_2^-, H_2O_2 and HOCl. Similarly, increased production of lipooxygenase and cyclooxygenase metabolites and/or the activation of cytokines linked with many cardiovascular diseases may produce reactive oxygen species. Destruction of heme proteins and subsequent release of iron may produce cytotoxic OH· radicals. Activation of phoslipases may cause a cascade of reactions potentiating the generation of oxygen free radicals. Irrespective of the mechanism(s), the generated oxygen species can initiate a new cascade of reactions, producing more cytotoxic agents, and cause further injury.

10. A number of cardiovascular diseases may be dealt with the antioxidant therapy. However, the mechanism(s) of free radical generation must be clearly understood before any potential antioxidant therapy, because the increased presence of oxidative stress may also be an epiphenomenon not directly linked with the actual disease process. On the other hand, it seems likely that antioxidant therapy may be beneficial in the management of many cardiovascular diseases.

11 ABBREVIATIONS

PMN:	polymorphonuclear leukocytes
MDA:	malonaldehyde
ACE:	angiotensin-converting enzyme
MDA-LM:	malonaldehyde-like material
LV:	left ventricle
GSH:	glutathione

SOD: superoxide dismutase
XO: xanthine oxidase
PRC: postrest contraction
LDL: low-density lipoprotein
HPLC: high-performance liquid chromatography
ESR: electron spin resonance
DMPO: dimethyl-pyrroline-N-oxide
TxB$_2$:   thromboxane B2
CK: creatine kinase
NO: nitric oxide
SH: thiol
ONOO$^-$:   peroxynitrite radical
Mb: myoglobin
MPG: N-(2-mercaptopropionyl)-glycine
DMTU: dimethyl-thiourea
PBN: phenyl-N-tert-butyl nitrone
VT: ventricular tachycardia
VF: ventricular fibrillation
GSH-Peroxidase:
                 glutathione peroxidase
GsH-Reductase:
                 gLutathione reductase
G-6-dehydrogenase:
                 glucose-6-phosphate dehydrogenase
RV: right ventricle

12 REFERENCES

1. Dzau VJ, Packer M, Lilly LS, Swartz SL et al. N Engl J Med 1984;310:345—352.
2. Graham DG, Tiffany SM, Bell WR, Gutknecht WF. Molec Pharmacol 1978;14:644—653.
3. Prasad K, Kalra J, Bharadwaj B. Br J Exp Pathol 1989;70:463—468.
4. Gervasi PC, Agrillo MR, Citti L, Danes R et al. Anticancer Res 1986;6:1231—1236.
5. Belch JJF, Bridges AB, Scott N, Chopra M. Br Heart J 1991;65:245—248.
6. Chidsey CA, Harrison DC, Braunwald E. N Engl J Med 1962;267:650—654.
7. Prasad K, Kalra J, Massey KL, Bharadwaj B. Angiology 1989;40:472—477.
8. Bagchi D, Iyengar J, Jones R, Stockwell P et al. Prostaglandins Leukotrients Essen Fat Acid 1989;38:145—150.
9. Sobotka PA, Brottman MD, Weitz Z, Birnbaum AJ et al. Free Radic Biol Med 1993;14: 643—647.
10. Singal PK, Kapur N, Dhillon KS, Beamish RE et al. Can J Physiol Pharmacol 1982;60: 1390—1397.
11. Haggaedal J, Jonsson L, Johansson G, Bjurrstron S et al. Acta Physiol Scand 1987;131: 447—452.
12. Edes I, Piros G, Forster T, Csanady M. Basic Res Cardiol 1987;82:551—556.
13. Tomlinson CW, Godin DV, Rabkin SW. Biochem Pharmacol 1985;34:4033—4041.
14. Myers CE, McGuire WP, Liss RH, Ifrim I et al. Science 1977;197:165—167.
15. Kobayashi A, Kaneko M, Fukuchi T, Yamazaki N. In: Nagano M, Takeda N, Dhalla NS (eds)

The Cardiomyopathic Heart. New York: Raven Press, 1994;165—173.

16. Sakanashi T, Sako S, Nozuhara A, Adachi K et al. Biochem Biophys Res Commun 1991;181: 145—150.
17. Fukuchi T, Kobayashi A, Kaneko M, Ichiyama A et al. Jpn J Heart 1991;32:655—666.
18. Jiang JP, Chen V, Downing SE. Am Heart J 1991;122:115—121.
19. Weglicki WB, Bloom S, Cassidy MM, Freedman AM et al. Am J Cardiovasc Pathol 1992;4: 210—215.
20. Cutilletta AF, Aumont MC, Nag AC, Zak R. J Molec Cell Cardiol 1975;7:767—780.
21. Dart CH, Holloszy JO. Circ Res 1969;25:245—253.
22. Bartsova D, Chvapil M, Korecky B, Poupa O et al. J Physiol (Lond) 1969;200:285—295.
23. Penney DG. In: Zak R (ed) Growth of the Heart in Health and Disease. New York: Raven Press, 1984;337—362.
24. Levitsky S. Ann Thorac Surg 1986;41:2—3.
25. Singal PK, Forbes M, Sperelakis N. Can J Physiol Pharmacol 1984;62:1239—1244.
26. Batist G, Mersereau W, Malashenko BA, Chiu RCJ. Circulation 1989;52(Suppl 3):10—13.
27. McCord JM. N Engl J Med 1985;312:159—163.
28. Hamrell BB, Alpert NR. Circ Res 1977;40:20—25.
29. Malaisse WJ, Malaisse-Lagae F, Sener A, Pipeleers DG. Proc Natl Acad Sci USA 1982;79: 927—930.
30. Rabinovitch A, Suarez WL, Thomas PD, Strynadka K et al. Diabetologica 1992;35:436—443.
31. Rabinovitch A, Suarez WL, Power RF. Life Sci 1992;51:1937—1943.
32. Sato Y, Hotta N, Sakamoto N, Matsuoka S et al. Biochem Med 1981;25:373—378.
33. Oberly L. Free Radic Biol Med 1988;5:113—124.
34. Karpen CW, Pritchard KA, Arnold JH, Cornell DG. Diabetes 1982;31:947—951.
35. Wohaieb SA, Godin DV. Diabetes 1987;36:1014—1018.
36. Imanaga I, Kamegawa Y. In: Nagano M, Takeda N, Dhalla NS (eds) The Cardiomyopathic Heart. New York: Raven Press, 1994;419—428.
37. Bouchard RA, Bose D. Am J Physiol 1991;260:H341—H354.
38. Parinandi NL, Thompson EW, Schmid HHO. Biochim Biophys Acta 1990;1047:63—69.
39. Tani M, Neely JR. Circ Res 1988;62:931—940.
40. Steinbrecher UP, Zhang H, Lougheed M. Free Radic Biol Med 1990;9:155—168.
41. Steinberg D. In: Shepherd J, Morgan HG, Packard CJ, Brownlie SM (eds) Atherosclerosis – Developments, Complications, and Treatment. Amsterdam: Elsevier, 1987;3—20.
42. Prasad K, Kalra J. Am Heart J 1993;125:958—973.
43. Haberland ME, Fong D, Cheng L. Science 1988;241:215—218.
44. Carew TE, Schwenke DC, Steinberg D. Proc Natl Acad Sci USA 1987;84:7725—7729.
45. Belch JJ, Chopra M, Hutchinson S, Lorimer R et al. Free Radic Biol Med 1989;6:375—378.
46. Morel DW, Hessler JR, Chisolm GM. J Lipid Res 1983;24:1070—1076.
47. Haberland ME, Fong D, Cheng L. Science 1989;241:215—218.
48. Sharma RC, Crawford DW, Kramsch DM, Sevanian A et al. Arterioscl Thromb 1992;12: 403—415.
49. Yla-Herttuala S, Palinski W, Rosenfeld ME, Parthasarathy S et al. J Clin Invest 1989;84:1086— 1095.
50. Steinbrecher UP, Parthasarathy S, Leake DS, Witztum JL et al. Proc Natl Acad Sci USA 1984;81:3883—3887.
51. White CR, Brock TA, Chang LY, Crapo J et al. Proc Natl Acad Sci USA 1994;91:1044—1048.
52. Gage JE, Hess OM, Murakami T, Ritter M et al. Circulation 1986;73:865—869.
53. Theroux P. Circulation 1987;75(Suppl 5):103—110.
54. Jayakumari N, Ambikakumari V, Balakrishnan KG, Iyer KS. Atherosclerosis 1992;94:183—190.
55. Das DK, Engelman RM. In: Das DK (ed) Pathophysiology of Reperfusion Injury. Florida: CRC Press, 1993;149—180.
56. Das DK, Maulik N. Meth Enzymol 1994;233C:601—610.

57. Tosaki A, Droy-Lefaix MT, Pali T, Das DK. Free Radic Biol Med 1993;14:361—370.
58. Otani H, Engelman RM, Rousou JA, Breyer RH et al. J Thorac Cardiovasc Surg 1986;91: 290—295.
59. Das DK, Engelman RM, Rousou JA, Breyer RH et al. Basic Res Cardiol 1986;81:155—166.
60. Tosaki A, Bagchi D, Pali T, Cordis GA et al. Biochem Pharmacol 1993;45:961—969.
61. Hearse DJ. In: Roberts AJ (ed) Pathophysiology of reperfusion injury. New York: Marcel Dekker, 1987;7—17.
62. Das DK, Cordis GA, Rao PS, Liu X et al. J Chromatogr A 1991;536:273—282.
63. Tosaki A, Haseloff RF, Hellegouarch A, Schoenheit K et al. Basic Res Cardiol 1992;87: 536—547.
64. Cordis GA, Maulik N, Bagchi D, Engelman RM et al. J Chromatogr A 1993;632:97—103.
65. Cordis GA, Bagchi D, Maulik N, Das DK. J Chromatogr A 1994;661:181—191.
66. Prasad R, Engelman RM, Clement R, Otani H et al. Can J Physiol Pharmacol 1988;66: 1518—1523.
67. Prasad MR, Engelman RM, Jones RM, Das DK. Biochem J 1989;263:731—736.
68. Das DK, Engelman RM. In: Das DK, Essman WB (eds) Oxygen Radicals: Systemic Events and Disease Processes. Basel: Karger, 1990;97—121.
69. Jolly SR, Kane WJ, Bailie MB, Abrams GD et al. Circ Res 1984;54:277—285.
70. Michael LH, Zhana Z, Hartley CJ, Bolli R et al. Circ Res 1990;66:1040—1044.
71. Tosaki A, Droy-Lefaix MT, Pali T, Das DK. Free Rad Biol Med 1993;14:361—370.
72. Otani H, Engelman RM, Rousou JA, Breyer RH et al. J Thorac Cardiovasc Surg 1986;91: 290—295.
73. Bilzer M, Lauterburg BH. J Hepatol 1991;13:84—89.
74. Massey KD, Burton KP. Am J Physiol 1989;256:H1192—1199.
75. Ferrari R, Curello S, Boffa GM, Condorelli E et al. Ann NY Acad Sci 1989;570:237—253.
76. Mickle DA, Li RK, Wiesel RD, Birnbaum PL et al. Ann Thorac Surg 1989;47:553—557.
77. Srimani BN, Engelman RM, Jones R, Das DK. Circ Res 1990;66:1535—1543.
78. Kimura Y, Iyengar J, Engelman RM, Das DK. J Cardiovasc Pharmacol 1990;16:992—999.
79. Das DK, Engelman RM, Clement R, Otani H et al. Biochem Biophys Res Commun 1987;148: 314—319.
80. van der Kraaij AMM, Mostert LJ, van Eljk HG, Koster JF. Circulation 1988;78:442—449.
81. Lesnefsky EJ, Repine JE, Horowitz LD. J Pharmacol Exp Ther 1990;253:1103—1109.
82. Vasilets LA, Mokh VP, Bogdanov GN, Guseva TI. Kardiologia 1987;27:83—87.
83. Ceconi C, Curello S, Cargnoni A, Boffa GM et al. Cardiovasc Sci 1990;1:191—198.
84. Boucher FR, Schatz CJ, Guez DM, deLeiris JG. Am J Hypertens 1992;5:22—25.
85. Giuseppe M, Campo F, Squadrito F, Ioculano M et al. Res Commun Chem Pathol Pharmacol 1992;76:287—303.
86. Rao PS, Liu X, Das DK, Weinstein GS et al. Ann Thorac Surg 1991;52:908—915.
87. Rudyk BI, Sabadyshin RA. Kardiologica 1991;31:52—54.
88. Tosaki A, Droy-Lefaix MT, Pali T, Das DK. Free Radic Biol Med 1993;14:361—370.
89. Kimura Y, Iyengar J, Subramanian R, Cordis GA et al. Basic Res Cardiol 1992;87:128—138.
90. Flack JE, Kimura Y, Engelman RM, Rousou JA et al. Circulation 1991;84(Suppl 3):369—374.
91. Das DK, Maulik N, Moraru II. J Molec Cell Cardiol 1995;27:181—193.
92. Das DK, Engelman RM, Kimura Y. Cardiovasc Res 1993;27:578—584.
93. Maulik N, Watanabe M, Engelman D, Engelman RM et al. Molec Cell Biochem 1995;144: 67—74.
94. Das DK, Maulik N, Engelman RM, P. Ray et al. Molec Cell Biochem (In press).
95. Maulik N, Yoshida T, Das DK. Free Radic Biol Med 1998;24:869—875.
96. Maulik N, Yoshida T, Engelman RM, Deaton D et al. Molec Cell Biochem (Focussed issue) (In press).
97. Maulik N, Engelman DT, Watanabe M, Engelman RM et al. Cardiovasc Res 1995;30:593—601.
98. Engelman DT, Watanabe M, Maulik N, Engelman RM et al. Surg Forum 1995;56:233—236.

99. Engelman DT, Watanabe M, Maulik N, Cordis GA et al. Ann Thorac Surg 1995;60:1275—1281.
100. Maulik N, Engelman D, Watanabe M, Engelman RM et al. Circulation 1996;94(Suppl 2): 398—406.
101. Galaris D, Cadenas E, Hochstein P. Arch Biochem Biophys 1989;273:497—504.
102. Hogg N, Rice-Evans C, Darley-Usmar V, Wilson MT et al. Arch Biochem Biophys 1994;314: 39—44.
103. Braunwald E, Kloner RA. Circulation 1982;66:1146—1149.
104. Przylenk K, Kloner RA. Circ Res 1986;58:148—156.
105. Bolli R, Zhu WX, Hartley CJ, Michael LH et al. Circulation 1987;76:458—468.
106. Triana JF, Li XY, Jamaluddin U, Thornby JI et al. Circ Res 1991;69:731—747.
107. Sun JZ, Kaur H, Halliwell B, Li XY et al. Circ Res 1993;73:534—549.
108. Li XY, McCay PB, Zughaib M, Jeroudi MO et al. J Clin Invest 1993;92:1025—1041.
109. Jeroudi MO, Triana FJ, Patel BS, Bolli R. Am J Physiol 1990;259:H889—H901.
110. Kaplinsky E, Ogawa S, Michelson EL, Dreifus LS. Circulation 1981;63:333—340.
111. Elharrar V, Zipes DP. Am J Physiol 1977;233:H329—H345.
112. Tennant R, Wiggers C. Am J Physiol 1935;112:351—362.
113. Ferdinandy P, Das DK, Tosaki A. J Molec Cell Cardiol 1993;25:683—692.
114. Bernier M, Hearse DJ, Manning AS. Circ Res 1986;58:331—340.
115. Hearse DJ, Tosaki A. J Cardiovasc Pharmacol 1987;9:641—650.
116. Tosaki A, Szerdahelyi P, Engelman RM, Das DK. J Pharmacol Exp Ther 1993;267:1045—1053.
117. Das DK, Flansaas D, Engelman RM, Rousou JA et al. Biol Neonate 1987;51:156—169.
118. Das DK, Engelman RM, Flansaas D, Otani H et al. Basic Res Cardiol 1987;82:36—50.
119. Sohal RS, Arnold LA, Sohal BH. Free Radic Biol Med 1990;10:495—500. Vega JA, Cavallotti C, Collier WL, Giuseppe DV et al. Mech Aging Devel 1992;64:37—48.
120. Harman D. The free radical theory of aging. In: Pryor WA (ed) Free Radicals in Biology, vol 6. New York: Academic Press, 1982;255—275.
121. Maulik N, Baker JE, Engelman RM, Das DK. Annals N.Y. Arad Sci 1996;793:439—448.
122. Otani H, Engelman RM, Rousou JA, Breyer RH et al. Circulation 1987;76(Suppl 5):161—167.
123. Maulik N, Engelman RM, Wei Z, Lu D et al. Circulation 1993;88(Part 2):387—394.
124. Kumar CT, Reddy VK, Prasad M, Thyagaraju K et al. Molec Cell Biochem 1992;111:109—115.
125. Davies KJA, Quintanilha T, Brooks GA, Packer L. Biochem Biophys Res Commun 1982;107: 1198—1205.
126. Dillard CJ, Litov RE, Savin WM, Dumelin EE et al. J Appl Physiol 1978;45:927—932.
127. Packer L. In: Benzi G, Packer L, Siliprandi (eds) Biochemical Aspects of Physical Exercise. Amsterdam: Elsevier, 1986;73—92.
128. Sumida S, Tanaka K, Kitao H, Nakadomo F. Int J Biochem 1989;21:835—838.
129. Kanter MM, Hamlin RL, Unverferth DV, Davies HW et al. J Appl Physiol 1985;59:1298—1303.
130. Singh VN. J Nutr 1992;122:760—765.
131. Jenkins RR. Sport Med 1988;5:156—170.
132. Ji LL. Med Sci Sports Exerc 1993;25:225—231.
133. De Scheerder IK, van de Kraay AMM, Lamers JMJ, Koster JF et al. Am J Cardiol 1991;69: 392—395.
134. Homans DC, Asinger R, Pavek T, Crampton M et al. Am J Physiol 1994;263:H392—H398.
135. Murohara Y, Yui Y, Hattori R, Kawai C. Am J Cardiol 1991;67:765—767.
136. Yoshiharu M, Yui Y, Hattori R, Kawai C. Am J Cardiol 1991;67:765—767.
137. Menasche P, Piwnica A. Ann Thorac Surg 1989;47:939—944.
138. Fantone JC, Ward PA. Am J Pathol 1982;107:397—402.
139. Shlafer M, Kane PF, Kirsh MM. J Thorac Cardiovasc Surg 1982;83:830—837.
140. Otani H, Engelman RM, Rousou JA, Breyer RH et al. J Molec Cell Cardiol 1986;18:953—961.
141. Myers CL, Weiss SJ, Kirsh MM, Shepard BM et al. J Thorac Cardiovasc Surg 1986;91:281—287.
142. Engelman RM, Rousou JA, Iyengar J, Das DK. Ann Thorac Surg 1991;52:918—926.
143. Ferreira R, Burgos M, Milei J, Llesuy S et al. J Thorac Cardiovasc Surg 1990;100:700—708.

144. Illes EW, Silverman NA, Krukenkamp IB, del Nido PJ et al. Circulation 1989;80(Suppl 3): 30—36.
145. Qayumi AK, Jamieson WRE, Godin DV, Lam S et al. J Invest Surg 1990;3:331—340.
146. Ytrehus K, Gunnes S, Myklebust R, Mjos CD. Cardiovasc Res 1987;21:492—499.
147. Gey KF, Puska P, Jordan P, Moser UK. Am J Clin Nutr 1991;53:3265—3345.
148. Gey KF. Bibl Nutr Dieta 1986;37:53—91.
149. Christman MF, Morgan RW, Jacobson FS, Ames BN. Cell 1985;41:753—762.
150. Lu D, Maulik N, Moraru II, Kreutzer DL et al. Am J Physiol 1993;33:C715—C722.
151. Maulik N, Moraru II, Das DK. Int J Toxicol Occ Env Health 1993;68.

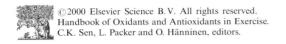
©2000 Elsevier Science B.V. All rights reserved.
Handbook of Oxidants and Antioxidants in Exercise.
C.K. Sen, L. Packer and O. Hänninen, editors.

Part IX • Chapter 25

Exercise-induced oxidative stress in the heart

Li Li Ji

The Biodynamics Laboratory, University of Wisconsin-Madison, 1141 Natatorium, 2000 Observatory Drive, Madison, WI 53706, USA. Tel.: +1-608-262-7250. Fax: +1-608-262-1656.
E-mail: ji@soemadison.wisc.edu

1 INTRODUCTION
2 FREE RADICAL PRODUCTION IN THE HEART
   2.1 Metabolic characteristics of the heart
   2.2 ROS production in the mitochondria
   2.3 Other sources of ROS generation
      2.3.1 Peroxisome
      2.3.2 Xanthine oxidase
      2.3.3 Catecholamine
      2.3.4 Neutrophils
3 MYOCARDIAL ANTIOXIDANT DEFENSE SYSTEMS
   3.1 Antioxidant enzymes
   3.2 Antioxidant vitamins
   3.3 Glutathione and other low-molecular weight antioxidants
4 EXERCISE-INDUCED MYOCARDIAL OXIDATIVE STRESS
   4.1 Does exercise increase ROS production in the heart
   4.2 Does exercise cause myocardial oxidative damage
5 FACTORS INFLUENCING HEART OXIDATIVE STRESS IN EXERCISE
   5.1 Antioxidant nutrients
   5.2 Drug metabolism
   5.3 Aging
6 SUMMARY
7 PERSPECTIVES
8 ACKNOWLEDGMENTS
9 ABBREVIATIONS
10 REFERENCES

1 INTRODUCTION

The role of reactive oxygen species (ROS) in heart toxicity and pathology can be dated back to the late 1920s when deficiency of the trace element selenium (Se) was discovered as a significant factor in causing microangiopathy (the Mulberry Disease) in livestock [1]. Epidemiological study of the relationship between Se and Keshan Disease in China is another example demonstrating that the heart is a vulnerable organ to oxidative damage when its antioxidant defense capacity is severely hampered due to nutritional and pathological disorders [2]. There is now increasing research and clinical evidence that the balance between ROS production and antioxidant defense in the heart is rather fragile. A slight tilt of this balance can cause significant oxidative stress and damage to the myocardium, as illustrated by heart ischemia-reperfusion (I-R) injury. In this chapter, the characteristics of ROS production and antioxidant defense in the heart will be outlined. Since the focus of this book is the relationship between oxygen toxicity and exercise, research evidence showing that strenuous physical exercise may lead to oxidative stress in the myocardium will be presented and critically reviewed. Further discussions will be directed to several factors influencing the susceptibility of the heart to oxidative damage.

2   FREE RADICAL PRODUCTION IN THE HEART

2.1 Metabolic characteristics of the heart

As a highly aerobic organ, the heart has one of the highest oxygen consumption rates among all body tissues. This metabolic characteristic has a significant impact on the rate of ROS generation. Table 1 contains the resting oxygen consumption rate in the heart compared to several major organs in the body, such as the kidney, brain, liver and skeletal muscle. The high oxygen consumption rate of the myocardium is due to the required energy output (ATP turnover) even in the resting condition. During maximal exercise in a human, the myocardial blood flow increases 4- to 5-fold as does the oxygen consumption [3]. To meet such metabolic demand the myocardium is equipped with efficient bioenergetic machinery, characterized by a high mitochondrial population and density. Mitochondrial protein content in the heart per g wet weight basis is 2- to 3-fold greater than in skeletal muscle [4]. The activities of enzymes involved in fatty acid metabolism, citric acid cycle and the electron transport chain (ETC) are also among the highest in the body. The rate of palmitate oxidation and the activities of citrate synthase (CS) and cytochrome c oxidase are 2- to 3-fold higher in the myocardium than in all major types of skeletal muscle [5].

The relationship between myocardial oxygen consumption, ROS generation and oxidative injury is elegantly demonstrated by the research of hyperthyroidism [6]. By supplying thyroxine (T4) in drinking water for 3 weeks, the investigators showed that a hyperthyroid rat hearts developed tachycardia, increased cyto-

Table 1. Oxygen consumption and ATP turnover rate in human tissues.

Tissue	O_2 Consumption (μmol/min/g wet wt)	Equivalent ATP Turnover (μmol/min/g wt)
Kidney	7.1	42.6
Heart	4.5	27.0
Brain	1.7	10.2
Liver	1.6	9.6
Skeletal Muscle (R)	0.08	0.5
Skeletal Muscle (E)	6.4	40.0

R: resting state; E: during marathon running [3].

chrome c oxidase activity and other signs of mitochondrial hypermetabolism. Associated with these changes were higher levels of the lipid peroxidation product malondialdehyde (MDA) and antioxidant enzyme activities. When the hyperthyroid animals were treated with β-blocking agents or α-tocopherol (vitamin E), these phenomena indicative of myocardial oxidative stress, were abolished or partially prevented.

2.2 ROS production in the mitochondria

The metabolic characteristics of heart influence the rate of ROS production in two ways:
1. the high mitochondrial volume and density provide increased sources for ROS production; and
2. the high oxygen flux in the mitochondria may favor a higher rate of electron leakage.

The steady state concentration of oxygen intermediates depends not only on the rate of production, but also the capacity of antioxidant systems. As will be discussed in the following section, the heart has an unfavorable ratio for the production and removal of ROS.

Mitochondria has long been recognized to be a major cellular site of ROS generation [7] and many early studies found that submitochondrial particles from the heart actively produce superoxide radicals ($O_2^{\bullet-}$). The work of Cadenas et al. [8] and Bovies et al. [9] showed that functional mitochondria have natural electron leakage due to the autoxidation of ubisemiquinone. The reduced ubiquinone serves as an electron donor for oxygen thus, forming $O_2^{\bullet-}$ under physiological conditions (Fig. 1). It was demonstrated that $O_2^{\bullet-}$ production involves NADH-ubiquinone reductase (complex I) and ubiquinone-cytochrome c reductase (complex III) of ETC, the transition sites from two- to one-electron transfer [8,10]. Furthermore, these findings point out a direct relationship between the steady state concentration of ubisemiquinone and the generation rate of $O_2^{\bullet-}$. With the catalysis of mitochondrial (Mn) superoxide dismutase (SOD), $O_2^{\bullet-}$ is readily reduced to H_2O_2. It is conceivable that as an organ, the heart is subjected to a higher rate of $O_2^{\bullet-}$ and H_2O_2 production due to its high mitochondrial protein content.

In isolated mitochondria, production rate of ROS depends primarily on the metabolic state [11]. It is interesting that H_2O_2 generation is greater in state 4 than in state 3 respiration. It is estimated that in rat or pigeon hearts, mitochondria: steady state production of H_2O_2 is $\sim 0.3-0.6$ nmol/min·mg^{-1} protein. This amount of H_2O_2 represents approximately 2% of the total oxygen consumption under the same conditions, or $\sim 3-6$ µmol/min·heart^{-1} in a 250 g human heart (assuming 40 mg heart mitochondrial protein/g wet weight). Furthermore, we can calculate using the above estimates that 4—8 mmol of H_2O_2 flushes through the heart everyday, equivalent to several bottles of 3% H_2O_2 solution sold in the drug store. Since intact mitochondria contain high levels of Mn

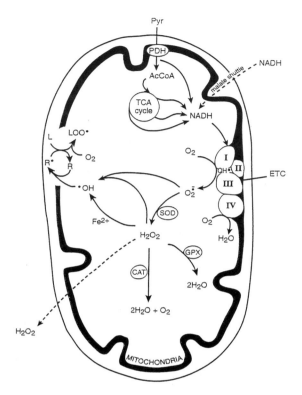

Fig. 1. Generation of reactive oxygen species (ROS) in the mitochondria. CAT: catalase; ETC: electron transport chain; GPX: glutathione peroxidase; LOO$^\bullet$: lipid peroxy radical; PDH: pyruvate dehydrogenase; QH$^\bullet$: semiquinone; R$^\bullet$: alkyl radical; SOD: superoxide dismutase. Reactions are not balanced stoichiometrically.

SOD which constantly removes $O_2^{\bullet-}$, submitochondrial particles washed of SOD were used to evaluate the rate of $O_2^{\bullet-}$ generation. In the presence of succinate and antimycin, $O_2^{\bullet-}$ production was measured to be 4—7 nmol/min·mg^{-1} protein, with an $O_2^{\bullet-}/H_2O_2$ ratio of 1.5:2.1 [9]. These values represent only the basal "leaks and spills" of ROS in the heart and they are likely to increase significantly when oxygen consumption increased due to metabolic demand.

2.3 Other sources of ROS generation

Although mitochondria are the major cellular site of ROS production, there are several other potential sources in the myocardial cell that can produce ROS. Some of them are active under normal physiological conditions, whereas others are activated only under special circumstances, such as I-R, certain pathogenic conditions and diseases, drug administration, and severe exercise.

2.3.1 Peroxisome

Peroxisomes are known to produce H_2O_2, but not $O_2^{\bullet-}$, under physiological conditions [11]. The major enzymes involved include D-amino acid oxidase, L-hydroxyacid oxidase, fatty acyl-CoA oxidase, and in nonprimates, urate oxidase. Although the liver is the primary organ where peroxisomal contribution to the overall H_2O_2 production is significant, other organs are also exposed to peroxisomal H_2O_2 generation [12]. In the heart, uric acid can be formed in significant amount from purine nucleotide degradation, particularly during ischemia, which may activate urate oxidase pathway. Peroxisomal oxidation of fatty acid may be a potentially important source of H_2O_2 production because fatty acids are the main energy substrate for the heart. Prolonged starvation has been shown to increase H_2O_2 generation mainly because of the increased fatty acid oxidation in peroxisomes [13]. Similar to starvation, fatty acids are the primary energy substrate for the myocardium and skeletal muscle during prolonged exercise. Thus, it would be interesting to evaluate the contribution of peroxisomes to the steady state production of H_2O_2 in this organ. Regardless of the route of production, most of the H_2O_2 produced in the peroxisomes are destroyed by catalase, a major antioxidant enzyme found in the peroxisomes and mitochondria. However, $10-40\%$ of H_2O_2 may diffuse to the cytosolic medium, where it may react with $O_2^{\bullet-}$ to form hydroxyl radicals ($^{\bullet}OH$) via the Haber-Weiss reaction, or with Fe^{+2} to form $^{\bullet}OH$ via the Fenton reaction [11].

2.3.2 Xanthine oxidase

Several cytosolic enzymes also contribute to the cellular generation of H_2O_2 in the heart. One that has received increasing attention in the past decade is xanthine oxidase (XO). This complex flavoprotein-containing enzyme is primarily located at the luminal surface of the endothelium. Under normal conditions, XO acts as a dehydrogenase transferring an electron from its substrate hypoxanthine (HX) to NAD^+. Since the concentration of HX in the resting heart is low (<0.2 µmol/g wet wt) [14,15], the enzyme has little significance in producing ROS. However, this pathway may become highly active during I-R of the myocardium. Details of this free radical generating system have been reviewed extensively [16,17], therefore, only a brief summary is given below (Fig. 2). In general, I-R results in two alterations in the myocardium which favor the formation of $O_2^{\bullet-}$ and H_2O_2. Firstly, ischemia causes degradation of adenine nucleotides (ATP, ADP and AMP), followed by an efflux of adenosine and inosine from myocytes to the interstitial space. The hydrolytic product of the latter two compounds, HX, is the substrate for XO. Secondly, I-R can convert XO from the dehydrogenase form to its oxidase form, either by a thio-disulfide redox mechanism, or by activating a Ca^{2+}-dependent protease [16,18,19]. XO then uses O_2 directly as an electron acceptor producing $O_2^{\bullet-}$ or H_2O_2. In addition to I-R, strenuous exercise has also been proposed to activate XO-catalyzed

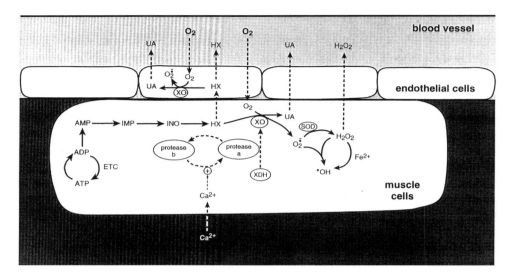

Fig. 2. The role of xanthine oxidase (XO) in free radical generation in the heart muscle and endothelial cells. ETC: electron transport chain; HX: hypoxanthine; UA: uric acid; XDH: xanthine dehydrogenase. Reactions are not balanced stoichiometrically.

reactions and generate ROS in skeletal muscle [20]. For example, large amount of HX and xanthine was found in the blood circulation after strenuous muscular contraction in men due to an insufficient supply and subsequent degradation of high-energy phosphates [21]. However, it needs to be pointed out that the presence of XO in the heart is highly species-specific. Rat, dog and pig hearts have active XO, whereas a rabbit heart apparently lacks XO activity. The current consensus supports an active role of XO in I-R induced myocardial damage in humans [17].

2.3.3 Catecholamine

The heart releases large amount of catecholamines from sympathetic nerve terminals under various stressful conditions, including ischemia [16], cold or heat exposure, and physical exercise [22]. Catecholamines are known to enhance myocardial metabolism via β-adrenergic receptor stimulation thereby increasing O_2 uptake. This can result in an increased mitochondrial ROS production by the mechanisms previously discussed. Administration of isoprenaline, a synthetic β-agonist that stimulates myocardial metabolism, has been reported to cause oxidative injury in Syrian hamsters [23]. On the other hand, β-adrenoceptor blocking agents reduce myocardial oxidative stress partly because the drugs decrease myocardial oxygen consumption [24]. Furthermore, autoxidation of epinephrine to adrenochrome is associated with the formation of $O_2^{\bullet-}$ [11]. This mechanism has been proposed to be a possible cause of I-R induced myocardial oxidative injury [16]. However, the quantitative significance of catecholamines as a source of ROS production remains unclear.

2.3.4 Neutrophils

Polymorphonuclear neutrophils (PMN) are blood-borne cells that play a critical role in defending organisms from viral and bacterial invasion. In response to initial tissue injury, whether caused by ROS or not, they migrate to the site of injury during the acute phase response and clear tissue debris by phagocytosis. The two primary factors PMN released are lysozymes and $O_2^{\bullet -}$ [25]. Lysozymes break down damaged tissue debris using proteases and peptidases, while $O_2^{\bullet -}$ is produced by a membrane-borne NADPH oxidase (Fig. 3). This is especially important when $O_2^{\bullet -}$ is involved in the initial oxidative injury since $O_2^{\bullet -}$ acti-

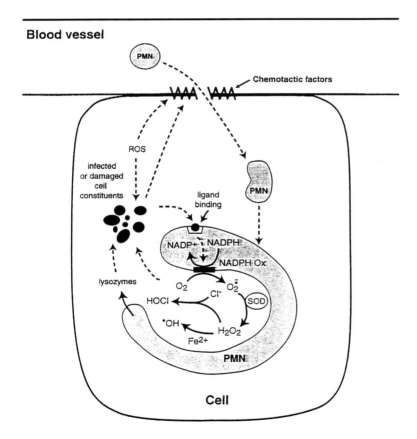

Fig. 3. The process of polymorphoneutrophil (PMN) infiltration and activation in the cell. NADPH Ox: NADPH oxidase; ROS: reactive oxygen species; SOD: superoxide dismutase. Reactions are not balanced stoichiometrically.

vates a chemotactic factor that attracts PMN [26]. While this is a desirable reaction in most circumstance, it may also provide a secondary source of ROS production causing further tissue injury. In the case of myocardial I-R injury, PMN have been identified as a potential damaging factor due to their infiltration into the endothelial cell region where initial oxidative attack is inflicted by ROS generated by other activated pathways, such as XO. It has been shown that anti-inflammatory drugs, such as ibuprofen and prostacycline, can independently reduce myocardial infarction size caused by I-R [16]. Use of antibodies to deplete PMN prior to I-R has also been found effective in preventing the heart from extensive oxidative injury [16]. These findings support the notion that PMN activation is probably an important etiologic mechanism for extended oxidative damage in the heart in certain pathological conditions.

3　MYOCARDIAL ANTIOXIDANT DEFENSE SYSTEMS

Postneonatal heart is a fixed postmitotic organ that normally has low rate of cell proliferation and a slow protein turnover. This genotypical characteristic suggests that the myocardium may have limited adaptability to acute and/or chronic oxidative stress, and to repair already-caused damage, therefore, antioxidant supplementation may deem critical under oxidative stress. However, recent literature indicates that the myocardium is still capable of upregulating its antioxidant enzyme systems.

3.1 Antioxidant enzymes

Heart is equipped with all the major antioxidant enzymes, i.e., SOD, catalase and glutathione peroxidase (GPX), as well as adequate levels of glutathione reductase (GR) and glutathione S-transferase. As an aerobic tissue, the myocardium has higher activities of all antioxidant enzymes compared with those in skeletal muscle (Table 2). However, the antioxidant enzyme activities are substantially lower in the heart than in the liver. Taking the high rate of oxygen consumption and

Table 2. Myocardial antioxidant enzyme activity compared to liver and skeletal muscle.

Tissue	SOD			GPX			CAT	GR	GST	CS
	Cu/Zn	Mn	Total	Cyto	Mito	Total				
Liver	500	50	14400	550	430	85	670	40.0	940.0	18
Myocardium	65	21	2610	150	70	17	39	1.3	2.1	72
Soleus	NA	NA	2050	NA	NA	12	37	1.3	1.1	40
Red vastus L.	21	8	1960	23	17	4	12	0.6	0.5	8

Activities for Cu/Zn and Mn SOD, unit/mg protein; SOD total, unit/g wet wt; cytosolic & mitochondrial GPX, nmol/min/mg protein; catalase, $K \times 10^{-2}$/g wet wt; unit for other enzymes, μmol/min/g wet wt. NA, not available [30,68,69].

ROS-producing potential into consideration, the capacity of the myocardium to remove ROS is rather limited. Using the activity of mitochondrial enzyme CS as an estimate of myocardial oxidative capacity, the ratios of the various antioxidant enzyme activities over that of CS may be indicative of the relative antioxidant potential of the tissue. As shown in Table 2, the activity ratios of SOD, catalase and GPX over CS are much lower in the heart than in either liver, soleus (an oxidative skeletal muscle with metabolic properties similar to those of the myocardium), or red vastus lateralis muscle. Therefore, when exposed to high levels of ROS the myocardium may not have sufficient reserve to cope with the increased oxidative stress thereby risking cell damage. This limitation of antioxidant enzymes in the heart has significant clinical implication as SOD and catalase are frequently supplemented during cardiac surgery in order to recover and enhance myocardial resistance to ROS due to I-R [16,17].

As a postmitotic tissue, the myocardium has a slow protein turnover that could have significant implication in antioxidant defense systems. In rats fed a Se-deficient diet, it takes longer for the myocardium to deplete its Se-dependent GPX activity, particularly in the mitochondria, as compared to other tissues such as liver and skeletal muscle [27]. It is not clear whether this was caused simply by a slower myocardial protein turnover or reflected an adaptive response in protection against potential oxidative stress due to Se deficiency. Endurance training, which is known to induce a number of mitochondrial oxidative and antioxidant enzymes in skeletal muscle, has limited effects on the heart [4,27,28]. SOD, GPX and catalase activities were reportedly decreased after an acute episode of hypoxia in the heart. This renders the myocardium more susceptible to subsequent ROS produced during reoxygenation [15,29]. Furthermore, several studies have shown that exercise training may even decrease antioxidant enzyme activities in the heart (see following sections).

However, recent research has proven it wrong to conclude that the heart cannot upregulate antioxidant enzyme defenses and, therefore, relies on exogenous antioxidants under oxidative stress. Our early work showed that Se-deficiency increased myocardial Mn SOD activity in the mitochondria, possibly as a compensation for the decreased GPX activity [27]. GSH depletion by the administration of buthionine sulfoximine (BSO) significantly increased myocardial SOD activity in mice [30]. Work by Cowan and co-workers [31] has demonstrated that hyperbaric oxygen induces myocardial GPX. Both GPX activity and mRNA levels were increased in cultured myocytes when PO_2 was elevated from 40 mmHg to 150 mmHg, suggesting a pretranslational activation of GPX gene expression [31]. It is interesting to note that chronic exposure of cultured myocytes to H_2O_2 enhanced catalase, but not SOD or GPX gene expression by a transcriptional mechanism [32]. Thus, it is clear that mild oxidative stress can induce myocardial antioxidant enzymes in a complex and specific manner.

Functional data are now available indicating that enhanced antioxidant enzyme defenses protect the heart from oxidants under various physiological and pathological conditions. Using isolated perfused hearts from transgenic mice, Das and co-workers have shown that overexpression of heart GPX protects against I-R injury [33]. In contrast, GPX knockout mice were shown to be more susceptible to I-R induced myocardial damage [34].

3.2 Antioxidant vitamins

Vitamin E (α-tocopherol) is the most important fat-soluble chain-breaking anti-oxidant in the body. Although it is incorporated into virtually all cell membrane bilayers, a major portion of the tissues vitamin E is concentrated in the inner mitochondrial membrane where the electron transport chain is located [35]. Vitamin E concentration in the cellular membrane is rather low, about one in several thousand molecules of phospholipid [36]. In the heart, vitamin E content was reported to be approximately 60–70 nmol/g wet weight, similar to those in the lung and liver, but 2- to 3-fold higher than in the skeletal muscle [35]. Despite the relatively low concentration, vitamin E levels in the tissue are relatively stable and difficult to deplete, particularly in the myocardium. This is because after vitamin E quenches an electron from a free radical species and is converted to a vitamin E radical, it can be reduced back to vitamin E by ascorbic acid (vitamin C), which is backed by a GSH redox system.

Vitamin E deficiency has not been consistently linked to cardiomyopathy, although some studies indicate that a higher incidence of cardiovascular disease is associated with lower levels of serum vitamin E [37]. For example, genetically cardiomyopathic Syrian hamsters (BIO 14.6) had significantly lower levels of vitamin E than normal values and the administration of vitamin E for ten days reversed myocardial lipid peroxidation and creatine kinase leakage shown in the defected animals [38]. Epidemiological and research evidence consistently supports the hypothesis that a higher vitamin E intake may prevent cardiovascular diseases by reducing the incidence of atherosclerosis, caused in part by the peroxidative modification of LDL [39]. However, randomized control trials of antioxidant (including vitamin E) supplementation failed to confirm this benefit in patients with coronary disease [40]. The mechanism by which vitamin E can attenuate atherosclerosis and prevent coronary heart disease remains to be established [41].

Ascorbic acid (vitamin C) is a water soluble antioxidant vitamin present in the cytosolic compartment of the cell and extracellular fluid. The spatial arrangement of vitamins E and C facilitates the efficient removal of free radicals generated in the membrane phase [42]. After donating an electron to the vitamin E radical, ascorbate is oxidized to a semidehydroascorbate (SDA) radical, a less reactive species. The latter goes through a disproportionation reaction to form dehydroascorbate. In the presence of GSH, the enzyme dehydroascorbate reductase catalyzes the regeneration of ascorbate. In animals, SDA radicals can also be directly converted to ascorbate by the enzyme SDA reductase, using NADH as the reducing power. Interestingly, the heart contains almost no activity of this enzyme [42].

3.3 Glutathione and other low-molecular weight antioxidants

The myocardium contains approximately $1-2$ mM of reduced glutathione (GSH), depending on the species. This concentration of GSH, among various organs, ranks only above that of skeletal muscle and is substantially lower than eye lens ($8-10$ mM), liver ($6-8$ mM), spleen ($4-5$ mM) and kidney ($3-4$ mM) [42]. The oxidative type of skeletal muscles, soleus, contains a higher level of GSH (~ 3 mM in rat) than the myocardium [43]. Nevertheless, GSH is regarded as the most important nonenzymatic antioxidant in the heart because of the limited antioxidant enzyme activity [44]. The general antioxidant properties of GSH are beyond the scope of this chapter [45,46], therefore, only a brief summary pertinent to the heart is provided.

GSH is a substrate for GPX which removes H_2O_2 and lipid peroxide. These two species are not free radicals but highly cytotoxic and have been proposed as the most dangerous species in the heart [29]. By accepting an electron from the peroxide, GSH is oxidized to glutathione disulfide (GSSG). GSSG can be reduced back to GSH by the flavin-containing enzyme GR. This important step ensures that cells are kept in the reduced environment that is essential for many enzymes and cofactors to function. The reducing power of the GR reaction comes from NADPH via the hexose monophosphate pathway or in some tissues is supplied by the isocitrate dehydrogenase catalyzed reaction. Together, these reactions make GSH a "recyclable" and "master" antioxidant in the cell. GSH is an efficient scavenger of $^{\bullet}OH$ and singlet oxygen [45]. In addition, GSH is involved in the recycling of vitamin E and SDA radicals [36]. When there is an excessive production of ROS that exceeds the recycling capacity of GR, GSSG levels will rise resulting in a decreased GSH/GSSG ratio. Therefore, the GSH/GSSG ratio is a sensitive index of the cellular redox status [47]. In order to maintain the GSH/GSSG ratio, cells are capable of exporting GSSG to alleviate oxidative stress [47].

Most of the de novo synthesis of GSH occurs in the liver, therefore, the myocardium, like many other tissues in the body, probably has to import GSH from the circulation via the γ-glutamyl cycle [48]. GSH is first cleaved by the membrane-bound enzyme γ-glutamyltranspeptidase (GGT) and its ingredient amino acid glutamate, cysteine and glycine are transported into the cell. GSH is synthesized by γ-glutamylcysteine synthetase (GCS) and GSH synthetase in a number of ATP-requiring steps. GCS is considered the rate-limiting step for GSH synthesis. It is interesting to note that the myocardium has lower activity of GGT compared to the kidney, liver and skeletal muscle in the dog and rat [49,50]. This may in part explain why the heart has a relatively low concentration of GSH. GGT activity was found to increase with endurance training in the skeletal muscle, but not in the myocardium, of beagle dogs [49]. Rigorous swim training has been found to increase GGT activity in the rat heart [51]. Furthermore, when GSH was depleted by BSO in a mouse heart, an acute bout of swimming increased heart GGT activity by 70% [30]. These findings indicate a cellular compensatory mechanism to enhance GSH import into the heart in face of a deteriorated GSH status during heavy exercise.

In addition to GSH, other low-molecular weight antioxidants such as dihydrolipoate, ubiquinone and uric acids have recently been recognized to have a "tocopherol-sparing effect" [52,53]. These compounds may facilitate the regeneration of ascorbate from the SDA radical, which is formed during the reduction of vitamin E radical [54]. For example, administration of α-lipoate (which is converted to dihydrolipoate in the cell) to rats attenuate hypoxic/reoxygenation and peroxidative damage in rat heart mitochondria [55].

4   EXERCISE-INDUCED MYOCARDIAL OXIDATIVE STRESS

Although an acute bout of strenuous exercise has been shown to cause oxidative cell injury in skeletal muscle and liver [56,57], there is no clear-cut evidence that a similar effect occurs in the myocardium as a result of exercise. Some early investigators reported ultrastructural damage and mitochondrial dysfunction in the heart following exhaustive exercise in rats [58,59], but ROS were not implicated in the observed damaging effects. Several later studies failed to confirm these findings and it was, therefore, concluded that there was no functional disorder in the myocardium due to metabolic stress [60]. For many years the well-known benefits of exercise training on cardiovascular function have probably overshadowed the fact that high intensity exercise can potentially be detrimental to the heart. In the past decade, the question as to whether or not the heart is susceptible to exercise-induced oxidative stress has been revisited. Available data now suggest that the heart is not devoid of the oxidative challenge imposed by acute or chronic exercise. Essential to resolving this controversy are the following two basic questions: 1) Does exercise increase ROS production in the heart? and 2) Is there evidence that the heart is oxidatively damaged by ROS?

4.1 Does exercise increase ROS production in the heart

Few studies have provided direct evidence that ROS production is increased in the heart during acute physical exertion that enhances myocardial work. Using electron paramagnetic resonance (EPR) spectroscopy, several laboratories have detected free radical signals indicative of semiquinone radicals (g = 2.004) and peroxyl radicals (g = $\parallel$ 2.030, g $\perp$ = 2.005) in rapidly frozen myocardium [15,61,62]. These free radical signals, however, were not found to increase significantly in the myocardia of acutely exercised rats (unpublished observation). However, Kumar et al. [63] showed that an acute bout of exhaustive endurance exercise increased the generation of free radical signals (R$^\bullet$) in the myocardium of female albino rats. Dietary supplementation of vitamin E for 60 days abolished the exercise-induced free radical production. Somani et al. [64] reported that the steady state concentration of ascorbic radicals significantly increased in rat myocardium pre-exposed to chronic exercise training. Using dichlorofluorescein

(DCFH) as a probe, we have recently investigated the effect of an acute bout of exhaustive exercise on ROS production in rat hearts and found no significant increase in the rate of ROS generation in either heart homogenate or isolated mitochondria [65]. These controversial findings may in part reflect a technical difficulty in detecting free radical species which could be rapidly converted to other ROS by free radical chain reaction and/or interact with intracellular scavengers [11]. Indeed, many scientists believe that $O_2^{\bullet-}$ does not increase its steady state concentration due to an acute oxidative burst, because of its short half-life (10^{-7} s) and the presence of SOD [11,42].

Despite the lack of direct evidence, there are sufficient "footprints" which indicate an enhanced ROS production as a result of strenuous myocardial work. The increases in the activities of myocardial SOD, GPX and catalase are often regarded as evidence that ROS production is increased during exercise, because within a wide range these enzymes are activated by high concentrations of their substrates [11,66]. Calderera et al. [67] reported that catalase activity in rat hearts, as well as in liver and skeletal muscle, was increased after an acute bout of exercise. However, later work by various investigators has not consistently supported this finding [68]. Ji et al. [69] found no appreciable alteration in the total activities of SOD, GPX or catalase in rat heart, after 1-h running on a treadmill, except for Cu-Zn SOD activity which was significantly increased. Furthermore, no significant exercise effect was observed in antioxidant enzyme activities in the heart of a rat immediately after an acute bout of maximal graded exercise and 30 min after recovery, except for Mn SOD activity (Cu-Zn SOD not measured) which increased [70]. However, Somani et al. [71] showed significant increases in Mn SOD, GPX and catalase in rat hearts after an acute bout of maximal exercise. Exercise intensity seems to be a key factor in revealing detectable effects of ROS on antioxidant enzymes in rodent hearts.

Another approach to evaluate whether the myocardium is exposed to excessive ROS is to investigate the response of antioxidant enzymes to chronic exercise stress. If there is an increase in ROS, then the myocardial antioxidant enzymes are expected to shown an adaptation, as occurs in the skeletal muscle [56,68]. There is considerable controversy in the literature regarding myocardial antioxidant enzyme response to training. Higuchi et al. [72] reported no alteration of myocardial antioxidant enzyme activity after training. This finding was consistent with the work of Ji et al. [27] in which rats consuming either a Se-adequate or deficient diet revealed no significant change in heart antioxidant enzymes after endurance training. Kihlstrom et al. [73,74] reported decreased activities of several antioxidant enzymes in rat hearts as a result of swimtraining. Venditti and Di Meo [75] also recently reported unchanged GPX and a decreased GR activities in rat hearts after 10 weeks swim training. Our two recent studies confirmed that neither moderate treadmill training [76] nor rigorous swim training [51] had an effect on myocardial antioxidant enzyme activities in the rat. In contrast to the above data, Kanter et al. [77] showed in an early study that although 9 weeks of swim training did not affect SOD, catalase or GPX activity in mouse hearts, all three enzymes were induced after 21 weeks. Powers et al. [78] reported an increase in SOD activity in the left ventricle of rat heart after training at various intensities and duration (Fig. 4). However, in the right ventricle only high intensity exercise with longer duration induced SOD. Activities of catalase and GPX did not change after training at any intensity or duration. Taken together, the above studies suggest that hearts working at high oxygen consumption rate are likely to be exposed to an increased ROS, particularly $O_2^{\bullet-}$. Further, normal levels of SOD may not be sufficient to remove increased $O_2^{\bullet-}$ production.

Exercise-induced ROS production has been shown to affect vitamin E reserve in the heart. Vitamin E concentration was found to decline in body tissues affected by endurance training [79]. More dramatic changes were observed when tissue vitamin E levels were expressed per unit of mitochondrial ubiquinone content [80]. Available data show that vitamin E content in the heart undergoes only a marginal decrease following treadmill training as compared to skeletal muscle [80,81]. Swim training was found to decrease vitamin E content in the endosubmyocardium of the left ventricle, but not the episubmyocardium or right ventricle, in rats [62]. The differences in the training response of vitamin E between heart and skeletal muscle may be explained by a higher myocardial vitamin E concentration (~ 70 nmol/g), which is next to the brown adipose tissue. Alternatively, vitamin E may be replenished more efficiently by other antioxidant systems, such as vitamin C and GSH, in the heart during exercise [54].

Exercise-induced ROS production may disturb myocardial GSH status. Leeuwenburgh et al. [30] showed that after an acute bout of exhaustive swimming GSH content in mouse hearts decreased from 0.9 to 0.7 µmol/g wet weight, whereas GSSG concentration also declined (Table 3). A significant amount of GSH ($\sim 20\%$) was probably oxidized to GSSG and exported out of the heart. This prudent exercise effect on myocardial GSH is also evident in a mouse previously depleted of GSH by BSO.

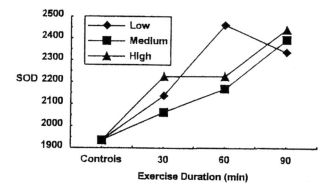

Fig. 4. Mean activity of SOD in left ventricular myocardium in control and trained groups at various intensity and duration. Enzyme activity, µmol of substrate/min^{-1}/100 mg.protein^{-1} [78].

Table 3. Heart glutathione status in response to exhaustive exercise in mice.

	N	GSH	GSSG	GSH/GSSG	GSH+GSSG
GSH-adequate					
Rest	8	0.9 ± 0.07	0.1 ± 0.01	8.8 ± 0.1	1.10 ± 0.09
Exercise	8	0.7 ± 0.03^a	0.08 ± 0.01^a	8.7 ± 0.5	0.87 ± 0.03^a
GSH-depleted					
Rest	8	0.09 ± 0.02^b	0.01 ± 0.002^b	12.1 ± 2.6	0.11 ± 0.02^b
Exercise	8	0.05 ± 0.004^a	0.004 ± 0.001^a	12.5 ± 1.7	0.06 ± 0.01^a

Values are mean $\pm$ SEM (μmol/g wet wt). [a]$p < 0.05$, Exercised vs. Rested; [b]$p < 0.05$, GSH-depleted vs. GSH-adequate [30].

4.2 Does exercise cause myocardial oxidative damage

Ultrastructural studies reveal that myocardia subjected to high levels of physical exercise exhibit some abnormalities, such as mitochondrial swelling, sarcotubular membrane disruption, fluid and/or ionic shifts, defects of Ca^{+2} transport, and occurrence of giant mitochondria [59,82—85]. It is difficult to determine whether these morphological alterations are caused by oxidative damage. There appears to be no functional alteration in the oxidative phosphorylation pathway of heart mitochondria following an acute bout of strenuous exercise [60]. Packer et al. [86] compared the oxidative capacity of isolated heart mitochondria from guinea pigs that had rest and those that had endurance exercise, it was that found that there was no significant difference between the two groups. Ji and Mitchell [70] showed that an acute bout of maximal graded exercise significantly increased heart mitochondrial state four respiration using either site one or site two substrates. Although state three respiration rates also increased, the increment was disproportional to that of state four, resulting in a decreased respiratory control index (RCI). These changes appeared similar to those observed in mitochondria isolated from skeletal muscle of rats exercised to exhaustion [77]. When the heart mitochondria were exposed to $O_2^{\bullet-}$ in vitro, the exercised and rested rats were not different in their susceptibility to $O_2^{\bullet-}$. However, it should be kept in mind that metabolic demand as indicated by heart rate and VO_2 do not increase in the rodent heart as much as in the human heart at a given workload, possibly because of the already high resting metabolic rate [87]. It seems that only very rigorous physical exertion may bring about oxidative stress in the rodent heart. For example, exhaustive exercise was shown to result in an increased cardiac lipid peroxidation along with augmented EPR signals in the rats [63]. Heart mitochondrial sarcoplasmic and endoplasmic latency was reportedly reduced in rats after swimming to exhaustion in a recent study [75]. Heart mitochondria isolated from rigorously swim-trained rats (6 h/day, 5 days/week for 6—7 weeks) showed decreased state three respiration and RCI using site one substrates [51]. After exposure to $O_2^{\bullet-}$ in vitro, state four and three respiration and RCI in trained animals exhibited greater reductions of respiratory function than the controls. Myocardial GSH content and GR activity were significantly decreased in trained rats [51]. It would be interesting to examine whether a human heart, which works at a greater workload during maximal physical exertion than rodent heart, is subjected to a higher level of oxidative stress.

5   FACTORS INFLUENCING HEART OXIDATIVE STRESS IN EXERCISE

While the previous sections have discussed ROS generation and oxidative stress during exercise in the normal heart, a number of physiological, pathological and nutritional factors can predispose the heart to increased levels of ROS and/or decreased antioxidant defenses. Age could also have an impact on the level of oxidative stress induced by exercise. Investigations of these factors may not only help us understand the mechanisms underlying an exercise-induced oxidative stress, but also provide potential therapeutic intervention against cell oxidative injury.

5.1 Antioxidant nutrients

Nutrition has an intimate impact on cellular antioxidant defense systems [53,88]. The effect of Se deficiency on the overall heart function has been well-recognized [89]. However, a causal relationship between Se deficiency and myocardial pathology has not been established. With adequate vitamin E in the diet, Se deficiency seems to be well tolerated by both sedentary and physically stressed experimental animals. Ji et al. [27] showed that rats fed a Se-deficient diet (< 0.01 ppm) and trained for 8 weeks did not display abnormal profiles in the heart in terms of lipid peroxidation and metabolic enzyme activities, whereas their heart mitochondrial and cytosolic GPX were reduced to 20 and 4%, respectively. Lang et al. [90] found that Se deficiency had no significant effect on endurance capacity in rats and did not exacerbate the exercise-induced GSSG level or loss of vitamin E in the plasma. However, when animals suffered from both Se and vitamin E deficiencies, the oxidative damage observed was more severe than deficiency of either antioxidant alone [91].

Vitamin E deficiency has been well documented to increase the susceptibility of skeletal muscle to exercise-induced lipid peroxidation and to decrease endurance time [35,57,92]. However, there is insufficient data to conclude whether normal physiological functions of the heart are impaired by vitamin E deficiency. Gohil et al. [35] reported that the myocardia of rats fed a vitamin E deficient diet displayed normal mitochondrial respiratory function using several electron donors, except for 2-oxoglutarate. They further demonstrated that an acute bout of exhaustive exercise had no significant effect on mitochondrial respiratory capacity in either vitamin E deficient or control rats. Tiidus [81], however, showed that rats fed a vitamin E-free diet for 8 and 16 weeks had increased lipid peroxidation in the heart as compared to rats fed the same diet but supplemented with 35 mg/kg vitamin E. An acute bout of exercise did not cause a significant increase in the thiobarbituric acid reactant substance (TBARS) in vitamin E-deficient rats at 8 weeks, but resulted in more than a 2-fold higher TBARS at 16 weeks. There have been numerous studies showing that vitamin E supplementation increases tissue resistance to oxidative stress, though insufficient data are available regarding its protection in the heart [92]. Scholz et al. [93] recently reported that a rat fed a high vitamin E diet showed a slower rate of heart mitochondrial lipid peroxidation under in vitro oxidative challenge. It is noteworthy that vitamin E supplementation may have a profound effect on plasma lipoprotein oxidative status, which directly affects cardiovascular health [94,95].

There is a paucity of data dealing with the effect of vitamin C deficiency on exercise-induced tissue oxidative damage in the heart. By reducing dietary vitamin C content to 10% of the normal values (0.2 g/kg), Packer et al. [86] demonstrated that the myocardial capacity of oxidize pyruvate, 2-oxoglutarate and succinate was significantly reduced in the vitamin C deficient guinea pigs than in the controls. Running time to exhaustion was also significantly shortened by vitamin C deficiency. Interestingly, a group of guinea pigs supplemented with twice as much as normal vitamin C in the diet also exhibited similar metabolic defects in the heart and early fatigue. Other tissues such as liver and skeletal muscle were not as susceptible as the heart. Compared with vitamin E, this study seems to indicate that vitamin C plays a critical role in defending against exercise-induced oxidative stress in the heart.

GSH deficiency is associated with a spectrum of physiological and biochemical disorders [45,46,48]. However, little is known about the consequence of GSH deficiency on exercise-induced oxidative stress in the heart. Leeuwenburgh et al. [30] have investigated the effect of GSH deficiency (BSO injection) on tissue GSH status, endurance capacity and antioxidant systems in mice subjected to an acute bout of exhaustive swimming. BSO treatment depleted the GSH and GSSG concentration in the mouse heart to 10% of the control values with no significant alteration in the GSH/GSSG ratio. Endurance performance was similar between GSH-depleted and adequate mice. In GSH-adequate mice, exhaustive swimming decreased GSH and GSSG by $\sim 20\%$ ($p < 0.05$) without altering the GSH/GSSG ratio. In GSH-depleted mice, swimming decreased GSH by 44% and GSSG by 60% (Table 3). However, the GSH:GSSG ratio was not altered and no enhanced lipid peroxidation was observed due to GSH deficiency.

5.2 Drug metabolism

Many drugs can produce free radicals in the process of being metabolized in the body [42]. Cigarette smoking, alcohol consumption, and environmental pollutants can also activate free radical generating mechanisms. The liver is the major organ to be exposed to the various sources of oxidants and to metabolize the toxins. However, it is well known that physical exercise can alter the pharmacokinetics (i.e., absorption, distribution and clearance) of a drug, thereby affecting its bioavailability and potency [96]. Hepatic blood flow decreases during exercise reducing the detoxification capacity of the liver, at least for the flow-limited drug [96]. This can theoretically increase the risk of other organs that have increased blood perfusion during exercise. Here the author intends to use Adriamycin (ADM, Doxorubicin) as an example.

ADM is a widely used anthracycline antitumor drug with a well-known side effect on the heart [42,97]. The possible mechanisms of ADM cardiotoxicity have been reviewed [98]. It has been shown in the bovine heart that ADM can accept an electron from the complex I (NADH reductase) of the mitochondrial ETC and be converted to an ADM free radical, and subsequently $O_2^{\bullet-}$ [99,100]. $O_2^{\bullet-}$ is then converted to H_2O_2 and $^{\bullet}OH$, which can act on the lipid membrane of the mitochondria and cause peroxidative damage. Heart is particularly sensitive to this damage because it has relatively low levels of antioxidant defense [100]. ADM is a flow-limited drug, therefore, an increase in blood perfusion to an organ would increase the unbound drug and hence the extraction of the drug from the blood. During maximal exercise in human, myocardial blood flow increases 3- to 4-fold above the resting levels, whereas the decreased hepatic blood flow reduces drug metabolism and clearance [96]. Thus, the interaction of ADM and exercise has raised concerns among some exercise physiologists [70,77,101].

Kanter et al. [77] investigated the effects of chronic ADM cardiotoxicity in mice undergoing swimming training. It was found that at a dose of 4 mg/kg body weight, 2 doses/week over 7 weeks, ADM inhibited the training-induced antioxidant enzyme adaptation in the blood, liver and myocardium. However, trained mice had a lesser degree of ultrastructural damage caused by ADM than the sedentary drug group. It was concluded that training alleviated some toxic effect caused by the drug because of the antioxidant enzyme adaptation.

The effects of ADM on the heart mitochondrial function were studied in rats that were exercised or rested [70]. 20% of the established cumulative toxic dose of ADM, 8 mg/kg was given within 24 h. The drug increased state four respiration, decreased RCI, and abolished an exercise-induced increase in state three respiration. However, heart mitochondria from ADM treated rats did not show enhanced susceptibility to exogenous oxidative challenge in either the rested or exercised group. The authors concluded that although ADM did not cause overwhelming myocardial damage, it might impair the ability of the heart mitochondria to produce sufficient ATP at high work loads. This conclusion seems to agree with several previous reports showing that ADM interferes with cardiovascular performance during physical exercise. For example, Langton et al. [101] showed that rabbits receiving ADM during a 8-week period of time suffered attenuated cardiac index and mean arterial pressure responses to exercise stimulus.

5.3 Aging

Aging influences both ROS production and cellular antioxidant defense systems in various organs and tissues, including the heart [53,66,68]. Therefore, aging is expected to alter the sensitivity of the myocardium to an exercise-induced oxidative stress. Nohl [102] has shown that the mitochondria in the heart from older rats produce more $O_2^{\bullet-}$ and H_2O_2 than those from the young rats. However, the rate of mitochondrial respiration does not increase with age in the heart [103]. The mechanism for an increased free radical production seems to be related to a defect of electron transfer in aging myocardium. Indeed, it was found that the ratios of ubiquinone, cytochrome b, and cytochrome c, respectively, over cytochrome aa_3 were increased in the older animals as compared to young ones [102]. This increased stoichiometry was proposed to facilitate the electron transfer out of sequence thereby producing $O_2^{\bullet-}$.

Age-related decrease of antioxidant enzyme activity can also put the senescent heart under oxidative stress. However, there is no clear consensus as to whether aging is associated with an increase or decrease of myocardial antioxidant capacity. Nohl et al. [104] showed that catalase and Se GPX activities were elevated in aged rat heart. Fiebig et al. [76] reported higher total activities of heart SOD, GPX, GR and GGT, as well as total GSH content in 26- vs. 4-month-old rats. Ji et al. [69] showed that Cu-Zn SOD, cytosolic GPX and catalase activities decreased in the aging heart, whereas Mn SOD and mitochondrial GPX increased. These differential antioxidant enzyme responses probably reflected an age adaptation to ROS production in the mitochondria. However, the antioxidant enzyme adaptation did not seem to prevent mitochondrial and tissue lipid peroxidation in the senescent heart [66,69,104]. So far, it is not clear whether the observed oxidative changes are directly related to the functional deterioration in aged heart such as excitation-contraction coupling, sarcoplasmic reticulum function, protein synthesis, and ATP generation [105].

To test the hypothesis that exercise-induced oxidative stress in the heart is exacerbated by aging, we have recently performed a study wherein young and old rats were subjected to an acute bout of treadmill running at similar relative workload (75% VO_2 max) and with similar duration (55 and 58 min) [65]. Myocardial ROS production measured by DCFH oxidation was increased by 25% ($p < 0.05$) in the aged heart, but only 11% ($p > 0.05$) in the young heart. Further, exercise increased heart MDA content in the old but not young rat. Thus, despite age adaptations of the antioxidant systems, aged hearts seem to produce more ROS and are more vulnerable to oxidative damage than young hearts at similar levels of metabolic stress.

6.0 SUMMARY

1. The heart is a highly aerobic organ characterized by a high density of mitochondria, a high rate of oxygen uptake, and a large energy turnover rate even at the resting state. These morphological and physiological properties favor a constant production of ROS as a byproduct of metabolism. During and shortly after maximal sustained myocardial work, ROS generation in the

heart is probably augmented due to an increased electron leakage from the respirator chain, activated xanthine oxidatase and enhanced catecholamine secretion. However, the heart possesses only moderate levels of antioxidant enzymes compared to other aerobic tissues, therefore, its ability to remove ROS is rather limited. The nonenzymatic antioxidants, i.e., antioxidant vitamins and GSH, may thus, be more important in the heart. The delicate balance between production and removal of ROS makes the heart vulnerable to oxidative stress.

2. There is both direct and indirect evidence that high intensity physical exercise increases ROS production in the heart. Intrinsic myocardial antioxidant systems seem to be capable of metabolizing most of these deleterious species, therefore, acute tissue oxidative damage due to exercise probably does not occur to normal healthy subjects. However, antioxidant reserves of vitamin E and GSH in the heart have been shown to deteriorate due to vigorous acute and chronic exercise. Furthermore, there is preliminary evidence that ROS may target specific cellular and subcellular components susceptible to oxidative injury, such as mitochondria. These areas require further investigations.

3. A number of physiological, pathological and nutritional factors are known to increase myocardial susceptibility to exercise-induced oxidative stress by either increasing ROS production, or weakening antioxidant defense, or both. Research concerning the interactions of antioxidant deficiency/supplementation, drug metabolism and aging with exercise can greatly enhance our understanding of the etiologic mechanism of oxidative stress in this vital organ.

7   PERSPECTIVES

Due to the importance of the heart, vast resources have been put into cardiovascular research over the years. Yet, our understanding on free radical-antioxidant balance during exercise in the heart is still quite limited. The following areas appear to need particular attention.

1. Although there is some evidence that ROS production is increase in the heart during exercise, data in this respect are sparse and sometime equivocal. We need to gain definitive information as to whether heavy exercise generates sufficient amount of ROS in the heart to overwhelm the intrinsic antioxidant defense system, and the cellular sources of the ROS.

2. As a postmitotic organ, the heart has demonstrated limited adaptive response to acute and chronic exercise. However, recent research shows that gene regulation in the myocardium is altered due to a variety of physiological, pathological and nutritional conditions. Whether exercise could modulate gene expression of antioxidant enzymes and other proteins related to antioxidant function is a research field that is still wide-open .

3. Increasing evidence points to an intimate relationship between the various cardiovascular diseases and oxidative injury. Exercise is a well-known preventive measure of cardiovascular diseases, but also produces some risk of oxida-

tive stress. This paradox requires further clarification using both epidemiological and experimental approaches. We need to consider the pros and cons of the various exercise modes, intensity and duration for different population to maximize the benefit while reducing the risks of exercise. This challenge has provided unlimited opportunity for future exercise physiologists and biochemists.

8 ACKNOWLEDGMENT

The author thanks the American Heart Association (AHA) National Center, AHA Illinois and Wisconsin Affiliates for supporting the research presented in the current chapter.

9 ABBREVIATIONS

ADM:	adriamycin
BSO:	buthionine sulfoximine
CS:	citrate synthase
DCFH:	dichlorofluorescein
EPR:	electron paramagnetic resonance
ETC:	electron transport chain
GCS:	γ-glutamylcysteine synthetase
GGT:	γ-glutamyltranspeptidase
GPX:	glutathione peroxidase
GR:	glutathione reductase
GSH:	glutathione
GSSG:	glutathione disulfide
HX:	hypoxanthine
I-R:	ischemia-reperfusion
MDA:	malondialdehyde
PMN:	polymorphonuclear neutrophil
RCI:	respiratory control index
ROS:	reactive oxygen species
SDA:	semidehydroascorbate
SOD:	superoxide dismutase
XO:	xanthine oxidase

10 REFERENCES

1. National Research Council. "Selenium: Its Biological Function." Washington DC: National Research Council, 1976;81–82.
2. Whanger PD. J Nutr 1989;119:1236–1239.
3. Newsholme EA, Leech AR. Biochemistry for the Medical Sciences. Chichester: John Wiley and Sons, 1983;144–146.
4. Ji LL, Stratman FW, Lardy HA. Biochem Pharmacol 1987;36:3411–3417.

5. Veerkamp JH. In: Busch FM, Jennekens GI, Scholte HR (eds) Mitochondria and Muscular Diseases. The Netherlands: Beetsterzwaag, 1981;29—50.
6. Asayama K, Dobashi K, Hayashibe H, Kato K. J Nutr Sci Vitaminol 1989;35:407—418.
7. Miquel J, Fleming J. In: Johnson J, Walford R, Harman D, Miquel J (eds) Biology of Aging. New York: Alan R. Liss, Inc., 1986;51—76.
8. Cadenas E, Boveris A, Ragan CI, Stoppani AOM. Arch Biochem Biophys 1977;180:248—257.
9. Boveris A. In: Reich M, Coburn R, Lahiri S, Chance B (eds) Tissue hypoxia and ischemia. New York: Plenum, 1977;67—82.
10. Loschen G, Flohe L, Chance B. FEBS Lett 1971;18:261—264.
11. Chance B, Sies H, Boveris A. Physiol Rev 1979;59:527—605.
12. Master C, Holmes R. Physiol Rev 1977;57:816—882.
13. Godin DV, Wohaieb SA. Free Radic Biol Med 1988;5:165—176.
14. Van Bilsen M, Van der Vusse GJ, Coumans WA, De Groot MJM et al. Am J Physiol 1989; 257:H47—H54.
15. Ji LL, Fu RG, Mitchell EW, Waldrop TG et al. Can J Physiol Pharmacol 1993;71:811—817.
16. Simpson PJ, Lucchesi BR. J Lab Clin Med 1987;110:13—30.
17. Downey JM. Ann Rev Physiol 1990;52:487—504.
18. Bindoli A, Cavallini A, Rigobello MP, Coassin M et al. Free Radic Biol Med 1988;4:163—167.
19. Hearse DJ, Manning AS, Downey JM, Yellon DM Acta Physiol Scand 1986;548:65—78.
20. Hellsten Y. Acta Physiol Scand 1994;621:1—73.
21. Sahlin K, Ekberg K, Cizinsky S. Acta Physiol Scand 1001;142:273—81.
22. Brooks GA, Fahey TD. Exercise Physiology. London: McMillan, 1985;290—291.
23. Freedman AM, Cassidy MM, Weglicki WB. Magn Reson 1991;4:185—189.
24. Pincemail J, Camus G, Roesgen A, Dreezen E, Bertrand Y, Lismonde M, Deby-Dupont G, Deby C. Eur J Appl Physiol Occ Physiol 1990;61:319—322.
25. Pyne DB. Sports Med 1994;17:245—58.
26. Petrone WF, English DK, Wong K, McCord JM. Proc Natl Acad Sci USA 1980;77:1159—1163.
27. Ji LL, Stratman FW, Lardy HA. J Am Coll Nutr 1992;11:79—86.
28. Schaible T, Scheuer J. Progr Cardiovas Dis 1985;27:297—324.
29. Dhaliwal H, Kirshenbaum LA, Randhawa AK, Singal AK. Am J Physiol 1991;261:H632—H638.
30. Leeuwenburgh C, Leichtweis S, Fiebig R, Hollander J, Gore M, Ji LL. Molec Cell Biochem 1996;156:17—24.
31. Cowan DB, Weisel RD, Williams WG, Mickle DAG. J Molec Cell Cardiol 1992;24:423—433.
32. Lai CC, Peng M, Huang L, Huang WH, Chiu TH. J Molec Cell Cardiol 1996;28:1157—1163.
33. Yoshida T, Watanabe M, Engelman DT, Engelman RM, Schley JA, Maulik N, Ho YS, Oberley TD, Das DK. J Molec Cell Cardiol 1996;28:1759—1767.
34. Yoshida T, Maulik N, Engelman RM, Ho YS, Magnenat JL, Rousou JA, Flack JE 3rd, Deaton D, Das DK. Circulation 1997;96(Suppl9):II—II21620.
35. Gohil K, Packer L, de Lumen B, Brooks GA et al. J Appl Physiol 1986;60:1986—1991.
36. Packer L. Am J Clin Nutr 1991;53:1050S—1055S.
37. Diplock AT. Am J Clin Nutr 1991;53:189S—193S.
38. Sakanashi T, Sako S, Nozuhara A, Adachi K et al. Biochem Biophys Res Comm 1991;181: 145—150.
39. Diplock AT. Free Radic Res 1997;26:565—583.
40. Rapola JM, Virtamo J, Ripatti S, Huttunen JK, Albanes D, Taylor PR, Heinonen OP. Lancet 1997;349:1715—1720.
41. Diaz MN, Frei B, Vita JA, Keaney JF Jr. N Engl J Med 1997;337:408—416.
42. Halliwell B, Gutteridge JMC. Free Radicals in Biology and Medicine. Oxford, UK: Clarendon Press, 1985,73—75,104—106.
43. Ji LL, Fu RG, Mitchell EW. J Appl Physiol 1992;73:1854—1859.
44. Ferrarri R, Ceconi C, Curello S, Cargnoni A et al. Am J Med 1991;91:95S—105S.

45. Meister A, Anderson ME. Ann Rev Biochem 1983;52:711—760.
46. Meister A. J Biol Chem 1988;263:17205—17208.
47. Flohe L. In: Pryor W (ed) Free Radicals in Biology, vol 5, New York: Academic Press, Inc., 1982;223—253.
48. Deneke SM, Fanburg BL. Am J Physiol 1989;257:L163—L173.
49. Sen CK, Marin E, Kretzchmar M, Hanninen O. J Appl Physiol 1992;73:1265—1272.
50. Leeuwenburgh C, Hollander J, Leichtweis S, Fiebig R, Gore M, Ji LL. Am J Physiol 1997;272: R363—R369.
51. Leichtweis S, Leeuwenburgh C, Chandwaney R, Ji LL. Acta Physiol Scand 1997;160:139—148.
52. Mascio PD, Murphy ME, Sies H. Am J Clin Nutr 1991;53:194S—200S.
53. Yu B P. Physiol Rev 1994;74:139—162.
54. Packer L. In: Cadenas E, Packer L (eds) Biological oxidants and antioxidants: New developments in research and health effects. Hippokrates: Verlag, 1993.
55. Scheer B, Zimmer G. Arch Biochem Biophys 1993;302:385—390.
56. Jenkins R.R. Sport Med 1988;5:156—170.
57. Davies KJA, Quintanilha TA, Brooks GA, Packer L. Biochem and Biophysical Research Communication 1982;107:1198—1205.
58. Banister EW, Tomanek RJ, Cvorkov N. Am J Physiol 1971;220:1935—1940.
59. King GA, Gollnick PD. Am J Physiol 1970;218:1150—1155.
60. Terjung RL, Klinkerfuss GH, Baldwin KM, Winder WW et al. Am J Physiol 1973;225:300—305.
61. Zweier JL, Flaherty JT, Weisfeldt ML. Proc Natl Acad Sci 1987;84:1404—1407.
62. Baker JE, Felix CC, Llinger GN, Kalyanaraman B. Proc Natl Acad Sci 1988;85:2786—2789.
63. Kumar CT, Reddy VK, Prasad M, Thyagaraju K et al. Molec Cell Biochem 1992;111:109—115.
62. Somani SM, Arroyo CM. Indian J Physiol Pharmacol 1995;39:323—329.
65. Ji LL, Bejma J, Ramires P, Donahue C. Med Sci Sports Exer 1998;30:5322.
66. Nohl H. Br Med Bull 1993;49:653—667.
67. Calderera CM, Guarnierri C, Lazzari F. Bull Italian Exp Biol Soc 1973;49:72—77.
68. Ji LL. Med Sci Sport Exer 1993;25:225—231.
69. Ji LL, Dillon D, Wu E. Am J Physiol 1991;261:R386—R392.
70. Ji LL, Mitchell EW. Biochem Pharmacol 1994;47:877—885.
71. Somani SM, Frank S, Rybak LP. Pharmacol Biochem Behav 1995;51:627—634.
72. Higuchi M, Cartier LJ, Chen M et al. J Gerontol 1985;40:281—286.
73. Kihlstrom M. J Appl Physiol 1990;68:1672—1678.
74. Kihlstrom M, Ojala J, Salminen S. Acta Physiol Scand 1989;135:549—554.
75. Venditti P, Di Meo S. Int J Sports Med 1997;18:497—502.
76. Fiebig R, Gore M, Chandwaney R, Leeuwenburgh C, Ji LL. Age 1996;19:83—89.
77. Kanter MM, Hamlin RL, Unverferth DV, Davis HW, Merola AJ. J Appl Physiol 1985;59: 1298—1303.
78. Powers SK, Criswell D, Lawler J, Martin D et al. Am J Physiol 1993;265:H2094—H2098.
79. Packer L, Slater TF, Rothfuss LM, Wilson DS. Ann NY Acad Sci 1989;570:311—321.
80. Gohil K, Rothfuss L, Lang J, Packer L. J Appl Physiol 1987;63:1638—1641.
81. Tiidus PM, Behrens WA, Madere R, Kim JJ et al. Nutr Res 1993;13:219—224.
82. Sohal RS, Sun SC, Colcolough HL, Burch GE. Lab Invest 1968;18:49—56.
83. Thomas DP, Marchall KI. Int J Sports Med 1988;9:257—260.
84. Pierce GN, Kutryk MJB, Djalla KS, Beamish RE et al. J Appl Physiol 1984;57:326—331.
85. Coleman R, Silbermann M, Gershon D, Reznick AZ. Gerontol 1987;33:34—39.
86. Packer L, Gohil K, DeLumen B, Terblanche SE. Comp Biochem Physiol 1986;83B:235—240.
87. Brooks GA, White TP. J Appl Physiol 1978;45:1009—1015.
88. Ji L L. Free Rad Biol Med 1995;6:1079—1086.
89. Konz KH, Haap M, Hill KE, Burk RF et al. J Molec Cell Cardiol 1989;21:789—795.
90. Lang JK, Gohil K, Packer L, Burk RF. J Appl Physiol 1987;63:2532—2535.
91. Oster O, Maham M, Oelert H, Prellwitz W. Clin Chem 1989;35:851—856.

92. Goldfarb AH. Med Sci Sports Exer 1993;25:232–236.
93. Scholz RW, Minicucci LA, Reddy CC. Biochem Molec Biol Int 1997;42:997–1006.
94. Diplock AT. Free Radic Res 1997;26:565–583.
95. Diaz MN, Frei B, Vita JA, Keaney JF Jr. N Engl J Med 1997;337:408–416.
96. Somani SM, Gupta SK, Frank S, Corder CN. Drug Develep Res 1990;20:251–275.
97. Arcamone F. Doxorubicin anticancer antibiotics. New York: Academic Press, 1981.
98. Olson RO, Mushlin PS. FASEB J 1990;4:3076–3086.
99. Davies KJA, Doroshow JH, Hochstein P. FEBS Lett 1983;153:227–230.
100. Davies KJA, Doroshow JH. J Biol Chem 1986;261:3060–3067.
101. Langton D, Jover B, McGrath BP, Ludbrook J. Cardiovasc Res 1990;24:959–968.
102. Nohl H. In: Johnson Jr. JE, Walford R, Harman D, Miquel J (eds) Free radicals, aging and degenerative diseases. New York: Alan R. Liss, Inc. 1986;77–98.
103. Hansford RG. Biochim Biophys Acta 1983;726:41–80.
104. Nohl H, Hegner D, Summer KH. Mech Aging Dev 1979;11:145–151.
105. Lakatta EG, Yin FC. Am J Physiol 1982;242:H927–H941.

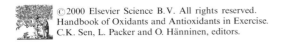
©2000 Elsevier Science B.V. All rights reserved.
Handbook of Oxidants and Antioxidants in Exercise.
C.K. Sen, L. Packer and O. Hänninen, editors.

Part IX • Chapter 26

Influence of exercise-induced oxidative stress on the central nervous system

Satu M. Somani and Kazim Husain

Department of Pharmacology, Southern Illinois University School of Medicine, P.O. Box 19230, Springfield, IL 62794-1222, USA. Tel.: +1-217-785-2196. Fax: +1-217-524-0145.
E-mail: SSomani@wpsmtp.siumed.edu

1 INTRODUCTION
   1.1 Oxygen and central nervous system
   1.2 Reactive oxygen species in the central nervous system
   1.3 Lipid peroxidation in the central nervous system
   1.4 Antioxidant system and central nervous system
2 OXYGEN-INDUCED CNS TOXICITY
   2.1 Antioxidant-system/lipid peroxidations
   2.2 Treatments
3 EXERCISE-INDUCED OXIDATIVE STRESS
   3.1 Acute exercise and central nervous system
   3.2 Exercise training and central nervous system
4 EXERCISE AND DRUG INTERACTION ON CNS
5 CENTRAL NERVOUS SYSTEM DISEASES: REACTIVE OXYGEN SPECIES/ANTIOXIDANT SYSTEM
   5.1 Alzheimer's disease
   5.2 Parkinson's disease
   5.3 Amyotrophic lateral sclerosis
   5.4 Down syndrome
   5.5 Multiple system atrophy
   5.6 Huntington disease
   5.7 Cerebrovascular injury
6 STRATEGIES TO IMPROVE CNS FUNCTIONS
   6.1 Antioxidant-supplementation
       6.1.1 Vitamins
       6.1.2 Glutathione
       6.1.3 Antioxidant-enzymes
       6.1.4 Other free radical scavengers
7 SUMMARY
8 PERSPECTIVES
9 ABBREVIATIONS
10 REFERENCES

1 INTRODUCTION

1.1 Oxygen and the central nervous system

Oxygen is essential to most higher organisms for their survival, however, concentrations of oxygen greater than those present in normal air have been proven harmful. The oxidative damage that results from high pressure oxygen is frequently experienced in professional diving, closed-circuit military underwater activity, hyperbaric oxygen (HBO) therapy for peripheral vascular ischemia, carbon monoxide (CO) poisoning, and severe localized infections [1]. Breathing highly pressurized oxygen can cause central nervous system (CNS) toxicity in humans with symptoms including nausea, paresthesia, tinnitus, twitching, tunnel vision, unconsciousness, and convulsions [2]. The convulsions of CNS oxygen toxicity, which resemble grand mal epileptic seizures, start in humans within a relatively short time of the oxygen exposure. Reactive oxygen species (ROS) that are produced in excess upon exposure to highly pressurized oxygen overwhelm the antioxidant system of the CNS and seem to mediate the hyperoxic injury [3].

The CNS is rich in lipids, and molecular oxygen dissolves 7- to 8-fold more in the nonpolar medium such as CNS than in the aqueous cell compartments. The brain's rate of oxygen metabolism is high, but the tissue oxygen stores are lacking. Neuronal cells are rich in mitochondria and have a high demand for adenosine triphosphate (ATP). Oxidative phosphorylation occurs extensively and involves ubiquinones, which are abundantly present in the CNS. Those ubiquinones auto-oxidize readily and are apparently involved in the production of ROS [4,5]. The microcirculatory blood vessels of the brain and spinal cord are frail and can be torn easily thus, resulting in the release of iron and copper into the tissues. These transition metals act as catalysts in the generation of ROS [6]. The gray and white matter of the CNS contain a high level of ascorbic acid [7]. These neuronal cells can concentrate ascorbate 100-fold more than the plasma because of the brain's particular active transport system for ascorbic acid. Although ascorbic acid is a powerful antioxidant, its high concentration in the CNS, in the presence of iron and copper (due to their release by CNS injury), could become pro-oxidant and produce ROS [8,9]. Thus, due to ROS produced by hyperoxic oxygen exposure the blood-brain-barrier breaks down and cerebral edema accumulates [10]. However, the prime site in the brain for ROS attack, which causes seizures is still obscure. Therefore, antioxidant therapy may provide protection against CNS oxygen injury.

Since exercise increases oxygen consumption and uptake in vital tissues of humans and animals, it also enhances ROS formation in the various tissues of animals [11—13]. We have shown that heart tissue from exercise-trained rats produces the ascorbyl-electroparamagnetic radical [14]. Since the brain's concentration of ascorbic acid is much higher in neuronal tissue than in the plasma, it is not known whether ascorbyl-electroparamagnetic radicals are produced in the brain specifically due to exercise training; but it would be interesting to study the effects of exercise intensity on ascorbyl radical formation in the CNS. Glucose interacts with proteins to produce oxygen radicals [15]. The brain utilizes glucose as its primary source of energy, and during exercise, there seems to be a greater demand for energy in the brain due to its increased oxygen consumption (uptake) and cerebral blood flow. Various brain regions utilize glucose differently and superoxides are produced during the oxidative metabolism of glucose.

1.2 Reactive oxygen species in the central nervous system

The CNS is particularly susceptible to the toxic effects of oxygen due to its generation of ROS. Among the various organ systems of the body, the CNS uses a disproportional 20% of the oxygen consumed by humans. However, brain constitutes about 2% of the body weight. Consequently, oxygen becomes harmful when it is converted to ROS. ROS are very reactive, short-lived and have been known to cause damage to blood vessels in the brain [16], as well as to the brain's parenchyma [17]. The sequential univalent reduction of oxygen produces superoxide anion radical (O_2-), hydrogen peroxide (H_2O_2), and free hydroxyl radicals ($\cdot OH$). O_2- radicals can be produced in the CNS from a variety of sources, such as the mitochondrial electron transport chain and by dihydroorotic dehydrogenase [18]; it is also generated by xanthine oxidase, which is concentrated primarily in the endothelium of the cerebral blood vessels [19,20]. Superoxide is also produced in the CNS by prostaglandin H synthase, lipoxygenase and cytochrome P-450 oxygenase pathways [21,22]. In addition, enzymatic and non-enzymatic oxidation of catecholamines, L-amino acids, and hemoglobin have all been shown to produce dangerous levels of superoxide and H_2O_2 in the CNS [23–25]. Activated polymorphonuclear leukocytes generate superoxide from nicotimnamide adenine dinucleotide phosphate reduced (NADPH) oxidase in the CNS [26,27] H_2O_2 is generated in the brain's mitochondria entirely from the dismutation of superoxide in the CNS [28–30], while hydroxyl radicals can be generated in the CNS by superoxide-driven Fenton reactions or metal-catalyzed Haber-Weiss reactions [31,32]. Finally, nitric oxide (NO) is also produced in specific neurons of the CNS and in the brain microvascular endothelium by NO synthase [33]. NO can react with superoxide radicals to produce peroxy nitrite anions (ONO), which can cause brain injury. For example, ROS generated in the CNS may interact with aromatic amino acids (tryptophan, phenylalanine, and tyrosine) and sulfur containing amino acids (cystine and cystein) present at the active sites of the enzymes. Glutamine synthase and $Ca^{++}ATPase$ have been shown to be inactivated in the CNS of animals due to ROS-induced oxidation [34,35].

1.3 Lipid peroxidation in the central nervous system

Reactive oxygen species generated in the CNS rapidly react with lipids, proteins and nucleic acids [36]. The CNS is particularly vulnerable to the damaging effects of ROS on membranous lipids [37] due to its following characteristics:
1. High rate of oxygen consumption
2. High rate of oxidative metabolic activity
3. High concentrations of readily oxidizable substrates, such as polyunsaturated fatty acids and catecholamines
4. High content of iron
5. Low levels of antioxidant enzymes and glutathione
ROS generated in the CNS can attack the unsaturated bonds of membrane lipids

and may undergo lipid peroxidation (LPO). Lipid peroxides may generate a peroxidation cascade that allows the peroxidative damage to spread to distant tissues and organelles. Transition metals, such as iron, seem to play an important role in the generation of ROS, as well as in the process of LPO in neuronal membranes. The impact of LPO on membrane lipids, membrane receptors and membrane-bound enzymes (ATPase and acetylcholinesterase) can alter the function, structure and fluidity of membranes and may result in an altered calcium influx [38,39]. The aldehydes that produced lipid peroxide fragmentations (malondialdehyde, 4-hydroxy alkenals) are cytotoxic [40,41]. A plethora of evidence indicated that enhanced LPO contributes to the pathogenesis of oxygen toxicity and thus, several neurodegenerative diseases. Therefore, it is essential to inhibit LPO reaction by different means: iron-chelating agents, spin-trapping agents, free radical scavengers and chainbreaking antioxidants.

1.4 Antioxidant system and central nervous system

Detoxification of ROS is one of the prerequisites of an aerobic life style. This detoxification is a part of the antioxidant defense system generated in the body. Oxidative stress results when the production of ROS exceeds the ability of the antioxidant system to eliminate them [12]. The antioxidant system includes antioxidant enzymes: superoxide dismutase (SOD), catalase (CAT), glutathione peroxidase (GSH-Px) and an ancillary enzyme, glutathione reductase (GR). There are also non-enzymatic antioxidants in this bodily system which include: glutathione, vitamin E, ubiquinol (coenzyme Q_{10}), ascorbic acid, thioredoxin, and α-lipoic acid. All of these are critical for protection against ROS. When the body's normal protective measures are active, oxygen consumed by the organs will form O_2-, which can be readily dismuted by SOD to H_2O_2 and singlet oxygen ($^1O_2$). H_2O_2 is then converted, by either CAT or GSH-Px, to H_2O and $^1O_2$. Finally reduced glutathione (GSH) consumed in the GSH-Px reaction is recycled back to its reduced form by GR.

These antioxidant enzymes and GSH are much lower in the CNS when compared to erythrocytes and peripheral tissues [42,43]. Glutathione, in its reduced state, plays an important role in protecting cells against free radical and oxyradical damage [44]. The turnover of GSH in the brain is considered to be slower than the turnover of GSH in the liver and kidney. The half-life of GSH in rat brains is estimated to be 70 h [45] as compared to the 29-min halflife of GSH [46] in mouse kidneys. Glutathione deficiency, induced by buthionine sulfoximine (inhibitor of glutathione synthesis), leads to the enlargement and degeneration of mitochondria in the rat brain. Such a glutathione deficiency probably causes accumulation of H_2O_2-damaging mitochondria [47].

The brain stem and the spinal cord are more vulnerable to ROS injury because of their inherent low levels of GSH compared to the cerebrum and cerebellum [48]. Low levels of glutathione were found in six regions of the brain compared to the liver levels of young adult, middle-aged and aged rats [49]. The exposure of brain mitochondria to oxidative stress (caused by butyl hydroperoxide) results in glutathione depletion and the formation of glutathione-protein mixed disulfide [50]. In particular, the substantia nigra neurons showed an exceptional vulnerability to oxidative stress. When malondialdehyde (MDA) levels are measured as an index of endogenous lipoperoxidation, which represent oxidative stress, different brain regions exhibit varying concentrations of MDA formation under normal physiological conditions [51,52]. Thus, these findings suggest that the CNS has a great vulnerablity to oxyradical toxicity, and that it may possess unique coping mechanism(s) to deal with oxidative stress.

Many pathologic conditions are caused by the nervous system's over production of ROS and the antioxidant system's lack of coping mechanisms: Parkinson's disease (PD), ischemic reperfusion injury, cataract formation, aging process, arthritis, amyotrophic lateral sclerosis, Huntington disease, cerebrovascular injury, asthma, carcinogenesis, Down syndrome (DS), Alzheimer's disease (AD), multiple system atrophy (MSA) and other ailments.

2   OXYGEN-INDUCED CNS TOXICITY

2.1 Antioxidant system/lipid peroxidation

CNS oxygen toxicity depends upon the exposure time to oxygen and the partial pressure of oxygen [53]. ROS have been implicated in oxygen toxicity and were first reported by Gershman et al. [54]. They reported that the formation of ROS and lipid peroxides in the CNS increases after exposure to oxygen at increased levels of pressure [51,55]. In addition, increased CNS glutathione oxidation has also been reported during HBO exposure [56–59]. These effects, showing hyperbaric hypoxia on the CNS antioxidant system and LPO are depicted in Table 1. Most of the studies in rats and guinea pigs show increased SOD activity in the brain [60,61], which indicates superoxide generation due to the presence of excess oxygen at high-pressure levels. Conversely, the activities of CAT and GSH-Px decreased in the brains of rats and guinea pigs due to HBO exposure [60], thereby reflecting the accumulation of H_2O_2 and lipid hydroperoxide in the animals' CNS. The levels of GSH and protein sulfhydryl groups were depleted in the cerebal cortex (CC) and brain of the rats at various time intervals of HBO exposure [56,62]. We suspect that the inhibition of antioxidant enzymes and the depletion of GSH in the CNS may be due to ROS-mediated inactivation of the brain's enzyme proteins and the oxidation of GSH to glutathione oxidized (GSSG). Jenkinson et al. [63] have reported that hyperbaric hyperoxia increases GR activity in the rat brains and this may be related to increases in GSSG levels during oxidative stress, thereby sending intracellular signals to induce GR production. Such studies in rats have also demonstrated an appreciable augmentation of LPO in the entire brain, as well as in various brain regions of rats [51,61].

Table 1. Oxygen toxicity: antioxidant system and lipid peroxidation in central nervous system.

Species	Condition	Duration	Brain / brain regions	% Change (+ increase; − decrease)					Reference
				SOD	CAT	GSH-Px	GSH/Protein-SH	LPO	
Rat (Sprague-Dawley)	Hyperbaric hyperoxia[b]	4 h 8.25 h	Brain Brain	+20% −2%	+17% −18%	+10% −27%	− −	− −	Harabin et al. [60]
Guinea pig	Hyperbaric hyperoxia[b]	6.25 h 11.25 h	Brain Brain	+14% −2%	+2% −28%	−17% −34%	− −	− −	Harabin et al. [60]
Rat (Wistar)	Normobaric hyperoxia[a]	12 h 36 h 48 h	Brain Brain Brain	− +30% +35%	− − −	− − −	− − −	+75% +99% +138%	Ahotupa et al. [61]
Rat (Wistar)	Normobaric hyperoxia[a]	1 h 3 h 5 h 8 h 24 h	Cerebral Cortex Cerebral Cortex Cerebral Cortex Cerebral Cortex Cerebral Cortex	− − − − −	− − − − −	− − − − −	−36% −45% −34% −24% −72%	− − − − −	Gordon and Gajkowska [56]
Rats (Sprague–Dawley)	Hyperbaric hyperoxia[b]	200 min	Brain	−	−	−	−1.5%	−	Jenkinson et al. [74]
Rats (Sprague–Dawley)	Hyperbaric hyperoxia[b]	200 min	Brain	−	−	−	+6%	−	Jenkinson et al. [63]
Rats (Sprague–Dawley)	Hyperbaric hyperoxia[b]	160 min 200 min	Brain Brain	−			−5% +4%		Peacock et al. [62]

(Continued.)

Table 1. Continued.

Species	Condition	Duration	Brain / brain regions	%Change (+ increase; – decrease)					Reference
				SOD	CAT	GSH–Px	GSH/Protein-SH	LPO	
Rat (Wistar)	Hyperbaric hyperoxia[b]	20 min	Brain	–	–	–	–	+22%	Noda et al. [51]
			Accumbens	–	–	–	–	+7%	
			Amygdala	–	–	–	–	+2%	
			Caudate Putamen	–	–	–	–	+15%	
			Cerebellum	–	–	–	–	+3%	
			Cerebral Cortex	–	–	–	–	+40%	
			Corpus Callosum	–	–	–	–	+19%	
			Globus Pallidus	–	–	–	–	+16%	
			Hippocampus	–	–	–	–	+20%	
			Hypothalamus	–	–	–	–	+11%	
			Inferior Colliculus	–	–	–	–	+18%	
			Olfactory Bulb	–	–	–	–	+27%	
		20 min for 7 days	Septum	–	–	–	–	+22%	
			Spinal Cord	–	–	–	–	+42%	
			Substantia Nigra	–	–	–	–	+13%	
			Brain	–	–	–	–	+20%	

[a] 100% O_2 at 1 or 2 atmospheric pressure; [b] 100% O_2 at 2–5 atmospheric pressure; SOD: superoxide dismutase; CAT: catalase; GSH-Px: glutathione peroxidase; GSH: reduced glutathione; LPO: lipid peroxidation.

2.2 Treatments

Excess reactive oxygen species that are produced upon exposure to high pressure oxygen and deplete the antioxidant system seem to mediate hyperoxic CNS damage [3,55]. The severity of CNS toxicity and the lack of effective protective agents led to the use of several different compounds for protection in animals [54,64—66]. However, the actual mechanisms of protection that these agents provide remain unclear. Since ROS are produced in excess and the CNS antioxidant system is suppressed in CNS oxygen toxicity, ROS scavengers and exogenous antioxidants have been attempted as means of protection. Studies have shown that superoxide and H_2O_2 generation increases in oxygen toxicity [3,55]. Therefore, it is essential to attenuate the onset of CNS oxygen toxicity by increasing the concentrations of CNS enzymatic antioxidants to combat superoxide and H_2O_2. Free SOD and CAT injections have not been proven successful against CNS oxygen toxicity [67,68] due to the short circulating halflife of these enzymes and their inability to cross the blood-brain-barrier. However, Yusa et al. [69] have shown that liposome-entrapped SOD and CAT (injected intravenously), significantly protected against oxygen-induced CNS toxicity in rats. Some modified SOD can cross blood-brain barrier and provide protection to the brain against ROS. The endogenous tripeptide glutathione (GSH) is a well-known detoxifier of ROS and protected both rats and mice from CNS hyperbaric hyperoxia [65,66]. However, GSH has not protected rats from normobaric hyperoxic exposure [64]. A selenium deficiency has been known to decrease tissue GSH-Px activity [70] and increase the toxicity of oxygen in rats [71—73]. Since exogenous GSH administration did not protect selenium-deficient rats from hyperbaric hyperoxia [74], it is likely that GSH-Px activity is required for GSH-induced protection from CNS hyperbaric hyperoxia. As GSH is a peptide which can be easily degraded in the body (after administration), it is suggested that esters of glutathione may be more appropriately used to prevent CNS oxygen toxicity. Clearly, GSH appears to be an important endogenous antioxidant, since the depletion of tissue GSH has been demonstrated to augments oxygen toxicity [75,76]. The intracellular transport of GSH is another crucial factor in determining its availability in the CNS to counteract ROS produced during oxygen toxicity [62]. The dietary antioxidant, β-carotene, has also been reported to protect the rats against CNS oxygen toxicity [77]. Subsequently, during antioxidant therapy, ROS types their origin and their mode of action, as well as lipophilic antioxidants such as vitamin E and lipoic acid, must be carefully evaluated against CNS oxygen toxicity.

3   EXERCISE-INDUCED OXIDATIVE STRESS

Physical exercise is associated with enhanced respiration and increased oxygen uptake in the body's vital organs/tissues by as much as 15- to 20-fold. The brain consumes 20% of the oxygen taken in by the body. Most of the oxygen consumed by cells is reduced to H_2O through mitochondrial electron transport chains; however, 2—5% of oxygen is converted into ROS via one electron reduction in the mitochondria. During the last decade, evidence has accumulated revealing the production of ROS and other free radicals during exercise and exerted oxidative stress on vital organs/tissues [11,13,78,79]. To protect themselves from ROS injury, cells contain several antioxidant defense mechanisms: endogenous antioxidants (glutathione, vitamins C, A, E, uric acid and iron binding protein) and antioxidant enzymes, such as superoxidase dismutase (SOD), CAT and glutathione peroxidase (GSH-Px). The AOE activities are well distributed in all organs of the body, which are dependent on oxygen consumption rate, metabolic rate, and metal ion and fatty acid amounts. AOE activities are prone to alteration with changes in bodily oxygen consumption (oxidative stress). Oxidative stress can be described as a disturbance in the antioxidant system rendering it unable to adequately scavenge free radicals/ROS and arrest LPO chain reactions. Antioxidant system responses to physical exercise are dependent on the type, mode, intensity, frequency, and duration of the exercise. The modulation of AOE activity depends primarily upon its substrate (ROS), cosubstrate production, nature of catalytic center, affinity of the enzyme to the substrate (K_m, Michaelis Menton constants), and selectivity and specificity of the substrate.

Exercise enhances the blood flow in most organs, but depletes the flow in the liver, which in turn influences the compartmentalization of GSH in the liver. Such changes in blood flow rates, during and after exercise may alter the transport of glutathione (extracellular and intracellular), and the synthesis or degradation of glutathione due to an increased uptake of oxygen in the blood. Consequently, the effectiveness of the antioxidant system varies after acute exercise and exercise training. Antioxidant activity in various tissues, specifically in different animal brain regions, is summarized in Table 2.

3.1 Acute exercise and central nervous systems

Recently, Somani et al. [52] investigated the effects of acute exercise (100% VO_{2max}, Maximum oxygen consumption) on antioxidant enzymes and LPO studied in specific areas of the Fisher-344 rat brain. The changes in antioxidant enzymes and LPO in specific areas of rat brains after acute exercise are depicted in Table 2.

Studies show that due to acute exercise, SOD activity decreased in the CC with no significant SOD changes in other brain regions. CAT activity increased, due to acute exercise, in the cerebal cortex and the corpus striatum (CS); whereas, GSH-Px activity increased profoundly in the cortex and decreased in the CS. GSH-Px activity increased profoundly in the cortex, a region with low basal activity. Perhaps to cope with the oxidative stress of exercise, this enzyme is activated in the cortex to eliminate hydroperoxides. Glutathione reductase activity, which controls endogenous levels of reduced glutathione (GSH), was decreased in the cortex, due to acute exercise, suggests an inadequate level of reducing equivalents

Table 2. Exercise-induced changes in antioxidant system/lipid peroxidation in the central nervous system.

Species	Exercise mode and duration	Brain/brain regions	% Change (+ increase; − decrease)						Reference
			SOD	CAT	GSH−Px	GR	GSH GSSG	orLPO	
Rats (Fisher-344)	Acute exercise/ treadmill (30 min)	Cerebral cortex	−26	+54	+147	−17	–	+66	Somani et al. [52]
		Cerebellum	NC	NC	+20	−15	–	NC	
		Corpus Striatum	−15	+40	−66	−10	–	+112	
		Hypothalamus	−18	NC	NC	NC	–	NC	
		Medulla	+8	NC	+26	−10	–	+22	
Rat (Fisher-344)	Exercise training/ treadmill (6.5 weeks)	Cerebral cortex	NC	NC	+33	+62	+13 Red +10 Oxi	−50	Somani and Husain [83]
		Cerebellum	−15	NC	−22	NC	NC	−25	
		Corpus striatum	+36	+25	+22	+214	NC	−31	
		Hypothalamus	−25	−29	+43	NC	–	−29	
		Medulla	−20	NC	+10	−20	NC	NC	
Rat (Sprague-Dawley)	Exercise training/ treadmill (7.5 weeks)	Brainstem	+30	–	NC	–	+9 Red +50 Oxi	–	Somani et al. [81]
		Corpus striatum	+30	–	−13	–	+10 Oxi	–	
		Cerebral cortex	NC	–	NC	–	+33 Oxi	–	
		Hippocampus	+10	–	NC	–	–	–	

SOD: superoxide dismutase; CAT: catalase; GSH-Px: glutathione peroxidase; GR: glutathione reductase; GSH: reduced glutathione; GSSG: oxidized glutathione; Red: reduced GSH; Oxi: oxidized GSSG; NC = no change.

NADPH and a failure to maintain GSH levels. Consequently, harm may incur as GSH is important in the regulation of brain function and is reportedly decreased during oxidative stress [50]. Acute exercise significantly increases LPO in the CS, which contains high basal MDA levels and controls motor activity. It is notable that LPO is inversely proportional to GSH-Px activity in the CS which has a high dopamine content [80]. Since dopamine is labile to auto-oxidation and may be transformed to toxic intermediates with the generation of ROS, acute exercise may cause peroxidative injury to the striatal membrane, alter neurotransmitters and may interupt motor function. Interestingly, acute exercise selectively inhibits striatal acetylcholinesterase (AChE) activity and such an inhibition is correlated with an increase in LPO, thereby resulting in perturbation of motor activity [38].

3.2 Exercise training and the central nervous system

Somani and co-workers' [81] investigation of the effects of exercise training (7.5 weeks) on the antioxidant system in brain regions of Sprague-Dawley rats, show the regional variations in cerebral GSH and GSSG levels and GSH-Px and SOD activities in sedentary control rats. These variations were enhanced in specific brain regions after exercise training. The brain regions of sedentary control rats showed: 1) GSH levels were lower in the brain stem (BS) than the CC and CS — the latter two were comparable; 2) GSSG levels were also lower in brain stem than the CC and CS; 3) The GSH/GSSG ratio was observed in the decreasing order CS > BS > CC. In sedentary control rats, GSH-Px activity was found in the decreasing order CS > BS > CC > hippocampus (H); however, SOD activity levels registered in reverse order: CC > BS > CS > H. Thus, SOD activity was stimulated in brain regions due to exercise training (Table 2). This pattern is interesting in the brain regions of sedentary control rats when compared to level of changes in exercised rats. BS and CS seem to be more sensitive to oxidative stress, and SOD was induced in these regions during exercise. Evidently exercise does not produce significant alterations in GSH-Px activity in the brain regions, but SOD activity increases significantly following exercise training (Table 2).

Examination of glutathione levels in each specific brain region of the rats showed that the cerebal cortex of sedentary controls has higher levels of GSH than other regions, and this suggests that this area may deal with oxidative stress better than other regions. The exercise training did not significantly change the GSH levels in this region, but the cerebral cortex showed a significant decrease in GSSG following exercise which indicates that the GSH to GSSG conversion did not occur due to exercise training. It seems, therefore, that exercise training results in a better redox ratio in this region and that the CC seems to be more capable of coping with oxidative stress because it has the highest concentration of GSH. This may be a biochemical correlation to the physical sensation of greater wellbeing and greater awareness following everyday exercise in humans. SOD and GSH-Px activity was not altered in this region due to exercise training

(Table 2).

The level of GSH is significantly low in the BS when compared to CC and CS, thereby potentially predisposing it to greater oxidative stress. However, GSH levels slightly increased in this region due to exercise training. But, GSSG levels significantly decreased in BS indicating the turnover of GSH caused by exercise training. The GSH/GSSG ratio was highest in the BS of the exercise-trained rat when compared to the sedentary control regions. This ratio suggests that exercise training may contribute to the BS becoming more resistant to oxidative stress. This region also shows increased activity of SOD in conjunction with exercise training possibly due to enzyme induction. The oxidative stress seems to be predominantly due to the production of superoxide radicals, which are then scavenged by SOD. Since GSH-Px activity in BS is identical in exercised rats and sedentary control rats, there is no further change in GSH-Px activity, which suggests that no significant peroxidation takes place in the BS. These results show exercise training greatly benefits this region. Since the brain stem is a very vital area in autonomic functioning, cardiovascular regulation and respiration, exercise training may improve this region and its functions, which include controlling the heart rate and blood pressure [82]. Such improvements in physical fitness could result in the improved cardiovascular function that typically accompanies regular exercise training.

The GSH levels and SOD activity in the CS region are comparable to levels in the CC region of sedentary control rats, although the size of the CS is much smaller than the CC [81]. However, the CS region has a significantly higher GSH-Px activity than the CC. Similarly, the CS region SOD activity increased, and GSSG levels increased slightly, after exercise training. The metabolic percentages of the corpus striatum (basal ganglia), in terms of O_2 consumption by these tissues on a per g basis, exceed that of the CC. Thus, the highest levels of GSH-Px activity and GSH concentration may help this part of the brain to cope with any oxyradicals formed during periods of high oxygen consumption such as exercise. The H has the lowest levels of GSH-Px and SOD among all the four brain regions studied [81]. Exercise training increases SOD activity, in this region, which scavenges the superoxides formed from the excess O_2 consumed during exercise. The BS and CS show a significant increase in SOD enzyme activity (30%) due to exercise training where as the CC did not show any change in this enzyme activity. Apparently, exercise training causes more oxidative stress in the BS and CS regions that have a better ability to induce antioxidant enzymes that can cope with the superoxides formed during exercise training. The BS and CS appear to be more sensitive to oxidative stress, due to levels of enzyme induction, whereas CC and H regions may have acquired more resistance to oxidative stress due to their higher levels of GSH. GSH was present 43% less in the BS than the CC. However, exercise training significantly increases GSH to GSSG ratios in BS and in CC, but this ratio does not change in the CS. Therefore, the benefit of exercise training is evident as GSSG levels decrease and GSH levels remain unaltered in these two regions in particular.

Recently, Somani and Husain [83] have reported the effects of exercise training (6.5 weeks) on the antioxidant system in various brain regions of Fisher 344 rats. In sedentary control rats, SOD activity decreases in the following order: cerebellum > medulla > cortex > striatum > hypothalamus. However, exercise training alters the decreasing order of SOD activity: cerebellum > striatum > medulla > cortex > hypothalamus. In other words, exercise training increase SOD activity only in the striatum, a deeper area of the brain which has low enzyme activity and controls motor function (Table 2). Perhaps the enzyme SOD is activated in the striatum to prevent superoxides in order to maintain and facilitate motor activity during exercise training. SOD activity is sensitive to tissue oxygenation, and its biosynthesis has been reported to be elevated in rats subjected to high oxygen tension [84]. Since the oxygen utilization has increased during exercise training, SOD activity is elevated in this brain region. Conversely, due to exercise training, SOD activity decreased in the medulla, cerebellum and hypothalamus, all superficial areas of the brain. Such a decrease in SOD activity may be due to either feedback inhibition of the enzyme or oxidative inactivation of enzyme proteins; feedback inhibition and oxidative inactivation of SOD have been documented by other investigators [85,86]. A significant augmentation of GSH-Px activity in the cortex and hypothalamus, which have low basal activity, is indicative of an efficient elimination of hydroperoxides after exercise training (Table 2). GSH-Px is a nonspecific enzyme for hydroperoxides, and this lack of substrate specificity extends its range of substrates from H_2O_2 to organic hydroperoxide [28]. A significant decrease in CAT activity, along with an increase in GSH-Px activity in the hypothalamus, suggests an enhanced removal of H_2O_2 due to exercise training. Additionally, GR activity, which controls the endogenous GSH levels, increased profoundly in the cortex and striatum, suggesting the maintenance of GSH due to exercise training. These results are consistent with our previous report on Sprague-Dawley rats [81]. Exercise training also causes a significant depletion of MDA in the cortex, striatum, cerebellum and hypothalamus which denotes an adaptive response to decreased LPO rates. No significant change in GSH and GSSG contents in brain regions (Table 2) is indicative of the regions adaptive response after exercise training, or a resistance to oxidative stress. Interestingly, exercise training selectively inhibits hypothalamic AChE activity, and the inhibition correlates with increased LPO, which indicates the perturbation of hypothalamic functions [87].

4. EXERCISE AND DRUG INTERACTION ON THE CNS

The biotransformation of chemicals can be both harmful and helpful to the body. Under normal, healthy conditions, a chemical can be safely biotransformed and excreted from the body. However, several metabolic pathways may form electrophilic intermediate metabolites that generate superoxides and free radicals. Chemicals that contain nitro, amine, iminium, or quinone functional groups usually form these electrophilic intermediate metabolites which can covalently

Table 3. Drugs and chemicals which produce CNS toxicity mediated via ROS/free radicals.

Drugs	Free radicals (ROS)	Reference
Cisplatin	ROS	Clerici et al. [209]
BCNU – carmustine	methylradical	Reed eet al. [210]
Procarbazine	free radical	Sinha [211]
Ethanol	α-hydroxy-ethyl radical	Reinke et al. [92]
Physostigmine	esroline to catechol to quinones	Somani et al. [212]
Quinones	reactive metabolites	Kochli et al. [213]
Morphine	covalent binding	Nagamatsu et al. [214]
Parathione	reactive metabolite	Chambers et al. [215]
6-Hydroxy dopamine	ROS/free radical	Aust et al. [216]

bind to macromolecules and produce tissue-specific toxicity. Table 3 summarizes the drug-induced neurotoxicity mediated via the production of ROS and free radicals. Two specific pathways that produce free radicals, or $^-O_2$, include NADPH-cytochrome P-450 reductase [88] and one electron reduction under low oxygen tension [89]. Once these reactive metabolites are generated, interaction with the ferrous ion could produce the hydroxy radical (^-OH), possibly leading to toxic effects. As exercise will increase the body's oxygen consumption and the levels of AOE, physical activity may reduce the toxicity of several chemicals. For example, ethanol and nicotine have been reported to induce cytochrome P-450 II E_1 in the brain of rats [90,91]. Ethanol has also been reported to generate α-hydroxyl ethyl radicals and exert oxidative stress [92]. We have recently demonstrated the interaction of exercise and ethanol on AOE activity in various brain regions of rats. In the brain, GSH-Px activity increases in the hypothalamus and striatum. CAT and GR activity also increased in the striatum, and a decrease in SOD activity in the striatum and medulla was shown. Malondialdehyde levels increases in all brain regions after a single dose of ethanol when combined with acute exercise (Table 4). It is suggested, therefore, that the combination of acute exercise and ethanol exerts significant oxidative stress on specified brain regions of rats [52]. In addition, acute physical stress has been reported to increase the permeability of the blood-brain-barrier [93,94]. Thus, excess ethanol might have penetrated into the brain regions of exercised rats and caused oxidative injury. Even peripherally acting drugs, such as pyridostigmine, have been reported to reach the brain and negatively affect the centrally controlled functions under stressful conditions [94].

The interaction of exercise training and chronic ethanol ingestion on the antioxidant system of rat brains has been recently studied [83]. The data indicate that SOD activity decreases significantly in the cortex, medulla, cerebellum and hypthalamus but increases in the striatum (Table 5). On the other hand, the GSH-Px activity significantly increases in the cortex, striatum and hypothalamus when intense exercise and alcohol are combined. GR activity profoundly increases in the cortex, striatum and cerebellum, whereas it decreases in the medulla under such conditions. (Table 5). MDA levels significantly decrease in the medulla and

Table 4. Interaction of acute exercise (AE) and single ethanol dose (Et) on antioxidant enzymes and lipid peroxidation in brain regions of rat.

	Cortex	Striatum	Medulla	Cerebellum	Hypothalamus
SOD					
AE	NC	NC	NC	NC	NC
Et	+33%	NC	−45%	NC	NC
AE + Et	+31%	−57%	−41%	NC	NC
CAT					
AE	NC	NC	NC	NC	NC
Et	−54%	+92%	+114%	NC	−57%
AE + Et	NC	NC	+42%	NC	−65%
GSH-Px					
AE	+147%	NC	NC	NC	NC
Et	NC	+138%	NC	NC	+189%
AE + Et	NC	+69%	NC	NC	+176%
GR					
AE	−17%	NC	NC	NC	NC
Et	NC	+52%	NC	NC	NC
AE + Et	NC	+37%	NC	NC	NC
MDA					
AE	NC	+112%	NC	NC	NC
Et	+73%	NC	NC	NC	NC
AE + Et	NC	NC	+58%	NC	NC

NC: no change; SOD: superoxide dismutase; CAT: catalase; GSH-Px: glutathione peroxidase; GR: glutathione reductase; MDA: malondialdehyde.

cerebellum in response to exercise training and chronic ethanol ingestion. The combination significantly depletes GSH levels in the cortex, striatum and medulla, whereas GSH/GSSG ratios decrease in the medulla only (Table 5). Therefore, we suggest that exercise training may protect certain brain regions from ethanol-induced oxidative injury.

5. CENTRAL NERVOUS SYSTEM DISEASES — REACTIVE OXYGEN SPECIES/ANTIOXIDANT SYSTEM

Recent evidences have shown that ROS and free radicals are implicated in the etiology and pathogenesis of CNS diseases such as Alzheimer's disease, Parkinson's disease, Amyotrophic Lateral Sclerosis, Down syndrome, Multiple System Atrophy, Huntington diseases, neuritis, stroke, epilepsy and other cerebrovascular and neurodegenerative disorders. During CNS disease processes, ROS are generated and react with proteins, lipids and nucleic acids. Damage to functional groups in biological molecules causes molecular and cellular oxidative damage that leads to CNS disease. Brain cells are endowed with an elaborate antioxidant defense system to scavenge ROS in the process of CNS diseases.

This section addresses the etiology of CNS diseases and changes in the antioxidant system during the development of specific CNS disorders.

Table 5. Interaction of exercise training (ET) and chronic ethanol ingestion (CEt) on antioxidant system and lipid peroxidation in brain regions of rat.

	Cortex	Striatum	Medulla	Cerebellum	Hypothalamus
SOD					
ET	NC	+36%	−20%	−15%	−25%
CEt	−75%	NC	−40%	−15%	−25%
ET + CEt	−31%	+58%	−41%	−53%	−32%
CAT					
ET	NC	NC	NC	NC	−23%
CEt	−34%	−44%	NC	NC	−42%
ET + CEt	NC	NC	NC	NC	NC
GSH-Px					
ET	+33%	NC	NC	−22%	+43%
CEt	NC	NC	NC	−22%	NC
ET + CEt	+41%	+42%	NC	NC	+64%
GR					
ET	+62%	+214%	−20%	NC	NC
CEt	+43%	+221%	−40%	+43%	NC
ET + CEt	+84%	+356%	−41%	+49%	NC
MDA					
ET	−50%	−31%	NC	−25%	−29%
CEt	+30%	NC	−34%	NC	+40%
ET +CEt	NC	NC	−40%	−31%	NC
GSH					
ET	NC	NC	NC	NC	ND
CEt	−17%	−42%	−59%	NC	ND
ET + CEt	−24%	−39%	−52%	NC	ND
GSSG					
ET	NC	NC	NC	NC	ND
CEt	NC	NC	NC	ND	
ET + CEt	NC	−33%	NC	NC	ND
GSH/GSSG Ratio					
ET	NC	NC	NC	NC	ND
CEt	NC	NC	−62%	−34%	ND
ET + CEt	NC	NC	−56%	NC	ND

NC: no change; ND: not detected; SOD: superoxide dismutase; CAT: catalase; GSH-Px: glutathione peroxidase; GR: glutathione reductase; MDA: malondialdehyde; GSH: reduced glutathione; GSSG: oxidized glutathione.

5.1 Alzheimer's disease (AD)

AD is a major neurodegenerative disorder. It is characterized by the gradual, progressive formation of neurofibrillary tangles, senile plaques and loss of selective neurons [95,96]. The most severe of all AD symptoms seen in humans is a gradual loss of memory, reasoning and orientation. Although a number of hypotheses have been put forward as to the cause of AD, the pathogenetic mechanism is still obscure. One hypothesis speculates that ROS play a pivotal role in the pathogenesis of AD [97]. It has been suggested that in AD, ROS interact with amyloid protein to form senile plaques, while amyloid protein itself may generate ROS within the membrane [98–100]. The activation of microglia by β-amyloid, and electron transport chain defects have also been proposed to generate ROS in AD [101,102]. The induction of heme-oxygenase-1 is associated with neurofibrilla tangles and senile plaques in AD [103]. Fibroblasts from AD patients have also shown increased sensitivity to ROS [104,105]. Thus, ROS can initiate LPO, an early stage of tissue damage implicated as one of the mechanisms by which oxidative damage occurs during the onset of AD [106]. Studies in humans have detected an increased LPO in diseased CNS tissues when they are compared with control samples (Table 6). Studies indicate that AD is associated with an increased basal and Fe^{++}-induced formation of MDA in the frontal cortex but not in cerebellum [107]. An increased Fe^{++}/H_2O_2-induced formation of MDA in the cortex, but not in the cerebellum, has been reported in AD studies [108]. Other studies, as shown in Table 5, have also indicated an increased LPO product in the cortex of AD patients [109–114].

The changes in CNS antioxidant systems of AD cases are summarized in Table 6. This data indicates that SOD activity typically increases in the brain, and in specific areas of the brain, of individuals with AD [110,111,115–118]. However, a few studies demonstrated a decrease in brain SOD activity and cerebrospinal fluid (CSF) in AD cases [109,119]. Since both decreases and increases in SOD protein levels were noticed in the brain regions of AD cases [120,121], superoxide influx is likely to be increased in specific brain regions of AD patients. Likewise, a trend of increases and decreases in CAT activity has been shown in specific brain areas of AD cases [110,111,115], while CAT protein levels only increase in the H plus parahippocampal gyri [121]. Both increases and decreases in GSH-Px and GR activity are seen in specific brain regions of AD cases [110]. Similarly, GSH and GSSG levels also fluctuate in particular brain regions of AD cases. Such studies of antioxidant system functioning during AD do not indicate consistency. Further correlative studies are required to resolve the issue of antioxidant enzyme activity, mRNA and protein levels in specific brain areas of AD patients and control subjects.

5.2 Parkinson's disease (PD)

PD is a major progressive movement disorder that occurs most commonly in the elderly, and is characterized by selective degeneration of nigral dopaminergic neurons projecting to the caudate-putamen [122]. The etiology of PD is unknown, however, recent evidence suggests the involvement of ROS and oxidative stress in the development of this disorder [123,124]. The current hypothesis speculates the formation of ROS, which may lead to neuronal damage due to oxidative stress [125,126]. Results form postmortem studies have provided evidence supporting the involvement of oxidative stress in the pathogenesis of PD. Neurotoxin 1-methyl-4-phenyl-1,2,3,6-tetrahydropyridine (MPTP) is selectively toxic to nigros-

Table 6. Central nervous system disorders and antioxidant system/lipid peroxidation.

CNS disorder	Species	Brain/brain regions	% Change (+ increase; - decrease)						References
			SOD	CAT	GSH-Px	GR	GSH or GSSG	LPO	
Alzheimer's disease	Human	Cortex gyrus cinguli	+12C	-	-	-	-	-	Marklund et al. [115]
			+10M						
		Hippocampus	-5C	-	-	-	-	-	
			+19M						
		Hypothalamus	+4C	-	-	-	-	-	
			+5M						
		Nucleus caudatus	+23C	-	-	-	-	-	
			+8M						
Alzheimer's disease	Human	Amygdala	+8	-29	-	-	-	-	Gsell et al. [116]
		Basal nucleus M.	+8	-7					
		Caudate nucleus	+19	-26					
		Entorhinal cortex	+6	-2					
		Frontal cortex	+11	-13					
		Hippocampus	+8	-6					
		Occipital cortex	+7	-8					
		Parietal cortex	+8	-24					
		Putamen	-2	-27					
		Temporal cortex	+15	-19					
Alzheimer's disease	Human	Cerebral cortex	-1 Cp	-	-	-	-	-	Kurobe et al. [120]
			-22 Mp						
Alzheimer's disease	Human	Cerebrospinal fluid	-35	-	-	-	-	-	Bracco et al. [119]
Alzheimer's disease	Human	Cerebellum	-25	-	-	-	-	-	Richardson [109]
		Frontal cortex	-35					+300	
		Hippocampus	-27						

(Continued.)

Table 6. Continued.

CNS disorder	Species	Brain/brain regions	% Change (+ increase; – decrease)						References
			SOD	CAT	GSH-Px	GR	GSH or GSSG	LPO	
Alzheimer's disease	Human	Amygdala	+55	-42	+5	+50	–	+112	Lovell et al. [110]
		Cerebellum	+14	+25	-38	+5	–	+5	
		Hippocampus	+51	+106	+61	+44	–	+140	
		Inferior parietal lobule	+21	+17	-5	+7	–	+6	
		Middle frontal gyrus	+28	-19	-36	+12	–	+8	
		Occipital pole	+15	+112	-33	+10	–	+93	
		Pyriform cortex	+120	+82	+10	+27	–	+500	
		Superior and middle temporal gyri	+150	+300	-80	-90	–	+40	
Alzheimer's disease	Human	Amygdala	+29	+100	–	–	+5	+5	Balaz and Leon [111]
		Cerebellum	-15	+6	–	–	-6	+6	
		Frontal lobe	+55	-5	–	–	+4	+43	
		Hippocampus	+22	+70	–	–	-21	+22	
		Motor cortex	+24	+16	–	–	-38	+32	
		Meynert N.	NC	+12	–	–	-30	+16	
		Olfactory bulb	-10	NC	–	–	+74	+27	
		Occipital lobe	+80	-15	–	–	-18	+75	
		Parahippocampal gyrus	+31	+21	–	–	-10	+18	
		Parolfactory gyrus	+7	-6	–	–	-24	+32	
		Prepyriformgyrus	+9	+45	–	–	-5	+53	
		Sensory cortex	+14	+50	–	–	-14	+40	
Alzheimer's disease	Human	Brain	+30	–	–	–	–	–	Zemlan et al. [117]
Alzheimer's disease	Human	Hippocampus plus parahippocampal gyri	+25P	+50P	–	–	–	–	Pappolla et al. [121]

(Continued.)

Table 6. Continued.

CNS disorder	Species	Brain/brain regions	% Change (+ increase; − decrease)						References
			SOD	CAT	GSH–Px	GR	GSH or GSSG	LPO	
Alzheimer's disease	Human	Frontal cortex	—	—	—	—	+12	—	Perry et al. [144]
		Hippocampus	—	—	—	—	+37	—	
		Occipital cortex	—	—	—	—	+21	—	
		Substantia innominta	—	—	—	—	+20	—	
		Substantia nigra	—	—	—	—	+6	—	
Alzheimer's disease	Human	Temporal cortex						+35	McIntosh et al. [112]
Alzheimer's disease	Human	Inferior parietal lobe	—	—	—	—	—	+12	Palmer and Burns [113]
		Inferior temporal gyrus	—	—	—	—	—	+40	
		Occipital cortex	—	—	—	—	—	+5	
		Sensory/motor cortex	—	—	—	—	—	+6	
		Superior frontal gyrus	—	—	—	—	—	+9	
		Superior temporal gyrus	—	—	—	—	—	+35	
Alzheimer's disease	Human	Temporal cortex	—	—	—	—	—	+42	Andorn et al. [114]
Alzheimer's disease	Human	Hippocampus plus associative cortex	+50C	—	—	—	—	—	Delacourte et al. [117]
Parkinson's disease	Human	Cerebrospinal fluid	−2	NC	+9	+12	—	—	Marttila et al. [139])
		Amygdala	−1C, −9M	+3	+13	−8	—	—	
		Caudatus	−7C, −15M	−12	−18	+11	—	—	
		Cerebellum	+33C, +40M	+10	+33	−9	—	—	
		C. semiovale	−2C, NC,M	+17	−7	+3	—	—	
		Frontal cortex	+22C, +11M	+31	+9	+15	—	—	
		Nucleus ruber	+38C, +9M	+18	NC	+57	—	—	
		Nucleus basalis	+97C, +2M	−23	+44	+10	—	—	
		Pallidum	+29C, −13M	−16	−1	+14	—	—	
		Putamen	+3C, NC,M	+29	+36	+13	—	—	
		Substantia nigra	+55C, −6M	−21	−1	+11	—	—	
		Temporal cortex	+55C, +15M	+3	+9	−5	—	—	
		Thalamus	+27C, +11M		−20		—	—	

Table 6. Continued.

CNS disorder	Species	Brain/brain regions	% Change (+ increase; – decrease)						References
			SOD	CAT	GSH-Px	GR	GSH or GSSG	LPO	
Parkinson's disease	Human	Caudate	–	–32	–50	–	–	–	Ambani et al. [140]
		Cerebellum	–	–25	NC	–	–	–	
		Frontal cortex	–	NC	–9	–	–	–	
		Globus pallidus	–	–40	–10	–	–	–	
		Hypothalamus	–	–27	+6	–	–	–	
		Occipital cortex	–	–21	–20	–	–	–	
		Putamen	–	–32	–45	–	–	–	
		Red nucleus	–	–30	+7	–	–	–	
		Substantia nigra	–	–35	–60	–	–	–	
		Temporal cortex	–	–20	NC	–	–	–	
		Thalamus	–	–25	–30	–	–	–	
		Vermis	–	–14	–10	–	–	–	
Parkinson's disease	Human	Cerebellum	–2.5 +4C –6M	–	–	–	–	–	Saggu et al. [137]
		Substantia nigra	+4 –1C +33M	–	–	–	–	–	
Parkinson's disease	Human	Caudate nucleus	–	–	–	–	–6	+20	Jenner et al. [130]
		Cerebellum	+4C –6M	–	–	–	–	+29	
		Cerebral cortex	–	–	–	–	–30	+10	
		Globus pallidus	–	–	–	–	–8	+19	
		Putamen	–	–	–	–	–38	+770	
		Substantia nigra	–1C +33M	–	–	–	–40	–	

(Continued.)

Table 6. Continued.

CNS disorder	Species	Brain/brain regions	% Change (+ increase; decrease)						Reference
			SOD	CAT	GSH-Px	GR	GSH or GSSG	LPO	
Parkinson's disease	Human	Striatum	–	–	–	–	–35	–	DiMonte et al. [142]
Parkinson's disease	Human	Caudate nucleus	–	–	–	–	–17	–	Perry and Yong [143]
		Cerebellar cortex	–	–	–	–	–16	–	
		Frontal cortex	–	–	–	–	–14	–	
		Occipital cortex	–	–	–	–	–14	–	
		Putamen	–	–	–	–	–19	–	
		Substantia nigra	–	–	–	–	–28	–	
Parkinson's disease	Human	Caudate nucleus	–	–	–	–	–6T	–	Perry et al. [144]
							+14		
		Cerebellar cortex	–	–	–	–	–20T	–	
							+24		
		Frontal cortex	–	–	–	–	–14T	–	
							–18		
		Occipital cortex	–	–	–	–	–14T	–	
							+9		
		Substantia nigra	–	–	–	–	–33T	–	
							–100		
Parkinson's disease	Human	Caudate	–	–	–7	–	–	–	Kish et al. [141]
		Frontal cortex	–	–	–20	–	–	–	
		Globus pallidus	–	–	–26	–	–	–	
		Putamen	–	–	–14	–	–	–	
		Substantia nigra	–	–	–19	–	–	–	
		Temporal cortex	–	–	–9	–	–	–	

(Continued.)

Table 6. Continued.

CNS disorder	Species	Brain/brain regions	% Change (+ increase; − decrease)						References
			SOD	CAT	GSH-Px	GR	GSH or GSSG	LPO	
Parkinson's disease	Human	Caudate	—	—	—	—	—	+11	Dexter et al. [129]
		Cerebellum	—	—	—	—	—	+24	
		Cortex	—	—	—	—	—	−6	
		Globus pallidus (L)	—	—	—	—	—	+21	
		Globus pallidus (M)	—	—	—	—	—	+11	
		Putamen (lateral)	—	—	—	—	—	+4	
		Putamen (medial)	—	—	—	—	—	+5	
		Substantial nigra	—	—	—	—	—	+35	
Parkinson's disease	Human	Substantia nigra	—	—	—	—	−47 Red / −26 Oxi	—	Sofic et al. [145]
Parkinson's disease	Human	Caudate nucleus	—	—	+17	—	—	—	
		Cerebral cortex	—	—	−7	—	—	—	
		Globus pallidus (L)	—	—	−5	—	—	—	
		Globus pallidus (M)	—	—	−16	—	—	—	
		Putamen	—	—	+10	—	—	—	
		Substantia nigra	—	—	+9	—	—	—	
Parkinson's disease	Human	Caudate nucleus	—	—	—	—	−4 Red / −17 Oxi	—	Sian et al. [123]
		Cerebral cortex	—	—	—	—	−20 Red / +11 Oxi	—	
		Globus pallidus (L)	—	—	—	—	−8 Red / +12 Oxi	—	
		Globus pallidus (M)	—	—	—	—	−8 Red / +2 Oxi	—	
		Putamen	—	—	—	—	−30 Red / +26 Oxi	—	
		Substantia nigra	—	—	—	—	−40 Red / +29 Oxi	—	

(Continued.)

Table 6. Continued.

CNS disorder	Species	Brain/brain regions	% Change (+ increase; – decrease)						References
			SOD	CAT	GSH-Px	GR	GSH or GSSG	LPO	
Parkinson's disease	Human	Brain	–	–	–	–	–48 to –90T	–	Riederer et al. [146]
Parkinson's disease	Human	Cerebrospinal fluid	+2C +60M	–	–	–	–	–	Yoshida et al. [138]
Amyotrophic lateral sclerosis	Human	Cerebrospinal fluid	+27C +100M	–	–	–	–	–	Yoshida et al. [138]
Amyotrophic lateral sclerosis	Human	Brain	–43C	–	–	–	–	–	Rosen et al. [151]
Amyotrophic lateral sclerosis	Human	Brain	+81C	–	–	–	–	+36	Feaster et al [153]
Amyotrophic lateral sclerosis	Human	Cerebrospinal fluid	–63	–	–	–	–	–	Bracco et al. [119]
Amyotrophic lateral sclerosis	Human	Brain	–38C, –1M (F) –10C, –7M (S)	–	–	–	–	–	Bowling et al. [150]
Down syndrome	Human	Cerebral cortex	+60C	–	–2	–	–	–	Brooksbank and Balazs [158]
Multiple system atrophy	Human	Caudate nucleus	–	–	–	–	+40 or NC	–	Sian et al. [123]
		Cerebral cortex	–	–	–	–	–25 or +25	–	
		Globus pallidus (L)	–	–	–	–	+96 or –60	–	
		Globus pallidus (M)	–	–	–	–	–10 or +25	–	
		Putamen (L)	–	–	–	–	–29 or –33	–	
		Putamen (M)	–	–	–	–	–30 or NC	–	
		Substantia nigra	–	–	–	–	–15 or +10	–	

(Continued.)

Table 6. Continued.

CNS disorder	Species	Brain/brain regions	% Change (+ increase; − decrease)						References
			SOD	CAT	GSH-Px	GR	GSH or GSSG	LPO	
Huntington's disease	Human	Cerebrospinal fluid	+50C +60M	—	—	—	—	—	Yoshida et al. [138]
Huntington's disease	Human	Caudate nucleus Cerebral cortex Substantia nigra	— — —	— — —	— — —	— — —	−10 or −50 −13 or −40 +5 or ND	— — —	Sian et al. [123]
Cerebrovascular injury	Human	Cerebrospinal fluid	+114	—	—	—	—	—	Gruener et al. [175]
Cerebrovascular injury	Rat	Cerebral cortex	+4C +63M	+23	+22	+56	—	+59	Singh and Pathak [181]
Cerebrovascular injury	Rat	Hippocampus	—	—	—	—	—	+913	Willmore et al. [180]
Cerebrovascular injury	Rat	Isocortex	—	—	—	—	—	+56	Willmore and Rubin [182]

SOD: superoxide dismutase; CAT: catalase; GSH-Px: glutathione peroxidase; GR: glutathione reductase; GSH: reduced glutathione; GSSG: oxidized glutathione; LPO: lipid peroxidation; C: CuZn-SOD; M: Mn-SOD; Mp: Mn-SOD protein; NC: no change; P: protein; T: total GSH + GSSG; Red: reduced glutathione; Oxi: oxidized glutathione; F: familial; S: sporadic; Cp: CuZn-SOD protein.

triatal dopaminergic neurons, thereby providing a model and a clue to the mechanism in PD [127]. Oxidative stress in PD may also arise from the slow metabolism rate of dopamine [128]. Studies have indicated that LPO is involved in the death of neurons in PD patients [129–132]. The finding of an inverted iron content in the substantia nigra of a Parkinson's brain further supports this phenomenon [129,133,134]. The nature of ROS responsible for cell death in PD implicates H_2O_2 and ·OH [135,136]. The alteration in antioxidant systems in select areas of the PD brain is summarized in Table 5. In most studies, manganese-superoxide dismutase (Mn-SOD) activity increased in the substantia nigra of PD cases [129,136] and also in the cerebrospinal fluid of PD patients [138] Both increases and decreases in CAT and GSH-Px activity has been reported in the substantia nigra of PD cases [123,139–141].

The consistent depletion of endogenous antioxidant GSH in the substantia nigra suggests that GSH plays a pivotal role in the pathogenesis of PD (Table 6). Such a depletion in human PD cases has been reported [123,129,142–145]. Other studies have also demonstrated a depletion of total glutathione and increased levels of oxidized glutathione (GSSG) [123,144,146]. Thus, the GSH depletion may initiate a cascade of events, such as enhanced LPO, leading to the destruction of nigrastriatal pathways. In addition, GSH depletion may also render the nigrostriatal pathway prone to a toxic insult. Such studies indicate that oxidative damage is present in the brain of PD.

5.3 Amyotrophic lateral sclerosis (ALS)

ALS is a motor neuron-degenerative disease that is usually fatal within 5 years of the onset of symptoms. The paralysis of the victim is due to the degeneration of motor neurons in the brain and spinal cord, however, the underlying etiology of the neurodegeneration is not clear. About 10% of ALS cases are familiar whereas 20% of ALS cases are familial (FALS). FALS is clinically defined as an age-dependent autosomal dominant trait [147,148]. Studies have demonstrated 11 distinct FALS-associated mutations in exon 2 and 4 of the gene encoding cyto-stolic copper zinc superoxide dismutase (CuZn-SOD). Additional mutations have also been reported [149]. SOD activity in the postmortem frontal cortex of FALS patients with missense mutations is significantly decreased, but the decrease in enzyme activity did not occur in patients with sporadic ALS nor in a FALS case without a missense mutation of CuZn-SOD [150]. Protein carbonyl content, a measure of protein oxidation, increase in patients with sporadic ALS vs. a control group, which suggests that oxidative stress is a common feature of ALS. Alterations in the activity of the human brain's antioxidant enzyme SOD and cerebrospinal fluid in ALS cases are depicted in Table 6.

Most studies indicate that CuZn-SOD activity in the brain and cerebrospinal fluid decrease in human ALS cases [119,150–152]. However, a few studies show an increase in brain CuZn-SOD activity [153], as well as an increase in CuZn-SOD and Mn-SOD activity in the cerebrospinal fluid of ALS patients [138]. It has been suggested that an altered, noval function of this enzyme, rather than a reduction of its activity, may be responsible for the pathogenesis of FALS [154]. Recent reports indicate that oxidative reactions that are catalyzed by mutant CuZn-SOD enzymes are likely to initiate the neuropathological changes in ALS patients [149,155]. Therefore, the antioxidant enzyme therapy may be useful for the treatment of ALS.

5.4 Down syndrome (DS)

DS is a neurodegenerative disease, similar to dementia of Alzheimer's [156,157]. DS patients possess additional genetic material typically, an extra chromosome 21, which has been linked to various physical abnormalities. The genetic abnormality in DS individuals with trisomy 21, resulting in mental retardation, is not understood scientifically. Possibly, an overexpression of SOD may result in the excess production of H_2O_2 which is then followed by excessive hydroxyl radical production and a subsequent attack of cellular constituents. Table 6 depicts the changes in antioxidant systems and LPO in the brain of DS cases. An increased SOD activity, but no significant rise in GSH-Px activity, has been reported in the DS fetal brain [158]. Similar studies demonstrate an increase in SOD and GSH-Px activity in the fibroblast of DS patients [153,159], along with an increase in LPO [158,160]. These studies suggest that oxidative stress is involved in the pathogenesis of DS, and antioxidant therapy may be useful in DS cases.

5.5 Multiple system atrophy (MSA)

Multiple system atrophy (MSA) is a neurodegenerative disorder similar to PD. Pathologically there is nigrostriatal degeneration with marked gliosis and cell loss in the substantia nigra, caudate nucleus and putamen [123]. Table 6 summarizes the changes in antioxidant systems in the brain regions and cerebrospinal fluid of MSA cases. The GSH content of the lateral globus pallidus in MSA patients increases as compared to control subjects, whereas the GSSG content decreases [123]. The GSH level also decreases in substantia nigra and putamen. The nigral GSH/GSSG ratio decreased in MSA patients when compared to controls, indicating an oxidative stress condition in MSA patients. Yoshida et al. [138] have observed that CuZn-SOD and Mn-SOD protein levels increased in the CSF of MSA patients. Such results tend to suggest that the blood-brain barrier may be destroyed in MSA patients and CuZn-SOD in the blood may affect their CuZn-SOD levels. However, the increase in Mn-SOD levels may be caused by an induction in damaged tissue, since inflammatory cells are known to induce the biosynthesis of Mn-SOD by cytokines (161). Apparently, more detailed studies are required to examine the complete antioxidant system to clarify the etiology of MSA in humans.

5.6 Huntington's disease (HD)

HD is a neurodegenerative and psychiatric disorder. It is characterized by atrophy with gliosis and marked neuronal loss in the caudate nucleus and putamen [123]. A number of hypotheses have been proposed, but the etiology of HD is still unclear. However, the oxidative stress hypotheses may be involved in the pathogenesis of this disease. Table 6 summarizes the alterations in the brain's antioxidant system and cerebrospinal fluid of HD patients. Sian et al. [123] demonstrated that GSH levels are slightly decreased in the CC and caudate nucleus, whereas GSSG levels were depleted in these regions of HD cases. Yoshida et al. [138] measured CuZn-SOD and Mn-SOD protein levels in the CSF of HD cases to find that both CuZn-SOD and Mn-SOD levels increase in the CSF of HD patients, thus, indicating the damage of the blood-brain barrier, inflammatory reactions in the damaged tissues, and the release of cytokines. The cytokines are known to involve the activation and biosynthesis of Mn-SOD [161]. Apparently, a complete analysis of antioxidant systems would yield more understanding of the mechanism involved in the pathogenesis of HD.

5.7 Cerebrovascular injury

Head and spinal cord injury, as well as cerebral ischemia and stroke, are very common in society [162]. The severity of CNS injury appears to correlate with the incidence of post-traumatic epilepsy. CNS trauma initiates a sequence of responses such as altered blood flow and vasoregulation, disruption of the blood-brain-barrier, increases in intracranial pressure, ischemia, hemorrhage, inflammation and necrosis [163]. The pathophysiological process underlying disorders of CNS injury are not well understood. However, recent studies have emphasized the effect of free radicals on the pathogenesis of cerebrovascular injuries. Demopolous et al. [164] first proposed the free radical hypothesis associated with CNS injuries and it has been subsequently supported by other investigators [165–167]. Severe elevation of the arterial blood pressure causes cerebrovascular injury, which has been demonstrated to be a result of excess superoxide generation [168]. Ischemia, induced by occlusion of the arterial supply to the CNS, causes neurological dysfunction [169]. Suppressing generation has also been demonstrated in cerebral vessels, as well as in the CSF, after ischemia [170,171]. Many investigators have reported increased LPO following cerebral ischemia injury [164,172]. There are evidences implicating ROS generation in cerebral hemorrhages due to the fact that hemoglobin is capable of releasing superoxides [25] and increasing LPO during cerebral hemorrhages [173]. It has also been shown that traumatic injury to the brain or to the spinal cord is mediated by the production of superoxide [174,175]. There are indirect evidences of ROS generation as evidenced by enhanced lipid-peroxidation after traumatic CNS injury [176,177]. The precise mechanism of post-traumatic epilepsy remains unknown, although it has been suggested that blood in contact with cortical tissue is associated with epileptogenesis. A contusion or cortical laceration causes the extravasation of red blood cells, with hemolysis and a deposition of hemoglobin within the neutrophil. Iron, liberated from hemoglobin and transferrin, can cause free radical generation and the initiation of LPO causing human post-traumatic epilepsy [178,179] and experimental epilepsy in animals [180,181]. Table 6 summarizes the changes in antioxidant systems following cerebrovascular injury in human and rats. Analysis of CSF from acute stroke patients reveals an increase in SOD contents indicating that superoxides are formed in these patients, and an increased synthesis of SOD protein may protect the oxidative damage of superoxide radicals [175]. Cerebrovascular injury in rats demonstrated an increase in antioxidant enzymes Mn-SOD, CAT, GSH-Px and GR in the cerebral tissues, as well as enhanced LPO [180—182]. These studies suggest that ROS are involved in the pathogenesis of cerebrovascular injury.

6   STRATEGIES TO IMPROVE CNS FUNCTIONS

6.1 Antioxidant supplementation

Recent studies suggest that ROS and free radical-induced oxidative stress is involved in CNS oxygen toxicity, both during exercise and in the pathogenesis of CNS disorders. Therefore, antioxidant nutrients may play a significant role in the prevention and management of CNS injuries brought on by oxidative stress. During antioxidant therapy, it is essential to consider the types of ROS and free radicals and their modes of action and origin, as well as the use of hydrophilic vs. lipophilic antioxidants. There is convincing evidence that oxidative damage in the CNS and its functions can be improved by exogenous antioxidant supplements.

6.1.1 *Vitamins*

Vitamin E is among the major lipid antioxidant vitamins and vitamin C is a major water-soluble antioxidant vitamin. Free radical-induced LPO has been shown to be suppressed in the CNS of animals during neuronal degeneration by vitamin E supplementation [165,183]. Vitamin E deficiencies enhance the effects of HBO on the CNS while vitamin E supplementation decreases it [59,60]. In experimental animals, iron-induced trauma was blocked by vitamin E and selenium [163,182]. Supplementing the body with vitamin E has proven to be most effective against Tardive dyskinesia [184]. Dietary vitamin E supplements in rats have also resulted in a reduction of LPO after swimming exercise [185]. In humans, dietary vitamin E supplementation for 2 weeks or a single dose reduced the extent of LPO caused by exercise-induced oxidative stress [78,186]. Unfortunately, however, vitamin E is an unsuitable therapy for acute CNS injury due to its low nervous system uptake levels [187]. Vitamin E supplements also decrease the incidence of intraventricular cerebrovascular injury [177] and cerebral ischemia [188]. Recently, vitamin E supplementation has been shown to be protective against neurodegeneration from PD [124]. More recently, it has been suggested that oral antioxidant supplementation may be preventive against LPO in the human brain [112]. However, as previously noted, vitamin E is less effective against acute brain injury and ischemia [189].

Vitamin C, or ascorbate, has dual effects. It acts as a pro-oxidant at low concentrations and as an antioxidant at higher concentrations [23]. Dietary administration of vitamin C has been shown to be effective in preventing exercise-induced oxidative stress [190]. The protective effect of vitamin C has also been demonstrated against oxidative injury in cerebral ischemia [188]. Preliminary data have revealed that ascorbic acid supplementation may improve the recovery of exercise-induced oxidative tissue injury. While there is no convincing evidence that oxidative damage in the CNS can be suppressed by vitamin C supplements, vitamin C can regenerate vitamin E, directly. Therefore, the combination of both may be more effective than ingesting either vitamin alone.

β-carotenes, apart from being the best source of vitamin A, have been reported to be free radical quenchers, $^1O_2$ scavengers, and inhibitors of LPO. β-carotene-rich diets have been shown to protect against CNS oxygen toxicity in rats [77]. It is suggested that β-carotene, or vitamin A, may also be beneficial to other CNS disorders.

6.1.2 Glutathione (GSH)

GSH is the most abundant thiol present in the cells. The roles of GSH include:
1) to serve as a cosubstrate for GSH peroxidase (GPX), wherein GSH is used as a hydrogen donor to reduce H_2O_2 and organic peroxide to water and alcohol, respectively;
2) to conjugate with exogenous and endogenous toxic compounds, catalyzed by GSH sulfur-transferase;
3) to reduce protein disulfide and GSH-protein mixed disulfide bonds, maintaining the sulfhydryl residues of certain proteins and enzymes in the reduced state;
4) to restore cysteine in a nontoxic form; and
5) GSH assumes a vital role in keeping α-tocopherol (vitamin E) and ascorbic acid (vitamin C) in reduced states.

GSH administration in rats has proven effective in protecting against hyperbaric CNS oxygen toxicity [62,63]. Exogenous GSH administration may not be able to reach CNS in sufficient concentrations because of its degradation in the blood and tissues. Therefore, GSH esters have been more effective against cisplatin-induced neurotoxicity [191]. GSH has been found to be effectively protective against CNS oxygen toxicity in rats and mice [62,63,65,74]. In addition, glutathione supplementation is also known to be protective against exercise-induced oxidative stress [192]. The depletion of GSH in PD brains suggests that GSH plays an important role in the disease's pathogenesis. Therefore, GSH, or its esters supplementations, have therapeutic inplications for the management and prevention of PD [144].

6.1.3 Antioxidant enzymes (AOE)

AOE are a significant defense mechanism for neuronal cells combating CNS oxygen toxicity [23]. Yusa et al. [69] have shown that treating rats with liposomes containing SOD and CAT, 2 h before HBO exposure, shifts the onset of convulsions. SOD has been reported to diminish reperfusion injury after spinal cord ischemia [193] and cerebral edema in rats [194]. Similarly, cerebrovascular injury caused by acute hypertension has been shown to be reversable with SOD and CAT treatment [168,195]. CNS traumatic injury has been reported preventable and reversable due to SOD and CAT administration [174]. Enzymatic antioxidants (SOD, CAT, and GSH-Px) usually act for only a short time, and have poor ability to cross the blood-brain-barrier and reach the specific site of injury. Therefore, more research is required to achieve maximum protective effects against CNS injury with antioxidant enzymes. Fortunately, Ebselen, a low molecular weight agent that has GSH-Px-like activity [183] and inhibits LPO. It has recently been shown to be otoprotective against cisplatin-induced ototoxicity [196].

6.1.4 Other free radical scavengers

Other therapies have been studied for their potential role in ROS/free radical-induced CNS diseases. For instance, cerebrovascular injury has reportedly been prevented by pretreatment with mannitol, a scavenger of hydroxyl radicals [195,197]. Evidently, Dimethyl sulfoxide (DMSO) prevents ischemic myelopathy and paresis in dogs subjected to ischemia of the spinal cord [198]. In addition, the use of chelating agents that prevent iron ions from participating in hydroxyl radical production and LPO has also been studied in association with CNS disorders. A new series of 21-amino steroids (Lazaroids) with built-in iron chelating activity has been developed for the acute treatment of CNS injury [199]. Such agents, with antioxidant properties, have been tested in head injury, spinal cord injury, stroke, neurotoxicity, hemorrhage, and reperfusion injury [189,200]. Free radical spin trappers such as N-tert-butyl%-phenyl nitrone (PBN) have also been tried as protectors against CNS disorders [34,201,202]. As a result of such studies, it is suggested that the derivatives of PBN will have therapeutic use in the future. Striatal lesions produced by malonate has reportedly been attenuated by coenzyme Q_{10} [203]. The administration of coenzyme Q_{10} for 1 month in HD patients reveals a significant protection against such lesions [204]. Nerve growth factor protects rat hippocampal and human cortical neurons against iron-induced injury [205]. Interestingly, endogenous cofactors %-lipoic acid and dihydrolipoic acid, which are well tolerated in humans are also neuroprotective against cerrebrovascular injury [206—208]. Recently, we have also demonstrated a dose-dependent protection of %-lipoic acid against cisplatin-induced ototoxicity [217].

It is suggested that the use of antioxidants and free radical scavengers in the treatment of neurodegenerative diseases requires more detailed studies.

7   SUMMARY

1. Breathing oxygen is essential for human and animal life, but at high levels of pressure, oxygen can cause central nervous system (CNS) toxicity. The generation of reactive oxygen species (ROS) and free radicals occurs due to an increase in oxygen pressure in the brain during exercise, as well as in the development processes of neurodegenerative diseases.
2. Several reports indicate that HBO exposure results in the formation of ROS and lipid peroxides in the CNS and depletes the antioxidant system. Studies show that exercise-induced oxidative stress commonly generates ROS and lipid peroxides and perturbs the antioxidant enzymes and glutathione in specific brain regions of animals. Recent evidences have also demonstrated perturbation of the CNS antioxidant system in many CNS disorders.
3. The combination of exercise training and alcohol ingestion on CNS antioxidant systems has also recently been studied. It is suggested that exercise training may protect certain brain regions against ethanol-induced oxidative injury. Even peripherally acting drugs pyridostigmine and others have been reported to cross the blood-brain-barrier and affect CNS functions during physical stress.
4. Antioxidant nutrients appear to play a significant role in the prevention and management of CNS injuries that are caused by oxidative stress. There is convincing evidence that oxidative damage in the CNS and its functions can be improved by exogenous antioxidant supplements, such as antioxidant vitamins, glutathione and antioxidant enzymes. Other therapies, such as the use of radical scavengers, iron chelators, free radical spin trappers and other endogenous antioxidant α-lipoic acids have also protected the brain against CNS injuries.
5. It is suggested that during any type of antioxidant therapy, as well as during the use of hydrophilic or lipophilic antioxidants, the types of ROS/free radicals and their origin and mode of action in the CNS must be considered.

8   PERSPECTIVES

The implication of ROS/free radicals in CNS oxygen toxicity, exercise and drug metabolism, as well as in the pathogenesis of several CNS disorders and injuries, has been studied. However, the roles of endogenous antioxidants, as well as exogenous supplementation in CNS disease processes and injuries have not been well explored. Since GSH plays a pivotal role in the maintenance of the intracellular redox status and AOE functions, during acute exercise and exercise training, it is essential to study results of the exercise performance and intracellular-interorgan homeostasis, especially in the CNS. Recent work on adenosine A_3 receptors, through which adenosine enhances the activity of antioxidant enzymes, has opened a door for studying the interactions of agonists and antagonists of adenosine on antioxidant enzymes and LPO in the CNS during exercise, HBO exposure and neurodegenerative processes. The use of more selective agonists and antagonists, of adenosine A_1 A_2 and A_3 receptors, will provide a better understanding of the mechanisms responsible for the activation or inhibition of antioxidant enzymes in the CNS during exercise, HBO exposure and during neurodegeneration. Exercise, oxygen exposure and CNS injuries may enhance the production of nitric oxide (NO) in cerebrovascular tissues. It is not known whether NO synthase inhibitors or activators would have antagonistic or synergistic effects on adenosine receptor-induced responses in CNS antioxidant systems. Both adenosine and NO may play a role during exercise, cerebrovascular oxygen exposure and during the development of CNS disorders. Therefore, the actions and interactions of both agents, through modulatory receptors on antioxidant systems would be an important future study. Moreover, it is likely that Ca^{++}-dependent enzymes, such as protein kinase C and NO synthase, may contribute to exercise, HBO and CNS injury-induced oxidative stress on cerebrovascular systems. The exploration of calcium channel-blockers, nucleoside transport blockers, protein kinase C and NO synthase inhibitors will provide a better understanding of adenosine receptor-mediated antioxidant responses in cerebrovascular tissues. In addition, further studies of the role of proto-oncogene Bcl-2, transcription factors activator protein-1 (AP-1) and nuclear factor -κB (NF-κB), and heat shock proteins may reveal the intracellular regulation that occurs in the CNS antioxidant defense system during exercise, HBO exposure, as well as during CNS disease processes.

9   ABBREVIATIONS

AChE:	Acetylcholinesterase
AP-1:	Activator protein-1
AD:	Alzheimer's disease
ALS:	Amyotrophic leteral sclerosis
AOE:	Antioxidant enzyme
ATP:	Adenosine triphosphate
BS:	Brain stem
C:	Copper zinc superoxide dismutase
CAT:	Catalase
Cp:	Copper zinc superoxide dismutase protein
CNS:	Central nervous system
CSF:	Cerebrospinal fluid
CC:	Cerebral cortex
CuZn-SOD:	Copper zinc-superoxide dismutase
CS:	Corpus striatum
CO:	Carbon monoxide

DMSO:	Dimethyl sulfoxide
DS:	Down syndrome
F:	Familial
FALS:	Familial amyotrophic lateral sclerosis
GSH:	Glutathione reduced
GSSG:	Glutathione oxidized
GSH-Px:	Glutathione peroxidase
GR:	Glutathione reductase
H:	Hippocampus
HD:	Huntington disease
H_2O:	Water
H_2O2:	Hydrogen peroxide
˙OH:	Hydroxy radical
HBO:	Hyperbaric oxygen
Km:	Michaelis menton constant
LPO:	Lipid peroxidation
M:	Manganese -superoxide dismutase
MDA:	Malondialdehyde
Mn-SOD:	Manganese-superoxide dismutase
MPTP:	1-methyl-4-phenyl-1,2,3,6-tetrahydropyridine
Mp:	Manganese-Superoxide dismutase protein
MSA:	Multiple system atrophy
NADPH:	Nicotimnamide adenine dinucleotide phosphate reduced
NF-kB:	Nuclear factor -kappa B
NO:	Nitric oxide
$^1O_2$:	Singlet oxygen
O_2˙−:	superoxide anion
Oxi:	Oxidized
ONOO-:	Peroxy nitrite anion
PBN:	N-tert-butyl-1-phenyl nitrone
P:	Protein
PD:	Parkinson's disease
Red:	Reduced
ROS:	Reactive oxygen species
S:	Sporadic
SOD:	Superoxide dismutase
T:	Total
VO2 max:	Maximum oxygen consumption

10 REFERENCES

1. Meyers RA, Baker T, Cowley RA. Hyperbaric Oxygen 1992;1:129—133.
2. Harabin AL, Survanshi SS, Homer LD. Toxicol Appl Pharmacol 1995;132:19—26.

3. Torbati D, Church DF, Keller JM, Pryor WA. Free Radic Biol Med 1992;13:101–106.
4. Boveris A, Cadenas E, Boveris A, Cadenas E, Stoppani AOM. Biochem J 1976;156:435–440.
5. Demopoulos HB, Flamma ES, Seligman ML, Jorgensen E, Ransohoff J. Acta Neurol Scand 1977;56(Suppl):152–153.
6. Halliwell B, Gutteridge JMC. Arch Biochem Biophys 1986;246:501–514.
7. Spector R. N Engl J Med 1977;296:1393–1398.
8. Schaefer A, Kumlos M, Seregi A. Biochem Pharmacol 1975;24:1781–1787.
9. Zaleski MM, Floyd RA. Neurochem Res 1985;10:397–410.
10. Lanse SB, Lee JC, Jacobs A, Brody H. Aviat Space Env Med 1978;49:890–898.
11. Davies KJA, Qintanilha AT, Brooks GA, Packer L. Biochem Biophys Res Commun 1982;107:1198–1205.
12. Jenkins RR, Goldfarb A. Med Sci Sports Exerc 1993;25:210–212.
13. Sjodin BY, Hellsten-Westling Y, Apple FS. Sports Med 1990;10:236–254.
14. Somani SM, Arroyo CM. Ind J Physiol Pharmacol 1995;39:323–329.
15. Wolff SP, Dean RT. Biochem J 1987;245:243–250.
16. Kontos HA. Circ Res 1985;57:508–512.
17. Chan DH, Yurko M, Fishman RA. J Neurochem. 1982;38:525–530.
18. Forman HJ Kennedy J. Arch Biochem Biophys 1976;173:219–225.
19. Betz AL. J Neurochem 1985;44:574–580.
20. Povlishock JT, Wei EP, Kontos HA. FASEB J 1988;2:A-835–839.
21. Kukreja RC, Kontos HA, Hess ML, Ellis EF. Circ Res 1986;59:612–618.
22. Kuthan H, Ullrich V. Eur J Biochem 1982;126:583–588.
23. Halliwell B, Gutteridge JMC. Trends in Neurosci 1985;378:22–26.
24. Heikkila RE, Cohen G. Science 1973;181:456–460.
25. Misra HP, Fridovich I. J Biol Chem 1972;247:6960–6967.
26. Blight AR. CNS Trauma 1985;2:299–303.
27. Badwey JA, Karnovsky ML. Ann Rev Biochem 1980;49:695–701.
28. Chance B, Sies H, Boveris A. Physiol Rev 1979;59:72–77.
29. Boveris A, Cadenas E. FEBS Lett 1975;54:311–316.
30. Freeman BA, Crapo JD. Lab Invest 1982;47:412–417.
31. McCord JM, Roy RS. Can J Physiol Pharmacol 1982;60:1346–1350.
32. McCord JM, Day ED. FEBS Lett 1978;86:139–144.
33. Garthwaite J. Trends in Neurosci 1991;14:60–67.
34. Oliver CN, Starke-Reed PE, Stradtman ER, Liu GJ, Carney JM, Floyd RA. Proc Natl Acad Sci USA 1990;87:5144–5147.
35. Carney JM, Starke-Reed PE, Oliver CN, Landum RW, Cheng MS, Wu JF, Floyd RA. Prod Natl Acad Sci USA 1991;88:3633–3636.
36. Ames BN, Shigenaga MK, Hagen TM. Proc Natl Acad Sci 1993;90:7915–7922.
37. Evans PH. Br Med Bull 1993;49:577–587.
38. Husain K. Somani SM. Prog Neuropsychopharmacol Biol Psychiat 1997;21:659–670.
39. Halliwell B, Chirico S. Am J Clin Nutr 1993;57:715–725.
40. Esterbauer H, Schaur RJ, Zollner H. Free Radic Biol Med 1991;11:81–128.
41. Mark RJ, Lovell MA, Markesbery WR, Uchida K, Mattson MP. J Neurochem 1997;68:255–264.
42. Husain K, Dube SN, Sugendran S, Singa R, DasGupta S, Somani SM. J Appl Toxicol 1996;16:245–248.
43. Somani SM, Husain K, Schlorff EC. Oxidants, Antioxidants and Free Radicals (eds) Baskin S, Salem H. Taylor Francis, Washington DC, 1997;125–141.
44. Werner P, Cohen G. Ann NY Acad Sci 1993;679:364–369.
45. Douglas GW, Mortensen RA. J Biol Chem 1956;222:581–585.
46. Sekura R, Meister A. Proc Natl Acad Sci USA 1974;71:2969–2972.
47. Jain A, Martensson J, Stole E, Auld PA, Meister A. Proc Natl Acad Sci 1991;88(5):1913–1917.

48. Kudo H, Kokunai T, Kondoh T, Tamaki N, Matsumoto S. Brain Res 1990;511(2):326—328.
49. Ravindranath V, Shivakumar BR, Anandatheerthavarada HK. Neurosi Lett 1989;101:187—190.
50. Ravindranath V, Reed DJ. Biochem Biophys Res Commun 1990;169:1075—1079.
51. Noda Y, McGeer PL, McGeer EG. J Neurochem 1983;40:1329—1332.
52. Somani SM, Husain K, Diaz—Phillips L, Lanzotti DJ, Kareti KR, Trammell GL. Alcohol 1996; 13:603—610.
53. Jamieson D, Chance B, Cadenas E, Boveris A. Ann Rev Physiol 1986;48:703—719.
54. Gerschman R, Gilbert DL, Nye SW, Dwyer P, Fenn WO. Science 1954;119:623—626.
55. Yusa T, Beckman JS, Crapo JD, Freeman BA. J Appl Physiol 1987;63(1):353—358.
56. Gordon-Majszak W, Gajkowska B. Exp Toxicol Pathol 1992;44:96—101.
57. Dirks RC, Faiman MD. Brain Res 1982:248:355—360.
58. Jerrett SA, Jefferson D, Mengel CE. Aerospace Med 1973;44:40—46.
59. Zirkle LG, Mengel CE, Horton BD, Duffy EJ. Aerospace Med 1965;36:1027—1030.
60. Harabin AL, Braisted JC, Flynn ET. J Appl Physiol 1990;69(1):328—335.
61. Ahotupa M, Mäntylä E, Peltola V, Puntala A, Toivonen H. Acta Physiol Scand 1992;145: 151—157.
62. Peacock MD, Schenk DA, Lawrence RA, Morgan JA, Jenkinson SG. J Appl Physiol 1994;76(3): 1279—1284.
63. Jenkinson SG, Jordan JM, Lawrence RA. J Appl Physiol 1988;256:2531—2536.
64. Gerschman R, Gilbert DL, Caccamise D. Am J Physiol 1958;192:563—571.
65. Sanders AP, Currie WD Woodhall B. Proc Soc Exp Biol Med 1969;130:1021—1027.
66. Sanders AP, Gellin RS, Kramer RS Currie WD. Aerospace Med 1972;43:533—536.
67. Block ER. Aviat Space Env Med 1977;48:645—648.
68. Hilton JG, Brown GL, Proctor PH. Toxicol Appl Pharmacol 1980;53:50—53.
69. Yusa T, Crapo JD, Freeman BA. J Appl Physiol Respirat Environ Physiol 1984;57(6):1674— 1681.
70. Lawrence RA, Burk RF. Biochem Biophys Res Commun 1976;71:952—958.
71. Jenkinson SG, Lawrence RA, Burk RF Gregory P. Toxicol Appl Pharmacol 1983;68:399—404.
72. Jenkinson SG, Long TH, Lawrence RA. J Lab Clin Med 1984;103:143—151.
73. Forman HJ, Rotman EI, Fischer AB. Lab Invest 1983;192:563—571.
74. Jenkinson SG, Jordan JM, Duncan CA. Am J Physiol 1989;257:393—L398.
75. Weber CA, Duncan CA, Lyons MJ Jenkinson SG. Am J Physiol 1990;258:L308—L312.
76. Suttorp N, Toepfer W, Roka L. Am J Physiol 1986;251:671—680.
77. Bitterman N, Melamed Y, Ben-amotz A. J Appl Physiol 1994;76(3):1073—1076.
78. Kanter MM, Nolte LA, Holloszy JO. J Appl Physiol 1993;74(2):965—969.
79. Leaf DA, Kleinman MT, Hamilton M Barstow TJ. Med Sci Sports Exerc 1997;29:1036—1039.
80. Matin MA, Husain K. Meth Find Clin Exptl Pharmacol 1985;7:79—81.
81. Somani SM, Rybak LP, Ravi RP. Pharmacol Biochem Behav 1995;50:635—639.
82. Murakami E, Hiwada K, Kokubu T. Jpn Circ J 1988;52:1299—1300.
83. Somani SM, Husain K. J Appl Toxicol 1997;17:329—336.
84. Fridovich I. Ann Rev Biochem 1975;44:147—159.
85. Pigeolet E, Corbisier P, Houbion A, Lambert D, Michiels C, Raes M, Zachary MD, Ramack J. Mech Ageing Devel 1990;51:283—297.
86. Sinet PM, Carber P. Arch Biochem Biophys 1981;212:411—416.
87. Husain K, Somani SM. Prog Neuropsychopharmacol Biol Psychiat 1998;22:411—423.
88. Ortiz deMontellano PR. In: Oxygen Activation and Transfer. Cytochrome P-450, Structure, Mechanism and Biochemistry, New York: Plenum Press 1986;217—220.
89. DeGroot H, Noll T. Hepatology 1983;3:601—606.
90. Anandatheerathavarada HK, Shanker SK, Bhamre S, Boyd MR, Song BJ, Ravindranath V. Brain Res 1993a;601:279—285.
91. Anandatheerthavarada HK, Williams JF, Wecker L. J Neurochem 1993b;60:1941—1944.
92. Reinke LA, Moore DR, Hange CM McCoy PB. Free Radic Res 1994;21:213—222.

93. Sharma HS, Cervos-Navarro J, Day PK. Neurosci Res 1991;10:211—221.
94. Friedman A, Kaufer D, Shemer J, Hendler I, Soreq H, Tur-Kaspa I. Nature Med 1996;2:1382—1385.
95. Davies CA, Mann DMA, Sumpter PQ, Yates PO. J Neurol Sci 1987;78:151—164.
96. Rogers J, Morrison JH. Neurosci 1985;5:2801—2808.
97. Volicer L, Crino PB. Neurobiol Age. 1990;11:567—571.
98. Mattson M, Goodman Y. Brain Res 1995;676:219—224.
99. Hensley K, Carney J, Mattson M, Aksenova M, Harris M, Wu J, Floyd R, Butterfield D. Proc Natl Acad Sci USA 1994;91:3270—3274.
100. Behl C, Davis JB, Lesley R, Schubert D. Cell 1994;77:817—827.
101. Klegeris A, Walker D, McGeer P. Biochem Biophys Res Commun 1994;199:984—991.
102. Parker W, Parks J, Filley C Kleinschmidt DB. Neurology 1994;44:1090—1096.
103. Smith MA, Kutty RK, Richey PL. Am J Pathol 1994;145:42—47.
104. Tesco G, Latorraca S, Piersanti P, Piancentini S, Amaducci L, Sorbi S. Mech Ageing Devel 1992;66:117—120.
105. Kumar U, Dunlop D, Richardson J. Life Sci 1994;54:1855—1860.
106. Crysta H, Dickson D, Flud P, Masur D, Scott R, Mehler M. Neurology 1988;38:1682—1687.
107. Subbarao KV, Richardson JS, Ang LC. J Neurochem 1990;55:342—345.
108. Hajimohammadreza I, Brammer M. Neurosci Lett 1990;112:333—337.
109. Richardson JS. Ann NY Acad Sci 1993;695:73—76.
110. Lovell MA, Ehmann WD, Butler SM, Markesberg WR. Neurology 1995;45:1594—1601.
111. Balazs L, Leon M. Neurochem Res 1994;19(9):1131—1137.
112. McIntosh LJ, Trush MA, Troncoso JC. Free Radic Biol Med 1997;23(2)183—190.
113. Palmer AM, Burns MA. Brain Res 1994;645:338—342.
114. Andorn, AC, Britton RS, Bacon BR. Neurobiol Age 1990;11:316—320.
115. Marklund SL, Adolfsson R, Gottfries CG, Winblad B. J Neurological Sci 1985;67:319—325.
116. Gsell W, Conrad R, Hickethier M, Sofic E, Frolich L, Wichart I, Jellinger K, Moll G, Ransmayr G, Beckmann H, Riederer P. J Neurochem 1995;64:1216—1223.
117. Zemlan FP, Thienhaus OJ, Bosmann HB. Brain Res 1989;476:160—162.
118. Delacourte A, Defossez A, Ceballos I, Nicole A, Sinet PM. Neurosci Letts 1988;92:247—253.
119. Bracco F, Scarpa M, Rigo A, Battistin L. P S E B M 1991;196:3641.
120. Kurobe N, Inagaki T, Kato K. Clin Chim Acta 1990;192:171—180.
121. Pappolla MA, Omar RA, Kim KS, Robakis NK. Am J Pathol 1992;140(3):621—628.
122. Cohen GJ. Neural Transm 1983;19:89—103.
123. Sian J, Dexter DT, Lees AJ, Daniel S, Agid Y, Javoy-Agid F, Jenner P, Marsden CD. Ann Neurol 1994;36:348—355.
124. Fahn S. Ann Neurol 1992;32:S128—S132.
125. Jenner P, Olanow CW. Neurology 1996;47(Suppl 3):S161—170.
126. Olanow CW. Ann Neurol 1992;32:S2—S9.
127. Singer TP, Castagnoli NJ, Ramsay RR Trevor AJ. J Neurochem 1987;49:1—8.
128. Olanow CW. Neurology 1990;40:32—37.
129. Dexter DT, Carter CJ, Wells FR, Javoy-Agid F, Agid Ym, Lees A, Jenner P, Marsden CD. J Neurochem 1989;52:381—389.
130. Jenner P, Dexter DT, Sian J, Schapira AHV, Marsden CD. Ann Neurol 1992;32:S82—S87.
131. Dexter DT, Holley AE, Flitter WD. Mov Disord 1994;9:92—97.
132. Yoritaka, A, Hatton, N, Uchida, K Mizuno Y. Proc Nat Acad Sci USA 1996;93:2696—2713.
133. Sofic E, Paulus W, Jellinger K, Riederer P, Youdim MBH. J Neurochem 1991;56:978—982.
134. Galazka FJ, Bauminger ER, Friedman A, Barcikowska M, Hechel D, Nowik I. Mov Disord 1996;11:8—16.
135. Obata T, Giueh CC. J Neurol Transm Gen Sect 1992;89:139—145.
136. Chiueh CC, Krishna G, Tulsi P. Free Radic Biol Med 1992;13:581—583.
137. Saggu H, Cooksey J, Dexter D, Wells FR, Lees A, Jenner P, Marsden CD. J Neurochem 1989;53:

692−697.

138. Yoshida E, Mokuno K, Aoki S, Takahashi A, Riku S, Murayama T, Yanagi T, Kato K. J Neurol Sci 1994;124:25−31.
139. Marttila RJ, Lorentz H, Rinne UK. J Neurol Sci 1988;86:321−331.
140. Ambani LM, Van Woert MH, Murphy S. Arch Neurol 1975;32:114−118.
141. Kish SJ, Morito C, Hornykiewicz H. Neurosci Letts 1985;58:343−346.
142. DiMonte DA, Chan P, Sandy MS. Ann Neurol 1992;32:S111−S115.
143. Perry TL, Yong VW. Neurosci Letts 1986;67:269−274.
144. Perry TL, Godin DV, Hansen S. Neurosci Lett 1982;33:305−310.
145. Sofic E, Lange KW, Jellinger K, Riederer P. Neurosci Letts 1992;142:128−130.
146. Riederer P, Sofic E, Rausch W-D, Schmidt B, Reynolds GP, Jellinger K, Youdim MBH. J Neurochem 1989;52:515−520.
147. Mulder DW, Kurland LT, Offord KP, Beard CM. Neurology 1986;36:511−517.
148. Rosen DR, Siddique T, Patterson D. Nature 1993;362:59−62.
149. Deng H-X, Hentati A, Tainer JA, Iqbal Z, Cayabyab A, Hung W-Y, Getzoff ED, Ping H, Herzfeldt B, Roos RP, Warner C, Deng G, Soriano E, Smyth C, Parge HE, Ahmed A, Roses AD, Hallewell RA, Pericak-Vance MA, Siddique TS. Science 1993;261:1047−1051.
150. Bowling AC, Schulz JB, Brown Jr., RH, Beal MF. J Neurochem 1993;61:2322−2325.
151. Rosen DR, Bowling AC, Patterson D, Usdin TB, Sapp P, Mezey E, McKenna-Yasek D, O'Regan J, Rahmani Z, Ferrante RJ, Brownstein MJ, Kowall NW, Beal MF, Horvitz HR, Brown RH Jr. Hum Mol Genet 1994;3(6):981−987.
152. Rothstein JD, Bristol LA, Hosler Bm, Brown RH Jr., Kuncl RW. Proc Natl Acad Sci USA 1994;91:4155−4159.
153. Feaster WW, Kwok LW, Epstein CJ. Am J Hum Genet 1977;29:563−570.
154. Bowling AC, Barkowski EE, McKenna-Yasek D, Sapp P, Horvitz HR, Beal MF, Brown RH Jr. J Neurochem 1995;64:2366−2369.
155. Wiedau-Pazos M, Goto JJ, Rabizadeh S, Gralla EB, Roe JA, Lee MK, Valentine JS, Bredesen DE. Science 1996;271:515−518.
156. Lai F, Williams RS. Arch Neurol 1989;46:849−853.
157. Oliver C, Holland AJ. Psychol Med 1986;16:307−322.
158. Brooksbank BWL, Balazs R. Devel Brain Res 1984;16:37−44.
159. Sinet P-M, Lejeune J, Jerome H. Life Sciences 1979;24:29−34.
160. Balazs R, Brooksbank BWL, J Mental Def Res 1985;29:1−14.
161. Asayama K, Urr IM. J Biol Chem 1985;260:2212−2217.
162. Annegers JF, Grabow JD, Grover RV, Laws ER, Elveback LR, Kurland LT. Neurology 1980; 30:683−689.
163. Willmore LJ. Epilepsia 1990;31(suppl 3):S67−S73.
164. Demopoulos HB, Flamm ES, Pietronnero DD, Seligman ML. Acta Physiol Scand 1980;492: 91−119.
165. Hall ED, Braughler JM. Free Radic Biol Med 1989;6:303−313.
166. Kontos HA. Chem Biol Interactions 1989;72:229−255.
167. Jesberger JA, Richardson JS. Int J Neurosic 1991;57:1−17
168. Wei EP, Christman CW, Kontos HA Povlischock JT. Am J Physiol 1985;248:157−163.
169. Jenkins LW, Povlishock JT, Becker DP, Miller JD, Sullivan HG. Acta Neuropathol 1979;48: 113−119.
170. Wei EP, Kontos HA. Physiologist 1987;30:122−128.
171. Kirsch JR, Phelan AM, Lange DG, Traystman RJ. Fed Proc 1987;46:799−803.
172. Kogure K, Watson BD, Busto R, Abe K. Neurochem Res 1982;7:437−442.
173. Ohta S, Saskaki S Kuwabara H. J Cereb Blood Flow Metab 1987;7:654−658.
174. Kontos HA, Wei EP. J Neurosurg 1986;64:803−808.
175. Gruener N, Gross B, Gozlan O, Barak M. Lifes Sci 1994:54(11):711−713.
176. Hall ED, Braughler JM. CNS Trauma 1986;3:281−286.

177. Saunders RD, Dugan LL, Demediuk P, Mean ED, Horocks LA, Anderson DK. J Neurochem 1987;49:24—28.
178. Payan H, Toga M, Berard-Badier M. Epilepsia 1970;11:81—94.
179. Penry JK, White BG, Brackett CE. Neurology 1979;29:600—601.
180. Willmore LJ, Triggs WJ, Gray JD. Brain Research 1986;382:422—426.
181. Singh R, Pathak PN. Epilepsia 1990;31(1):15—26.
182. Willmore LJ, Rubin JJ. Exp Neurol 1984;83:62—70.
183. Muller A, Cadenas E, Graft P, Sies H. Biochem Pharmacol 1984;33:3235—3239.
184. Dabiri LM, Pasta D, Darby JK, Mosbacher D. Am J Psychiatry 1994;151:925—926.
185. Brady PS, Brady LJ, Ullrey DE. J Nutr 1979;109:1103—1109.
186. Dillard CJ, Litov RE, Savin WM, Mumelin EE Tappel AL. J Appl Physiol 1978;45:927—932.
187. Maxwell SRJ. Drugs 1995;49(3):345—361.
188. Suzuki J, Fujimoto, S Mizoi K, Oba M. Stroke 1984;15:672—680.
189. Hall ED, Braughler JM, Yonkers PA, Smith SL, Linseman KL, Means ED, Scherch HM, Von Voigtlander PF, Lahti RA, Jacobsen EJ. J Pharmacol Exp Ther 1991;258(2):688—694.
190. Sastre J, Asensi M, Gasco E, Pallardo FV, Ferrero JA, Furukawa T, Vina J. Am J Physiol 1992; 263:992—995.
191. Hamers FPT, Brakkee JH, Cavalletti F, Tedeschi M, Marmouti L, Pezzoni G, Neijt JP, Gispen WH. Cancer Res 1993;53:544—549.
192. Sen CK, Atalay M, Hanninen OJ. Appl Physiol 1994;77:2177—2181.
193. Agee JM, Flanagan T, Blackbourne LH, Kron IL, Tribble CG. Ann Thorac Surg 1991;5:911—915.
194. Chan PH, Longar S, Fishman RA. Ann Neurol 1987;21:540—546.
195. Kontos HA, Wei EP, Dietrich WD, Navari RM, Povlishock JT, Ghatak VR, Ellis EF, Patterson JL. Am J Physiol 1981;240:511—516.
196. Ryback LP, Husain K, Morris C, Whitworth C, Somani SM. Am J Otology 1999 (In Press).
197. Mizoi K, Yoshimoto T, Suzuki J. Acta Neurochem 1981;56:157—162.
198. Coles JC, Ahmed M, Mehta HU Kaufman JCE. Ann Thorac Surg 1986;41:551—560.
199. Braughler JM, Hall ED, Jacobsen EJ, McCall JM, Means ED. Drugs Future 1989;14:143—152.
200. Naftchi NE. Int J Devel Neurosci 1991;9(2):113—126.
201. Cao X, Phillis JW. Brain Res 1994;644:267—272.
202. Smith CD, Carney JM, Starke-Reed PE. Proc Natl Acad Sci USA 1991;88:10540—10543.
203. Beal MF, Henshaw R, Jenkins BG. Ann Neurol 1994;36:882—888.
204. Koroshetz W, Jenkins B, Rosen B. Neurology 1993;43:334.
205. Zhang Y, Tatsuno T, Carney JM. J Cereb Blood Flow Metab 1993;13:378—288.
206. Greenamyre JT, Garcia OM, Greene JG. Neurosci Lett 1994;171:17—20.
207. Packer L, Wih EH, Tritschler HJ. Free Radic Biol Med 1995;19:227—250.
208. Prehn JH, Karkoutly C, Nuglisch J, Peruche B, Krieglstein J. J Cereb Blood Flow Metab 1992; 12:78—87.
209. Clerici WJ, Hensley K, DiMartino DL. Hear Res 1996; 98:116—124.
210. Reed DJ, Mary HE, Boorse RB, Gregory KM, Beilstein MA. Cancer Res 1985;35:568—372.
211. Sinha BK. Biochem Pharmacol 1984;33:2777—2782.
212. Somani SM, Kutty RK, Krishna G. Toxicol Appl Pharmacol 1990;106:28—34.
213. Kochli HW, Wermurth B, VonWartburg JP. Biochem Biophys Acta. 1980;616:133—139.
214. Nagamastu K, Kido Y, Terao T, Ishida T, Toki S. Drug Metab Dispos 1983;11:190—196.
215. Chambers JE, Munson JR, Chambers HW. Biochem Biophys Res Commun 1989;165:327—334.
216. Aust SD, Chignell CF, Bray TM, Kalyanaraman B, Mason RP. Toxicol Appl Pharmacol 1993; 120:168—178.
217. Rybak LP, Husain K, Whitworth C, Somani SM. Toxicol Sci 1999;47:195—202.

Part X

Aging

© 2000 Elsevier Science B.V. All rights reserved.
Handbook of Oxidants and Antioxidants in Exercise.
C.K. Sen, L. Packer and O. Hänninen, editors.

Part X • Chapter 27

Oxidants and aging

Kenneth B. Beckman and Bruce N. Ames

*Department of Molecular and Cell Biology, 401 Barker Hall, University of California at Berkeley,
CA 94720—3202, USA. Tel.: +1-510-642-5163. Fax: +1-510-643-7935.
E-mail: kbeckman@uclink4.berkeley.edu*

1   INTRODUCTION
2   AN OVERVIEW OF THE FREE RADICAL THEORY OF AGING
   2.1   The origins of the free radical theory
   2.2   Sources of oxidants
   2.3   Targets of oxidants
   2.4   Antioxidant defenses
   2.5   Repair of oxidative damage
   2.6   Synthesis: the interaction of oxidant generation, oxidative damage, and repair
3   REFINEMENTS AND COROLLARIES OF THE FREE RADICAL THEORY
   3.1   Oxygen radicals and evolutionary theories of aging
   3.2   Oxygen radicals and the somatic mutation theory of aging
   3.3   Oxygen radicals and mitochondrial theories of aging
4   OXIDATIVE PHENOMENOLOGY: AGE-ASSOCIATED TRENDS
   4.1   Accumulation of oxidative end-products
   4.2   Steady-state levels of oxidative modification
   4.3   Oxidative depletion of biochemical pools
   4.4   Age-associated trends in antioxidant defenses and repair
   4.5   Age-associated trends in oxidant generation
5   INTERSPECIES COMPARISONS
   5.1   Oxidative damage and maximum life span potential
   5.2   Antioxidant defenses and maximum life span potential
   5.3   Generation of reactive oxygen species and maximum life span potential
6   ENVIRONMENTAL MANIPULATION AND LIFE SPAN
   6.1   Dietary restriction
   6.2   Activity restriction
   6.3   Oxygen tension
7   SUPPLEMENTATION AND LIFE SPAN
   7.1   Dietary antioxidants
   7.2   Pharmacological supplements
8   SUMMARY
9   PERSPECTIVES
   9.1   Nitric oxide
   9.2   Regulatory roles for oxidants and antioxidants: signal transduction
   9.3   Oxidants and apoptosis
   9.4   Exercise and life span
10   ACKNOWLEDGEMENTS
11   ABBREVIATIONS
12   REFERENCES

1   INTRODUCTION

The study of aging has been characterized by a huge phenomenological literature, and at the same time, the lack of established primary causes. The diverse life histories of animal species, which manifest aging in very different ways, have been an obstacle to testing unified theories. In order for experimental gerontology to provide more than a catalog of age-related changes, it has been necessary to define the alterations that are common to most old cells, tissues, and animals, while simultaneously respecting that there is not a single phenomenon of aging or a single cause. This has taken some time, and from the outside it may have appeared that the field has been mired in phenomenology.

Throughout this time, though, there has never been a shortage of unified theories attempting to reduce aging to something more tractable. In fact, gerontologists have been prolific in this regard [1,2]. Whereas some researchers have believed that a small number of random, deleterious mechanisms could explain degenerative senescence, others have opted for theories of "programmed" aging, in which senescence is the final destination in a developmental pathway. In the course of these debates, a number of scientists have rallied around a set of ideas called the free radical theory of aging — loosely, the belief that damage by reactive oxygen species is critical in determining life span. This theory inspired many experiments in which evidence of oxidative damage in aged animals was sought.

In the last 10 years or so, the nature of aging research has changed dramatically; one might say that the field has entered early adulthood. The tools of molecular biology are now sophisticated and accessible enough that researchers within gerontology have adopted them. At the same time, molecular biologists situated on the edge of aging research have made inroads, and have discovered that fruit flies and nematodes are amenable to the study of aging. Also, medical researchers investigating human diseases of aging, such as Alzheimer's disease and inherited progerias, have overcome long-standing roadblocks.

It has been gratifying, therefore, that many of the preliminary studies in what might be called "molecular gerontology" lend credibility to the free radical theory. Results from disparate experimental systems have recently shown that oxygen radicals play a role in degenerative senescence, and the pace of discoveries is quickening. The likely result of this combination of approaches will be the unraveling of the physiological tangle of aging, and it seems safe to say that one of the important knots will turn out to be oxidative stress.

However, there is a danger that in the excitement of theoretical confirmation, certain nuances are lost. For instance, the revelation that oxygen radicals may be involved in neurodegeneration does not mean that oxidative stress determines life span. The free radical theory has sought not only to explain the mechanisms of senescence, but it has also attempted to explain differences between species' life spans in terms of oxidants. So although many recent studies indicate that oxygen radicals play some kind of role in aging, only a small number of these support the more ambitious version of the free radical theory. On the other hand, there is no reason to cling to such a stringent version of the free radical theory, and it is becoming apparent that whether or not they determine life span, oxygen radicals are certainly important players in aging's pathophysiology. In other words, the scope of the free radical theory of aging should include aging-associated oxidative stress in general, rather than limiting itself to those oxidative events which may determine life span. In fact, many current articles indicate that such a blurring of distinctions has already occurred and that as it is commonly used, "free radical theory" encompasses a broad set of ideas. Therefore, our first purpose here is to delineate these different conceptions of the free radical theory.

Due to the recent popularity of free radical research, a large number of reviews have addressed various aspects of the interplay between oxidants and aging [3—40]. Rather than merely updating this literature, our aim in this chapter is to provide a systematic categorization of the types of experiments that have been performed. The phenomenon and study of aging are incredibly diverse, and although it is a diversity of evidence which makes the free radical theory appealing, the menagerie of animals and techniques used can be confusing. By breaking the literature down into smaller pieces, we hope to make it easier to digest.

In this chapter, then, we will briefly outline the evolution of the free radical theory, and then describe the different areas of evidence. We will focus on recent experiments, and point to the areas which we feel are most likely to provide future insights. The way in which we have categorized the literature is outlined in Table 1. Although any such system is somewhat arbitrary, we hope that ours will make it easier to assimilate the existing literature and envision future experiments.[1]

2 AN OVERVIEW OF THE FREE RADICAL THEORY OF AGING

2.1 The origins of the free radical theory

In 1956, Denham Harman suggested that free radicals produced during aerobic respiration cause cumulative oxidative damage, resulting in aging and death. He noted parallels between the effects of aging and of ionizing radiation, including mutagenesis, cancer, and gross cellular damage [41,42]. At the time, it had recently been discovered that radiolysis of water generates hydroxyl radical (•OH) [43], and early experiments using paramagnetic resonance spectroscopy had identified the presence of •OH in living matter [44]. Harman, therefore, hypothesized that endogenous oxygen radical generation occurs in vivo, as a by-

---

[1]   In reviewing as broad a topic as the free radical theory, we have been forced to limit both the content and the number of references cited. Although we have done our best to include recent work, omissions were inevitable. We apologize to all authors whose work we have not managed to include, and direct readers to other recent reviews for material we have left out.

Table 1. A categorization of the strengths and weaknesses of approaches to the testing of the free radical theory of aging.

Experimental approach	Chapter section	Strengths of the approach	Weaknesses of the approach
Oxidative phenomenology	4.0	Simplicity. Large existing data set. Elucidation of the basic biochemistry of oxidative stress. Technical foundation for other approaches. Negative result may be instructive.	Results are merely correlative (oxidative damage may be a consequence of ageing). Negative results, considered uninteresting, may fail to appear in the literature.
Interspecies comparisons	5.0	Specific testable predictions. Deviations from predictions may refine theory. Use of different species avoids conclusions that are species- or strain-specific. Negative results may be instructive.	Logistical problems in animal handling. Quantitative comparisons complicated by qualitative interspecies differences in oxidative defenses and/or repair.
Dietary restriction	6.1	Very well established model of life span extension. Straightforward methodology. Probably relevant to human aging and cancer.	Results are somewhat correlative (alterations in oxidative stress may be consistent with but incidental to a more fundamental cellular switch).
Activity restriction	6.2	A direct test of the rate of living theory, with specific testable predictions. Straightforward methodology.	To date, limited to relatively simple organisms, such as invertebrates.
Manipulation of oxygen concentration	6.3	A direct test of the rate of living theory, with specific testable predictions. Straightforward methodology.	Results hard to interpret. Are positive results (life span attenuation by hyperoxia, extension by hypoxia) relevant to normoxic aging? Not applicable to most mammals.
Supplementation with dietary antioxidants	7.1	(Potentially) a test of the free radical theory.	Results hard to interpret, due to unknown fates of supplements, potential adverse effects, complexity of overall antioxidant defenses.
Administration of pharmacological antioxidants	7.2	(Potentially) a test of the free radical theory.	Results hard to interpret, due to unknown fates of supplements, potential adverse effects, complexity of overall antioxidant defenses.

product of enzymatic redox chemistry. He ventured that the enzymes involved would be those "involved in the direct utilization of molecular oxygen, particularly those containing iron". Finally, he hypothesized that traces of iron and other metals would catalyze oxidative reactions in vivo, and that peroxidative chain reactions were possible, by analogy to the principles of in vitro polymer chemistry. All of these predictions have been confirmed during the past 40 years.

The theory gained credibility with the identification in 1969 of the enzyme superoxide dismutase (SOD) [45], which provided the first compelling evidence of in vivo generation of superoxide anion ($O_2\bullet^-$), and from the subsequent elucidation of elaborate antioxidant defenses [46]. The use of SOD as a tool to locate subcellular sites of $O_2\bullet^-$ generation led to a realization which buttressed the free radical theory, namely, that mitochondria are a principal source of endogenous oxidants [47]. Gerontologists had long observed that species with higher metabolic rates have shorter maximum life span potential (MLSP): they age faster [48]. In fact, it had been proposed at the turn of the century that energy consumption per se was responsible for senescence, a concept referred to as the "rate of living" hypothesis [48–50]. The realization that energy consumption by mitochondria may result in $O_2\bullet^-$ production linked the free radical theory and the rate-of-living theory irrevocably: a faster rate of respiration, associated with a greater generation of oxygen radicals, hastens aging. By now, the two concepts have essentially merged.

2.2 Sources of oxidants

Ground state diatomic oxygen, ($^3\Sigma g^- O_2$ or more commonly, O_2), despite being a radical species and the most important oxidant in aerobic organisms, is only sparingly reactive itself due to the fact that its two unpaired electrons are located in different molecular orbitals and possess "parallel spins". As a consequence, if O_2 is simultaneously to accept two electrons, these must both possess antiparallel spins relative to the unpaired electrons in O_2, a criterion which is not satisfied by a typical pair of electrons in atomic or molecular orbitals (which have opposite spins according to the Pauli exclusion principle). As a result, O_2 preferentially accepts electrons one at a time from other radicals (such as transition metals in certain valences). Thus, in vivo, typical two- or four-electron reduction of O_2 relies upon coordinated, serial, enzyme-catalyzed one-electron reductions, and the enzymes which carry these out typically possess active-site radical species such as iron. One- and two-electron reduction of O_2 generates superoxide ($O_2\bullet^-$) and hydrogen peroxide (H_2O_2), respectively, both of which are generated by numerous routes in vivo, as discussed below. In the presence of free transition metals (in particular iron and copper), $O_2\bullet^-$ and H_2O_2 together generate the extremely reactive hydroxyl radical ($\bullet OH$). Ultimately, $\bullet OH$ is assumed to be the species responsible for initiating the oxidative destruction of biomolecules. In addition to $O_2\bullet^-$, H_2O_2, and $\bullet OH$, two energetically excited species of O_2 termed "singlet oxygens" can result from the absorption of energy, (for instance, from ultraviolet light). Designated by the formulas $^1\Delta gO_2$ and $^1\Sigma g^+O_2$, both of these species differ from the triplet ground state ($^3\Sigma g^-O_2$) in having their two unpaired electrons in opposite spins, thereby eliminating the spin restriction of ground-state O_2 and enabling greater reactivity. The chemistry of oxygen and its derivatives has been extensively discussed elsewhere [51,52]. Since all of these species ($O_2\bullet^-$, H_2O_2, $\bullet OH$, $^1\Delta gO_2$, and $^1\Sigma g^+O_2$), by different routes, are involved in oxygen's toxicity, we will collectively refer to them as "oxidants".

It is now beyond doubt that oxidants are generated in vivo and can cause significant harm [27,46,47,53—55]. There are numerous sites of oxidant and oxygen radical generation, four of which have attracted much attention: mitochondrial electron transport, peroxisomal fatty acid metabolism, cytochrome P450 reactions, and phagocytic cells (the "respiratory burst"). Before discussing the potential contributions of different sources of oxidants, it is worthwhile briefly to outline them.

In the textbook scheme of mitochondrial respiration, electron transport involves a coordinated four-electron reduction of O_2 to H_2O, the electrons being donated by NADH or succinate to complexes I and II, respectively, of the mitochondrial electron transport chain (ETC). Ubiquinone (coenzyme Q, or UQ), which accepts electrons from complexes I (NADH dehydrogenase) and II (succinate dehydrogenase), undergoes two sequential one-electron reductions to ubisemiquinone and ubiquinol (the Q cycle), ultimately transferring reducing equivalents to the remainder of the electron transport chain: complex III (UQ-cytochrome C reductase), cytochrome c, complex IV (cytochrome c oxidase), and finally, O_2 [51]. However, it appears mitochondrial electron transport is imperfect, and one-electron reduction of O_2 to form $O_2\bullet^-$ occurs. The spontaneous and enzymatic dismutation of $O_2\bullet^-$ yields hydrogen peroxide (H_2O_2), and so a significant by-product of the actual sequence of oxidation-reduction reactions may be the generation of $O_2\bullet^-$ and H_2O_2.

How much $O_2\bullet^-$ and H_2O_2 do mitochondria generate? In classic experiments during the 1970s, measurements of H_2O_2 generation by isolated mitochondria indicated that it is maximal when ADP is limiting and the electron carriers are consequently reduced ("state 4" respiration) [56]. Estimates of state 4 H_2O_2 generation by pigeon and rat mitochondrial preparations amounted to $1-2\%$ of total electron flow [56,57]. One problem with this estimate of mitochondrial H_2O_2 generation is its reliance on the use of buffer saturated with air (20% O_2). In vivo, the partial pressure of O_2 is about 5%, and so these calculations may overestimate the flux of oxidants in vivo. Even disregarding the use of air-saturated buffer, the initial estimate of percentage ETC flux leading to H_2O_2 can be challenged on the grounds that in these experiments, the concentrations of substrates fed to mitochondria were higher than occurs physiologically [58,59]. When H_2O_2 is measured with more physiological concentrations, the flux is about 10-fold lower [58], and experiments using subcellular fractions of SOD-deficient *E. coli* suggest in vivo leakage of 0.1% from the respiratory chain [59].

What proportion of mitochondrial H_2O_2 ultimately derives from ETC $O_2\bullet^-$

generation? Unfortunately, the measurement of $O_2\bullet^-$ generation by intact mito-chondria is prevented by the presence of mitochondrial SOD (mSOD). Therefore, the isolation of submitochondrial particles from which mSOD has been removed (by sonication of the intact organelles followed by extensive washing), was used for the detection of ETC $O_2\bullet^-$. In these experiments, stoichiometric estimates of the ratio of $O_2\bullet^-$ generation (by submitochondrial particles) to H_2O_2 generation (by the intact organelles) fell between 1.5 and 2.1 [60—64]; since two $O_2\bullet^-$ mol-ecules dismutate, (either spontaneously or with the help of mSOD), to form one molecule of H_2O_2, such results suggest that virtually all mitochondrial H_2O_2 may originate as $O_2\bullet^-$ [65]. Moreover, as most cellular H_2O_2 originates from mitochondria, $O_2\bullet^-$ from the ETC may be a cell's most significant source of oxi-dants [47].

In a recent discussion of the classic in vitro work [66], some of the original experimenters take issue with the idea that free $O_2\bullet^-$ exists in mitochondria as a result of normal flux through the ETC. They point out that in addition to having removed mSOD from mitochondria, the sonication they employed also resulted in the loss of cytochrome c, which rapidly scavenges $O_2\bullet^-$ in vitro and is present in mitochondria at local concentrations from 0.5 to 5 mM. In mitochondria, they argue, mSOD and cytochrome c rapidly scavenge $O_2\bullet^-$ (in the matrix and intermembrane spaces, respectively). More to the point, the authors stress that unless the ETC was poisoned with inhibitors such as antimycin A, $O_2\bullet^-$ genera-tion was not detected in their experiments [60,61]. Arguing that mSOD should act to increase the rate of $O_2\bullet^-$ generation in vivo (by accelerating product removal by dismutation to H_2O_2) they suggest that the actual role of mSOD in vivo may be to increase hydrogen peroxide generation (with $O_2\bullet^-$ as a rapidly consumed intermediate) [66]. Ultimately, there remains a good deal of uncer-tainty surrounding the mechanisms, quantity, and meaning of mitochondrial $O_2\bullet^-$ generation in vivo [67], a mystery which is deepened by recent reports of enzymatic nitric oxide (NO$\bullet$) generation in mitochondria [68—70]. Since $O_2\bullet^-$ and NO$\bullet$ react to form the oxidant peroxynitrite (ONOO$^-$), mitochondrial $O_2\bullet^-$ generation may soon need to be considered in the light of its ability to destroy NO$\bullet$ and form ONOO$^-$, as is discussed below.

A second source of oxygen radicals is peroxisomal β-oxidation of fatty acids, which generates H_2O_2 as a by-product. Peroxisomes possess high concentrations of catalase, and so it is unclear whether or not leakage of H_2O_2 from peroxi-somes contributes significantly to cytosolic oxidative stress under normal cir-cumstances. However, a class of nonmutagenic carcinogens, the peroxisome pro-liferators, which increase the number of hepatocellular peroxisomes and result in liver cancer in rodents, also cause oxidative stress and damage [71—74]. Inter-estingly, during the regeneration of the liver following partial hepatectomy, there exist peroxisomes which do not stain for catalase activity [75], hinting that during rapid cell proliferation, oxidant leakage from peroxisomes may be enhanced.

Microsomal cytochrome P450 enzymes metabolize xenobiotic compounds, usually of plant origin, by catalyzing their univalent oxidation or reduction.

Although these reactions typically involve NADPH and an organic substrate, some of the numerous cytochrome P450 isozymes directly reduce O_2 to $O_2\bullet^-$ [76,77], and may cause oxidative stress. An alternative route for cytochrome P450-mediated oxidation involves redox cycling, in which substrates accept single electrons from cytochrome P450 and transfer them to oxygen. This generates $O_2\bullet^-$ and simultaneously regenerates the substrate, allowing subsequent rounds of $O_2\bullet^-$ generation [51]. Although it is unclear to what extent cytochrome P450 side-reactions proceed under normal conditions, it is possible that such chronic $O_2\bullet^-$ generation by cytochrome P450 is the price animals pay for their ability to detoxify acute doses of toxins [9].

Lastly, phagocytic cells attack pathogens with a mixture of oxidants and free radicals, including $O_2\bullet^-$, H_2O_2, nitric oxide, and hypochlorite [78–80]. Although the massive generation of oxidants by immune cells differs from the above three sources of free radicals to the extent that it is the result of pathology, it is, nevertheless, a normal and unavoidable consequence of innate immunity. Chronic inflammation is, however, unique among the endogenous sources of oxidants because it is mostly preventable [81–83].

In addition to these four sources of oxidants, there exist numerous other enzymes capable of generating oxidants under normal or pathological conditions, often in a tissue-specific manner [51]. To give a single relevant example: the deamination of dopamine by monoamine oxidase generates H_2O_2, in some neurons, and has been implicated in the etiology of Parkinson's disease [84]. Lastly, the widespread catalytic generation of the radical nitric oxide (NO$\bullet$), achieved by various isozymes of nitric oxide synthase and central to processes as diverse as vascular regulation, immune responses, and long-term potentiation, increases the potential routes for destructive oxidative reactions [85]. The interaction between $O_2\bullet^-$ and NO$\bullet$ results in $ONOO^-$, which is a powerful oxidant.

As originally articulated by Harman, the free radical theory of aging does not distinguish between different sources of oxidants. However, the rate of living hypothesis clearly singles out mitochondrial $O_2\bullet^-$ and H_2O_2 generation, as it is the mitochondrial respiration rate which negatively correlates with MLSP. Also, many other established sources of oxidants are tissue specific (associated with hepatic, neuronal, and other specialized functions), and are less likely to explain aging across a broad range of species. For this reason, mitochondrial $O_2\bullet^-$ and H_2O_2 have captured the lion's share of attention. However, it may turn out that for some age-associated disorders, nonmitochondrial oxidants are critical. In the expanded sense of the free radical theory, any oxidants, mitochondrial or not, may play a role. Therefore, despite the great number of intracellular sources of oxidant that have been identified in a qualitative way, in terms of ranking their relative importance the field is in its infancy.

2.3 Targets of oxidants

What are the targets of endogenous oxidants? The three main classes of biological molecules; lipids, nucleic acids, and proteins, are susceptible to free radical attack, and there is plenty of evidence to suggest that all suffer oxidative damage in vivo. Although it is well beyond the scope of this review to treat the biochemistry of oxidative damage in any great depth, the area has been expertly reviewed [51]. A synopsis of the better known pathways of oxidative damage, however, is warranted and the most familiar end-products are described here.

The earliest research on the destruction of biological molecules by oxidants involved lipids [86]. Food chemists have long understood that the rancidity of fats results from peroxidative chain reactions in lipids ("autoxidation"): a lipid hydroperoxyl radical abstracts a hydrogen atom from the double bond of a neighboring unsaturated lipid, forming a hydroperoxide and an alkyl radical, the latter which combines with O_2 to regenerate a lipid hydroperoxyl radical capable of initiating another round of oxidation. Ultimately, intramolecular reactions and decomposition yield cyclic endoperoxides and unsaturated aldehydes, the latter of which are reactive and may act as mutagens [87], inactivate enzymes [88,89], or operate as endogenous fixatives, reacting with proteins and nucleic acids to form heterogeneous cross-links [90]. Moreover, a primary effect of lipid peroxidation is decreased membrane fluidity, which alters membrane properties and can significantly disrupt membrane-bound proteins [91].

Oxidative damage to nucleic acids includes adducts of base and sugar groups, single- and double-strand breaks in the backbone, and cross-links to other molecules. The spectrum of adducts in mammalian chromatin oxidized in vitro and in vivo includes more than 20 known products, including damage to all four bases and thymine-tyrosine cross-links [92—94]. The electrochemical properties of the adduct 8-oxoguanine (8-oxogua) and the deoxynucleoside 8-oxo-2,7-dihydro-2'-deoxyguanosine (8-oxodG), which have permitted the coupling of extremely sensitive electrochemical detection to HPLC chromatography, have resulted in hundreds of studies concerning its formation, accumulation, and excretion [95]. The identification of specific enzymatic repair of oxidative lesions has recently provided both proof of the significance of oxidative DNA damage, as well as tools to manipulate the load of damage in vivo by genetic knockout [95—100].

The oxidation of proteins is less well characterized, but several classes of damage have been documented, including oxidation of sulfhydryl groups, reduction of disulfides, oxidative adduction of amino acid residues close to metal-binding sites via metal-catalyzed oxidation, reactions with aldehydes, protein-protein cross-linking, and peptide fragmentation [101,102]. A particularly intriguing recent development has been the realization that a number of enzymes possessing active-site iron-sulfur clusters are acutely sensitive to inactivation by $O_2\bullet^-$ [103,104]. For example, *E. coli* aconitase is inactivated by $O_2\bullet^-$ with a rate constant of 10^9 M^{-1} s^{-1} [105,106]. Mammalian mitochondrial aconitase is inactivated in vitro and in vivo by treatments which increase mitochondrial $O_2\bullet^-$ generation, such as growth under hyperbaric conditions [107,108]. Since aconitase participates in the citric acid cycle, its inhibition would be expected to have pleiotropic effects. Moreover, the mechanism of aconitase inhibition by $O_2\bullet^-$ has been demonstrated to involve the release of free iron from the enzyme [103]. Free iron atoms catalytically exacerbate oxygen stress (see below), and it has been proposed that superoxide's genotoxicity is a function of its ability to liberate protein-bound iron [109,110].

Unlike lipids and nucleic acids, proteins represent a very diverse target for oxidative damage. Although protein oxidation has been demonstrated at the level of the peptide backbone and amino acids, there has been relatively little scrutiny of differences between proteins in their sensitivities. A detailed quantitative comparison of bovine serum albumin and glutamine synthase has shown susceptible residues of the former (methionine and the aromatic amino acid residues) to be oxidized about twice as fast as those on the latter, implicating all four levels of protein structure in relative susceptibility [111]. A study of the oxidation sensitivities of various cloned K^+ channels from T lymphocytes, cardiac cells, and neurons, revealed that whereas five of the cloned channels were highly sensitive to oxidation, an equal number were resistant [112]. Differential sensitivities raise the possibility that the loss of homeostasis which is a hallmark of aging could result from the selective oxidation of proteins.

In the context of aging, a particularly relevant aspect of oxygen's toxicity is its promotion by some metals and by elevated O_2 partial pressure. Iron and copper catalyze the homolytic cleavage of ROOH (the Fenton reaction), leading to the generation of $\bullet OH$ [51]. It is $\bullet OH$ which is the most reactive oxidant, reacting at diffusion-limited rates. The catalytic properties of iron and copper explains why cells possess metal chelating proteins such as ferritin and transferrin, which reduce the concentration of redox-active metals [113,114]. In humans, the body's content of iron increases with age (in men throughout their lives, and in women after menopause), and it has been suggested that this accumulation may increase the risk of oxidative damage with age [115,116]. Lastly, oxidative stress in vivo is aggravated by increasing O_2 partial pressure, due to a more pronounced flux of mitochondrial $O_2\bullet^-$ [47]. Consequently, the manipulation of O_2 partial pressure is a relatively simple tool that has been used to test the free radical theory.

2.4 Antioxidant defenses

Cells are equipped with an impressive repertoire of antioxidant enzymes, as well as small antioxidant molecules mostly derived from dietary fruits and vegetables [46,117]. These include:

(i) enzymatic scavengers such as SOD, which hastens the dismutation of $O_2\bullet^-$ to H_2O_2, and catalase and glutathione peroxidase (GPX), which convert H_2O_2 to water;

(ii) hydrophilic radical scavengers such as ascorbate, urate, and glutathione (GSH);

(iii) lipophilic radical scavengers such as tocopherols, flavonoids, carotenoids, and ubiquinol;

(iv) enzymes involved in the reduction of oxidized forms of small molecular anti-oxidants, (GSH reductase, dehydroascorbate reductase), or responsible for the maintenance of protein thiols (thioredoxin reductase); and

(v) the cellular machinery which maintains a reducing environment, (e.g., glu-cose-6-phosphate dehydrogenase, which regenerates NADPH).

The complement of defenses deployed differs not only between organisms or tis-sues, but even between cellular compartments. For instance, GPX plays an impor-tant role in mammals but is absent from flies and nematodes [118,119], and there exist in humans three forms of SOD (cytosolic Cu,Zn-SOD, mitochondrial Mn-SOD, and extracellular SOD), encoded and regulated independently [55].

As far as supporting the free radical theory of aging is concerned, the univer-sality of antioxidant defenses is good news. Although the nature of these defenses varies between species, the presence of some type of antioxidant defense is uni-versal. In fact, some antioxidants, such as SOD, are very highly conserved. Clearly, an indifference to oxygen free radicals is inconsistent with life, underlin-ing the centrality of oxidative damage. Moreover, the fact that antioxidant defenses are not uniform has been incorporated into the free radical theory; dif-ferences in antioxidant defenses between species have been put forth to explain differences in life span. Although there is something uncomfortably ad hoc in these two different interpretations of the data, they are not inconsistent. Whereas aerobic life requires organisms to cope with oxidation to some extent, different evolutionary pressures appear to have selected for more or less investment in these defenses, as is discussed in section 3 below.

Lastly, a persistent problem in testing the free radical theory is that antioxi-dants are both parallel, (different antioxidants can play similar roles, e.g., catalase and GPX), and serial, (enzymes operate in tandem to decompose radicals to harmless products, e.g., SOD and catalase). Consequently, measurements of indi-vidual antioxidant activities do not have great relevance. In fact, as is discussed below, measurements of age-related changes in individual antioxidants have led to conflicting results [14]. For this reason, aggregate assays have been devised, such as the susceptibility of crude cellular homogenates to in vitro oxidation by ionizing radiation [120,121]. Although these assays do not provide any informa-tion about the specific mechanisms of defense, they conveniently measure overall effectiveness.

2.5 Repair of oxidative damage

Unlike defenses against oxidants, which have been extensively characterized, the machinery for repairing oxidative damage is relatively unexplored. Nevertheless, it is clear that cells repair oxidized lipids, (e.g., phospholipase A_2 cleaves lipid peroxides from phospholipids) [122], oxidized nucleic acids (e.g., glycosylases specifically recognize and excise oxidized bases from double-stranded DNA) [97,123—125], and oxidized proteins [126—129]. The comparative biochemistry of cellular repair is very fertile ground for the free radical theory.

2.6 Synthesis: the interaction of oxidant generation, oxidative damage and repair

The existence of multiple intracellular sources of oxidants and complex defenses has led to refinements of the free radical theory. For example, it is clear that the metabolism of oxygen radicals is dynamic, with damage resulting from an increase in oxidant generation or a decrease in antioxidant defenses. Consequently, a difference in life span between species or individuals could be due to different rates of living, or to different "rates of scavenging" [3,10]. The picture has been further complicated by the discovery of specific enzymatic repair of oxidative damage, leading to "repair" or "fidelity" versions of the theory, in which life span is determined by the failure to correct oxidative damage [122,130].

The relationship between these three components of oxidative stress; oxidant generation, antioxidant protection, and repair of oxidative damage, and the way in which they have been investigated in testing the free radical theory, is illustrated schematically in Fig. 1. Increases in oxidant generation, and decreases in antioxidant protection and repair systems, are amongst the theory's testable predictions, and have been examined both as a function of age in individuals of the same species, as well as between species of differing MLSP.

Lastly, an extremely important, (if experimentally recalcitrant), aspect of the interactions between oxidants, antioxidants, and repair are feedback loops, positive and negative, between them. Antioxidant defenses and cellular repair systems have been shown to be induced in response to oxidative challenges [131—133], and are of course potential targets of oxidative destruction [134]. Also, the generation of oxidants may be enhanced by the malfunctioning of oxidatively damaged molecules [135,136]. Therefore, by examining Fig. 1 it is not difficult to envision ways in which primary oxidative destruction of any target, (e.g., the components of the mitochondrial ETC, scavenging enzymes such as SOD, or DNA repair enzymes), might promote further oxidative damage in what is frequently called a "catastrophic vicious cycle."

Although such cycles are intuitively appealing, their documentation awaits future work and will be extremely difficult from a technical standpoint. An alternative to lab-based approaches, namely the computational modeling of these complex interactions in what has been termed a "Network Theory of Ageing," is being pursued by theoretical gerontologists [137]. Ultimately, a question of obvious importance is whether or not such cycles, if they exist, could be broken, and modeling may help pinpoint weak links for therapeutic intervention.

3   REFINEMENTS AND COROLLARIES OF THE FREE RADICAL THEORY

As the free radical theory has gained ground, it has incorporated other ideas. For example, as mentioned above, the rate of living hypothesis dovetailed with the free radical theory once mitochondrial free radical generation was confirmed.

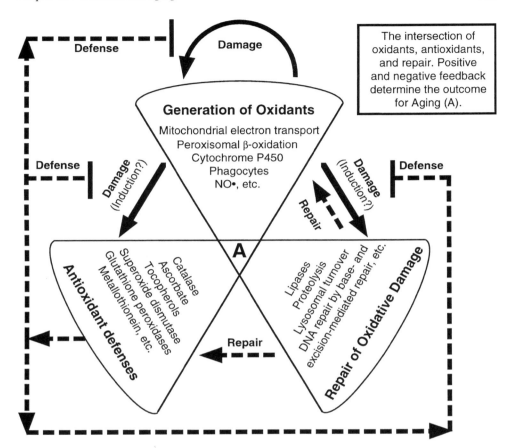

Fig. 1. The ultimate outcome of oxidative stress is a function of: (a) oxidant generation, (b) antioxidant defenses, and (c) repair of oxidative damage. Bolds arrows denote damage by oxidants, and dashed arrows routes for its prevention or repair. Due to the ways in which these processes may interact, (e.g., mitochondrial oxidants may damage the enzymes responsible for repairing oxidized mitochondrial components, thereby worsening mitochondrial oxidant generation), multiple positive and negative feedback loops are possible. Aging (A) is situated at the intersection of these processes. In testing the free radical theory, changes in a−c have been measured both as a function of age, and as a function of species maximum life span potential. The similarity of the figure to the international emblem of radiation is not a coincidence; the free radical theory has its roots in radiation biology.

Three other ideas that have been influential are the evolutionary concept of antagonistic pleiotropy, the somatic mutation theory of aging, and the mitochondrial theory of aging.

3.1 Oxygen radicals and evolutionary theories of aging

The intracellular generation of oxidants capable of limiting life span may appear paradoxical. It seems reasonable to expect that natural selection might have devised aerobic cells which do not leak toxic by-products. Evolutionary biologists have contributed to the free radical theory by suggesting why physiologically harmful generation of oxygen radicals occurs. They have argued that natural selection favors genes that act early in life and increase reproduction, rather than genes which act to preserve nongerm cells (the "disposable soma"), a principle called "antagonistic pleiotropy" [138—142].

   The concept of antagonistic pleiotropy stresses that in the wild, reproductive success is principally a function of external factors. With the exception of modern-day humans, individuals do not usually die of old age, but are eaten, parasitized, or out-competed by others. Therefore, preserving the cells of the "disposable soma", otherwise known as the body, may be disadvantageous if it detracts from more pressing problems. The toxicity of respiratory burst oxidants, for instance, cannot easily be eliminated by evolution, since this would result in death from childhood infection. Similarly, an investment in improved antioxidant defenses maximizes fitness only if the resources are not better invested in strength, beauty, speed, and so on. The potential relevance of this concept to exercise-associated oxidative damage is clear-cut. The human capacity for strenuous exercise at peak performance, a product of evolution, was probably "selected for" because it served short-term goals, such as hunting, escaping predators or conflict, sexual display, etc. In other words, the hypothesis that exercise might have a toxicological "cost" is well in line with current evolutionary theory.

3.2 Oxygen radicals and the somatic mutation theory of aging

The somatic mutation theory holds that the accumulation of DNA mutations is responsible for degenerative senescence [97,143—146]. In the case of cancer, which results from both point mutations in oncogenes and the loss of tumor suppressor gene function, (often by deletion), the role of mutations is unquestionable [117]. It remains to be seen whether or not the argument is equally valid for non-proliferative senescence. For instance, whereas significant age-related increases in somatic mutations in a reporter transgene (lacZ) have been measured in a mitotic tissue of transgenic mice, (the liver), no increase was detected in the largely post-mitotic brain of the same animals [147], suggesting that neurodegeneration, at least, is unlikely to be the result of accumulated somatic mutations in nuclear DNA. Moreover, the accumulation of mutations in the liver tissues was not dramatic, suggesting that mutagenesis may be of little functional consequence to mitotic tissues as well [148]. In light of these data, what evidence is there that somatic mutations are related to aging? A compelling argument for the somatic mutation theory of aging was provided years ago in the discovery that DNA repair ability correlates with species-specific life span [149], a phenomenon which has recently been reconfirmed [150]. However, it has been noted that DNA repair, which is necessary for the prevention of tumorigenesis, is necessary but not sufficient for longevity [150]. Ultimately, arguments about the physiological significance of somatic mutations hinge upon how disruptive a given mutational burden is to a cell or animal; with current methods, this is an unanswerable question.

In any case, it has been demonstrated in numerous studies with prokaryotes, yeast, and mammalian cells that oxidants are mutagens, against which cells actively protect their genetic material [151,152]. Although it is not yet clear what fraction of mutations can be attributed to oxidative damage, the characterization and cloning of defense genes against oxidative mutagenesis [95], and the development of in vivo mutagenesis assays [153], has finally opened up avenues for definitive experiments.

3.3 Oxygen radicals and mitochondrial theories of aging

The mitochondrion has also long attracted attention as one of the cell's weak links, an organelle whose dysfunction has profound negative pleiotropic effects [154]. Mitochondria supply ATP and also sequester potentially toxic Ca^{2+} ions and yet, due to their generation of $O_2\bullet^-$ and H_2O_2, they are on the front lines of respiratory oxidative stress. The idea that the mitochondrion is, therefore, uniquely vulnerable was embraced early on by proponents of the free radical theory [155]. In the early 1980s, Miquel and his colleagues proposed that oxidative damage to mitochondrial DNA in postmitotic cells would lead to mutations and blocks to replication, and consequently to mitochondrial dysfunction and physiological decline [143,156,157]. This "mitochondrial DNA mutation hypothesis of aging", which incorporates free radicals, somatic mutations, and the central role of mitochondria in homeostasis, is presently under intense scrutiny [16,158–171]. Of course, the fact that aerobic exercise exerts profound effects on muscle mitochondria makes these mitochondrial theories of aging of particular relevance to the topic of this volume.

4   OXIDATIVE PHENOMENOLOGY: AGE-ASSOCIATED TRENDS

The phenomenological approach to the free radical theory has involved looking for traces of oxidative damage in vivo. Phenomenology is not well suited to critically testing the free radical theory, since the data, (which are voluminous and generally supportive), mainly represent correlations. Documented increases in oxidative damage, no matter how impressive, may be a consequence of a primary, nonoxidative event. Nevertheless, phenomenology is the foundation upon which more powerful experiments depend, since the analytical methods developed for it have been used to compare species, genetic mutants, and populations with differing life spans. In fact, almost all of the biomarkers of oxidative stress described in this section have been found to accumulate at a faster rate in short-lived species, and in many cases, this rate correlates with O_2 consumption. Familiarity with the most frequently measured endpoints is a prerequisite to assessing the free radical theory.

If oxidative damage is a significant cause of cellular degeneration, then one expects to see more of it in older individuals. Oxidative damage has been described in terms of "accumulation, modification and depletion"; accumulation of end-products of oxidative damage (such as lipofuscin), modification of existing structures (such as oxidative adducts in DNA) and depletion (such as the loss of enzymatic activity or reduced thiols).

4.1 Accumulation of oxidative end-products

The gradual and steady accumulation of intracellular yellow-brown fluorescent pigments, referred to as lipofuscin, occurs in numerous phyla. Lipofuscin arises prominently in postmitotic cells, where it is argued that it remains undiluted by rounds of cell division [172], and is located in small granules in secondary lysosomes. Lipofuscin is structurally complex and variable, consisting mostly of cross-linked lipid and protein residues [172–174], and is ubiquitous, documented in species as diverse as nematodes, fruit flies, rats, bees, crab-eating monkeys, crayfish. Most important, it is abundant in aged tissues, where it may occupy more than half of the volume of the cell [38].

Early on, it was discovered that incubation of amino acids with the lipid peroxidation product malonaldehyde under acidic conditions leads to the formation of lipofuscin-like fluorophores [90]. The plausibility of such a reaction, given the contents and low pH of lysosomes, suggested that lipid peroxidation in vivo leads to the formation of lipofuscin [91]. Other in vitro studies of lipid peroxidation have since uncovered a great number of routes to fluorescent, cross-linked products via promiscuous oxidative chemistry, which suggests that lipofuscin is a biomarker of lipid peroxidation [38,172,175].

Despite extensive in vitro experiments, it is not known with certainty how lipofuscinogenesis occurs in vivo, nor how lipofuscin comes to accumulate with age. Lipid peroxidation could occur throughout the cell and be followed by lysosomal phagocytosis and cross-linking of peroxidative by-products, in which case an age-related increase in lipofuscin content could be seen as the result of oxidative damage. Alternatively, an age-associated decline in lysosomal activity, (due to something besides oxidation), might increase the residence time of phagocytosed material enough to enhance lipofuscinogenesis in situ from constant amounts of peroxides [176]. In support of the latter possibility, infusion into rat brains of lysosomal proteinase inhibitors leads to the rapid accumulation of lipofuscin-like granules [177]. This scenario suggests that lipofuscinogenesis may be a consequence, not a cause, of aging.

Experiments with cultured cardiac myocytes have established roles for both oxidative damage and lysosomal turnover [136]. Lipofuscin accumulates in these cells in culture, and growth under increasing O_2 partial pressure from 5% to

40% markedly enhances its accumulation [178]. Inclusion of iron in the growth medium further increases lipofuscinogenesis, and the iron chelator desferal depresses it, suggesting that Fenton reaction-generated •OH is an initiator [179]. Lastly, antioxidants inhibit lipofuscin formation in cultured cardiomyocytes, whereas lysosomal protease inhibitors increase it [180−182].

Even if oxidative damage is primarily responsible for depositing lipofuscin in the lysosomes of senescing animals, is it more than a biomarker of aging? It has been theorized that lipofuscin accumulation is likely to impair autophagy, as more lysosomal volume is occupied by the indigestible material [136]. As lysosomes are responsible for the recycling of materials and organelles, their failure may include the following:

(i) a delay in mitochondrial turnover (with a concomitant decrease in mitochondrial efficiency or an increase in mitochondrial oxidant generation);
(ii) an accumulation of oxidatively modified proteins and lipids in the cytosol awaiting degradation (potentially aggravating cytosolic lipid peroxidation);
(iii) an accumulation of lipofuscin-bound iron in a redox-active form (which might promote further intralysosomal lipid peroxidation); and
(iv) the disruption of lysosomal membranes (and the spillage of hydrolytic enzymes into the cytosol).

Although these speculations [136] remain to be substantiated, it has been shown that when treated with sublethal doses of H_2O_2, cultured cells display lysosomal disruption, and leakage of the lysosomal compartment into the cytosol [183]. Also, it has been demonstrated that the sensitivity of cultured primary hepatocytes to oxidation, which was associated with a loss of GSH and an influx of calcium ions, was prevented by the iron chelator desferal [184]. What is intriguing about these results is the fact that whereas desferal stabilized the lysosomes, it did not prevent the loss of GSH nor the increase in intracellular calcium, and so it may be that it is lysosomal leakage per se, rather than peroxidative damage, which is the actual lethal step in this model of oxidative killing.

4.2 Steady-state levels of oxidative modification

Unlike cytosolic proteins whose half-lives are measured in minutes or hours, some extracellular proteins are rarely recycled, and oxidative modification of these old macromolecules occurs. A class of fluorescent cross-linked molecules that is distinct from lipofuscin forms on long-lived proteins such as collagen and lens crystallin [185]. These modifications are initiated by the reaction of reducing sugars with free amino groups (glycation), a chemical sequence which is unrelated to oxidation and results in a molecule known as an Amadori product. Further nonoxidative rearrangements result in stable, cross-linked "advanced glycation end products" (AGEs) [186], whose absolute abundance appears to be an excellent biomarker of age [187]. Recently, it was discovered that oxidation is one fate of the Amadori product. Pentosidine, the name given to a cross-link involving arginine, lysine and pentose moieties, is one such a "glycooxidation product," the formation of which requires the presence of O_2 [188]. It appears as if Amadori products themselves are a source of H_2O_2 in vitro, which then accelerates glucose-mediate fluorogenic collagen cross-linking in a catalase-sensitive fashion, although it is unclear to what extent this occurs in vivo [187,189]. As is the case with other AGEs, the tissue burden of pentosidine is elevated in diabetics, as a consequence of hyperglycemia.

Pentosidine has been found to accumulate as a function of age in shrews, rats, dogs, cows, pigs, monkeys, and humans, yielding equivalently shaped curves in all cases [190]. It is not clear, however, how glycooxidative modifications might contribute to degeneration. It has been proposed that cross-linking in cartilage is related to its decreased elasticity and relative resistance to proteolysis in old animals [191]. However, the absolute amount of collagen pentosidine cross-links attained at death is much higher in long-lived than in short-lived species: 6—7 pmol/mg in 3.5-year-old shrews, 15—18 pmol/mg in 25-year-old monkeys, and 50—100 pmol/mg in 90-year-old humans [190]. In other words, it appears that the rate of pentosidine accumulation may merely be a measure of more rapid oxidative damage in short-lived species, rather than an actual cause of dysfunction.

An intriguing twist to this story has been the cloning of a specific cellular receptor for AGE, called RAGE, (Receptor for AGE), that belongs to the immunoglobulin superfamily and is expressed by mononuclear cells and the vascular endothelium [192,193]. One of the effects of AGE binding by RAGE is the generation, (in mononuclear cells), of intracellular oxidants, the activation of the oxidant-sensitive transcription factor NF-$\kappa\beta$, and the induction of downstream events linked to atherogenesis [194,195]. It has recently been shown that RAGE, which is highly expressed by microglial cells in the brain [196], is a receptor for amyloid-β-peptide (Aβ). RAGE binding of Aβ results in oxidant generation, implicated in the etiology of Alzheimer's disease [20,197].

Several amino acid residues in proteins are susceptible to oxidative modification, forming side chain carbonyl derivatives [102]. The development of sensitive methods for the analysis of protein carbonyls by Stadtman and his co-workers [198] enabled them to study oxidative modification in human brain tissue and cultured fibroblasts, as well as in rat liver. They found a 2- to 3-fold rise in protein carbonyl content between a young and old age and an increase from 10% to about 30% of the total protein pool [8]. The increase was exponential and correlated well with decreased activity of the oxidation-sensitive enzyme glucose-6-phosphate dehydrogenase (G6PD). By comparison, the rise in protein oxidation in the mongolian gerbil was less dramatic, increasingly significantly in brain, heart, and testis, but not in kidney. As in human tissues, trends for the activity of G6PD correspond to the increased damage, falling in brain and heart but not in kidney [121]. Similar results have been reported in an insect model. An age-associated 2.5-fold increase in the protein carbonyl content of old vs. young houseflies has also been documented [199]. As in the case of humans, the increase occurs exponentially during the life span. The similarity of the degree and pattern of increase in insects and mammals is striking, considering the enormous difference in their MLSP, (40 days vs. 100 years). Moreover, protein carbonyl levels increase similarly in mitochondrial extracts from the thoracic flight muscles of these animals [135]. Mitochondrial aconitase is particularly prone to oxidative modification during aging in vivo, and was identified by the immuno-blotting of housefly mitochondrial protein extracts with a monoclonal antibody designed to detect protein carbonyls [200]. Carbonylation of this key citric acid cycle enzyme increased in parallel with a decline in its activity.

Somewhat stronger evidence that protein oxidation may play a causative role in senescence comes from comparisons of "crawlers" vs. "fliers" of the same aging cohort. Although the two groups share the same chronological age, crawlers are phenotypically senescent individuals which have lost the ability to fly and have a shorter remaining average life span than fliers, (e.g., 9.0 days vs. 13.3 days for 10-day-old crawlers and fliers, respectively). The protein carbonyl content of crawlers was 29% higher than that of fliers [199], reflecting their greater pheno-typic age, as was the degree of carbonyl modification of mitochondrial (but not cytosolic) aconitase [200]. Humans suffering from Werner's syndrome, a disease characterized by premature senescence, are individuals whose phenotypic aging is also accelerated, and they too appear to have more extensive protein oxidation. Fibroblasts from Werner's patients of all ages have a level of protein carbonyls equivalent to that in 80-year-old controls [201]. In a creative study attempting to correlate protein oxidation to a physiologically relevant endpoint, it was shown that in old mice, inter-animal variation in protein carbonyl content of two differ-ent areas of the brain, (cerebral cortex vs. cerebellum), was associated with paral-lel inter-animal variation in memory and motor function deficits [202].

Are protein carbonyls physiologically relevant, or are they merely markers? What are the actual consequences of protein modification? Unfortunately, there is little quantitative data with which to answer this question, although qualitative data exists. The fate of oxidized proteins may depend upon the form of damage. For example, metal-catalyzed oxidation of G6PD by iron/citrate results in a ther-molabile enzyme which is a better substrate for proteolysis than is the native enzyme [203]. Rapid turnover of metal-oxidized G6PD may, therefore, proceed efficiently. On the other hand, G6PD modification by 4-hydroxy-2-nonenal, a lipid peroxidation product, also inactivates the enzyme, but does not render the enzyme thermolabile or increase its degradation by proteases [88]. This difference exists despite the fact that in both cases, the same lysine residue is affected. To make matters more complex, the cross-linking of G6PD multimers by 4-hydro-xy-2-nonenal, (which predictably results in a product with lipofuscin-like fluores-cence), produces a molecular species which actually inhibits the multicatalytic protease [204]. The cost to a cell of protein oxidation is presently an unknown quantity.

The appearance of protein-bound 3,4-dihydroxyphenylalanine (DOPA) on •OH-damaged proteins has been characterized. When converted to a quinone, protein bound DOPA can undergo redox cycling, generating $O_2 \bullet^-$. It has, there-fore, been proposed that protein oxidation may contribute to the progression of aging not merely by the loss of protein function, but also by an acceleration of the flux of oxidants [63,205–209].

The oxidative modification of DNA has also been studied in animals of different ages, with conflicting results. Although some studies have reported a modest increase in specific oxidative adducts, single-strand breaks and abasic sites, others have been negative [97,210–213]. The failure to detect an age-related increase in oxidative adducts by the analytical chromatographic techniques typically employed may have been due to the difficulty of working close to the limit of sensitivity [95]. In fact, it has become apparent that the measurement of the adduct 8-oxodG is frequently plagued by artifacts [214–218], and that these may have compromised some published experiments. Of particular concern are measurements of 8-oxodG in mitochondrial DNA (mtDNA) [219], which have generally been higher than in nuclear DNA, but which may be particularly prone to artifacts associated with the analysis of small samples [216,219]. Moreover, it is noteworthy that even among the highly variable published estimates of 8-oxodG in mtDNA are values that are equivalent to the lowest measured values of 8-oxodG in nuclear DA [220]. Due to the small number of studies of mtDNA, and the high variability between the measured values, it is not yet possible to conclude that mtDNA is, in fact, more heavily oxidized than nDNA. Encouragingly, alternative PCR-based methods for measuring oxidative damage have recently been used to compare oxidation of mtDNA and nDNA by exogenous oxidants, with the result that the former appears more sensitive than the latter [221,222], although these studies could not quantify baseline values of damage. With methodological improvements, future experiments may be more conclusive. For instance, the use of single-cell gel electrophoresis, (the comet assay), to measure single-strand breaks and abasic sites in whole rat hepatocytes in situ, revealed a statistically significant 1.5-fold increase in old rats compared with young rats [223], (although this experiment did not distinguish between oxidative and non-oxidative damage).

In any case, even if the burden of oxidative adducts does increase with age, there is virtually no information about the likely effect of oxidative DNA damage in vivo, apart from the knowledge that it leads to mutations and cancer. The fact that there is active DNA repair in post-mitotic tissues (in which the danger of mutation due to replication is nonexistent), and that such repair is often targeted to transcribed regions of the genome, suggests that DNA damage itself interferes with gene expression, and is not tolerated [224,225]. This important question deserves more attention.

4.3 Oxidative depletion of biochemical pools

The oxidative depletion of molecules with increasing age has not been well documented in senescent animals, since the destruction of molecules does not often leave traces. Luckily, some pathways of oxidative damage do leave biochemical fingerprints. The loss of integrity of lipid bilayers due to peroxidation is one of the most salient effects of oxidative damage [91], and results in the generation of aldehydes and alkanes. Unfortunately these are not easily measured, the widespread use of the simple and nonspecific thiobarbituric acid test notwithstanding [86]. Nevertheless, countless studies have reported an increase in thiobarbituric acid-reactive substances (TBARS) with age. Combined with other more reliable assays, these have demonstrated that there is a greater degree of lipid peroxidation in older animals [226]. The measurements of exhaled ethane and pentane is a technique that has the advantage of being applicable to humans [227]. Unlike lipofuscin and TBARS, which measure the size of a pool of destroyed molecules and require a tissue biopsy, the assay of exhaled hydrocarbons measures the rate of damage, and is noninvasive. Breath pentane has been found to increase significantly with age in humans, suggesting that increased lipid turnover occurs with age due to peroxidation [228–230]. Refinement of the technique and elimination of the associated artifacts [231] should facilitate further testing of the free radical theory in humans.

The loss of activity of several oxygen-sensitive enzymes, (G6PD, glutamate synthetase), has been reported in mammalian models of aging [8]. In houseflies, a decline in G6PD, glutamate synthetase and alcohol dehydrogenase activities has also been documented, and coincides with a dramatic loss of protein sulfhydryls [232]. Another commonly reported age-related loss is an increase in the ratio of oxidized to reduced glutathione, which may reflect a disruption of the cell's redox state [37,233].

4.4 Age-associated trends in antioxidant defenses and repair

What is the cause of age-related oxidative damage? It could result from less active antioxidant defenses and repair, but studies which have measured age-related changes in antioxidant defenses have generated conflicting results. Recent measurements of antioxidants in mongolian gerbils [121] and mice [233] are representative of the types of patterns which have been uncovered in many other studies [28,234–241]. In various tissues of gerbils, there was not a consistent pattern of change; increases in SOD and decreases in GSH were observed, whereas GPX was equivalent at different ages and catalase increased or decreased, depending upon the tissues and the age at analysis. In mouse brain, on the other hand, significant decreases in SOD, catalase, and GSH reductase were observed, although GPX levels were unchanged.

Another complication is that defenses are induced in response to stress. Therefore, a higher level may indicate better protection, or alternatively, greater need for antioxidant defenses due to an increase in oxidant generation. Studies of antioxidants in rat heart and skeletal muscles illustrate this point. In heart, decreases in cytosolic SOD and GPX and increases in mitochondrial SOD and GPX were noted in older animals, and several indices of oxidative damage were also elevated [242]. From these results, it was concluded that although overall myocardial antioxidant defenses were weakened in the older animals, they were induced in mitochondria as a compensatory response. In skeletal muscles, in contrast, increases were observed in both cytosolic and mitochondrial forms of all of the enzymes studied [243], despite the fact that indices of lipid peroxidation were again elevated. In this case, it was concluded that both cytosolic and mitochondrial antioxidants were induced. The credibility of these hypotheses is not in question, but it is hard to see how they could be disproved. When these and similar studies of age-related antioxidant levels are combined, what remains is a confusing assemblage of ambiguous trends.

Of course, interactions between antioxidants are complex, which aggravates the problem. In order to avoid the problems posed by assays of individual antioxidants, aggregate measures of antioxidant defenses have been devised. A crude but integrative measure of antioxidant defenses, for instance, is the susceptibility of a homogenate to induced oxidation. X-irradiation of a whole body homogenate of houseflies results in a linear, dose-dependent increase in protein carbonyls. When homogenates of old and young flies are compared, the rate of induction of protein carbonyls by X-irradiation is 45% higher in 14-day-old than 5-day-old flies. This suggests that the antioxidant defenses in older flies are less able to cope with oxidative stress. Moreover, the activity of G6PD, an enzyme known to be sensitive to oxidation, decreases upon X-irradiation of living flies, and does so to a greater extent in old than young animals [120]. When this assay was applied to the gerbil samples described above, in which no overall change in antioxidants was seen, a clear difference between young and old tissues emerged. Whereas 6 krad of X-irradiation induced a 20—38% increase in protein carbonyls in 5-month-old animals, it induced a 152—211% increase in 26-month old animals [121]. Similarly, although synaptosomes from young and old mice contain equivalent amounts of ATP and GSH, those of old mice were far more sensitive to GSH depletion by the diethyl maleate than those from young mice [244]. Lastly, reperfusion injury is a well-established model of oxidative stress associated with the re-establishment of blood flow following ischemia, and it causes greater oxidative damage to heart tissues of old rats than young ones [245]. The use of a polyclonal antiserum specific for adducts between lipid peroxidation end-products and proteins detected such covalent modifications of mitochondrial proteins from old but not young animals, which was associated with a more dramatic loss of respiratory capacity in the former. Whereas the baseline mitochondrial respiratory parameters (before ischemia-reperfusion) did not differ between young and old animals, the administration of a physiologically relevant stress revealed a probable age-related decline in antioxidant defenses.

Another alternative to measuring absolute levels of antioxidants in old vs. young animals is to investigate the ability of animals of different ages to induce antioxidants, an approach that has been applied to the analysis of SOD in the nematode C. elegans [246]. Whereas in young animals, challenge with hyperoxia or the redox cycling compound plumbagin resulted in an increase in SOD activity. In middle-aged or old animals it actually resulted in a net loss of activity.

What about repair of oxidative damage? Does its activity decrease with age?

The bulk of evidence suggests that there is probably not an overall age-associated change in the intrinsic ability of cells to degrade damaged proteins [247,248]. Although a dramatic decrease in the activity of the oxidized protein-specific alkaline protease has been reported in old rat hepatocytes [101], no change in this activity was measured in the heart or brain of 25-month-old vs. 5-month-old gerbils [121]. In a separate work, a 50% age-related decline in a single activity (peptidylglutamyl-peptide hydrolase activity) of the hepatic multicatalytic protease was associated with its selective sensitivity, (relative to the multicatalytic protease's other activities), to metal-catalyzed oxidation, suggesting that resistance to oxidants may, (logically), characterize the proteases responsible for degrading damaged proteins [249].

Although the intrinsic protease activity may not decrease with age, there is evidence that repair of oxidized proteins may be less easily induced in response to an oxidative insult in old animals. For instance, exposure of young and old rats to 100% O_2 increased the content of protein carbonyls in both groups over a 48 h period. Between 48 and 54 h of exposure, however, alkaline protease activity was induced in young animals, with a corresponding decrease in protein carbonyls to initial levels. In old animals, on the other hand, no increase in activity was observed, and protein carbonyl levels continued to rise throughout the time course [101].

There is circumstantial evidence from mutagenesis studies that either antioxidant defenses or repair of oxidative DNA damage (or both) are less efficient in old mice. The induction of somatic mutations in mice by γ-irradiation is from 2.3- to 3.6-fold higher in old rather than in young animals, depending upon the dose [250]. The induction of mutations in young and old animals was reduced by feeding the animals a cocktail of dietary antioxidants, confirming that oxidants played a mutagenic role in these experiments. Therefore, the more pronounced induction of mutations in older mice is indirect evidence of decreased antioxidant defenses and repair [250]. Later experiments employing peripheral lymphocytes from young and old human subjects resulted in similar results [251]. The ability of human peripheral lymphocytes to repair oxidative DNA damage induced by H_2O_2 has also been found to be less efficient in cells from older donors [252].

Altogether, the results above suggest that older cells may be less able to prevent oxidative damage from occurring, and less effective at removing the damage once it has occurred. There is a clear need for more and better data about age-related trends in defenses and repair.

4.5 Age-associated trends in oxidant generation

The accumulation of oxidative damage could also result from an age-associated increase in the primary generation of oxidants, and some research suggests that this is the case. Generation of H_2O_2 and $O_2\bullet^-$ by isolated mitochondria and sub-mitochondrial particles from 25-month-old gerbils, for instance, is about

150—200% that of 5-month-old animals [121], and that of aged rat heart [235] and brain [253] have also been reported to be elevated. On the other hand, a recent study which paid specific attention to maintaining physiological substrate concentrations during in vitro mitochondrial incubations failed to detect an age-related increase in mitochondria H_2O_2 output [58]. Recent measurements of oxidant generation in carefully isolated rat hepatocytes from young and old animals, employing an intracellular dye which fluoresces upon oxidation, have confirmed under conditions which preserve cellular integrity that cellular oxidant generation appears to increase [171]. A similar increase in oxidant generation documented in flight muscle mitochondria of houseflies was associated with increases in the activities of every measured component of the electron transport chain except for the content of UQ [254], suggesting that an imbalance in electron transport may be the cause of aberrant reduction of oxygen. In another experiment, a population of chronologically identical 12-day-old flies was separated into phenotypically older "crawlers" and younger "fliers" as described above. Mitochondrial H_2O_2 generation was twice as high in the crawlers than in the fliers, reflecting their greater phenotypic age.

Interestingly, oxidative damage to mitochondrial membranes and proteins has itself been implicated in enhanced oxidant generation; exposure of isolated mitochondria to the free radical generator 2,2-azobis (2-aminopropane) dihydrochloride or the cross-linking agent glutaraldehyde resulted in mitochondria which were more able to generate H_2O_2 when fed exogenous substrate [254]. When these in vitro studies are combined with the above evidence of increased oxidative damage, the picture that emerges is a potentially "vicious cycle" of oxidative damage and oxidant generation.

5   INTERSPECIES COMPARISONS

All of the data discussed in the previous section identify age-related differences within a given species. A complementary, and in some ways more powerful approach, is to compare species that have different MLSP. Comparative biochemistry and physiology, inspired by the rate of living hypothesis, has played a key role in establishing the free radical theory. Several representative studies are described below.

5.1 Oxidative damage and maximum life span potential

The accumulation of cardiac lipofuscin in the monkey correlates with its cumulative O_2 consumption, starting at sexual maturation [255]. Comparisons between rodents, dogs, and primate species also revealed a close correlation between specific metabolic rate and lipofuscin accumulation [256,257]. The accumulation of the glycooxidation product pentosidine is similar. Short-lived species such as the shrew, (MLSP = 3.5 years), or rat, (MLSP = 3 years), with high specific metabolic rates, accumulate pentosidine in collagen at a rate of about 0.3—0.5 pmol/

mg annually. Longer-lived primates such as monkeys and humans accumulate pentosidine at about a tenth as fast [190].

Interspecies comparisons of protein oxidation mirror these results. The protein carbonyl content of 15-day-old individuals of five species of fly correlated negatively with mean life span; the longest-lived species, (*Drosophila melanogaster*, mean life span = 65.5 days), had roughly a third of the level of protein oxidation as shortest-lived species, (*Phaenicia sericata*, mean life span = 29.5 days) [258]. The content of protein carbonyls was 20% higher in the heart, and about 50% higher in the brain, of 3.5-month-old individuals of *Mus musculus* (MLSP = 3.5 years) than in 3.5-month-old individuals of *Peromyscus leucopus* (MLSP = 8 years) [259].

The excretion of the oxo8gua and 8-oxodG in urine is a reflection of whole body oxidative hits to DNA [260]. The validity of its use to measure in vivo oxidative hits is strengthened by a recent study of 33 women, in which both O_2 consumption and excretion of 8-oxodG were measured. There was a highly significant positive correlation, (p = 0.00007, r = 0.64), between O_2 consumption and excretion of adducts [261]. When the urinary output of the oxidative DNA repair products oxo8gua. thymine glycol and thymidine glycol were compared in mice, rats, and humans, they were found to correlate with species-specific metabolic rate [260,262].

5.2 Antioxidant defenses and maximum life span potential

One version of the free radical theory proposes that the differences in life span between species are due to species-specific antioxidant capacity. Early work by Cutler and his colleagues tested this association; MLSP correlated positively with SOD but negatively with catalase and GPX [3]. Recently other groups have revisited this hypothesis, with similar results. Comparisons between SOD, catalase, GPX and GSH in brain, liver and heart from mice, rats, guinea pigs, rabbits, pigs, and cows were carried out and revealed that:
(i)   SOD and catalase activities correlated positively with MLSP;
(ii) GSH activity correlated negatively with MLSP; and
(iii) GPX correlated positively with MLSP in the brain and negatively in the liver and heart [263].
Interspecies comparisons between more distantly related vertebrate Classes found either no correlation or a negative correlation between antioxidants and MLSP. For instance, in the liver of fish, frogs, birds, and mammals, strongly significant negative correlations were found for catalase, GPX, and GSH, whereas all other measured antioxidants, (SOD, GSH reductase, ascorbate, urate, GSH), failed to correlate with MLSP [264]. When the same antioxidants were measured in brain and lung tissues of the same species, virtually identical results were obtained [265,266].

Comparisons between two very closely related species of mice; the house mouse, (*Mus musculus*), and the white-footed mouse, (*Peromyscus leucopus*), which lives twice as long, have revealed higher levels of SOD, catalase, and GPX in brain and heart extracts of the latter, with the differences in GPX being the most dramatic. Also, when brain homogenates of the two species were challenged with X-irradiation, protein carbonyls accumulated at a 3-fold higher rate in shorter-lived *M. musculus* than longer-lived *P. leucopus* [259].

Altogether, these results suggest that the evolution of longevity has not been associated with a clear-cut increase in antioxidant capacity, at least across the broad sweep of evolution. (The comparisons between *M. musculus* and *P. leucopus* invites the speculation that the more recent radiation of long-lived species may be associated with the coordinate upregulation of antioxidant defenses). In any case, what emerged from the comparative biochemistry of free radical defenses is a fascinating paradox: birds, which typically have much longer long life spans than rodents, have lower activities of antioxidants and higher metabolic rates. This paradox has inspired the interspecies comparisons of mitochondrial oxidant generation discussed below.

5.3 Generation of reactive oxygen species and maximum life span potential

The rate of living hypothesis identified an inverse correlation between metabolic rate and life span, and the free radical theory supplied a convenient mechanistic link: the mitochondrial generation of oxidants. Appealing as it is, one of the problems with the rate of living hypothesis is the conspicuous lack of fit of a few groups, notably birds and primates. Both of these groups live longer than their specific metabolic rate would predict. As a result, the total lifetime oxygen consumption of these groups are quite a bit higher than other groups, (e.g., during their MLSP, pigeons and canaries consume 465 and 1,222 liters of O_2 per gram, respectively, whereas mice, rats, guinea pigs, and trout consume 77, 28, 48, and 26 liters of O_2, respectively) [240,266]. However, it cannot be assumed that the generation of oxidants is a direct function of metabolic rate, as mitochondria of different species (or even tissues) may exhibit different rates of intrinsic oxidant generation. These lines of reasoning by two laboratories have led to a similar line of experimentation, the results of which suggest that longevity is associated with a lesser capacity for mitochondrial oxidant generation [258,259,267−269].

For example, isolated pigeon mitochondria from brain, liver, or heart consume from 2- to 3-fold as much oxygen as isolated rat mitochondria from the same tissues. However, pigeon mitochondria generate only a third to a half as much H_2O_2 as rat mitochondria under the same conditions. As a result, the calculated percentage of O_2 converted to $O_2 \bullet^- /H_2O_2$ by mitochondria from lung, liver, and brain is about 10-fold lower in pigeons than in rats. This lower rate of oxidant generation corresponds with the roughly 10-fold longer life span of pigeons [269]. A second, independent comparison of mitochondrial oxidant generation by pigeons and rats found similar results [268]. Detailed respiratory comparisons have shown that generation of oxidants from both complex I and complex III of the mitochondrial electron transport chain is lower in pigeons than rats [270].

In fact, the earliest interspecies study of mitochondrial oxidant production compared liver mitochondria of five mammalian species and thoracic muscle mitochondria of two species of fly [271], and also found that longer MLSPs were associated with lower mitochondrial oxidant generation. The mitochondria from flies produced from 6-fold more to 300-fold more oxidants than those from mammals. In a more recent comparison of heart tissues of eight diverse mammalian species of widely varying life span, sub-mitochondrial particles of the short-lived species were found to generate more $O_2\bullet^-$ than those of long-lived species, a property correlated directly with the concentration of CoQ_9, (coenzyme Q possessing nine isoprene units in its isoprenoid tail), and inversely with CoQ_{10}, (although experiments intended to demonstrate a direct relationship between $CoQ_9{:}CoQ_{10}$ ratio and $O_2\bullet^-$ generation failed to do so) [272].

Interestingly, it appears as if the concept of intrinsic mitochondrial radical generation may also partially explain longevity differences between more closely related species. Measurements of $O_2\bullet^-$ and H_2O_2 generation by isolated mitochondria from the mouse species *M. musculus* and *P. leucopus* revealed that the former, which live half as long as the latter, also generate 48—74% more $O_2\bullet^-$ and 300—500% more H_2O_2. (As is the case with rats and pigeons, long-lived *P. leucopus* has the higher specific metabolic rate of the two species [259]). Lastly, a comparison of five species of dipteran fly whose mean life spans vary by 2-fold also showed that the rate of generation of mitochondrial $O_2\bullet^-$ and H_2O_2 correlated negatively with life span [258].

Altogether, interspecies comparisons of oxidative damage, antioxidant defenses, and oxidant generation provide some of the most compelling evidence that oxidants are one of the most significant determinants of life span.

6   ENVIRONMENTAL MANIPULATION AND LIFE SPAN

6.1 Dietary restriction

Limiting the dietary intake of mammals is a well established way to extend life span [273]. Interestingly, early expectations that DR would lower metabolic rate per se have not been confirmed, and so if DR attenuates oxidative damage, it is not via a simple reduction in oxygen consumption [32,274]. Rather, there is now convincing evidence that dietary restriction (DR) may act by decreasing oxidative stress and increasing antioxidant defenses and repair [275]. For example, mice whose caloric intake was restricted by 40% (DR) compared to ad libitum (AL) fed controls, and who lived 43% longer on average, had a less rapid accumulation of protein carbonyls in brain, heart, and kidney. Moreover, the generation of H_2O_2 and $O_2\bullet^-$ by mitochondria and sub-mitochondrial particles from DR animals was lower than from AL animals, and also increased less with advancing age. In this study, however, DR did not appear to enhance antioxidant defenses [235]. In another study, 40% DR of rats increased the activities of SOD, catalase, and GPX at older ages; free radical damage, as measured by thiobarbituric acid-reactive material and lipofuscin accumulation, was correspondingly lower [276]. In a third study, focusing on mitochondrial oxidant generation and membrane properties of synaptosomal preparations, 40% DR reduced mitochondrial oxidant generation in both young and old samples, and prevented the age-dependent decline in membrane fluidity, despite the fact that increases in the cholesterol/phospholipid ratio were common to both groups of animals [277]. Other experiments have been recently reviewed [33,275].

Dietary restriction also delays cancer incidence, which may be a reflection of fewer mutations induced by oxidants in DR animals. Dietary restriction has been shown to strengthen DNA repair, [278], although few studies have focused specifically on repair of oxidative lesions. Not only caloric restriction, but also restriction of protein intake, can forestall the occurrence of cancer in rodent models. Although the mechanism by which protein restriction operates is not clear, enhanced protection against cellular degeneration, including oxidative damage, is a likely candidate. It is, therefore, interesting that the level of protein carbonyls in animals fed a low-protein diet was significantly lower than in animals fed standard lab chow, and that treatment of the animals with γ-irradiation induced a greater increase in protein carbonyls in high- than in low-protein animals [279].

6.2 Activity restriction

The metabolic activity of caged houseflies can be reduced by limiting the space available for flight, ("low activity = LA" vs. "high activity = HA"). It is expected that the LA flies should live longer due to lower O_2 consumption and generation of oxidants, and this is in fact observed. LA flies exhibit more than a 2-fold increase in both mean life span and MLSP. Measurements of protein carbonyls in 14-day-old LA and HA flies, which have not yet begun to die, revealed an elevation of more than 50% in HA flies relative to LA flies in both whole-body extracts [199] and in mitochondria [135].

Under unfavorable conditions, the nematode *C. elegans* may undergo a morphological transformation to form a "dauer larva", a resting stage that does not feed, exhibits altered metabolic activity, and can survive for several times the MLSP of adult nematodes before returning to the adult stage. Interestingly, dauer larvae have also been found to have increase SOD activity [280].

6.3 Oxygen tension

Another experimental manipulation which modulates life span is growth under different O_2 tensions. The growth of houseflies in an atmosphere of 100% oxygen, for example, markedly reduces their mean and MLSPs, and also increases the rate of accumulation of protein carbonyls in whole body extracts [199] and in isolated mitochondria [135]. Similarly, elevated atmospheric O_2 decreased, and subnormal oxygen increased, the mean and maximum life spans of nematodes

[281]. Of course, the principal drawbacks of this type of experiment are its in-applicability to mammals, and the fact that elevations or decreases in ambient O_2 in such species will be likely to be confound by the overt pathology of hypo- or hyperoxia.

7 SUPPLEMENTATION AND LIFE SPAN

7.1 Dietary antioxidants

As one of the most intuitive approaches to testing the free radical theory, nutritional supplementation has been attempted with numerous species and compounds, with the result that mean life span has been extended in some instances [282]. In mammals, results have been mixed. To cite recent studies, life-long oral supplementation of rats with UQ was without effect on mortality [283], whereas supplementation of the Senescence Accelerated Mouse strain with "β-CATE-CHIN", a commercial supplement with antioxidant activities [284,285] resulted in life extension [286]. Negative results from the feeding of antioxidants have been rationalized by arguing that many of the antioxidants fed to mammals interfere with mitochondrial respiration, and so the failure of antioxidant trials to extend MLSP may have been due to their toxicity [287].

Although no large-scale human nutritional intervention trials have been aimed specifically at the study of aging, a few have been undertaken in the hopes that dietary antioxidants might help prevent cancer. Three similar and heavily scrutinized studies are the α-Tocopherol, β-Carotene (ATBC) Prevention Study [288], the Physicians' Health Study [289] and the β-Carotene and Retinol Efficacy Trial (CARET) [290], all of which were designed to assess the effect of antioxidants on lung cancer risks. Although the details of these enormous experiments are not important to this discussion, the overall result was instructive: there was either no decrease or a modest increase in lung incidence and mortality with β-carotene administration.

These negative results, as well as negative results described above using laboratory rodents, should not be taken as evidence that the free radical theory of aging is flawed. In fact, they prove merely that a complex organism like a human or rodent is unlikely to respond predictably to crude manipulations such as supplementation with one or a small number of compounds [291], as well as that a single endpoint, (such as lung cancer), is not equivalent to aging. Since the time when the results of these human trials were announced, a number of explanations have been forwarded to explain the paradoxical promotion of cancer by β-carotene [292], which indicates that the ultimate value of these trials may be a more precise understanding of this antioxidant. Ultimately, what these experiments prove is that until the biochemistry of dietary and cellular antioxidants is better understood, supplementation trials in laboratory animals or humans in which longevity or the incidence of a single disease is the endpoint will remain unreliable; molecular gerontology should focus on more instructive experiments.

For example, in a recent short-term feeding experiment, the thiol donor N-acetyl-cysteine, which increases intracellular glutathione concentrations, was found to markedly improve mitochondrial ETC complex activity in rats [293], a parameter of physiological function which has been noted to decrease with age, and short-term feeding with a complex antioxidant-containing plant extract attenuated oxidative damage in rat mitochondria [294]. Similarly, the nutritional supplement (R)-α-lipoic acid, which serves as both a coenzyme and antioxidant in mitochondria in vivo, attenuated an age-related loss of ascorbic acid recycling and increase in sensitivity to oxidant challenge [295].

7.2 Pharmacological supplements

Dramatic antiaging effects have been observed by Floyd and co-workers with the free radical spin trap N-tert-butyl-α-phenylnitrone (PBN). Initial studies used PBN as a spin trap to measure radical generation during ischemia/reperfusion injury of gerbil brain [296]. During reperfusion, the appearance of protein carbonyls correlated well with the loss of glutamine synthetase activity, and the appearance of PBN-dependent nitroxide radical. Interestingly, it was also discovered that pretreatment with PBN attenuated protein oxidation and loss of glutamine synthetase activity, as well as reduced lethality.

In a subsequent study which investigated the effect of PBN on spontaneous protein oxidation, it was discovered that twice-daily administration of PBN to old gerbils (32 mg/kg) reversed age-related oxidative damage [297]. For example, during normal aging of gerbils the level of brain protein carbonyls increased 185% and glutamine synthetase activity declined by about 35%. A marked drop in neutral protease activity was also observed. Old animals administered PBN for 2 weeks, however, experienced a reversal of these trends: protein carbonyls dropped, and glutamine synthetase and neutral protease activities were virtually restored. This effect was reversible, as over a 2-week period following cessation of PBN treatment, the oxidation of proteins increased, and the activities of glutamine synthetase and neutral protease fell. Most impressive, however, was the performance of the PBN-treated old gerbils in a test of short-term memory: whereas the old gerbils were twice as likely to make errors as young gerbils, the old animals treated with PBN performed as well as the young [297].

Although these preliminary results held great promise, not only for the study of aging, but also for its therapeutic treatment, subsequent experiments reported that the results were irreproducible [298,299]. Further follow-up work from a third laboratory confirmed the initial findings in gerbil brain, but at the same time found no effect of PBN in lowering the level of protein carbonyls in gerbil heart or mouse brain [300]. The chronic treatment of aged rats with PBN was found to reverse age-related cognitive impairment [301]. Lastly, the administration of PBN from age 20 weeks throughout the life of a short-lived strain of mouse, (the senescence accelerated mouse), increased its life span from 42 to 56 weeks, (an increase of 33%) [302]. As was above argued to be the case for experiments with dietary intervention, maximum worth will be derived from pharmacological experiments when they include not only endpoint mortality measurements but more focused studies of cellular effects.

8 SUMMARY

Above, we have outlined a few of the major experimental approaches to testing the free radical theory of aging. In Table 1, the strengths and weaknesses of different modes of experimentation are assessed. How powerful are different types of experiment? Has the free radical theory been supported?

Before discussing the merits of individual experiments, it should be stressed that if one is to judge them by their abilities to falsify the free radical theory, they are all bound to fail, for the simple reason that the free radical theory is very hard to falsify. The absence of a predicted outcome, (for instance, life span extension by antioxidant supplementation), may often be explained by (justifiable) ad hoc reasoning. The physiology of oxidative stress, being a complex interaction of endogenous and exogenous factors, generally permits the "explanation" of negative results. How then shall one judge the different types of experiment and the theory itself? In fact, as the results discussed above illustrate, the momentum gathering behind the free radical theory is not due to any single experiment or approach, but rather derives from the extraordinarily multidisciplinary nature of current research. Although no single line of reasoning alone permits definitive conclusions, together they present a compelling case. (This philosophy, that the study of aging should employ a combination of different approaches, has been convincingly espoused before [1]).

Age-related oxidative phenomenology continues to provide evidence that senescence is associated with increased oxidant generation, a decline in the robustness of defenses and repair, and an accumulation of end-products of oxidative damage. Although these trends are only correlations, the study of age-related changes has been rewarded with surprises such as the receptor for AGE (RAGE), which turns out to be involved in the etiology of Alzheimer's disease, and evidence that lysosomal lipofuscin may directly disrupt cells in vivo and in vitro. In fact, oxidative phenomenology has focused efforts on understanding the interplay between the components of oxidative stress outlined in Fig. 1. The search for evidence of age-related DNA and protein oxidation has stimulated research into DNA repair, proteolytic salvage pathways, mitochondrial defenses, and so on.

Interspecies comparisons have better potential directly to test the free radical theory. As predicted, differences between long- and short-lived species have been documented in all components of oxidative stress. Perhaps most instructive, however, have been results that initially appeared contradictory, such as the fact that birds are an outlier group in rate of living calculations. Attempts to account for the discrepancy have led to promising ad hoc hypotheses about the role of mitochondrial oxidant generation in aging. Unfortunately, relatively few researchers are familiar with or prepared to handle a variety of experimental animals, despite the research potential of a diverse menagerie.

In contrast, the model of dietary restriction has appeal precisely because it is so well-established, homogeneous, and relevant to specific human diseases. Although early predictions that DR would result in a lower metabolic rate have proved unfounded [32], the discovery that oxidative defenses are enhanced by DR have strengthened both the free radical theory and the concept of antagonistic pleiotropy [303]. Although currently, results from DR studies are merely consistent with the free radical theory, future experiments may reveal specific pathways whereby DR upregulates defenses and repair.

Manipulation of metabolic activity and oxygen concentration are interesting systems, if of somewhat questionable relevance to normal aging. One drawback of such experiments is that they have generally been limited to invertebrates; the manipulation of metabolism in mammals is less straightforward. In the future, transgenic mouse models may allow a specific manipulation of metabolic rate in a consistent genetic background.

Attempts to manipulate life span with nutritional and pharmacological antioxidants obviously hold great appeal, as direct and intuitive tests of the theory. Although until recently, they have not quite lived up to their promise (at least in mammals), this may have been due to a lack of the appropriate compounds. The serendipitous discovery of PBN's pharmacological properties appears to have opened up new avenues.

The answer to the question of whether or not the free radical theory has yet been confirmed depends upon one's conception of what the theory predicts. In its broader sense, ("oxidants contribute significantly to the process of degenerative senescence"), the theory has clearly been validated. In the more strict sense of the theory "oxidants determine MLSP", the data are not yet conclusive, although a large body of consistent data has been generated.

9 PERSPECTIVES

Lastly, we here briefly mention aspects of oxidative physiology which are likely to receive much more attention in years to come, and we end with a discussion of the complex, (and as yet virtually unstudied), ways in which exercise may affect the process of senescence.

9.1 Nitric oxide

A topic of great importance, which we have here largely omitted, is the role of nitric oxide (NO●), both as a damaging oxidant in its own right (via its reaction with O_2), and as a signaling molecule which is susceptible to oxidative scavenging. NO●, the chemical previously known as endothelium-derived relaxation factor, is generated enzymatically by isozymes of nitric oxide synthase, and is involved in vascular tone, innate immunity, and neuronal signal transduction.

Moreover, NO reacts with $O_2\bullet^-$ to form peroxynitrite (ONOO$^-$), itself a powerful oxidant. Therefore, not only must nitric oxide synthase be seen as a potential source of damaging oxidants [304,305], but $O_2\bullet^-$ may now be considered physiologically relevant scavengers of the free radical signaling molecule NO$\bullet$ [26].

9.2 Regulatory roles for oxidants and antioxidants: signal transduction

The discovery that NO$\bullet$ could serve as a signaling molecule has foreshadowed a more general recognition that radical species are more than by-products. As mentioned above, the interaction between $O_2\bullet^-$ and NO$\bullet$ indicates that both may be regulatory molecules [26]. In other ways, the relationship between oxidants and signaling is surfacing. For instance, the nitration of tyrosine residues on a synthetic peptide substrate of cell cycle kinases destroyed its ability to be phosphorylated, which illustrates a mechanism for an individual amino acid adduct to exert an amplified effect [306]. At a more physiological level, it has been shown that the sensitivity of hippocampal brain slices to muscarinic acetylcholine receptor agonists, which falls in an age-related fashion, can be restored by various antioxidant treatments, and is potentiated (in old animals) by NO$\bullet$ generating systems [307].

Perhaps most intriguing have been discoveries, such as the potential regulation of aconitases by $O_2\bullet^-$ [106,107] and the realization that cell signaling via the *ras* -family of tyrosine kinases involves oxidants [308], which suggest that oxidants play a role in signal transduction by design. These discoveries strengthen the free radical theory for the following reason. If the regulated, enzymatic generation of oxidants play a role in signaling pathways ("legitimate oxidants"), then even a small increase in oxidant generation by nonregulated pathways ("illegitimate oxidants") may have an exaggerated impact, by mimicking the "legitimate" process. The arrival of "redox regulation" as a viable field of inquiry, as evidenced by numerous topical recent reviews [309–311], may usher in a period when oxidants are seen as molecules of central physiological importance, in much the same way as are (for instance) lipid metabolites. As far as acceptance of the free radical theory is concerned, such a paradigm shift will probably lead to de facto acceptance of its broader conception, (the idea that oxidants play a role in the process of aging). After all, if it turns out that oxidants and oxidative reactions are central to physiology, then how could they not be central to aging as well? If the free radical theory once lacked appeal because oxidants appeared to be stoichiometrically minor by-products, those days may soon be over.

On the other hand, in its more narrow conception ("oxidants define MLSP"), the free radical theory still lacks experimental confirmation. A hypothetical example will illustrate this point. Even if mitogenic stimulation by ras, for instance, were to involve oxidant generation in mice and humans, and the disregulation of ras signaling by "illegitimate" oxidants in aged individuals were shown to be important in degenerative senescence, the different life spans of these organisms still beg an explanation; it still would remain to be explained why the process of oxidative disregulation takes so much longer to occur in humans than in mice. In conclusion, despite the growing consensus that the oxidants and oxygen free radicals are involved in degenerative senescence, there remain countless mechanistic questions to be uncovered, as well as a central outstanding unknown: do oxidants determine maximum life span, in humans and other organisms?

9.3 Oxidants and apoptosis

Another topic we have decided to omit, because of space limitations and because this is an extremely fast-moving and frequently reviewed area, is the role of oxidants and mitochondria in apoptosis. Suffice it to mention that in the previous year or two there have appeared dozens of experiments documenting either the loss of mitochondrial membrane potential [312], the release of mitochondrial cytochrome c [313], (or an "apoptosis inducing factor" [312]), into the cytosol, or the generation of oxidants by mitochondria during apoptosis [312]. Combined with the mitochondrial localization of the Bcl-2 family of anti-apoptosis proteins, and copious evidence that oxidant challenges can induce apoptosis [314–316], these experiments have shown that mitochondria are central to the process of cell suicide [312,313]. Despite this general consensus, however, there exist a number of disagreements about the details of the mitochondrion's role in the process [317], and even greater uncertainty about the role of oxidants. An equally complex problem will be defining the role of apoptosis itself in aging [148]. For instance, by eliminating neuronal cells, apoptosis may contribute to neurodegeneration, yet effective apoptosis is also clearly critical in preventing (age-related) tumorigenesis. In short, both the machinery and impact of apoptosis are still incompletely understood; conclusions about the interplay between oxidants, apoptosis and aging will have to await further experimentation [148].

9.4 Exercise and life span

Although the predictive power of the free radical theory is far from established, one can still speculate about the way in which exercise-related oxygen toxicity might affect the process of aging, and life span itself. In our minds, this question centers around the interactions outlined in Fig. 1. In other words, exercise induces tremendous cellular adaptation, often in response to cellular damage, (e.g., as in the case of muscle building). Presumably, oxygen toxicity from exercise could, therefore, cause either long-term oxidative damage, (from increased oxidant generation by mitochondrial respiration) or, due to the upregulation of inducible antioxidant defenses, it could protect cells from the endogenous oxidative insults of ordinary metabolism. Discovering whether, and in what direction, exercise affects the basic processes of senescence will be an interesting question to attack. (Of course, for the average modern human, who runs a fairly high risk of dying from diseases linked to a sedentary lifestyle, the prescription for a longer and healthier life is almost certainly to exercise more!).

10 ACKNOWLEDGEMENTS

We would like to thank Caleb Finch for critically reading the manuscript, and Irwin Fridovich for offering numerous detailed and useful comments. This chapter is a modified version of an article which appeared in Physiological Reviews 1998;78:547—581. B.N.A. is indebted to the National Cancer Institute (Outstanding Investigator Grant CA39910) and the National Institute of Environmental Health Sciences (Grant ESO1896).

11 ABBREVIATIONS

Aβ:	amyloid β-peptide
AGE:	advanced glycation end-product
ATP:	adenosine triphosphate
CoQ_9:	coenzyme Q (chain length = 9)
CoQ_{10}:	coenzyme Q (chain length = 10)
DOPA:	3,4-dihydroxyphenylalanine
DR:	dietary restriction
ETC:	electron transport chain
GPX:	glutathione peroxidase
GSH:	glutathione
G6PD:	glucose-6-phosphate dehydrogenase
HA:	high-activity
LA:	low-activity
MLSP:	maximum life span potential
mSOD:	mitochondrial superoxide dismutase
mtDNA:	mitochondrial DNA
NADH:	nicotinamide adenine dinucleotide, reduced form
NADPH:	nicotinamide adenine dinucleotide phosphate, reduced form
8-oxodG:	8-oxodeoxyguanosine
8-oxogua:	8-oxoguanine
PBN:	N-tert-butyl-α-phenylnitrone
RAGE:	receptor for advanced glycation end-products
ROOH:	alkyl hydroperoxide
SOD:	superoxide dismutase
TBARS:	thiobarbituric acid-reactive substances

12 REFERENCES

1. Finch CE. Longevity, Senescence, and the Genome. Chicago: Univ. of Chicago Press; 1990.
2. Medvedev ZA. Biol Rev Camb Philos Soc 1990;65:375—398.
3. Cutler RG. Am J Clin Nutr Suppl 1991;53:373S—379S.
4. Fleming JE, Reveillaud I, Niedzwiecki A. Mutat Res 1992;275:267—279.
5. Floyd RA, Carney JM. Ann Neurol Suppl 1992;32:S22—27.
6. Harman D. Mutat Res 1992;275:257—266.

7. Sohal RS, Orr WC. Ann N Y Acad Sci 1992;663:74—84.
8. Stadtman ER. Science 1992;257:1220—1224.
9. Ames BN, Shigenaga MK, Hagen TM. Proc Natl Acad Sci USA 1993;90:7915—7922.
10. Feuers RJ, Weindruch R, Hart RW. Mutat Res 1993;295:191—200.
11. Harman D. Drugs Aging 1993;3:60—80.
12. Matsuo M. Comp Biochem Physiol 1993;105:653—658.
13. Nohl H. Br Med Bull 1993;49:653—667.
14. Sohal RS. Aging Clin Exp Res 1993;5:3—17.
15. Harman D. Ann N Y Acad Sci 1994;717:1—15.
16. Shigenaga MK, Hagen TM, Ames BN. Proc Natl Acad Sci USA 1994;91:10771—10778.
17. Warner HR. Free Radic Biol Med 1994;17:249—258.
18. Beal MF. Ann Neurol 1995;38:357—366.
19. Knight JA. Ann Clin Lab Sci 1995;25:1—12.
20. Smith MA, Sayre LM, Monnier VM, Perry G. Trends Neurosci 1995;18:172—176.
21. King CM, Barnett YA. Biochem Soc Tranc 1995;23:375S.
22. Yu BP, Yang R. Ann N Y Acad Sci 1996;786:1—11.
23. Benzi G, Moretti A. Neurobiol Aging 1995;16:661—674.
24. Carney JM, Smith CD, Carney AM, Butterfield DA. Ann N Y Acad Sci 1994;738:44—53.
25. Cortopassi G, Liu Y, Hutchin T. Exp Gerontol 1996;31:253—265.
26. Darley-Usmar V, Wiseman H, Halliwell B. FEBS Lett 1995;369:131—135.
27. Davies KJ. Biochem Soc Symp 1995;61:1—31.
28. De La Paz MA, Zhang J, Fridovich I. Curr Eye Res 1996;15:273—278.
29. Hensley K, Butterfield DA, Hall N, Cole P et al. Ann N Y Acad Sci 1996;786:120—134.
30. Reiter RJ, Pablos MI, Agapito TT, Guerrero JM. Ann N Y Acad Sci 1996;786:362—378.
31. Schapira AH. Neuropathol Appl Neurobiol 1995;21:3—9.
32. Sohal RS, Weindruch R. Science 1996;273:59—63.
33. Wachsman JT. Mutat Res 1996;350:25—34.
34. Zorov DB. Biochim Biophys Acta 1996;1275:10—15.
35. Harman D. Ann N Y Acad Sci 1996;786:321—336.
36. Martin GM, Austad SN, Johnson TE. Nature Genet 1996;13:25—34.
37. Sastre J, Pallardo FV, Vina J. Age 1996;19:129—139.
38. Yin D. Free Radic Biol Med 1996;21:871—888.
39. Goto S, Nakamura A. Age 1997;20:81—89.
40. Gilchrest BA, Bohr VA. FASEB J 1997;11:322—330.
41. Hempelmann LH, Hoffman JG. Ann Rev Nuclear Sci 1953;3:369—389.
42. Harman D. J Gerontol 1956;2:298—300.
43. Stein G, Weiss J. Nature 1948;161:650.
44. Commoner B, Townsend J, Pake GE. Nature 1954;174:689—691.
45. McCord JM, Fridovich I. J Biol Chem 1969;244:6049—6055.
46. Yu BP. Physiol Rev 1994;74:139—162.
47. Chance B, Sies H, Boveris A. Physiol Rev 1979;59:527—605.
48. Rubner M. Das problem der Lebensdauer und seine Beziehungen zu Wachstum und Ernährung. Munich: R. Oldenburg, 1908.
49. Pearl R. The rate of living. London: University of London Press, 1928.
50. Sohal RS. In: Witler R (ed) Cellular Aging: Concepts and Mechanisms. Basel: Karger, 1976: 25—40.
51. Halliwell BH, Gutteridge JMC. Free Radicals in Biology and Medicine, 3rd edn. Oxford: Oxford University Press, 1999.
52. Wood PM. Biochem J 1988;253:287—289.
53. Halliwell B. Br J Exp Pathol 1989;70:737—757.
54. Beyer W, Imlay J, Fridovich I. Prog Nucl Acids Res 1991;40:221—253.
55. Fridovich I. Annu Rev Biochem 1995;64:97—112.

56. Boveris A, Chance B. Biochem J 1973;134:707—716.
57. Nohl H, Hegner D. Eur J Biochem 1978;82:563—567.
58. Hansford RG, Hogue BA, Mildaziene V. J Bioenerg Biomembr 1997;29:89—95.
59. Imlay JA, Fridovich I. J Biol Chem 1991;266:6957—6965.
60. Forman HJ, Kennedy JA. Biochem Biophys Res Commun 1974;60:1044—1050.
61. Loschen G, Azzi A, Richter C, Flohe L. FEBS Lett 1974;42:68—72.
62. Boveris A, Cadenas E. FEBS Lett 1975;54:311—314.
63. Dionisi O, Galeotti T, Terranova T, Azzi A. Biochim Biophys Acta 1975;403:292—300.
64. Boveris A, Cadenas E, Stoppani AO. Biochem J 1976;156:435—444.
65. Boveris A, Oshino N, Chance B. Biochem J 1972;128:617—630.
66. Forman HJ, Azzi A. FASEB J 1997;11:374—375.
67. Nohl H, Gille L, Schonheit K, Liu Y. Free Radic Biol Med 1996;20:207—213.
68. Ghafourifar P, Richter C. FEBS Lett 1997;418:291—296.
69. Giulivi C, Poderoso JJ, Boveris A. J Biol Chem 1998;273:11038—11043.
70. Tatoyan A, Giulivi C. J Biol Chem 1998;273:11044—11048.
71. Kasai H, Okada Y, Nishimura S, Rao MS et al. Cancer Res 1989;49:2603—2605.
72. Ockner RK, Kaikaus RM, Bass NM. Hepatology 1993;18:669—676.
73. Lake BG. Annu Rev Pharmacol Toxicol 1995;35:483—507.
74. Arnaiz SL, Travacio M, Llesuy S, Boveris A. Biochim Biophys Acta 1995;1272:175—180.
75. Oikawa I, Novikoff PM. Am J Pathol 1995;146:673—687.
76. Goeptar AR, Scheerens H, Vermeulen NP. Crit Rev Toxicol 1995;25:25—65.
77. Koop DR. FASEB J 1992;6:724—730.
78. Chanock SJ, el BJ, Smith RM, Babior BM. J Biol Chem 1994;269:24519—24522.
79. Moslen MT. Adv Exp Med Biol 1994;366:17—27.
80. Robinson JM, Badwey JA. Immunol Ser 1994;60:159—178.
81. Parsonnet J, Friedman GD, Vandersteen DP, Chang Y et al. N Engl J Med 1991;325:1127—1131.
82. Correa P, Chen VW. Cancer Surv 1994;20:55—76.
83. Ohshima H, Bartsch H. Mutat Res 1994;305:253—264.
84. Fahn S, Cohen G. Ann Neurol 1992;32:804—812.
85. Liu RH, Hotchkiss JH. Mutat Res 1995;339:73—89.
86. Gutteridge JM, Halliwell B. Trends Biochem Sci 1990;15:129—135.
87. Marnett LJ, Hurd HK, Hollstein MC, Levin DE et al. Mutat Res 1985;148:25—34.
88. Szweda LI, Uchida K, Tsai L, Stadtman ER. J Biol Chem 1993;268:3342—3347.
89. Chen JJ, Yu BP. Free Radic Biol Med 1994;17:411—418.
90. Chio KS, Tappel AL. Biochem 1969;8:2821—2826.
91. Tappel AL. In: Trump BF, Arstila AU (eds). Pathobiology of cell membranes. New York: Academic Press, 1975:145—170.
92. Dizdaroglu M. Mutat Res 1992;275:331—342.
93. Dizdaroglu M. Int J Radiat Biol 1992;61:175—183.
94. Halliwell B, Dizdaroglu M. Free Radic Res Commun 1992;16:75—87.
95. Beckman KB, Ames BN. J Biol Chem 1997;272:19633—19636.
96. Epe B. Rev Physiol Biochem Pharmacol 1996;127:223—249.
97. Bohr VA, Anson RM. Mutat Res 1995;338:25—34.
98. Lu R, Nash HM, Verdine GL. Curr Biol 1997;7:397—407.
99. Rosenquist TA, Zharkov DO, Grollman AP. Proc Natl Acad Sci USA 1997;94:7429—7434.
100. Slupska MM, Baikalov C, Luther WM, Chiang JH et al. J Bacteriol 1996;178:3885—3892.
101. Starke-Reed PE, Oliver CN. Arch Biochem Biophys 1989;275:559—567.
102. Stadtman ER, Oliver CN. J Biol Chem 1991;266:2005—2008.
103. Flint DH, Tuminello JF, Emptage MH. J Biol Chem 1993;268:22369—22376.
104. Kuo CF, Mashino T, Fridovich I. J Biol Chem 1987;262:4724—4727.
105. Gardner PR, Fridovich I. J Biol Chem 1992;267:8757—8763.
106. Gardner PR, Fridovich I. J Biol Chem 1991;266:19328—19333.

107. Gardner PR, Raineri I, Epstein LB, White CW. J Biol Chem 1995;270:13399—13405.

108. Gardner PR, Nguyen DD, White CW. Proc Natl Acad Sci USA 1994;91:12248—12252.

109. Keyer K, Gort AS, Imlay JA. J Bacteriol 1995;177:6782—6790.

110. Liochev SI, Fridovich I. Free Radic Biol Med 1994;16:29—33.

111. Berlett BS, Levine RL, Stadtman ER. J Biol Chem 1996;271:4177—4182.

112. Duprat F, Guillemare E, Romey G, Fink M et al. Proc Natl Acad Sci USA 1995;92:11796—11800.

113. Halliwell B, Gutteridge JM. Arch Biochem Biophys 1986;246:501—514.

114. Minotti G, Aust SD. Chem Phys Lipids 1987;44:191—208.

115. Koster JF, Sluiter W. Br Heart J 1995;73:208—209.

116. Vercellotti GM. Clin Chem 1996;42:657.

117. Ames BN, Gold LS, Willett WC. Proc Natl Acad Sci USA 1995;92:5258—5265.

118. Vanfleteren JR. Biochem J 1993;292:605—608.

119. Sohal RS, Agarwal A, Agarwal S, Orr WC. J Biol Chem 1995;270:15671—15674.

120. Agarwal S, Sohal RS. Biochem Biophys Res Commun 1993;194:1203—1206.

121. Sohal RS, Agarwal S, Sohal BH. Mech Ageing Devel 1995;81:15—25.

122. Pacifici RE, Davies KJ. Gerontology 1991;37:166—180.

123. Croteau DL, Bohr VA. J Biol Chem 1997;272:25409—25412.

124. Cunningham RP. Curr Biol 1997;7:R576—579.

125. Tchou J, Kasai H, Shibutani S, Chung MH et al. Proc Natl Acad Sci USA 1991;88:4690—4694.

126. Rivett AJ. Essays Biochem 1990;25:39—81.

127. Giulivi C, Pacifici RE, Davies KJ. Arch Biochem Biophys 1994;311:329—341.

128. Pacifici RE, Kono Y, Davies KJ. J Biol Chem 1993;268:15405—15411.

129. Stadtman ER. Methods Enzymol 1995;258:379—393.

130. Holmes GE, Bernstein C, Bernstein H. Mutat Res 1992;275:305—315.

131. Dennog C, Hartmann A, Frey G, Speit G. Mutagenesis 1996;11:605—609.

132. Hardmeier R, Hoeger H, Fang-Kircher S, Khoschsorur A et al. Proc Natl Acad Sci 1997;94:7572—7576.

133. Storz G, Tartaglia LA, Farr SB, Ames BN. Trends Genet 1990;6:363—368.

134. Hu JJ, Dubin N, Kurland D, Ma B-L et al. Mutat Res 1995;336:193—201.

135. Sohal RS, Dubey A. Free Radic Biol Med 1994;16:621—626.

136. Brunk UT, Jones CB, Sohal RS. Mutat Res 1992;275:395—403.

137. Kowald A, Kirkwood TB. Mutat Res 1996;316:209—236.

138. Kirkwood TBL. Nature 1977;270:301—304.

139. Kirkwood TB, Rose MR. Phil Trans E Soc Lond B 1991;332:15—24.

140. Kirkwood TB. Am J Clin Nutr 1992;55:1191S—1195S.

141. Rose MR, Finch CE. Genetics and Evolution of Aging. Dordrecht: Kluwer, 1994.

142. Williams GC, Nesse RM. Q Rev Biol 1991;66:1—22.

143. Miquel J. Mutat Res 1992;275:209—216.

144. Vijg J, Gossen JA. Comp Biochem Physiol 1993;104:429—437.

145. Evans DA, Burbach JP, van Leeuwen FW. Mutat Res 1995;338:173—182.

146. Morley AA. Mutat Res 1995;338:19—23.

147. Dolle ME, Giese H, Hopkins CL, Martus HJ et al. Nat Genet 1997;17:431—434.

148. Warner HR, Johnson TE. Nat Genet 1997;17:368—370.

149. Hart RW, Setlow RB. Proc Natl Acad Sci USA 1974;71:2169—2173.

150. Cortopassi GA, Wang E. Mech Ageing Devel 1996;91:211—218.

151. Feig DI, Reid TM, Loeb LA. Cancer Res 1994;54:1890S—1894S.

152. Grollman AP, Moriya M. Trends Genet 1993;9:246—249.

153. Martus HJ, Dolle ME, Gossen JA, Boerrigter ME et al. Mutat Res 1995;338:203—213.

154. Luft R. Proc Natl Acad Sci USA 1994;91:8731—8738.

155. Harman D. J Am Geriatr Soc 1972;20:145—147.

156. Miquel J, Economos AC, Fleming J, Johnson JJ. Exp Geront 1980;15:575—591.

157. Fleming JE, Miquel J, Cottrell SF, Yengoyan LS et al. Gerontology 1982;28:44−53.
158. Richter C, Park JW, Ames BN. Proc Natl Acad Sci USA 1988;85:6465−6467.
159. Bandy B, Davison AJ. Free Radic Biol Med 1990;8:523−539.
160. Nagley P, Mackay IR, Baumer A, Maxwell RJ et al. Ann N Y Acad Sci 1992;673:92−102.
161. Schapira AH, Cooper JM. Mutat Res 1992;275:133−143.
162. Muller HJ. Brain Pathol 1992;2:149−158.
163. Richter C. Mutat Res 1992;275:249−255.
164. Wei YH. Mutat Res 1992;275:145−155.
165. Arnheim N, Cortopassi G. Mutat Res 1992;275:157−167.
166. Bittles AH. Mutat Res 1992;275:217−225.
167. Wallace DC, Shoffner JM, Trounce I, Brown MD et al. Biochim Biophys Acta 1995;1271:141−151.
168. Ozawa T. Biochim Biophys Acta 1995;1271:177−189.
169. Richter C. Int J Biochem Cell Biol 1995;27:647−653.
170. Cortopassi G, Liu Y. Mutat Res 1995;338:151−159.
171. Hagen TM, Yowe DL, Bartholomew JC, Wehr CM et al. Proc Natl Acad Sci U S A 1997;94:3064−3069.
172. Sohal RS. Age Pigments. Amsterdam: Elsevier, 1981.
173. Tsuchida M, Miura T, Aibara K. Chem Phys Lipids 1987;44:297−325.
174. Porta EA. Arch Gerontol Geriatr 1991;12:303−320.
175. Kikugawa K, Kato T, Hayasaka A. Lipids 1991;26:922−929.
176. Hochschild R. Exp Geront 1971;6:153−166.
177. Ivy GO, Schottler F, Wenzel J, Baudry M et al. Science 1984;226:985−987.
178. Sohal RS, Marzabadi MR, Galaris D, Brunk UT. Free Radic Biol Med 1989;6:23−30.
179. Marzabadi MR, Sohal RS, Brunk UT. Mech Ageing Devel 1988;46:145−157.
180. Marzabadi MR, Jones C, Rydstrom J. Mech Ageing Devel 1995;80:189−197.
181. Marzabadi MR, Sohal RS, Brunk UT. APMIS 1991;99:416−426.
182. Marzabadi MR, Sohal RS, Brunk UT. Anal Cell Pathol 1990;2:333−346.
183. Brunk UT, Zhang H, Dalen H, Ollinger K. Free Radic Biol Med 1995;19:813−822.
184. Ollinger K, Brunk UT. Free Radic Biol Med 1995;19:565−574.
185. Monnier VM, Cerami A. Science 1981;211:491−493.
186. Cerami A. J Am Geriatr Soc 1985;33:626−634.
187. Monnier VM, Glomb M, Elgawish A, Sell DR. Diabetes 1996;45(Suppl 3):S67−S72.
188. Thorpe SR, Baynes JW. Drugs Aging 1996;9:69−77.
189. Elgawish A, Glomb M, Friedlander M, Monnier VM. J Biol Chem 1996;271:12964−12971.
190. Sell DR, Lane MA, Johnson WA, Masoro EJ et al. Proc Natl Acad Sci USA 1996;93:485−490.
191. Baker GTd, Sprott RL. Exp Gerontol 1988;23:223−239.
192. Schmidt AM, Hori O, Brett J, Yan SD et al. Arterioscl Thromb 1994;14:1521−1528.
193. Schmidt AM, Hori O, Cao R, Yan SD et al. Diabetes 1996;45(Suppl 3):S77−S80.
194. Schmidt AM, Yan SD, Brett J, Mora R et al. J Clin Invest 1993;91:2155−2168.
195. Schmidt AM, Hori O, Chen JX, Li JF et al. J Clin Invest 1995;96:1395−1403.
196. Hori O, Brett J, Slattery T, Cao R et al. J Biol Chem 1995;270:25752−25761.
197. Yan SD, Chen X, Fu J, Chen M et al. Nature 1996;382:685−691.
198. Levine RL, Garland D, Oliver CN, Amici A et al. Meth Enzymol 1990;186:464−478.
199. Sohal RS, Agarwal S, Dubey A, Orr WC. Proc Natl Acad Sci USA 1993;90:7255−7259.
200. Yan LJ, Levine RL, Sohal RS. Proc Natl Acad Sci USA 1997;94:11168−11172.
201. Oliver CN, Ahn BW, Moerman EJ, Goldstein S et al. J Biol Chem 1987;262:5488−5491.
202. Forster MJ, Dubey A, Dawson KM, Stutts WA et al. Proc Natl Acad Sci USA 1996;93:4765−4769.
203. Friguet B, Szweda LI, Stadtman ER. Arch Biochem Biophys 1994;311:168−173.
204. Friguet B, Stadtman ER, Szweda LI. J Biol Chem 1994;269:21639−21643.
205. Dean RT, Gebicki J, Gieseg S, Grant AJ et al. Mutat Res 1992;275:387−393.

206. Dean RT, Gieseg S, Davies MJ. Trends Biochem Sci 1993;18:437—441.
207. Gieseg SP, Simpson JA, Charlton TS, Duncan MW et al. Biochemistry 1993;32:4780—4786.
208. Davies MJ, Fu S, Dean RT. Biochem J 1995;305:643—649.
209. Gebicki JM. Redox Report 1997;3:99—110.
210. Mullaart E, Lohman PH, Berends F, Vijg J. Mutat Res 1990;237:189—210.
211. Wang YJ, Ho YS, Lo MJ, Lin JK. Chem-Biol Interact 1995;94:135—145.
212. Kaneko T, Tahara S, Matsuo M. Mutat Res 1996;316:277—285.
213. Hirano T, Yamaguchi R, Asami S, Iwamoto N et al. J Gerontol A Biol Sci Med Sci 1996;51:
     B303—B307.
214. Cadet J, Douki T, Ravanat JL. Environ Health Perspect 1997;105:1034—1039.
215. Collins A, Cadet J, Epe B, Gedik C. Carcinogenesis 1997;18:1833—1836.
216. Helbock HJ, Beckman KB, Shigenaga MK, Walter PB et al. Proc Natl Acad Sci USA 1998;95:
     288—293.
217. Kasai H. Mutat Res 1997;387:147—163.
218. Pflaum M, Will O, Epe B. Carcinogenesis 1997;18:2225—2231.
219. Beckman KB, Ames BN. Meth Enzymol 1996;264:442—453.
220. Higuchi Y, Linn S. J Biol Chem 1995;270:7950—7956.
221. Salazar JJ, Van Houten B. Mutat Res 1997;385:139—149.
222. Yakes FM, Van Houten B. Proc Natl Acad Sci USA 1997;94:514—519.
223. Higami Y, Shimokawa I, Okimoto T, Ikeda T. Mutat Res 1994;316:59—67.
224. Hanawalt PC. Mutat Res 1995;336:101—113.
225. Hanawalt PC, Gee P, Ho L, Hsu RK et al. Ann N Y Acad Sci 1992;663:17—25.
226. Meydani SN, Wu D, Santos MS, Hayek MG. Am J Clin Nutr 1995;62:1462S—1476S.
227. Kneepkens CM, Lepage G, Roy CC. Free Radic Biol Med 1994;17:127—160.
228. King CM, Bristow-Craig HE, Gillespie ES, Barnett YA. Mutat Res 1997;377:137—147.
229. Mendis S, Sobotka PA, Euler DE. Clin Chem 1994;40:1485—1488.
230. Zarling EJ, Mobarhan S, Bowen P, Kamath S. Mech Ageing Devel 1993;67:141—147.
231. Springfield JR, Levitt MD. J Lipid Res 1994;35:1497—1504.
232. Agarwal S, Sohal RS. Mech Ageing Devel 1994;75:11—19.
233. Mo JQ, Hom DG, Andersen JK. Mech Ageing Devel 1995;81:73—82.
234. Sawada M, Carlson JC. J Cell Biochem 1990;44:153—165.
235. Sohal RS, Ku HH, Agarwal S, Forster MJ et al. Mech Ageing Devel 1994;74:121—133.
236. Sohal RS, Arnold LA, Sohal BH. Free Radic Biol Med 1990;9:495—500.
237. Sohal RS, Arnold L, Orr WC. Mech Ageing Devel 1990;56:223—235.
238. Rao G, Xia E, Richardson A. Mech Ageing Devel 1990;53:49—60.
239. Uejima Y, Fukuchi Y, Teramoto S, Tabata R et al. Mech Ageing Devel 1993;67:129—139.
240. Perez-Campo R, Lopez-Torres M, Rojas C, Cadenas S et al. Mech Ageing Devel 1993;67:
     115—127.
241. Rodriguez-Martinez MA, Ruiz-Torres A. Mech Ageing Devel 1992;66:213—222.
242. Ji LL, Dillon D, Wu E. Am J Physiol 1991:R386—392.
243. Ji LL, Dillon D, Wu E. Am J Physiol 1990:R918—R923.
244. Martinez M, Ferrandiz ML, Diez A, Miquel J. Mech Ageing Devel 1995;84:77—81.
245. Lucas DT, Szweda LI. Proc Natl Acad Sci USA 1998;95:510—514.
246. Darr D, Fridovich I. Free Radic Biol Med 1995;18:195—201.
247. Sahakian JA, Szweda LI, Friguet B, Kitani K et al. Arch Biochem Biophys 1995;318:411—417.
248. Gafni A. Annu Rev Gerontol Geriatr 1990;10:117—131.
249. Conconi M, Szweda LI, Levine RL, Stadtman ER et al. Arch Biochem Biophys 1996;331:
     232—240.
250. Gaziev AI, Podlutsky A, Panfilov BM, Bradbury R. Mutat Res 1995;338:77—86.
251. Gaziev AI, Sologub GR, Fomenko LA, Zaichkina SI et al. Carcinogenesis 1996;17:493—499.
252. Barnett YA, King CM. Mutat Res 1995;338:115—128.
253. Gabbita SP, Butterfield DA, Hensley K, Shaw W et al. Free Radic Biol Med 1997;23:191—201.

254. Sohal RS, Sohal BH. Mech Ageing Devel 1991;57:187—202.
255. Nakano M, Mizuno T, Katoh H, Gotoh S. Mech Ageing Devel 1989;49:41—48.
256. Nakano M, Gotoh S. J Gerontol 1992;47:B126—B129.
257. Nakano M, Mizuno T, Gotoh S. Mech Ageing Devel 1993;66:243—248.
258. Sohal RS, Sohal BH, Orr WC. Free Radic Biol Med 1995;19:499—504.
259. Sohal RS, Ku HH, Agarwal S. Biochem Biophys Res Commun 1993;196:7—11.
260. Shigenaga MK, Gimeno CJ, Ames BN. Proc Natl Acad Sci USA 1989;86:9697—9701.
261. Loft S, Astrup A, Buemann B, Poulsen HE. FASEB J 1994;8:534—537.
262. Adelman R, Saul RL, Ames BN. Proc Natl Acad Sci 1988;85:2706—2708.
263. Sohal RS, Sohal BH, Brunk UT. Mech Ageing Devel 1990;53:217—227.
264. Lopez-Torres M, Perez-Campo R, Rojas C, Cadenas S et al. Mech Ageing Devel 1993;70: 177—199.
265. Barja G, Cadenas S, Rojas C, Lopez-Torres M et al. Comp Biochem Physiol Biochem Mol Biol 1994;108:501—512.
266. Perez-Campo R, Lopez-Torres M, Rojas C, Cadenas S et al. J Comp Physiol 1994;163:682— 689.
267. Ku HH, Sohal RS. Mech Ageing Devel 1993;72:67—76.
268. Ku HH, Brunk UT, Sohal RS. Free Radic Biol Med 1993;15:621—627.
269. Barja G, Cadenas S, Rojas C, Perez-Campo R et al. Free Radic Res 1994;21:317—327.
270. Herrero A, Barja G. Mech Ageing Devel 1997;98:95—111.
271. Sohal RS, Svensson I, Brunk UT. Mech Ageing Devel 1990;53:209—215.
272. Lass A, Agarwal S, Sohal RS. J Biol Chem 1997;272:19199—19204.
273. Weindruch R, Walford RL, Fligiel S, Guthrie D. J Nutr 1986;116:641—654.
274. Weindruch R, Sohal RS. N Engl J Med 1997;337:986—994.
275. Yu BP. Free Radic Biol Med 1996;5:651—668.
276. Rao G, Xia E, Nadakavukaren MJ, Richardson A. J Nutr 1990;120:602—609.
277. Choi JH, Yu BP. Free Radic Biol Med 1995;18:133—139.
278. Haley ZV, Richardson A. Mutat Res 1993;295:237—245.
279. Youngman LD, Park JY, Ames BN. Proc Natl Acad Sci USA 1992;89:9112—9116.
280. Larsen PL. Proc Natl Acad Sci USA 1993;90:8905—8909.
281. Honda S, Ishii N, Suzuki K, Matsuo M. J Gerontol 1993;48:B57—B61.
282. Harman D. Proc Natl Acad Sci USA 1981;78:7124—7128.
283. Lonnrot K, Metsa-Ketela T, Alho H. Gerontology 1995;41(Suppl 2):109—120.
284. Kumari MV, Yoneda T, Hiramatsu M. Biochem Mol Biol Int 1996;38:1163—1170.
285. Yoneda T, Hiramatsu M, Sakamoto M, Togasaki K et al. Biochem Mol Biol Int 1995;35: 995—1008.
286. Kumari MV, Yoneda T, Hiramatsu M. Biochem Mol Biol Int 1997;41:1005—1011.
287. Harman DH. Age 1987;10:58—61.
288. Albanes D, Heinonen OP, Huttunen JK, Taylor PR et al. Am J Clin Nutr 1995;62:1427S—1430S.
289. Hennekens CH, Buring JE, Manson JE, Stampfer M et al. N Engl J Med 1996;334:1145—1149.
290. Omenn GS, Goodman GE, Thornquist MD, Balmes J et al. J Natl Cancer Inst 1996;88: 1550—1559.
291. Block G. Am J Clin Nutr 1995;62(suppl):1517S—1520S.
292. Potter JD. Cancer Lett 1997;114:329—331.
293. Miquel J, Ferrandiz ML, De Juan E, Sevila I et al. Eur J Pharmacol 1995;292:333—335.
294. Sastre J, Millan A, Garcia de la Asuncion J, Pla R et al. Free Radic Biol Med 1998;24:298—304.
295. Lykkesfeldt J, Hagen TM, Vinarsky V, Ames BN. FASEB J 1998.
296. Oliver CN, Starke-Reed PE, Stadtman ER, Liu GJ et al. Proc Natl Acad Sci USA 1990;87: 5144—5147.
297. Carney JM, Starke-Reed PE, Oliver CN, Landum RW et al. Proc Natl Acad Sci USA 1991;88: 3633—3636.
298. Cao G, Cutler RG. Arch Biochem Biophys 1995;320:106—114.

299. Cao G, Cutler RG. Arch Biochem Biophys 1995;320:195—201.
300. Edamatsu R, Mori A, Packer L. Biochem Biophys Res Commun 1995;211:847—849.
301. Socci DJ, Crandall BM, Arendash GW. Brain Res 1995;693:88—94.
302. Dubey A, Forster MJ, Sohal RS. Arch Biochem Biophys 1995;324:249—254.
303. Kenyon C. Cell 1996;84:501—504.
304. Poderoso JJ, Carreras MC, Lisdero C, Riobo N et al. Arch Biochem Biophys 1996;328:85—92.
305. Schulz JB, Matthews RT, Henshaw DR, Beal MF. Neuroscience 1996;71:1043—1048.
306. Kong SK, Yim MB, Stadtman ER, Chock PB. Proc Natl Acad Sci USA 1996;93:3377—3382.
307. Joseph JA, Villalobos-Molina R, Denisova N, Erat S et al. Ann N Y Acad Sci 1996;786:
     112—119.
308. Irani K, Xia Y, Zweier JL, Sollott SJ et al. Science 1997;275:1649—1652.
309. Suzuki YJ, Forman HJ, Sevanian A. Free Radic Biol Med 1997;22:269—285.
310. Demple B. Gene 1996;179:53—57.
311. Sen CK, Packer L. FASEB J 1996;10:709—720.
312. Zamzami N, Hirsch T, Dallaporta B, Petit PX et al. J Bioenerg Biomemb 1997;29:185—193.
313. Reed JC. Cell 1997;91:559—562.
314. Dypbukt JM, Ankarcrona M, Burkitt M, Sjoholm A et al. J Biol Chem 1994;269:30553—30560.
315. Johnson TM, Yu ZX, Ferrans VJ, Lowenstein RA et al. Proc Natl Acad Sci USA 1996;93:
     11848—11852.
316. Slater AF, Nobel CS, Orrenius S. Biochim Biophys Acta 1995;1271:59—62.
317. Jacobson MD. Trends Biochem Sci 1996;83—86.

©2000 Elsevier Science B.V. All rights reserved.
Handbook of Oxidants and Antioxidants in Exercise.
C.K. Sen, L. Packer and O. Hänninen, editors.

Part X • Chapter 28

Caloric restriction, exercise and aging

Roger J.M. McCarter

Department of Physiology, University of Texas Health Science Center, 7703 Floyd Curl Drive, San Antonio, TX 78284, USA. Fax: +1-210-567-4410.

1   INTRODUCTION
    1.1   Aging processes
    1.2   Caloric restriction (CR)
    1.3   Physical activity
    1.4   Inter-relationships between caloric restriction and exercise
    1.5   Questions to be addressed
2   CALORIC RESTRICTION AND AGING
    2.1   Different regimens
    2.2   Physiologic and metabolic effects
    2.3   Effects of CR on pathology
    2.4   Mechanisms of action
3   EXERCISE AND AGING
    3.1   Types of exercise
    3.2   Physiologic and metabolic effects
    3.3   Effects on longevity
    3.4   Mechanisms of action
4   CR, EXERCISE AND AGING
    4.1   Overview
    4.2   Experimental results
    4.3   Insights from combined effects of CR and exercise
5   SUMMARY
    5.1   CR and aging
    5.2   Exercise and aging
    5.3   CR, exercise and aging
6   PERSPECTIVES
    6.1   Hormesis
    6.2   CR, exercise and hormesis
7   ABBREVIATIONS
8   REFERENCES

1   INTRODUCTION

1.1 Aging processes

Despite more than a century of very active investigation, identification of mechanisms underlying the aging of multicellular organisms remains elusive [1,2]. Recent insight from evolutionary biologists indicates one reason for this surprising deficiency: a variety of different mechanisms may be involved in limiting the life span of different organisms. For example, animals not limited to terrestrial living such as birds and flying lemurs are protected from many predators and stresses. Such animals may have evolved greater longevity and an array of mechanisms of aging different from their earth-bound counterparts of a similar size [3]. Another reason for the lack of understanding is the scarcity of the experimental techniques with which the rate of aging, and in turn longevity, may be manipulated reproducibly. In particular, it should be noted that manipulations which shorten the life span are not especially helpful for gaining insight into aging processes. Such manipulations may simply shorten life by damaging organs and/or promoting disease processes, rather than by modulating aging processes. In this regard caloric restriction (CR) and exercise are of special importance for probing the aging processes. This is because these two manipulations represent strategies which have been demonstrated to improve function and to extend life expectancy in a variety of species. Since extreme CR and intense physical exertion are known to be harmful, it is important to establish the characteristics of restriction and exercise which are beneficial. Also of importance, is to establish criteria for determining whether or not the beneficial effects of these manipulations are the result of slowing aging or due to changes unrelated to aging.

Since mechanisms of aging have not yet been precisely identified there is little current agreement regarding definitions in this area. Medawar [4] pointed out that aging is used to describe almost all changes with time in biological properties. These changes are usually assumed to be deleterious although many properties either do not change with age or the changes which occur may not be detrimental to survival. Due to these difficulties most gerontologists focus on the survival of cohorts born at similar times and, in particular, on the exponential increase in rate of mortality which occurs with advancing postmaturational life. The survival time at which 50% mortality occurs, the median life span, is termed the life-expectancy of the group. This quantity is influenced by many factors, including protection from the environment and the presence or absence of disease. For example, the life-expectancy of men and women in the USA has increased dramatically during the present century, in association with decreased infant mortality and improved public health and sanitation, among other factors, as shown in Fig. 1 [5]. In contrast, the maximum life span (or time of survival of the 10% longest-lived members of the cohort) is a more robust quantity and less susceptible to change. For example, there is no evidence that the maximum human life span (about 120 years) has changed over recorded time. Extending the maximum life span, therefore, is one criterion used by gerontologists as evidence that a given manipulation has retarded aging processes [6]. Finch et al. [7] point out that the maximum life span is determined by few data points in often small cohort sizes. These authors suggest the rate of mortality doubling following attainment of sexual maturity (the mortality rate doubling time (MRDT)) may be a more reliable indicator of the rate of aging. Even this criterion is complicated by data showing that the rate of mortality does not continue to increase exponentially with age at advanced ages in cohorts of large numbers [8]. Due to these complications there is no single generally agreed upon test for establishing rates of aging. However, there is general agreement that functional decline and increased pathology are

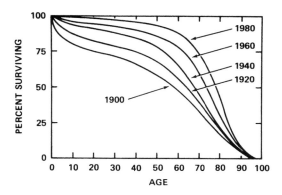

Fig. 1. Survival curves for the US population, 1900–1980. Reproduced with permission from the W.H. Freeman and Company from [5].

characteristic features of aging [9]. On this basis, therefore, many gerontologists accept that manipulations retarding aging processes should satisfy at least three criteria. They should:
1) increase the MRDT or some measure of maximum life span,
2) slow the age-related decline of physiological function, and
3) reduce the severity or prevent the incidence of age-related pathology.

1.2 Caloric restriction (CR)

Early studies by McCay and colleagues [10,11] established that feeding rats only enough food to permit maintenance of weight or small increases in weight resulted in increased longevity compared with similar rats fed ad libitum. Subsequent studies by others demonstrated decreased incidence of age-related diseases associated with reduced intake of food [12]. Systematic investigation and characterization of this effect have more recently been carried out by Walford and colleagues in mice [13], by Masoro and colleagues in rats [14], and by many others in a wide variety of species [13]. These studies have consistently demonstrated increased median and maximum life span, increased MRDT, decreased rates of functional decline and reduced age-related pathology in animals fed less food than those fed ad libitum. Thus, the CR (or food restriction, or diet restriction) paradigm is widely accepted as one which acts to retard aging processes. Mechanisms responsible for this effect are under intense investigation. Attempts to uncover the underlying mechanisms have thus far been unsuccessful. A major reason for this failure is the fact that this simple nutritional manipulation is associated with a very large number of molecular, organ and systemic changes. One such change, which has been well documented in rodents, is a surprising increase in physical activity in animals eating less food, when compared with those fed ad libitum.

1.3 Physical activity

Regular physical activity is widely regarded as an effective strategy to maintain psychological and physiological status with advancing age [15]. As noted above for CR, exercise training results in a very large number of compositional and physiological changes, many of which are in a direction counter to those associated with advancing age. Increased life-expectancy has also been found in both rodent and human studies associated with lifelong physical activity. Of the many different possible types of physical activity, only aerobic or endurance-type exercise has been systematically studied with respect to survival [16]. It should be noted, however, that resistance or strength training is widely believed to also exert beneficial effects, especially with respect to maintenance of muscle function with age [17]. In contrast, lengthening of active muscles in so-called eccentric exercise is known to damage muscle fibers and may have more widespread systemic effects [18]. For any given type of exercise there exist age-related levels of intensity which are necessary to induce training effects. The intensity of endurance exercise is most often assessed by measuring the oxygen consumption required to sustain the exercise as a fraction of maximum oxygen consumption ($\dot{V}_{O_{2max}}$). In contrast, intensity of resistance exercise is assessed by measuring the load lifted as a fraction of the maximum load which can be lifted once only (1RM, or one repetition maximum). Lifelong effects of habitual physical activity would then be expected to be a function of both the duration and intensity of exercise, as well as the type of exercise undertaken.

1.4 Inter-relationships between caloric restriction and exercise

Both of these manipulations are known to induce a large number of changes in body composition and function. Many of the changes result in the organism exhibiting a physiologically more youthful status at a given age. It is especially of note that both of these manipulations result in the organism having greater ability to maintain homeostasis in the face of most, but not all, challenges. Since reduced ability to respond to challenge is a characteristic feature of advancing age, it is tempting to explore the possibility that sustained physical activity is part of the mechanism by which CR retards aging processes. Alternatively, since both CR and exercise constitute metabolic challenges, perhaps the beneficial effects of these regimens may share a common basis in providing a chronic low level stress capable of inducing sustained mobilization of cellular defense systems. The more modest effects on longevity of regular exercise in comparison with those of CR may then be viewed in terms of the more specific nature of the metabolic challenge presented by exercise to some, but by no means all tissues. Both of these manipulations result in a reapportioning of available energy supplies away from growth, so that CR and exercising animals would be expected to exhibit lower body weights and altered body composition, if food intake is not altered.

1.5 Questions to be addressed

The primary goal of this work is to evaluate the use of CR and exercise as strategies to gain insight into mechanisms of aging. What insights may be gained from determining the shared effects of CR and habitual physical activity? Secondly, since CR results in increased physical activity, does increased physical activity play a role in the anti-aging effects of CR? Finally, both of these manipulations represent metabolic challenges to the organism. Possibly an altered metabolic rate is a factor in the retardation of aging by CR and does the increased metabolic rate of exercise reduce the otherwise beneficial effects of CR? These questions will be addressed by examining data obtained mainly in laboratory rodents, but some information is available in species ranging from fruit flies to non-human primates and in aging men and women. Discussions will cover CR and exercise separately, then in combination.

2   CALORIC RESTRICTION AND AGING

2.1 Different regimens

As noted previously there is widespread agreement that CR extends longevity by retarding aging processes. The effect is indeed robust since increased longevity with CR has been demonstrated in species ranging from worms to rats, in diets of variable nutrient composition and using a variety of different regimens [13]. Studies are also currently underway to determine the validity of the effect in non-human primates and in men and women [19–21]. It should be noted that CR initiated in adulthood might not be beneficial in humans. The results of Lee and Paffenbarger [22] demonstrate increased risk of all cause mortality for individuals experiencing weight loss of even 1 kg during a 10-year period. In contrast, the data of Bergman [23], analyzed by Jones [24], suggest no difference in the rate of aging of Australian prisoners of war held in concentration camps during World War II, in comparison with that of Australian civilians of similar age. The ubiquitous presence of the anti-aging effect of CR suggests that it acts by altering fundamental aging processes. The possibility exists that this effect may have evolved in response to sporadic food shortages in nature [25]. Thus, the effect of CR on longevity may be different or may not occur in species which have evolved under conditions of plentiful supplies of food. Such conditions would exist for example in moist tropic latitudes for plant-eating animals [25]. However, for almost all species examined to date under laboratory conditions, restriction of caloric intake has resulted in retardation of aging [1] as demonstrated in Fig. 2. The power of this simple nutritional strategy to affect aging processes may be assessed from the variety of different regimens under which it has been observed. The effect has been most systematically studied in rodents, so subsequent discussion focuses mainly on results obtained using laboratory rodents. Another important factor is the health of the animals. Conventional

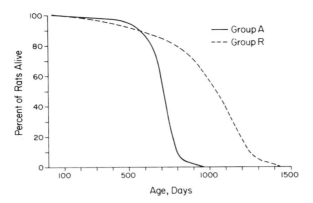

Fig. 2. Survival curves for male Fischer 344 rats fed ad libitum (group A, n = 115) and fed 40% less than ad libitum (group R, n = 115). Reproduced with permission from the Gerontological Society of America from [27].

rodent facilities are often compromised by the spread of infectious agents amongst animal colonies. Analysis of such facilities vs. barrier-type facilities indicates improved health and longevity in rodents maintained under specific pathogen free (SPF) conditions [26]. In order to eliminate the possibility that CR increases longevity simply by protecting against the effects of infectious pathogens, rather than by modulating aging processes, most modern studies have been conducted with rodents that were maintained under barrier protected SPF conditions [27]. In many of these studies restriction of food intake was initiated immediately after weaning and then extended over the life span. Significant extension of life has also been demonstrated to occur even when restriction was initiated in adulthood, or when restriction was carried out only during the phase of rapid growth, i.e., from 6 weeks of age to 6 months of age in Fischer 344 rats. These effects are shown in Fig. 3, from the work of Yu et al. [28]. Restriction of food was always by 40% of ad libitum intake in these rats. Degree of extension of median life span depended upon the duration of restriction (i.e., group 2 > group 4 > group 3). However, it is of interest that maximum life spans of groups 2 and 4 rats were similar (1,226 and 1,177 days, respectively), i.e., restriction of food from 6 months of age onwards was as effective as restriction of food from 6 weeks of age in extending maximum life span. Similar effects were found in two long-lived mouse strains (B10C3F$_1$ and C57BL/6J) by Weindruch and Walford [29], who initiated restriction (about 20% below ad libitum feeding) at 12 months of age.

   Widely different degrees of CR have been used by different investigators, ranging from a mild restriction of 10% to severe restriction of 70% less than ad libitum levels [30]. Many studies are compromised by the absence of complete survival data or by the use of non-SPF animals and the short life span of control animals, suggesting the possibility of unhealthy conditions. However, most stud-

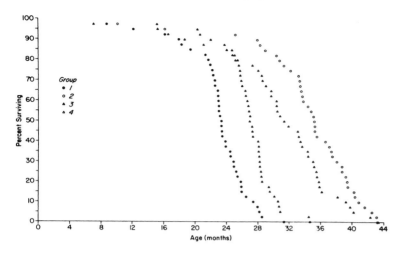

Fig. 3. Survival of male SPF Fischer 344 rats with caloric restriction at different times. Group 1 was fed ad libitum. Group 2 rats were fed 40% less food than group 1 from 6 weeks of age. Group 3 rats were fed 40% less food than group 1 from 6 weeks to 6 months of age. Group 4 rats were fed ad libitum to 6 months of age, then fed 40% less food than group 1 rats from that point onwards. Reproduced with permission from Gerontological Society of America from [28].

ies suggest a direct relationship between degree of restriction and the extension of life. Data from four separate studies in rats and mice with varying degrees of restriction from 25 to 65% of ad libitum intake are shown in Fig. 4. Such results indicate that retardation of aging processes depends upon the level of restriction of food intake. Taken together with the previous discussion of duration of restriction, the data suggest that both intensity and duration are important factors in the action of CR on aging, at least in laboratory rodents.

In contrast, several other variables appear to be unimportant in this action, e.g., the method of restricting calories appears uncritical, since several studies involving every-other-day (EOD) feeding, meal feeding or even periodic fasting, found increased longevity [13]. Variations in composition of the diet, such as by altering protein, fat and mineral levels similarly did not affect the anti-aging action [9]. The conclusion to be drawn from a large body of data from different laboratories using various rodent strains and diets is that it is the reduced intake of calories which is the critical factor in the anti-aging action. The important question then is how the aging processes are coupled to caloric intake. Identification of this coupling would be expected to yield valuable insights regarding mechanisms of aging. The search for this coupling was initiated by identifying physiological processes and pathologies which are affected by the reduced input of calories.

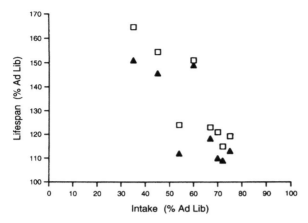

Fig. 4. Extension of lifespan vs. degree of restriction of caloric intake, when caloric restriction was initiated early in life. Open squares: median lifespan; solid triangles: maximum lifespan. Reproduced with permission from Clinics in Geriatric Medicine from [30].

2.2 Physiologic and metabolic effects

Identification of mechanisms by which CR retards aging is complicated by the very large number of changes in body composition and function which accompany the chronic reduction of food intake. A list of some of the many parameters which are known to vary with age and which are modulated by CR is given in Table 1. (Additional information is given in references [1,9,13,14].)

Particular examples of aging changes which are modulated by CR are shown in Figs. 5 and 6. In these, age-related changes in Fischer 344 rats fed ad libitum are compared with changes in similar rats fed 40% less than ad libitum from 6

Table 1. Modulation of age-related changes in physiological parameters by caloric restriction (Modified from the Society for Experimental Biology and Medicine from [31]).

Serum cholesterol and triglycerides
Plasma glucose levels
Hormone levels
Hormone receptor sensitivity
Protein turnover
Collagen crosslinking
Immune function
Reproductive activity
Bone metabolism
DNA synthesis and repair
Membrane composition and fluidity
Gene expression and transcription
Memory and neuronal function
Physical activity
Oxidative stress

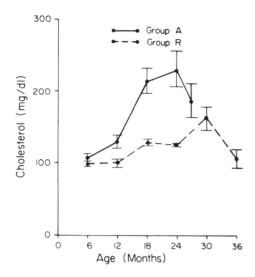

Fig. 5. Variation of serum cholesterol with age in rats fed ad libitum (group A) or fed 40% less than ad libitum from 6 weeks of age onwards (group R). Values are mean ± SEM. Reproduced with permission from the American Physiological Society from [32].

weeks of age onwards. The results demonstrate:
1) decreased plasma cholesterol levels at a given age in restricted vs. ad libitum fed rats [32]; and
2) delayed loss of mass of gastrocnemius muscles with age in restricted vs. ad libitum fed rats [27].
In contrast, Fig. 7 demonstrates that spontaneous movement of rats around their

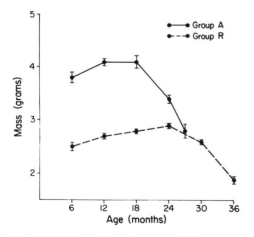

Fig. 6. Variation with age in mass of the two gastrocnemius muscles combined in male F344 rats fed ad libitum (group A) or fed 40% less than ad libitum from 6 weeks of age (group R). Values are mean ± SEM. Reproduced with permission from the Gerontological Society of America from [27].

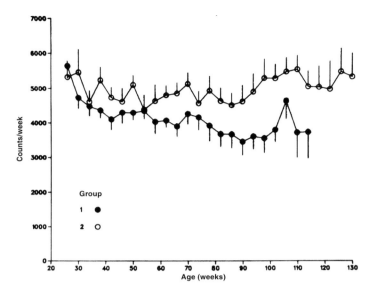

Fig. 7. Spontaneous activity of rats in their cages with age. Measurements represent the number of interruptions of intersecting light beams recorded over a 24-h period. Solid circles refer to rats fed ad libitum; open circles refer to rats restricted to eating 60% of the food consumed by rats fed ad libitum. Values are mean ± SEM. Reproduced with permission from Gerontological Society of America from [28].

cages is sustained with age in CR rats but declines with age in rats fed ad libitum [28]. Figure 8 demonstrates that metabolic rate of the whole body (measured over 24 h under usual living condition and expressed in terms of lean mass)

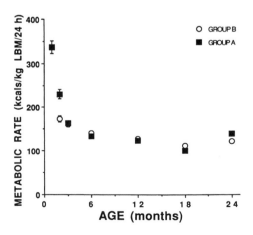

Fig. 8. Variation of daily metabolic rate with age, in rats fed ad libitum (group A) and rats fed 40% less than ad libitum intake from 6 weeks of age onwards (group B). Values are mean ± SEM. Reproduced with permission from the American Physiological Society from [33].

does not changed over most of the life span [33]. This latter result is surprising in view of the very extensive literature documenting decreased metabolic rate following reduction of food intake [34]. Indeed, documentation of this effect is so extensive that Garrow has stated, "There is no investigator who has looked for this effect and failed to find it" [35]. Reduction in metabolic rate is in fact observed in CR, but was shown to be a transient effect in the usual rodent paradigm of initiating CR at 6 weeks of age [36]. This reduction of metabolic rate and its subsequent normalization is consistent also with food consumption data demonstrating the same food consumption over most of the life span measured per unit body weight in restricted vs. ad libitum fed rats [37]. Similar results have also been demonstrated by Duffy et al. in rats [38].

The fact that longevity is increased in CR rats without lifelong reduction in a specific metabolic rate is in disagreement with one of the most popular theories of aging, the "Rate of Living" theory of Pearl and Rubner [39,40]. This will be expanded upon later in this chapter. Of immediate interest is the fact that metabolic rate is sustained in CR rats at the same intensity as in rats fed ad libitum, but under conditions of decreased oxidative stress. Indeed, one of the most remarkable metabolic aspects of CR is that it is associated with decreased levels of oxidative free radical damage and altered levels of antioxidant protection [41]. Chipalkatti et al. [42] were the first to note decreased levels of lipofuscin and malondialdehyde in brains of CR vs. ad libitum fed mice of a similar age. Koizumi et al. [43] found decreased levels of lipid peroxidation in liver homogenates of CR vs. ad libitum fed mice of similar age. Extensive studies by Yu and colleagues (e.g., [44]) have demonstrated similar effects in tissues of CR vs. ad libitum fed rats of various ages. Consistent with these results, Matsuo et al. [45] found that CR suppresses age-dependent increases in levels of expired pentane (a putative marker of tissue lipid peroxidation) in rats. The effects of CR on antioxidant defenses are more difficult to interpret. Measurements in mice (e.g., [43]) and rats (e.g., [46]) demonstrate increased activity of some compounds (such as catalase) and decreased levels of others (such as vitamin E) in a tissue-specific manner. In general, however, many independent studies have demonstrated a protective effect of CR against the presence of oxidative tissue damage [41]. The clear implication of these results, taken together with those on specific metabolic rate, is that CR enables appropriate rates of tissue metabolism to occur under conditions less damaging to the survival of the organism [47]. If CR modulates aging processes by exerting broadly protective effects against intrinsic and extrinsic damaging agents then, at any given age, there should be decreased incidence of tissue pathology. This should be especially apparent for advanced ages, when exponentially increasing levels of pathology are frequently observed. The following section examines evidence for such effects in CR vs. ad libitum fed animals.

2.3 Effects of CR on pathology

As impressive as are the effects of CR in extending life and in slowing the rate of functional decline, its effect on age-related pathology is of much greater practical significance. One example from rodent studies will illustrate this point: in a series of experiments the San Antonio group demonstrated that chronic nephropathy is a major age-associated disease in ad libitum fed male Fischer 344 rats [48]. Renal failure was the primary contributor to death in more than 50% of the rats fed ad libitum. In contrast, this disease was almost never seen in CR rats, most of which died at much greater ages [48]. The incidence of the disease was found to be significantly reduced also by replacing casein in the semisynthetic diet with soy protein, or by reducing the protein content of the diet without restricting calories. However, neither of these strategies was as effective as CR in virtually eliminating the disease in old animals [49]. In these studies it was also shown that CR greatly reduced the incidence of cardiomyopathy and also delayed, but it did not prevent, the occurrence of neoplastic diseases. Of practical interest was the finding that CR initiated in adulthood (6 months of age) was just as effective in retarding this broad spectrum of diseases as was CR initiated just after weaning (6 weeks of age) [48]. Other investigators have demonstrated similar effects in mice and in other rat strains. For example, Cheney et al. [50] demonstrated decreased prevalence of tumors in CR vs. ad libitum fed B10C3F$_1$ hybrid mice; Fernandes et al. [51] found significant reduction of renal disease due to autoimmune processes in NZB hybrid mice; and Loyd [52] demonstrated decreased age-related diseases in SHR rats, in which major diseases are associated with the hypertensive condition. Figure 9 shows the effect of CR on the incidence of tumors in male and female mice at the time of sacrifice ([53] based on the data of Bronson and Lipman, and [54]).

There is indeed abundant evidence that CR retards or prevents a broad spec-

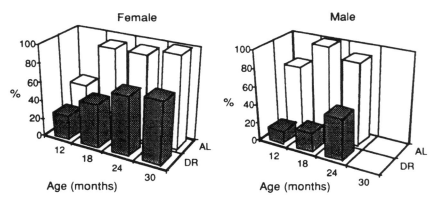

Fig. 9. Percentage of male and female mice of mixed strains exhibiting pathological lesions at the time of sacrifice. AL: mice fed ad libitum. DR: mice fed 60% of food consumed by AL mice. Reproduced with permission from CRC Press from [53].

trum of age-related diseases [13]. It should be noted that these effects were observed more than 50 years ago, particularly with regard to the growth of tumors, including in the classic studies of McCay et al. [55,56]. This effect of CR on pathology is consistent with the broadly protective actions of CR on metabolic and physiologic parameters. Thus, CR promotes continued metabolic and other cellular functions under conditions less damaging to cellular homeostasis. The new metabolic and physiologic status brought about by CR in turn leads to decreased tissue pathology at any age and to increased longevity. The important question then is: what mechanisms underlie these broadly protective effects of CR? In addition, are these mechanisms accessible by strategies other than CR? The latter is important as well, since there seems little likelihood that human populations will be convinced to consume fewer calories on a chronic basis, even if benefits of reduced disease in old age can be demonstrated in long-lived species such as non-human primates.

2.4 Mechanisms of action

Given the profoundly beneficial actions of CR it is not surprising that intense activity has been directed towards uncovering the underlying mechanisms. McCay's initial studies focussed on the notion that retardation of growth was the key factor [10,11]. Subsequent studies by this group attempted to identify dietary components (such as protein content) which might extend longevity independent of decreased food consumption [57]. More recent studies in rats and mice [as described previously] have essentially ruled out these possibilities, given the successful anti-aging action of CR initiated even in adulthood and using diets of widely differing compositions [13,14,28,29]. Indeed most current gerontologists agree that CR retards aging processes as a consequence of the reduced input of calories rather than by the reduction of any single nutrient, and most agree that this effect occurs when initiated in adulthood, as well as when initiated during development [9,13]. Another popular hypothesis was based on the reduced adiposity associated with CR and the well-known problems of function, disease and mortality associated with obesity in men and women. This view has been discounted on the basis of data generated in mice and rats by Harrison et al. [58] and by Yu et al. [27], respectively. These studies demonstrated the extension of life by CR even under conditions of high body fat content, and found no correlation between degree of adiposity and longevity in ad libitum fed animals. Interestingly, in CR rats there was a positive correlation between longevity and the degree of adiposity [27].

By far the most popular explanation of the mechanism action of CR, however, is that retardation of aging as a consequence of reduction in metabolic rate, in accordance with the Rate of Living theory of aging. This hypothesis was advanced in 1977 by Sacher [6] and continues to have an influence [59,60]. Sacher based this conclusion on the widely accepted Rate of Living theory of Pearl [39] and on one of the best documented findings in nutritional science, namely that reduction of food intake leads to a decrease in metabolic rate which is not accounted for by a corresponding decrease in metabolic mass [35]. The Rate of Living theory assumes that metabolic rate is a major factor in determining life span and, indeed, that maximum life span is inversely related to the intensity of metabolism, i.e., to the metabolic rate per unit metabolic mass. Experimental support for this view came from the early data of Rubner [40], who found that the oxygen consumption per unit body mass over the adult life span was approximately the same in five different species of domestic animals (about 200 kcal/g body weight/life span). Support also came from studies on the life span of insects and other poikilotherms raised at different temperatures [61] and from many studies demonstrating inverse relationships between maximum life span and specific metabolic rate [62]. The interpretation of all of these data remains controversial [3,63]. Despite a large body of evidence against this theory [3], it remains a popular framework for examining age-related changes and for developing mechanisms of aging [34]. Sacher's view then was that CR reduces the metabolic rate and, in accordance with the Rate of Living theory, longevity is thereby increased. Evidence against this view first came from a study by Masoro et al. [37] demonstrating that food consumed per gram of body weight over the life span was similar in rats fed ad libitum and fed the life-prolonging restricted diet. Direct measurements of oxygen consumption and carbon dioxide production were used by McCarter and Palmer [33] to compare metabolic rates of rats under usual living conditions. These measurements were conducted over 24-h periods with rats in their usual cages and, following measurement, the lean body mass of each rat was determined. The results were clear, as shown in Fig. 8. Over most of the life span the specific metabolic rate of CR rats was not less than that of rats fed ad libitum. Similar results were found for 18-month-old rats by Duffy et al. [38]. Decreased metabolic rate was indeed observed in CR rats for about 6 weeks following initiation of CR in young animals [36]. Following this initial transient, however, the body weight of CR rats adapted to the decreased nutrient intake, so that specific metabolic rates of CR and ad libitum fed animals were similar. Two important points should be made regarding these data: firstly, results were obtained under conditions in which extended longevity is known to occur, i.e., with rats in their usual living environment. Secondly, it is certainly possible that other species may respond to CR in a different manner with respect to metabolic rate, as suggested by the evolutionary analysis of Masoro and Austad [25]. For example, some species when faced with restricted food intake might respond by entering a state of hibernation, or torpor, and exhibit a profound and sustained decrease in metabolic rate. Regardless of these possible differences in response, it is clear that Fischer 344 rats subjected to CR from 6 weeks of age onwards demonstrate retarded aging in the absence of a sustained decrease in specific metabolic rate. It seems likely, therefore, that decreased rate of metabolism is not a necessary condition of the action of CR in extending life. Also, retardation of aging by CR probably does not occur as a consequence of decreased rate of living, and the effect does not provide experimental support for the Rate of Living theory of aging. (Further examination of this issue can be found in [34].)

The discussion thus far has focussed on theories which have been subjected to experimental tests and have been largely discounted. Several other possibilities remain and are under active investigation. These include: the glucocorticoid hypothesis, based on findings of elevated levels of corticosterone in CR vs. ad libitum fed rodents (for review, see [64]); the oxidative stress hypothesis (e.g., reference [65]) based on findings of decreased free radical damage in tissues of CR rodents as discussed previously; and the free radical—glycation/maillard reaction hypothesis, suggesting the possibility that CR may inhibit synergistic interactions between oxidative free radical damage and damage induced by the nonenzymatic glycation of macromolecules [66]. This theory is supported by the recent results of Sell et al. [67] showing an inverse relation between rates of accumulation of tissue glycoxidation products and species life span. The authors also demonstrated decreased rates of accumulation of glycoxidation products with CR in several species, consistent with the plasma glucose-lowering effects known to occur in CR [68]. In the present context, however, another important possibility is that increased physical activity associated with CR may play a role in the action of CR on aging. Increased levels of physical activity are widely believed to provide protection against disease and to reduce age-related decline in function. It seems possible, therefore, that the broadly protective effects of CR may be due in part to increased levels of physical activity. Tests of this hypothesis will be described following a general examination of the effects of exercise on parameters of aging. In particular, effects of exercise on longevity and function will be discussed.

3   EXERCISE AND AGING

Habitual physical activity is widely regarded as an essential strategy to combat the diseases and frailty of old age [69]. The current positive view of exercise is in contrast to earlier views that strenuous exercise such as competitive rowing would decrease life expectancy [16]. Emphasis on the deleterious aspects of exercise was supported by both experimental data and theories of aging. Early studies by Slonaker [70] and by Benedict and Sherman [71] in rodents found decreased longevity in rats forced to exercise in drums; the Rate of Living theory of aging [39] predicts decreased longevity with increased metabolic rate in exercise. The outcomes of these earlier studies may have been determined in large part by the presence of infectious disease in non-SPF animal facilities [72], but contemporary studies also suggest deleterious metabolic aspects [73] and increased risk of mortality [74] with strenuous exercise. In marked contrast, the sedentary lifestyle characteristics of many individuals in developed countries has been described by Holloszy and Khort [72] as a state of severe "exercise deficiency". Astrand [69] points out that successful evolutionary development and survival of the hominid species has been associated with a physically active lifestyle. Furthermore, the current lifestyle of physical inactivity is a major risk factor for development of frailty and age-related diseases [69].

Decline in physical activity with age is in fact a characteristic feature in many species: Sohal and Buchan [75] found decreased flying activity of houseflies with age. Holloszy [76] demonstrated that voluntary wheel running in female Long-Evans rats decreased from 8 to 2 km/day, from 4 to 34 months of age, as shown in Fig. 10. McGandy et al. [77] estimated a linear decrease in physical activity of about 25% in men and women in the age range 28–80 years. Such decreases in activity would be expected to have deleterious consequences independent of any aging effects. This is because relative inactivity has been demonstrated to have a broad range of adverse functional consequences, including decreased appetite [78], muscle atrophy associated with inhibition of protein synthesis and increased rates of protein degradation [79], glucose intolerance and decreased responsiveness to insulin [69], and decreased rate of maximal oxygen consumption ($\dot{V}_{O_{2max}}$) [72]. Regular physical activity may then be viewed as a stress necessary on a repeated basis for continued wellbeing. As in the case of CR, effects of exercise will depend upon the duration and intensity. While the anti-aging effects of CR appear to depend only on the amount and duration of restriction of calories, beneficial effects of exercise depend also upon the nature of the exercise. This will determine the degree of stress, the specific muscle groups being activated and the type of contractile activity in these muscle groups.

3.1 Types of exercise

As indicated earlier, most data on the effects of exercise on aging have been obtained using endurance or aerobic-type activity. There is an important emerging literature on resistance-type exercise in aging, especially related to the maintenance of muscle mass and bone density in men and women [17]. In addition to these two major types, exercise can also be performed under isometric condi-

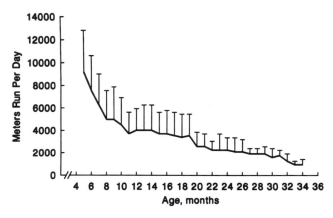

Fig. 10. Voluntary wheel running with age of female Long-Evans rats fed ad libitum. Results are mean ± SD. Reproduced with permission from the Gerontological Society of America from [76].

tions when little or no shortening occurs, and under conditions of active lengthening, such as in walking down stairs, lowering weights, etc. There are large
differences between effects of these activities on muscle metabolism and damage.
For example, shortening of muscles under lightly loaded conditions consumes
less energy than shortening under heavily loaded conditions. Both of these contractions consume more energy than when tension is developed but no shortening occurs (as under isometric conditions). Consequently, muscle metabolism is
stimulated much more by contractions in which large amounts of external work
are done, as in intense resistance exercise [80]. Not surprisingly, therefore, benefits related to maintenance of muscle mass are associated with this type of activity, whereas benefits of aerobic activity are associated more with cardiovascular
fitness than with altered muscle function [17]. The most surprising effects, however, are associated with active-lengthening, or eccentric-type contractions.
Stretching active muscles greatly reduces the energy consumed by these muscles
during contraction [81]. Despite the reduction in metabolic rate, however, this
type of activity results in by far the greatest damage to muscle fibers of any activity. The effect is thought to be mediated by free radicals and may stimulate
increased turnover of proteins in muscle fibers [18,82]. Most bodily movements
involve muscle groups working in pairs, as agonists and antagonists. Usual movements, therefore, will result in active shortening of some muscle fibers and active
lengthening of others. The reduced metabolic cost and increased protein turnover
of active lengthening enables the control of limb movements at low energy cost,
as well as promoting protein turnover.

3.2 Physiologic and metabolic effects

Some of the large number of effects of regular physical activity, which will include
all of the above types of exercise under usual living conditions, are indicated in
Table 2. It should be noted that many age-related physiological declines are attenuated by regular physical activity, such as the loss of muscle strength, decreased
($\dot{V}_{O_{2max}}$), decreased glucose tolerance, decreased heat tolerance, etc. In some cases,
the rate of physiologic decline is not altered by exercise. Rather, the function
occurs at a more favorable set-point. This is illustrated in Fig. 11, with respect to
pulmonary function [83]. Habitual athletes experience loss with age of the ability
to expire air maximally in 1 s ($FEV_{1.0}$ or forced expiratory volume in 1 s) at the
same rate as do sedentary individuals. However, at any given age the athletes

Table 2. Effects of regular physical activity (modified from the American Journal of Clinical Nutrition
from [69]).

Increased:	Maximal oxygen uptake; muscle strength; metabolic rate; capillary density in skeletal muscle; cardiac efficiency; endurance; function of joints, tendons, ligaments; tolerance to heat; HDL/LDL ratio
Decreased:	Blood pressure; heart rate at given oxygen consumption; risk of cardiac morbidity and mortality; risks of obesity, glucose intolerance, osteoporosis

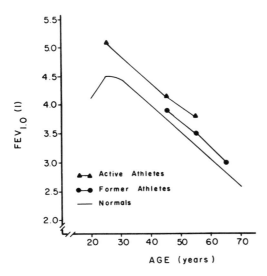

Fig. 11. Variation in forced expiratory volume in 1 s (FEV$_{1.0}$) with age in active athletes, formerly active athletes and sedentary individuals. Reproduced with permission from Georg Thieme Verlag from [83].

have greater FEV$_{1.0}$ than do sedentary individuals [83]. This ability of exercise to reset the status, or set-point, of a physiological parameter is strikingly similar to some changes in function observed with CR. Examples and implications of such resettings of physiological status with age have been explored by Richardson and McCarter [84].

In addition to slowing the decline of physiologic and metabolic parameters with age, exercise has also been viewed as an effective strategy for the prevention and treatment of age-associated diseases such as non-insulin-dependent (type 2) diabetes mellitus, coronary heart disease, colon cancer, hypertension and osteoporosis [85,86]. The conclusion is that exercise modulates many deleterious aspects of aging, including deterioration of function and increased incidence and severity of disease [86]. On this basis, exercise is a potential agent for retarding aging processes. The remaining criterion is, however, a critical factor: evidence is required that exercise modulates life span. This will now be examined in detail.

3.3 Effects on longevity

The earliest studies correlating physical activity and longevity were those documenting rates of mortality associated with professions and competitive sports [87,88]. In general, the data suggested lower risk of mortality with increasing levels of physical activity. Systematic investigation of the effects of exercise on longevity were first undertaken by Paffenbarger and colleagues in an extended series of studies, summarized by Lee et al. [86]. Perhaps the best known of these, the Harvard Alumni Health Study, involved 16,936 male alumni whose activities were followed from 1962 and 1966 until 1978 [89]. The age range at baseline was 35—74 years and all subjects were free of physician-diagnosed coronary heart disease. Estimates were made of the amounts of energy expended weekly on all types of physical activity, from walking to competitive sports, and mortality was then followed. In all age groups those expending up to 3,500 kcal/week on physical activity exhibited decreased risk of mortality than those expending less than 500 kcal/week. The inverse relation between risk of mortality and level of physical activity was present regardless of the presence of other risk factors such as cigarette smoking, high body mass index, hypertension, etc. The investigators concluded that the risk of inactivity was only slightly less than that associated with cigarette smoking for these individuals. The data suggested that vigorous physical activity delayed mortality by about 2 years [89]. Other studies in different, mostly male populations, suggest that the benefit of exercise is in delaying mortality rather than in extending the maximum life span [90,91]. Emerging data suggest similar effects in women and this benefit can be realized even when exercise is initiated late in life (65 years and older) [86]. Thus, a large number of studies provides evidence that regular, vigorous exercise increases life expectancy in humans but may not extend maximum life span. Extension of maximum life span has been used as a criterion for establishing that aging processes are retarded by a given manipulation. In order to establish whether or not the beneficial effects of exercise involve retardation of aging, it is essential to measure effects on maximum life span. This is difficult to establish in men and women. Investigations involving laboratory animals have been used for this purpose.

The use of animal models includes both advantages and disadvantages. The age of onset of exercise and type of exercise can be controlled and precise measurement of effects on survival can be determined. However, the relevance of the outcomes to theories of aging and to effects in men and women must be carefully evaluated. For example, early animal studies frequently involved conditions inducing stress, such as in forced treadmill running or in forced swimming of rodents during daylight hours, when these nocturnal animals would usually be asleep [16]. Studies in flies have involved removing wings and/or housing conditions which prevented usual physical activity [92]. Housing conditions of rodent colonies may have involved the presence of infectious disease in many animals [72]. Interpretation of data from earlier studies is thus, difficult because of the presence of factors known to influence survival, in addition to the possible effects of exercise. Systematic studies relating survival to exercise in laboratory animals have been conducted using endurance-type training. The important variables in these studies are:

1) the use of forced or voluntary exercise, such as in treadmill running and swimming vs. voluntary wheel running;
2) the age of onset of exercise, usually following weaning, during adulthood or in late middle-age;
3) the intensity of exercise, since physiological adaptations to exercise are known to involve threshold levels of activity [93];

4) gender, since female and male rats respond differently to exercise, with females increasing food intake but males exhibiting no change in food intake when exercising [76]; and

5) strain, not just species of animal, since different rat strains exhibit large differences in willingness or desire to exercise [16].

The earliest published work in this area apparently is that of Slonaker [70], who demonstrated decreased longevity in rats with voluntary wheel running. This result was supported by subsequent studies involving forced treadmill exercise or running in drums, by McCay et al. [56] and by Benedict and Sherman [71]. The results were viewed as confirming the Rate of Living theory of aging, in that the presumed increased daily metabolic rate associated with exercise would lead to a more rapid consumption of the fixed lifetime metabolic energy potential. In contrast, later studies by Retzlaff et al. [94] found that 10 min of daily walking (11.5 m/min) increased both median and maximum life span of Sprague-Dawley rats. As pointed out by Holloszy and Khort [72], data of this study are unusual in many respects, such as in exercising rats being heavier than sedentary control rats and, importantly, because the sedentary control animals were remarkably short-lived. Similar results were obtained by Edington et al. [95], who demonstrated increased longevity in rats executing treadmill walking for 20 min/day at 10 m/min. Again, however, variable survival of control rats raised questions regarding the possible presence of disease in these animals. This possibility was also suggested by the finding of increased mortality when the exercise was initiated in old rather than in young rats.

Most of these earlier studies, therefore, provide conflicting data and are compromised by questions related to experimental design and to the health of the animals. The issue was more directly addressed by Goodrick and colleagues in a series of studies involving male and female Wistar rats, running voluntarily in cages with wheels attached from 6 weeks of age. The data demonstrated increased median and maximum life span of running vs. sedentary rats [96,97]. The conclusion drawn was that, as in the case of CR, exercise acted as a retardation of growth and so extended life, as originally postulated by McCay et al. [10]. When exercise was initiated at later ages (10.5 or 18 months of age) there were no effects on survival [97]. In this case, the authors suggested the data were consistent with the existence of an "age threshold" for beneficial effects of exercise, as originally postulated by Edington et al. [95]. However, an alternative explanation is that the low levels of running activity of the older rats were not sufficient to induce physiological adaptations, regardless of age [72]. A similar explanation may attend the absence of longevity effects following long-term swimming activity in rats, as found by Beauchenne et al. [98]. The first studies utilizing animals known to be free of infectious disease (using SPF rats) were conducted by Holloszy and colleagues. These studies also provided the first data on pathology present at death so that an assessment could be made of whether or not the exercise modulated age-related disease. Holloszy et al. [99] used SPF male Long-Evans rats. Exercise was initiated at 6 months of age and the rats initially ran vigorously

— about 7 km per day. After 3—6 months running activity declined but the authors found that decreasing food intake by about 8% below ad libitum consumption resulted in sustained lifetime running. A control group of rats fed 8% less than ad libitum demonstrated no longevity effects due to this mild CR. There was a significant increase in median life span of running rats in comparison with that of sedentary rats (1,012 ± 138 days vs. 923 ± 160 days, respectively). However, there was no significant effect of running activity on maximum life span, in contrast to that found by Goodrick [96]. Moreover, histopathological analysis of tissues at death revealed no significant differences in the causes of death between exercising and sedentary rats, in contrast to food-restricted, paired weight controls, which exhibited significantly reduced neoplasms [99]. Similar results were later found in the case of female Long-Evans rats [100] for running activity initiated at 4 months of age: significant increase in median but not maximum life span in runners vs. sedentary rats. In these rats, the complication of decreased caloric intake to sustain running activity of the previous study [98] was avoided. The extensive and declining running with the age of the female Long-Evans rats is shown in Fig. 10. Holloszy et al. [99] suggested the difference between their results and those of Goodrick [96] might be due to the use of SPF vs. nonbarrier protected rats, i.e., that the control Wistar rats of Goodrick's study may have had increased mortality because of the presence of infectious disease and that exercise protected the running rats, resulting in the apparent extension of both median and maximum life span. This conclusion is strongly supported by subsequent studies involving both lifelong exercise and CR.

3.4 Mechanisms of action

Existing literature provides evidence for all possible outcomes of the effects of exercise on longevity, ranging from no effect to the extension of both median and maximum life span. It is important to bear in mind that these studies deal only with endurance-type exercise and that physiological adaptations to this type of exercise are known to involve threshold levels of intensity [93]. Lack of effects on longevity may thus be a consequence of insufficient levels of exercise. Conversely, strenuous exercise is known to be deleterious in the presence of disease, so shortened life span may be related to the presence of multiple stresses (disease and exercise) rather than to aging effects. These issues, therefore, complicate interpretation of existing data. However, in the most rigorously controlled studies [99,100] consistent results were obtained. The studies suggest that beneficial physiological adaptations resulting from voluntary wheel running afford protection from disease and early death but do not slow the rate of aging. This results in an increased median but not a maximum life span, i.e., it seems that endurance-type exercise may not retard aging processes, despite its CR-like action in decreasing the fraction of consumed energy available for growth, proliferation and/or the maintenance of homeostasis. A further test of this conclusion comes from studies combining CR and voluntary wheel running.

4   CR, EXERCISE AND AGING

4.1 Overview

The initial metabolic response to reduced food intake appears entirely appropriate to enable the animal to conserve limited energy resources, i.e., there is an acute reduction in resting and daily energy expenditure and a reduction in the thermal effect of food [36,101]. On the other hand, several studies demonstrate that CR does not result in reduced spontaneous activity of rats in their cages [28,101,102] as might be expected to further conserve energy resources. On the contrary, providing rodents (whose food intake has been reduced) with running wheels results in a substantial increases in voluntary wheel running with age [102,103]. If CR and exercise separately exert beneficial effects, it may be possible then for additive benefits to be realized by combining these two manipulations. Alternatively, if increased physical activity plays a role in the beneficial effects of CR, then increasing levels of exercise might further extend the beneficial effects of CR. Several investigators have tested these hypotheses.

4.2 Experimental results

This was first done by McCay et al. [56] using middle-aged "albino" rats (200—450 days old) running 2 h per day in barrels and eating a restricted diet, such that weights of sedentary rats were 10% less than those of sedentary rats eating ad libitum. Median life span was greatest in restricted running rats, but maximum life span of these rats was less than that of restricted sedentary rats. Goodrick et al. [97] initiated voluntary wheel running at 6 weeks of age in male Wistar rats fed ad libitum or fed every other day (EOD). Using this regimen, body weights of sedentary EOD rats were 20% less than those of sedentary ad libitum fed rats. Both ad libitum fed and EOD rats ran voluntarily throughout life (about 2 km/day). Voluntary running increased maximum life span in ad libitum fed rats (10th percentile survivors) from 88 to 115 weeks for sedentary vs. running rats respectively. In contrast, running activity decreased maximum life span in EOD rats from 158 to 145 weeks. Thus, both of these early studies suggested deleterious effects of exercise on age-related benefits of CR. However, the studies did not employ SPF animals and the data may be interpreted as an effect of exercise in possibly exacerbating effects of chronic disease in these conventionally housed animals. The first use of SPF rats was the study of Holloszy and Schechtman [103]. These authors initiated voluntary wheel running in male Long-Evans rats at 3 months of age and utilized CR of about 30% less than ad libitum. Both ad libitum fed and CR rats ran extensively throughout life, with CR rats exhibiting higher levels of daily activity, averaging about 3 km/day. Running activity decreased median life span in CR rats but there was no significant effect on maximum life span when compared with sedentary CR rats. The increased mortality between 20 and 30 months of age in the restricted runners suggests that effects of exercise might diminish benefits of CR, as suggested by the work of Skalicky et al. [104]. However, subsequent work by Holloszy [72] resulted in no early deaths in restricted runners. These effects have been recently investigated in the author's laboratory using male SPF Fischer 344 rats with CR of 40% and voluntary wheel running initiated at 6 weeks of age [102]. There were four groups of rats: A, sedentary, fed ad libitum; AE, fed ad libitum and provided with wheels in their cages; B, sedentary, fed 40% less food than A rats; BE, fed same amount of food as B rats and provided with running wheels in cages. Figure 12 illustrates the profound effect of CR on voluntary wheel running: there were immediate and large difference in running activity of AE vs. BE rats (about 1 vs. 6 km/day, respectively). AE rats greatly reduced their running activity with age. Remarkably, BE rats exhibited high, sustained running with age such that these rats were running almost 5 km/day at a time when all AE and A rats had died. Running activity significantly reduced body weights of BE rats and even the low activity levels of AE rats reduced their peak body weights (Fig. 13) and decreased oxidative stress in cardiac and liver tissues [105,106]. Despite the intense wheel running, the spontaneous movement of BE rats around their cages was not less than that of sedentary B rats or sedentary A rats. Figure 14 demonstrates that the low level of running had no effect on the survival of ad libitum fed animals (AE vs. A rats). In contrast, the high levels of running of BE rats did increase median life span but did not increase maximum life span (BE vs. B rats). No effect of intense running activity on early mortality was found, in contrast to the earlier results of Holloszy and Schechtman in Long-Evans rats [103]. Pathology at death was measured in all rats (40 rats in each of the four groups). Even low levels of exercise significantly reduced the incidence of severe nephropathy in ad libitum fed rats (AE vs. A rats) but had no effect on the incidence of pituitary tumors and lymphomas. In BE rats, exercise resulted in a sig-

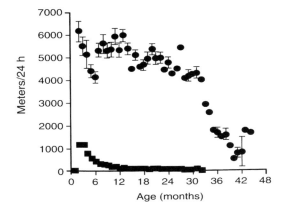

Fig. 12. Voluntary wheel running with age in male F344 rats, fed ad libitum (squares) or fed 40% less than ad libitum (circles) from 6 weeks of age onwards. Data are mean ± SEM. Reproduced with permission from Editrice Kurtis s.r.l. from [102].

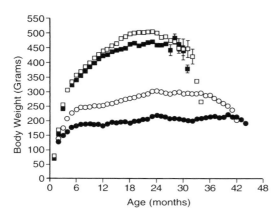

Fig. 13. Variation in body weight with age in male F344 rats. Open squares: group A rats, sedentary and fed ad libitum; solid squares: group AE rats, fed ad libitum and having running wheels in cages; open circles: group B rats, sedentary and fed 40% less than group A rats; solid circles: group BE rats, fed 40% less than group A rats and having running wheels in cages. Values are mean ± SEM. Reproduced with permission from Editrice Kurtis c.r.l. from [102].

nificant increase in cardiomyopathy and did not affect the incidence of other tissue pathologies. In this study, daily metabolic rates were also measured over 24 h, with rats in their cages and under usual living conditions. Metabolic rate was expressed relative to metabolic mass (body weight to the power 0.75), since lean mass could not be determined because of the extensive tissue pathology

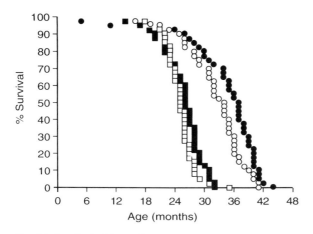

Fig. 14. Survival with age in male F344 rats. Open squares: group A rats, sedentary and fed ad libitum; solid squares: group AE rats, fed ad libitum with running wheels in cages; open circles: group B rats, sedentary, fed 40% less than group A rats; solid circles: group BE rats, fed 40% less food than group A rats with running wheels in cages. There were 40 rats in each group at the start of the experiment. Reproduced with permission from Editrice Kurtis s.r.l. from [102].

assays conducted on all rats. Over the life span the specific metabolic rate of BE rats was significantly greater than that of other rats. It is of some interest that these rats also exhibited the greatest median life span and had maximum life span similar to that of B rats. A more recent study utilized male SPF Fischer 344 rats restricted by only 10% less than ad libitum (unpublished data). Running activity of these rats was sustained over most of the life span, as shown in Fig. 15, and falls between the extensive activity of the 40% CR group (BE) and the very low activity of the ad libitum fed rats (AE). There was a remarkable effect on longevity of this combined intermediate running and mild CR. Median life span (but not maximum life span) of these rats was similar to that of sedentary, 40% restricted rats. Maximum life span was significantly greater than that of ad libitum fed rats, but less than that of 40% restricted rats. However, studies recently concluded by my colleague Dr H. Bertrand (personal communication) demonstrate that this effect is attributable to the 10% restriction of food, rather than to the concomitant moderate running activity. It seems, therefore, that a reduction in food intake of even 10% in male Fischer 344 rats is sufficient to induce significant effects on longevity, in contrast to the Long-Evans rats utilized by Holloszy and colleagues [99,103].

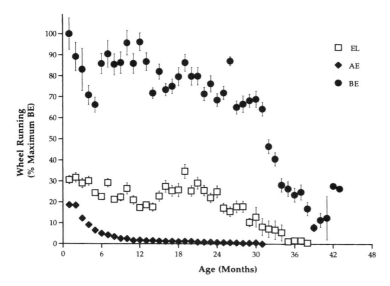

Fig. 15. Variation of wheel running with age and different levels of restriction in male F344 rats. Solid diamonds: rats fed ad libitum; open squares: rats fed 10% less than ad libitum; solid circles: rats fed 40% less than ad libitum. Values are mean ± SEM, n = 40, with wheel running expressed as a percentage of maximum running activity of BE rats. Reproduced with permission from Editrice Kurtis s.r.l. from [102].

4.3 Insights from combined effects of CR and exercise

Studies using conventionally housed rats [56,97] demonstrated increased mortality when CR and exercise were combined. In contrast, more recent studies employing barrier maintained SPF rats found no change in maximum life span when these two manipulations were combined [102,103]. Since the rats of the later studies were known to be free of infectious disease, the data suggest that aging processes are not further retarded by combining CR with lifelong running activity. Rather, the addition of running activity to possibly unhealthy rats provided sufficient stress to promote mortality in the earlier studies. It should be pointed out that the combination of CR and exercise did result in reduction of oxidative stress in some tissues (cardiac mitochondria and liver microsomes [105,106]) but also increased the incidence of cardiomyopathy present at death [102]. Thus, lifelong intense exercise in the BE Fischer 344 rats produced both beneficial and adverse effects. Also, the small size (Fig. 13) and high levels of exercise (Fig. 12) of these BE rats resulted in the highest metabolic rate per unit mass of all rats. Despite having significantly higher specific metabolic rates over the life span than other rats, these BE rats also exhibited the highest average survival rate (Fig. 14). Thus, the life-prolonging actions of CR were not reduced by increased specific metabolic rate. These data, together with those of earlier studies [34], therefore, argue strongly against the role of metabolic rate in the action of CR on aging. The increased median longevity of BE rats over B rats (Fig. 14) is consistent with the results of many studies in exercising men and women [86], i.e., sustained exercise increases life expectancy. This result is in disagreement with those of earlier rodent studies [97,103], but suggests that when exercise of sufficient intensity is sustained over a life span in healthy animals and in healthy men and women, life expectancy, but not maximum life span is increased. The impressive extension of median and maximum life span produced by only 10% restriction of calories is of interest. This result in Fischer 344 rats is in contrast to the absence of longevity effects of an 8% restriction in the study of Holloszy and Schechtman [103]. The difference may be related to intensity of running or to different rat strains — Fischer 344 vs. Long-Evans. If the latter, this would be consistent with the suggestion of Masoro and Austad [25] that differences in evolutionary history might change the physiological response to CR, with some genetic types being more sensitive to this nutritional challenge than others. The protective effects of exercise against early mortality may be viewed in terms of protection against disease without retardation of aging. The results also suggest that increased physical activity is not an important component of the mechanism by which aging is retarded in CR. The broadly protective effects of CR apparently are not additive with the limited protection provided by sustained exercise. The data suggest that mechanisms related to the mobilization of cellular defenses against stress merit investigation, since it seems possible that both CR and exercise may act by mobilizing processes protective of cellular homeostasis. In particular, CR and exercise may act by initiating hormetic effects [107] as first suggested by Lindell [108] and extended by Masoro [109]. These possibilities will be explored in the final section.

5 SUMMARY

5.1 CR and aging

There are currently no, generally, agreed upon definitions of aging and the molecular basis of aging remains undetermined. However, there is acceptance of criteria for establishing that a given manipulation has slowed the aging processes, whatever these processes may be. These criteria include experimental demonstration of:
1) increased maximum life span or increased MRDT,
2) decreased rate of functional decline, and
3) decreased incidence or severity of pathology.
CR is widely viewed as the only manipulation known to reliably retard aging processes in mammals because it satisfies all three of these criteria. The work of many investigators demonstrates that the anti-aging effects of CR depend on the restriction of energy intake rather than on restriction of any particular dietary component. Also, this action is not related to developmental effects, since it is successful even when initiated in adulthood. Identification of mechanisms underlying this action have been unsuccessful, in part due to the very large number of functional changes which occur in long-term CR. Despite this, current research has enabled many suggested mechanisms of action to be rendered unlikely. These mechanisms include: the reduction of metabolic rate, retarded growth and reduction of adiposity. A focus point of the present discussion is the possibility that increased lifelong physical activity plays an important role in the anti-aging action of CR.

5.2 Exercise and aging

There is considerable evidence that long-term endurance exercise and resistance exercise result in adaptations that are counter to many of the usual deleterious consequences of aging. These include maintenance of muscle mass, decreased adiposity and improved cardiovascular and pulmonary function. Habitual exercise also decreases the risks of developing cardiovascular disease, type 2 diabetes and osteoporosis. There is evidence that intensity, as well as duration of exercise is important in causing physiological adaptations. Thresholds of intensity may exist for producing particular beneficial effects, such as in maintenance of muscle mass, and effects on longevity. However, even low intensities of exercise have been shown to induce beneficial metabolic changes in animal studies. Also, epidemiological studies demonstrate that inactivity, or a sedentary life style, is by far the greatest modifiable risk factor for many age-associated diseases.

Regarding effects on longevity, there is evidence in studies of men and women that life-expectancy or median life span may be extended by lifelong exercise of moderate intensity. Animal studies have produced equivocal results. However, in many of these studies it is not clear that the animals were healthy and free of disease. More recent work using SPF rats known to be free of infectious disease has produced consistent results: long-term voluntary wheel running of moderate to high intensity was associated with extension of median, but not maximum life span. These results have been interpreted to indicate that such exercise does not alter aging processes, but rather exerts protective effects, which enables a larger fraction of the population to live longer.

5.3 CR, exercise and aging

Animal studies employing CR and exercise in combination have also produced equivocal results. Some of these studies indeed indicate detrimental effects of exercise on benefits derived from CR. The same caveats described previously regarding the importance of the animal's health apply to these results. More recent work using SPF rats has consistently demonstrated no significant effect (positive or negative) of exercise on the extension of maximum life span by CR. The absence of an effect on maximum life span is particularly striking in view of the intense running of the rats (about 4 km/24 h) over most of the life span. Data from this study [102] suggest that both physical activity and specific metabolic rate are not important components of the anti-aging action of CR. This conclusion is strengthened by recent data showing even mild (10%) CR can exert significant anti-aging effects with or without simultaneous voluntary running. In summary, studies to date suggest that both CR and exercise may act to mobilize cellular protective actions. The different characteristics of mobilization of protective mechanisms induced by CR and exercise may provide valuable insight into the anti-aging mechanism of CR and into aging processes themselves.

6   PERSPECTIVES

6.1 Hormesis

Several authors have suggested that CR may exert beneficial effects because it imposes a metabolic stress on the organism resulting in the mobilization of protective mechanisms [108–110]. There is indeed an extensive literature documenting the fact that organisms across wide phylogenetic lines respond to low levels of stress by improving their functional status. Organisms subjected to such low levels of stress exhibit enhanced function, less susceptibility to environmental challenge and increased longevity, whereas high levels of the same stress result in death [107]. The phenomenon was first identified and defined as hormesis by Southam and Ehrlich in studies of naturally occurring inhibitors of fungal growth [111]. Later studies in laboratory animals extended the concept to effects of radiation and chemical agents. These were shown to induce beneficial effects, including life span extension at low doses but were lethal at higher doseages [112]. It is now generally accepted that this phenomenon may be present in all cells and has been conserved throughout evolutionary development [107]. Masoro [109] has pointed out that severe reduction of caloric intake causes damage and probable death, whereas low to moderate levels of CR induce a wide range of beneficial effects including life span extension. As such, CR may represent another example of hormesis. Similar reasoning can be applied to increased levels of physical activity. Moderate levels of exercise are known to induce beneficial effects, including increased life expectancy. Both CR and exercise represent metabolic challenges to the organism and, therefore, might be expected to result in adaptive, possibly protective, mechanisms. To what extent are the life prolonging effects of CR and exercise examples of hormesis?

6.2 CR, exercise and hormesis

This discussion will focus on the increased longevity associated with hormesis. The extent to which known effects of CR and exercise are consistent with the large body of data available from studies of laboratory animals exposed to low doses of radiation and chemical agents will be examined. Neafsey [113] has pointed out that increased longevity in hormesis is unrelated to decreased caloric intake, in that food intake and weight gain are often normal or increased under these conditions. Analysis of survival curves by Sacher [6] indicates that hormesis in the absence of toxic effects would not alter the rate of aging, i.e., in a plot of the logarithm of mortality rate vs. age there is no change of slope (designated α by Sacher) and, therefore, no change in the MRDT. Rather, extension of life by hormetic effects results from a reduction in the "vulnerability" parameter, a measure of the initial vulnerability of the population to causes of disease and mortality. This parameter (designated G_o by Sacher) represents the intercept on the mortality rate axis of the regression of the logarithm of mortality rate vs. age. Analysis of data from several studies of CR demonstrates the effect of CR on survival is to decrease α (decreased slope, increased MRDT) without affecting G_o, in such plots [113]. Thus, Sacher's analysis suggests hormetic effects provide protection by reducing initial vulnerability without altering aging processes. CR, on the other hand exerts protective actions by slowing aging processes, without altering the initial vulnerability. A further important point is that even relatively brief periods of CR result in life span extension [28] whereas termination of exposure to an hormetic agent does not result in longevity benefits for surviving organisms [113]. Further study is, therefore, needed before equating the effects of CR and hormesis on longevity. In particular it remains possible that the protective effects of these two phenomena arise from different molecular mechanisms. Effects of exercise apparently are in better agreement with hormetic phenomena, since exercise is viewed as extending life by mechanisms not related to aging processes, i.e., exercise prolongs life by reducing vulnerability (G_o) but does not reduce the aging rate constant (α). It should be noted that functional benefits of exercise (such as on pulmonary function) are not fully preserved after the termination of exercise [83], consistent with the absence of benefits extending beyond termination of low level stress in hormesis [113].

Molecular mechanisms associated with cellular protection and life extension in CR have been attributed to daily periods of moderate hyperadrenocorticism [109], to enhanced synthesis of mRNA [108], to decreased oxidative and glycation stress [66], and to enhanced immune function, amongst other possibilities [13]. The beneficial effects of exercise on increased longevity are not clearly related to events at the molecular level in all cells, other than by increasing rates of protein turnover in working muscle cells and in cells subserving the increased energy needs of the exercise. However, the net result is a decreased risk of mortality from all causes whatever the molecular mechanisms involved may be [74]. Molecular mechanisms of life extension in hormesis are likewise not known. Suggestions include upregulation of the heat shock (or stress) response, enhanced prostaglandin synthesis and/or increased cell proliferation, amongst other possibilities [113]. Identification of molecular mechanisms underlying the different protective effects exerted by CR and exercise promises to yield valuable insights into aging processes. As suggested by Masoro [109], one approach to achieving this end may be to investigate the involvement of hormesis in these effects.

7　ABBREVIATIONS

CR:	caloric restriction
EOD:	every-other-day
FEV:	forced expiratory volume
MRDT:	mortality rate doubling time
RM:	repetition maximum
SPF:	specific pathogen free
$\dot{V}_{O_{2max}}$:	maximal oxygen consumption

8　REFERENCES

1. Finch CE. Longevity, Senescence and the Genome. Chicago: University of Chicago Press, 1990; 1−662.
2. Comfort A. The Biology of Senescence. New York: Elsevier, 1979.
3. Austad SN, Fischer KE. J Gerontol 1991;46:B47−B53.
4. Medawar PB. An Unsolved Problem of Biology. London: HK Lewis Publisher, 1952.
5. Fries JF, Crapo LM. Vitality and Aging. San Francisco: WH Freeman Publishers, 1981.
6. Sacher GA. Life table modification and life prolongation. In: Finch C, Hayflick L (eds) Handbook of the Biology of Aging. New York: Van Nostrand Reinhold, 1977:582−638.
7. Finch CE, Pike C, Whitten M. Science 1990;249:902−903.
8. Carey JR, Liedo P, Orozco D, Vaupel J. Science 1992;258:457−458.
9. Masoro EJ. J Gerontol 1988;43:B59−B64.
10. McCay CM, Cromwell MF, Maynard LA. J Nutr 1935;10:63−79.
11. McCay CM, Maynard LA, Sperling G, Barnes L. J Nutr 1939;18:1−13.
12. Saxton JA. Biol Symp 1945;11:177−196.

13. Weindruch R, Walford RL. The Retardation of Aging and Disease by Dietary Restriction. Springfield, IL: Charles C. Thomas, 1988;1—337.
14. Yu BP. Rev Biol Res Aging 1990;4:349—371.
15. McAuley E, Cournea KS, Lettunich J. Gerontologist 1991;31:534—539.
16. McCarter R. Ann Rev. Gerontol Geriatr 1995;15:187—228.
17. Evans WJ. Nutr Rev 1996;54:535—539.
18. Zerba E, Komorowski TE, Faulkner JA. Am J Physiol 1990;258:C429—C435.
19. Kemnitz J, Roecker EB, Weindruch R, Olsen DF, Baum ST, Bergman RN. Am J Physiol 1994; 266:E540—E547.
20. Lane MA, Ingram DK, Cutler RG, Knapka J, Barnard DE, Roth GS. NY Acad Sci 1992;673: 36—45.
21. Hass, SB, Lewis SM, Duffy PH, Erschler W, Feuers RJ et al. Mech Ageing Devel 1996;91: 79—94.
22. Lee IM, Paffenbarger R. J Am Med Assoc 1992;268:2045—2049.
23. Bergman RN. J Gerontol 1948;3:14—20.
24. Jones HB. The relation of human health to age, place and time. In: Birren JE (ed) Handbook of Aging and the Individual. Chicago: University Chicago Press, 1959:336—363.
25. Masoro EJ, Austad SN. J Gerontol 1996;51A:B387—B391.
26. Weisbroth SH. Exp Gerontol 1972;7:417—425.
27. Yu BP, Masoro EJ, Murata I, Bertrand H, Lynd FT. J Gerontol 1982;37:130—141.
28. Yu BP, Masoro EJ, McMahan CA. J Gerontol 1985;40:657—670.
29. Weindruch RH, Walford RL. Science 1982;215:1415—1418.
30. McCarter R. Clin Geriatr Med 1995;11:553—565.
31. Yu BP. Proc Soc Exp Biol Med 1994;205:97—105.
32. Liepa GU, Masoro EJ, Bertrand HJ, Yu BP. Am J Physiol 1980;238:E253—E254.
33. McCarter R, Palmer J. Am J Physiol 1992;263:E448—E452.
34. McCarter R. Energy Utilization. In: Masoro EJ (ed) Handbook of Physiology, vol 2, Aging. New York: Oxford University Press, 1995:95—118.
35. Garrow JS. Energy Balance and Obesity in Man. London: Elsevier-North Holland, 1978: 1—195.
36. McCarter R, McGee J. Am J Physiol 1989;254:E175—E179.
37. Masoro EJ, Yu BP, Bertrand HA. Proc Natl Acad Sci USA 1982;79:4239—4241.
38. Duffy PH, Fevers RJ, Leakey JA et al. Mech Ageing Dev 1989;48:117—133.
39. Pearl R. The Rate of Living. New York: Alfred Knopf, 1928;1—185.
40. Rubner M. Das problem der Lebensdauer und seine Beziehung-en zum Wachstum under Ehr-narung. Munich: Oldenburg, 1908:1—204.
41. Yu BP. Physiol Rev 1994;74:139—163.
42. Chipalkatti S, De A, Aiyer AS. J Nutr 1983;113:944—950.
43. Koizumi A, Weindruch R, Walford R. J Nutr 1987;117:361—367.
44. Yu BP. Free Radic Biol Med 1996;21:651—668.
45. Matsuo M, Gomi F, Kuramoto K, Sagal M. Gerontology 1993;48:133—138.
46. Laganiere S, Yu BP. Mech Ageing Devel 1989;48:221—230.
47. Masoro EJ, McCarter R. Ageing 1991;3:117—128.
48. Maeda H, Gleiser CA, Masoro EJ, Murata I, MacMahan CA, Yu BP. J Gerontol 1985;40: 671—688.
49. Iwasaki K, Gleiser CA, Masoro EJ, McMahan CA, Seo E, Yu BP. J Gerontol 1988;43:B5—B12.
50. Cheney KE, Liu RK, Smith GS, Meredith P, Mickey MR, Walford R. J Gerontol 1983;38: 420—430.
51. Fernandes G, Friend P, Yunis E, Good RA. Proc Natl Acad Sci USA 1978;75:1500—1504.
52. Loyd T. Life Sci 1982;34:625—635.
53. Shimokawa I, Higami T. Effect of dietary restriction on pathological processes. In: Yu BP (ed) Modulation of Aging Processes by Dietary Restriction. Boca Raton: CRC Press, 1994:247—266.

54. Bronson RT, Lipman RD. Growth Dev Aging 1991;55:169.
55. Moreschi C. Z Immunitatsforsch 1909;2:651—659.
56. McCay C, Sperling C, Barnes L. Arch Biochem Biophys 1943;2:469.
57. McCay CM, Maynard LA, Sperling G, Osgood HS. J Nutr 1941;21:45.
58. Harrison DE, Archer JR, Ascle CM. Proc Natl Acad Sci USA 1984;81:1835—1838.
59. Gonzalez-Pacheco DM, Buss WC, Koehler KM, Woodside WF, Alpert SS. J Nutr 1993;123: 90—97.
60. Lynn WS, Wallwork JC. J Nutr 1992;122:1917—1918.
61. Sohal RS, Allen RG. Adv Free Radic Biol Med 1986;2:117—160.
62. Cutler R. Anti—oxidants, aging and logevity. In: Pryor WA (ed) Free Radicals in Biology, vol 6. Orlando: Academic Press, 1984:381—383.
63. Lints FA. Gerontology 1989;35:36—57.
64. Nelson JF. Neuroendocrine involvement in the retardation of aging by food restriction: A hypothesis. In: Yu BP (ed) Modulation of Aging Processes by Dietary Restriction. Boca Raton, Florida: CRC Press Handbook, 1994:37—55.
65. Yu BP. Modulation of oxidative stress as a means of life-prolonging action of dietary restriction. In: Cutler RG Parker L, Bertram J, Mori (eds) Oxidative Stress and Aging. Basel: Birkhauser Verlag, 1995:331—341.
66. Kristal BS, Yu BP. J Gerontol 1992;47:B107—B114.
67. Sell DR, Lane MA, Johnson WA et al. Proc Natl Aca Sci USA 1996;93:485—490.
68. Masoro EJ, McCarter RJ, Katz MS, McMahan CA. J Gerontol 1992;47:B202—B208.
69. Astrand P. Am J Clin Nutr 1992;55:1231S—1236S.
70. Slonaker JR. J Anim Behav 1912;2:20—42.
71. Benedict FG, Sherman HC. J Nutr 1937;14:179—198.
72. Holloszy JO, Khort W. Exercise. In: Masoro EJ (ed) Handbook of the Physiology of Aging. New York: Oxford University Press, 1995:633—666.
73. Ji LL. Med Sci Sports Ex 1993;25:225—231.
74. Paffenbarger RS, Hyde RT, Wing AL, Hsieh C. N Engl J Med 1986;314:605—613.
75. Sohal RS, Buchan PB. Exp Gerontol 1981;15:137—142.
76. Holloszy JO. J Gerontol 1993;48:B97—B100.
77. McGandy RG, Barrows CH, Spania A, Meredith A, Stone JK, Norris AH. J Gerontol 1966;21: 581—587.
78. Altman DF. Gastroenterol Clin North Am 1990;19:227—234.
79. Musacchia X, Steffen J, Fell R. Ex Sports Sci Rev 1988;16:61—87.
80. McCarter R. Effects of Exercise and Dietary Restriction on Energy Metabolism and Longevity. In: Yu BP (ed) Modulation of Aging Processes by Dietary Restriction. Boca Raton: CRC Press, 1994:157—174.
81. Curtin N, Davies R. J Mechanochem Cell Motil 1975;3:147—154.
82. Evans WJ, Cannon JG. The metabolic effects of exercise—induced muscle damage. In: Holloszy JO (ed) Exercise and Sports Sciences Reviews. Baltimore: Williams and Wilkins, 1991:99—126.
83. Skinner JS. Age and performance. In: Keul J (ed) Limiting Factors of Physical Performance. Stuttgart: Georg Thieme Publishers, 1973:271—282.
84. Richardson A, McCarter R. Mechanism of food restriction: Change of rate or change of set point? In: Ingram, DK, Baker GT, Shock NW (eds) The Potential for Nutritional Modulation of Aging Processes. Trumbull, Connecticut: Food and Nutrition Press, 1991:177—192.
85. Bouchard C, Shephard RJ, Stephens T. Physical activity, fitness and health: International Proceedings and Consensus Statement. Champaign, Illinois: Human Kinetics Publishers, 1994.
86. Lee IM, Paffenbarger RS, Hennekens CH. Ageing 1997;9:2—11.
87. Smith E. Report on the sanitary conditions of tailors in London. Report of the Medical Officer. London: The Privy Council, 1864:416—430.
88. Hartley PHS, Llewellyn GF. Br Med J 1939;1:657—662.
89. Paffenbarger RS, Hyde RT, Wing AL, Hsieh C. N Engl J Med 1986;315:399—401.

90. Pekkanen J, Marti B, Nissimen A, Tuomilehto J, Punsar S, Karvonen M. Lancet 1987;1: 1473−1477.
91. Lindsted KD, Tonstad S, Kuzma JW. J Clin Epidemiol 1991;44:355−364.
92. Sohal RS, Buchan PB. Exp Gerontol 1981;16:157−162.
93. Fitts RH, Booth FW, Winder WW, Holloszy JO. Am J Physiol 1975;228:1029−1033.
94. Retzlaff EJ, Fontaine J, Futura W. Geriatrics 1966;21:171−177.
95. Edington DW, Cosmas A, McCafferty WB. J Gerontol 1972;27:341−343.
96. Goodrick CL. Gerontology 1980;26:22−23.
97. Goodrick CL, Ingram DK, Reynolds J, Freeman R, Cider NL. J Gerontol 1983;38:36−45.
98. Beauchenne RE, Dellwo W, Darabian P, Haley-Zitlin V, Wright DL. Abstr of Biological Effects of Dietary Restriction, An International Conference, Washington, DC, 1990.
99. Holloszy JO, Smith EK, Vining M, Adams S. J Appl Physiol 1985;59:826−831.
100. Holloszy JO. J Gerontol 1993;48:B97−B100.
101. Boyle PC, Storlien LH, Harper AE, Keesey RE. Am J Physiol 1982;241:R392−R397.
102. McCarter R, Shimokawa I, Ikeno Y, Higami Y, Hubbard G, Yu BP, McMahan, CA. Ageing 1997; 9:73−79.
103. Holloszy JO, Schechtman KB. J Appl Physiol 1991;70:1529−1535.
104. Skalicky MG, Hofecker G, Kment G, Niedermuller H. Mech Ageing Develop 1980;14: 361−377.
105. Kim JD, Yu BP, McCarter RJ, Lee SY, Herlihy JT. Free Radic Biol Med 1996;20:83−88.
106. Kim JD, McCarter RJ, Yu BP. Ageing 1996;8:123−129.
107. Furst A. Health Phys 1987;52:527−530.
108. Lindell A. Life Sci 1982;31:625−630.
109. Masoro EJ. Exp Gerontol 1998;33:61−66.
110. Totter JR. Health Phys 1987;52:549−551.
111. Southam JM, Ehrlich J. Phytopathology 1943;33:517−524.
112. Calabrese EJ, McCarthy ME, Kenyon E. Health Phys 1987;52:531−541.
113. Neafsey PJ. Mech Ageing Devel 1990;51:1−31.

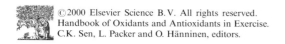
©2000 Elsevier Science B.V. All rights reserved.
Handbook of Oxidants and Antioxidants in Exercise.
C.K. Sen, L. Packer and O. Hänninen, editors.

Part X • Chapter 29

Oxidative stress and the pathogenesis of sarcopenia

M.E. Lopez[1], T.A. Zainal[2], S.S. Chung[1], J.M. Aiken[1] and R. Weindruch[3,4]
Departments of
[1] *Animal Health and Biomedical Sciences,*
[2] *Nutritional Sciences, and*
[3] *Medicine, University of Wisconsin, Madison, WI 53706, USA.*
[4] *Wisconsin Regional Primate Research Center, University of Wisconsin and Geriatric Research, Education and Clinical Center, Wm. Middleton VA Medical Center (GRECC-11G), 2500 Overlook Terrace, University of Wisconsin at Madison, Madison, WI 53705, USA. E-mail: rhweindr@facstaff.wisc.edu*

1   INTRODUCTION
2   CHANGES IN SKELETAL MUSCLES WITH AGING
    2.1   Morphological changes
    2.2   Changes in muscle function
    2.3   Changes in metabolic capacity
3   POSSIBLE CAUSES OF SARCOPENIA
    3.1   Denervation-reinnervation process
    3.2   Contraction-induced injury
    3.3   Satellite cell changes
4   OXIDATIVE STRESS AND SARCOPENIA
    4.1   Hypothesis
    4.2   Mitochondria, oxygen radicals and aging
    4.3   Mitochondrial myopathies and encephalomyopathies
    4.4   Age-associated abnormalities of mtDNA and the electron transport system
    4.5   Oxidative damage
    4.6   Antioxidant status
5   INTERVENTIONS
    5.1   Exercise
    5.2   Antioxidant supplementation
    5.3   Caloric restriction
6   SUMMARY
7   PERSPECTIVES
8   ACKNOWLEDGEMENTS
9   ABBREVIATIONS
10 REFERENCES

1   INTRODUCTION

A loss of motor ability occurs with senescence in mammals and in other classes of animals. In humans, physical frailty increases markedly with old age leading to a myriad of medical and social problems such as injuries, lack of independence and institutionalization [1,2]. The annual costs imposed by physical frailty in the USA in 1990 were estimated at nearly US$80 billion and, by 2030, this could exceed US$130 billion (in 1990 dollars) unless interventions are found [3].

Although deleterious changes with age in the nervous and cardiovascular systems, among others, contribute to physical frailty, endogenous alterations occurring in skeletal muscle may underlie muscle loss and dysfunction.

The loss of skeletal muscle mass during aging, often referred to as sarcopenia, is reflected by decreases of 25–50% in the cross-sectional area of several limb muscles due to muscle fiber atrophy and loss [4] (Fig. 1). Muscle mass appears to be the main determinant of the loss of strength with aging [5]. Because of the enormity and universality of sarcopenia, it is important to understand the underlying mechanisms so that interventions can be rationally designed. Several hypotheses have been proposed to explain the causes of sarcopenia, including cumulative effects of contraction-induced injuries [6], decline in the recruitment of satellite cells to replace damaged muscle fibers [7], decline in the number of motor units [8] and increased oxidative stress/damage [9]. This latter hypothesis is one of the main focuses of this article.

The essential feature of the oxidative stress hypothesis of aging is that under normal physiological conditions, the use of oxygen by cells generates toxic reactive oxygen species (ROS) and their metabolites (ROM), which cause macromolecular damage [10,11] (Fig. 2). Some oxidative damage is irreversible, progressively accumulating with age, and is postulated to be the main cause for the decline in physiological vigor with aging. Besides causing molecular damage, ROM also influence normal cellular functions (e.g., transcriptional control, signal transduction and apoptosis [12,13,14]). Therefore, increases in oxidative stress with aging may alter key pathways which control cellular functions.

Although the oxidative stress hypothesis has garnered some support, its validity has not been broadly tested, especially in relation to functional losses such as those occurring in skeletal muscle. Skeletal muscle, brain and heart, which are largely composed of postmitotic cells dependent on oxidative energy metabolism, are logical sites where oxidative damage may accrue, irreversibly damaging cells and thereby being especially problematic.

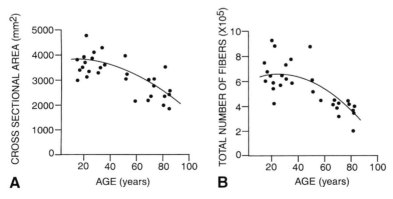

Fig. 1. Relationship between age of men and either the cross-sectional area of the vastus lateralis (VL) (**A**) or the total number of fibers in the muscle (**B**). (Redrawn from Lexell et al. [18].)

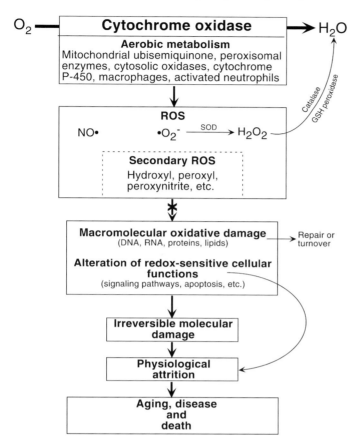

Fig. 2. Proposed involvement of oxidative stress and damage in aging. An X indicates the interdiction by nonenzymatic antioxidant defense mechanisms. SOD = superoxide dismutase. (Modified from Weindruch and Sohal [234].)

If the oxidative stress hypothesis is valid, it should explain the mechanism of the decreased stamina and strength associated with aging. Stamina depends on the steady supply of adenosine triphosphate (ATP), the main source of which is the mitochondrion. Mitochondria are not only the main producers of ATP, but also the main consumers of oxygen and generators of ROM. Accordingly, mitochondria may also be the victims of the ROM that they generate. Self-inflicted damage to mitochondria may represent the primary factor for loss in muscle mass and be the hallmark of senescence.

This chapter first provides a noncomprehensive overview of sarcopenia by summarizing age-associated morphological, functional and metabolic changes which occur in skeletal muscles. Next, the possible causes of sarcopenia are discussed. This is followed by a more detailed appraisal of one suggested cause: oxidative stress of mitochondrial origin. The development of interventions to attenuate the progression of sarcopenia is an important area of inquiry and the final topic surveyed.

2   CHANGES IN SKELETAL MUSCLE WITH AGING

2.1 Morphological changes

A gradual decrease in muscle fiber diameter, degeneration of sarcoplasm and replacement of muscle fibers by fat and connective tissue are some of the changes that occur with age in skeletal muscles. The result is an age-associated decrease in the percentage of fat-free mass and an increase in the percentage of body fat [15—17]. Three prominent age-associated morphological changes which contribute to this phenotype are discussed herein: muscle atrophy, changes in fiber type and denervation.

2.1.1 Muscle atrophy

Both muscle fiber loss and atrophy may contribute to sarcopenia [18]. A consequence of senile muscle atrophy is reduced muscle strength, which lowers the ability of older persons to engage in physical activity. In humans, muscle atrophy has been evaluated by measuring the cross-sectional area (CSA) of the muscle using ultrasound, computerized transaxial tomography or magnetic resonance. CSA and volume of plantar flexor muscle were, 12 and 18% lower in 58- to 68-year-old persons compared to 21- to 33-year-olds, respectively, [15]. When whole vastus lateralis (VL) cross-sections were studied, both the muscle area and the total fiber number decreased by $\sim 40\%$ in people from 20 to 80 years of age [18] (Fig. 1). It was concluded that muscle CSA loss begins as early as 25 years, leading to about a 10% decrease by age 50 and then continues at an accelerated rate.

As capillary beds provide oxygen and energy substrates to muscle fibers and remove the byproducts of muscle activity (e.g., lactate), vascularization might influence the functional performance of muscle fibers. However, age-related changes in the number of capillaries around a fiber have not been reported in old rats for the soleus, flexor digitorum longus (FDL) and extensor digitorum longus (EDL) [19—21]. In humans, no differences with age occurred (but only up to 65 years) in the capillary ratio of the VL [17]. These data suggest that decreased capillarity is not a major contributor to the deleterious changes observed in skeletal muscle with aging.

One advantage of animal models (e.g., laboratory rodents), is that whole muscles from healthy old animals can be obtained, weighed and fiber numbers and types determined. There exist several reports describing age-associated decreases in muscle weight in old rats, three of which are summarized in Table 1 and Fig. 3. These data show muscle-specific decreases in mass of 11—38% in rats at variable stages of senescence. Findings on the influence of age on muscle fiber num-

Table 1. Decreases in muscle weight in senescent rats.

Ages (months)	Muscle	% Decrease	Reference
10, 29	Gastrocnemius	27	[36]
	Plantaris	27	
	Quadriceps	27	
	Soleus	11	
6, 36	Gastrocnemius	38	[24]
	Plantaris	37	
	Soleus	18	
	EDL	16	
9, 31	Gastrocnemius	25	[232]
	Plantaris	22	
	EDL	15	
	Soleus	13	

ber in rats are somewhat contradictory. We observed a 26% drop in VL fiber number in 4- vs. 32-month-old male Wistar rats [22]. When studying rat soleus, Larsson and Edstrom [23] found a 13% decrease in fiber number in marginally old rats ($\sim$ 22 months), when compared to young (6 months). However, several other investigators have reported no age-related changes (Table 2). Thus, the effects of aging may be muscle-specific and depend on whether the muscle is weight-bearing. For example, soleus is a weight-bearing muscle while EDL is not.

Only limited attention has been given to studying sarcopenia in very old rats and mice (> 30 months old). Thus, laboratory rodents appear underutilized as models of sarcopenia in very old (> 80 years) people. Mice and rats from long-lived strains at 20 and 30 months of age are, respectively, 50% and 75% through the $\sim$ 40-month maximum life span typically attained. Thus, based on mortality characteristics, they would most closely resemble people less than 80 years of

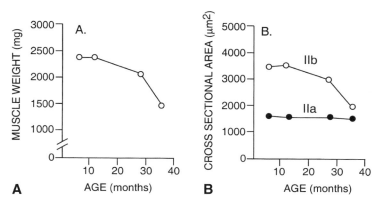

Fig. 3. Weight and fiber size of the gastrocnemius muscle in male FxBNF$_1$ rats at 6, 12, 28 and 36 months. (Drawn from data of Brown and Hasser [24].)

Table 2. Evidence for no age-dependent changes in fiber number in rat skeletal muscles.

Ages (months)	Muscle	Reference
3, 30	EDL	[34]
	Soleus	
6, 22	EDL	[23]
	Tibialis	
6, 24	EDL	[39]
	Soleus	
3, 22	EDL	[19]
	Soleus	
7, 27	FDL	[20]
5, 21	EDL	[37]

age. The study of muscle atrophy in very old FxBNF$_1$ rats, now limited to Brown and Hasser's data [24] deserves attention as the rate and consequences of muscle atrophy increase in the "oldest old". Indeed, these investigators conclude that the "marked reduction in peak tetanic tension, fiber area and muscle mass between 28 and 36 months indicates an accelerated age-related decline in this time period".

2.1.2 Muscle fiber type

Skeletal muscles are composed of different fiber types. Based on their actin-activated myosin ATPase activity, they can be classified into type I (slow) and type II (fast) fiber types [25]. Myosin ATPase activity is positively correlated with muscle contraction velocity. Thus, the measure of ATPase activity can be used as an indication of contraction speed. Type I fibers have lower ATPase levels and contract more slowly than do type II fibers. ATPase activity, together with acid or alkaline conditions, has been used to characterize fibers into subtypes [26–28]. Type II fibers have been subclassified based on the abundance of energy metabolism enzymes (glycolytic and oxidative pathways). When both contractile and metabolic characteristics are taken into account, muscle fibers can be classified as slow oxidative (SO or type I), fast oxidative glycolytic (FOG or type IIa) or fast glycolytic (FG or type IIb) [29,30]. In addition, each fiber type contains a specific isozyme for the contractile protein myosin (e.g., MHC I, IIa, IIb, IIx) [31].

　　Some investigators describe a change in muscle fiber type proportions with age in humans. There is a transition in fiber type from fast to slow in VL with an increase in the percentage of slower contracting fibers [18]. This situation could arise from either a conversion of type II to type I fibers and/or the preferential loss of type II fibers. However, no changes in fiber type ratio were observed in two other studies comparing the VL of 20- to 30-year-olds with 50- to 70-year-old people [17,32]. In addition, no changes in fiber type proportions were observed when comparing 4- to 31-year-old rhesus monkeys [33].

The influence of age on skeletal muscle fiber type in rats is well studied (Table 3). Several investigators describe increases in the percentages of type I fibers with age in soleus, diaphragm and plantaris muscles [34—37]. These same investigators have reported decreases in type IIa fibers in the same muscles. However, other investigators have not found any age-related changes in muscle fiber type composition in soleus, FDL, tibialis [19,20,23,38], EDL [19,21,23,34,39]. These discrepancies might be due to many factors including age, strain, diet, cage size and differences in the fiber type composition of the muscle types studied. For example, the EDL, gastrocnemius, VL and tibialis contain many fast-twitch fibers, whereas soleus is largely a slow-twitch muscle.

The reduction with age in fiber CSA in human VL appears to be greater for type II than for type I fibers [17,32]. Also, Proctor et al. [17] found type IIa fibers to be 31% smaller and type IIb fibers 40% smaller in the VL from 50- to 65-year-old individuals compared to those 20—30 years of age.

As shown in Table 4, decreases with age in fiber CSA in rat muscles are described by some (but not all) investigators and are related to fiber type. However, not all reports describe decreases in the CSA of muscle fibers from old rats. For example, the CSA of the EDL did not change in rats from 6 to 22 months of age [23]. Furthermore, Hegreberg and Hamilton [33] saw no changes in fiber diameter of the masseter, soleus, triceps and biceps femoris of rhesus monkeys 4 years of age when compared to 31 years of age.

Table 3. Influence of age on fiber type composition in rat skeletal muscles.

Ages (months)	Muscle	Fibre type	Change	Reference
3, 30	Soleus	Type I	85% → 94%	[34]
2, 24	Soleus	Type I	71% → 99%	[35]
5, 21	Soleus	Type I	80% → 96%	[37]
3, 30	Diaphragm	Type I	34% → 38%	[34]
9, 29	Plantaris	Type I	15% → 26%	[36]
3, 30	Soleus	Type IIa	9% → 3%	[34]
6, 22	Soleus	Type IIa	10% → 0%	[23]
2, 22	Soleus	Type IIa	14% → 0%	[35]
3, 30	Diaphragm	Type IIa	30% → 23%	[34]
9, 29	Plantaris	Type IIa	31% → 16%	[36]
3, 22	Soleus	Type IIa	No change	[19]
7, 27	FDL	Type IIa	No change	[20,38]
6, 22	Tibialis	Type IIa	No change	[23]
3, 30	EDL	Type IIb	No change	[34]
6, 22	EDL	Type IIb	No change	[23]
6, 24	EDL	Type IIb	No change	[39]
9, 27	EDL	Type IIb	No change	[21]
3, 22	EDL	Type IIb	No change	[19]

Table 4. Decreases in muscle fiber cross-sectional area in old rats are greater in type II fibers.

Ages (months)	Muscle	Change	Reference
18, 27	Lateral omohyoideus (type II)	↓ 30%	[233]
6, 22	Soleus (type II)	↓ 55%	[23]
10, 29	Plantaris (type IIb)	↓ 37%	[36]
6, 22	Soleus (type I)	↓ 23%	[37]
12, 36	Gastrocnemius (type IIb)	↓ 49%	[24]
6, 22	EDL Tibialis	↔	[23]
7, 27	FDL	↔	[20]
12, 36	Gastrocnemius (type IIa)	↔	[24]

2.1.3 Denervation

A denervated fiber can be reinnervated and thus, regenerate into a normal fiber. If the fiber remains denervated, it will undergo atrophy and/or disappear [7]. When a fiber is denervated, it loses cytoplasmic volume, as well as many of its nuclei. As skeletal muscle is a postmitotic tissue, satellite cell division has to contribute to the loss in nuclei in order to reverse the fiber atrophy. Satellite cells, which are localized within the basal lamina that surrounds the muscle fiber, display a decreased ability to proliferate with age such that the capacity of an atrophied fiber to regenerate may decrease with age [7].

The number of active motor units decreases with age (reviewed in Roos et al. [40]). Some muscle fibers from the lost motor unit become reinnervated by the other remaining motor units [8,40]. This motor unit reorganization by reinnervation increases the number of muscle fibers per motor unit. Edstrom and Larsson [41] reported a 34% increase in the innervation ratio of motor units (= number of muscle fibers/motor unit) in the soleus from 22- vs. 5-month-old motor units of rats. Kadhiresan et al. [42] reported age-related changes in the innervation ratio in rat medial gastrocnemius and these changes were fiber type-dependent. The innervation ratio in type I fibers of old rats was 86% of the value for adult rats, while for type II fibers it was 289% of the adult value.

As previously discussed, in many muscles there is an age-associated increase in the type I:type II ratio. This may occur due to type II fiber denervation which then become reinnervated by axonal ramification from slow fibers [8]. Therefore, these signs of motor unit fiber rearrangement (i.e., increased innervation ratio and motor unit size), indicate that the muscle fiber population undergoes a denervation and reinnervation process with aging. Muscle denervation is subsequently considered as a causative explanation for sarcopenia.

2.2 Changes in muscle function

2.2.1 Strength

Strength represents the maximal force or tension that can be developed by a muscle. Muscle strength is well known to decrease with age and appears due, in large part, to muscle atrophy (reviewed by Mazzeo et al. in [43]). Reduced muscle strength is defined as decreased force per unit of muscle fiber CSA. Strength is measured either by maximal voluntary contraction or the ability to lift free weights. A 25–35% decrease in muscle strength was observed in 80-year-old individuals compared to 70-year-old people [44]. Winegard et al. [45] conducted a longitudinal study in older individuals, (average 71 years), who were studied for 12 years. Losses of 7% in voluntary strength of the dorsiflexors ankle muscles and 28% for plantarflexors were observed. More recently, Hurley et al. [46] reported a 30% decrease in strength of quadriceps in old (average 72 years), when compared to young (average 23 years) men.

These declines in strength with age are associated with changes in muscle contractile properties. Longer contraction and half-relaxation times were reported to occur in the soleus [35] and tibialis [23] from old rats. However, no age-related changes were reported in contraction time in FDL of 7-month-old vs. 27-month-old rats [20] or in the half-relaxation time of tibialis of 6-month-old vs. 22- to 32-month-old rats [23,47]. Contraction time and half-relaxation time of the muscle twitch depend on the capacity of the sarcoplasmic reticulum for calcium release and recapture. Delbono et al. [48] have shown that calcium available for triggering mechanical responses decreases with age in human VL. Therefore, a slower return to resting contractile function may involve a slower rate at which Ca^{2+} ions are transported back into the sarcoplasmic reticulum lumen, as well as slower cross-bridge detachment.

Based on the known decrease in muscle mass and reduced size and number of fibers in some muscles, one would predict a decrease in peak tetanic tension in aged skeletal muscle. Larsson and Edstrom [23] observed age-related decreases in twitch force in soleus and tibialis when comparing 6-month-old vs. 22-month-old rats. A decrease in tetanus force was reported in soleus of old rats [23,35]. However, no changes with age were seen in rat tibialis [23] or FDL [20].

2.2.2 Endurance

Muscular endurance is a measure of its functional capacity. Endurance is measured by the work capacity of a muscle and is evaluated as work performed or VO_2max. Maximal aerobic capacity is usually measured with the subject on a treadmill, progressively increasing the velocity and grade until oxygen consumption per unit time reaches a plateau. Endurance refers to the length of time a subject can work at a given power output. VO_2max represents the cardiovascular system's capacity to deliver oxygen to working muscles and the muscle's capacity to use it.

Not surprisingly, an age-associated decrease in muscle endurance occurs in humans (reviewed in Bemben [49]) with the maximal aerobic capacity (VO_2max) decreasing at an average rate of 1% per year after the third decade [50]. Coggan et al. [15] reported a 45% lower VO_2max in older (58—68 years) when compared to younger (21—33 years) untrained men. A decrease in VO_2 max has been reported in VL of older (average 73 years) when compared to younger (average 24 years) people [51]. When older persons (average 63 years) were compared to young (average 25 years), endurance-trained subjects, VO_2max was 24% higher in the younger group [52]. Similarly, a 31% decrease in VO_2max has been found in old (70—83 years) vs. young (20—29 years) individuals [53].

2.3 Changes in metabolic capacity

2.3.1 Glycolytic

The two major fuels used by muscle are carbohydrates (glucose) and free fatty acids. While glycolysis can supply energy for short periods of time, oxidative metabolism is required to maintain the necessary ATP levels for endurance exercise. It has been proposed that age-associated decline in muscular endurance may be related to a preferential usage of glycolytic pathways [54]. Some age-related changes in glycolytic capacity have been observed and decreases in oxidative capacity do occur in humans.

There appears to be only limited information on the influence of age on glycolytic enzyme activities in human skeletal muscle. One report [44] described no changes in the levels of lactate dehydrogenase (LDH) (glycolytic enzyme) in VL of old humans when compared to young. Another study in the VL comparing men (average 25 vs. 71 years) did not find any age-related changes in the activity of phosphofructokinase or LDH [55]. The levels of key glycolytic enzymes (glycogen phosphorylase, phosphofructokinase and pyruvate kinase) were 2-fold lower in VL muscle of young persons (average 20 years) and older people (average 70 years) compared to individuals of middle age (30—60 years) [56]. LDH activity decreased about 20% in VL of old men (average 80 years) from previous measurements on these individuals four years earlier, while the activity of this enzyme did not change in the biceps brachii [57]. No changes in LDH or myokinase were detected in a follow-up study of men (ages 73—83 years) after 7 years in the VL [58].

Most of the gerontological data on activities of glycolytic enzymes derive from studies of rats and reveal no influences of age. Comparing 10-month-old to 24-month-old rats, Holloszy et al. [36] found no influence of age on hexokinase activity in soleus, VL or plantaris. Similarly, gastrocnemius of 24-month-old rats had the same hexokinase activity as that of 6-month-old animals [59]. Also, no age-associated change in phosphofructokinase activity (a key regulatory enzyme for glycolysis) was observed in soleus [36] or gastrocnemius [59] of old rats. The activity of glycogen phosphorylase, a rate-limiting enzyme for glycogenolysis, was stable with age in soleus, VL and quadriceps of rats [36,60].

However, the activities of some glycolytic enzymes do change with age. For example, LDH activity was 22—38% lower in the soleus, VL and plantaris of 29-month-old compared to 6- to 10-month-old rats [36,61]. Further, pyruvate kinase activity decreased in soleus (13%), VL (31%) and plantaris (42%) of rats from 10—29 months of age [36]. Thus, a selective age-associated decrease occurs in glycolytic enzyme activities which could ultimately affect muscle performance.

2.3.2 Oxidative

A cell's ability to produce ATP aerobically depends on its oxidative enzyme activity. Mitochondrial respiratory capacity, as judged by citrate synthase (CS) activity, may be impaired with age. Some investigators have found CS activity to decline with age in skeletal muscles in humans. For example, Coggan et al. [15] found CS activity in gastrocnemius to be 20% lower in older (58—68 years) than in younger (21—33 years) people. In addition, Rooyackers et al. [51] found decreased (18%) CS activity in VL of 73-year-old compared to 24-year-old subjects. These investigators also report a 31% decrease in Cytochrome c oxidase (COX) activity and a 40% decline in muscle mitochondrial protein synthesis. However, Proctor et al. [17] did not observe an influence of age on CS activity of VL when comparing young (20—30 years) to late middle age (50—65 years) individuals. In addition, no changes in oxidative enzyme activities, (for example CS, 3-hydroxy-CoA-dehydrogenase, an enzyme in the β oxidation pathway of fatty acid oxidation), were found in human VL when comparing 20-year-old with 76-year-old individuals [44].

In rats, Holloszy et al. [36] studied 10-month-old vs. 29-month-old animals and observed decreases in CS activity in the soleus (22%) and plantaris (24%). The latter finding was confirmed by Powers et al. [61]. Furthermore, CS activity decreased by $\sim 20\%$ in gastrocnemius from 10—25 months of age [59,62]. Activities of other oxidative enzymes have been studied in relation to age. Decreases of 15—23% in succinate dehydrogenase (SDH) and fumarase activities in plantaris and soleus occur with aging [36]. The activities of other ETS enzymes in skeletal muscle of rodents and humans also decline with age [63—66] and are discussed below (Section 4.4, Age-associated abnormalities of mtDNA and the electron transport system).

3   POSSIBLE CAUSES OF SARCOPENIA

Although the cause of sarcopenia remains unknown, several explanations have been proposed (e.g., [6—9,67,68]). As is the case for many pathophysiological changes which occur with aging, the true mechanism of sarcopenia may prove to be multifactorial, including contributions of some, or even all, of the proposed explanations discussed herein. Other factors that are not discussed here are probable contributors to sarcopenia, such as disuse atrophy, which is increasingly common in very old people. We hypothesize, however, that oxidative stress may be a primary underlying mechanism. Arguably, none of the explanations discussed in this section exclude the contributions of oxidative stress as the causal agent in senile muscle and nerve degeneration.

3.1 Denervation-reinnervation process

As discussed above, sarcopenia is characterized by the loss of muscle mass and muscle fiber number. Other changes that occur in skeletal muscle with age are altered proportions of type I and type II fibers, as well as the presence of whole groups of atrophied fibers [8,18,41]. These characteristics have led to the proposal that the denervation-reinnervation process plays an important role in sarcopenia [8,67]. It is hypothesized that muscle groups (i.e., fascicles and their associated nerves), become more susceptible to denervation and less able to reinnervate successfully. The predicted result is muscle fiber atrophy and loss.

The motor unit consists of the motor neuron and the skeletal muscle fibers it innervates. Each motor neuron is comprised of a cell body, located within the spinal cord and the axons which innervate the muscle fibers. A study examining the influences of age on numbers of lumbosacral motor neurons (limb motor neurons) found that, while no loss was observed in people before 60 years of age, a decline occurred thereafter [69]. Similarly, Galea [70] observed a progressive loss of motor units in the distal muscles of the arm (thenar group and extensor digitorum brevis) in subjects older than 60 years of age. However, no influence of age was found in the biceps brachii (proximal muscle of the arm). In old rats (31 months), Hashizume et al. [71] observed a 19% decrease in medial gastrocnemius motor axon number compared with 12-month-old animals. This decrease was accompanied by a 22% decrease in the total number of motor neurons (especially α-neurons). These data accord with the observations of Kadhiresan et al. [42] who observed a 16% decrease in the number of motor units of the medial gastrocnemius in old (~ 25 months) when compared to young (~ 11 months) rats. Interestingly, this decrease occurred in type II fibers which is consistent with the selective loss of fast motor neurons. Consistent with the denervation-reinnervation hypothesis, these data suggest fewer motor units innervate the skeletal muscle fibers of old rats and people.

The influence of age on the neuromuscular junction has also been investigated. Oda [72] found a positive correlation between length of endplate and age in individuals 32—76 years of age. Increased branching of preterminal axons and a greater number of small conglomerates of acetylcholine receptors in the endplate were also observed in the older subjects. In rats, Rosenheimer and Smith [73] described a decreased number of nerve terminal branches per endplate in diaphragm, EDL and soleus muscles in 31-month-old vs. 25-month-old animals. They also reported an age-associated increase in end-plate area. Taken together, these data suggest a focal destabilization of neuromuscular junctions with age which may contribute to the denervation process.

3.2 Contraction-induced injury

Faulkner et al. [6] suggest that contraction-induced injury may explain both age-associated muscle atrophy and decreased strength. They propose that skeletal muscles are continually assaulted with minute injuries resulting from normal contractions. Further, with aging, the number of susceptible fibers increases whilst repair capacity decreases. This contraction-induced damage appears to be confined to single fibers [74].

Contraction-induced injuries have been described after exercise protocols which lengthen the muscles during contractions (eccentric contractions), as opposed to those which shorten the muscles (concentric contractions) [75]. When studying 25-year-old people subjected to an exercise protocol of eccentric contractions, Friden et al. [76] reported a disorganization of myofilaments in sarcomeres originating from the myofibrillar Z-bands. These changes were focal (localized to individual sarcomeres) and occurred in 32% of the fibers examined 1 h after exercise, 52% after 3 days of exercise and 12% after 6 days of exercise. Newham et al. [75] also studied young volunteers and observed that 40% of the fibers were damaged immediately after exercise and that the damage became more pronounced (57% of the fibers affected) 1—2 days after exercise.

The cause of the injury is unknown. Morgan [77] hypothesized that during contractions, "weak" sarcomeres (the longest) undergo a loss of thick and thin filament overlap that results in a rapid uncontrolled elongation. In contrast, "strong" sarcomeres (the shortest), maintain filament overlap. Macpherson et al. [78] reported that the sarcomeres with the longest length before a stretch contain the majority of damage after a stretch. Talbot and Morgan [79] found that after eccentric contractions, 8% of sarcomeres examined were overextended to beyond filament overlap and that these were distributed randomly throughout the muscle. Upon relaxation, nearly all sarcomeres returned to their original filament overlap pattern ($<1\%$ failed to reinterdigitate properly). These changes did not occur in muscles after isometric (no change in length) contraction.

Faulkner's group [80] has defined two distinct injuries (as measured by force deficit) which occur in muscles from mice following contraction. The primary injury (measured at 10 min and 3 h post contraction), is initiated by the mechanical disruption of the ultrastructure of specific sarcomeres. This damage can give rise to a delayed secondary injury (studied at 3 days) characterized by an inflammatory response and degeneration of severely damaged fibers. The damage caused by the secondary injury was somewhat more severe than that caused by the primary injury (e.g., 53% force deficit after 3 days vs. 38% force deficit after 3 h), in young mice (3—4 months). Also, the number of missing and damaged fibers peaked at 3 days.

Other observations from these investigators suggest that free radical damage may be involved in the secondary injury [81]. Young and old mice treated with 1,000 units/kg superoxide dismutase (SOD) coupled to polyethylene glycol (PEG) for 3 days prior to and after contraction protocols, displayed less severe secondary injuries than did nontreated controls. Free radical damage, however, could not account for the entire force deficit created by the secondary injury. The authors speculated that the remaining force deficit may be due to incomplete free radical protection, other unknown factors or incomplete recovery.

An age-associated increase in damage after contraction-induced injury has been reported. McCully and Faulkner [82] developed a method to examine muscle contractions and their subsequent repair in situ. By stimulating the peroneal nerve to contract the EDL muscles of anesthetized mice, the duration, force and number of contractions could be controlled. Compared to young mice, old animals were more susceptible to damage and recovered less successfully. Using a similar protocol, Zerba et al. [81] used force deficit as an indicator of the extent of damage and found that old mice (~ 26 months) had somewhat greater damage than 2-month-old mice. Also, Brooks and Faulkner [83] measured the force deficit in EDL from mice of different ages 1 min after single stretches of the contracting muscle. Greater force deficits were observed in older (~ 26 months) compared with younger (5–12 months) animals.

Incomplete recovery is the other component of the contraction-induced injury theory. Brooks and Faulkner [84] have shown that, 28 days after the contraction protocol, the EDL from young mice is completely recovered. In contrast, old mice displayed a 16% force deficit. The inability of the EDL muscle in old animals to completely recover after 28 days is thought to result from less successful fiber regeneration because of a decrease with age in the rate of reinnervation (rather than the ability of the muscle itself to regenerate) [85,86]. Two experimental approaches were taken to study age-related changes in muscle regeneration capacity. In the first one (absence of innervation), muscle grafts were used to study fibers regenerating in the absence of nerves. In the second approach (presence of innervation), the muscle was treated with Marcaine which causes severe muscle fiber damage without interrupting the motor nerve fibers. In the presence of innervation (Marcaine injection), there were no differences between animals of different ages. However, when regenerating muscles were dependent on innervation by regenerating nerves, muscle mass and tetanic force were lower in regenerating old (24 months) when compared to young (4 months) muscle.

3.3 Satellite cell changes

Satellite cells are mononucleated cells which are closely associated with the surface of skeletal muscle fibers. These cells are essential for both normal muscle growth and regeneration following injury. When fibers increase in size (i.e., increase cytoplasmic mass), the associated satellite cells divide and fuse with the fiber. The nuclei of satellite cells are the only sources available for the DNA required for fiber growth. In the event of injury, the surviving (and possibly damaged) fibers activate the satellite cells and begin the regeneration process.

At birth, 32% of the total nuclei in rat subclavius muscle are from satellite cells and this percentage plummets to 4% at 6 months of age [87]. Satellite cell percentages also decrease from 10 to 5% and from 7 to 2% in rat soleus and EDL muscles, respectively, between 1 and 24 months of age [88]. Rodrigues and Schmalbruch [89] also observed that the percentage of satellite cells decline in soleus and EDL muscles from 3 to 10 months of age. Since satellite cells provide the primary means of increasing fiber size, this decline may be a significant factor in the reduced regenerative capacity of injured muscle fibers from older organisms (as reviewed by Carlson [7]).

Little appears to be known about the regenerative capacity of satellite cells in vivo, however, some in vitro data exist. Satellite cells from old rats (> 30 months) can proliferate in vitro [90], albeit at a lower proliferative potential [91]. The decline in proliferative potential was most pronounced during the first weeks of life and continued at a lower rate thereafter.

The reduced number and proliferative potential of satellite cells are hypothesized to explain the low regenerative potential of muscle with age. Several studies have examined muscle recovery after denervation (e.g., [92, 93]). In the muscles which are reinnervated, the degree of recovery depends on the ability of the nerve to support the fibers, as well as the ability of the fibers to respond to the nerve. Muscle mass has been shown to decrease more than 50% within one month of denervation [92], such that the time to reinnervation also affects the degree of recovery. Immediately after denervation, there is an increase in the number of satellite cells, presumably in response to the muscle injury; however, after about 2 months, the number of satellite cells decreases [89,93]. A significant question raised by Carlson [7], is whether satellite cells from aged muscles are in sufficient numbers and have the regenerative capacity to restore the cytoplasmic volume of the muscle fibers. If not, satellite cell changes with age may play an important role in the fiber loss and atrophy.

4 OXIDATIVE STRESS AND SARCOPENIA

Although the above hypotheses provide compelling evidence for important roles of neurons, satellite cells and injury in sarcopenia, they do not exclude a causal role of oxidative stress in muscle loss. For example, what molecular events lead to age-associated motor neuron loss and sarcomere weakening? What causes satellite cell number decline and reduced in vitro proliferative capacities with age? Could these age-associated changes result from oxidative damage over time? Consistent with this scenario is the observation by Zerba et al. [81] that the secondary injury after repeated muscle contractions was diminished by SOD treatment, implicating oxidative damage as mediating the injury. The possible contributions of oxidative stress/damage to the three hypotheses of sarcopenia just considered have not been closely evaluated. There exists, however, evidence which argues for independent contributions of oxidative stress/damage in sarcopenia.

4.1 Hypothesis

We are investigating the contributions of oxidative stress of mitochondrial origin to sarcopenia (Fig. 4). Our hypothesis is that oxidative stress, originating principally from normal cellular respiration, damages mitochondria, the sites of the electron transport system (ETS). The ROS and ROM, which are generated as abnormal byproducts of the ETS, damage diverse macromolecules (lipids, proteins and nucleic acids). This damage results in a less efficient, "leaky" ETS which produces less ATP and more ROS, further damaging mitochondria. With age, cells would have an accumulation of oxidatively damaged mitochondria which cannot generate sufficient ATP. The ultimate consequence may be cellular death. Since skeletal muscle and nervous tissues are mostly postmitotic and therefore, have limited regenerative capacities, they would appear to be quite vulnerable to such damage. Accordingly, we hypothesize that the loss of skeletal muscle fibers and perhaps motor neurons may result, in part, from mitochondrial ROS and ROM generation.

There are reasons to believe that this scenario may contribute to the development of sarcopenia. Free radicals have been proposed as contributing to other situations of muscle damage, such as that occurring after exercise or in muscular dystrophy, malignant hyperthermia, ischemia/reperfusion damage and alcoholic and inflammatory myopathies [94]. Skeletal muscle accounts for a large share of the body's total oxygen consumption at rest, due to its large mass, and most of the oxygen consumption during vigorous physical activity. Also, as noted, skeletal muscle, as a postmitotic tissue, has low repair capacities that occur in more mitotically active tissues. Here we consider the contributions of mitochondria and oxidative stress/damage to the development of sarcopenia.

4.2 Mitochondria, oxygen radicals and aging

The mitochondrion is unique to mammalian cellular organelles in that it contains its own ∼16.5 kb double-stranded circular DNA genome. It encodes 22 tRNAs, 2 rRNAs and 13 polypeptides of the ETS (Fig. 5). The genome is abundant in every nucleated cell with two to 10 copies per mitochondrion [95] and 10s to 100s of mitochondria per cell, depending on the cells energy requirements [96]. The enzyme complexes of the ETS are encoded by both nuclear and mitochondrial genes (Fig. 6). Complex I (NADH dehydrogenase) and complex IV (COX) contain the largest number of mitochondrial subunits, with mtDNA encoding seven of approximately 40 subunits of complex I and three of the 13

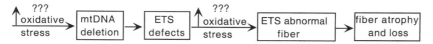

Fig. 4. Hypothesized mechanism for the involvement of oxidative stress in skeletal muscle fiber atrophy and loss during aging. Whether or not oxidative damage causes mtDNA deletions is uncertain.

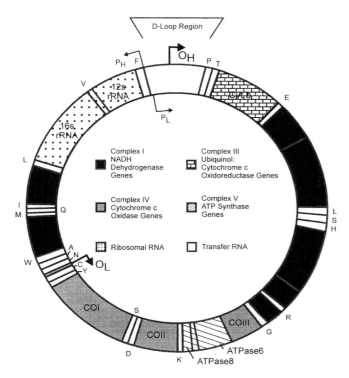

Fig. 5. Organization of mammalian mitochondrial genome. Letters indicate tRNA genes. O_H and O_L are heavy and light strand origins of replication, respectively.

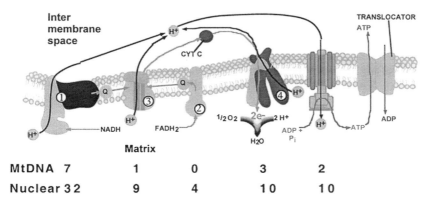

MtDNA	7	1	0	3	2
Nuclear	32	9	4	10	10

Fig. 6. Complexes of the ETS and oxidative phosphorylation in the mitochondrial inner membrane. Complex numbers are circled. The number of subunits contributed by either the mitochondrial or nuclear genome is indicated below each complex. (Adapted from Wallace [235].)

subunits of complex IV. Complex II (SDH) is entirely nuclear encoded while complex III (ubiquinol cytochrome c reductase) has one of its 10 peptide subunits encoded by mtDNA. Age-associated damage to the mtDNA encoding these subunits, therefore, may reduce the enzymatic activities of the complexes [97].

The mitochondrion, as the site of cellular oxidative respiration, has an interior rich in oxygen. It has been estimated that $\sim 90\%$ of cellular oxygen is consumed in mitochondria and $\sim 2\%$ of that oxygen is converted to superoxide free radicals by complexes of the ETS in the mitochondrial inner membrane [98]. High levels of ROM may damage mitochondrial (and nonmitochondrial) macromolecules such as lipids, proteins and DNA. Accordingly, mitochondria represent potential hotspots for damage and, therefore, several investigators have postulated a mitochondrial role in aging. Harman [99] originally proposed the free radical theory of aging which focused on cellular damage via lipid peroxidation. Soon thereafter, Szilard [100] hypothesized a somatic mutational theory of aging, arguing that the aging process is the result of an accumulation of mutational hits in the nuclear DNA over time. The theory has subsequently been extended to include the idea that, compared to nuclear genome, mtDNA is more susceptible to oxidative damage due to the presence of higher levels of ROS, a lack of protective histones and less efficient DNA repair [11,101,102].

4.3 Mitochondrial myopathies and encephalomyopathies

Support for the mitochondrial/oxidative stress hypothesis of sarcopenia derives from the occurrence of mtDNA abnormalities in human neuromuscular diseases. Histological evaluation of mitochondrial enzymatic activities has revealed abnormalities in a broad class of neuromuscular disorders known as mitochondrial myopathies and encephalomyopathies (reviewed in [97,103,104]. The disorders include myoclonic epilepsy and ragged red fiber (RRF) disease, mitochondrial encephalopathy with lactic acidosis and stroke-like episodes (MELAS), Kearns-Sayre syndrome and Leber's hereditary optic neuropathy (LHON). These diseases are, clinically and biochemically, a diverse group of disorders, affecting primarily those tissues having the highest energy demands: brain, skeletal muscle and heart. The mitochondrial abnormalities associated with these diseases range from point mutations in the case of LHON [105] and MELAS [106] to large mtDNA deletions in the mitochondrial encephalomyopathies (reviewed in [103,104]).

RRFs, so named because of their appearance when stained with Gomori trichrome [107], occur at high levels in skeletal muscle from mitochondrial myopathy patients. RRFs result from an abnormal accumulation of mitochondria causing hyperreactive staining for the ETS's entirely nuclear-encoded complex II (designated SDH^{++} fibers). Fibers negative for COX activity (designated COX$^-$ fibers) also occur in myopathy patients.

These two enzymatic defects can co-localize within the same fiber [104, 108–110]. Mitochondrial DNA abnormalities have been linked to these oxidative defects in skeletal muscle from myopathy patients [109,111,112]. For these studies, in situ hybridization, using probes to normal and mutant mtDNA, was combined with histochemical techniques for the localization of COX and SDH activities. These studies have shown that most of the affected fibers contain increased levels of mutant mtDNA, with a corresponding decrease in levels of wild type mtDNA. These results indicate that mtDNA abnormalities can localize in diseased muscle fibers where they may cause oxidative defects.

4.4 Age-associated abnormalities of mtDNA and ETS

Mitochondria may be causally involved in the aging process [10,113,114]. The number of mitochondrial genomes containing large deletions increases with age in several tissues [115—118]. These age-associated mtDNA deletions assume multiple forms in humans [115,116,119—121]. Studies of age-associated mtDNA deletions have also been performed in animal models, with multiple deletions detected in skeletal muscles of rhesus monkeys [122,123], as well as in several tissues of mice [124—127] and rats [22,128,129]. Most of these studies detected the highest deletion levels in nervous tissue, heart and skeletal muscle.

The physiological importance of the age-associated occurrence of mtDNA deletions remains unclear. Analysis of skeletal muscle homogenates has detected very low levels of these age-associated mtDNA deletions (typically $< 0.1\%$ of total mitochondrial genomes) [64,130,131] compared to the levels observed in the mitochondrial myopathy diseases (20—80% of mitochondrial genomes) [132,133]. However, by analyzing defined numbers of muscle fibers from rhesus monkeys, we discovered that the calculated abundance of specific mtDNA deletions was dependent upon the number of fibers analyzed. In samples containing thousands of fibers (such as in tissue homogenates), many deletion products were detected but the abundance of these individual products was always low ($< 0.1\%$). In contrast, samples containing 10 muscle fibers displayed few deletion products, however, the abundance of the few individual products was much higher ($4—13\%$) [134]. Thus, as the number of fibers assayed decreased, the calculated deletion abundance increased which led to two main conclusions:
1. Deleted mitochondrial genomes may accumulate to high levels within individual fibers.
2. Deleted mitochondrial genomes are not distributed equally among all fibers. These data, in addition to in situ hybridization studies of human muscle [108,110] and rhesus monkeys [135], show the focal nature of age-associated mtDNA deletions in skeletal muscle.

Just as mtDNA deletions increase with age, so do ETS enzyme defects as measured biochemically and histologically. Biochemical measures of ETS complex activities in homogenates of several tissue types derived from humans, rhesus monkeys, rats and mice have been performed. In general, age-associated decreases have occurred in the activities of complex I and IV. Those tissues in which robust biochemical declines have been most consistently detected are, again, the highly oxidative, nonreplicating tissues such as skeletal muscle, heart and brain (reviewed in [66,136]). Enzymatic declines of complex I or IV are usually not seen in tissues with replicative capacities such as liver [137—141] or kidney [140,141].

Abnormalities of ETS enzymatic activities, such as COX$^-$ fibers and RRFs, have been identified histologically in aged human muscle [142—144]. As noted, RRFs occur at high levels (up to 32% of fibers) in skeletal muscle from mitochondrial myopathy patients [104], but also occur at lower levels in normal aged muscle (e.g., 0.7% of human quadriceps muscle fibers) [144]. Subsequent histochemical studies on muscle tissue from nonhuman primates [135,145] and rats [22] also described increases with age in these ETS abnormalities.

Our group recently described an age-related increase in the relative abundance of COX$^-$/SDH^{++} fibers in quadriceps from rhesus monkeys (n = 14, 2—39 years) [135]. A single section (8 µm) was analyzed from each animal, with each section containing thousands of fibers. Muscle from the older monkeys (> 20 years) contained individual fibers which were COX$^-$, SDH^{++} or both COX$^-$ and SDH^{++}. No such abnormal fibers were seen in 2- to 16-year-old animals. COX$^-$ fibers that were not SDH^{++} appeared first in 20- and 22-year-old animals, while fibers which were both COX$^-$ and SDH^{++} were detected more frequently in animals over 25 years of age. The relative abundance of fibers (i.e., those within a single section of a muscle biopsy) which displayed abnormal enzyme activities increased with age, ranging from 0.04% COX$^-$ fibers in a 20-year-old to 0.47% COX$^-$/SDH^{++} fibers in the 39-year-old.

The cause(s) of the loss of COX activity or the proliferation of mitochondria in these fibers is unknown, but has been correlated histologically with mtDNA deletions by in situ hybridizations in many of the affected fibers in aged humans [108,110] and rhesus monkeys [135]. Brierley et al. [146] screened muscle samples from aged humans for the so-called "common deletion" (mtDNA^{4977}) and found that about 6% of the COX$^-$ fibers had high levels of the deletion.

In our study of rhesus monkeys [135], we sought to determine whether mitochondrial genomes containing large deletions occur in fibers with ETS abnormalities and performed in situ hybridizations on sections containing these fibers. The expression of five different mitochondrially encoded genes (12s rRNA, ND2, COX I, ND4 and Cyt b) was analyzed to determine if deleted mitochondrial genomes were present in the COX$^-$/SDH^{++} fibers. A strong association between the occurrence of deleted mitochondrial genomes and enzymatic abnormalities was detected. Of the 26 COX$^-$/SDH^{++} fibers that were examined by in situ hybridization, 23 fibers (89%) contained deleted mitochondrial genomes (Fig. 7). It is possible that the remaining 11% of the COX$^-$/SDH^{++} fibers which were not associated with deleted mitochondrial genomes may result from smaller mtDNA deletions, point mutations, as well as defects in nuclear-encoded factors. The majority of these 23 fibers had regions deleted from the major arc of the mitochondrial genome (nts 5,742 to 16,569 in human mtDNA) [147]. However, four of the 23 fibers (17%) displayed evidence of deletions involving

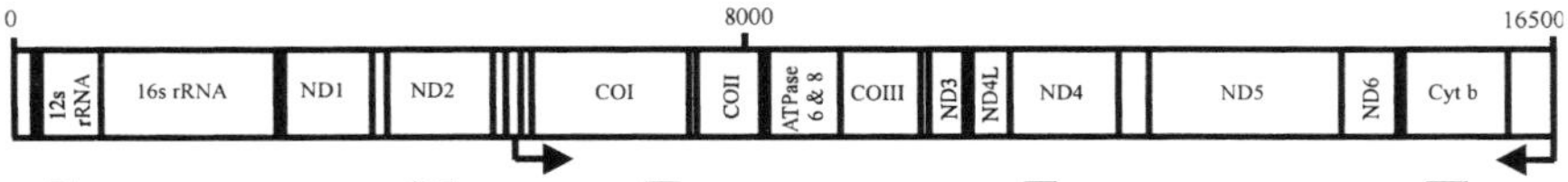

	1	2	3	4	5
8 of 26	+	+	+	−	−
11 of 26	+	+	+	−	+
4 of 26	−	−	−	+	+
3 of 26	+	+	+	+	+

Fig. 7. Summary of in situ hybridization experiments utilizing five mitochondrial RNA antisense probes as performed on 26 COX$^-$/SDH^{++} fibers from seven different rhesus monkeys (22–32 years of age). A '+' indicates reactivity while a '−' indicates very little or no reactivity. Controls using sense strand probes indicated very little nonspecific hybridization and that the probes were specific for mitochondrial RNA (data not shown). (From Lee et al. [135].)

genes located in the minor arc of the mitochondrial genome and the light strand origin of replication (nts 1 to 5752 in human mtDNA) [147]. Taken together, the in situ hybridization experiments suggest a strong association between the presence of mtDNA-deleted molecules and histological abnormalities of complexes II and IV.

Histological analysis of single cross-sections provides an estimate of enzymatic abnormalities through only one plane of the muscle. Several investigations of ETS enzymatic activities in myopathy patients [148,149] and aging individuals [146] have shown that the ETS abnormalities occur in small regions along the length of the fiber (i.e., they are segmental). Therefore, this "single cross section approach" provides little information on the total number of enzymatic abnormalities in the entire muscle fiber.

Accordingly, we took a "longitudinal approach" for the detection of fibers with ETS abnormal regions [135]. Ninety fibers bearing ETS abnormalities were identified in quadriceps samples from 20-, 25-, 26- and 32-year-old monkeys when followed longitudinally for distances of 350–1,600 μm. As might be expected, data from the cross-sectional analysis markedly underestimated the number of abnormal fibers. For example, in examining single cross-sections of fibers from 25-year-old quadriceps, only 0.05% of the fibers in a single section were determined to be COX$^-$/SDH^{++}; however, 6-fold more fibers (0.31%) contained COX$^-$/SDH^{++} regions when these same fibers were examined over a distance of 350 μm. Similarly, the percentage of fibers exhibiting the COX$^-$/SDH^{++} phenotype in the sample from the 32-year-old monkey more than doubled from 0.27% (cross-sectional) to 0.60% when examined over a 580-μm region.

Quadriceps samples from a 25-year-old monkey were more thoroughly studied longitudinally so as to more accurately assess the occurrence of ETS abnormal fiber regions [135]. Serial sections containing 4,177 fibers were followed for a total length of 1.6 mm leading to the identification of 46 fibers with ETS abnormal regions. The abnormal regions averaged ∼285 μm and were segmental, with most of the abnormalities beginning and ending within the 1.6-mm region examined. Extrapolation to the average length of a rhesus monkey quadriceps (100—200 mm) would predict a total of 2,875—5,750 fibers with ETS-abnormal regions. This would suggest that, at some point in the length of the quadriceps, each fiber would have at least one ETS abnormal region. An accurate assessment of the abundance of these ETS abnormal regions, therefore, requires a systematic characterization of muscle fibers along their length.

A significant finding from the longitudinal analysis was that many of the COX$^-$/SDH^{++} fibers displayed considerable atrophy. Thirteen of the 90 fibers (14%) with ETS abnormalities exhibited progressive decreases in fiber size over the 350- to 1,600-μm distances examined (Fig. 8). The CSA of the 13 atrophying COX$^-$/SDH^{++} fibers decreased by 50—83%, while measurements of the 27 randomly selected, ETS-normal fibers (from the same sections) indicated their areas changed an average of $8.5 \pm 0.3\%$ over the same distances, demonstrating that the atrophy was specific for the COX$^-$/SDH^{++} fibers. The difference in cross-sectional area of the ETS abnormal and normal fibers was statistically significant ($p < 0.001$).

Our recent data further define the role of dysfunctional mitochondria in senescent muscle atrophy. Since mtDNA deletions were associated with the large majority of COX$^-$/SDH^{++} fibers and were not detected in fibers with normal COX and SDH activities, strong support exists for a causal relationship between mtDNA deletions and the subsequent appearance of ETS enzymatic abnormalities. Furthermore, because 14% of the ETS abnormal fibers followed for distances up to 1,600 μm showed atrophic changes, support is provided for an etiologic role of mtDNA deletions and ETS dysfunctions in sarcopenia.

4.5 Oxidative damage

Applied to sarcopenia, the oxidative stress hypothesis of aging would predict that loss of mass and functional performance of skeletal muscle with age is correlated with increased levels of oxidative damage to biomolecules such as lipid, DNA and protein with aging. As shown in Table 5, there is substantial evidence to support the notion of increased oxidative damage in aged skeletal muscle.

ROS are molecules that contain oxygen and have higher reactivity than ground state molecular oxygen. Superoxide radical, the first reactive metabolite generated in the reduction of molecular oxygen to water, leads to the formation of ROM, including hydrogen peroxide and hydroxyl radical. Intracellular ROS are generated from the auto-oxidation of small molecules such as reduced flavins and thiols, and from the activity of certain oxidases, cyclo-oxygenases, lipoxygenases, dehydrogenases and peroxidases. For example, plasma membrane NADPH oxidase-mediated production of ROS occurs in phagocytic cells [150] and ischemia promotes conversion of xanthine dehydrogenase to ROS-generating xanthine oxidase in the cytosol [151]. In addition, oxidative phosphorylation in mitochondria [152], fatty acid oxidation in peroxisomes [153] and cytochrome

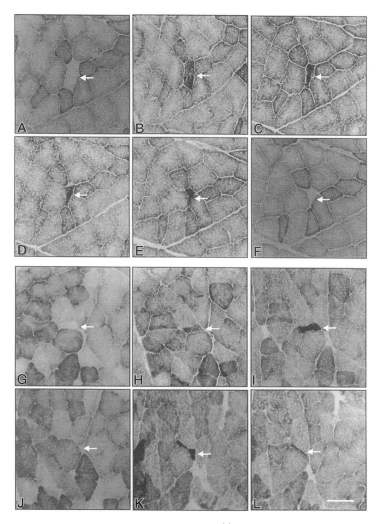

Fig. 8. Fiber atrophy occurs in COX$^-$/SDH^{++} fibers. COX (A,F,G,J) and SDH (B-E,H,I,K,L) stains from a 25-year-old (A-F) and 32-year-old (G-L) rhesus monkey. Arrows indicate a representative atrophic fiber in pictures A-F and another in pictures G-L. Total fiber length examined from A to F is 624 μm and from G to L is 448 μm. (From Lee et al. [135].)

P450 electron transport in the endoplasmic reticulum [154] are all fundamental and continuous sources of ROS. As we discuss elsewhere, mitochondria are presumed to be the primary cellular sites of ROS production and oxidative damage incurred during aging. We now review evidence supporting the accumulation of oxidative damage in mammalian skeletal muscle lipid, DNA and protein during aging.

Table 5. Oxidative damage increases with age in skeletal muscle.

Observation	Species	Muscle	Ages	Reference
Lipofuscin	Rat	Soleus	29 months	[162]
	Human	VL	17–76 years	[55]
	Rat	Tibialis	2, 11, 30 months	[163]
TBARS	Rat	Gastrocnemius	12, 24 months	[156]
	Rat	VL	4,26, 31 months	[157]
	Rat	Soleus	4, 24 months	[158]
	Rat	Soleus VL	5, 15, 27 months	[159]
	Mouse	Hindlimb	3, 31 months	[160]
	Human	VL	25–93 years	[161]
MtDNA deletions	Monkey	VL	6–27 years	[122]
	Mouse	Hindlimb	5, 16, 25 months	[124]
8-OHdG	Mouse	Hindlimb	8, 27 months	[169]
	Human	VL	25–93 years	[161]
Carbonyls	Rat	Hindlimb	5, 28 months	[177]
	Mouse	Hindlimb	3–31 months	[160]
	Human	VL	25–93 years	[161]
Sulfhydryls	Rat	Hindlimb	5, 28 months	[177]
	Mouse	Hindlimb	3–31 months	[160]
Dityrosine	Mouse	Hindlimb	4, 14, 30 months	[179]
3NT	Rat	Hindlimb	5, 28 months	[189]

4.5.1 Lipid peroxidation

Many studies have examined the effect of aging on various measures of lipid per-oxidation in mammalian tissues. Most of these studies have measured the tissue content of thiobarbituric acid reactive substances (TBARS) as a marker of endogenous lipid peroxidation, and the results have been contradictory [155]. Unlike other tissues, ample evidence shows that TBARS content increases with age in skeletal muscle [156–161]. Comparing gastrocnemius muscle from 24- vs. 12-month-old male Fischer 344 rats, Starnes et al. [156] reported that TBARS content increased with aging. Formation of TBARS, measured as malondialdehyde (MDA), was found to be elevated in both skeletal muscle crude homogenate and mitochondrial fractions from rats aged 26 and 31 months vs. 4-month-old animals [157] and in soleus muscle, but not in gastrocnemius muscle, when comparing 24- with 4-month-old rats [158]. Furthermore, MDA concentrations increased in rat soleus and VL muscles at 15 and 27 months vs. 5 months of age [159]. Recently, studying mitochondria isolated from upper hindlimb skeletal muscle, Lass et al. [160] demonstrated that TBARS content increases markedly with age in male C57BL/6Nia mice between 3 and 31 rather than 30 months of age. Comparing vastus medialis or lateralis muscle from 66 people aged 25–93 years, there was a significant age-dependent increase in levels of MDA [161].

In addition to TBARS content, several investigators [55,162–165] have examined age-related alterations in skeletal muscle levels of lipofuscin, a byproduct of the oxidative polymerization of lipids. Following a report by Gutmann et al. [162] describing accumulation of lipofuscin with aging in rat skeletal muscle, Orlander et al. [55] measured lipofuscin in skeletal muscle from 16- to 76-year-old men. Lipofuscin was found more frequently in biopsies from older men. However, comparative fine-structural analysis of lipofuscin in skeletal muscle of rats of different ages (2, 11 and 30 months of age) revealed no significant age-associated changes in the presence of lipofuscin [163]. More recently, Beregi et al. [164] utilized electron microscopy to examine skeletal muscle cells isolated from humans and CBA mice and reported that the presence of lipofuscin in mitochondria was greater in older people and mice. Lastly, no age-related increase in lipofuscin was observed in skeletal muscle from male NMRI mice at 20 months vs. 1 month of age [165].

4.5.2 DNA oxidation

Although numerous oxidative lesions occur in DNA, 8-hydroxylation of the guanine base is the most abundant [102]. A major mutagenic lesion, 8-hydroxydeoxyguanosine (8-OHdG) produces predominantly G $\rightarrow$ T transversion mutations [166]. This type of alteration has previously been shown to generate point mutations in mitochondrial DNA (mtDNA) due to mispairing [103]. Additionally, 8-OHdG accumulates in DNA exposed to ROS [167]. Taken together, these studies support the notion of 8-OHdG as a useful marker for estimating age-induced DNA damage. For example, Fraga et al. [168] reported an age-related increase in the 8-OHdG concentration in the intestine, kidney and liver of Fischer rats between 1 and 24 months of age. However, the role of DNA oxidation in aging skeletal muscle is less well established. Also using 8-OHdG as an indicator of DNA oxidative damage, Sohal et al. [169] demonstrated that the concentration of 8-OHdG in skeletal muscle was greater in 27-month-old rather than 8-month-old C57BL/6 male mice, suggesting an age-related increase. Comparing vastus medialis or lateralis skeletal muscle from 66 subjects aged 25–93 years, there was a significant age-dependent increase in levels of 8-OHdG [161]. Lastly, as discussed elsewhere in this review, multiple mtDNA deletions have been reported to increase with aging in skeletal muscle [122,124]; however, the etiology of these deletions is unclear but could involve DNA oxidative damage [125].

4.5.3 Protein oxidation

Typically, protein oxidation results in the generation of various amino acid residue modifications. For example, site-specific, metal-catalyzed oxidation of arginine, lysine, proline and threonine amino acid residues results in the production of carbonyl derivatives [170,171]. In addition, carbonyl groups may be introduced into proteins by reactions with aldehydes, such as MDA and 4-hydroxy-2-nonenal (HNE), produced during lipid peroxidation [172,173]. Therefore, carbonyl derivatives provide a reliable marker of oxidative damage. Cysteine and methionine residues are particularly sensitive to oxidation by almost all forms of ROS. Cysteine residues are converted to disulfides while methionine residues are oxidized to methionine sulfoxide; however, repair systems can convert the oxidized forms of cysteine and methionine residues back to their normal state. Accordingly, a decrease in the amount of protein sulfhydryl group provides a useful marker of cysteine oxidation. Another protein oxidative modification that may be used as an indicator of oxidative damage involves formation of dityrosine from tyrosine [174,175]. Since dityrosine is not typically found in proteins, it provides an excellent marker for measuring protein oxidative damage in skeletal muscle with aging.

Protein oxidative damage is particularly detrimental with aging because of the vital role of proteins in biology. Protein carbonyl content has been shown to increase with age in mouse heart, liver and kidney [176]. However, investigations of age-related changes in protein carbonyl content in mammalian skeletal muscle is sparse. Using mitochondria isolated from upper hindlimb skeletal muscle, Lass et al. [160] demonstrated that protein carbonyl content increases 2-fold with age when comparing male C57BL/6 mice between 3 and 31 rather than 30 months of age, suggesting that mitochondria in skeletal muscles accumulate significant oxidative damage with aging. In addition, it should be noted that caloric restriction (CR) prevented the age-related increase in carbonyl content [160]. Comparing vastus medialis or lateralis skeletal muscle from 66 subjects aged 25—93 years, there was a significant age-dependent increase in protein carbonyl levels [161]. Viner et al. [177] reported that levels of carbonyl groups per mole of Ca-ATPase in sarcoplasmic reticulum vesicles isolated from hindlimb muscles of male Fischer 344 rats aged 5 or 28 months slightly increased with aging.

Investigations into age-related changes in skeletal muscle protein sulfhydryl content is lacking. A comparison of total sulfhydryl content in sarcoplasmic reticulum vesicles isolated from hindlimb muscles of male Fischer 344 rats aged 5 or 28 months, revealed an age-related decrease [177]. In addition, Viner et al. [177] reported that sarcoplasmic reticulum Ca-ATPase from old as compared to young rats demonstrated a lower content of sulfhydryl groups. Specifically, based on a total of 24 cysteine residues, the difference in protein thiols corresponds to a loss of 1.5 mol cysteine/mol Ca-ATPase during aging. It should be noted that an age-related modification of cysteine residues in skeletal muscle has also been established for other proteins such as phosphoglycerate kinase [178]. Using mitochondria isolated from upper hindlimb skeletal muscle, Lass et al. [160] demonstrated that protein sulfhydryl content decreased with age when comparing male C57BL/6 mice between 3 and 31 rather than 30 months of age. Again, CR prevented the age-related loss of protein sulfhydryl content [160]. These studies indicate an age-related loss of protein sulfhydryl content in skeletal muscle.

Tyrosyl radicals, which are generated by peroxidases and other heme proteins, can react with each other to form dityrosine, a stable end product. Since these residues are not typically found in proteins, their detection in skeletal muscle with aging would suggest increased tyrosyl radical-induced oxidative damage with age. Similar to protein sulfhydryl content, a gap currently exists in the literature concerning formation of dityrosine radicals with age. In a study comparing hindlimb skeletal muscle from three groups of male C57BL/6 mice (4, 14 and 30 months of age), levels of dityrosine were increased at 30 months compared to 4 months of age when using an isotope dilution gas chromatography-mass spectrometry (GC/MS) method [179]. These investigators suggest that the accumulation of dityrosine with age in skeletal muscle is consistent with the idea that tyrosyl radical plays a role in age-related protein oxidation. Interestingly, CR prevented the increase in dityrosine levels in skeletal muscle with age [179].

Nitric oxide (NO) is a free radical generated enzymatically by nitric oxide synthase (NOS), an enzyme that exists in three isoforms [180]. These isoforms include type I NOS (neuronal constitutive or nc-NOS), type II NOS (inducible or i-NOS) and type III NOS (endothelial constitutive or ec-NOS). Nitric oxide is synthesized by each isoform of NOS as it catalyzes the oxidation of L -arginine to L -citrulline, a reaction requiring molecular oxygen and nicotinamide adenine dinucleotide phosphate (NADPH) as cosubstrates and producing citrulline as a by-product. Essential co-factors include flavin adenine nucleotide (FAD), flavin mononucleotide (FMN), tetrahydrobiopterin and calmodulin. Synthesis of NO by nc-NOS and ec-NOS, two constitutive isoforms of NOS, is regulated by calcium-dependent calmodulin binding; however, i-NOS is transcriptionally regulated.

Production of NO in skeletal muscle is functionally important for vascular control, muscle metabolism and contractile function [181]. Type I NOS is expressed by muscle fibers and by neuronal axons in the muscle tissue. Immunohistochemical staining has shown that type I NOS is localized to the sarcolemma of fast-twitch fibers [182,183]. Interestingly, immunohistochemical labeling has demonstrated that type III NOS co-localizes with SDH [184]. Calcium-dependent NOS activity is enriched in the mitochondrial fraction of muscle homogenates [184], further supporting an association of type III NOS with mitochondria. These findings are significant to aging research since mitochondria are hypothesized to be the most important cellular sites of age-associated oxidative stress/ damage. Immunohistochemical analysis demonstrated that type II NOS, in response to an inflammatory challenge, could be upregulated in skeletal muscle myocytes, as well as endothelial cells and macrophages within the muscle [185].

Nitric oxide reacts with superoxide anions to generate peroxynitrite (ONOO⁻), one of the most reactive free radical species in biological systems and a recognized mediator of oxidative injury [186]. Methionine and cysteine protein residues are very susceptible to oxidation by peroxynitrite, while tryptophan and tyrosine are selective targets for peroxynitrite-dependent nitration. Peroxynitrite, along with other reactive nitrogen species (RNS) generated as a result of the interaction between oxygen and NO, catalyzes the nitration of protein tyrosine residues to form 3-nitrotyrosine. The nitration of tyrosine residues by these RNS inhibits cyclic interconversion of protein tyrosine residues between phosphorylated and

unphosphorylated forms [187]. Therefore, peroxynitrite-induced nitration compromises various cell regulation and signal transduction pathways mediated by
phosphorylation within the cell. The accumulation of nitrotyrosine-modified
proteins as detected by immunohistochemical staining with antisera against 3-
nitrotyrosine has been shown to be a convenient marker of peroxynitrite-induced
oxidative damage [188]. Therefore, techniques designed to measure the accumulation of 3-nitrotyrosine with age in skeletal muscle may provide a tool to better
understand the role of oxidative stress and damage in the etiology of sarcopenia.

Unlike the situation for ROS, investigation of the involvement of RNS in sarcopenia has been limited [189,190]. 3-Nitrotyrosine may provide a good marker of
oxidative damage because it is not normally found in proteins. In order to test
the hypothesis that proteins damaged by RNS accumulate in skeletal muscle
with age, Leeuwenburgh et al. [190] utilized GC-MS techniques to measure 3-
nitrotyrosine in skeletal muscle from 9- and 24-month-old female Long-Evans/
Wistar hybrid rats. They observed no influence of age on levels of protein-bound
3-nitrotyrosine in VL.

However, a recent study has demonstrated that certain proteins are oxidized
selectively in vivo. After isolating sarcoplasmic reticulum vesicles from hindlimb
muscles of male Fischer 344 rats, Viner et al. [189] reported that the level of nitration of the SERCA2 a slow-twitch isoform of Ca-ATPase in these vesicles was
greater in aged (28 months) than adult (5 months) rats. Specifically, these investigators found approximately one and four nitrotyrosine residues per young and
old Ca-ATPase, respectively. Further, they reported that nitration was undetectable in a closely related form of Ca-ATPase, strongly suggesting that certain isoforms are selectively modified by RNS. Therefore, analysis of 3-nitrotyrosine in
whole tissue homogenates, as performed by Leeuwenburgh et al. [190], may fail
to detect a selective increase in the oxidation of specific proteins by RNS. These
studies suggest that, as a result of their interaction with RNS, only certain proteins accumulate oxidative damage during aging.

4.6 Antioxidant status

In considering the oxidative stress/damage hypothesis of sarcopenia, it is important to examine the contributions that cellular antioxidant defenses may play in
attenuating the process. Elaborate cellular defense mechanisms involving both
enzymatic and nonenzymatic antioxidant systems are present in mammals to
contend with oxidative stress. For example, primary enzymatic antioxidants in
the cell include SOD, catalase (CAT) and glutathione peroxidase (GPX) [98].
Glutathione (GSH) and α-tocopherol (vitamin E) are considered to be the major
cellular nonenzymatic antioxidants [191]. Investigations into whether or not
these enzymatic and nonenzymatic antioxidant systems change with age in skeletal muscle, as described in Table 6, may help elucidate the etiology of sarcopenia.

Skeletal muscle has been widely studied for the effects of aging on the enzymatic
antioxidant system [61,157—160,165,192—199] and on GSH status [159,199]. In

Table 6. Antioxidant enzyme activities increase with age in skeletal muscle.

Enzyme	Species	Muscle	Ages (months)	Reference
SOD	Rat	Biceps brachii Extensor Gastrocnemius Plantaris Sternomastoideus	3, 19, 23	[192]
	Rat	VL	4, 26, 31	[157]
	Rat	VL	5, 15, 27	[179]
	Rat	Soleus	4, 24	[197]
	Mouse	Hindlimb	2, 26	[198]
CAT	Rat	Gastrocnemius	4, 15, 27	[193]
	Rat	VL	4, 26, 31	[157]
	Rat	VL	5, 15, 27	[159]
	Rat	Hindlimb	11, 26, 34	[196]
	Rat	Soleus	4, 24	[197]
GPX	Mouse	Hindlimb	1, 7, 20	[165]
	Rat	Gastrocnemius	4, 15, 27	[193]
	Rat	VL	4, 26, 31	[157]
	Rat	Diaphragm	4, 24	[62]
	Rat	Gastrocnemius Soleus	4, 24	[158]
	Rat	Soleus VL	5, 15, 27	[159]
	Rat	Hindlimb	11, 26, 34	[196]
	Rat	Soleus	4, 24	[197]

general, an age-associated increase in the level of the enzymatic and nonenzymatic antioxidant systems occurs in aging skeletal muscle. Ji et al. [157] proposed that increased antioxidant enzyme activity levels in older animals may be a response to elevated cellular production of free radicals during the aging process. Oh-Ishi et al. [197] have suggested that the changes observed in antioxidant enzymatic activity with age are directly correlated with the oxidative potential of the muscle. Compared to their glycolytic fast-twitch muscle counterparts, oxidative slow-twitch muscles may have increased susceptibility to age-related oxidative stress and damage as a result of their greater oxidative capacity.

4.6.1 Superoxide dismutase

Superoxide dismutase, which catalyzes the conversion of superoxide to oxygen and hydrogen peroxide, is one of the most important enzymes in the antioxidant enzymatic system found in skeletal muscle. There are two major forms of SOD, a copper and zinc containing enzyme (CuZnSOD), localized in the cell nucleus and cytoplasm [200], as well as a manganese containing enzyme (MnSOD) found specifically in mitochondria [201].

Despite considerable investigation into the influence of age on total SOD,

CuZnSOD and MnSOD activity levels [157—160,192—198], definitive conclusions are difficult to reach because the data show either no change or increased activity with age. This discrepancy may derive from differences in muscle fiber type, assay methods, diet and/or animal sex and strain.

In the first report on the SOD status in aging skeletal muscle, total SOD, CuZnSOD and MnSOD activities were determined in various skeletal muscles from male rats between 3 and 23 months of age [192]. In this study, total SOD activity increased progressively with age in nearly all muscles sampled. The activity levels of CuZnSOD and MnSOD were found by others [157] to be greater in VL from old male Wistar rats (26 and 31 months) than in 4-month-old rats. An age-related increase in total SOD activity in both soleus and VL muscles was observed when two groups of male Fischer 344 rats, 5 and 27 months of age, were compared [159]. In addition to greater activity and content of CuZnSOD in both soleus and EDL muscles of older male Fischer rats, Oh-Ishi et al. [197] saw an age-related increase in MnSOD activity normalized to CS activity in soleus muscle. These investigators also found no influence of age on the expression of mRNAs for SOD isoenzymes. Furthermore, CuZnSOD and MnSOD content, as well as CuZnSOD, but not MnSOD activity, were increased with aging when comparing diaphragms from mice aged 2 months and 26 months [198].

Unlike these studies demonstrating increased SOD activity with age, Vertechy et al. [193] found no change in either CuZnSOD and MnSOD activity or content with age in gastrocnemius muscle from male albino rats aged 4, 15, or 27 months. Ji et al. [194] demonstrated no age-related change in total SOD activity in VL muscle when comparing rats 5 and 27.5 months of age. Furthermore, Lawler et al. [158] confirmed that total SOD activity in both gastrocnemius and soleus muscles did not change with age when comparing 4- and 24-month-old female Fischer 344 rats. These investigators also showed that SOD activity in diaphragm was unaffected by aging in these rats whilst Luhtala et al. [196] reported that total and MnSOD activities were unaltered in rat hindlimb skeletal muscle between 11 and 34 months of age. Also using mitochondria isolated from upper hindlimb skeletal muscle, Lass et al. [160] demonstrated that SOD activity remained unaltered with age when comparing male C57BL/6Nia mice between 3 and 31 rather than 30 months of age. These reports suggest that age-related changes in SOD activity require further investigation using parallel studies in order to avoid such variables as muscle fiber type, assay methods and/or animal's sex and strain. Clarification of possible age-related changes in SOD activity is necessary since increased SOD activity has been shown to be accompanied by increased formation of hydrogen peroxide [202]. In response to elevated hydrogen peroxide levels, CAT and GPX activity would be expected to increase with aging.

4.6.2 Catalase

Catalase plays a major role in the cell's enzymatic antioxidant defense system by converting hydrogen peroxide to water and oxygen. Catalase is localized to peroxisomes and cytoplasm [203].

Several studies have shown that an age-dependent increase in CAT activity occurs in skeletal muscle [157,159,193,196,197] although, as with SOD, evidence exists which disputes this notion [160,194,198]. Vertechy et al. [193] found that CAT activity increased in gastrocnemius muscle when comparing 15- or 27-month-old male rats with animals aged 4 months. Furthermore, CAT activity was doubled in rat VL at 31 months compared with 4 months of age [157] and in rat soleus and VL muscles at 15 and 27 months but not at 5 months of age [159]. Interestingly, Luhtala et al. [196] reported that CAT activity in mitochondria- and peroxisome-enriched fractions from rat skeletal muscle homogenates increased progressively with age between 11 and 34 months of age, whereas the cytosolic fractions showed no significant alteration. Furthermore, the increase in CAT activity was attenuated by CR [196]. Catalase activity increased in rat soleus muscle with aging, but not in EDL muscle when comparing two groups of rats 4 and 24 months of age [197]. However, no age-related change in CAT activity was observed in rat VL muscle between 5 and 27.5 months of age [194] and in diaphragm when comparing two groups of mice 2 and 26 months of age [198]. Employing mitochondria isolated from upper hindlimb skeletal muscle, Lass et al. [160] demonstrated that catalase activity was unaltered with age when comparing male C57BL/6 mice aged 3–31 rather than 30 months. Therefore, data describing age-dependent changes in catalase have been inconsistent.

4.6.3 Glutathione system

Glutathione is one of the major nonenzymatic antioxidant defenses in the cell and is one of the most effective scavengers of oxygen radicals. Glutathione peroxidase utilizes GSH to reduce peroxides. Glutathione is oxidized to glutathione disulfide (GSSG) as a result of these cellular functions and is regenerated by the enzyme glutathione reductase (GR). The reducing power of NADPH from the hexose monophosphate shunt is required for the reduction of GSSG back to GSH. The rate-limiting enzyme for the hexose monophosphate shunt is glucose-6-phosphate dehydrogenase (G-6-PDH). Glutathione is also utilized by glutathione S-transferase (GST) which catalyzes the conjugation of GSH with a variety of organic peroxides in order to increase their water solubility and promote excretion. Lastly, transport of GSH across cell membranes requires that GSH be cleaved into its constitutive amino acids, whose transport across the membrane requires the enzyme γ-glutamyltranspeptidase (GGT).

In the first report to investigate the effect of aging on GPX in skeletal muscle, an age-related increase in GPX activity was detected in skeletal muscle from male NMRI-mice at 20 months of age vs. 1-month-old animals [165]. Following this first study, substantial evidence has confirmed this age-dependent increase in GPX activity in skeletal muscle [61,157–159,193,196,197]. However, a few studies have reported no age-related change in GPX activity [160,195,198] or decreased GPX activity with age [194]. Vertechy et al. [193] reported that GPX activity was greater in rat gastrocnemius muscle at 15 and 27 months of age compared with 4 months. Glutathione peroxidase activity was found to be elevated in both cytosolic and mitochondrial fractions from skeletal muscle of rats aged 26 and 31 months vs. 4-month-old animals [157] and in rat soleus and VL muscles when comparing 15- and 27-month-old animals with rats aged 5 months [159]. Increased GPX activity with age was also reported in rat diaphragm [61] and in gastrocnemius and soleus muscles [158] in 24- but not 4-month-old female Fischer 344 rats.

However, Luhtala et al. [196] reported that GPX activity in mitochondria and peroxisome enriched fractions of rat skeletal muscle homogenates increased progressively with age between 11 and 34 months of age, whereas the cytosolic fractions demonstrated no significant alteration. As was the case for catalase, the increase in GPX activity with aging was prevented by CR. GPX activity was also found to increase in rat soleus muscle with aging, but not in the EDL, when comparing rats at 4 and 24 months of age [197], suggesting that the increased oxidative capacity of the slow-twitch soleus muscle may underlie this difference. No age-related change in GPX activity was observed in rat [195] or mouse diaphragm [198]. Using mitochondria isolated from upper hindlimb skeletal muscle, Lass et al. [160] demonstrated that GPX activity remained unaltered with age when comparing male C57BL/6 mice between 3 and 31 rather than 30 months of age. In contrast, decreased GPX activity was observed in rat VL at 27.5 months of age when compared to animals 5 months of age [194]. As with GPX activity, GR activity is increased in rat gastrocnemius muscle when comparing 27-month-old rats with those aged 4 months [193].

Much information on the glutathione system in aging rat muscle has been provided by Ji's laboratory. They first reported [157] that GR, GST and G-6-PDH activities were increased in VL muscle of rats at 26 and 31 months of age compared with 4 months. Increased activity of GR and GST were observed at 15 and 27 months in both soleus and VL muscles of male Fischer 344 rats when compared to 5-month-old animals [159]. Investigation of GST activity in rat VL muscle revealed increased activity in 27.5-month-old compared to 5-month-old animals [194]. Leeuwenburgh et al. [159] also demonstrated that the activity of GGT, a key enzyme for the uptake of GSH by skeletal muscle, increased with aging in VL but not soleus muscle.

Leeuwenburgh et al. [159] have shown that the concentration of GSH, as well as the GSH/GSSG ratio in soleus muscle increased significantly with age in male rats at 15 and 27 months of age compared with 5 months, however, these parameters did not change in VL muscle. Since VL muscle is composed predominantly of fast-twitch fibers while soleus muscle is a slow-twitch oxidative muscle, these data support the hypothesis that the functional deterioration of mitochondria with age contributes to the increased production of free radicals observed during aging. Ohkuwa et al. [199] also reported that the concentration of GSH and the GSH/GSSG ratio in gastrocnemius and soleus muscle of female Wistar rats increases at 25 weeks compared to 8 weeks of age. However, as found also by Leeuwenburgh et al. [159], GSSG levels did not demonstrate an age-related change. In contrast to these studies, Noy et al. [204] reported that decreased skeletal muscle concentrations of GSH, NADH and NADPH concentrations in rats between 4 and 6 months and 28 and 32 months of age were accompanied by corresponding increases in their oxidized forms.

4.6.4 Vitamin E

Vitamin E is considered to be an important nonenzymatic defense against lipid peroxidation. This molecule is embedded within membranes and clearly has an antioxidant role [205]. Comparing gastrocnemius muscle from 24-month vs. 12-month-old male Fischer 344 rats, Starnes et al. [156] reported that levels of α-tocopherol did not change with age. However, these same investigators revealed that levels of α-tocopherol quinone, the oxidized form of α-tocopherol, increased in the older rats. Since oxidation of α-tocopherol precedes lipid peroxidation, detection of α-tocopherol quinone is considered to be a sensitive estimate of cellular oxidant stress. These increased quinone levels with age suggest that older animals must oxidize more vitamin E than younger animals to prevent lipid peroxidation.

5   INTERVENTIONS

Sarcopenia is a natural, age-associated phenomenon which compromises the independence and well being of older individuals. However, several lines of evidence suggest that the progression of sarcopenia can be attenuated or partially reversed by one or more candidate interventions. These include exercise training, antioxidant supplementation and CR.

5.1 Exercise

Both resistance and endurance training have beneficial effects on skeletal muscle in older persons. Resistance training can lead to increased muscle mass and strength, mainly by increasing fiber CSA. Endurance training has a positive effect on oxidative enzyme activities. In addition, it increases the level of activity of older individuals. Taken together, exercise training, primarily strength training, has positive effects in reversing or preventing the age-associated loss of muscle mass.

5.1.1 Strength training

There is solid evidence that healthy older people respond favorably to strength-training programs, defined as training in which the resistance against the muscle is progressively increased over time (reviewed in [43,206,207]). Exercise designed to increase strength emphasizes high force development with relatively short durations of exercise. Resistance training intensity is generally reported as a percentage of one repetition maximum (1 RM), the maximum amount of force that a muscle group can generate with one single contraction. Studies employing high training intensities in older subjects result in very substantial improvements in strength. A high-intensity (80% of 1 RM) strength training program performed by men between 60 and 72 years of age for 12 weeks resulted in an average increase in knee flexor and extensor strength of 227% and 107%, respectively [208]. When older women (average 72 years) were subjected to strength training for 6 months, a 50% increase in strength of quadriceps was reported [209]. In a similar study, older subjects (average 75 years) showed an increase in strength in all muscles except those of the ankle region [210].

Resistance training can lead to increased muscle mass and strength in old humans, primarily by increasing fiber CSA. Frontera et al. [208] reported that strength training led to an 11% increase in midthigh CSA in 60- to 72-year-olds, as assessed by computed tomography. This increase may have been due to a 34% increase in type I and 28% increase in type II fiber area. Furthermore, a 4% increase in quadriceps CSA was found in a group of elderly women (average 72 years) when subjected to strength training for 6 months [209].

Strength training programs can be beneficially applied to frail older persons. When Fiatarone et al. [211] subjected very old individuals (86—96 years) to a strength training program for 8 weeks, a 174% increase in strength and 11% increase in CSA of the quadriceps resulted. In another study of frail, older (72—98 years) persons on strength training for 10 weeks, increases in muscle strength (113%) and CSA (3%) were obtained [212]. A third study of frail, (determined by being unable to descend stairs step over step without holding the railing), older people (average 78 years) trained for 10 weeks led to increases in strength of 9—16% [213].

Although strength training has the potential to increase functional independence of and to decrease injury risk in older individuals, it appears necessary to continue the training as long as possible. For example, a group of elderly women (average 83 years) who had been subjected to a strength training program for 8 weeks were followed up a year thereafter [214]. Quadriceps isometric strength had dropped $\sim 25\%$ compared to the subjects' post-training values and $\sim 10\%$ from the pretraining values. Also, the functional mobility improvements gained from this resistance exercise had also been lost.

Increases in strength and muscle mass obtained with strength training programs also increase the ability to perform activities of daily life (e.g., stair climbing, walking, chair rising) [209,213]. These exercise programs also reduce the risk of falling. Buchner et al. [210] found a decrease in the fall rate in the 18-month period of follow-up after a 6-month resistance training protocol applied to old subjects (average 75 years). Furthermore, an increase in maximal aerobic capacity (VO_2 max) was reported after strength training in older men, suggesting that increased muscle mass can increase maximal aerobic power [215].

5.1.2 Endurance training

Several studies show that older persons favorably respond to aerobic exercise (reviewed in [43]). Unlike resistance training, endurance training requires long sessions repeated at least three times per week and involves high repetition muscle contractions. Endurance training leads to minimal strength gains, however, it results in increased maximal aerobic capacity (VO_2max).

A 6-week endurance training program resulted in an increase in VO_2max in a group of older men (average 64 years) [216]. Elderly subjects (average 75 years) who participated in an endurance training program for 6 months showed a 9% increase in aerobic capacity (VO_2max) [210]. For endurance training to be beneficial, it has to be performed on a regular basis. For example, older women and men (average 62 years) who had exhibited a 15% increase in VO_2max after a 4-month endurance training program were studied. After 4 months of detraining, VO_2max returned to its original pretraining value [217].

Some adaptations may occur in skeletal muscle due to prolonged endurance training. Endurance-trained older men show a higher percentage of type I fibers and a lower percentage of type IIb fibers than normal, fit individuals. In addition, fiber CSA of type I fibers in the VL muscle was 16% greater in trained vs. untrained subjects [17]. However, Freyssenet et al. [216] did not find any changes in the distribution and CSA of type I, IIa and IIb fibers in the VL after older subjects (average 64 years) were subjected to a 6-week endurance training program.

Other changes have been described in the muscles from endurance-trained older persons. An increase in capillary density in skeletal muscle is one of the first changes to occur during endurance training. Proctor et al. [17] found 25–30% higher values in the VL of trained vs. untrained in both young and old subjects. Also studying the VL, Freyssenet et al. [216] reported an increase in the number of capillaries/fiber, especially of those in contact with type I fibers. Endurance-trained older individuals (from 50 to 65 years) displayed 37% higher CS activity in the VL when compared to untrained [17]. In addition, CS activity is higher in the gastrocnemius of trained older people when compared to untrained [15]. Taken together, these studies indicate that, in healthy older persons, exercise programs can substantially improve strength and endurance.

5.2 Antioxidant supplementation

The use of antioxidants has been shown to reduce oxidative stress in skeletal muscle (Table 7). As discussed earlier, the injury caused by lengthening the EDL muscles of mice was lessened by treatment with PEG-SOD [81]. Vitamin E supplementation decreased levels of carbon-centered and hydrogen radicals in homogenates of rat soleus [218]. Vitamin E (30 mg/kg) injected into immobilized, atrophying soleus muscles from young rats was found to reduce levels of TBARS in [219]. Also, vitamin E treatment can inhibit exercise-induced protein oxidation in rats [220] and lipid peroxidation in people [221].

Table 7. Lowered oxidative stress in skeletal muscles after antioxidant supplementation.

Situation	Antioxidant	Species	Muscle	Reference
Force generation (P_0) (postinjury)	SOD	Mouse	EDL	[81]
Free radical levels	Vitamin E (in vitro)	Rat	Soleus	[218]
Lipid peroxidation (immobilization atrophy)	Vitamin E	Rat	Soleus	[219]
Protein oxidation (postexercise)	Vitamin E	Rat	Several	[220]
Lipid peroxidation (postexercise)	Vitamin E	Human	VL	[221]

Not all data support the efficacy of antioxidants in lowering oxidative damage in skeletal muscles. For example, when 5 month old rats were fed a diet supplemented with ascorbic acid, α-tocopherol, β-carotene and a synthetic antioxidant, no influence of diet was seen on levels of oxidative damage (o-tyrosine and 3-nitrotyrosine) in the VL were observed at 9 and 24 months of age [190]. Together, these data support the necessity of testing the influence of long-term administration of antioxidant nutrients or enzymes on the progression of sarcopenia.

5.3 Caloric restriction

The restriction of calorie intake when conducted without essential nutrient deficiency extends maximum life span and retards both the rate of biological aging and the development of late-life diseases in mice and rats [222,223]. Caloric restriction also extends life span in water fleas, rotifers, spiders and fish [222]. Two long-term studies are ongoing to determine if CR retards diseases and aging in a primate species (rhesus monkeys) [224,225].

One hypothesis to explain the beneficial effects of CR is that it lowers oxidative stress/damage [10,222,226,227]. Several lines of evidence support this hypothesis. In laboratory rodents, CR decreases the steady-state concentrations of the products of oxidative damage to protein, lipids and DNA in several tissues including skeletal muscles [169,176,228,229]. This effect may involve decreased mitochondrial production of ROS and ROM [176].

As summarized in Table 6, old rodents show consistent increases in antioxidant enzyme activities in skeletal muscle. We measured muscle mass and antioxidant enzyme activities in hindlimb skeletal muscle samples from male Brown-Norway × Fischer $344F_1$ rats of various ages fed normally or subjected to CR at 14 weeks of age [196]. We found that the total muscle mass recoverable from the upper hindlimb muscles of CR rats was ~ 30% less than that of ad libitum fed controls at 11 months of age. However, CR countered the 50% loss of muscle mass observed in very old (34 months) ad libitum fed rats. These data on muscle mass loss partially agree with those of Yu et al. [230] who studied the effect of CR on the weight of the gastrocnemius in male Fischer 344 rats. They found that muscle mass of the CR rats averaged 60% that of controls until 18 months of age when the ad libitum rats began to lose mass. At 25 months of age, muscle mass did not differ between groups but the CR group progressively lost mass thereafter. Our data differ from these in showing no loss of muscle mass between 11 and 34 months in rats on CR; however, this disparity may reflect longevity differences between the two rat strains.

As for the antioxidant enzyme activities in our study [196], there was no influence of age or CR on SOD activity, but clear age-associated increases in the activities of GPX and CAT were observed in the $1,000 \times g$ supernatant and $12,000 \times g$ fraction (which is enriched in mitochondria) in ad libitum fed rats and these increases were attenuated by CR. A logical speculation is that antioxidant enzyme induction in muscle from old ad libitum fed rats is driven by an age-related increase in ROS as was suggested by Ji et al. [157].

A recent collaborative study with Sohal's laboratory focused on the age-associated accrual of oxidative damage to mitochondrial macromolecules in mouse hindlimb skeletal muscles [160]. The influences of CR initiated at 4 months of age on these measures were also evaluated. The level of mitochondrial protein carbonyls was 150% greater in 29-month-old when compared to 7-month-old mice. When mitochondrial protein sulfhydryl content was analyzed, 18-month-old mice had 50% lower levels when compared to 3-month-old mice. In addition, TBARS levels were increased 2.5-fold in mice 12—14 months old when compared to young. Furthermore, the rate of superoxide radical generation was 41% higher in older mice when compared to young. None of these age-associated changes were seen in mice subjected to CR. In ad libitum fed mice, there was no influence of age on activities of antioxidant enzymes such as SOD, CAT and GPX; however, CR mice showed an age-associated increase in CAT activity. Taken together, these data demonstrate an increase in oxidative damage to mitochondrial macromolecules with age which is attenuated by CR.

The previous study focused on the effects of early-onset CR. Additional data from our laboratory indicate that CR does not have to be started early in life to attenuate the development of sarcopenia. We studied skeletal muscles in rats subjected to CR in late middle age (at 17 months) [22]. A decrease in the number of muscle fibers in the control-fed animals (3—4 months compared to 30—32 months) was found with age in the VL. However, late-onset CR prevented this age-associated loss of muscle fibers and attenuated the loss in type I fibers. The increase with aging in mtDNA deletion products in soleus and ADL was lessened by CR. Furthermore, when histological studies were performed, fewer ETS abnormal fibers were found in CR rats.

The data from this latter study [22] suggest that CR started in late middle age can ameliorate age-associated mitochondrial abnormalities associated with sarcopenia. Accordingly, CR can be viewed as an intervention that may potentially be applied later on in life to retard the progression of sarcopenia. It is also possible that the way by which CR attenuates the development of sarcopenia can be discovered and pharmacologically mimicked. An optimistic scenario would involve treating an individual with the "CR mimetic" which retards sarcopenia's progression in the face of a normal caloric intake.

6   SUMMARY

1. Sarcopenia, an important contributor to senile physical frailty, is character-ized by age-dependent changes in muscle mass, fiber type composition and innervation.
2. Changes in muscle function, such as decreased strength and endurance and metabolic capacity also occur in aging skeletal muscle.
3. Hypothesized causes of sarcopenia include denervation-reinnervation, con-traction-induced injury, satellite cell changes and oxidative stress/damage.
4. Oxidative stress of mitochondrial origin may contribute to the age-dependent development of sarcopenia in a focal way.
5. Understanding the mechanism by which caloric restriction attenuates the development of sarcopenia may result in effective clinical therapy.

7   PERSPECTIVES

Sarcopenia is an important topic because it universally afflicts older persons and causes physical frailty. Accordingly, studies designed to elucidate the etiology and pathogenesis of sarcopenia are important to pursue as they will provide insights into preventive strategies and therapies. Recent advances in stem cell biology [231], which have suddenly provided new opportunities for the replace-ment of dead and atrophic muscle fibers, are worthy of vigorous pursuit. Optimis-tically, these lines of research will eventually produce sarcopenia-specific inter-ventions which will contribute to an increased span of robust health for humans.

8   ACKNOWLEDGEMENTS

Our research is supported by NIH grants from the National Institute on Aging (P01 AG11915, R01 AG11604 and T32 AG00213), the National Center for Research Resources (Primate Research Center Program RR00167). The authors gratefully acknowledge the assistance of Ms. Jennifer Christensen in preparing this article. This is publication #99−08 from the Madison Geriatric Research, Education and Clinical Center and #38−031 from the Wisconsin Regional Pri-mate Research Center.

9   ABBREVIATIONS

8-OHdG:	8-hydroxydeoxyguanosine
ATP:	adenosine triphosphate
Ca-ATPase:	calcium-ATPase
CAT:	catalase
COX:	cytochrome C oxidase
CR:	caloric restriction
CS:	citrate synthase
CSA:	cross-sectional area
CuZnSOD:	Copper, ZincSOD
EDL:	extensor digitorum longus
ETS:	electron transport system
FAD:	flavin adenine nucleotide
FDL:	flexor digitorum longus
FG:	fast glycolytic
FMN:	flavin mononucleotide
FOG:	fast oxidative glycolytic
G-6-PDH:	glucose-6-phosphate dehydrogenase
GC/MS:	gas chromatography-mass spectrometry
GGT:	γ-glutamyl transpeptidase
GPX:	glutathione peroxidase
GR:	glutathione reductase
GSH:	glutathione
GSSG:	glutathione disulfide
GST:	glutathione S-transferase
HNE:	4-hydroxy-2-nonenal
LDH:	lactate dehydrogenase
LHON:	Leber's hereditary optic neuropathy
MDA:	malondialdehyde
MELAS:	mitochondrial encephalopathy with lactic acidosis and stoke-like episodes
MHC:	major histocompatibility complex
MnSOD:	manganese-containing enzyme
mtDNA:	mitochondrial DNA
NADH:	nicotinamide adenine dinucleotide
NADPH:	nicotinamide adenine dinucleotide phosphate
NO:	nitric oxide
NOS:	nitric oxide synthase
$ONOO^-$:	peroxynitrite
PEG:	polyethylene glycol
PEG-SOD:	polyethylene glycol adsorbed superoxide dismutase
RM:	repetition maximum
RNS:	reactive nitrogen species

ROM: reactive oxygen metabolites
ROS: reactive oxygen species
RRFs: ragged red fibers
SDH: succinate dehydrogenase
SERCA2:   sarcoplasmic endoplasmic reticular calcium ATPase 2
SOD: superoxide dismutase
SO: Slow Oxidative
TBARS: thiobarbituric acid reactive substances
VL: vastus lateralis
VO_2max: maximal O_2 consumption

10 REFERENCES

1. Weindruch R (ed). Reducing Frailty and Falls in Older Persons. Springfield, IL: CC Thomas, 1991.
2. Fried LP. Frailty. In: Hazzard WR (ed) Principles of Geriatric Medicine and Gerontology, 3rd edn. New York: McGraw-Hill Inc., 1994;1149—1156.
3. NIH. Physical Frailty, A Reducible Barrier to Independence for Older Americans. NIH Report to Congress, September 1991;91—397.
4. Lexell J. Human aging, muscle mass, and fiber type composition. J Gerontol Biol Sci 1995;50: 11—16.
5. Evans WJ. Exercise, nutrition and aging. Clin Geriatr Med 1995;11:725—734.
6. Faulkner JA, Brooks SV, Zerba E. Muscle atrophy and weakness with aging: contraction-induced injury as an underlying mechanism. J Gerontol Biol Sci 1995;50A:124—129.
7. Carlson BM. Factors; Influencing the repair and adaptation of muscles in aged individuals: satellite cells and innervation. J Gerontol Biol Sci 1995;50A:96—100.
8. Larsson L. Motor units: remodeling in aged animals. J Gerontol Biol Sci 1995;50A:91—95.
9. Weindruch R. Interventions based on the possibility that oxidative stress contributes to sarcopenia. J Gerontol Biol Sci 1995;50A:157—161.
10. Sohal RS, Weindruch R. Oxidative stress, caloric restriction, and aging. Science 1996;273: 59—63.
11. Beckman KB, Ames BN. The free radical theory of aging matures. Physiol Rev 1998;78: 547—581.
12. Sen CK, Packer L. Antioxidant and redox regulation of gene transcription. FASEB J 1996;10: 709—720.
13. Sun Y, Oberley LW. Redox regulation of transcriptional activators. Free Radic Biol Med 1996; 21:335—348.
14. Kroemer G, Zamzami N, Susin SA. Mitochondrial control of apoptosis. Immunol Today 1997; 18:44—51.
15. Coggan AR, Abduljalil AM, Swanson SC, Earle MS, Farris JW, Mendenhal LA et al. Muscle metabolism during exercise in young and older untrained and endurance-trained men. J Appl Physiol 1993;75:2125—2133.
16. Baumgartner RN, Stauber PM, McHugh D, Koehler KM, Garry PJ. Cross-sectional age differences in body composition in persons 60+ years of age. J Gerontol Biol Sci 1995;50:M307—316.
17. Proctor DN, Sinning WE, Walro JM, Sieck GC, Lemon PW. Oxidative capacity of human muscle fiber types: effects of age and training status. J Appl Physiol 1995;78:2033—2038.
18. Lexell J, Taylor CC, Sjostrom M. What is the cause of the ageing atrophy? Total number, size and proportion of different fiber types studied in whole vastus lateralis muscle from 15- to 83-year-old men. J Neurol Sci 1988;84:275—294.

19. Mitchell ML, Byrnes WC, Mazzeo RS. A comparison of skeletal muscle morphology with training between young and old Fischer 344 rats. Mech Ageing Dev 1991;58:21—35.
20. Walters TJ, Sweeney HL, Farrar RP. Aging does not affect contractile properties of type IIb FDL muscle in Fischer 344 rats. Am J Physiol 1990;258:C1031—1035.
21. Brown M, Ross TP, Holloszy JO. Effects of ageing and exercise on soleus and extensor digitorum longus muscles of female rats. Mech Ageing Dev 1992;63:69—77.
22. Aspnes LE, Lee CM, Weindruch R, Chung SS, Roecker EB, Aiken JM. Caloric restriction reduces fiber loss and mitochondrial abnormalities in aged rat muscle. FASEB J 1997;11: 573—581.
23. Larsson L, Edstrom L. Effects of age on enzyme-histochemical fibre spectra and contractile properties of fast- and slow-twitch skeletal muscles in the rat. J Neurol Sci 1986;76:69—89.
24. Brown M, Hasser EM. Complexity of age-related change in skeletal muscle. J Gerontol Biol Sci 1996;51A:B117—123.
25. Brooke MH, Kaiser KK. Some comments on the histochemical characterization of muscle adenosine triphosphatase. J Histochem Cytochem 1969;17:431—432.
26. Brooke MH, Kaiser KK. Three "myosin adenosine triphosphatase" systems: the nature of their pH lability and sulfhydryl dependence. J Histochem Cytochem 1970;18:670—672.
27. Guth L, Samaha FJ. Procedure for the histochemical demonstration of actomyosin ATPase. Exp Neurol 1970;28:365—367.
28. Samaha FJ, Guth L, Albers RW. Phenotypic differences between the actomyosin ATPase of the three fiber types of mammalian skeletal muscle. Exp Neurol 1970;26:120—125.
29. Peter JB, Barnard RJ, Edgerton VR, Gillespie CA, Stempel KE. Metabolic profiles of three fiber types of skeletal muscle in guinea pigs and rabbits. Biochemistry 1972;11:2627—2633.
30. Armstrong RB, Phelps RO. Muscle fiber type composition of the rat hindlimb. Am J Anat 1984; 171:259—272.
31. Pette D, Staron RS. Mammalian skeletal muscle fiber type transitions. Int Rev Cytol 1997;170: 143—223.
32. Hortobagyi T, Zheng D, Weidner M, Lambert NJ, Westbrook S, Houmard JA. The influence of aging on muscle strength and muscle fiber characteristics with special reference to eccentric strength. J Gerontol Biol Sci 1995;50A:B399—B406.
33. Hegreberg GA, Hamilton MJ. An age series study of skeletal muscle morphology of rhesus monkeys. In: Davis RT, Leathers CW (eds) Behavior and pathology of aging in rhesus monkeys. New York: A.R Liss, 1985;327—334.
34. Eddinger TJ, Moss RL, Cassens RG. Fiber number and type composition in extensor digitorum longus, soleus, and diaphragm muscles with aging in Fischer 344 rats. J Histochem Cytochem 1985;33:1033—1041.
35. Ansved T, Larsson L. Effects of ageing on enzyme-histochemical morphometrical and contractile properties of the soleus muscle in the rat. J Neurol Sci 1989;93:105—24.
36. Holloszy JO, Chen M, Cartee GD, Young JC. Skeletal muscle atrophy in old rats: differential changes in three fiber types. Mech Ageing Dev 1991;60:199—213.
37. Ansved T. Effects of immobilization on the rat soleus muscle in relation to age. Acta Physiol Scand 1995;154:291—302.
38. Walters TJ, Sweeney HL, Farrar RP. Influence of electrical stimulation on a fast-twitch muscle in aging rats. J Appl Physiol 1991;71:1921—1928.
39. Brown M. Change in fibre size, not number, in ageing skeletal muscle. Age Ageing 1987;16: 244—248.
40. Roos MR, Rice CL, Vandervoort AA. Age-related changes in motor unit function. Muscle Nerve 1997;20:679—690.
41. Edstrom L, Larsson L. Effects of age on contractile and enzyme-histochemical properties of fast- and slow-twitch single motor units in the rat. J Physiol 1987;392:129—145.
42. Kadhiresan VA, Hassett CA, Faulkner JA. Properties of single motor units in medial gastrocnemius muscles of adult and old rats. J Physiol 1996;493:543—552.

43. Mazzeo RS, Cavanagh P, Evans WJ, Fiatarone M, Hagberg J, McAuley E et al. Exercise and physical activity for older adults. Med Sci Sport Exerc 1998;30:992—1008.
44. Grimby G. Muscle performance and structure in the elderly as studied cross-sectionally and longitudinally. J Gerontol Biol Sci 1995;50:17—22.
45. Winegard KJ, Hicks AL, Sale DG, Vandervoort AA. A 12-year follow-up study of ankle muscle function in older adults. J Gerontol Biol Sci 1996;51:B202—207.
46. Hurley MV, Rees J, Newham DJ. Quadriceps function, proprioceptive acuity and functional performance in healthy young, middle-aged and elderly subjects. Age Ageing 1998;27:55—62.
47. McBride TA, Gorin FA, Carlsen RC. Prolonged recovery and reduced adaptation in aged rat muscle following eccentric exercise. Mech Ageing Dev 1995;83:185—200.
48. Delbono O, O'Rourke KS, Ettinger WH. Excitation-calcium release uncoupling in aged single human skeletal muscle fibers. J Membr Biol 1995;148:211—222.
49. Bemben MG. Age-related alterations in muscular endurance. Sports Med 1998;25:259—269.
50. Astrand I. Aerobic work capacity in men and women with special reference to age. J Appl Physiol 1960;169:1—92.
51. Rooyackers OE, Adey DB, Ades PA, Nair KS. Effect of age on in vivo rates of mitochondrial protein synthesis in human skeletal muscle. Proc Natl Acad Sci USA 1996;93:15364—15369.
52. Proctor DN, Joyner MJ. Skeletal muscle mass and the reduction of VO₂max in trained older subjects. J Appl Physiol 1997;82:1411—1415.
53. Taylor DJ, Kemp GJ, Thompson CH, Radda GK. Ageing: effects on oxidative function of skeletal muscle in vivo. Mol Cell Biochem 1997;174:321—324.
54. Cartee GD. Influence of age on skeletal muscle glucose transport and glycogen metabolism. Med Sci Sports Exer 1994;26:577—585.
55. Orlander J, Kiessling KH, Larsson L, Karlsson J, Aniansson A. Skeletal muscle metabolism and ultrastructure in relation to age in sedentary men. Acta Physiol Scand 1978;104:249—261.
56. Schlenska GK, Kleine TO. Disorganization of glycolytic and gluconeogenic pathways in skeletal muscle of aged persons studied by histometric and enzymatic methods. Mech Ageing Dev 1980;13:143—154.
57. Aniansson A, Grimby G, Hedberg M. Compensatory muscle fiber hypertrophy in elderly men. J Appl Physiol 1992;73:812—816.
58. Aniansson A, Hedberg M, Henning G-B, Grimby G. Muscle morphology, enzymatic activity, and muscle strength in elderly men: a follow-up study. Muscle Nerve 1986;9:585—591.
59. Larkin L, Leiendecker ER, Supiano M, Halter J. Glucose transporter content and enzymes of metabolism in nerve-repair grafted muscle of aging Fischer 344 rats. J Appl Physiol 1997;83:1623—1629.
60. Johnson P, Hammer JL. Cardiac and skeletal muscle enzyme levels in hypertensive and aging rats. Comp Biochem Physiol 1993;104:63—67.
61. Powers SK, Lawler J, Criswell D, Lieu FK, Dodd S. Alterations in diaphragmatic oxidative and antioxidant enzymes in the senescent Fischer 344 rat. J Appl Physiol 1992;72:2317—2321.
62. Farrar RP, Monnin KA, Fordyce DE, Walters TJ. Uncoupling of changes in skeletal muscle β-adrenergic receptor density and aerobic capacity during the aging process. Aging Clin Exp Res 1997;9:153—158.
63. Trounce I, Byrne E, Marzuki S. Decline in skeletal muscle mitochondrial respiratory chain function: possible factor in ageing. Lancet 1989;1(8639):637—639.
64. Cooper JM, Mann VM, Schapira AHV. Analyses of mitochondrial respiratory chain function and mitochondrial DNA deletion in human skeletal muscle: effect of ageing. J Neurol Sci 1992;113:91—98.
65. Boffoli D, Scacco SC, Vergari R, Solarino G, Santacroce G, Papa S. Decline with age of the respiratory chain activity in human skeletal muscle. Biochim Biophys Acta 1994;1226:73—82.
66. Desai VG, Weindruch R, Hart RW, Feuers RJ. Influences of age and dietary restriction on gastrocnemius electron transport system activities in mice. Arch Biochem Biophys 1996;30:145—151.

67. Lexell J. Evidence for nervous system degeneration with advancing age. J Nutr 1997;127(Suppl 5):1011S—1013S.
68. Loeser FR, Delbono O. Aging and the musculoskeletal system. In: Hazzard W, Blass JP, Ettinger WHJ, Halter JB, Ouslander JG (eds) Principles of Geriatric Medicine and Gerontology, 4th edn. New York: McGraw-Hill, 1999;1097—1111.
69. Tomlinson BE, Irving D. The numbers of limb motor neurons in the human lumbosacral cord throughout life. J Neurol Sci 1977;34:213—219.
70. Galea V. Changes in motor unit estimates with aging. J Clin Neurophysiol 1996;13:253—260.
71. Hashizume K, Kanda K, Burke RE. Medial gastrocnemius motor nucleus in the rat: age-related changes in the number and size of motoneurons. J Comp Neurol 1988;269:425—430.
72. Oda K. Age changes of motor innervation and acetylcholine receptor distribution on human skeletal muscle fibres. J Neurol Sci 1984;66:327—338.
73. Rosenheimer JL, Smith DO. Differential changes in the end-plate architecture of functionally diverse muscles during aging. J Neurophysiol 1985;53:1567—1581.
74. Jones DA, Newham DJ, Round JM, Tolfree SE. Experimental human muscle damage: morphological changes in relation to other indices of damage. J Physiol 1986;375:435—448.
75. Newham DJ, McPhail G, Mills KR, Edwards RH. Ultrastructural changes after concentric and eccentric contractions of human muscle. J Neurol Sci 1983;61:109—122.
76. Friden J, Sjostrom M, Ekblom B. Myofibrillar damage following intense eccentric exercise in man. Int J Sport Med 1983;4:170—176.
77. Morgan DL. New insights into the behavior of muscle during active lengthening. Biophys J 1990; 57:209—221.
78. Macpherson PC, Dennis RG, Faulkner JA. Sarcomere dynamics and contraction-induced injury to maximally activated single muscle fibres from soleus muscles of rats. J Physiol 1997; 500:523—533.
79. Talbot JA, Morgan DL. Quantitative analysis of sarcomere non-uniformities in active muscle following a stretch. J Musc Res Cell Mot 1996;17:261—268.
80. Faulkner JA, Jones DA, Round JM. Injury to skeletal muscles of mice by forced lengthening during contractions. Q J Exp Physiol 1989;74:661—670.
81. Zerba E, Komorowski TE, Faulkner JA. Free radical injury to skeletal muscles of young, adult, and old mice. Am J Physiol 1990;258:C429—C435.
82. McCully KK, Faulkner JA. Injury to skeletal muscle fibers of mice following lengthening contractions. J Appl Physiol 1985;59:119—126.
83. Brooks SV, Faulkner JA. The magnitude of the initial injury induced by stretches of maximally activated muscle fibres of mice and rats increases in old age. J Physiol 1996;497:573—580.
84. Brooks SV, Faulkner JA. Contraction-induced injury: recovery of skeletal muscles in young and old mice. Am J Physiol 1990;258:C436—442.
85. Carlson BM, Faulkner JA. Muscle transplantation between young and old rats: age of host determines recovery. Am J Physiol 1989;256:C1262—1266.
86. Carlson BM, Faulkner JA. The regeneration of noninnervated muscle grafts and marcaine-treated muscles in young and old rats. J Gerontol Biol Sci 1996;51:B43—49.
87. Allbrook DB, Han MF, Hellmuth AE. Population of muscle satellite cells in relation to age and mitotic activity. Pathology 1971;3:223—243.
88. Gibson MC, Schultz E. Age-related differences in absolute numbers of skeletal muscle satellite cells. Muscle Nerve 1983;6:574—580.
89. Rodrigues AdC, Schmalbruch H. Satellite cells and myonuclei in long-term denervated rat muscles. Anat Rec 1995;243:430—437.
90. Allen RE, McAllister PK, Masak KC. Myogenic potential of satellite cells in skeletal muscle of old rats. A brief note. Mech Ageing Dev 1980;13:105—109.
91. Schultz E, Lipton BH. Skeletal muscle satellite cells: changes in proliferation potential as a function of age. Mech Ageing Dev 1982;20:377—383.
92. Gutmann E. The denervated muscle. Prague: Publishing House of Czechoslovakian Academy of

Science, 1962.

93. Lu D-X, Carlson BMA. A quantitative study of satellite in long-term denervated rat extensor digitorum longus muscles (Abstract). Anat Rec 1993;1(Suppl):78.

94. Jackson MJ, O'Farrell S. Free radicals and muscle damage. Br Med Bull 1993;49:630—641.

95. Clayton DA. Replication of animal mitochondrial DNA. Cell 1982;28:693—705.

96. Robin ED, Wang R. Mitochondrial DNA molecules and virtual number of mitochondria per cell in mammalian cells. J Cell Physiol 1988;136:507—513.

97. Wallace DC. Mitochondrial diseases in man and mouse. Science 1999;283:1482—1488.

98. Chance B, Sies H, Boveris A. Hydroperoxide metabolism in mammalian organs. Pysiol Rev 1979;59:527—603.

99. Harman D. Aging: a theory based on free radical and radiation chemistry. J Gerontol 1956;11: 298—300.

100. Szilard L. On the nature of the aging process. Proc Natl Acad Sci USA 1959;45:30.

101. Harman D. The aging process. Proc Natl Acad Sci USA 1981;78:7124—7128.

102. Ames BN. Endogenous oxidative DNA damage, aging and cancer. Free Radic Res Commun 1989;7:121—128.

103. Wallace DC. Diseases of the mitochondrial DNA. Ann Rev Biochem 1992b;61:1175—1212.

104. DiMauro S. Mitochondrial encephalomyopathies. In: Rosenberg RN, Prusiner SB, DiMauro S, Barchi RL, Kunkel LM (eds) Molecular and Genetic Basis of Neurological Disease. Boston: Butterworth-Heinemann, 1993;665—694.

105. Wallace DC, Singh G, Lott MT, Hodge JA, Schurr TG, Lezza AM et al. Mitochondrial DNA mutation associated with Leber's hereditary optic neuropathy. Science 1988;242:1427—1430.

106. Kobayashi Y, Momoi MY, Tominaga K, Momoi T, Nihei K, Yanagisawa M et al. A point mutation in the mitochondrial tRNA(Leu(UUR) gene in MELAS (mitochondrial myopathy, encephalopathy, lactic acidosis and stroke-like episodes). Biochem Biophys Res Commun 1990; 173:816—822.

107. Engel WK, Cunningham GG. Rapid examination of muscle tissue: an improved trichrome method for fresh-frozen biopsy sections. Neurology 1963;13:919—923.

108. Müller-Höcker J, Seibel P, Schneiderbanger K, Kadenbach B. Different in situ hybridization patterns of mitochondrial DNA in cytochrome c oxidase-deficient extraocular muscle fibres in the elderly. Virchows Arch A Pathol Anat 1993;422:7—15.

109. Prelle A, Fagiolari G, Checcarelli N, Moggio M, Battistel A, Comi GP et al. Mitochondrial myopathy: correlation between oxidative defect and mitochondrial DNA deletions at single fiber level. Acta Neuropathol 1994;87:371—376.

110. Johnston W, Karpati G, Carpenter S, Arnold D, Shoubridge EA. Late-onset mitochondrial myopathy. Ann Neurol 1995;37:16—23.

111. Moraes C, Ricci E, Bonilla E, DiMauro S, Schon EA. The mitochondrial tRNA(Leu(UUR)) mutation in mitochondrial encephalomyopathy, lactic acidosis, and stroke-like episodes (MELAS): genetic, biochemical, and morphological correlations in skeletal muscle. Am J Hum Genet 1992;50:934—949.

112. Sciacco M, Bonilla E, Schon EA, DiMauro S, Moraes CT. Distribution of wild-type and common deletion forms of mtDNA in normal and respiration-deficient muscle fibers from patients with mitochondrial myopathy. Hum Mol Genet 1994;3:13—19.

113. Linnane AW, Marzuki S, Ozawa T, Tanaka M. Mitochondrial DNA mutations as an important contributor to ageing and degenerative diseases. Lancet 1989;1:642—645.

114. Wallace DC. Mitochondrial genetics: a paradigm for aging and degenerative diseases? Science 1992;256:628—632.

115. Cortopassi GA, Arnheim N. Detection of a specific mitochondrial DNA deletion in tissues of older humans. Nucl Acids Res 1990;18:6927—6933.

116. Cortopassi GA, Shibata D, Soong N-W, Arnheim NA. A pattern of accumulation of a somatic deletion of mitochondrial DNA in aging human tissues. Proc Natl Acad Sci USA 1992;89: 7370—7374.

117. Linnane AW, Baumer A, Maxwell RJ, Preston H, Zhang C, Marzuki S. Mitochondrial gene mutation: The ageing process and degenerative diseases. Biochem Int 1990;22:1067—1076.
118. Yen T-C, Su J-H, King K-L, Wei Y-H. Ageing-associated 5 kb deletion in human liver mitochondrial DNA. Biochem Biophys Res Commun 1991;178:124—131.
119. Linnane AW, Zhang C, Baumer A, Nagley P. Mitochondrial DNA mutation and the ageing process: bioenergy and pharmacological intervention. Mutat Res 1992;275:195—208.
120. Corral-Debrinksi M, Horton T, Lott MT, Shoffner JM. Mitochondrial DNA deletions in human brain: regional variability and increase with advanced age. Nature Genet 1992;2:324—329.
121. Zhang C, Baumer A, Maxwell RJ, Linnane AW, Nagley P. Multiple mitochondrial DNA deletions in an elderly human individual. FEBS Lett 1992;297:34—38.
122. Lee CM, Chung SS, Kaczkowski JM, Weindruch R, Aiken JM. Multiple mitochondrial DNA deletions associated with age in skeletal muscle of rhesus monkeys. J Gerontol Biol Sci 1993; 48:B201—205.
123. Lee CM, Eimon P, Weindruch R, Aiken JM. Direct repeat sequences are not required at the breakpoints of age-associated mitochondrial DNA deletions in rhesus monkeys. Mech Ageing Devel 1994;75:69—79.
124. Chung SS, Weindruch R, Schwarze SR, McKenzie DI, Aiken JM. Multiple age-associated mitochondrial DNA deletions in skeletal muscle of mice. Aging 1994;6(3):193—200.
125. Chung SS, Eimon PM, Weindruch R, Aiken JM. Analysis of age-associated mitochondrial DNA deletion breakpoint regions from mice suggests a novel model of deletion formation. Age 1996; 19:117—128.
126. Brossas JY, Barreau E, Courtois Y, Treton J. Multiple deletions in mitochondrial DNA are present in senescent mouse brain. Biochem Biophys Res Commun 1994;202(2):654—659.
127. Tanhauser SM, Laipis PJ. Multiple deletions are detectable in mitochondrial DNA of aging mice. J Biol Chem 1995;270:24769—24775.
128. Van Tuyle GC, Gudikote JP, Hurt VR, Miller BB, Moore CA. Multiple, large deletions in rat mitochondrial DNA: evidence for a major hot spot. Mutat Res 1996;349:95—107.
129. Gudikote JP, Van Tuyle GC. Rearrangements in the shorter arc of rat mitochondrial DNA involving the region of the heavy and light strand promoters. Mutat Res 1996;356:275—286.
130. Simonetti S, Chen X, DiMauro S, Schon EA. Accumulation of deletions in human mitochondrial DNA during normal aging: analysis by quantitative PCR. Biochim Biophys Acta 1992; 1180:113—122.
131. Lee CM, Weindruch R, Aiken JM. Age-associated alterations of the mitochondrial genome. Free Radic Biol Med 1997;22:1259—1269.
132. Holt IJ, Harding AE, Morgan-Hughes JA. Deletions of muscle mitochondrial DNA in patients with mitochondrial myopathies. Nature 1988;331:717—719.
133. Schon EA, Hirano M, DiMauro S. Mitochondrial encephalomyopathies: clinical and molecular analysis. J Bioenerg Biomemb 1994;26:291—299.
134. Schwarze S, Lee CM, Chung SS, Roecker EB, Weindruch R, Aiken JM. High levels of mitochondrial DNA deletions in skeletal muscle of old rhesus monkeys. Mech Ageing Dev 1995;83: 91—101.
135. Lee CM, Lopez ME, Weindruch R, Aiken JM. Association of age-related mitochondrial abnormalities with skeletal muscle fiber atrophy. Free Radic Biol Med 1998;25:964—972.
136. Papa S. Mitochondrial oxidative phosphorylation changes in the life span. Molecular aspects and physiopathological implications. Biochim Biophys Acta-Bioenerg 1996;1276:87—105.
137. Torii K, Sugiyama S, Takagi K, Satake T, Ozawa T. Age-related decrease in respiratory muscle mitochondrial function in rats. Am J Respir Cell Mol Biol 1992;6:88—92.
138. Sugiyama S, Takasawa M, Hayakawa M, Ozawa T. Changes in skeletal muscle, heart and liver mitochondrial electron transport activities in rats and dogs of various ages. Biochem Mol Biol Int 1993;30:937—944.
139. Takasawa M, Hayakawa M, Sugiyama S, Hattori K, Ito T, Ozawa T. Age-associated damage in mitochondrial function in rat hearts. Exp Geront 1993;28:269—280.

140. Gold PH, Gee MV, Strehler BL. Effect of age on oxidative phosphorylation in the rat. J Gerontol 1968;23:509—512.

141. Abu-Erreish GM, Sanadi DR. Age-related changes in cytochrome concentration of myocardial mitochondria. Mech Ageing Dev 1978;7:425—432.

142. Müller-Höcker J. Cytochrome c oxidase deficient fibres in the limb muscle and diaphragm of man without muscular disease: An age-related alteration. J Neurol Sci 1990;100:14—21.

143. Müller-Höcker J. Progressive loss of cytochrome c oxidase in the human extraocular muscles in ageing — A cytochemical-immunohistochemical study. Mutat Res 1992;275:115—24.

144. Rifai Z, Welle S, Kamp C, Thornton CA. Ragged red fibers in normal aging and inflammatory myopathy. Ann Neurol 1995;37:24—29.

145. Müller-Höcker J, Schafer S, Link TA, Possekel S, Hammer C. Defects of the respiratory chain in various tissues of old monkeys — a cytochemical-immunocytochemical. Mech Ageing Dev 1996;86:197—213.

146. Brierley EJ, Johnson MA, Lightowlers RN, James OF, Turnbull DM. Role of mitochondrial DNA mutations in human aging: implications for the central nervous system and muscle. Ann Neurol 1998;43:217—223.

147. Anderson S, Bankier AT, Barrell BG, de Bruijn MHL, Coulson AR, Drouin J et al. Sequence and organization of the human mitochondrial genome. Nature 1981;290:457—465.

148. Shoubridge EA, Karpati G, Hastings KE. Deletion mutants are functionally dominant over wild-type mitochondrial genomes in skeletal muscle fiber segments in mitochondrial disease. Cell 1990;62:43—49.

149. Shoubridge EA. Mitochondrial DNA diseases: Histological and cellular studies. J Bioenerg Biomemb 1994;26:301—310.

150. Weiss SJ, LoBuglio AF. Phagocyte-generated oxygen metabolites and cellular injury. Lab Invest 1982;47:5—18.

151. McCord JM, Roy RS. The pathophysiology of superoxide: roles in inflammation and ischemia. Can J Physiol Pharmacol 1982;60:1346—1352.

152. Bandy B, Davison AJ. Mitochondrial mutations may increase oxidative stress: implications for carcinogenesis and aging? Free Radic Biol Med 1990;8:523—539.

153. Masters C, Holmes R. Peroxisomes: new aspects of cell physiology and biochemistry. Physiol Rev 1977;57:816—882.

154. Estabrook RW, Werringloer J. Cytochrome P450: Its role in oxygen activation for drug metabolism. In: Donald MJ, Robert RG (ed) Drug Metabolism Concepts. Washington DC: American Chemical Society, 1976.

155. Rikans LE, Ardinska V, Hornbrook KR. Age-associated increase in ferritin content of male rat liver — implication for diquat-mediated oxidative injury. Arch Biochem Biophys 1997;344:85—93.

156. Starnes JS, Cantu G, Farrar RP, Kehrer JP. Skeletal muscle lipid peroxidation in exercised and food-restricted rats during aging. J Appl Physiol 1989;67:69—75.

157. Ji LL, Dillon D, Wu E. Alteration of antioxidant enzymes with aging in rat skeletal muscle and liver. Am J Physiol 1990;258:R918—923.

158. Lawler JM, Powers SK, Visser T, Van Dijk H, Kordus MJ, Ji LL. Acute exercise and skeletal muscle antioxidant and metabolic enzymes: effects of fiber type and age. Am J Physiol 1993;265:R1344—1350.

159. Leeuwenburgh C, Fiebig R, Chandwaney R, Ji LL. Aging and exercise training in skeletal muscle: responses of glutathione and antioxidant enzyme systems. Am J Physiol 1994;267:R439—R445.

160. Lass A, Sohal BH, Weindruch R, Forster MJ, Sohal RS. Caloric restriction prevents age-associated accrual of oxidative damage to mouse skeletal muscle mitochondria. Free Radic Biol Med 1998;25:1089—1097.

161. Mecocci P, Fano G, Fulle S, MacGarvey U, Shinobu L, Polidori MC et al. Age-dependent increases in oxidative damage to DNA, lipids, and proteins in human skeletal muscle. Free

Radic Biol Med 1999;26:303—308.

162. Gutmann E. Muscle. In: Finch CE, Hayflick L (eds) Handbook of the Biology of Aging. New York: Van Nostrand Reinhold, 1977;445—469.

163. Ikeda H, Tauchi H, Sato T. Fine structural analysis of lipofuscin in various tissues of rats of different ages. Mech Ageing Dev 1985;33:77—93.

164. Beregi E, Regius O, Huttl T, Gobl Z. Age-related changes in the skeletal muscle cells. Zft Gerontol 1988;21:83—86.

165. Salminen A, Saari P, Kihlstrom M. Age- and sex-related differences in lipid peroxidation of mouse cardiac and skeletal muscles. Comp Biochem Physiol 1988;89B:695—699.

166. Cheng KC, Cahill DS, Kasai H, Nishimura S, Loeb LA. 8-Hydroxyguanine, an abundant form of oxidative DNA damage, causes G $\rightarrow$ T and A $\rightarrow$ C substitutions. J Biol Chem 1992;267: 166—172.

167. Kasai H, Nishimura S. Hydroxylation of guanine in nucleosides and DNA at the C-8 position by heated glucose and oxygen radical-forming agents. Environ Health Perspect 1986;67:111—116.

168. Fraga CG, Shigenaga MK, Park JW, Degan P, Ames BN. Oxidative damage to DNA during aging: 8-hydroxy-2'-deoxyguanosine in rat organ DNA and urine. Proc Natl Acad Sci USA 1990;87:4533—4537.

169. Sohal RS, Agarwal S, Candas M, Forster MJ, Lal H. Effect of age and caloric restriction on DNA oxidative damage in different tissues of C56BL/6 mice. Mech Ageing Dev 1994;76: 215—224.

170. Farber JM, Levine RL. Sequence of a peptide susceptible to mixed-function oxidation. Probable cation binding site in glutamine synthetase. J Biol Chem 1986;261:4574—4578.

171. Amici A, Levine RL, Tsai L, Stadtman ER. Conversion of amino acid residues in proteins and amino acid homopolymers to carbonyl derivatives by metal-catalyzed oxidation reactions. J Biol Chem 1989;264:3341—3346.

172. Esterbauer H, Schaur RJ, Zollner H. Chemistry and biochemistry of 4-hydroxynonenal, malonaldehyde and related aldehydes. Free Radic Biol Med 1991;11:81—128.

173. Uchida K, Stadtman ER. Covalent attachment of 4-hydroxynonenal to glyceraldehyde-3-phosphate dehydrogenase. A possible involvement of intra and intermolecular cross-linking reaction. J Biol Chem 1993;268:6388—6393.

174. Huggins TG, Wells-Knecht MC, Detorie NA, Baynes JW, Thorpe SR. Formation of o-tyrosine and dityrosine in proteins during radiolytic and metal-catalyzed oxidation. J Biol Chem 1993; 268:12341—12347.

175. Wells-Knecht MC, Huggins TG, Dyer DG, Thorpe SR, Baynes JW. Oxidized amino acids in lens protein with age. Measurement of o-tyrosine and dityrosine in the aging human lens. J Biol Chem 1993;268:12348—12352.

176. Sohal RS, Ku H-H, Agarwal S, Forster MJ, Lal H. Oxidative damage, mitochondrial oxidant generation and antioxidant defenses during aging and in response to food restriction in the mouse. Mech Ageing Dev 1994b;74:121—133.

177. Viner RI, Ferrington DA, Aced GI, Miller-Schlyer M, Bigelow DJ. In vivo aging of rat skeletal muscle sarcoplasmic reticulum Ca-ATPase. Chemical analysis and quantitative simulation by exposure to low levels of peroxyl radicals. Biochim Biophys Acta 1997;1329:321—335.

178. Cook LL, Gafni A. Protection of phosphoglycerate kinase against in vitro aging by selective cysteine methylation. J Biol Chem 1988;263:13991—13993.

179. Leeuwenburgh C, Wagner P, Holloszy JO, Sohal RS, Heinecke JW. Caloric restriction attenuates dityrosine cross-linking of cardiac and skeletal muscle proteins in aging mice. Arch Biochem Biophys 1997;346:74—80.

180. Knowles RG, Moncada S. Nitric oxide synthases in mammals. Biochem J 1994;298:249—258.

181. Reid MB. Role of nitric oxide in skeletal muscle: synthesis, distribution and functional importance. Acta Physiol Scand 1998;162:401—409.

182. Kobzik L, Reid MB, Bredt DS, Stamler JS. Nitric oxide in skeletal muscle. Nature 1994;372 (6506):546—548.

183. Grozdanovic Z, Nakos G, Dahrmann G, Mayer B, Gossrau R. Species-independent expression of nitric oxide synthase in the sarcolemma region of visceral and somatic striated muscle fibers. Cell Tis Res 1995;281:493—499.

184. Kobzik L, Stringer B, Balligand JL, Reid MB, Stamler JS. Endothelial type nitric oxide synthase in skeletal muscle fibers: mitochondrial relationships. Biochem Biophys Res Commun 1995;211:375—381.

185. Thompson M, Becker L, Bryant D, Williams G, Levin D, Margraf L et al. Expression of the inducible nitric oxide synthase gene in diaphragm and skeletal muscle. J Appl Physiol 1996;81: 2415—2420.

186. Freeman B. Free radical chemistry of nitric oxide. Looking at the dark side. Chest 1994;105: 79S—84S.

187. Hunter T. Protein kinases and phosphatases: the yin and yang of protein phosphorylation and signaling. Cell 1995;80:225—236.

188. Beckman JS, Koppenol WH. Nitric oxide, superoxide, and peroxynitrite — the good, the bad, and the ugly. Am J Physiol 1996;40:C1424—1437.

189. Viner RI, Ferrington DA, Huhmer AF, Bigelow DJ, Schoneich C. Accumulation of nitrotyrosine on the SERCA2a isoform of SR Ca-ATPase of rat skeletal muscle during aging: a peroxynitrite-mediated process. FEBS Lett 1996;379:286—290.

190. Leeuwenburgh C, Hansen P, Shaish A, Holloszy JO, Heinecke JW. Markers of protein oxidation by hydroxyl radical and reactive nitrogen species in tissues of aging rats. Am J Physiol Regul Integr Comp Physiol 1998;43:R453—461.

191. Machlin LJ, Bendich A. Free radical tissue damage: protective role of antioxidant nutrients. FASEB J 1987:441—445.

192. Lammi-Keefe CJ, Swan PB, Hegarty PVJ. Copper-zinc and manganese superoxide dismutase activities in cardiac and skeletal muscles during aging in male rats. J Gerontol 1984;30: 153—158.

193. Vertechy M, Cooper MB, Ghirardi O, Ramacci MT. Antioxidant enzyme activities in heart and skeletal muscle of rats of different ages. Exp Geront 1989;24:211—218.

194. Ji LL, Dillon D, Wu E. Myocardial aging: antioxidant enzyme systems and related biochemical properties. Am J Physiol 1991;26:R386.

195. Lawler JM, Powers SK, Van Dijk H, Visser T, Kordus MJ, Ji LL. Metabolic and antioxidant enzyme activities in the diaphragm: effects of acute exercise. Respir Physiol 1994;96:139—149.

196. Luhtala TA, Roecker EB, Pugh T, Feuers RJ, Weindruch R. Dietary restriction attenuates age-related increases in rat skeletal muscle antioxidant enzyme activities. J Gerontol Biol Sci 1994; 49:B231—238.

197. Oh-Ishi S, Kizaki T, Yamashita H, Nagata N, Suzuki K, Taniguchi N et al. Alterations of superoxide dismutase iso-enzyme activity, content, and mRNA expression with aging in rat skeletal muscle. Mech Ageing Dev 1995;84:65—76.

198. Oh-ishi S, Toshinai K, Kizaki T, Haga S, Fukuda K, Nagata N et al. Effects of aging and/or training on antioxidant enzyme system in diaphragm of mice. Respir Physiol 1996;105: 195—202.

199. Ohkuwa T, Sato Y, Naoi M. Glutathione status and reactive oxygen generation in tissues of young and old exercised rats. Acta Physiol Scand 1997;159:237—244.

200. McCord JM, Fridovich I. Superoxide dismutase. An enzymic function for erythrocuprein (hemocuprein). J Biol Chem 1969;244:6049—6055.

201. Weisiger RA, Fridovich I. Mitochondrial superoxide dismutase. Site of synthesis and intramito-chondrial localization. J Biol Chem 1973;248:4793—4796.

202. Scott MD, Meshnick SR, Eaton JW. Superoxide dismutase-rich bacteria. Paradoxical increase in oxidant toxicity. J Biol Chem 1987;262:3640—3645.

203. Peeters-Joris C, Vandevoorde AM, Baudhuin P. Subcellular localization of superoxide dismutase in rat liver. Biochem J 1975;150:31—39.

204. Noy N, Schwartz H, Gafni A. Age-related changes in the redox status of rat muscle cells and

their role in enzyme-aging. Mech Ageing Dev 1985;29:63—69.

205. Horton AA, Fairhurst S. Lipid peroxidation and mechanisms of toxicity. Crit Rev Toxicol 1987; 18:27—79.

206. Fielding RA. The role of progressive resistance training and nutrition in the preservation of lean body mass in the elderly. J Am Coll Nutr 1995;14:587—594.

207. Frischknecht R. Effect of training on muscle strength and motor function in the elderly. Reprod Nutr Dev 1998;38:167—174.

208. Frontera WR, Meredith CN, O'Reilly KP, Knuttgen HG, Evans WJ. Strength conditioning in older men: skeletal muscle hypertrophy and function. J Appl Physiol 1988;64:1038—1044.

209. Welsh L, Rutherford OM. Effects of isometric strength training on quadriceps muscle properties in over 55-year-olds. Eur J Appl Physiol Occ Physiol 1996;72:219—223.

210. Buchner DM, Cress ME, de Lateur BJ, Esselman PC, Margherita AJ, Price R et al. The effect of strength and endurance training on gait, balance, fall risk, and health services use in community-living older adults. J Gerontol Biol Sci 1997;52:M218—224.

211. Fiatarone MA, Marks EC, Ryan ND, Meredith CN, Lipsitz LA, Evans WJ. High-intensity strength training in nonagenarians. Effects on skeletal muscle. JAMA 1990;263:3029—3034.

212. Fiatarone MA, O'Neill EF, Ryan ND, Clements KM, Solares GR, Nelson ME et al. Exercise training and nutritional supplementation for physical frailty in very elderly people. N Engl J Med 1994;330:1769—1775.

213. Chandler JM, Duncan PW, Kochersberger G, Studenski S. Is lower extremity strength gain associated with improvement in physical performance and disability in frail, community-dwelling elders? Arch Phys Med Rehab 1998;79:24—30.

214. Connelly DM, Vandervoort AA. Effects of detraining on knee extensor strength and functional mobility in a group of elderly women. J Orthop Sports Phys Ther 1997;26:340—346.

215. Frontera WR, Meredith CN, O'Reilly KP, Evans WJ. Strength training and determinants of VO_2max in older men. J Appl Physiol 1990;68:329—333.

216. Freyssenet D, Berthon P, Denis C, Barthelemy JC, Guezennec CY, Chatard JC. Effect of a 6-week endurance training programme and branched-chain amino acid supplementation on histomorphometric characteristics of aged human muscle. Arch Physiol Biochem 1996;104:157—162.

217. Pickering GP, Fellmann N, Morio B, Ritz P, Amonchot A, Vermorel M et al. Effects of endurance training on the cardiovascular system and water compartments in elderly subjects. J Appl Physiol 1997;83:1300—1306.

218. Hiramatsu M, Velasco RD, Packer L. Decreased carbon centered and hydrogen radicals in skeletal muscle of vitamin E supplemented rats. Biochem Biophys Res Commun 1991;179:859—864.

219. Kondo H, Miura M, Itokawa Y. Oxidative stress in skeletal muscle atrophied by immobilization. Acta Physiol Scand 1991;142:527—528.

220. Reznick AZ, Witt E, Matsumoto M, Packer L. Vitamin E inhibits protein oxidation in skeletal muscle of resting and exercised rats. Biochem Biophys Res Commun 1992;189:801—806.

221. Meydani M, Evans WJ, Handelman G et al. Protective effect of vitamin E on exercise-induced oxidative damage in young and older adults. Am J Physiol 1993;264:R992—R998.

222. Weindruch R, Walford RL. The Retardation of Aging and Disease by Dietary Restriction. Springfield, IL: CC Thomas, 1988.

223. Yu BP (ed). Modulation of Aging Processes by Dietary Restriction. Boca Raton, FL: CRC Press, 1994.

224. Ingram DK, Cutler RG, Weindruch R, Renquist DM, Knapka JJ, April M et al. Dietary restriction and aging: The initiation of a primate study. J Gerontol Biol Sci 1990;45:B148—B163.

225. Kemnitz JW, Weindruch R, Roecker EB, Crawford K, Kaufman PL, Ershler WB. Dietary restriction of adult male rhesus monkeys: Design, methodology, and preliminary findings from the first year of study. J Gerontol Biol Sci 1993;48:B17—B26.

226. Weindruch R, Cheung MK, Verity MA, Walford RL. Modification of mitochondrial respiration by aging and dietary restriction. Mech Ageing Dev 1980;12:375—392.

227. Yu BP, Langaniere S, Kim J-W. Influence of life-prolonging food restriction on membrane lipo-peroxidation and antioxidant states. In: Simic MG, Taylor KA, Ward JF, von Sonntag T (eds) Oxygen Radicals in Biology and Medicine. New York: Plenum, 1989;1067—1073.
228. Laganiere S, Yu BP. Antilipoperoxidation action of food restriction. Biochem Biophys Res Commun 1987;145:1185—1191.
229. Chung MH, Kasai H, Nishimura S, Yu BP. Protection of DNA damage by dietary restriction. Free Radic Biol Med 1992;12:523—525.
230. Yu BP, Masoro EJ, Murata I, Bertrand HA, Lynd FT. Life span study of SPF Fischer 344 male rats fed ad libitum or restricted diets: longevity, growth, lean body mass and disease. J Gerontol 1982;37:130—141.
231. Solter D, Gearhart J. Putting stem cells to work. Science 1999;283:1468—1470.
232. Cartee GD, Bohn EE, Gibson BT, Farrar RP. Growth hormone supplementation increases skeletal muscle mass of old male Fischer 344/Brown Norway rats. J Gerontol Biol Sci 1996;51A: B214—219.
233. McCarter RJM, Masoro EJ, Yu BP. Rat muscle structure and metabolism in relation to age and food intake. Am J Physiol 1982;242:R89—93.
234. Weindruch R, Sohal RS. Caloric intake and aging. N Engl J Med 1997;337:986—994.
235. Wallace DC. Mitochondrial DNA in aging and disease. Sci Am 1997;277:40—47.

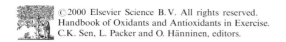

©2000 Elsevier Science B.V. All rights reserved.
Handbook of Oxidants and Antioxidants in Exercise.
C.K. Sen, L. Packer and O. Hänninen, editors.

Part X • Chapter 30

Molecular mechanisms of oxidative stress in aging: free radicals, aging, antioxidants and disease

Michael Pollack and Christiaan Leeuwenburgh

University of Florida, Aging Biochemistry Laboratory, Center for Exercise Science, College of Health and Human Performance, P.O. Box 118206, Gainesville, Florida 32611, USA. Tel.: +1-352-392-0584. E-mail: cleeuwen@ufl.edu

1 INTRODUCTION
2 SOURCES OF OXIDANTS
   2.1 Mitochondria
        2.1.1 Mitochondria and aging
   2.2 Phagocytes
        2.2.1 Phagocytes and aging
3 AGING AND ANTIOXIDANT DEFENSES
4 PROTEIN OXIDATION AND AGING
5 REPAIR AND TURNOVER OF OXIDATIVELY DAMAGED PROTEINS
6 PHYSIOLOGICAL RELEVANCE OF OXIDATION
7 LIFE-PROLONGING INTERVENTIONS
   7.1 Dietary restriction
   7.2 Chronic adapted exercise
   7.3 Antioxidant therapy
        7.3.1 Natural and synthetic antioxidants
8 ANTIOXIDANTS IN HUMAN HEALTH AND DISEASE
   8.1 Cardiovascular disease
   8.2 Neurodegenerative diseases
        8.2.1 Alzheimer's
        8.2.2 Parkinson's
9 SUMMARY
10 PERSPECTIVES
11 ACKNOWLEDGEMENTS
12 ABBREVIATIONS
13 REFERENCES

1 INTRODUCTION

The aging process has been shown to result in an accelerated functional decline. The exact mechanisms that cause this functional decline are unclear. The free radical theory of aging, however, has gained strong support because it is able to explain some of the processes that occur with aging and the degenerative diseases of aging. This theory proposes that an increase in oxygen radical production with age by mitochondria produce an increase in cellular damage [1–4].

Indeed, researchers have shown that oxygen utilization by mitochondria of aerobic organisms can generate several reactive radicals, such as superoxide (O_2^{-}), hydrogen peroxide (H_2O_2), and possibly hydroxyl radical ($HO^{\bullet}$; [5–7]).

In addition, nitric oxide (NO·) is also produced by mitochondria [8] and may have implications for the aging process and several disease states associated with aging. Phagocytes are another potent source of oxidant production, and they produce O_2^-, H_2O_2, HO·, NO·, and hypochlorous acid (HOCl; [7,9−10]). HOCl is an inflammatory mediator and a strongly oxidizing and chlorinating compound that can form other reactive metabolites, such as nitryl chloride (NO_2Cl) and nitrogen dioxide ($NO_2·$), in the presence of nitrite [11]. Recently, scientists have shown that activated human polymorphonuclear neutrophils convert nitrite into NO_2Cl and $NO_2·$ metabolites, which can significantly contribute to the formation of potentially harmful compounds [12]. The potentially deleterious effects of reactive oxygen, reactive nitrogen, and chlorinating species — for simplicity, referred to as oxidants or radicals — can affect the aging process.

Aerobic organisms are well-protected against oxidative challenges by sophisticated antioxidant defense systems. However, it appears that during the aging process an imbalance between oxidants and antioxidants balance may occur, referred to as oxidative stress. Oxidative stress induced by oxidant species occurs under conditions when antioxidant defenses are depleted or when the rate constants of the radical reactions are greater than the antioxidant defense mechanisms [13]. As we age the defense mechanisms preventing oxidation may decline in specific tissues, and accelerated oxidative damage could, therefore, trigger a deterioration in physiological function. We will critically look at this interrelationship.

Oxidative damage of biomolecules increases with age and is postulated to be a major causal factor of cellular biochemical senescence [14−20]. There is much support for this hypothesis, including the following observations: Studies by Sohal and coworkers using transgenic *Drosophila* in which the antioxidant enzymes, superoxide dismutase (SOD) and catalase (Cat) — two enzymes that scavenge the highly reactive oxidants, superoxide and hydrogen peroxide, respectively — are overexpressed this showed increases in the average and maximum life span and a reduction in oxidative damage [21,22]. Also, several aged species produce a significantly greater amount of reactive oxygen species compared to their younger counterparts [19,20,23]. Moreover, caloric restriction intervention, — that is, a restriction of 60% of the caloric intake of the ad libitum regimen without malnutrition — extends the life span of rodents by 40% [24,25]. In addition, other species such as invertebrates and fish also show remarkable increases in life span with caloric restriction [25−28]. The postulated mechanism is that a reduction in oxygen consumption, with a concomitant reduction in metabolic rate and body temperature in caloric restricted animals, lowered the chronic oxidative stress with age. In addition, caloric restriction also retards a variety of age-related deleterious biochemical and physiological changes, such as the development of cancer and diabetes [25,28]. Furthermore, caloric restriction attenuates protein oxidation, DNA damage, and lipid peroxidation in several housefly and animal models [21−30].

Other evidence that links oxidant generation and aging is provided by the strong inverse correlation between the rate of mitochondrial oxidant generation and the maximum life span among different species, i.e., animals with high mito-chondrial metabolism have a short life span since they have higher oxygen con-sumption and therefore higher oxidant production [27,28]. In addition, there is a strong correlation between maximum life span of a species and its SOD activity (the first defense against reactive oxygen species). For example, the activity of human SOD is approximately 16-fold greater than that of mice. The increase in SOD activity may provide more protection against superoxide radicals. This would strongly suggest that life span may, in part, depend on the activity of this enzyme [27,31].

We will review several potent sources of oxidant formation and the potentially deleterious effect of oxygen, nitrogen, and chlorinating species on cellular bio-molecules. The mitochondria and phagocytes will be highlighted in relationship to biological aging and selected diseases of aging.

2   SOURCES OF OXIDANTS

The oxygen molecule in its diatomic ground state ($^3\Sigma g^- O_2$) is essential for the production of energy. By itself it qualifies as a radical species since it has two unpaired electrons, each of which is located in a different π antibonding orbital. These two electrons also have parallel spins, i.e., they both share the same spin quantum number. Consequently, ground state oxygen is sparingly reactive: so far to oxidize O_2 another molecule by accepting an electron pair, both electrons would have to possess antiparallel spins relative to the unpaired electrons in O_2, according to Pauli's exclusion principle. This criterion is seldom met in a typical electron pair, so oxygen tends to accept electrons one at a time.

In vivo, multielectron reduction of O_2 is carried out by a coordinated series of enzymes that reduce O_2 1-electron at a time. If O_2 accepts a single electron, the electron must enter an antibonding orbital producing the superoxide radical O_2^-. Two-electron reduction of O_2, with the addition of $2H^+$, generates hydrogen peroxide (H_2O_2). Most O_2^- is metabolized by SOD to H_2O_2 and oxygen. In reactions catalyzed by free transition metals such as Fe^{2+}, O_2^- and H_2O_2 can generate the extremely reactive hydroxyl radical (HO·). This molecule is believed to be the major cause of damage to proteins, lipids, and DNA. Oxidative damage to these biomolecules seems to depend on hydrogen peroxide and a reduced tran-sition metal. Therefore, molecules that contain transition metals, such as aconi-tase (a Krebs cycle enzyme), are likely to undergo oxidative damage [17,18,32−34].

2.1 Mitochondria

The main function of mitochondria is energy production. During oxidative phos-phorylation, however, highly reactive oxygen radicals are generated. It has been estimated that the release of reactive intermediates accounts for about 2% of the oxygen consumed during respiration. One major site of oxidant production occurs in the mitochondrial electron transport chain in which O_2 is reduced to H_2O (Fig. 1). In this process, electrons from NADH are donated to complex I (NADH dehydrogenase complex), and electrons from succinate are donated to complex II (succinate dehydrogenase complex). Ubiquinone, also known as co-enzyme Q or UQ, accepts electrons from both complexes and is sequentially reduced, one electron at a time, to ubisemiquinone and ubiquinol. Ultimately, electrons are transferred through complex III (UQ-cytochrome c reductase), cytochrome c, and complex IV (cytochrome-c oxidase) with the result of reducing O_2 to H_2O. Mitochondrial electron transport, however, is imperfect and results in the production of O_2^- from the one-electron reduction of O_2. Some speculate that this electron comes from the free radical ubisemiquinone: instead of accepting another electron and proton to form ubiquinol, one of the electrons may leak from ubisemiquinone and reduce O_2 to O_2^-. Enzymatic dismutation of O_2^- then leads immediately to H_2O_2, another important biological oxidant [7].

How much O_2^- and H_2O_2 is generated during mitochondrial respiration? In state four respiration, which is characterized by a high degree of reduction of the electron carriers and a limiting supply of ADP, H_2O_2 production is at its maximum. It has been estimated that under these conditions the release of reactive intermediates accounts for 2% of the oxygen consumed during respiration [5].

Ultimately how much of this mitochondrial H_2O_2 is derived from dismutation of O_2^- in the electron transport chain? Measurement of O_2^- production cannot be accomplished in intact mitochondria because it is dismutated by mitochondrial SOD (mSOD). However, by isolating submitochondrial fractions and by removing mSOD by sonication and washing, it is possible to detect electron transport chain O_2^- production. In experiments done in the 1970s, it was found that submitochondrial particles produce from 4- to 7- nmol O_2^-/min per mg of protein, resulting in O_2^-/H_2O_2 ratios of 1.5–2.1 [6]. Since two O_2^- anions dis-

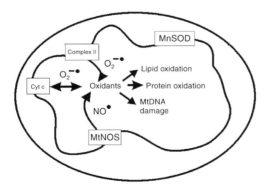

Fig. 1. Mitochondrial oxidant production; MnSOD: manganese superoxide dismutase; MtNOS: mitochondrial nitric oxide synthase.

mutate to form one H_2O_2 molecule, these results indicate that O_2^- is almost certainly a precursor of mitochondrial H_2O_2 (Fig. 1).

The enzyme nitric oxide synthase (NOS), which produces the free radical gas NO· from L-arginine, has been primarily investigated in endothelial cells. However, recent experiments have been performed which indicate that NOS in mitochondria produce NO· (Fig. 1). First, several studies using immunohistochemical techniques showed that skeletal muscle expresses endothelial-type nitric oxide synthase (ec-NOS). These studies also show that there is a strong correlation of ec-NOS expression to mitochondrial content visualized histochemically by succinate dehydrogenase [35]. In addition Bates et al. [36,37] have demonstrated localization of NO· synthase in mitochondria isolated from heart, skeletal muscle, kidney, and brain using a monoclonal antibody against the ec-NOS. Recently, mitochondria have been unambiguously identified as sources of NO·, using electron paramagnetic resonance with spin-trapping techniques. Giulivi et al. isolated NOS from Percoll-purified rat liver mitochondria [38]. Several different mitochondrial preparations, such as toluene-permeabilized mitochondria, mitochondrial homogenates, and a crude preparation of NOS, were incubated with the spin trap N-methyl-D-glucamine-dithiocarbamate-Fe II which produced a signal ascribed to the NO· spin adduct [8]. The intensity of the signal increased with time, protein concentration, and L-arginine, and decreased with the addition of the NOS inhibitor N^G-monomethyl-L-arginine. Kinetic parameters, molecular weight, requirement of cofactors, and cross-reactivity to monoclonal antibodies against macrophage NOS suggest similarities to the inducible form. However, the constitutive expression of this NOS enzyme and its membrane localization may indicate a distinctive isoform [8]. These findings suggest that mitochondrial NOS and NO· production may not only have an important role as a cellular transmitter, messenger, or regulator, but also as an active player in oxidative metabolism [8,34–38]. Since NO· and O_2^- react to produce another very reactive oxidant, peroxynitrite ($ONOO^-$), it is clear that mitochondria are a major source of free radicals and oxidants.

2.1.1 Mitochondria and Aging

Several studies have investigated if there is an age-associated increase in the generation of oxidants by mitochondria. An experiment using mongolian gerbils (*Meriones unguiculatus*) found that O_2^- and H_2O_2 production increased with age, especially in isolated mitochondria and submitochondrial particles from the aged heart [39]. In another study using whole hepatocytes of older rats, it was found that older hepatocytes had a decrease in the mitochondrial membrane potential of 30% and an increase in mitochondrial hydrogen peroxide generation of 23%. H_2O_2 levels within the liver cells were also increased [40]. Furthermore, another study on intact, isolated rat hepatocytes reached the same conclusion: cellular oxidant generation by mitochondria increases with age [41].

Similarly, experiments using intact muscle mitochondria from house flies has shown that the rate of H_2O_2 generation progressively increases 2-fold as the house fly ages [42]. On the other hand, an experiment which attempted to maintain proper physiological substrate concentrations during in vitro mitochondrial incubations detected no difference in H_2O_2 generation by rat heart mitochondria when comparing 24-month-old rats (senescent adults) and 6-month-old rats (young adults) [43].

The enhanced generation of oxidants by older mitochondria may itself be caused by oxidative damage to mitochondrial membranes and proteins. In one experiment, when isolated mitochondria were exposed to oxidant generators like glutaraldehyde (an intermolecular cross-linking agent) or 2,2-azobis-di-hydrochloride, the mitochondria generated H_2O_2 at an increased rate [42]. This evidence, along with the above studies, paints a vicious cycle of mitochondrial oxidant damage and oxidant generation.

In connection with such findings, Miquel and his colleagues [44,45] have widely promulgated the mitochondrial mutation theory of aging. In this theory, senescence is linked to mutations of mitochondrial DNA (mtDNA) in differentiated cells. As discussed earlier, isolated mitochondria from aged animals have an increased production of reactive oxygen species compared to young animals. This observation may be of key importance because it is likely to increase the rate at which proteins and DNA are oxidized. Since these mutations occur in postmitotic cells and mtDNA lacks excision and recombination repair mechanisms, it has been postulated that these mutations would lead to problems in replication, leading to a decline in physiological performance and the pathogenesis of many age-related diseases [44,45]. In addition, mtDNA is not protected by histones or DNA-binding proteins and, therefore, is directly exposed to a high steady-state level of reactive oxygen and nitrogen species. Thus, oxidative modification and mutation of mtDNA may occur with great ease. Mutations in mtDNA can lead to the production of less functional respiratory chain proteins, resulting in increased free radical production and possibly more mtDNA mutations. This vicious cycle operates in different tissues at variable rates and leads to differential accumulation of oxidatively modified mtDNA. This may ultimately reduce energy output and contribute to the common signs of normal aging.

In this context, one study by Yakes et al. [46] compared whether mtDNA accumulates more oxidative DNA damage relative to nuclear DNA; it also investigated whether there were differences in repair between nuclear and mtDNA. Specifically, the researchers investigated the formation and repair of H_2O_2-induced DNA damage in a 16.2 kb mitochondrial fragment and a 17.7 kb fragment flanking the β-globin gene. Fibroblasts treated with a relatively high dose of hydrogen peroxide exhibited 3-fold greater damage to the mitochondrial fragment compared with the nuclear fragment. Furthermore, damage to the nuclear fragment was completely repaired within 1.5 h; whereas, no DNA repair in the mitochondrial fragment was observed [46]. These data suggest that mtDNA is more susceptible to oxidants, and mitochondrial repair mechanisms may be nonexistent or less efficient.

2.2 Phagocytes

Phagocytic cells are another major source of oxidants. Neutrophils and other phagocytes attack pathogens using a mixture of oxidants – for example, O_2^-, $NO·$, H_2O_2, and HOCl. The process of phagocytosis begins when the neutrophil travels to a site of infection as directed by certain chemotactic signals that are generated at the infection site. When foreign microbes, which may be bound by serum-derived glycoproteins (i.e., opsonized), perturb the plasma membrane of a neutrophil, a dormant pyridine-nucleotide-dependent oxidase is activated. This pyridine nucleotide oxidase is believed to be a reduced nicotinamide adenine dinucleotide phosphate oxidase (NADPH oxidase) or a reduced nicotinamide adenine dinucleotide oxidase (NADH oxidase), whose action might involve a b type cytochrome [7,10]. This process initiates a "respiratory burst", which lasts for 15 to 20 min and reduces O_2 to O_2^- (a one-electron reduced product) and H_2O_2 (a two-electron reduced product). It also serves as the first source of oxidant production in phagocytes.

Simultaneously, the plasma membrane of the phagocyte invaginates around the foreign particle, surrounding it and subsequently pinching off to become a phagosome. Also during this time period, degranulation occurs: granular lysosomes migrate toward the phagosome, fuse with it, and empty their granular contents into it; after fusion with lysosomes, the phagosome becomes a phagolysosome. The contents of the lysosomes primarily include digestive enzymes like acid hydrolases, neutral proteases, and alkaline phosphatases. These lysosomes also contain cationic proteins, lipopolysaccharides, lactoferrin, myeloperoxidase (MPO), and biopolymers that might be involved in bactericidal reactions. This entire process occurs extremely rapidly taking no longer than a few minutes [7,10].

Inside the phagolysosome, the heme containing enzyme MPO forms an enzyme-substrate complex with H_2O_2 that can then catalyze the two-electron oxidation of halides like Cl^-, Br^-, and I^- by H_2O_2. The oxidation of the halides, particularly Cl^-, forms a toxic agent with potent antimicrobial properties. In the case of chloride, the oxidation product is HOCl, which subsequently kills the ingested microorganism. The H_2O_2 needed for this process is generated in the respiratory burst and can be detected in the phagosome [9]. Furthermore, a recent study on the MPO-hydrogen-peroxide-chloride system showed that MPO also generates Cl_2 gas and that human neutrophils employ chlorine gas as an oxidant during phagocytosis [47].

2.2.1 Phagocytes and aging

Currently it is unclear if there are age-associated trends in oxidant production by phagocytes. Age-dependent oxidant generation is relevant because it is very common for older individuals to suffer from inflammatory-related conditions such as arthritis. Some studies have indicated that oxidant production is a function of age; in fact, several experiments have shown that older macrophages produce a decreased amount of O_2^-, H_2O_2, NO· and other oxidants [48−50]. In a study on rat peritoneal macrophages by Alvarez et al., production of O_2^- was decreased by 50% and H_2O_2 by 75% in older macrophages [49]. NO· production was also reduced to 40% with age [48]. In a study done on human monocytes by Alvarez et al., they found that superoxide production was age and sex dependent. It decreased 45% in men and 70% in women during aging [51].

Other studies have shown that oxidant production is age-dependent, but in these studies the generation of reactive oxygen species appeared to increase with age. In a study by Lavie et al., they found a 2-fold increase in oxidant production by senescent peritoneal macrophages after being stimulated by latex and zymosan [52]. Also, a study on patients with obliterative atherosclerosis of the lower legs showed an increase in superoxide anion production by polymorphonuclear leukocytes (PMNLs) under basal conditions. After stimulating these PMNLs with formyl-methionin-leucyl-phenylalanine and calcium ionophore, the researchers found that the PMNLs of the atherosclerotic patients had an increased ability to release myeloperoxidase and elastase than PMNLs of healthy, middle-aged subjects [53]. Moreover, in a recent study there was an increased concentration of hydrogen peroxide, following stimulation by formyl peptide, in individual neutrophils from older volunteers (ages 65 and older) compared to neutrophils from younger volunteers (aged 21−34 years). By analyzing enzyme kinetics, the researchers concluded that the age-associated accumulation of H_2O_2 in stimulated neutrophils could be accounted for by impaired glutathione peroxidase (GPX) [54]. Further studies are warranted to investigate whether age causes an increase or decrease in oxidant production by PMNLs and whether aging-associated human diseases significantly affect oxidant production.

3   AGING AND ANTIOXIDANT DEFENSES

The possibility that oxidative stress and aging is mainly due to a decline in antioxidant defenses is still not clear. In fact, most researchers would argue that antioxidant defenses are, in general, not different between young and old animals. We will briefly discuss the general trends of several major organs, the effects of age on each of the major antioxidant systems, and the effect of selected antioxidants on age. This topic has been extensively reviewed by Matsuo [55], and we will discuss some of the general findings on the antioxidant enzymes − SOD, Cat, and GPX. We will also discuss the major trends involving the changes, if any, in water soluble and lipid soluble antioxidants, mainly focusing on vitamin C, GSH, and vitamin E, realizing that there are a multitude of other known and possibly unknown antioxidant defenses which may change with age.

SOD is a cytosolic (copper/zinc) and a mitochondrial (manganese) isoenzyme, which dismutates the superoxide radical to oxygen and hydrogen peroxide. The majority of the studies, which investigated total SOD activity in the brains of rats and mice, have found little change in the enzyme's activity with age [55].

(One study, in fact, actually found an increase in mitochondrial SOD activity in the brain of rats with age, which is not what one would expect if decreased antioxidant enzymes were a major factor in aging) [56]. Furthermore, the majority of the studies investigating the liver of mice also showed no change in total SOD. In contrast, many studies in rats showed a decrease in liver SOD activity [55]. This discrepancy is unclear, but could give an indication of variable adaptations between species. Most studies show that SOD activity in the heart of both mice and rats does not change with age [55]. Skeletal muscle SOD, however, does increase with age in old rats compared to either young or middle-aged rats (Table 1, [57—60]). Some of the inductions of SOD with age could reflect a chronic adaptation to the increase in superoxide production.

Gluthathione peroxidase is the major hydrogen peroxide scavenger enzyme, and it is found in both the cytosol and mitochondria. Together with its substrate GSH (discussed later), they form a formidable defense against hydrogen peroxides and lipid peroxides. Rat brain shows no change with age in this important reactive oxygen species scavenging enzyme [55]. Both the liver and the heart GPX show about an equal number of studies reporting either no change or a decrease in enzyme activity; thus, there is no consistent pattern of change with this enzyme [55]. Again, skeletal muscle GPX activity increased with age in rats, indicating an adaptive change to reduce oxidative stress in this tissue (Table 1 [57]).

Another H_2O_2 metabolizing enzyme is Cat. It metabolizes hydrogen peroxide to oxygen and water. This enzyme is primarily found in the peroxisomes, but it is also located, less abundantly, in mitochondria. The literature shows no consistent trend in changes of Cat activity in brain tissues with aging; an equal amount of studies show an increase or a decrease in activity [55]. This may reflect difficulties in the measurement of Cat activity. Cat activity in the liver seems to decline consistently in aging rats. In striking contrast, Cat activity increases in the heart and skeletal muscle of aging rats [55,57]. For example, Leeuwenbugh et al. found that skeletal muscle Cat activity increased by a large margin of 150% comparing 4.5-month-old rats with 26.5-month-old rats, and there was a 40% increase com-

Table 1. Activities of antioxidant enzymes in deep vastus lateralis (DVL) skeletal muscle of young and old rats [56].

	GPX DVL	CAT DVL	SOD DVL
Young	4.25 ± 0.29	15.8 ± 2.2	1960 ± 143
Adult	5.70 ± 0.34^a	29.4 ± 3.8^b	2190 ± 118
Old	5.88 ± 0.36^a	39.6 ± 4.2^b	2510 ± 120^a

Values are means ± SE; GPX: glutathione peroxidase; SOD: superoxide dismutase (units/g wet weight); CAT: catalase ($K \times 10^{-2}$/g wet weight); GSH: glutathione µmol/g wet weight; Young = 4.5 months; Adult = 14.5 months; Old = 26.5 months. $^ap < 0.05$, Adult or Old vs. Young; $^bp < 0.001$, Adult or Old vs. Young. (Adapted from [57].)

paring middle-aged animals (14.5 months) with the very old animals ([57] Table 1).

Vitamin C is a critical water soluble antioxidant interacting with GSH and vitamin E in maintaining a reduced intracellular environment [61]. This antioxidant shows a consistent decline with age in various species. For example, researchers from Sweden determined that the nucleus accumbens in 3-, 6- and 18-month-old Sprague-Dawley rats revealed a significant age-related decrease in basal extracellular vitamin C concentration [62]. Several studies show that there is a significant decline in vitamin C levels in the liver of rats [63,64]. Vitamin C content also decreases with age in toad skeletal muscle [65]. One complexity is that these data are difficult to translate to humans since humans lack the enzymes to synthesize vitamin C and are dependent on acquiring vitamin C from their diets. Many epidemiological studies clearly show that inadequate vitamin C levels correlate highly with diseases such as cancer and cataracts [14], providing cogent evidence that this antioxidant has strong anti-aging properties.

GSH (L-γ-glutamyl-L-cysteinyl-glycine; GSH) is a tripeptide (Fig. 2) found in virtually all animal cells. It is an important reducing agent that maintains enzyme activity and functions to maintain compounds like dehydroascorbate (vitamin C) and α-tocopherol (vitamin E, Fig. 3) in the reduced state.

GSH has several characteristics that determine its metabolism and antioxidant function. One is that glutamate and cysteine peptide linkage is linked through a γ-carboxyl group of glutamate instead of the more common α-carboxyl peptide linkage [66—68]. This unique characteristic makes the γ-carboxyl bond resistant to all peptidases except γ-glutamyltranspeptidase, which is bound to the external surface of the cell membrane. Therefore, GGT does not effect the intracellular breakdown of GSH [66—68]. Most importantly, the moiety of GSH is the cysteinyl reactive thiol group, which is responsible for many of the antioxidant functions of GSH metabolism (Fig. 2).

These characteristics, along with the fact that GSH is the most abundant non-protein thiol source and antioxidant in the cell, give GSH multiple functions for antioxidant defense, such as the following:

1) GSH provides a substrate for GSH peroxidase wherein GSH is used to reduce hydrogen and organic peroxides to water and alcohol;
2) GSH conjugates with harmful exogenous and endogenous toxic compounds;
3) GSH reduces disulfide linkage of proteins and other molecules maintaining glycolytic and antioxidant enzymes in the reduced state;

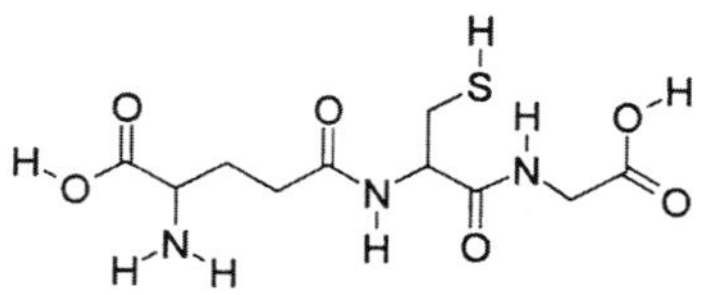

Fig. 2. Glutathione.

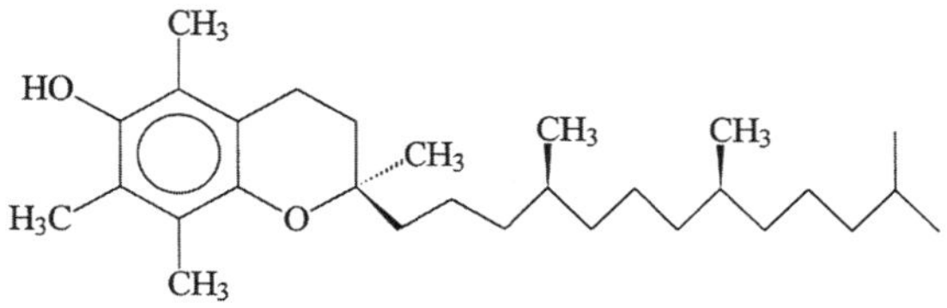

Fig. 3. Vitamin E.

4) GSH is a major thiol source maintaining essential redox status of the cell;
5) GSH is a major nontoxic storage form of cysteine providing a vehicle for transport between organs; and
6) GSH plays an important role in the reduction of ribonucleotides to deoxy-ribonucleotides [66–68].

There are several papers that discuss the effect of age and GSH levels. We will discuss some of the findings in brain, liver, heart, and skeletal muscle tissues. One study investigated GSH and several major antioxidant enzymes. In contrast to what one might expect, a significant increasing pattern of GSH content was found in the mice cerebellum and brain stem with age [69]. They also reported that mouse brain Cat activity did not show a significant change in any of the regions of the brain except in the cerebellum; whereas, SOD and GPX activity increased with age in most regions of the brain, suggesting that overall antioxidant defenses were not impaired with increasing age in mouse brain [69]. Most studies are in agreement that there is no significant decline in GSH concentration in the brain. Other reports found an increase [70] in GSH in the brain, while another found no change in GSH content in brains of senescent rats [71]. These studies reported increases in plasma, heart, and liver GSH concentration in old rats [70,71]. There are, however, some reports that show a decrease in brain GSH levels [72,73]. These studies found no change or an increase in liver GSH concentration [63,70,72,73]. Liver GSH is critical since it supplies GSH to all tissues. The liver contains the highest GSH concentration and continuously exports GSH to extrahepatic tissues.

GSH levels in skeletal muscle have also been investigated with age. Leeuwenburgh et al. found no difference in GSH concentration in deep vastus lateralis muscle and a significant increase in GSH content in the soleus muscle (Table 2 [57]), indicating that aging does not result in a significant decline in this antioxidant and that there are fiber-specific adaptations of the GSH system in skeletal muscle with age (Table 2).

These studies at least indicate that there is no overall decline of this important antioxidant. Some studies report increases in GSH content such as in skeletal muscle [57]; while others show reduction in GSH content such as in the eye lens [63]. Thus, in most tissues GSH is unlikely a limiting antioxidant for proper antioxidant protection with aging. In contrast, studies investigating subcellular components and changes of GSH content with age have found that GSH may decline

Table 2. Content the antioxidant glutathione (GSH) in deep vastus lateralis (DVL) and in soleus skeletal muscle of young and old rats (56).

	GSH DVL	GSH Soleus
Young	1.94 ± 0.21	2.10 ± 0.13
Adult	1.91 ± 0.16	2.64 ± 0.06
Old	1.76 ± 0.15	2.88 ± 0.11[a]

Values are means ± SE; GPX: glutathione peroxidase; SOD: superoxide dismutase (units/g wet weight); CAT: catalase ($K \times 10^{-2}$/g wet weight). GSH: glutathione µmol/g wet weight. Young = 4.5 months; Adult = 14.5 months; Old = 26.5 months. [a]$p < 0.001$, Adult or old vs. young (adapted from [57]).

with aging. One such study investigating GSH in rat cerebral cortex synaptosomes as a function of age found a decrease in GSH content [74]. Another study investigating mitochondrial GSH content showed a general decline in GSH levels with aging in rats and mice in the liver, kidney, and brain [75]. This would suggest that there may be differences in GSH content among compartments within cells during the aging process. These changes may not have been detected when looking at the overall levels of GSH in tissues in some of the previously selected studies. Therefore, there is a need to investigate specific organelles within the cell to determine changes in antioxidant levels.

The lipid soluble antioxidant vitamin E refers to at least eight structural isomers of tocopherol and tocotrienols [76–83]. Among these, RRR-α-tocopherol possesses the highest antioxidant activity. Vitamin E is often used to attenuate oxidative stress in many pathophysiological conditions [77–83]. For example, in an often-cited study by Stephens et al., patients with angiographically proven symptomatic coronary atherosclerosis who receive α-tocopherol treatment have a significantly diminished risk for cardiovascular disease. These patients show a substantial reduction in the rate of nonfatal MI after 1 year of vitamin E treatment [84].

As an antioxidant, vitamin E is important because of its ability to convert several free radicals such as superoxide, hydroxyl, and lipid peroxyl radicals into "repairable" radical forms [13,83]. Moreover, vitamin E is the primary antioxidant in cell membranes and often acts as a chain breaking antioxidant attenuating further lipid peroxidation [13,61,83]. Also, vitamin E has a relatively long biological half-life and has limited side effects even when administered in high doses [80–82]. When vitamin E scavenges a radical, a vitamin E radical is formed. This vitamin E radical is not capable of scavenging additional radicals but can be "recycled" back to its native state by several other antioxidants such as vitamin C [13,61,83]. Thus, investigators often use both vitamin E and vitamin C in an attempt to achieve maximal antioxidant protection.

We will discuss the major trends that occur during aging and their effects on vitamin E levels. One study investigated the antioxidant enzymes (SOD, Cat and

GPX activities) and vitamin E concentration in rats. They found little change in these antioxidant defense systems throughout the life span of the rats. In fact, vitamin E concentration in lung and liver tissues increased with age [85]. Moreover, concentrations of tocopherols in selected areas of rat brains increased significantly with age in the medulla and spinal cord, with no changes in other regions of the brain [86]. Heart vitamin E did not decline in this study [86]. De et al. found that plasma levels of vitamin E and ascorbic acid decreased in serum, but there were no changes in liver concentration [64]. In another study, serum vitamin E increased markedly with age, but there was little change in membrane vitamin E content in ad libitum fed rats [87]. Sawada et al. reported no significant changes in blood vitamin E levels with age in rats [88].

In general, there is no dramatic overall decline with age of the major antioxidant defense systems or a decline in vitamin E concentration in ad libitum fed animals. In fact, some tissues actually show significant increases of vitamin E in senescence animals and upregulations of antioxidant enzymes, for example, in skeletal muscle [57]. Vitamin C shows a general decline with aging, which may not be relevant to humans since vitamin C concentration in humans is entirely dependent on dietary vitamin C intake. Lower concentrations of vitamin C in most tissues with age could partly explain the increase in oxidative damage which occur during in vitro oxidative challenges. Researchers often challenge tissues of young and old rats with free radicals in vitro and these studies often show that tissues from old animals are more susceptible to free radical damage than tissues from young animals [39,89,90].

Another potentially protective antioxidant in brain tissues is melatonin, and it is probably more influential than vitamin C in affecting the outcome of in vivo oxidative challenges in the brain. The brain rapidly takes up this pineal hormone, which declines with advancing age. Melatonin is more effective than GSH in scavenging the highly toxic hydroxyl radical in in vitro experiments, and it also has been found to be more efficient than vitamin E in neutralizing the peroxyl radical [91]. Besides melatonin, there may be a plethora of other potent antioxidants and antioxidant systems present. Alterations in these systems could have far greater relevance than vitamin E, vitamin C, and the primary antioxidant enzyme systems.

4   PROTEIN OXIDATION AND AGING

During the aging process, protein oxidation is increased in a wide variety of human and animal tissues. The exact pathways for oxidative cellular damage are poorly understood because the reactive metabolites are very short-lived and difficult to detect directly in vivo. The quantification of oxidative damage to proteins has been studied almost exclusively by assessing the total carbonyl content [92,93]. The oxidants responsible for carbonyl formation within the proteins in vivo are believed to be radicals, such as, hydroxyl radicals. Indeed, hydroxyl radicals can be generated by metal-catalyzed oxidation systems [18,89,94,95], and different metal-catalyzed oxidation systems convert several amino acid residues to carbonyl derivatives [18,89,94,95].

The assessment of protein oxidation using the reactive protein carbonyl assay does provide a good indication of overall oxidation; however, it also reflects covalent adduct formation from lipid peroxidation products [96]. Moreover, several oxidative pathways and products from lipid peroxidation and glycooxidation can generate carbonyls from proteins [96—99]. These pathways consist of both oxidative and nonoxidative pathways besides metal catalyzed oxidation, and they are efficient in generating reactive protein-carbonyls [96—99]. The oxidants and non-oxidant modifications are generated by HOCl, peroxynitrite, aldehydes, glucose, ribose, and the strongly oxidizing enzyme myeloperoxidase [96—99].

There is a large amount of literature available which clearly shows a consistent increase in protein-bound carbonyls with advanced age and in several degenerative diseases of aging. We will discuss some of these findings. For example, protein-bound carbonyls are present at low levels in dermal fibroblasts isolated from young to middle-aged humans, but they are increased 2-fold in fibroblasts from people over 60 years of age [100]. Furthermore, there are age-related increases in the carbonyl content of proteins in human brain [101], gerbil brain [102], rat hepatocytes [103], and in flies [104]. These studies show a consistent pattern of increasing protein oxidation in old age.

Recently, other radical species, besides the hydroxyl radical, have been implicated in oxidative protein damage. Radicals, such as NO· are implicated in several disease states such as cardiovascular disease and neurodegenerative diseases, but few studies to date have investigated the role of NO· on protein oxidation and aging. Since NO· is the only biological molecule produced in high enough concentrations to out-compete SOD for superoxide — consequently reacting with superoxide to form $ONOO^-$ — it could be a very relevant compound in aging.

Some studies investigating the deleterious effects of NO· metabolites and aging suggest that certain proteins are oxidized selectively in vivo. This may be possible because $ONOO^-$, formed from NO· and superoxide, reacts relatively slowly with most biological molecules, which makes it a selective oxidant [105—107]. $ONOO^-$ modifies tyrosine in proteins and generates 3-nitrotyrosines, a fairly specific marker detectable in vivo. For example, the level of nitration of the SERCA2a isoform of calcium-ATPase in sarcoplasmic reticulum vesicles isolated from rat skeletal muscle increases with age; there are approximately one and four nitrotyrosine residues per young and old Ca-ATPase, respectively [108]. In addition, nitration was undetectable in a closely related form of the protein [109], which strongly suggests that certain calcium-ATPases are selectively modified by reactive nitrogen species. In vitro studies suggest that this level of protein oxidation may alter the function of SERCA2a in vivo [109]. These observations raise the possibility that specific proteins accumulate oxidative damage during aging. Therefore, it is plausible that an increases in NO· and/or superoxide production with age, in mitochondria could become deleterious to mitochondrial respiratory enzymes.

In a recent study, very specific and sensitive analytical methods were used to measure the levels of some of these "fingerprints" of oxidative damage in tissue proteins of aging rats [110,111]. We found that specific markers for protein oxidation, such as o-tyrosine (a marker for hydroxyl radicals) and 3-nitrotyrosine (a marker for reactive nitrogen species) do not increase in skeletal muscle, heart, and liver of aging rats. This suggests that proteins damaged by hydroxyl radical and reactive nitrogen do not accumulate with aging in these tissues. This was surprising because previous studies using non-specific measures had suggested that proteins damaged by hydroxyl radical accumulate in the tissues of old animals. This study does strongly suggest that hydroxyl radical and reactive nitrogen species damage proteins during biological aging; however, the accumulation of these amino acids may have been prevented by removal mechanisms for these markers in these specific tissues [110]. Thus, proteolytic degradation of intracellular proteins may account in part for the relatively constant level of amino acid oxidation products seen in this study. Also, since the average level of protein oxidation in tissue was measured, it may have missed detecting a marked increase in protein oxidation in a few selected proteins or in specific organelles such as the mitochondria.

Protein oxidation and protein nitration has been also detected in Progeria's disease and in several other human disease states. Fibroblasts obtained from patients with diseases of accelerated aging (Progeria or Werner's syndrome) have dramatically higher levels of protein carbonyls [100] compared to that of age-matched controls. Leeuwenburgh et al. [112] and Beckman et al. [113] found that nitrated proteins are abundant in low density lipoproteins (LDL) and plaque isolated from patients with atherosclerosis. In these studies it is unclear whether peroxynitrite or other reactive nitrogen species were responsible for tyrosine nitration. Peroxynitrite is a source of hydroxyl radical-like species, but also of nitrogen dioxide. It is nitrogen dioxide that most likely has the ability to directly oxidize proteins and other macromolecules in vitro. Other pathways that generate reactive nitrogen species are mediated by myeloperoxidase and may be responsible for tyrosine nitration [11,12].

Peroxynitrite has also been implicated in neurodegenerative diseases and the generation of carbonyls from side-chain and peptide-bond cleavage. It also nitrates tyrosine residues. In brain tissue from patients with Alzheimer's disease, scientists found increased 3-nitrotyrosine in neurons including neurofibrillary tangles, whereas 3-nitrotyrosine was undetectable in the cerebral cortex of age-matched control brains [114]. In Alzheimer's brain, using in situ 2,4-dinitrophenylhydrazine labeling linked to an antibody system, Smith et al. describes protein-bound carbonyl reactivity [115]. Tissues from disease-related, intraneuronal lesions and other neurons showed significant increases in reactive carbonyls. In striking contrast, carbonyls were not found in neurons or glia in age-matched control cases. They concluded that oxidative stress is a key element in the pathogenesis of Alzheimer's disease. These findings strongly suggest that reactive oxygen species and possibly peroxynitrite are involved in the oxidative damage of

Alzheimer's disease.

In subjects with Parkinson's disease, protein carbonyls were assessed in post-mortem brain tissue and age-matched controls. In brain areas associated with Parkinson's, such as the substantia nigra, caudate nucleus, and the putamen, there was a significant increase in protein-bound carbonyl levels [116]. Other markers of protein oxidation are also affected with amyotrophic lateral sclerosis. Researchers investigated amyotrophic lateral sclerosis and found elevated levels of free 3-nitrotyrosine [117].

In summary, these results suggest that levels of oxidized proteins increase with age and in several neurodegenerative aging-associated diseases. Metal-catalyzed oxidation reactions could be partly responsible for protein oxidation; however, there are multitudes of other oxidative reactions, which can generate protein carbonyls and other oxidative modifications in proteins and amino acids. Reactive nitrogen species could nitrate proteins and have major physiological consequences on normal protein function. Thus, reactive metabolites from oxygen and nitrogen metabolism could be active players in aging and the degenerative diseases of aging.

5 REPAIR AND TURNOVER OF OXIDATIVELY DAMAGED PROTEINS

Oxidative damage repair mechanisms are a critical component in maintaining intracellular homeostasis. Oxidative DNA damage, which forms unnatural adducts, can be removed by a variety of mechanisms including endonucleases and glycosylases [83,118]. Protein damage will be recognized by specific proteases and degradation will follow [17,18,83]. Oxidized lipids can be repaired or removed by the GSH-GPX systems or by phospholipases [13,83,118,119]. We will briefly discuss the interplay between several factors underlying the accumulation and removal of oxidized proteins and oxidized amino acids in the cell.

In general, the level of oxidized proteins in a tissue reflects the balance between the relative rates of protein oxidation and clearance. For example, lens or collagen proteins turn over extremely slowly and thus, should accumulate products of oxidative damage over time. In contrast, intracellular proteins in liver and muscle turnover continuously with half-lives ranging from a few hours to $7-10$ days, since a mechanism exists for the continuous removal of these oxidized proteins. In general, one can predict that the accumulation of oxidized proteins is dependent upon the balance between pro-oxidant, antioxidant, and removal mechanisms. The interactions between several of these components are depicted schematically (Fig. 4).

Isolated mitochondria from old animals showed increased production of reactive oxygen species compared to young animals. This observation may be of key importance because it is likely to increase the rate at which proteins are oxidized. Thus, the significant age-related increases in the generation of superoxide and hydrogen peroxide by mitochondria in various tissues may have led to an increased accumulation of oxidized proteins observed by many researchers. Also, species-specific differences in metabolic rate may exist and could also influence the formation of oxidized macromolecules differently. Other factors affecting protein oxidation include changes in tissue specific antioxidant defenses with age (discussed in previous sections), which either, decline modestly, show no change, or increase. A final factor that may affect the accumulation and the removal of oxidized proteins are several proteolytic systems.

Starke-Reed, Stadtman and co-workers [17,103] have performed several pioneering studies addressing how proteins are oxidized and subsequently proteolytically degraded and how these systems may change with age. They found that with age there is less efficient removal of oxidized proteins through proteolytic cleavage, which may cause the accumulation of protein carbonyls with aging [17,103]. Several proteolytic enzymes responsible for degrading oxidized proteins decline with age in tissues [17,103]. These proteases rapidly degrade oxidized enzymes but do not effect native unoxidized enzymes. Several multicatalytic proteases provide

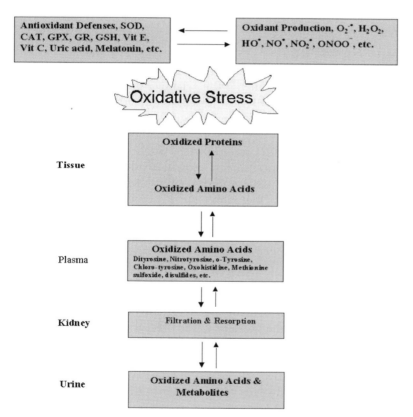

Fig. 4. Several distinct aspects of free radical biology eventually determine the accumulation of oxidized proteins: 1) oxidant production, 2) antioxidant protection, 3) oxidative damage, 4) repair of oxidative damage, and 5) removal of oxidative damage.

major intracellular pathways for protein degradation [120—129]. Recently, Cuervo and Dice discussed various proteolytic systems, such as ubiquitin-proteasome, calpain pathways, and multiple lysosomal pathways and the effect of age [120].

The existence of specific mitochondrial proteolytic systems that can recognize and degrade oxidatively damaged proteins is currently under investigation [121]. Investigators have found that mitochondria have their own proteolytic system, probably because the mitochondria possess both an inner and outer membrane, making them quite impermeable (especially the inner membrane) to cytosolic proteases and peptidases [121]. The presence of a mitochondrial proteolytic system indicates the need for removal of oxidized proteins and amino acids from the mitochondria. There is little known about the removal of oxidized proteins from mitochondria, but it is likely that small peptides and unnatural oxidized amino acids are removed. It is feasible that unnatural oxidized amino acids in mitochondria, such as o,o'-dityrosine (see section 6), are recognized and proteolytically removed, after which they are released into the plasma and then excreted into the urine. One indication of this possibility is provided by a study of Guilivi and Davies [129].

These scientists found that one such oxidation product, o,o'-dityrosine produced in red blood cells, was released after being exposed to a continuous flux of hydrogen peroxide [129]. The proteasome macroxyproteinase appears to be responsible for o,o'-dityrosine release during the selective degradation of oxidatively modified proteins [129]. We will now discuss how to monitor specific unnatural amino acids as markers for protein oxidation and turnover.

We have used gas chromatography and mass spectrometry (GC-MS) for the determination of unnatural oxidized amino acids, such as dityrosine. This approach could be very useful in monitoring protein oxidation and turnover. This analytical technique can detect trace amounts of unnatural oxidized amino acids, and it aids in identifying and elucidating the structure of unknown, new molecules. This approach can monitor stable end products such as o-tyrosine, m-tyrosine, o,o'-dityrosine, 3-chlorotyrosine and 3-nitrotyrosine using a combination of stable isotope dilution GC-MS [47,110—112,130].

Several oxidized amino acids and their oxidative pathways are depicted in Fig. 5. The hydroxyl radical (HO·) converts phenylalanine to o-tyrosine and m-tyrosine ([130]; Fig. 5). Another important free radical mechanism involves protein oxidation by tyrosyl radicals. Tyrosyl radicals can be generated by hydroxyl radicals, as well as by peroxidases and other heme proteins in the presence of hydrogen peroxide and tyrosine [130]. This reaction generates tyrosyl radicals which can cross-link tyrosine-residues on proteins to form protein-bound o,o'-dityrosine, an unnatural isomer and stable end-product of protein oxidation. Another potential mechanism for protein oxidation involves NO•, a long-lived radical that plays a critical role in cellular signaling and cytotoxic host defense mechanisms [131]. The interaction of NO• with superoxide yields peroxynitrite. Protonated peroxynitrite rapidly decomposes to generate several other reactive nitrogen species, including the nitronium ion (NO_2^+) and nitrogen dioxide ($NO_2^·$) [132]. Reactive

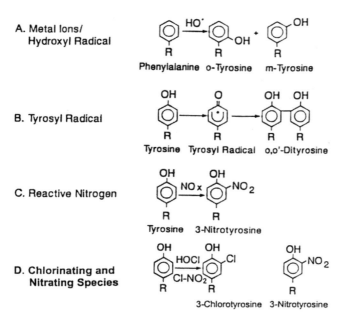

A. Metal Ions/ Hydroxyl Radical

Phenylalanine   o-Tyrosine   m-Tyrosine

B. Tyrosyl Radical

Tyrosine   Tyrosyl Radical   o,o'-Dityrosine

C. Reactive Nitrogen

Tyrosine   3-Nitrotyrosine

D. Chlorinating and Nitrating Species

3-Chlorotyrosine   3-Nitrotyrosine

Fig. 5. Formation of unnatural amino acids. Reaction pathways for the oxidation of protein-bound aromatic amino acids by (**A**) hydroxyl radical (HO•), (**B**) tyrosyl radical, (**C**) reactive nitrogen intermediates (NOx), such as peroxynitrite, and (**D**) hypochlorous acid (HOCl) and the recent discovered gas nitryl chloride (Cl-NO2). HO• reacts with phenylalanine residues in proteins to generate o-tyrosine and m-tyrosine (**A**), unnatural tyrosine isomers. Following a hydrogen abstraction, tyrosine becomes a highly reactive tyrosyl radical (**B**). Two tyrosyl radicals can cross-link to generate o,o'-dityrosine (**B**). The interaction of nitric oxide (NO•) with superoxide yields peroxynitrite (ONOO-). Protonated peroxynitrite rapidly decomposes to generate several other reactive nitrogen species, including the nitronium ion (NO2+) and nitrogen dioxide (NO2•) to generate 3-nitrotyrosine (**C**). Hypochlorous acid generates 3-chlorotyrosine and nitryl chloride (Cl-NO2) forms both 3-nitrotyrosine and 3-chlorotyrosine.

nitrogen species derived from NO• generate 3-nitrotyrosine in vitro and in vivo (Fig. 5). Moreover, scientists have recently shown that nitrite and HOCl present in physiological concentrations generate several nitrating and chlorinating species [11,12]. These in vitro studies demonstrate that the intermediate product nitryl chloride (CL-NO2) may well be of greater physiological importance than peroxynitrite (ONOO⁻) in protein modification [11,12]. Moreover, interactions of carbon dioxide-catalyzed oxidation of tyrosine by peroxynitrite may also be relevant in oxidative injury [133,134] (Fig. 5).

It is unclear yet if the unnatural amino acids generated by these oxidative pathways could be incorporated into cytosolic or mitochondrial proteins and thus interfere with normal physiological functions. The structures of the unnatural amino acids are very similar to their native forms making this a strong possibility (Fig. 5). However, these products have been detected in biological tissues under normal and pathophysiological conditions. For example, Wells-Knecht et al.

found that there were no significant changes in levels of *o*-tyrosine in human eye lens with age. In contrast, there was a significant increase in dityrosine in lens proteins of approximately 33% between the age of 1 and 78 [135]. Also, Leeuwen-burgh et al. found increases in skeletal muscle and heart dityrosine content in mice with age and showed that caloric restriction attenuated this increase [136].

3-nitrotyrosine has been detected in a variety of disease states such as cardio-vascular disease and in neurodegenerative diseases [112—114,117]. 3-chlorotyro-sine was detected by Hazen and Heinecke in human atherosclerotic lesions indi-cating that chlorinating reactions catalyzed by the myeloperoxidase system of phagocytes were one pathway for protein oxidation in vivo [137]. Thus, these spe-cific products can be used as markers for specific oxidation pathways in vivo.

In a recent study, we supplemented rats with specific antioxidants and found a significant reduction of protein-bound *o,o'*-dityrosine in skeletal muscle by approximately 50%. In contrast, antioxidant therapy minimally affected *o*-tyrosine levels in this tissue. Levels of the oxidized amino acids in urine samples mirrored those of skeletal muscle proteins. The antioxidant therapy produced a striking 50% decline in *o,o'*-dityrosine levels but barely changed *o*-tyrosine levels. Quantification of the levels of oxidized amino acids in urine may thus serve as an integrated, noninvasive measure of oxidative stress in vivo because they change in parallel with levels of protein-bound oxidized amino acids in skeletal muscle (Fig. 4) [138].

6 PHYSIOLOGICAL RELEVANCE OF OXIDATION

Since oxidative stress has been shown to have important implications in the aging process, it is beneficial to understand the role oxidants play in several selected physiological processes. That is, how do reactive oxygen species modify the func-tion of a biochemical system? and what mechanisms are involved in this change of function?

One interesting example concerns the effects of oxidation on cell surface recep-tors. Research on the transferrin receptor regulation process showed that free radical-induced oxidative stress generated by menadione, a known free radical inducer, was capable of rapidly downmodulating the membrane transferrin receptor due to blocking the recycling of the receptor on the cell surface. It is believed that the mechanism underlying such a change is related to the thiol group oxidation of cytoskeletal proteins and the disruption of calcium homeo-stasis, both of which are caused by menadione [139].

In another study on receptors, it was found that human erythrocyte insulin receptor processing was similarly impaired by menadione-induced oxidative stress. Insulin-induced downregulation is a model used to investigate cell surface regulative phenomena and how such processes are affected by the plasma mem-brane and the cytoskeleton. It was found that free radical-induced damage decreased the insulin-induced downregulation process, as measured by binding assays. In addition, there were slight alterations in the ultrastructure of the plasma membrane due to oxidative damage, but there were significant alterations in the cytoskeletal protein assembly. It is hypothesized that modifications in specific cytoskeletal elements by oxidative stress could lead to the observed decrease in the insulin-induced downregulation process. This hypothesis is supported by the fact that there were changes in the electrophoretic pattern of cytoskeletal proteins like spectrin [140].

In another study, it was observed that oxidative-induced stress to K562 cells altered the microfilament system and the microtubular network. The researchers hypothesized that oxidative imbalance modified the cytoskeleton, leading to impairment of the expression of receptors [141]. These cases are theorized to be specific examples of a more general mechanism in which the expression of cell surface receptors and their recycling are impaired by oxidant-induced modification of the cytoskeleton and intracellular molecules.

Moreover, modification of tyrosine residues in receptor molecules has been shown to impair signaling pathways. For example, a specific modification, such as nitration of a tyrosine residue would compromise one of the most important mechanisms of cellular regulation, the cyclic interconversion between the phosphorylated and unphoshorylated form of tyrosine [142]. This possibility is underscored by the demonstration that nitration of tyrosine residues in model substrates prevents the phosphorylation of these residues by protein tyrosine kinases [143,144]. It is postulated that the nitration of tyrosine residues is an irreversible process and can, therefore, lock the enzyme into a relatively inactive form.

A specific example concerns the platelet-derived growth factor (PDGF) receptor. This receptor has five known tyrosine autophosphorylation sites. Mutations in specific tyrosine residues in the receptor — e.g., tyrosines 1009 and 1021 — prevent the binding and activation of phosopholipase C-γ (PLC-γ), an important signaling protein. If PLC-γ does not bind to the tyrosine residues, then the inositol phospholipid signaling pathway is not activated [145]. Thus, a site-specific modification of a single amino acid by an oxidant could result in the decline of a protein's activity.

There are many other physiological effects of reactive oxygen species. For example, the free radical gas NO$^{\bullet}$ has been shown to have a wide variety of biological effects, including the ability to act as an inhibitor of mitochondrial electron transport [146]. Furthermore, NO$^{\bullet}$ binds reversibly to cytochrome oxidase and can completely inhibit mitochondrial oxygen consumption [146]. Another example concerns mitochondrial aconitase, a key enzyme in the citric acid cycle, which is a major target of superoxide and peroxynitrite mediated disruption of the (4Fe-4S) prosthetic group. This results in significant losses of aconitase activity [32—34]. Interestingly, aconitase activity declines as a function of age [147]. Therefore, oxidation may be a mechanism by which enzyme function declines with age.

7   LIFE-PROLONGING INTERVENTIONS

Since free radical reactions are postulated as a major cause of aging and degenerative diseases, much research has been done to develop life-prolonging interventions to slow down these chemical reactions. We will discuss several intervention therapies and their effect on attenuating oxidative stress and increasing life span.

7.1 Dietary restriction

Laboratory observations that rats on caloric-restricted diets live longer has been confirmed in a series of studies that show an inverse relationship between caloric intake and life span in mice. Restricting the caloric intake of rats by 30 to 60 percent has led to remarkable increases in the average life span and the maximal life span by similar amounts [148,149]. In one study, after decreasing the caloric intake of rats by 40% while maintaining normal levels of micronutrients, the average life span of the rats increased by 40% and the maximum life span by 49% [150].

In another study, groups of mice were fed different amounts of calories beginning one month after birth. There was a direct proportional relationship between the degree of caloric restriction (up to the point of frank starvation) and the increase in average and maximal life spans. Restricting calories in middle-aged mice (12 months) also resulted in an increased life span, but to a lesser degree. This finding refuted the contention that caloric restriction increased life spans by extending the developmental period [151].

A study was done comparing the concentrations of markers for oxidative damage (*o,o'*-dityrosine and *o*-tyrosine) between mice that had access to unlimited calories with those that were restricted to 60% of the caloric intake of the ad libitum regimen. In mice fed ad libitum, levels of *o,o'*-dityrosine increased with age in cardiac and skeletal muscle but not in liver or brain, and levels of *o*-tyrosine did not rise with age in any of the tissues examined. Caloric restriction prevented the increase in *o,o'*-dityrosine levels in cardiac and skeletal muscle but this did not influence *o*-tyrosine levels in any of the four tissues. Thus, caloric restriction was shown to attenuate an increase in certain aging markers vs. a regimen of ad libitum caloric intake [136].

Why does reducing caloric intake result in longer life spans and decreased oxidative damage? First, it is important to note that $2-3\%$ of the oxygen consumed by mammals is believed to result in the generation of superoxide anion and H_2O_2. Since decreased food intake results in proportionally less oxygen being utilized in mitochondrial respiration, reducing caloric intake will also result in less free radical generation. In support of this theory, there have been repeated findings that dietary restriction depresses body temperature, and a decrease in body temperature indicates a reduced rate of oxygen consumption [152]. For example, in caloric restricted mice housed at room temperature $(20-22°C)$, it was found that their body temperature cycles from $\sim 37°C$ to $23°C$ to $27°C$ daily [153]. The body temperature in caloric restricted rats also decreases, but by lesser amounts [154]. Moreover, a study by Lane et al. found that a 30% reduction in calories (compared with age-matched monkeys feeding ad libitum) decreased core (rectal) body temperature in rhesus monkeys by $\sim 0.5°C$ [155].

Harman, who proposed the free radical theory of aging in 1954, believes that food restriction increases life span by decreasing free radical reaction initiation rates [156]. Since less free radicals are generated, there will be less injury to the mitochondria and their DNA, which overall should reduce aging and age-associated diseases. For example, one study on the effects of caloric restriction on the rates of mitochondrial superoxide anion generation and hydrogen peroxide production in the brains of mice showed that O_2^- and H_2O_2 generation were reduced in the caloric restricted rats by 50% or more [157].

Alternatively, caloric restriction may cause more efficient electron transport chain coupling, resulting in less leakage of electrons and therefore a decreased generation of oxidants. Moreover, the beneficial effects of caloric restriction also involve increased antioxidant defenses. Lifelong caloric restriction increased the expression of SOD and Cat in liver tissue from 18-month-old rats; that is, there were higher mRNA levels and higher rates of nuclear transcription for SOD and Cat in the dietary restricted animals [158]. Similarly, another study found that dietary restriction (40% restriction of intake) in male Fischer F344 rats increased the activities of SOD by 24—38% and Cat by 64—75% in liver at 21 and 28 months of age. Also, at 28 months of age, GPX activity in the liver of caloric restricted rats was 37% higher than rats fed ad libitum [159]. These findings indicate an overall upregulation of antioxidant defenses.

Others believe that decreased food intake serves to lower the metabolic rate, which has been shown to be inversely proportional to life span in studies on mammals and cold-blooded animals. Two studies have found that the metabolic rate decreased in rhesus monkeys and rats after a lengthy period of caloric restriction [160, 161], but such findings were not confirmed in a third study [162]. In fact, in a study in which the metabolic rate of rats on an ad libitum diet was kept the same as those on restricted diets, the researchers found major increases in life span among the rats on a restricted diet without a decrease in metabolic rate [150,163].

Another hypothesis holds that caloric restriction increases longevity by slowing the rate of cell division in many tissues. Given that cancer is defined as the uncontrolled proliferation of cells, decreased cell division provides an explanation why the incidence of late-life lymphomas, breast, and prostate cancers is dramatically reduced in caloric restricted rats [28,164,165]. Alternatively, some argue that the longevity-increasing effects of caloric restriction are due to the fact that caloric restriction reduces glucose levels. Decreased blood glucose levels result in less sugar being accumulated on long-lived proteins, which reduces the overall deleterious buildup of glycoxidation products [166].

7.2 Chronic adapted exercise

Another potent life-prolonging intervention is regular physical exercise. Numerous studies have been done which show that regular exercise reduces aging changes and increases average life expectancy modestly (approximately 9% in rats) [167], but this leaves the maximum life span unchanged. On the other hand, acute exercise may result in increased oxidative stress since more O_2 is consumed. More oxygen consumption results in an increased generation of oxidants from electron leakage in the mitochondrial electron transport chain. In fact, overtraining is known to be injurious to organisms and can result in muscle damage, in the form of decreased mitochondrial respiratory control, increased levels of markers of protein oxidation, and the loss of the structural integrity of sarcoplasmic reticulum [168].

Protection from exercise-induced oxidative stress has been achieved in rats by diligent endurance training. Quintanilha and Packer, working with Bantin-Kingman female rats, found that endurance training raised the levels of antioxidant enzymes in both skeletal and cardiac muscle [169]. Leeuwenburgh et al. found that a 10-week exercise training program increased GPX and SOD activities in the deep portion of the deep vastus lateralis muscle (DVL) in young rats [170]. In another study, Leeuwenburgh et al. found that endurance trained rats had a 33% increased GSH content in DVL. They also found that trained rats had a 62% higher GPX activity and 27% higher SOD activity [171]. Therefore, although exercise results in increased oxidant levels, long-term exercise counters this effect by increasing the activity of antioxidants and antioxidant enzymes.

The following is a typical example of the moderating effects of physical exercise on aging. This study examined the effect of exercise on the tendons of male Sprague-Dawley rats, from 5 to 23 months of age. After training these rats in a treadmill, the researchers compared their tail tendons to those of a sedentary group. Overall, the tail tendon collagen of the exercise group had a lower thermal stability, and other biomechanical parameters with respect to maximum stress were also lowered in the trained group. Thus, it was concluded that physical exercise deterred aging effects on rat connective tissue [172].

Previous studies have found that male rats given access to voluntary wheel running showed an increase in average life span. However, since the male runners did not increase their food intake, it was not possible to determine whether the longevity-increasing effect was due to less energy being available for cell growth and proliferation or whether another exercise effect was involved. A study by Holloszy resolved the issue by studying female rats, who increase their caloric intake in response to wheel running. The female runners ate approximately 20% more (37% more from 5 to 10 months of age) than the sedentary rats, with both groups attaining similar peak body weights. The runners had a statistically significant increase in average life span without an increase in maximal life span, which shows that exercise can increase the average life span of rats independent of the concomitant decease in energy availability for cell activities [173].

7.3 Antioxidant therapy

Since free radical damage to biological molecules has been implicated as the primary cause of aging, many attempts have been made to attenuate free radical reactions through exogenous antioxidants. By abating these harmful reactions, scientists theorized that aging-associated diseases and the aging process itself would be slowed down, ultimately extending life span. Table 3 summarizes a selection of interventions and their effect on median and maximum life span [21,22,29,174–181] (Table 3).

Antioxidant enzymes, such as SOD, GPX, and Cat, have been shown to have higher levels of activity in longer lived strains of species. For example, such findings were obtained in studies of *Neurospora crassa* [178], *Drosophila melanogaster* [179], and *Caenorhabditis elegans* [180]. Therefore, genetically manipulating the antioxidant enzyme defense systems could prolong life (Table 3). Indeed, studies with *Drosophila* in which both SOD and Cat were overexpressed resulted in extension of the life span by a maximum of one-third and a reduction in protein oxidative damage [21,22]. Cat alone was ineffective in increasing life span [175].

Deprenyl, a MAO-B inhibitor, may be effective for creating symptoms of Parkinson's disease. Treatment of old male rats with deprenyl caused a significant increase in average life expectancy by 34% compared to saline-treated control animals (Table 3). This may be due to an upregulation of SOD and Cat activities, which may have provided protection of catecholaminergic neurons [176,177].

Table 3. The effect of antioxidants and antioxidant enzymes on median and maximum life span.

Antioxidants of diet (%)	Increase in life span (%)		Species
	Median	Maximum	
2-Mercaptoethylamine			
0.05%	12.8		Mice
1.00%	29.2		
Santoquin (0.5%)	18.1		Mice
Tocopherol-*p*-chloro-phenoxyacetate	13.0	13.0	Drosophila
d-Tocopherol	31.4	23.2	Nematodes
Vitamin E	16.8	15.4	Rotifer
Sulfhydryl agent	28.0		Rotifer
N-acetylcysteine		26.6	Drosophila
Antioxidant Enzymes			
Catalase only	No change		Drosophila
Catalase and Superoxide Dismutase	33.0+		Drosphilia
Deprenyl	34.0+[a]		Rats

[a]Deprenyl induces SOD and Cat antioxidant enzymes activity; 34.0% mean increase in [176,177] life span + specific strain maximum. (Adapted from [29,21,22,174–181].)

7.3.1 Natural and synthetic antioxidants

Besides antioxidant enzymes, there are a large number of antioxidant compounds that attenuate free radical reactions by breaking propagation chain reactions. The results, however, of these compounds are difficult to interpret since some of the antioxidants have unknown fates and perhaps potentially adverse effects.

Many antioxidant compounds have been shown to increase the average or mean life span of an organism. For example, in a study on the effect of adding *N*-acetylcysteine (NAC, an antioxidant and cysteine source to increase GSH levels) to the diet of *Drosophila melanogaster*, it was found that NAC results in a dose-dependent increase in median and maximum life span. Flies fed 1 mg/ml NAC food live 16.6% longer; those fed with 10 mg/ml NAC food live 26.6% longer [181].

Also, a study by Harman on vitamins C and E found that vitamin C did have some life-extending effects, and vitamin E produced a marginal increase on median life span with no influence in maximum life span [182]. Other studies using synthetic antioxidants achieved similar results: a synthetic antioxidant, butyl hydroxytoluene (BHT) was examined by Clapp et al. [183]. These researchers found that both sexes of BALB/c mice receiving 0.75% by weight BHT showed extended life spans. However, BHT at levels above 0.5% by weight have been shown to be toxic because at this level BHT adversely interferes with mitochondrial respiration [184]. A study examining a free radical scavenger, thiazolidine-4-carboxylic acid, found that intake at concentrations greater than 400 µM resulted in a significant increase in the median life span, but not the maximum life span. And Harman found in 1968 that adding 1.00% by weight of 2-mercapto-ethylamine to the diet of LAF_1 mice, shortly after they were weaned, resulted in increases in the average life span by 29.2%; on average these mice lived to 31.6 months vs. the previous average of 24.5 months [185].

Unfortunately, some of these studies have a shortcoming in that they lack food intake data. Without monitoring food intake, some of the increases in life span may have been due to the effect of caloric restriction and not that of the antioxidant. In studies where food intake was monitored, there was an associated decrease in body weight of up to 10—15% with the intake of various antioxidants [185,186]. Why antioxidants have this effect is not clear: some hypothesize that antioxidants adversely effect mitochondrial function, decreasing ATP formation by uncoupling aspects of mitochondrial respiration. Perhaps under these circumstances both body weight and superoxide anion and hydrogen peroxide levels will be decreased.

Regarding mice, there are a number of antioxidant compounds that will increase the average life span; for example, 2-mercaptoethylamine [185] and ethoxyquin [186]. However, there are only three known compounds that have been shown to increase the maximum life span in mice; they are 2-mercaptoethanol (2-ME) [187], and two pyridine derivatives [188,189]. The study on 2-ME by Heidrick et al. is the only study of the three that carefully monitored body weight and food intake. It showed that dietary supplementation at the level of 0.25% by weight of 2-ME increases average life span by 13% and maximum life span by 12%, without reducing caloric intake. Also, the total incidence of tumors was decreased 29% in the group taking 2-ME [187]. In contrast to mice, antioxidant supplementation increased mean, as well as maximum life spans in *Drosophila* [190,191] and nematodes [192].

However, why do so few antioxidants fail to raise the maximum life span in mouse models? Many scientists believe that these antioxidants are not added in significant concentrations to slow down the free radical damage to mitochondria or perhaps are not added in optimal combinations.

In addition to natural and synthetic antioxidants, there are a number of pharmacological spin traps, which can serve as antioxidants. Spin traps are nitrones or nitroso compounds that react with free radicals to form stable nitroxides, which are then quickly reduced to hydroxylamines (Fig. 6).

Nitroxide derivatives of spin traps such as *N-tert*-butyl-α-phenylnitrone (PBN) have been shown to have dramatic anti-aging effects and serve as excellent inhibitors of free radical reactions (Fig. 7). In one study on protein oxidation, old gerbils were given twice-daily intraperitoneal injections of PBN over a 2-week period. Their performance in running a radial-arm maze test was compared with that of young gerbils; at 32 mg/kg PBN the old gerbils performed nearly as well as the young gerbils. This result was accompanied by reversed age-related oxidative damage: levels of protein carbonyls dropped, glutamine synthetase and neutral protease activity increased, and unoxidized to oxidized ratios of proteins rose. Most impressive was the pronounced effect PBN had on the short-term memory of the older gerbils: untreated older gerbils made twice as many short-term memory errors as young gerbils, but treated older gerbils performed almost as well as the younger gerbils. The effect was also reversible: after stopping the treatment, glutamine synthetase and neutral protease activity fell and oxidation of proteins increased [193]. It is believed that these pronounced effects are due to the free radical scavenging effect of PBN and the inhibitory effect PBN has on the initiation of free radical reactions (Fig. 7).

Two subsequent studies with PBN were unable to confirm such results [194,195], but a third study did partially confirm the results of Carney et al.

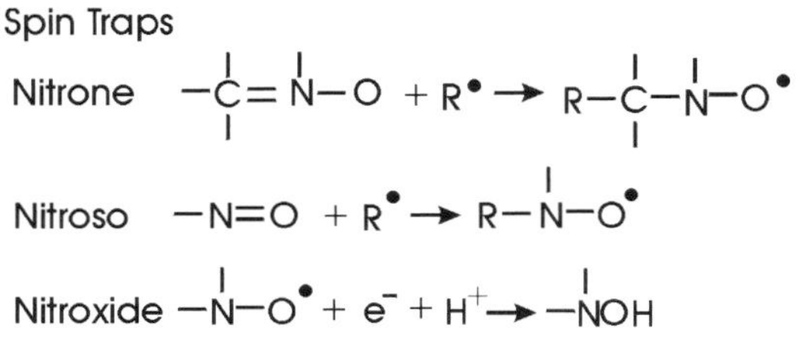

Spin Traps

$$-\overset{|}{\underset{|}{C}}=\overset{|}{N}-O \;+\; R^\bullet \;\longrightarrow\; R-\overset{|}{\underset{|}{C}}-\overset{|}{N}-O^\bullet$$

Nitrone

$$-N=O \;+\; R^\bullet \;\longrightarrow\; R-\overset{|}{N}-O^\bullet$$

Nitroso

$$-\overset{|}{N}-O^\bullet \;+\; e^- \;+\; H^+ \;\longrightarrow\; -\overset{|}{N}OH$$

Nitroxide

Fig. 6. Nitroso compounds and nitrones can react with free radicals to form nitroxides, which subsequently can be reduced to hydroxylamines [24].

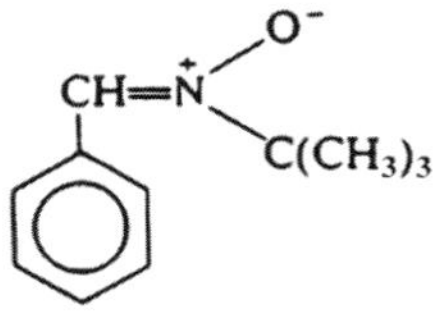

*Fig. 7. N-tert-*butyl-α-phenylnitrone (PBN) [265].

These scientists confirmed that protein carbonyl content decreased in gerbil brain cortex, but similar effects were not observed in the gerbil heart or the mouse brain cortex. Thus, the effects of PBN on protein carbonyls are variable depending upon tissue and species [196]. PBN has also been found to reverse age-related cognitive deficits in aged rats [197]. Lastly, it was found that daily intraperitoneal injections of 30 mg/kg of PBN in a strain of senescence-accelerated mice (SAM-P8) dramatically increased their mean life span: the control mice had a 50% mean survival rate of 42 weeks, but the PBN group's mean survival rate was increased to 56 weeks [198].

8   ANTIOXIDANTS IN HUMAN HEALTH AND DISEASE

Free radical damage to biological systems have been implicated in a large number of aging-associated diseases, from eye disorders such as cataracts and retrolental fibroplasia to cardiovascular disease and diabetes. Since there is such a myriad of aging-associated diseases, this review will limit its focus to cardiovascular disease and neurodegenerative diseases and the effect of antioxidant therapy.

8.1 Cardiovascular disease

Since cardiovascular disease is the primary cause of death in the USA, it is of chief importance to understand the etiology of atherosclerosis. Atherosclerosis is a disease of the arteries in which the innermost parts of the vessels, the intima, thicken. One of the primary types of thickening consists of fatty, slightly raised, narrow, yellow streaks. These streaks are rich in foam cells, which are distorted cells with a high lipid concentration that come from endogenous smooth muscle cells and from macrophages. These fatty streaks are likely the precursors of fibrous plaques, which have the effect of obstructing the arterial lumina. These plaques are also composed of various cellular debris, cholesterol crystals, and lipid deposits. They cause disease by limiting blood flow to the body organs. Heart attacks (myocardial infarction) and strokes (cerebral ischaemia) result when an arterial lumen is totally occluded, often with a thrombus forming at the plaque site.

What role does cholesterol play in developing atherosclerosis? The leading theory holds that the vascular endothelium produces lesions when damaged by mechanical and chemical reactions. Localized injured areas have increased permeability, resulting in a localized increase in the subendothelial space in concentrations of serum components such as LDL. With increased serum concentrations, more monocytes will attach to the subendothelial space, infiltrate, and develop into macrophages. Activated monocytes and macrophages cause damage to the endothelial cells by secreting O_2^-, H_2O_2, HOCl, NO· and hydrolytic enzymes. Other damaging compounds are continuously being produced in the subendothelial space by the reaction of O_2 with polyunsaturated substances present there [199—201].

Macrophages normally possess some LDL receptors, but if the LDL is peroxidized then the LDL is recognized by another type of receptor on the macrophage, the acetyl-LDL receptors or scavenger receptors. When bound to these receptors, LDL is rapidly engulfed by the macrophages resulting in a high intracellular concentration of cholesterol, which tends to convert the macrophage into a foam cell. In addition, since macrophages, smooth muscle cells, and arterial endothelial cells are known to oxidize LDL, this process of macrophage ingurgitation is increased [201].

Since oxidants have been implicated as a major cause of atherogenesis, it is reasonable to conclude that therapies which decrease the oxidation rate of serum components and vessel wall lipids and/or the permeability of the endothelial space should have a beneficial effect. Numerous studies have been conducted to test if the above hypothesis is correct, and much work is currently being done in this area. A few of the more significant and interesting results are reviewed below.

For example, a study on vitamin E supplementation found that men and women who supplemented their diets with 100 mg of vitamin E for two years or more had approximately a 40% decrease in the risk of coronary heart disease [202,203]. A study on vitamin C (ascorbate) found that human vascular endothelial cells, enriched with vitamin C, lowered their ability to modify LDL. The data also showed that extracellular vitamin C strongly inhibited metal ion-dependent, endothelial cell mediated atherogenic modification of LDL [204]. Vitamin C may also be important in the health of blood vessels due to its interaction with NO·. NO· has been shown to have vasodilatory effects, but it may be inactivated by reactive oxygen species such as superoxide radicals. Researchers have found that in essential hypertensive patients, impaired dilation of the blood vessels was significantly improved by vitamin C. Interestingly, this effect was reversed by N^G–monomethyl-L-arginine, a potent inhibitor of nitric oxide synthase [205] (Fig. 8).

Another example concerns the drug probucol; it is used clinically to lower blood cholesterol levels, but it is also a potent antioxidant. In a recent experiment, atherosclerotic lesions in Watanabe heritable hyperlipidemic rabbits regressed when treated with probucol, and this anti-atherogenic effect was far greater than expected merely from its cholesterol-lowering capability. Thus, the researchers suggested that its antioxidant properties contributed to its anti-atherogenic effect [206]. A study devoted to determining if probucol would decrease vascular O_2^- production confirmed that it does decrease vascular superoxide production in cholesterol-fed rabbits. Probucol treatment, in choles-terol-fed rabbits, normalized both O_2^- production and endothelium-dependent relaxation to acetylcholine. Thus, the researchers suggested that probucol may prevent O_2^- induced inactivation of endothelium-derived NO· [207].

Another recent study done on antioxidants and their anti-atherogenic effects concerns the Chinese herb, Salvia miltiorrhiza Bunge (SMB), which is widely used for the treatment of atherosclerosis-related disorders. The water-soluble polyphenolic antioxidant, Salvianolic acid B (Sal B), was isolated from the roots of this plant and was found to scavenge 1,1-diphenyl-2-picrylhydrazyl radicals and inhibit LDL oxidation more effectively than probucol. In an experiment using rabbits fed on a high cholesterol diet, endothelial damage at 6 weeks was found to be reduced by 53% in the SMB group. "SMB treatment also reduced the atherosclerotic area in the abdominal aorta significantly by 56% and choles-terol deposition in the thoracic aorta by 50%" [208].

Lastly, very exciting results have been obtained in rabbits undergoing diet sup-plementation with flaxseed oil. Flaxseed is a rich source of omega-3 fatty acids and lignans and is known to have antioxidant effects since it suppresses the pro-duction of oxygen free radicals by PMNLs and monocytes. Flax seed also supresses interleukin-1 (IL-1), tumor necrosis factor (TNF), leukotriene B4 (LTB4), and platelet activating factor (PAF). Since these compounds are known to stimulate PMNLs to produce oxygen free radicals, suppressing their produc-tion will also decrease levels of free radicals. In a well-designed experiment, flax-seed (type I flaxseed) reduced hypercholesterolemic atherosclerosis by 46% with-out significantly lowering serum lipids [209]. In a follow-up study on type II flaxseed (2−3% α-linolenic acid), it was found that this type of flaxseed reduced the development of atherosclerotic plaque by 69% [210].

8.2 Neurodegenerative diseases

Since the brain is one of the body's most metabolically active organs — consuming oxygen at a rate of 35 ml/min/kg, compared to the heart's oxygen consumption rate of 59 ml/min/kg [211,212], it is highly susceptible to damage from free radical processes. The brain is also unique in that it generates oxidants in ways that are for-eign to other body systems. For example, metabolism of excitatory amino acids and neurotransmitters generates reactive oxygen species, and the constant use of oxygen by neural mitochondria results in high superoxide levels by processes dis-

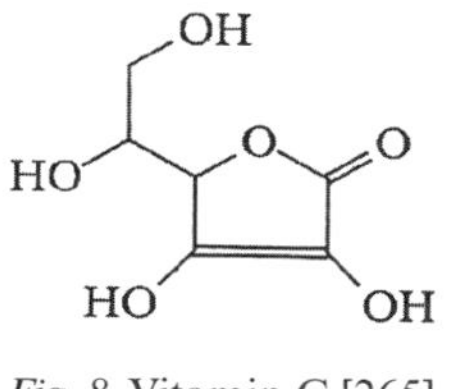

Fig. 8. Vitamin C [265].

cussed earlier in this paper [213]. Recently, it has been found that endogenous gua-nidino compounds like guanidinoglutaric acid can form highly reactive species such as superoxide and hydroxyl radical in aqueous solution [214].

The brain also appears to be particularly vulnerable to free radical damage because it lacks or has localized many of the antioxidant enzymes. For example, SOD is localized primarily in neurons [215], and GSH and GPX are localized in astrocytes [216,217]. Also, there appears to be very little activity of Cat in the brain [218].

The hypothesis that age-associated, chronic neurodegenerative diseases like Alzheimer's disease and Parkinson's disease are related to oxidative stress is well-supported by many findings. First, there are numerous reports in the litera-ture that patients with neurodegenerative diseases have damaged mitochondria coupled with high levels of oxidative damage [219—221]. Second, there are reports that in the cerebrospinal fluid there is free, nonprotein bound Fe^{3+} [222]. The brain normally has particularly high levels of iron in the globus pallidus and substantia nigra [223,224], which is believed to be due to the necessity of iron for the correct binding of neurotransmitters and receptors. However, in Alzheimer's disease there are increased neuronal iron concentrations due to increased neurofibrillary tangles [225]. In Parkinson's disease, it was discovered that the total iron content of the substantia nigra was 77% higher than other brain regions [226]. These findings are significant because nonprotein bound Fe^{3+}, through the Haber-Weiss reaction, can be reduced by superoxide to become Fe^{2+}. Fe^{2+} can then, in turn, react with hydrogen peroxide to form the highly reactive hydroxyl radical. These effects are believed to contribute to high levels of oxidative stress and the concomitant rapid peroxidation of highly abundant un-saturated brain lipids [227,228].

8.2.1 Alzheimer's disease

The role reactive oxygen species play in the etiology of Alzheimer's disease is cur-rently an area of intense research. It is well-known that Alzheimer's disease is clinically associated with the development of amyloid plaques. It is believed that these plaques are caused by the inproper folding and processing of amyloid β-precursor protein (AβPP). Aggregation of AβPP may involve free radicals [229], and it was found that AβPP can itself generate peptidyl free radicals [230]. These findings are supported by the discovery that the synthetic, in vitro formation of amyloid plaques from AβPP can be accelerated by the presence of oxygen; in fact, these amyloid plaques themselves appear to stimulate the production of reactive oxygen species [231].

At this point in time, much work is being done in developing antioxidant thera-pies for Alzheimer's disease. For example, researchers discovered that melatonin can protect neurons against AβPP toxicity and resistance to proteolysis. It was found that melatonin interacts with Aβ-40 and Aβ-42 to inhibit the formation of β-sheets and amyloid fibrils, the formation of which determines the toxicity and proteolytic resistance of AβPP [232]. Researchers in Germany are examining the protective effects of vitamin E and estrogen to limit oxidative stress in the long run [233]. Also under investigation in idebenone, a synthetic free radical scavenger which traps electrons, lazaroids (21-aminosteroids), pyrrolpyrimidines, NO· blockers, selegiline [234], and α-lipoic acid [213].

There is also evidence that extracts of ginkgo biloba are useful in the treatment of Alzheimer's disease. It has previously been demonstrated that extracts of ginkgo biloba confer give protection for neuronal cells against conditions of impaired oxidative phosphorylation [235]. This herb also can act as a free radical scavenger [236], and it has the capability to prevent peroxidation of lipid membranes by oxidants [237]. Recently, researchers in Germany conducted a clinical, double-blind, placebo-controlled study on 20 outpatients given oral doses of 240 mg/day of a specially manufactured ginkgo biloba extract, EGb 761, for three months. The purpose was to determine if the extract could stabilize cognitive performance or delay the progression of Alzheimer's related dementia. Using various psychometric tests, there was found to be a statistically significant improvement between the baseline values and final values for these tests among the group being actively treated with EGb 761 [238]. Another study on EGb 761 achieved similar results: in this year-long study, one group of Alzheimer patients took 40 mg of EGb 761 three times a day, while a second group of patients received a placebo. On the "Geriatric Evaluation by Relative's Rating Instrument" test, the ginkgo group improved daily living and social behavior by 37%, compared to 23% by those in the placebo group. Also, over the course of the study, the condition of only 19% of the ginkgo group patients deteriorated, compared to 40% of the placebo group. In conclusion, the researchers summarized that EGb 761 could stabilize and, in some cases, improve the cognitive performance and the social functioning of Alzheimer patients for 6 months to 1 year [239].

8.2.2 *Parkinson's disease*

Dopaminergic neurons are uniquely vulnerable to damage and disease. Their loss in humans is associated with diseases of the aged, most notably, Parkinson's disease. Parkinson's disease involves the loss of dopaminergic neurons, especially in the midbrain area called the substantia nigra. Oxidative stress is known to play a major role in the destruction of these neurons. For example, since Fe^{+3} is increased in the substantia nigra [226] and hydrogen peroxide is also produced during dopamine metabolism in the dopaminergic neurons [240], there is the possibility of Fe^{3+} catalyzed production of hydroxyl radicals which will result in significant damage to these neurons. Hydroxyl radical production is also increased when the mitochondrial respiratory chain dysfunctions, as has been found in diverse tissues of Parkinson's patients [241]. Other free radicals are generated when dopamine undergoes autoxidation or is enzymatically oxidized by monoamide oxidase [242]. Hydrogen peroxide produced in such reactions could then react with the free iron to form hydroxyl radicals, which react to damage biomolecules and could lead to the loss of dopaminergic neurons. Another source of neurotoxicity may be the release of copper ions in the presence of L-DOPA; it has been demonstrated that L-DOPA and dopamine can damage DNA by oxidizing it in the presence of copper ions and hydrogen peroxide [243]. Furthermore, research has shown that there is an increased production of superoxide in the mitochondria of the substantia nigra along with increased levels of activity of SOD [244]. In fact, the severity of Parkinson's symptoms has been correlated with the degree to which malondialdehyde [245] and hydroperoxides are increased and GSH levels are decreased [246,247].

Moreover, many studies have been done on the toxic metabolite 1-methyl-phenyl pyridium (MPP+) of the neurotoxin 1-methyl-4-phenyl-1,2,3,6 tetrahydropyridine (MPTP). In monkeys and other animal models, MPP+ induced Parkinson's disease-like symptoms and caused neuronal loss in the substantia nigra [248,249]. It was also found that MPP+ inhibits the mitochondria's respiratory chain complex I [250,251]. This intensively researched animal model for Parkinson's disease is being actively used to examine the role oxidants play in MPTP toxicity.

The loss of the dopaminergic neurons results in decreased dopamine production in various regions of the brain, including the cortex, nucleus accumbens, striatum, and thalamus [252]. Since these areas are involved in controlling voluntary movement, loss of dopamine results in improper signaling which causes the characteristic clinical symptoms: jerky movements, trembling of the hands and lips, muscle rigidity, body tremors, a shuffling gait, and eventually loss of the ability to control voluntary movements [253].

Many of the antioxidant therapies employed in the treatment of Alzheimer's disease are also being used to treat Parkinson's disease, e.g., melatonin. Low doses of 6-hydroxydopamine (6-OHDA) are known to induce apoptosis of undifferentiated and differentiated PC12 cells by generating free radicals, and this system has been proposed as an experimental model for Parkinson's disease. Significantly, melatonin was found to prevent apoptosis by 6-OHDA in neuronal cells, perhaps by scavenging free radicals and increasing the mRNA levels and the activity of antioxidant enzymes [254]. Melatonin and its precursor, *N*-acetyl-serotonin (normelatonin), have also been found to protect human neuroblastoma SK-N-MC cells and primary cerebellar granular neurons against oxidative stress [255]. Another study investigated the effects of melatonin on rescuing dying cells (100% tau+ neurons), including tyrosine hydroxylase immunopositive dopamine neurons. Apotosis was prevented in these cell lines, and this effect was dose and time dependent and was mimicked by other antioxidants such as 2-iodomelatonin and vitamin E. Melatonin also prevented the usual 50% loss of dopamine neurons caused by neurotoxic injury induced by 1-methyl-4-phenylpyridine. These remarkable results indicate that melatonin possesses a tremendous ability to rescue neurons from cell death [256] (Fig. 9).

Studies using other experimental models of Parkinson's disease found that inhibition of monoamine oxidase B (MAO-B), the enzyme responsible for the oxidation of dopamine, reduces oxidative stress on the dopaminergic neurons and can prevent neuronal degeneration [257]. In mutant mice lacking the gene for MAO-B, researchers found that these mice were resistant to the neurodegenerative effects of MPTP [258]. Moreover, in a double-blind study using selegiline (deprenyl) to inhibit MAO-B, it was established that selegiline can delay the need to be treated with L-DOPA by 10 months [259]. More recent studies have confirmed this antioxidant effect. For example, a study examining the effect of tocopherol and deprenyl on the progression of Parkinson's disease discovered that deprenyl (10 mg per day) but not tocopherol (2000 IU per day) delays the onset of disability associated with early Parkinson's disease [260].

Also under much investigation are thiol antioxidants, such as GSH, *N*-acetylcysteine (NAC), and dithiothreitol (DTT). These antioxidants and metal chelators, along with vitamin C, have been shown to prevent dopamine autooxidation; they also act to inhibit dopamine-induced apoptosis [261]. Other potential antioxidant treatments include α-lipoic acid [213], lazaroids [262], bromocriptine [263], and estrogen. Recently, estrogen replacement therapy has been shown to be protective against the development of Parkinson's disease-associated dementia [264] (Fig. 10).

9 SUMMARY

1. Major discoveries in free radical biology have been made in the past few decades substantiating the free radical theory of aging. Moreover, a large amount of scientific papers and a multitude of scientific disciplines have established a strong relationship between free radical biology and pathophysiology.
2. We discussed several major sources of free radical oxidant production in vivo and their relationship to aging and several degenerative diseases of aging. The mitochondria and phagocytes are potent sources of oxidant formation and may cause damage to DNA, lipids, and proteins generating unnatural structures.
3. Broadly, the altered biomolecules may play a critical role in the development of degenerative diseases and the aging process itself. Specific protein modifications can alter enzyme function or cell signaling ability. Furthermore, certain altered biomolecules that accumulate can affect protein function.
4. Scientific evidence has shown that several interventions such as dietary restriction, chronic exercise, and antioxidant therapies can attenuate the aging process and disease states.

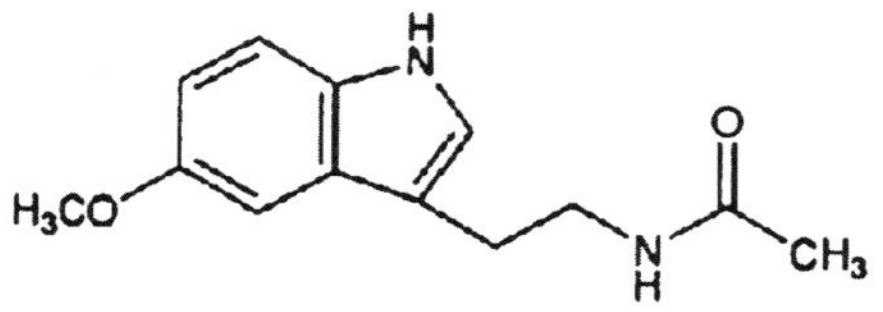

Fig. 9. Melatonin [265].

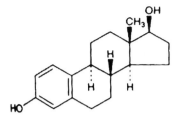

Fig. 10. Estradiol [265].

5. Therapies have been developed to reduce oxidative stress and therefore protect against the development of degenerative diseases such as atherosclerosis, Alzheimer's disease, and Parkinson's disease.

10 PERSPECTIVE

Aging has a strong genetic component, but it can be viewed partly as a degenerative process dictated by free radical reactions, possibly increasing the incidence of several degenerative disease states. The exact interrelationship is unclear, but there is a weighty amount of evidence that free radicals are involved. Free radicals increase with age, alter physiological function, increase disease states and accelerate pathophysiological conditions. This review describes a multitude of studies which clearly show the tremendous power of certain antioxidant interventions and other scientific advances in free radical biology, which will surely continue. However, the difficulties in preventing oxidative damage in vivo partly stem from our lack of understanding which reactive oxidants are active during the aging process and what specific antioxidant therapy provides optimal protection.

11 ACKNOWLEDGEMENTS

We would like to thank Sandy Drashin, Nicole Marek, and Cassandra Williams for their technical assistance with this manuscript, and Dr Powers and Jared Wilsey for their critical reading of this manuscript.

12 ABBREVIATIONS

SOD:	superoxide dismutase
Cat:	catalase
GPX:	glutathione peroxidase
NO·:	nitric oxide
ONOO⁻:	peroxynitrite
NO_2^+:	nitronium ion
$NO_2^•$:	nitrogen dioxide
Cl-NO₂:	nitryl chloride

HO·:   hydroxyl radical
PBN: *N-tert*-butyl-α-phenylnitrone
GSH: glutathione
NAC: *N*-acetyl-cysteine
DTT: dithiothreitol
MAO-B: monoamine oxidase B
6-OHDA: 6-hydroxydopamine
MPTP: 1-methyl-4-phenyl-1,2,3,6 tetrahydropyridine
MPP+:   1-methyl-4-phenyl pyridium
AβPP: β-precursor protein
PMNL: polymorphonuclear leukocytes
LDL: low-density lipoproteins
SAM-P8:   senescence-accelerated mice
2-ME: 2-mercaptoethanol
BHT: butyl hydroxytoluene
PDGF: platelet-derived growth factor
HOCl: hypochlorous acid
mtDNA: mitochondrial DNA
$O_2^{\cdot-}$:   superoxide
H_2O_2:   hydrogen peroxide
GC-MS: gas chromatography and mass spectrometry

13 REFERENCES

1. Harman D. J Gerontol 1956;11:298—300.
2. Harman D. J Am Geriatr Soc 1972;20:145—147.
3. Harman D. Molec Cell Biochem 1998;84:155—161.
4. Harman D. Ann NY Acad Sci 1996;786:321—336.
5. Boveris A, Chance B. Biochem J 1973;134:707—716.
6. Boveris A, Cadenas E, Stoppani AO. J Biochem 1976;156:435—444.
7. Chance B, Sies H, Boveris A. Phsyiol Rev 1979;59:527—609.
8. Giulivi C, Poderoso JJ, Boveris A. J Biol Chem 1998;272(18):11038—11043.
9. Klebanoff SJ. Ann Int Med 1980;93:480—489.
10. Hurst JK, Barrette WC Jr., Vihinen M, Mantsala P. Crit Rev Biochem Molec Biol 1989;24(4): 270—304.
11. Eiserich JP, Cross CE, Jones AD, Halliwell B, Van der Vliet A. J Biol Chem 1996;271: 19199—19208.
12. Eiserich JP, Hristova M, Cross CE, Jones DA, Freeman BA, Halliwell B, Van der Vliet A. Nature 1997;391:393—397.
13. Buettner GR. Arch Biochem Biophys 1993;300:535—543.
14. Ames BN, Shigenaga MK, Hagen TM. Proc Natl Acad Sci USA 1993;90:7915—7922.
15. Dean RT, Fu S, Stocker R, Davies MJ. Biochem J 1997;324:1—18.
16. Beckman KB, Ames B. Physiol Rev 1998;78:547—581.
17. Stadtman ER. Science 1992;257:1220—1224.
18. Lett BS, Stadtman E. J Biol Chem 1997;272:20313—20316.
19. Sohal RS, Weindruch R. Science 1996;273:59—63.
20. Sohal RS, Brunk UT. Mutat Res 1992;275:295—304.

21. WC, Sohal RS. Science 1994;263:1128—1130.
22. Sohal RS, Agarwal A, Agarwal S, Orr WC. J Biol Chem 1995;270:15671—15674.
23. Sohal RS, Sohal BH, Orr WC. Free Radic Biol Med 1995;19(4):499—504.
24. McCay CM, Crowell MF, Maynard LA. J Nutr 1995;10:63—79.
25. Weindruch R, Walford RL. The Retardation of Aging and Disease by Dietary Restriction. Springfield, Ill: Charles C. Thomas, 1988.
26. Weindruch R, Sohal RS. N Eng J Med 1997;337:986—994.
27. Esser K, Martin GM. Molecular aspect of aging. Chichester: J. Wiley and Sons, 1995.
28. Yu BP. Modulation of aging processes by dietary restriction. Boca Raton: CRC Press, 1994.
29. Yu BP. Free Radic Biol Med 1996;21:651—668.
30. Youngman LD, Kim Park JY, Ames BN. Proc Natl Acad Sci USA 1992;89:9112—9116.
31. Tolmasoff JM, Ono T, Cutler RG. Proc Natl Acad Sci USA 1980;77(5):2777—2781.
32. Castro L, Rodriquez M, Radi R. J Biol Chem 1994;269:29409—29415.
33. Gardner PR, Nguyen DD, White CW. Proc Natl Acad Sci USA 1994;91:12248—12252.
34. Hausladen A, Fridovich I. J Biol Chem 1994;269:29405—29408.
35. Kobzik L, Stringer B, Balligand JL, Reid MB, Stamler JS. Biochem Biophys Res Comm 1995; 211:375—381.
36. Bates TE, Loesch A, Burnstock G, Clark JB. Biochem Biophys Res Comm 1995;213:896—900.
37. Bates TE, Loesch A, Burnstock G, Clark JB. Biochem Biophys Res Comm 1995;218:40—44.
38. Tatoyan A, Giulivi C. J Biol Chem 1998;273(18):11044—11048.
39. Sohal RS, Agarwal S, Sohal BH. Mech Ageing Devel 1995;81(1):15—25.
40. Hagen TM, Yowe DL, Bartholomew JC, Wehr CM, Do KL, Park JY, Ames BN. Proc Natl Acad Sci USA 1997;94:3064—3069.
41. Sastre J, Pallardo FV, Pla R, Pellin A, Juan G, O'Connor JE, Estrela JM, Miquel J, Vina J. Hepatol 1996;24(5):1199—1205.
42. Sohal RS, Sohal BH. Mech Ageing Devel 1991;57(2):187—202.
43. Hansford RG, Hogue BA, Mildaziene V. Biomembrane 1997;1:89—95.
44. Miquel J, Fleming JE. Exp Gerontol 1984;19(1):31—36.
45. Miquel J. Exp Gerontol 1998;33(1—2):113—126.
46. Yakes MF, Van Houten B. Proc Natl Acad Sci USA 1997;94:514—519.
47. Hazen SL, Hsu FF, Mueller DM, Crowley JR, Heinecke JW. J Clin Invest 1996;98(6): 1283—1289.
48. Santa Maria C, Alvarez E, Machado A, Sobrino F. Cell Immunol 1996;169(1):152—155.
49. Alvarez E, Conde M, Machado A, Sobrino F. Biochem J 1995;312(2):555—560.
50. Biasi D, Carletto A, Dell'Agnola C, Caramaschi P, Montesanti F, Zavateri G, Zeminian S, Bellavite P, Bambara LM. Inflammation 1996;20(6):673—681.
51. Alvarez E, Santa Maria C. Mech Ageing Devel 1996;90(2):157—161.
52. Lavie L. Mech Ageing Devel 1996;90(2):157—161.
53. Mohacsi A, Kozlovszky B, Kiss I, Seres I, Fulop, Jr T. Biochem Biophys Acta 1996;1316(3): 210—216.
54. Ito Y, Kajkenova O, Feuers RJ, Udupa KB, Desai VG, Epstein J, Hart RW, Lipschitz DA. J Gerontol 1998;53(3):M169—M175.
55. Matsuo M. In: Yu BP, editor. Free radicals in Aging. Boca Raton: CRC Press, 1993.
56. Vanella A, Geremia E, D'Urso G, Tiriolo P, Di Silvestro I, Grimaldi R, Pinturo R. J Gerontol 1982;28(2):108—113.
57. Leeuwenburgh C, Fiebig R, Chandwaney R, Ji LL. Am J Phys 1994;267:R439—R445.
58. Ji LL. Med Sci Sports Exerc 1993;25(2):225—231.
59. Ji LL, Dillon D, Wu E. Am J Physiol 1990;258(4):R918—R923.
60. Oh-ishi S, Toshinai K, Kizaki T, Haga S, Fukuda K, Nagata N, Ohno H. Respir Physiol 1996; 105(3):195—202.
61. Yu BP. Physiol Rev 1994;74(1):139—162.
62. Svensson L, Wu C, Hulthe P, Johannessen K, Engel JA. Brain Res 1993;609(1—2):36—40.

63. Rikans LE, Moore DR. Biochem Biophys Acta 1988;966(3):269—275.
64. De AK, Darad R. Mech Ageing Devel 1991;59(1—2):123—128.
65. Panda AK, Ruth RP, Padhi SN. Exp Gerontol 1984;19(2):95—100.
66. DeLeve LD, Kaplowitz N. Sem Liv Dis 1990;10(4):251—266.
67. DeLeve LD, Kaplowitz N. Pharmacol Ther 1991;52(3):287—305.
68. Meister A. Meth Enzymol 1995;251:3—7.
69. Hussain S, Slikker, Jr W, Ali SF. Int J Dev Neurosci 1995;13(8):811—817.
70. Ohkuwa T, Sato Y, Naoi M. Acta Physiol Scand 1997;9(3):237—244.
71. Barja de Quiroga G, Perez-Campo R, Lopez Torres M. Biochem J 1990;272(1):247-250.
72. Ravindranath V, Shivakumar BR, Anandatheerthavarada HK. Neurosci Lett 1989;101(2):
    187—190.
73. Farooqui MY, Day WW, Zamorano DM. Comp Biochem Physiol 1987;88(1):177—180.
74. Favilli F, Iantomasi T, Marraccini P, Stio M, Lunghi B, Treves C, Vincenzini MT. Neurobiol
    Aging 1994;15(4):429—433.
75. De la Asuncion JG, Millan A, Pla R, Bruseghini L, Esteras A, Pallardo FV, Sastre J, Vina J.
    FASEB J 1996;10(2):333—338.
76. Meydani M, Meisler JG. Postgrad Med 1997;102(2):199—207.
77. Meydani M. Lancet 1995;345:170—175.
78. Meydani M, Evans WJ, Handelman G, Biddle L, Fielding RA, Meydani SN, Burrill J, Fiatarone
    MA, Blumberg JB, Cannon JG. Am J Physiol 1993;33:R992—R998.
79. Meydani SN, Meydani M, Blumberg JB, Leka LS, Siber G, Loszewski R, Thompson C, Pedrosa
    MC, Diamond RD, Stollar BD. JAMA 1997;277:1380—1386.
80. Meydani SN, Meydani M, Rall LC, Morrow F, Blumberg JB. Am J Clin Nutr 1994;60:704—709.
81. Kappus H, Diplock AT. Free Radic Biol Med 1992;13:55—74.
82. Tsai AJ, Kelley B, Peng, Cook N. Am J Clin Nutr 1978;31:831—837.
83. Halliwell B, Gutteridge JMC. Free Radicals in Biology and Medicine, 2nd edn. Oxford: Oxford
    University Press, 1995.
84. Stephens NG, Parsons A, Schofield PM, Kelly F, Cheeseman K, Mitchinson MJ. Lancet 1996;
    347(9004):781—786.
85. Matsuo M, Gomi F, Dooley MM. Mech Ageing Devel 1992;64(3):273—292.
86. Vatassery GT, Angerhofer CK, Knox CA. J Neurochem 1984;43(2):409—412.
87. Laganiere, Yu BP. Mech Ageing Devel 1989;48(3):207—219.
88. Sawada M, Carlson JC. Mech Ageing Devel 1987;41(1—2):125—137.
89. Desole MS, Esposito G, Enrico P, Miele M, Fresu L, De Natale G, Miele E, Grella G. Neurosci
    Lett 1993;159(1—2):143—146.
90. Cini M, Moretti A. Neurobiol Aging 1995;6(1):53—57.
91. Reiter RJ. FASEB J 1995;9(7):526—533.
92. Levine RL, Williams JA, Stadtman ER, Shacter E. Meth Enzymol 1991;233:346—356.
93. Reznick AZ, Packer L. Meth Enzymol 1994;233:357—362.
94. Stadtman ER, Oliver CN. J Biol Chem 1991;266(4):2005—2008.
95. Stadtman ER. Free Radic Biol Med 1990;9:315—325.
96. Burcham P, Kuhan Y. Biochem Biophys Res Comm 1996;220:996—1001.
97. Leeuwenburgh C, Simcox S, Williams MV, Holloszy JO, Heinecke J. Multiple pathways for the
    generation of 2,4—dinitrophenylhydrazine reactive moieties in vitro: implications for protein
    carbonyls as specific markers of oxidation in vivo. (In Preparation.)
98. Eiserich JA, Van der Vliet A, Handelman G, Halliwell B, Cross CE. Am J Clin Nutr 1995;62:
    1490S—1500S.
99. Ischiropoulos H, Al—Mehdi AB. FEBS Lett 1995;364:279—282.
100. Oliver CA, Ahn B, Moerman EJ, Goldstein S, Stadtman ER. J Biol Chem 1987;262:
    5488—5491.
101. Smith CD, Carney JM, Starke-Reed PE, Oliver CN, Stadtman ER, Floyd RA, Markesbery WR.
    Proc Natl Acad Sci USA 1991;88:10540—10543.

102. Carney JM, Starke-Reed PE, Oliver CN, Landum RW, Cheng MS, Wu JF, Floyd RA. Proc Natl Acad Sci USA 1991;88:3633—3636.
103. Starke-Reed PE, Oliver CN. Arch Biochem Biophys 1989;275:559—567.
104. Sohal RS, Agarwal S, Dubey A, Orr WC. Proc Natl Acad Sci USA 1993;90:7255—7259.
105. Beckman JS. The physiological and pathological chemistry of nitric oxide. In: Lancaster JR Jr (ed) Nitric Oxide: Principles and Actions. San Diego: Academic Press, Inc., 1996;1—82:
106. Beckman JS, Beckman TW, Chen J, Marshall PA, Freeman BA. Proc Natl Acad Sci USA 1990; 87:1620—1624.
107. Beckman JS, Chen J, Ischiropoulos H, Crow JP. Meth Enzymol 1994;233:229—240.
108. Viner RI, Ferrington DA, Huhmer AFR, Bigelow DJ, Schoneich C. FEBS Lett 1996;379: 286—290.
109. Viner RI, Ferrington DA, Huhmer AFR, Bigelow DJ, Schoneich V. Free Radic Res 1996;24: 243—259.
110. Leeuwenburgh C, Hansen P, Shaish A, Holloszy JO, Heinecke JW. Am J Phys 1998;274(2Pt 2): R453—461.
111. Crowley JR, Yarasheski K, Leeuwenburgh C, Turk J, Heinecke JW. Anal Chem 1998;259(1): 127—135.
112. Leeuwenburgh C, Dory MM, Hazen S, Wagner P, Oh-ishi S, Steinbrecher UP, Heinecke JW. J Biol Chem 1997;272:1433—1436.
113. Beckman JS, Ye YZ, Anderson PJ, Chen J, Accavitti MA, Tarpey MM, White CR. Biol Chem Hopp-Seyler 1994;375:81—88.
114. Smith MA, Richey Harris PL, Sayre LM, Beckman JS, Perry G. J Neurosci 1997;17(8): 2653—2657.
115. Smith MA, Sayre LM, Anderson VE, Harris PL, Beal MF, Kowall N, Perry G. J Histochem Cytochem 1998;46(6):731—735.
116. Alam ZI, Daniel SE, Lees AJ, Marsden DC, Jenner P, Halliwell B. J Neurochem 1997;69(3): 1326—1329.
117. Bruijn LI, Beal MF, Becher MW, Schulz JB, Wong PC, Price DL, Cleveland DW. Proc Natl Acad Sci USA 1997;94:7606—7611.
118. Pacifici RE, Davies KJ. Gerontology 1991;37(1—3):166—180.
119. Janero DR. Free Radic Biol Med 1990;9:515—540.
120. Cuervo AM, Dice JF. Front Biosci 1998;3:d25—43.
121. Marcillat O, Zhang Y, Lin SW, Davies KJA. Biochem J 1988;254:677—683.
122. Pacifici RE, Davies KJ. Meth Enzymol 1990;186:485—502.
123. Ursine F, Davies KJA. Protein Metabolism in Aging. New York: Wiley-Liss, 1990;373—380.
124. Davies KJ. J Biol Chem 1987;262:9895—9901.
125. Davies KJA, Delsignore ME, Lin SW. J Biol Chem 1987;262:9902—9907.
126. Davies JA, Delsignore ME. J Biol Chem 1987;262:9908—9913.
127. Davies JA, Lin SW, Pacifici RE. J Biol Chem 1987;262:9914—9920.
128. Giulivi C, Davies KJA. Meth Enzymol. 1969;233:363—371.
129. Giuliviv C, Davies KJA. J Biol Chem 1993;268:8752—875.
130. Leeuwenburgh C, Rasmussen JE, Hsu FF, Mueller DM, Pennathur S, Heinecke JW. J Biol Chem 1997;272(6):3520—3526.
131. Moncade S, Palmer RM, Higgs EA. Pharmacol Rev 1991;43:109—142.
132. Beckman JS, Koppenol WH. Am J Physiol 1996;271(5):C1424—C1437.
133. Lymar SV, Hurst JK. Chem Res Toxicol 1996;9:845—850.
134. Lymar SV, Jiang Q, Hurst JK. Biochem 1996;35:7855—7861.
135. Wells-Knecht MC, Huggins TG, Dyer DG, Thorpe SR, Baynes JW. J Biol Chem 1993;268(17): 12348—12352.
136. Leeuwenburgh C, Wagner P, Holloszy JO, Sohal RS, Heinecke JW. Arch Biochem Biophys 1997; 346(1):74—80.
137. Hazen SL, Heinecke JW. J Clin Invest 1997;99(9):2075—2081.

138. Leeuwenburgh C, Hansen P, Holloszy JO, Heinecke JW. Oxidized amino acids in urine. Am J Physiol 1999;276:R218—R135.
139. Malorni W, Iosi F, Santini MT, Testa U. Cell Sci 1993;106(1):309—318.
140. Malorni W, Masella R, Santini MT, Iosi F, Samoggia P, Cantafora A, Merrell D, Peterson SW. Exp Cell Res 1993;206(2):195—203.
141. Malorni W, Rainaldi G, Rivabene R, Santini MT, Peterson SW, Testa U, Donelli G. Eur J Histochem 1994;38(Suppl 1):91—100.
142. Hunter T. Cell 1995;80:225—236.
143. Kong SK, Yim MB, Stadtman ER, Chock PB. Proc Natl Acad Sci USA 1996;93:3377—3382.
144. Gow AJ, Duran D, Malcolm S, Ischiropoulos H. FEBS Lett 1996;385:63—66.
145. Alberts B, Bray D, Lewis J, Raff M, Roberts K. Molecular Biology of the Cell. 3rd edn. New York: Garland, 1994;P655—683.
146. Brown GC, Cooper CE. FEBS Lett 1994;356:295—298.
147. Yan LJ, Levine RS, Sohal RS. Proc Natl Acad Sci USA 1997;94:11168—11174.
148. Weindruch R, Walford RL. The retardation of aging and disease by dietary restriction. Springfield, IL: Charles C Thomas, 1988.
149. Weindruch R, Walford RL, Fligiel S, Guthrie D. J Nutr 1986;116(4):641—654.
150. Yu BP, Masoro EJ, Murata EJ, Bertrand HA, Lynd FT. J Gerontol 1982;37:130—141.
151. Weindruch R, Walford RL. Science 1982;215(4538):1415—1418.
152. Prosser CL. Temperature. In: Prosser CL (ed) Comparative Animal Physiology, 3rd edn. Philadelphia: WB Saunders, 1973;362—428.
153. Koizumi A, Tsukada M, Wada Y, Masuda H, Weindruch R. J Nutr 1992; 122: 1446—53.
154. Duffy PH, Feuers R, Nakamura KD, Leakey J, Hart RW. Chronobiol Int 1990;7:113—24.
155. Lane MA, Baer DJ, Rumpler WV, Weindruch R, Ingram DK, Tilmont EM, Cutler RG, Roth GS. Proc Natl Acad Sci USA 1996;3(9):4159—4164.
156. Harman D. Exp Gerontol 1998;33:95—112.
157. Sohal RS, Agerwal S, Candas M, Forster MJ, Lal H. Mech Ageing Devel 1994;76:215—224.
158. Semsei I, Rao G, Richardson A. Biochem Biophys Res Commun 1989;164(2):620—625.
159. Rao G, Xia E, Nadakavukaren MJ, Richardson A. J Nutr 1990;120(6):602—609.
160. Dullo AG, Girardier L. Int J Obes Relat Metab Disord 1993;17(2):115—123.
161. Ramsey JJ, Roecker EB, Weindruch R, Kemnitz JW. Am J Physiol 1997;272(5):E901—E907.
162. McCarter R, Masoro EJ, Yu BP. Am J Physiol 1985;248:E488—E490.
163. Harman D. Age 1994;17:119—146.
164. Weindruch R. Sci Am 1996;49:46—52.
165. Fishbein L. Biological Effects of Dietary Restriction. New York: Springer-Verlag, 1991.
166. Cefalu WT, Bell-Farrow AD, Wang ZQ, Sonntag WE, Fu MX, Baynes JW, Thorpe SR. J Gerontol 1995;50(6):B337—B341.
167. Holloszy JO. Mech Ageing Devel 1998;100(3):211—219.
168. Davies KJ, Quintanilha AT, Brooks GA, Packer L. Biochem Biophys Res Commun 1982;107(4):1198—1205.
169. Quintanilha AT, Packer L. Ciba Found Symp 1983;101:56—69.
170. Leeuwenburgh C, Fiebig R, Chandwaney R, Ji LL. Am J Physiol 1994;267(2):R439—R445.
171. Leeuwenburgh C, Hollander J, Leichtweis S, Griffiths M, Gore M, Ji LL. Am J Physiol 1997; 272(1Pt 2):R363—R369.
172. Viidik A, Nielsen HM, Skalicky M. Mech Ageing Devel 1996;88(3):139—148.
173. Holloszy JO. J Gerontol 1993;48(3):B97—B100.
174. Bozovic V, Enesco H. Age 1986;9:41—45.
175. Orr WC, Sohal RS. Arch Biochem Biophys 1992;297(1):35—41.
176. Kitani K, Miyasaka K, Kanai S, Carrillo MC, Ivy GO. Ann NY Acad Sci 1996;786:391—409.
177. Kitani K, Kanai S, Carrillo MC, Ivy GO. Ann NY Acad Sci 1994;717:60—71.
178. Munkers KD, Rana RS, Goldstein E. Mech Ageing Devel 1984;24:83—100.
179. Dwyer S, Berrios A, Arking R. Gerontol 1989;29:186a.

180. Johnson TE, Lithgow GJ. J Am Geriatr Soc 1992;40:936—945.
181. Brack C, Bechter-Thuring E, Labuhn M. Cell Molec Life Sci 1997;53(11—12):960—966.
182. Harman D. Age 1978;1:145—152.
183. Clapp NK, Satterfield LC, Bowels ND. J Gerontol 1979;34:497—501.
184. Horrum MA, Harman D, Tobin RB. Age 1987;10:58—61.
185. Harman D. J Gerontol 1968;23:476—482.
186. Comfort A. Nature 1971;229:254—255.
187. Heidrick ML, Hendricks LC, Cook DE. Mech Ageing Devel 1984;27:341—358.
188. Emanuel NM. Q Rev Biophys 1976;9:283—308.
189. Emanuel NM, Duburs G, Obukhov LK, Uldrikis J. Chem Abstr 1981;94:9632a.
190. Miquel J, Johnson, Jr JE. Gerontologist 1975;15:25.
191. Miquel J, Economos AC, Bensch KG, Atlam H, Johnson, Jr JE. Age 1979;2:78—88.
192. Epstein J, Gershon D. Mech Ageing Devel 1972;1:257—264.
193. Carney JM, Starke-Reed PE, Oliver CN, Landum RW, Cheng MS, Wu JF, Floyd RA. Proc Natl Acad Sci USA 1991;88:3633—3636.
194. Cao G, Cutler RG. Arch Biochem Biophys 1995;320:106—114.
195. Cao G, Cutler RG. Arch Biochem Biophys 1995;320:195—201.
196. Dubey A, Forster MJ, Sohal RS. Arch Biochem Biophysa 1995;324(2):249—254.
197. Socci DJ, Crandall BM, Arendash GW. Brain Res 1995;693:88—94.
198. Edamatsu R, Mori A, Packer L. Biochem Biophys Res Commun 1995;211:847—849.
199. Harman D. Free radical theory of aging: Role of free radicals in the origination and evolution of life, aging, and disease processes. In: Johnson JE Jr, Walford R, Harman D, Miquel J (eds) Free Radicals: Aging, and Degenerative Diseases. New York: Alan R. Liss, 1986: 3—49.
200. Heinecke JW. Curr Opin Lipidol 1997;8(5):268—274.
201. Brown MS, Goldstein JL Annu Rev Biochem 1983;52:223—261.
202. Rimm EB, Stampfer MJ, Ascherio A, Giovannucci E, Colditz GA, Willett WC. N Engl J Med 1993;328:1450—1456.
203. Stampfer MJ, Hennekens CH, Mason JE, Colditz GA, Rosner B, Willett WC. N Engl J Med 1993;328:1444—1449.
204. Martin A, Frei B. Arterioscl Thromb Vasc Biol 1997;17(8):1583—1590.
205. Taddei S, Virdis A, Ghiadoni L, Magagna A, Salvetti A. Circulation 1998;97(22):2222—2229.
206. Oshima R, Ikeda T, Watanabe K, Itakura H, Sugiyama N. Atherosclerosis 1998;137(1):13—22.
207. Inoue N, Ohara Y, Fukai T, Harrison DG, Nishida K. Am J Med Sci 1998;315(4):242—247.
208. Wu YJ, Hong CY, Lin SJ, Wu P, Shiao MS. Arterioscl Thromb Vasc Biol 1998;18(3):481—486.
209. Prasad K. Atherosclerosis 1997;132(1):69—76.
210. Prasad K, Mantha SV, Muir AD, Westcott ND. Atherosclerosis 1998;136(2):367—375.
211. McArdle WD, Katch KI, Katch VL. Exercise Physiology: Energy, Nutrition, and Human Performance. Philadelphia: Lea and Febiger, 1986.
212. Diem K, Lentner C. Documenta Geigy Scientific Tables. Basle, Switzerland: JR Geigy SA, 1970.
213. Packer L, Tritschler HJ, Wessel K. Free Radic Biol Med 1997;22(1):359—378.
214. Mori A, Kohno M, Masumizu T, Packer L. Biochem Mol Biol Int 1995;37:371—374.
215. Delacourte A, Defossez A, Ceballos I, Nicole A, Sinet PM. Neurosci Lett 1988;92:247—253.
216. Damier P, Hirsch EC, Zhang P, Agid YA, Javoy—Agid F. Neurosci 1993;52:1—6.
217. Benzi G, Moretti A. Free Radic Biol Med 1995;19:77—101.
218. Marklund SL, Westman NG, Lundgren E, Roos G. Cancer Res 1982;42:1955—1961.
219. Jenner P, Dexter DT, Sian J, Schapiro AH, Marsden CD. Ann Neurol Suppl 1992;32:S82—S87.
220. Dexter DT, Holley AE, Flitter WD, Slater TF, Wells FR, Daniel SE, Lees AJ, Jenner P, Marsden, CD. Mov Disord 1994;9:92—97.
221. Volicer L, Crino PB. Neurobiol Aging 1990;11:567—571.
222. Halliwell B, Gutteridge JM. Biochem J 1984;21:1—14.
223. Youdim MBH. Mt Sinai J Med 1988;55:97—101.

224. Gerlach M, Ben–Shachar D, Riederer P, Youdim MBH. J Neurochem 1994;63:793–807.
225. Good PF, Perl DP, Bierer LM, Schmeidler J. Ann Neurol 1992;31:286–292.
226. Sofic E, Riederer P, Heinsen H, Beckmann H, Reynolds GP, Hebenstreit G, Youdim MB. J Neural Transm 1988;74:199–205.
227. Stocks J, Gutteride JMC, Sharp RJ, Dormandy TL. Clin Sci 1974;47:223–233.
228. Mohanakumar KP, De Bartolomeis A, Wu RM, Yeh KJ, Sternberg L, Peng SY, Murphy DL, Chiueh CC. Ann NY Acad Sci 1994;738:392–399.
229. Dyrks T, Dyrks E, Hartmann T, Masters C, Beyreuther K. J Biol Chem 1992;267:18210–18217.
230. Hensley K, Carney JM, Mattson MP, Aksenova M, Harris M, Wu JF, Floyd RA, Butterfield DA. Proc Natl Acad Sci USA 1994;91:3270–3274.
231. Smithy MA, Sayre LM, Monnier VM, Perry G. Trends Neurosci 1995;18:172–176.
232. Pappolla M, Bozner P, Soto C, Shao H, Robakis NK, Zagorski M, Frangione B, Ghiso J. J Biol Chem 1998;273(13):7185–7188.
233. Behl C, Holsboer F. Fortschr Neurol Psychiatr 1998;66(3):113–121.
234. Parnetti L, Senin U, Mecocci P. Drugs 1997;53(5):752–768.
235. Spinnewyn B, Blavet N, Clostre F. La Presse Medicale 1986;15:1511–1515.
236. Barth SA, Inselmann G, Engemann R, Heidemann HT. Biochem Pharmacol 1991;41: 1521–1526.
237. Dorman DC, Cote LM, Buck WB. Am J Vet Res 1992;53:138–142.
238. Maurer K, Ihl R, Dierks T, Frolich L. J Psychiatr Res 1997;31(6):645–655.
239. Le Bars PL, Katz MM, Berman N, Itil TM, Freedman AM, Schatzberg AF. JAMA 1997;278 (16):1327–1332.
240. Ben-Shachar D, Riederer P, Youdim MBH. J Neurochem 1991;57:1609–1614.
241. Shoffner JM, Watts RL, Juncos JL, Torroni A, Wallace DC. Ann Neurol 1991;30:332–339.
242. Hirsch EC. Ann Neurol 1992;32:S88–S93.
243. Spencer JPE, Jenner A, Butler J, Aruoma OI, Dexter DT, Jenner P, Halliwell B. Free Radic Res 1996;24:95–105.
244. Saggu H, Cooksey J, Dexter D, Wells FR, Lees A, Jenner P, Marsden CD. J Neurochem 1989;53: 692–697.
245. Jenner P, Dexter DT, Sian J, Schapira AH, Marsden CD. Ann Neurol Suppl 1992;32:S82–S87.
246. Riederer P, Sofic E, Rausch WD, Schmidt B, Reynolds GP, Jellinger K, Youdim MB. J Neurochem 1989;52:515–520.
247. Perry TL, Godin DV, Hansen S. Neurosci Lett 1982;33:305–310.
248. Chiueh CC, Miyake H, Peng MT. Adv Neurola 1993;60:251–258.
249. Nicklas WJ, Vyas I, Heikkila RE. Life Sci 1985;36:2503–2508.
250. Obata T, Chiueh CC. J Neural Transm 1992;89:139–145.
251. Chiueh CC, Krishna G, Tulsi P, Obata T, Lang K, Huang SJ, Murphy DL. Free Radic Biol Med 1992;13:581–583.
252. Graybiel AM, Hirsch EC, Agid Y. Adv Neurol 1990;53:17–29.
253. Fisher LJ, Gage FH. Nature Med 1995;3:201–202.
254. Mayo JC, Sainz RM, Uria H, Antolin I, Esteban MM, Rodriguez C. J Pineal Res 1998;24(3): 179–192.
255. Lezoualc'h F, Sparapani M, Behl C. J Pineal Res 1998;24(3):168–178.
256. Iacovitti L, Stull ND, Johnston K. Brain Res 1997;768(1–2):317–326.
257. Gotz ME, Kunig G, Riederer P, Youdim MBH. Pharmacol Ther 1994;63:37–122.
258. Grimsby J, Toth M, Chen K, Kumazawa T, Klaidman L, Adams JD, Karoum F, Gal J, Shih JC. Nature Genet 1997;17(2):206–210.
259. N Engl J Med.1989;321:1364–1371.
260. N Engl J Med 1993;328(3):176–183.
261. Offen D, Ziv I, Sternin H, Melamed E, Hochman A. Exp Neurol 1996;141(1):32–39.
262. Nakao N, Frodl EM, Duan WM, Widner H, Brundin P. Proc Natl Acad Sci USAa 1994;91(26): 12408–12412.

263. Di Paola R, Uitti RJ. Drugs Aging 1996;9(3):159—168.
264. Marder K, Tang MX, Alfaro B, Mejia H, Cote L, Jacobs D, Stern Y, Sano M, Mayeux R. Neurology 1998;50(4):1141—1143.
265. Budvari S. The Merck Index, 12th edn. Whitehouse Station, New Jersey: Merck and Co., Inc., 1996.

Part XI

Disease processes

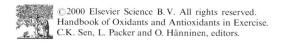
Part XI • Chapter 31

Oxidative stress, antioxidants and cancer

Mariette Gerber

Groupe d'Epidémiologie Métabolique, Centre de Recherche en Cancérologie, INSERM-CRLC, 34298 Montpellier Cedex 5, France. Tel.: +33-6761-3005. Fax: +33-6752-2901.

1   INTRODUCTION
2   INITIATION OF CARCINOGENESIS
    2.1   Oxidative stress
    2.2   Antioxidants
3   PROMOTION OF CARCINOGENESIS
    3.1   Cell cycle and its control
    3.2   Oxidative stress
    3.3   Antioxidants
4   TUMOR GROWTH AND PROGRESSION
    4.1   Experimental studies
    4.2   Apoptosis and *bcl*-2 genes
5   OXIDATIVE STRESS, ANTIOXIDANTS AND CANCER IN HUMANS
    5.1   Epidemiological observational studies
        5.1.1   Inverse association of antioxidants and cancer
        5.1.2   Modification of pro-oxidant-antioxidant balance
    5.2   Intervention studies
        5.2.1   Intermediate endpoints
        5.2.2   Precancerous state endpoint
        5.2.3   Cancer endpoint
    6   SUMMARY
    6.1   Mechanisms
    6.2   Epidemiological findings
    6.3   Public health implications
    7   PERSPECTIVES
8   ACKNOWLEDGMENTS
9   ABBREVIATIONS
10 REFERENCES

1   INTRODUCTION

One may wonder why it is necessary to write again on oxidative stress, antioxidants and cancer when so many reviews have already been dedicated to the topic [1,2]. Most of these reviews, however, were published when a rather simplistic concept of carcinogenesis prevailed: in the beginning is oxidative stress, and antioxidants are the savior.

Increasing knowledge of tumor biology led to more sophisticated concepts. The multistep process of carcinogenesis was taken into account, together with the specific mechanisms through which free radicals were at work in the various stages of carcinogenesis [3]. However, antioxidants still have the same role as before. Change occurred after the findings of the intervention study conducted in Finland, the ATBC study [4]. ATBC stands for α-tocopherol β-carotene, indicating supplementation with α-tocopherol, β-carotene or both. These results showed an increase in lung cancer incidence in the subjects supplemented with β-carotene and no effect in the subjects supplemented with vitamin E. The CARET study, a β-carotene and retinol intervention study [5] showed the same type of results, confirming the unexpected findings of the ATBC study and reinforcing the need to re-evaluate the relationship between oxidative stress, antioxidants and cancer.

Up to now, the approach used to examine the relationship between antioxidants and cancer has been first to report the results of epidemiological studies and then to propose mechanisms to explain the findings. However, the intervention studies, which were expected to confirm this approach, failed in fact to do so. The body of knowledge pertaining to oxidative stress, antioxidants and cancer has also increased over the last few years. Therefore, I now propose to turn the examination of this relationship on its head and first analyze the relationship of oxidative stress and antioxidants in the context of the natural history of cancer as depicted for several cancers [6—8]: initiation, promotion, tumor growth and progression. I shall then examine where and how findings from human studies can be inserted in the multistep process. Hypotheses and speculative mechanisms will be proposed to reconcile the protective effect of antioxidants in some situations with their deleterious role in others.

2   INITIATION OF CARCINOGENESIS

2.1 Oxidative stress

It is generally recognized that free radical processes, responsible for mutagenic and genotoxic events, occur at initiation [2]. Several radicals can be directly genotoxic, the more dangerous being the peroxy radicals because their reactivity is more selective, consequently they are longer-lived and further-reaching in biosystems than hydroxyl radicals, which are characterized by an indiscriminate reactivity, wasting their oxidative potential on inconsequential components, and travel on average no further than 1 nm, disappearing in under 1 ns [2]. Products from lipid peroxidation such as malondialdehyde (MDA) or 4-hydroxynonenal are also mutagenic [9]. In addition to direct genetic damage, radicals may also activate some procarcinogens [10].

In humans, inflammatory states, which are characterized by high concentrations of endogenous radicals such as superoxide, are associated with tumor development [11,12]. High-energy radiation induces tumors through cell water radiolysis and the production of hydroxyl radicals. It has been suggested that the increasing incidence of cancer with age might be due to the increasing rate of free radical production in elderly persons [13]. However, it might also be due to the increasing risk of encountering the environmental factors necessary if the multistep process of carcinogenesis is to continue. These data are summarized in Fig. 1.

2.2 Antioxidants

The main antioxidants considered here are β-carotene, vitamin E, vitamin C and selenium.

There are about 600 natural carotenoids with a comparable structure, a C40 isoprenoid skeleton. Carotenes are either acyclic (lycopene) or bicyclic (β-carotene) hydrocarbons. Oxygenated carotenoids are called xanthophylls (e.g., astaxanthin, cathaxanthin). Fifty carotenoids act as provitamin A (e.g., α- and β-carotene, β-cryptoxanthin). They are cleaved at the central bond [15] to give retinal. Eccentric cleavages can occur in tissues, leading to direct formation of retinoic acid [14]. Through the long conjugated polyene chain, all carotenes have the capacity to interact with singlet excited species, the most important being the

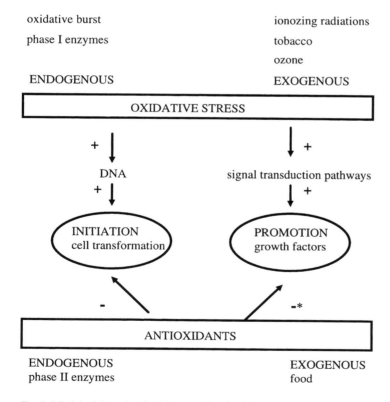

Fig. 1. Model of the role of oxidants and antioxidants at the initiation and promotion phases of carcinogenesis; + indicates a carcinogenic effect, – indicates an anticarcinogenic effect. *: In some situations β-carotene may act as a pro-oxidant; in some models antioxidants protect the transformed cell from the deleterious effect of the reactive oxygen species (see text).

singlet oxygen, $^1O_2$ [15,16]. Carotenes have also been shown to interact with reactive oxygen species and inhibit lipid peroxidation [15–18].

β-Carotene is the carotenoid most consistently studied in human and animal studies. More recently attention has been drawn to other carotenoids, such as α-carotene, β-cryptoxanthin, lycopene and lutein. Lycopene has been shown to modulate cytochrome P450 2E1 [19].

Natural vitamin E is made up of eight nutrients, tocopherols α β γ δ and tocotrienols α β γ δ. α-Tocopherol is found in the largest amounts in most animal species and displays the highest peroxidation chain-breaking capacity: vitamin C reduces oxidized vitamin E, suggesting that a deficit in vitamin C might leave oxidized vitamin E with a pro-oxidant capacity. Vitamin E metabolism is strongly associated with plasma lipids, primarily with LDL cholesterol, as vitamin E is distributed to cells through the LDL receptor. Vitamin E deficiency is not found in the developed countries. Although vitamin E is excreted in feces when the transfer protein is saturated, high doses may be deleterious: it has been shown that vitamin E interferes with the leucocyte capacity to lyse bacteria and with the vitamin K concentration necessary to ensure coagulation [20].

The active forms of vitamin C are ascorbic acid and ascorbates. These are hydrosoluble and sensitive to oxidation. The main sources are fresh fruit, especially citrus fruit. Vitamin C is a redox agent, antioxidant in certain situations (and probably so at the concentrations found in plants) but also capable of free radical generation in other circumstances, such as in the presence of transition metal [21].

The main role of selenium in the organism is to be a part of the active site of the enzyme glutathione peroxidase (GSHpx), which is responsible for protecting the organism against lipid peroxidation. Other roles have been suggested: detoxication of xenobiotics, modulation of inflammatory and immune responses and of the cyclooxygenase pathway [22].

At the initiation step, different forms of defense against oxidant-induced genetic damage operate, via various mechanisms:

1) oxidative stress can be prevented by antioxienzymes, including the seleno-dependent GSHpx;
2) enzymatic repair of DNA negates the damage resulting from oxidative stress; and
3) vitamin E, as a chain-breaking antioxidant, inactivates peroxyradicals in the membrane. Carotenes can play the same role.

Ascorbate and NADH are expected to be the primary inactivators of peroxyradicals in the cytosol [2]. These data are summarized in Fig. 2.

If antioxidants have been ineffective against the oxidative stress damage and any genetic damage to the cells has not been repaired, the latter become initiated cells.

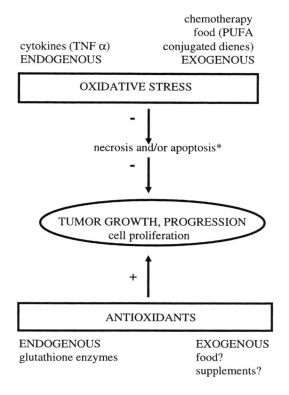

cytokines (TNF α)
ENDOGENOUS

chemotherapy
food (PUFA
conjugated dienes)
EXOGENOUS

OXIDATIVE STRESS

-

necrosis and/or apoptosis*

-

TUMOR GROWTH, PROGRESSION
cell proliferation

+

ANTIOXIDANTS

ENDOGENOUS
glutathione enzymes

EXOGENOUS
food?
supplements?

Fig. 2. Model of the role of oxidants–antioxidants at the tumor growth/progression phase of carcinogenesis. + indicates a carcinogenic effect; – indicates an anticarcinogenic effect. *: necrosis has been shown in animal and in vitro model. Apoptosis is hypothesized because it has been shown to be oxidative stress-induced in several models and because the bcl/2 gene product, antagonist of p53 has been mimicked by antioxidants (see text).

3 PROMOTION OF CARCINOGENESIS

3.1 Cell proliferation and its control

Cell cycle is traditionally described in four phases: G1, S, G2 and M. Quiescent cells are in a distinct phase called G0 from which cells will progress through the cycle. Cyclins are the key components of the cell progression machinery. In combination with their respective cyclin-dependent protein-kinases (CDKs), cyclins form the holoenzymes that phosphorylate different sets of proteins at consecutive stages of the cell cycle, thereby driving the cell through the different phases of the cycle.

When growth-related genes (c-fos, c-myc etc.) of G0 cells are stimulated, the D-type cyclins are expressed and launch the cell in the G1 phase by activation of the CDK4. The complex phosphorylates the retinoblastoma tumor suppressor gene protein (pRB). Phosphorylation of pRB releases E2F factor which activates components of the DNA replication thereby committing the cell to the S phase. The association of cyclin E with CDK2 is also essential for cell entrance to S phase. It is cyclin A, associated with either CDK1 or CDK2, which drives the cell through S and G2. After DNA synthesis is completed, it is the G2 phase. During this phase, cyclin B1 activates CDK1, forming the maturation promoting factor of which kinase activity is essential for cell entrance to M phase, the mitotic phase.

Under physiological conditions, cell proliferation is arrested upon a finite number of divisions with a G1 DNA content. The holoenzyme CDK4 is inhibited by p16 and p21 thus, pRB remains in its under phosphorylated form and blocks commitment of the cell to the S phase. In tumor cells, expression of D type cyclins is not restricted to early G1 cells. Consequently, it is likely that phosphorylation of pRB continues throughout the cell cycle, resulting in continuous proliferation.

Cell regulation is coupled to the alternative pathway of the cell, the programmed cell death, or apoptosis, which eliminates nonfunctional or abnormal cells, is controlled by p53. Tumour cells escape this mechanism by deregulation of the *bcl*-2 gene, among other possible mechanisms (Section 4.3).

3.1 Oxidative stress

Initiated cells may stay dormant until another genetic event triggers clonal proliferation. Increased cellular concentrations of active oxygen and radical peroxides can act as a second growth factor signal [24] and promote initiated cells to neoplastic growth [23]. It has been suggested that reactive oxygen species might be involved in the signal transduction pathway leading to NF-κB activation [25].

Mutations activate or deactivate several classes of proteins, mainly resulting in deregulation of the cell cycle [26].

3.2 Antioxidants

At this stage, the antioxidants can oppose the effect of radicals via the same mechanisms as described for the initiation step. Antioxidants are, therefore, theoretically, also protective at this step, via the same mechanisms as for initiation. However, complex interactions occur at this stage between radicals, antioxidants and the natural history of cancer.

Cerutti [27] reported on the difference between a promotable and a nonpromotable mouse cell clone: the promotable clone showed a higher level of antioxidant enzyme activities and concentration than the nonpromotable one. Promotion by reactive oxygen species was thus, only possible in this model if the initiated cell developed the capability of defense against the oxidative stress of the radicals which is required for growth factor synthesis. Vitamin E has been shown to promote tumors in an animal model [28], possibly by mimicking the antioxienzymes described in Cerutti's model.

The situation for β-carotene appears to be different. The antioxidant properties are determined not only by the chemical reactivity of the compound but also by the fate of the resulting antioxidant-derived radical, by the reactivity of the compound with other antioxidants present and by its reactivity with molecular oxygen. This is crucial to the initiation of the pro-oxidative pathways in the process of free radical scavenging by carotenoids [29]. Radical-cations and adduct-radicals are probably incapable of exerting pro-oxidative effects in lipid-rich environments such as biomembranes. However, all carotenoid adduct-radicals (but not the cation-radicals) can theoretically initiate a pro-oxidative pathway in tissues exposed to high O_2 pressure, such as lungs. In the case of NO_2 scavenging by β-carotene, nonradical products unlikely to exhibit pro-oxidative effects are generated. If glutathione is present, however, conversion occurs to glutathione thiyl radicals, which may produce a shift from carotenoid radical-cations to adduct-radicals capable of initiating a pro-oxidative pathway. Besides, carotenes appear to be more prone than xanthophylls to propagate as peroxyl radicals. In the situations described above (formation of radical adducts plus reaction with molecular oxygen) the antioxidant properties of carotenoids are, therefore, reversed resulting in opposed interactions with the natural history of cancer: the increased pro-oxidant state of the cell can facilitate promotion [23].

4 TUMOR GROWTH AND PROGRESSION

The phases of progression to tumor growth and of metastasis present a more complex picture. Point mutations may take place to reach the next phase (e.g., mutation of p53), hence one can assume that antioxidants have a protective role as in initiation phase. However, as foreseen by Szent-Georgy [30], oxidative stress, which was shown to play a role in cell signaling towards growth factor synthesis, may also regulate proliferation of rapidly dividing cells.

4.1 Experimental studies

It was shown first that tumor cells are characterized by a lower proportion of polyunsaturated fatty acid and a higher vitamin E content in their membranes than their normal counterparts [31], and the hypothesis of an appropriate oxidant/antioxidant balance in cell proliferation has been developed from models opposing polyunsaturated fatty acids and vitamin E [32]. The deleterious effect of peroxidation for cell proliferation was shown first: in two comparable tumor lines in vitro [33,34], then on different tumor lines and animal models with the addition of various polyunsaturated fatty acids [35—38]. Addition of polyunsaturated fatty acids showed a comparable inhibitory effect on rapidly dividing normal cells [39,40].

Other types of oxidative stress were also shown to inhibit tumor cell proliferation. Hypoxanthine and xanthine oxidase in an in vivo model significantly suppressed tumor growth at the point where they were infused [41], and Schwartz et al. [42] demonstrated that β-carotene inhibited tumor growth in conditions where it acted as a pro-oxidant. In a short-term fish oil feeding trial with patients treated for adenoma, cell proliferation decreased in the colonic mucosa [43]. More recently it was shown that a shift of the pro-oxidant/antioxidant balance toward the pro-oxidant state after androgen exposure at physiological doses induced growth arrest of an androgen-responsive prostate carcinoma cell line [44].

Antioxidants, especially vitamin E, were capable of opposing the deleterious effect of peroxidation in vitro [37,45] or in vivo [46,47].

4.2 Apoptosis and *bcl*-2 genes

For a long time these experimental findings appeared paradoxical, but they should now be considered in the light of the concept of apoptosis. Such programmed cell death is supposed to eradicate cells which deviate from the normal proliferating behavior. One might think that initiated cells promoted to proliferation would be the first targets of the apoptotis mechanism. Apoptosis is most often induced by an oxidative stress [48] and is usually less pronounced in tumor cells. The *bcl*-2 gene activity, which is related to an antiapoptosis effect and enhanced cell proliferation, decreases reactive oxygen species [49] and can be mimicked by antioxidants [50]. It has been suggested that the appropriate balance of oxidants and antioxidants is important for cell proliferation in the context of clonal expansion and apoptosis [12,51], strongly suggesting that increasing its antioxidant defenses gives the tumor cell a selective growth advantage.

5   OXIDATIVE STRESS, ANTIOXIDANTS AND CANCERS IN HUMAN STUDIES

Antioxidants showed several effects in human studies: a decreased cancer risk in many epidemiological observational studies, some paradoxical observations in case-control studies and a deleterious β-carotene effect in some intervention studies. These discrepancies can be better understood if we consider the findings in the context of the natural history of cancer.

5.1 Epidemiological observational studies

5.1.1   *Inverse association of antioxidants with cancer risk*

Prospective studies based on biological markers of antioxidants, or their intake, and case-control studies based on retrospective antioxidant nutrient intake are the epidemiological methods used to analyze the relationship between antioxidants and cancer. These studies tend to refer to the first stages of the carcinogenesis process. The first few studies, which were prospective studies based on biological markers, present the best methodology to show a causal relationship and to assess the level of exposure to antioxidant. Preference will, therefore, be given to the findings of such studies, when they exist.

5.1.1.1 β-Carotene. Several prospective studies were conducted based on plasma measurement. Their results are summarized in Table 1, which includes those using the baseline plasma levels of the intervention studies.

When they considered all sites, prospective studies based on biochemical markers showed inconsistent results, because the effect of β-carotene is regularly observed in some cancers and practically never in others.

The results are very consistent for lung cancer and also for cancers of the upper aerodigestive tract. They are also consistent for cervical cancer, but only few studies addressed this site. They are consistently negative for breast cancer (in one study the assessment was performed on adipose tissue [52]) and cancer of the colon. They are also negative for prostate and bladder cancers.

Some studies also assessed other carotenoids: one on 6,860 men of Japanese ancestry [53] showed that the reduction in upper aerodigestive tract cancers was also inversely associated with α-carotene and β-cryptoxanthin. All carotenoids were inversely associated with cervical cancers in the study of Batieha [54]. In the last analysis of the Washington County study performed after 17 years of follow-up of 25,802 subjects, all carotenoids other than lycopene were inversely

Table 1. Summary of results for serum or plasma concentrations of carotenoids and cancers in prospective studies.[a]

Cancer site	No of studies	No with inverse association[b]	No with dose-response association[c]
All	8	6	2/2
Lung	12	11	1/1
Upper aerodigest tr.	6	5	1/2
Stomach	5	2	1/1
Colorectum	9	0	
Pancreas	3	1	1/1
Liver	1	0	
Skin	7	1	1/1
Breast	3	0	
Ovary	1	0	
Endometrium	1	0	
Cervix	2	1	1/1
Prostate	4	0	
Bladder	4	0	
Kidney	1	1	1/1
Leukem/lymphoma	2	0	
Brain/CNS	2	0	

[a]Adapted from [120]; [b]Inverse association, a 30% or greater reduction in cancer risk or significantly reduced mean carotene level; [c]Dose-response association; a significant gradient; x/x: number of studies reporting a gradient per number of studies investigating a gradient.

associated with lung cancer, whereas the latter was the only one showing an effect on pancreatic cancer in a small study [55]. In the Hokkaido study only β-carotene reduced stomach cancer risk, with α-carotene and lycopene having no effect [56].

Prospective studies based on intake are in agreement with the ones based on biomarkers, with the additional finding that lycopene had a protective effect for prostate cancer [57]. The negative findings for colon and breast cancer were extended to lycopene and lutein.

5.1.1.2 Vitamin E. Several prospective studies have been performed based on vitamin E assessment but many of them did not control for lipid parameters, which are highly correlated to vitamin E, nor was storage adequate (–20°C). The Basel study [58] met both requirements and showed an increased risk for lung cancer and prostate cancer after 17 years of follow-up of smokers with low plasma levels of vitamin E.

Finally, it is important to note that in the heavy smoker sample of the ATBC study [4] vitamin E plasma levels were significantly lower in the subjects who developed lung cancer: the incidence was 61.4 for the bottom quartile of plasma vitamin E and 40.6 for the top quartile.

Most of the prospective studies based on vitamin E intake, reviewed by Knekt [59], report insignificant results either for all sites or for specific sites: lung, thyroid, colon, rectum or breast [60,61]. The more recent Netherlands cohort study [62] showed no association between vitamin E intake and breast cancer.

Contradictory findings appear for lung cancer in the two large studies recently reported: the NHANES study [63] showed a protective effect for vitamin E which was stronger in smokers, whereas the Zutphen study [64] did not reveal any association. No benefit was detected from supplementation rather than nutritional intake.

The Iowa Women's Health Study [65] showed that compared to nonsupplemented women, supplemented women showed a significantly lower incidence of cancer of the colon. Two further US studies consider the effect of supplementation. The one studying oropharyngeal cancers [66] showed that only vitamin E supplements protect against cancer incidence (OR = 0.5; CI 95%: 0.4–0.6). In the other study, on the role of β-carotene in nonsmokers with regard to lung cancer [67], it was shown that vitamin E supplementation reduced the risk of lung cancer, but there was no indication of a dose-response (OR = 0.55; CI 95%: 0.35–0.85).

Finally, two Italian case-control studies showed a significant reduction of risk, one for stomach cancer [68] and the other for breast cancer [69].

5.1.1.3 Vitamin C. Out of the 46 studies considering the effect of vitamin C intake on cancer mortality, 33 reported significant protection [70]. However, several sites are more consistently associated with vitamin C, whereas in others no risk modification is observed.

Protection was clear against stomach cancer [64,70]. In addition to the antioxidant activity countering the formation of nitrosamine, vitamin C was thought to protect against Helicobacter pylori, a major risk factor for stomach cancer. Vitamin C also protected against oropharyngeal and esophageal cancers in nine out of ten epidemiological studies devoted to these topics, and also against the rare salivary gland cancer [71]. Subjects with oral leucoplasia have lower vitamin C plasma levels than their normal counterparts [72].

Less consistent was the inverse association with lung cancer. However, recent major prospective studies demonstrated significantly lower lung cancer risk in subjects with lower plasma levels of vitamin C (the Basel study [58]) or of vitamin C intake (the NHANES study [63]). The latter showed that the effect was modified by the intensity of exposure to cigarettes. The Zutphen study [64] insisted on the stability of the vitamin C intake over several years.

About one-half of the studies considering the relationship between vitamin C intake and invasive carcinoma of the cervix showed a reduction of risk with a high intake. Low plasma levels were found to be associated with dysplasias of the cervix [70].

With colorectal cancer, we come to the group of cancers which are protected by vegetable and fruit intake but for which it is difficult to pinpoint the responsible nutrients. About 25% of the studies showed that vitamin C had a protective effect against cancer of the colon [70,73], but it is difficult to ascertain whether this observation was related specifically to vitamin C rather than to another fruit and/or vegetable microcomponent.

The results are even less substantial with hormone-dependent cancers, especially breast cancer. Although meta-analysis of 12 case-control studies showed an association of vitamin C intake with breast cancer, all prospective studies displayed negative findings [62,74,75].

5.1.1.4 Selenium. Most studies are based on the selenium plasma or cell content. The oldest studies [76,77] showed a higher risk for all cancers associated with low levels of selenium. This was not confirmed in more recent prospective studies [78,79]. After a large review [80], the authors conclude that selenium may be protective for pancreas and stomach cancers. It is interesting to note that most of the studies showing a reduced risk of cancers of various sites in subjects classified in the upper quartile of selenium level distribution were conducted in men [81−85]. In women, results are mostly negative [80,85−88].

5.1.2 Modification of pro-oxidant-antioxidant balance

Studies conducted with cancer patients are the ones relevant to this topic, as such patients are very likely at the step of tumor growth and progression.

5.1.2.1 Decrease in peroxidable substrate. Verreault et al. [89] reported that breast cancer patients with a high intake of polyunsaturated fat showed less invaded nodes than breast cancer patients with a lower intake of polyunsaturated fatty acids or a high intake of saturated fatty acids. It has been shown that a decrease in breast cancer risk was associated with an increased level of polyunsaturated fatty acids in erythrocyte membranes [90]. In a corollary fashion, tumor cells from poor prognosis breast cancers showed a lower level of polyunsaturated fatty acids than tumor cells from better prognosis breast cancers [91]. However, in 70 patients with early breast cancer, the lipoperoxide content of the breast adipose tissue was higher than that of 30 patients with benign breast disease [92]. But this does not prejudice the tumor cell content.

Plasma of cancer patients with less aggressive tumors display lower levels of MDA, a product of lipid peroxidation, than the control subjects after controlling for age and other confounding factors [93,94]. It was speculated that increased production of free radicals with aging could explain the lower severity of tumors in elderly patients compared to younger ones [95].

5.1.2.2 Antioxidant increase. Higher levels of plasma vitamin E were found in women with gynecological cancers than in controls [96—99]. The difference was significant moreover, after controlling for lipid parameters [100,101]. However, in 70 patients with early breast cancer, the vitamin E content of the breast adipose tissue was lower than in 30 patients with benign breast disease [92]. But this does not prejudice the tumor cell content. There was no significant difference between the concentration of vitamin E measured in the gluteal adipose tissue of postmenopausal breast cancer cases compared to population controls [52].

A report on women with estrogen receptor positive breast cancer showed that patients with a higher fat and vitamin E intake and a low vitamin C intake had a poorer prognosis than those with the opposite nutritional characteristics [102]. Multivariate analysis showed that a risk of therapeutic failure of 1.19 (CI 95%: 1.03—1.37) was associated with each intake of 1 mg of vitamin E per 10 megajoules.

5.2 Intervention studies

Intervention studies will be classified by endpoints selected for treatment evaluation, as an early marker like micronuclei in bronchial washings will indicate an early stage of carcinogenesis, possibly initiation, whereas hyperplasia or a benign tumor is close to the promotional stage and cancer incidence close to tumor growth.

5.2.1 *Intermediate endpoints*

β-carotene supplementation was shown to be beneficial when used to treat early markers of cancer risk prior to the hyperproliferation phase. It decreased the number of micronuclei in smokers' sputum [103]. On the other hand, McLarty [104] found that β-carotene associated with vitamin A had no effect on serial sputum cytology in a trial with subjects who had previously worked in asbestos factories.

β-carotene-induced regression of dysplasias of the oral cavity and the cervix [105]. It should be mentioned that in this study, vitamin A was even more protective than β-carotene (probably through differentiation induction), suggesting that the effect of β-carotene may rely on its provitamin A properties.

In a smaller sample of the Linxiang study 3,318 subjects with esophageal dysplasia took a single supplement with 26 vitamins and minerals, including β-carotene (15 mg). No marked benefit could be demonstrated during the 6 years of follow-up.

5.2.2 Precancerous states

Recently, an Indian study was conducted to treat progression of precancerous oral lesions [106]. The supplements consisted of vitamin A, riboflavine, zinc and selenium. After 1 year there was a significant difference in the regression or progression of lesions between supplemented and nonsupplemented subjects, and those with an improvement displayed significantly higher selenium levels compared with the unimproved subjects. The assay was neither randomized nor double-blinded, however.

Rectal cell proliferation was measured in 23 patients who had colorectal adenomas removed completely. After removal of the adenomas, they were randomized into a supplemented group (30,000 IU of vitamin A, 70 mg of vitamin E and 1 g of ascorbic acid) and a placebo group [107]. Biopsies were performed at 3 and 6 months after treatment. Supplementation was effective in reducing abnormal proliferation in the upper crypt, which the authors interpreted as an effect on a possible precancerous state.

Patients in the colon adenoma intervention assay [108] 751 completed a 4-year clinical trial. They were randomized into a 2 × 2 factorial design with four groups treated daily with placebo, β-carotene (25 mg), vitamin C (1 g) and vitamin E (400 mg), or β-carotene plus vitamins C and E. The primary endpoint was new adenomas. None of the antioxidants alone or combined modified adenoma recurrence. A significant increase in new adenomas in the right colon was observed (OR = 1.35 CI: 1.04−1.77) in subjects supplemented with vitamins E and C, but the authors interpreted the result as a chance finding.

In the Australian Polyp Prevention project, about 400 subjects were randomized into four groups: low fat (25% calories from fat), fiber supplement (11 g/day from wheat bran), β-carotene (20 mg/day). No treatment had any effect on adenoma recurrence, but there was a nonsignificantly increased risk in the β-carotene group. However, colonoscopy was not performed in 25% of participants and this large loss of endpoint data may bias the findings.

5.2.3 Cancers as an endpoint

5.2.3.1 The Quidong study. This assay was conducted to prevent the development of primary liver cancer [109] in a region were the incidence of this cancer is high and selenium serum levels low. One assay was conducted on 226 subjects presenting HB antigen. After 4 years five cancers developed in the selenium-supplemented sample (200 mg selenium per day) and none in the placebo sample. The second assay consisted of 2,474 subjects from the families of liver cancer patients. After 2 years liver cancer was diagnosed in 0.69% of the supplemented subjects (200 mg selenium per day) against 1.26% in the nonsupplemented subjects.

5.2.3.2 The Linxiang study. The assay was conducted in China and intended to evaluate mortality and incidence of esophageal and gastric cancers in 29,584 men from the general population which was globally deficient in micronutrients (β-carotene at baseline was 59 µg/l). They were randomized into a complex 2×4 design, using four different nutrient combinations including one consisting of β-carotene (15 mg), vitamin E (50 mg) and selenium (30 mg). After 5 years of follow-up, none of the combinations had produced any major reduction in esophageal or gastric cancers. Supplementation with β-carotene, vitamin E and selenium significantly decreased cancer mortality (by 13%) and stomach cancer mortality and incidence (by 21%). The reduction in cancer mortality appeared after 2 years of supplementation [110].

5.2.3.3 The ATBC study. This study involved 29,133 male heavy smokers in Finland [4]. They were randomized into a 2×2 factorial design with three treatment groups: dl-α-tocopherol acetate (50 mg/day), β-carotene (20 mg/day), β-carotene plus α-tocopherol, and placebo. After 7.5 years of follow-up there was an 16% excess of cumulative lung cancer incidence in the β-carotene group compared with the non-β-carotene group. The increase started after 3 years of follow-up. The increase was concentrated in the heaviest smokers (over 20 cigarettes/day) and those drinking over 11 g of alcohol per day. The incidence of prostate and stomach cancers were higher also, whereas there was no change in bladder and colorectal cancers. Vitamin E alone or combined with β-carotene had no effect on cancer mortality, but there was a decrease in prostatic cancer incidence.

5.2.3.4 The CARET study. The trial involved 14,254 current or former smokers and 4,060 asbestos-exposed workers in the US [5]. They were randomized into a treatment group (30 mg β-carotene and 25000 IU retinyl palmitate) and a placebo group. Analysis of all data [111] gave the results described in Table 2.

The increase in risk started after 18 months of treatment. Among non-asbestos-exposed patients it is concentrated in smokers, but asbestos-exposed smokers showed an increased risk whether they were smokers or not.

5.2.3.5 The Physicians Health study. The study involved 22,071 US male physicians [112]. At baseline, 11% were current smokers and 39% former smokers. Average baseline plasma levels of β-carotene were 0.56 mmol/l, almost twice as high as in the ATBC and CARET studies. The subjects were randomized in a

Table 2. Lung cancer risk in the treatment group of the CARET study.

Classes	OR	CI
All subjects	1.36	1.07—1.73
Asbestos exposed	1.82	1.16—2.84
Current smokers	1.40	1.04—1.86
Former smokers[a]	0.80	0.44—1.45
Former smokers[b]	2.34	1.17—4.68
Nondrinkers	1.21	0.80—1.23
Drinkers > 30 g ethanol	2.02	1.07—3.80

[a]Asbestos nonexposed; [b]Asbestos-exposed.

2×2 factorial trial of β-carotene (50 mg on alternate days), aspirin (325 mg on alternate days), both, or placebo. The aspirin component was stopped after 6 years because of favorable results in the prevention of myocardial infarction. The β-carotene component was followed for 12 years. No modification of risk was observed in this trial.

5.2.3.6 Interpretation of intervention studies. The reasons for a lack of effect might lie in the fact that antioxidants are only markers of certain foods and that such foods contain the effective components. Plants contain many compounds likely to protect against cancers (glucosinolates, isothiocyanates, S-methyl cysteine, allyl sulfurs, phytates, phyto-estrogens) some of which demonstrate antioxidant properties (phenolic compounds, flavonoids).

Interest focused on them when it became obvious that the protective effect of vegetables and fruit intakes was larger than that of the nutrients usually evaluated as components of the ingested fruit or vegetables. The failure of intervention studies with β-carotene and vitamin E enhanced this trend. Witte et al. [113] demonstrated it elegantly by further adjusting for potentially anticarcinogenic constituents of fruit and vegetables (namely antioxidants and fiber) the OR showing a decreased risk of colorectal adenomas in persons with a high intake of fruit and vegetables. None of the associations was decreased by adjusting for the relevant antioxidant nutrients, indicating that protective effects might reflect unmeasured constituents in these foods, at least for colorectal adenomas (only risk reduction with whole grain was decreased by adjusting for fiber, indicating that this particular reduction was fiber-dependent).

Knowledge of the precise content of these compounds in food and of their metabolism and physiological role is scarce, however, especially with regard to adsorption through the intestinal barrier and the chemistry of their derived metabolites in human and animal organisms. The study conducted by Hertog et al. [114] is of special interest because it was preceded by analytical work on several foods to identify and quantitate the main flavonoids present in the diet of the surveyed population. The intake of quercetine and kaempferol was not associated with cancer incidence (whereas it was shown to be protective against cardiovascular diseases). A more recent prospective study using the same database as Hertog et al. [114] showed a reduction of risk for cancer [115]. The follow-up of 9,959 Finnish men and women over 24 years showed a reduction for all sites (0.80, CI: 0.67–0.96), mainly reflecting the strong effect on lung cancer (0.54, CI: 0.34–0.87).

Experimental studies using such nonnutrient plant components are essentially conducted in vitro thus, avoiding the question of absorption. What is more, they generally pertain to properties other than antioxidant ones, such as the effect on the cell cycle [116,117].

Although it is possible that β-carotene is only a marker of other beneficial plant components, this does not explain the increased risk observed with supplementation.

One essential reason for the increased risk appears to be the situation of the subjects with regard to the natural history of cancer. In the ATBC [4] and CARET [5,111] studies, the particular local conditions may be responsible for implementing the pro-oxidant capacities of β-carotene: NO_2, which is known to interfere with β-carotene, is provided by current smoking, and molecular oxygen at atmospheric pressure is provided by breathing.

The CARET study permits further interpretation, because the asbestos- and tobacco-exposed subgroups have different point estimates for relative lung cancer risk (though with overlapping confidence intervals). Serum β-carotene above the median at baseline does not reduce lung cancer risk in asbestos-exposed subjects (RR = 0.95; 95% CI: 0.60, 1.49 vs. RR = 0.62; 95% CI: 0.46, 0.82 in heavy smokers). Besides, in asbestos-exposed subjects there is no difference in relative lung cancer risk between former and current smokers (Table 2). It is, therefore, likely that NO_2 does not play a part in the oxidative stress to which asbestos workers are subject. The NO_2 pathway transforming β-carotene into pro-oxidant described above thus, does not operate in this situation. β-Carotene can, therefore, react with another pro-oxidant, the anion superoxide of the inflammatory reaction caused by asbestos, enhancing carcinogenesis. Or it can act by another mechanism, the high level of antioxidant, protecting proliferation of transformed cells. However, the β-carotene plasma levels for the supplemented group were no higher in the lung cancer cases than in the cancer-free subjects.

6   SUMMARY

6.1 Mechanisms

The study of the mechanisms at work during the natural history of cancer strongly suggests that antioxidants can oppose transformation of normal cells by mutagenic oxidative stress. They probably also play a part at the promotion stage as reactive oxygen species act as second messengers in transcellular signaling systems, although antioxidant effects have been ambiguous in some models. This ambiguity might result from two situations, either:

1) antioxidants become pro-oxidants because of particular conditions (β-carotene, and atmospheric pressure of oxygen and NO_2 stress), or because of lack of regeneration (deficit in vitamin C to regenerate vitamin E); or
2) antioxidants allow promotion by reactive oxygen species because they protect the DNA replication process in the cells from oxidative stress.

The shift of the oxidant-antioxidant balance toward the antioxidant side observed in several tumor cells might also take place at the stage of tumor growth and facilitate carcinogenesis. But the shift is more probably the result of genetic instability in the regulation of apoptosis and of overexpression of antioxidant enzymes, rather than of exogenous antioxidants (except perhaps in the case of very high dosage supplementation).

The natural history of cancer and the chemistry of antioxidants suggest factors or mechanisms which might explain the increased risk of lung cancer in the population at risk covered by the ATBC and the CARET studies, although these are still speculative at present:

1) the presence of initiated cells in the populations at risk;
2) antioxidants possibly becoming antioxidants in specific situations;
3) high dosages of β-carotene; and
4) a shift in the pro-oxidant/antioxidant balance.

6.2 Epidemiological findings

Findings of epidemiological studies (prospective and retrospective case-control studies) support the protective role of antioxidants in the early stages of carcinogenesis. This is not true of all cancers, however: the only cancers which are consistently inversely associated with antioxidants are epithelial cancers in which carcinogens come into direct contact with the target cells: tobacco and the buccal epithelium; asbestos, benzo-pyrene, NO_2 and the epithelium of the lung; nitrosamines and the gastric epithelium; polyomavirus and the epithelium of the cervix. The other cancer sites do not appear to benefit from the protective effect of antioxidants.

The effect of each antioxidant varies with the cancer site: β-carotene and vitamin C share a risk-reducing effect for upper respiratory and digestive tract cancers and for cervical cancer. But there is stronger evidence of an association between lung cancer and carotenoids than between lung cancer and vitamin C, and of an association between gastric cancer and vitamin C rather than with carotenoids. This might reflect a specificity with regard to carcinogens. Vitamin E possibly decreases lung, stomach and cervical cancer risks, and selenium possibly lung and stomach cancers, but the findings are less consistent than for β-carotene and vitamin C. It is noteworthy that vitamin E and selenium seem to have a common effect and that this effect is mainly observed in men, as this might indicate that they react with carcinogens such as alcohol and tobacco. Prostatic cancer appears to be a special case, in that it has been inversely associated with lycopene intake [57] and vitamin E supplementation [4].

6.3 Public health implications

Antioxidant nutrients are never as risk-reducing as the food they come from, essentially fruit and vegetables. However, it should be noted that fruit and vegetables are not the main contributors of vitamin E, which has been found to be protective in several studies.

We, therefore, cannot be sure that these antioxidant nutrients, which are consistently inversely associated with some cancers, are effective by themselves. They might alternatively be markers for another risk-reducing component. This would explain the lack of protective effect of supplementation in intervention studies in the population not at risk (the Physician Health Study). Concomitant intake of synergic nutrients, such as provided by fruit and vegetables might be necessary: this would explain the moderate success of the Linxiang study, where a severely deficient population was supplemented with three antioxidants.

One can therefore conclude that antioxidants are not the magic bullet capable of protecting against all cancers at all stages of carcinogenesis.

7   PERSPECTIVES

In the short term, we can await the findings of on-going intervention studies. Such studies are usually based on a combined treatment. A study into antioxidants, Helicobacter pylori and stomach cancer is being conducted in Venezuela to evaluate the progression rate of precancerous lesions of the stomach [118]. It combines vitamin C (250 mg), vitamin E (200 mg) and β-carotene (6 mg). In France, the SUVIMAX study [119] provides daily supplementation with vitamin C (120 mg), β-carotene (6 mg), vitamin E (30 mg), selenium (100 mg) and zinc (20 mg), a combination equal to 1 to 3 times the recommended dietary allowances. If the combined supplementation provides no protection, this might instead indicate the role of other plant food components, such as glucosinolates, isothiocyanates, phenolic compounds, flavonoids, fiber etc.)

The agenda for further research is marked by the uncertainties and the speculative hypothesis developed above.

Is β-carotene the marker of increased risk through a lowered defense mechanism or through greater exposure to a specific carcinogen? Metabolism of carotenoids in situations relevant to human conditions must be investigated with special attention to doses, oxygen pressure and cell antioxidant environment.

If β-carotene is the marker of risk reduction only for upper aerodigestive tract cancers, which is/are the component(s) responsible? Intense research into the various components of fruit and vegetables is already in progress to answer this question, but models relevant to human situations have still to be designed. In the meantime reanalysis of the many epidemiological observational studies should be carried out using recently acquired information on food composition.

Should vitamin E always be studied in conjunction with vitamin C, keeping in mind that the main contributor of vitamin E is sunflower oil and mayonnaise, which are generally used with raw vegetables.

Such biochemical and epidemiological studies need to be supplemented by genetic and molecular studies to shed more light on the shift in the pro-oxidant/antioxidant balance occurring in the proliferating tumor cells.

The main question is: should intervention studies be continued, mainly with β-carotene? Taking into consideration the risk level of the population sample, keeping doses at nutritional levels and combining several antioxidants may be not deleterious, but may also not provide much more helpful guidelines for prevention than the usual one of four to five helpings of fruit and vegetables per day.

Even if we think it impossible to influence human food habits and lifestyles, it is essential that research be continued, with the aim of defining which combination of antioxidants will contribute to better health, and for which population: the whole population or the population at risk.

8 ACKNOWLEDGMENTS

The author thanks Robert Goulevitch for his help in literature search and editing.

9 ABBREVIATIONS

ATBC:	α-tocopherol β-carotene
CARET:	carotene retinol
CDK:	cyclin-dependent protein kinase
CI:	confidence interval
DNA:	desoxyribonucleic acid
GSHpx:	glutathione peroxidase
LDL:	light density lipoprotein
MDA:	malondialdehyde
NADH:	nicotinic amine dehydrogenase
OR:	odds ratios
pRB:	retinoblatoma protein

10 REFERENCES

1. Ames BN, Gold LS, Willett WC. Proc Nat Acad Sci USA 1995;92:5258—5265.
2. Simic MG. Mutat Res 1988;202:377—386.
3. Pryor WA. Environ Health Perspect 1997;105:875—882.
4. ATBC, The α-Tocopherol, β-Carotene Cancer Prevention Study GR. N Engl J Med 1994;330: 1029—1035.
5. Omenn GS, Goodman GE, Thornquist MD, Balmes J, Cullen MR, Glass A, Keogh JP, Meyskens FL, Valanis B, Williams JH, Barnhart S, Hammar S. N Engl J Med 1994;334:1150—1155.
6. Hill MJ, Morson BC, Bussey HJR. Lancet 1978;1:245—247.
7. Ponten J, Holmberg L, Trichopoulos D et al. Int J Cancer 1990;S5:5—21.
8. Vogelstein B, Fearon EF, Hamilton SR et al. N Engl J Med 1988;319:525—532.
9. Esterbauer H, Zollner H, Schaur RJ. ISI Atlas Sci Biochem 1988;1:311—317.
10. Cavalieri E, Rogan E, Roth R. In: Floyd RA (ed) Free Radicals and Cancer. New York: Marcel

Dekker, 1982:117—158.

11. Kensler TW, Egner PA, Moore KG, Taffe BG, Twerkok LE, Trush MA. Toxicol Appl Pharmacol 1987;90:337—346.
12. Cerutti PA. The Lancet 1994;344:862—863.
13. Harman D. In: Emerit I, Chance B (eds) Free Radicals and Aging. Basel, Switzerland: Birkhäuser Verlag, 1992:1—10.
14. Wang XD, Russel RM, Liu C, Stickel F, Smith DE, Krinsky NY. J Biol Chem 1996;271:26490—26498.
15. Krinsky NI. In: Preventive Med 1989;18:592—602.
16. Krinsky NI. Free Rad Biol Med 1989;7:617—635.
17. Burton GW, Ingold KU. Science 1984;224:569—573.
18. Palozza P, Krinsky NI. Methods in Enzymology 1992;213:403—420.
19. Astorg P, Gradelet S, Berges R, Suschetet M. Nutr Cancer 1996;25:27—34.
20. Halliwell B, Gutteridge JMC. In: Halliwell B, Gutteridge JMC (eds) Free Radicals in Biology and Medecine. Oxford, England: Clarendon Press, 1985.
21. Herbert V. Am J Clin Nutr 1994;60:157-158.
22. Neve J. Experientia 1991;47.
23. Cerutti PA. Science 1985;227:375—381.
24. Gerber M, Dornand J. In: C Pasquier, Olivier RY, Auclair C, Packer L (eds) Oxidative Stress, Cell Activation and Viral Infection. Basel, Switzerland: Birkhäuser Verlag, 1994.
25. Packer L, Suzuki YJ. In: Pasquier C et al. (eds) Oxidative Stress, Cell activation and Viral Infection. Basel/Switzerland: Birkhäuser Verlag, 1994:113—130.
26. Clurman BE, Roberts JM. J Nat Cancer Inst 1995;87:1499—1501.
27. Cerutti PA. Env Health Persp 1989;81:39—43.
28. Mitchel REJ, McCann R. Carcinogenesis 1993;14:659—662.
29. Everett SA, Dennis MF, Patel KB, Maddix S, Kundu SC, Willson R. J Biol Chem 1996;271:3988—3994.
30. Szent-Gyorgyi A, Egyud LG, McLaughlin JA. Science 1967;155:539—541.
31. Burton GW, Traber MG. Ann Rev Nutr 1990;10:357—382.
32. Slater T, Benedetto C, Burton GW, Cheeseman KH, Ingold KU, Nodes JT. In: Thaler-Dao H, Paoletti R, Crastes de Paulet A (eds) Icosanoids and Cancer. New York: Raven Press, 1984: 21—29.
33. Cheeseman KH, Collins M, Proudfoot K et al. Biochem J 1986;235:507—514.
34. Cheeseman KH, Emery S, Maddix SP et al. Biochem J 1988;250:247—252.
35. Masotti L, Casali E, Galeotti T. Free Radical Biol Med 1988;4:377—386.
36. Szabados GY, Tretter L, Horvath I. Free Rad Res Comm 1989;7:161—170.
37. Begin ME, Ells G, Horrobin DF. J Natl Cancer Inst 1988;80:188—194.
38. Najid A, Beneytout J-L, Tixier M. Cancer Lett 1989;46:137—141.
39. Cogrel P, Morel I, Lescoat G, Chevanne M, Brissot P, Cillard P, Cillard J. Lipids 1993;28: 115—119.
40. Southgate J, Pitt E, Trejdosiewicz LK. Br J Cancer 1996;1996:728—734.
41. Yoshikawa T, Kokura S, Tainaka K, Naito Y, Kondo M. Cancer Res 1995;55:1617—1620.
42. Schwartz JL, Antionades DZ, Zhao S. Ann NY Acad Sci 1993;680:262—278.
43. Anti M, Marra G, Franco A, Bartoli GM, Ficonelli R. Gastroenterology 1992;103.
44. Ripple MO, Henry WF, Rago RP, Wilding G. J Natl Cancer Inst 1997;89:40—48.
45. Gonzales MJ, Schemmel RA, Gray JI, Dugan L, Sheffield LG, Welsh CW. Carcinogenesis 1991; 12:1231—1235.
46. Gerber M, Richardson S, Favier F, Crastes de Paulet A. In: Emerit I et al. (eds) Antioxidants in Therapy and Preventive Medicine. New York: Plenum Press, 1990.
47. Lhuillery C, Cognault S, Germain E, Jourdan ML, Bougnoux P. Cancer Lett 1997;114: 233—234.
48. Buttke TM, Sandstrom PA. Immunol Today 1994;15:7—10.

49. Kane DJ, Sarafian TA, Anton R, Hahn H, Gralla EB, Valentine JS, Ord T, Bredesen DE. Science 1993;262:1274—1277.
50. Hockenbery DM, Oltvai ZN, Yin XM, Milliman CL, Korsmeyer SJ. Cell 1993;75:241—251.
51. Burdon RH. Free Rad Med 1995;18:775—794.
52. Van 't Veer P, Strain JJ, Fernandez-Crehuet J, Martin BC, Thamm M, Kardinaal AF, Kohlmeier L, Huttunen JK, Martin-Moreno JM, Kok FJ. Cancer Epidemiol Biom Prev 1996;5:441—447.
53. Nomura A, Heilbrun LK, Stemmermann GN. J Natl Cancer Inst 1985;74:319—323.
54. Batieha AM, Armenian HK, Norkus EP, Morris JS, Spate VE, Comstock GW. Cancer Epidemiol Biom Prev 1993;2:335—339.
55. Burney PGJ, Comstock GW, Morris JS. Am J Clin Nutr 1989;49:895—900.
56. Ito Y, Suzuki S, Yagyu K, Sasaki R, Suzuki K and Aoki K. J Epidemiol 1997;7:1—8.
57. Giovanucci E. Cancer 1995;75:1766—1777.
58. Eichholzer M, Stahelin HB, Gey KF, Ludin E, Bernasconi F. Int J Cancer 1996;66:145—150.
59. Knekt P. Ann Med 1991;23:3—12.
60. Howe GR et al. J Natl Cancer Inst 1991;83:336—340.
61. Willett WC, Manson JE, Colditz GA, Stampfer MJ, Rosner B. N Engl J Med 1993;329:234—240.
62. Verhoeven DTH, Assen N, Goldbohm RA, Dorant E, Van Ot Veer P, Sturmans F, Hermus RJJ, Van Den Brandt PA. Br J Cancer 1997;75:149—155.
63. Yong LC, Brown CC, Schatzkin A, Dresser CM, Slesinski MJ, Cox CS, Taylor PR. Am J Epidemiol 1997;146:231—243.
64. Ocke MC, Bas Bueno-de-Mesquita H, Feskens EJM, Van Staveren WA, Kromhout D. Am J Epidemiol 1997;145:358—365.
65. Bostick RM, Potter JD, McKenzie DR, Kushi LH, Steinmetz KA. Cancer Res 1993;53:4230—4237.
66. Gridley G, McLaughlin JK, Block G, Blot W, Gluch M, Fraumeni JF Jr. Am J Epidemiol 1992;135:1083—1092.
67. Taylor Mayne S, Janerich DT, Greenwald P, Chorost Stucci C, Zaman MB, Melamed MR, Kiely M, McKneally MF. J Natl Cancer Inst 1994;86:33—38.
68. Buiatti E, Palli D, Decarli A et al. Int J Cancer 1989;44:611—616.
69. Negri E, La Vecchia C, Franceschi S, D'Avanzo B, Talamini R, Parpinel M, Ferraroni M, Filiberti R, Montella M, Falcini F, Conti E, Decarli A. Int J Cancer 1996;65:140—144.
70. Block G. Am J Clin Nutr 1991;54:1310S—1314S.
71. Horn-Ross PL, Morrow M, Ljung BM. Am J Epidemiol 1997;146:171—176.
72. Ramaswamy G, Rao UR, Kumaraswamy SV, Anantita N. Eur J Cancer 1996;32B:120—122.
73. La Vecchia C, Braga C, Negri E, Franceschi S, Russo A, Conti E, Falcini F, Giacosa A, Montella M, Decarli A. Intern J Cancer 1997;73:525—530.
74. Graham S, Zielezny M, Marshall J, Priore R, Freudenheim J, Brasure J, Haughey B, Nasca P, Zdeb M. Am J Epidemiol 1992;136:1327—1337.
75. Hunter DJ, Manson JA, Colditz GA, Stampfer MJ, Rosner BA, Hennekens CH, Speizer FE, Willet WC. N Engl J Med 1993;329:234—240.
76. Willett W, Polk BF, Morris JS, Stampfer MJ, Pressel S, Rosner B, Taylor JO, Schneider K, Hames CG. Lancet 1983;2:130—134.
77. Salonen JT, Salonen R, Lappetelainen R, Maenpaa P, Alfthan G, Puska P. Br Med J 1985;290:417—420.
78. Ringstad J, Jacobsen BK, Tretli S, Thomassen Y. J Clin Pathol 1988;41:454—457.
79. Coates RJ, Weiss NS, Daling JR, Morris JS, Labbe RF. Am J Epidemiol 1988;128:515—523.
80. Comstock GW, Bush TL, Helzlsouer K. Am J Epidemiol 1992;13:511—521.
81. Kok F, de Bruijn AM, Hofman A, Vermeeren R, Valkenburg HA. Am J Epidemiol 1987;125.
82. Nomura A, Heilbrun LK, Morris JS, Stemmermann GN. J Natl Cancer Inst 1987;79:103—108.
83. Helzlsouer KJ, Comstock GW, Morris S. Cancer Res 1989;49:6144—6148.
84. Knekt P, Aromaa A, Maatela J, Alfthan G, Aaran RK, Hakama M, Hakulinen T, Peto R, Teppo

L. J Natl Cancer Inst 1990;82:864—868.

85. Van Den Brandt PA, Goldbohm A, Van 't Veer P, Bode P, Dorant E, Hermus RJJ, Sturmans F. Am J Epidemiol 1994;140:20—26.
86. Van Noord P, Collette HJA, Maas MJ, de Waard F. Intern J Epidemiol 1987;16:318.
87. Hunter DJ, Morris JS, Stampfer MJ, Colditz GA, Speizer FE, Willett WC. JAMA 1990;264: 1128—1131.
88. Garland M, Morris JS, Stampfer MJ, Colditz GA, Spate VL, Baskett CK, Rosner B, Speizer FE, Willett WC, Hunter DJ. J Natl Cancer Inst 1995;87:497—505.
89. Verreault R, Brisson J, Deschenes L, Naud F, Meyer F, Belanger L. J Natl Cancer Inst 1988;80: 819—825.
90. Zaridze DG, Chevchenko VE, Levtshuk AA, Lifanova YE, Maximovitch DM. Int J Cancer 1990;45:807—810.
91. Lanson M, Bougnoux P, Besson P, Lansac J, Hubert B, Couet C, Le Floch O. Br J Cancer 1990;61:776—778.
92. Chajes V, Lhuillery C, Sattler W, Kostner GM, Bougnoux P. Int J Cancer 1996;67:170—175.
93. Gerber M, Astre C, Segala C, Saintot M, Scali J, Simony-Lafontaine J, Grenier J, Pujol H. J Nutr 1996;126:1201S—1207S.
94. Saintot M, Astre C, Pujol H, Gerber M. Carcinogenesis 1996,17:1267—1271.
95. Gerber M, Segala C. In: Emerit I, Chance B (eds) Free Radicals and Aging. Basel: Birkhäuser Verlag, 1992:235—246.
96. Heinonen PK, Koskinen T, Tuimala R. Arch Gynecol 1985;237:37—40.
97. Heinonen PK, Kuoppala T, Koskinen T, Punnonen R. Arch Gynecol Obstet 1987;241:151—156.
98. Knekt P, Aromaa A, Maatela J, Alfthan G, Aaran RK, Nikkari T, Hakama M, Hakulinene T, Teppo L. Am J Epidemiol 1991;134:356—361.
99. Rougereau A, Person O, Rougereau G. Intl J Vit Nutr Res 1987;57:367—373.
100. Gerber M, Cavallo F, Marubini E et al. Int J Cancer 1988;42:489—494.
101. Gerber M, Richardson S, Salkeld R, Chappuis P. Cancer Inv 1991;9:421—428.
102. Holm LE, Nordevang E, Hjalmar ML, Lidbrink E, Callmer E, Nilsson B. J Natl Cancer Inst 1993;85:32—36.
103. Van Poppel G, Kok FJ, Hermus RJJ. Br J Cancer 1992;66:1164—1168.
104. McLarty JW, Holiday DB, Girard WM, Yanagihara RH, Kummet Td, Greenberg SD. Am J Clin Nutr 1995;62S:1431S—1438S.
105. Stich HF, Mathew B, Sankaranarayanan R, Nair MK. Cancer Detect Prev 1991;15:93—98.
106. Krishnaswany K, Prasad MPR, Krishna TP, Annapurna VV, Amarendra A, Reddy G. Eur J Cancer 1995;31B:41—48.
107. Paganelli GM, Biasco G, Brandi G, Santucci R, Gizzi G, Villani V, Cianci M, Miglioli M, Barbara L. J Natl Cancer Inst 1992;84:47—51.
108. Greenberg RE, Baron JA, Tosteson TD, Beck GJ, Freeman DH Jr, Bond JH, Frankl HD, Colacchio TA, Coller JA, Haile RW, Mandel JS, Nierenberg DW, Rothstein R, Snover DC, Stevens MM, Summers RW, Van Stolk RU. N Engl J Med 1994;331:141—147.
109. Yu H, Harris RE, Gao YT et al. Int J Epidemiol 1991;20:76—81.
110. Blot WJ, Li JY, Tailor PR, Guo W, Dawsey S, Wang GQ, Yang CS, Zheng SF, Gail M Li GY, Yu Y, Liu BQ, Tangrea J, Sun YH, Liu F, Fraumeni JF Jr, Zhang YH, Li B. J Natl Cancer Inst 1993;85:1483—1492.
111. Omenn GS, Goodman GE, Thornquist MD, Balmes J, Cullen MR, Glass A, Keogh JP, Meyskens FL, Valanis B et al. J Natl Cancer Inst 1996;88:1509—1604.
112. Hennekens CH, Buring JE, Manson JE, Stampfer M, Rosner B, Cook NR, Belanger C, La Motte F, Gaziano JM, Ridker PM, Willet W and Peto R. N Engl Med 1996;334:1145—1149.
113. Witte JS, Longnecker MP, Bird CL, Lee ER, Franki HD, Haile RW. Am J Epidemiol 1996; 144:1015—1025.
114. Hertog MGL, Feskens EJM, Hollman PCH, Katan MB, Kromhout D. Lancet 1993;342: 1007—1101.

115. Knekt P, Jarvinen R, Seppanen R, Heliovaara M, Teppo L, Pukkala E, Aromaa A. Am J Epidemiol 1997;146:223—230.
116. Matsukawa Y, Marui N, Sakai T, Satomi Y, Yoshida M, Matsumoto K, Nishino H, Aoike A. Cancer Res 1993;53:1328—1331.
117. Fotsis T, Pepper MS, Aktas E, Breit S, Rasku S, Adlercreutz H, Wahala K, Montesano R, Schweigerer L. Cancer Res 1997;57:2916—2921.
118. De Sanjose S, Munoz N, Sobala G, Vivas J, Peraza S, Cano E, Castro D, Sanchez V, Andrade O, Tompkins D, Schorah CJ, Axon AT, Benz M, Oliver W. Eur J Cancer Prev 1996;5:57—62.
119. Hercberg S, Galan P, Preziosi P, Roussel A-M, Arnaud J, Richard MJ, Malvy D, Paul-Dauphin A, Briancon S, Favier A. Intern J Vitam Nutr Res 1998;68:3—20.
120. IARC. Handbooks of cancer prevention vol 2. Carotenoids publ Int Ag Cen Res Lyon:1998.

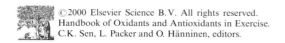
©2000 Elsevier Science B.V. All rights reserved.
Handbook of Oxidants and Antioxidants in Exercise.
C.K. Sen, L. Packer and O. Hänninen, editors.

Part XI • Chapter 32

Alcohol and oxidative stress

Charles S. Lieber

Mount Sinai School of Medicine and Alcohol Research and Treatment Center, Section of Liver Disease and Nutrition, Bronx Veterans Affairs Medical Center (151—2), 130 West Kingsbridge Rd, Bronx, NY 10468, USA. Tel.: +1-718-579-1646. Fax: +1-718-733-6257. E-mail: liebercs@aol.com

1   INTRODUCTION
2   METABOLISM OF ETHANOL
   2.1   Alcohol dehydrogenase pathway
   2.2   Microsomal ethanol-oxidizing system (MEOS)
      2.2.1   Role of MEOS in ethanol metabolism
      2.2.2   Oxidative stress, xenobiotic and retinoid toxicity and carcinogenicity
   2.3   Role of catalase
3   TOXICITY OF ACETALDEHYDE, INCLUDING ITS ADVERSE EFFECTS ON ANTIOXIDANT SYSTEMS
   3.1   Elevated acetaldehyde and mechanisms of toxicity
   3.2   Alterations of antioxidant systems and phospholipids
      3.2.1   Depletion of glutathione and S-adenosylmethionine
      3.2.2   Vitamin E deficiency
      3.2.3   Phosphatidylcholine depletion
4   SUMMARY
5   PERSPECTIVES
6   ACKNOWLEDGMENTS
7   ABBREVIATIONS
8   REFERENCES

1   INTRODUCTION

Alcohol-induced oxidative stress predominates in the liver because of its link to the oxidation of ethanol which occurs predominantly in that organ. Each of the three pathways of ethanol metabolism contributes in a unique manner. In addition, they all produce acetaldehyde which can cause peroxidation. The link between oxidative stress and the specific steps in the metabolism of alcohol will be reviewed for each pathway separately, followed by a more general discussion of the action of acetaldehyde and the alterations in defense mechanisms against oxidative stress. Finally, associative organ damage and possible therapeutic approaches will be reviewed. Specific pathologic alterations linked to a given aspect of the oxidative stress are discussed in connection with the corresponding disorders, while some more general pathologic consequences (e.g., fibrosis) are addressed in a separate chapter.

2   METABOLISM OF ETHANOL

The hepatocyte's three main pathways for ethanol metabolism are each located in different subcellular compartments:
1) the alcohol dehydrogenase (ADH) pathway is in the cytosol (or soluble fraction of the cell;
2) the microsomal ethanol-oxidizing system (MEOS) in the endoplasmic reticulum; and
3) catalase in the peroxisomes (Fig. 1).

2.1 Alcohol dehydrogenase pathway

The main pathway of ethanol metabolism proceeds via ADH, with transfer of hydrogen from the substrate to the co-factor nicotinamide adenine dinucleotide (NAD), converting it to its reduced form (NADH), and allowing for the produc-

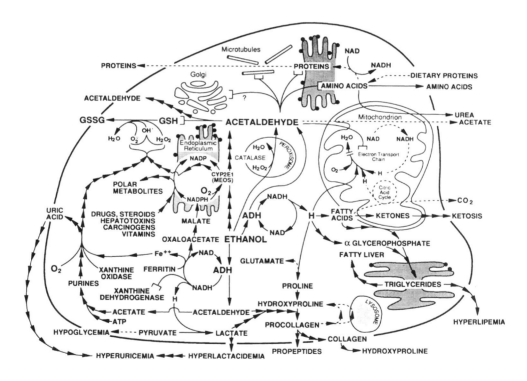

Fig. 1. Oxidation of ethanol in the hepatocyte. Many disturbances in intermediary metabolism and toxic effects can be linked to (i) ADH-mediated generation of NADH; (ii) the induction of the activity of microsomal enzymes, especially the MEOS containing P4502E1 (CYP2E1); and (iii) acetaldehyde, the product of ethanol oxidation. GSH: reduced glutathione; GSSG: oxidized glutathione; - - -, pathways that are depressed by ethanol; → → → → stimulation or activation; -[, interference or binding [1].

tion of acetaldehyde (Fig. 1). This first step generates an excess of reducing equivalents in the cytosol, NADH, with a shift in the redox potential, as measured by changes in the lactate/pyruvate ratio [2]. The reducing equivalents can also be transferred to NADP, the increased nicotinamide adenine dinucleotide phosphate-reduced form (NADPH) being utilized for synthetic pathways in the cytosol and microsomes (vide infra).

Some of the hydrogen equivalents formed in this reaction are transferred from the cytosol into the mitochondria. Since the mitochondrial membrane is impermeable to NADH, the reducing equivalents enter the mitochondria via shuttle mechanisms, such as the malate cycle, fatty acid elongation, and α-glycerophosphate cycles. Normally, fatty acids are reduced via β-oxidation in the citric acid cycle of the mitochondria, which serves as a "hydrogen donor" for the mitochondrial electron transport chain. When ethanol is reduced, the generated hydrogen equivalents, which are shuttled into the mitochondria, supplant the citric acid cycle as a source and the mitochondria are shifted to a more reduced redox state, as measured by changes in the ratio of β-hydroxybutyrate to acetoacetate [2].

The altered redox state is responsible for a variety of metabolic abnormalities: the increased lactate/pyruvate ratio results in hyperlactacidemia because of both decreased utilization [3] and enhanced production of lactate by the liver. The hyperlactacidemia contributes to the acidosis and also reduces the capacity of the kidney to excrete uric acid, leading to secondary hyperuricemia [4].

Another possible consequence of enhanced purine degradation increases production of activated oxygen species by xanthine oxidase (XO) (vide infra), as indicated by the protective effect of allopurinol against the alcohol-induced lipid peroxidation [5]. Other metabolic consequences include enhanced lipogenesis, depressed lipid oxidation, and hypoglycemia [6].

The increased NADH/NAD ratio raises the concentration of α-glycerophosphate which favors hepatic triglyceride accumulation by trapping fatty acids. In addition, excess NADH may promote fatty acid synthesis [7]. Theoretically, enhanced lipogenesis can be considered a means for disposing of the excess hydrogen. The activity of the citric acid cycle is depressed, partly because of a slowing of the reactions of the cycle that require NAD; the mitochondria will use the hydrogen equivalents originating from ethanol, rather than those derived from the oxidation of fatty acids that normally serve as the main energy source of the liver. The decreased fatty acid oxidation, whether it is a function of reduced citric acid cycle activity is secondary to the altered redox potential (vide supra), or as a consequence of permanent changes in mitochondrial structure and functions [6], results in the hepatic accumulation (as triglycerides) of fatty acids of different sources, lead to the development of a fatty liver.

A characteristic feature of liver injury in the alcoholic is the predominance of steatosis and other lesions in the perivenular zone, also called the centrilobular or zone three of the hepatic acinus. Multiple mechanisms for this zonal selectivity of toxic effects have been proposed. The hypoxia hypothesis originated from the observation that liver slices from rats fed alcohol, chronically consume more oxygen than those of the controls. It was then postulated that the enhanced consumption of oxygen would increase the gradient of oxygen tension along the sinusoids to the extent of producing anoxic injury of perivenular hepatocytes [8]. Indeed both in human alcoholics [9] and in animals fed extensive amounts of alcohol [10,11], there was a decrease in hepatic venous oxygen saturation (PO_2) [9,10], and in the tissue oxygen tension [11]; these have been found during the withdrawal state. However, these changes in hepatic oxygenation disappeared [10,12] or decreased [11] when alcohol was present in the blood. Acute ethanol administration increased splanchnic oxygen consumption in naive baboons, but the consequences of this effect on oxygenation in the perivenular zone were offset by an increased blood flow resulting in unchanged hepatic venous oxygen tension [10]. Ethanol actually induced an increase in portal hepatic blood flow [10,12—15]. In cats [3] and baboons [15] that were fed alcohol chronically, defective oxygen utilization rather than lack of blood oxygen supply characterized liver injury, that was produced by high concentrations of ethanol. The low oxygen tension normally prevailing in perivenular zones exaggerates the redox shift produced by ethanol [10]. By increasing NADH, hypoxia may occur and in turn inhibit the activity of NAD^+-dependent xanthine dehydrogenase (XD), thereby favoring that of oxygen-dependent XO [5]. Purine metabolism via XO leads to the production of oxygen radicals which can mediate toxic effects towards liver cells, including peroxidation. Physiological substrates for XO, hypoxanthine xanthine and AMP, significantly increased in the liver after the presents of ethanol, together with an enhanced urinary output of allantoin (a final product of xanthine metabolism). Allopurinol pretreatment resulted in 90% inhibition of XO activity, and also significantly decreased ethanol-induced lipid peroxidation [5].

In addition to the redox change, a main mechanism whereby ADH-mediated ethanol metabolism affects oxidative stress is through the production of acetaldehyde (vide infra).

ADH is also present in extra hepatic tissues such as the kidney and the stomach but their isozyme composition differs from that of the liver and the impact of ethanol metabolism on the redox level and the oxidative stress in these tissues has not been well chartered as yet.

2.2 Microsomal ethanol-oxidizing system (MEOS)

2.2.1 *Role of MEOS in ethanol metabolism*

That a cytochrome P450 enzyme system can also metabolize ethanol was demonstrated in liver microsomes in vitro and the system was found to be inducible by chronic alcohol feeding in vivo [16]; it was named the microsomal ethanol oxidizing system (MEOS) [16,17]. Its distinct nature was shown by:
a) isolation of a P-450 containing fractions from liver microsomes which, although devoid of any ADH or catalase activity, could still oxidize ethanol,

as well as higher aliphatic alcohols (e.g., butanol, which is not a substrate for catalase) [18,19]; and

b) reconstitution of ethanol-oxidizing activity using NADPH-cytochrome P-450 reductase, phospholipids, and either partially purified or highly-purified microsomal P-450 from untreated [20] or phenobarbital-treated [21] rats.

That chronic ethanol consumption results in the induction of a unique P-450, was also shown by Ohnishi and Lieber [20] using a liver microsomal P-450 fraction isolated from ethanol-treated rats. An ethanol-inducible form of P-450, purified from rabbit liver microsomes [22], catalyzed ethanol oxidation at rates much higher than other P-450 isozymes, and also had an enhanced capacity to oxidize 1-butanol, 1-pentanol and aniline [23], acetaminophen [24], CCl_4 [23], acetone [25,26], and N-nitrosodimethylamine (NDMA) [27]. The purified human protein (now called CYP2E1 or 2E1) was obtained in a catalytically active form, with a high turnover rate for ethanol and other specific substrates [28]. MEOS has a relatively high K_m for ethanol (8–10 mM compared to 0.2–2 mM for hepatic ADH) but, contrasting with hepatic ADH, which is not inducible in primates, as well as most other animal species. A 4-fold induction of 2E1 was found in biopsies of recently drinking subjects, using the Western blot technique with specific antibodies against this 2E1 [29].

The presence of 2E1 was also shown in extrahepatic tissues [30] and in nonparenchymal cells of the liver, including Kupffer cells [31]. In rats, ethanol treatment caused a 7-fold increase in CYP2E1 content of Kupffer cells. It also increased the hydroxylation of p-nitrophenol, a relatively specific substrate for CYP2E1, demonstrating that the induced CYP2E1 was catalytically active.

2.3 Oxidative stress, xenobiotic and retinoid toxicity and carcinogenicity

There is increased evidence that ethanol toxicity may be associated with an enhanced production of reactive oxygen intermediates. Numerous experimental data indicate that free radical mechanisms contribute to ethanol-induced liver injury. Increased generation of oxygen- and ethanol-derived free radicals occurs at the microsomal level, especially through the intervention of the ethanol-inducible 2E1 [32]. This induction is associated with proliferation of the endoplasmic reticulum (vide supra), which is accompanied by an increased oxidation of NADPH, with resulting H_2O_2 generation [33]. There is also increased superoxide radical production (Fig. 1) [34]. In addition, the 2E1 induction contributes to the well-known lipid peroxidation associated with alcoholic liver injury. DiLuzio [35,36] was one of the first to report that ethanol produces increased lipid peroxidation in the liver and that the ethanol-induced fatty liver could be prevented by antioxidants. Lipid peroxidation correlated with the amount of CYP 2E1 in liver microsomal preparations, and it was inhibited by antibodies against 2E1 in the control and ethanol-fed rats [37,38]. Indeed, 2E1 is rather "leaky" and its operation results in a significant release of free radicals, including 1-hydroxyethyl-free radical intermediates [39,40], confirmed by detecting the hydroxyethyl radicals in vivo [41].

Ethanol can also be converted to acetaldehyde by liver microsomes through a nonenzymatic pathway involving the presence of hydroxyl radicals originating from the iron-catalyzed degradation of H_2O_2 [42]. The production of ethanol-free radicals may be due to an oxidizing species bound to cytochrome P450 and abstracting a proton from the alcohol α-carbon [43]. Since hydroxyethyl radicals appear to be involved in the alkylation of hepatic proteins, they may contribute to the damaging effects of ethanol. Furthermore, an in vitro-produced hydroxyethyl radical forms stable adducts with albumin or fibrinogen [44], and patients with alcoholic cirrhosis have increased serum levels of both immunoglobulin G (IgG) and immunoglobulin A (IgA) reacting with proteins of liver microsomes incubated with ethanol and NADPH [44], which do not cross react with the epitopes derived from acetaldehyde-modified proteins.

Much of the medical significance of MEOS, and its ethanol-inducible 2E1, results not only from the oxidation of ethanol and from the unusual and unique capacity of 2E1 to generate reactive oxygen intermediates, but also from the activation of many xenobiotic compounds to their toxic metabolites, often free radicals. This pertains to carbon tetrachloride and other industrial solvents such as bromobenzene [45] and vinylidene chloride [46], as well as anesthetics such as enflurane [47] and halothane [48]. Ethanol also markedly increases the activity of the microsomal low K_m benzene-metabolizing enzymes [49] and this aggravates the hemopoietic toxicity of benzene. Enhanced metabolism (and toxicity) also pertains to a variety of prescribed drugs, including isoniazid and phenylbutazone [50], and some over-the-counter medications such as acetaminophen (paracetamol, *N*-acetyl-*p*-aminophenol) all of which are substrates for, or inducers of, cytochrome P4502E1 (CYP2E1). Therapeutic amounts of acetaminophen (2.5 to 4 g/day) can cause hepatic injury in alcoholics. In animals given ethanol for long periods, hepatotoxic effects peak after withdrawal [51] when ethanol is no longer competing for the microsomal pathway and when levels of the toxic metabolites are at their highest. Thus, heavy drinkers are most vulnerable to the toxic effects of acetaminophen shortly after the cessation of chronic drinking.

There is an association between alcohol misuse and an increased incidence of upper alimentary and respiratory tract cancers [52]. Many factors have been incriminated, one of which is the effect of ethanol on enzyme systems involved in the cytochrome P-450-dependent activation of carcinogens. This effect has been demonstrated with the use of microsomes derived from a variety of tissues, including the liver (the principal site of xenobiotic metabolism [53,54], the lungs [53,54], and intestines [30,55], the chief portals of entry for tobacco smoke and dietary carcinogens, respectively, and the esophagus [56], where ethanol consumption is a major risk factor in the development of cancer. Alcoholics are commonly heavy smokers, and a synergistic effect of alcohol consumption and smoking on cancer development has been described, as reviewed elsewhere [52]. Indeed, long-term ethanol consumption was found to enhance the mutagenicity of tobacco-derived products [52].

Alcohol may also influence carcinogenesis in many other ways [57], one of which involves severe vitamin A depletion which is associated with alcoholic liver disease already at early stages [58,59]. Depressed hepatic levels of vitamin A were observed even when alcohol was given with diets containing large amounts of vitamin A [60]. New hepatic enzyme pathways of retinol metabolism, inducible by either ethanol or drug administration, have been discovered [61,62]. Depletion in hepatic vitamin is associated with lysosomal lesions [63] and decreased detoxification of NDMA [64]. Although vitamin A deficiency might adversely affect the liver [63], an excess of vitamin A is also known to be hepatotoxic [65]. Long-term ethanol consumption enhances this effect, resulting in striking morphologic and functional alterations of the mitochondria [66], along with hepatic necrosis and fibrosis [59]. Hypervitaminosis A itself can induce fibrosis and even cirrhosis, as reviewed elsewhere [65]. Thus, alcohol abuse narrows the therapeutic window for vitamin A, which hinders it therapeutic use.

Retinol is an antioxidant but it is a weak one and, as noted earlier, its use is complicated by its intrinsic hepatotoxicity, exacerbated by ethanol. Unlike retinol, its precursor β-carotene is considered to lack toxicity. Furthermore, in addition to acting as a retinol precursor, β-carotene is also an efficient quencher of singlet oxygen and can function as a radical-trapping antioxidant. Moreover, β-carotene has been shown to have the potential of acting as a more efficient antioxidant than retinol. Carotenoids were found to inhibit free radical-induced lipid peroxidation [67–69]. However, in a study in rats, Alam and Alam [70] reported no change in either blood or tissue lipid peroxides following ingestion of β-carotene (180 mg/kg/day), for a period of 11 weeks and carotenoids did not protect against peroxidation in choline deficient rats [71]. By contrast, a study in guinea pigs noted a protective effect against in vivo lipid peroxidation when animals were pretreated with β-carotene [72].

Furthermore, Palozza and Krinsky [73] reported that β-carotene inhibited malondialdehyde production in a concentration-dependent manner and delayed the radical-initiated destruction of endogenous α- and γ-tocopherol in the rat, and Kim-Jun [74] reported inhibitory effects of β-carotene on lipid peroxidation in mouse epidermis. Mobarhan et al. [75] also showed that subjects replenished with β-carotene had a decreased level of circulating lipid peroxides, but it was not reported whether this could be achieved in individuals who continue to drink, and at a dose of β-carotene that has no toxicity in the presence of alcohol. One may wonder whether the combination of alcohol and β-carotene, at the dose used for replenishment, can be useful in terms of preventing lipid peroxidation, without producing some signs of toxicity. Indeed, enhanced hepatic toxicity of β-carotene in the presence of ethanol has been observed with the possible existence of a defect in utilization and/or excretion associated with liver injury and/or alcohol abuse [76,77].

In addition, in men, heavy drinking was associated with a relative increase in serum β-carotene [78], and relatively moderate drinking in women also has a similar effect [79]. It is noteworthy that β-carotene increased pulmonary cancer and cardiovascular complications in smokers [80]. This effect was confirmed in a study by Omenn et al. [81], and was found to be related to the amount of alcohol consumed [82], confirming the suspicion [83] that the toxicity resulted from an alcohol β-carotene interaction. Thus, vitamin A or β-carotene supplementation must be used cautiously in alcoholics, especially if β-carotene is given in beadlets, which potentiate the toxic alcohol-β-carotene interaction [84].

2.4 Role of catalase

Catalase can oxidize alcohol in vitro in the presence of an H_2O_2-generating system [85] (Fig. 1), and its interaction with H_2O_2 in the intact liver has been demonstrated [86]. However, its role is limited by the small amount of H_2O_2 generated [87]. Under physiological conditions, catalase thus appears to play no major role in ethanol oxidation.

The catalase contribution might be enhanced if significant amounts of H_2O_2 become available through β-oxidation of fatty acids in peroxisomes [88]. However, the peroxisomal enzymes do not oxidize short chain fatty acids such as octanoate; peroxisomal β-oxidation was observed only in the absence of ADH activity. In its presence, the rate of ethanol metabolism is reduced by adding fatty acids [89], and conversely, the ß-oxidation of fatty acids is inhibited by NADH produced from alcohol metabolism via ADH [89]. Similarly, the generation of reducing equivalents from ethanol by ADH in the cytosol inhibits H_2O_2 generation leading to significantly diminished rates of peroxidation of alcohols via catalase [90]. Furthermore, aminotriazole (a catalase inhibitor) has little, if any, effect on alcohol oxidation in vivo, as reviewed by Takagi et al. [91] and Kato et al. [92,93]. Thus, despite the considerable controversy that originally surrounded this issue, it was agreed by the principal contenders involved that catalase cannot account for microsomal ethanol oxidation [94,95]. However, catalase could contribute to fatty acid oxidation. Indeed, long-term ethanol consumption is associated with increases in the content of a specific cytochrome (P4504A1), this promotes microsomal ω-hydroxylation of fatty acids which may compensate, at least in part, for the deficit in fatty acid oxidation due to the ethanol-induced injury of the mitochondria [6]. Products of ω-oxidation increase liver cytosolic fatty acid-binding protein (L-FABPc) content and peroxisomal β-oxidation [96], an alternate but modest pathway for fatty acid disposition.

3. TOXICITY OF ACETALDEHYDE, INCLUDING ITS ADVERSE EFFECTS ON ANTIOXIDANT SYSTEMS

Due to the inducibility of 2E1, chronic excessive alcohol consumption results in enhanced acetaldehyde production that, in turn, aggravates the oxidative stress directly, as well as indirectly, by impairing defense systems against it.

3.1 Elevated acetaldehyde and mechanism of toxicity

Acetaldehyde, the product of ethanol oxidation, is highly toxic but is rapidly metabolized to acetate, mainly by a mitochondrial low K_m aldehyde dehydrogenase (ALDH). However, the activity of ALDH is significantly reduced by chronic ethanol consumption [97]. The decreased capacity of mitochondria of alcohol-fed subjects to oxidize acetaldehyde, associated with unaltered or even enhanced rates of ethanol oxidation (and therefore acetaldehyde generation because of MEOS induction; vide supra), results in an imbalance between production and disposition of acetaldehyde. The latter causes the elevated acetaldehyde levels observed after chronic ethanol consumption in humans [98] and in baboons, with a tremendous increase of acetaldehyde in hepatic venous blood [15], reflected high tissue levels.

The toxicity of acetaldehyde is due, in part, to its capacity to form protein adducts, resulting in antibody production, enzyme inactivation, [99] and decreased DNA repair [15,100]. It is also associated with a striking impairment of the capacity of the liver to utilize oxygen.

3.2 Alterations of antioxidant systems and phospholipids

3.2.1 Depletion of glutathione and S-adenosylmethionine

Acetaldehyde promotes glutathione (GSH) depletion, resulting in free radical-mediated toxicity, and lipid peroxidation. Indeed, in isolated perfused livers acetaldehyde was shown to cause lipid peroxidation [101,102]. In vitro, metabolism of acetaldehyde via XO or aldehyde oxidase may generate free radicals, but the concentration of acetaldehyde required is much too high for this mechanism to be of significance in vivo. However, another mechanism to promote lipid peroxidation is via GSH depletion. One of the three amino acids of this tripeptide is cysteine. Binding of acetaldehyde with cysteine and/or glutathione (GSH) may contribute to a depression of liver GSH [103]. Rats fed ethanol chronically have significantly increased rates of GSH turnover [104]. Acute ethanol administration inhibits GSH synthesis and produces an increased loss from the liver [105]. GSH is selectively depleted in the mitochondria [106] and may contribute to the striking alcohol-induced alterations of that organelle. GSH offers one of the mechanisms for the scavenging of toxic-free radicals, as shown in Fig. 2, which also illustrates how the ensuing enhanced GSH utilization (and thus, turnover) results in a significant increase in α-amino-*n*-butyric acid [108] (Fig. 3). The latter can serve to assess semiquantitatively the increased GSH turnover in vivo.

Although GSH depletion per se may not be sufficient to cause lipid peroxidation, it is generally agreed upon that it may favor the peroxidation produced by other factors. It is important in the protection of cells against electrophilic drug injury in general, and against reactive oxygen species in particular, especially in primates, which are more vulnerable to GSH depletion than rodents [110]. Iron

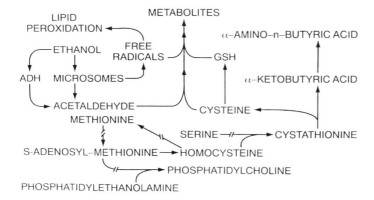

Fig. 2. Link between accelerated acetaldehyde production and increased free radical generation by "induced" microsomes, resulting in enhanced lipid peroxidation. Metabolic blocks due to alcohol, folate deficiency, and/or alcoholic liver disease are illustrated with possible beneficial effects of GSH, its precursors (including S-adenosylmethionine), and phosphatidylcholine [107].

overload may play a contributory role, as chronic alcohol consumption results in an increased iron uptake by hepatocytes [111]; iron exposure accentuates the changes of lipid peroxidation and of the glutathione status in the liver cell induced by acute ethanol intoxication [112].

Therapeutic use of GSH itself is complicated by the fact that its replenishment

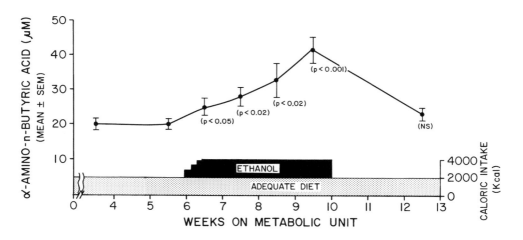

Fig. 3. Effect of alcohol consumption on plasma α-amino-*n*-butyric acid. Consumption of 4 g of ethanol/kg/day in addition to an adequate diet in three human volunteers resulted in a doubling of plasma α-amino-*n*-butyric acid after 2—4 weeks which was reversed after cessation of drinking. A similar trend was observed for the branched-chain amino acids. This increase was not observed when fat was substituted isocalorically by ethanol [109].

through supplementation is hampered by its lack of penetration into the hepato-cytes, except for its ethyl derivative, which is not suitable for the treatment of an alcoholic liver injury. Cysteine is one of the three amino acids of GSH, and the ultimate precursor of cysteine is methionine (Fig. 2). Methionine deficiency has been incriminated in alcoholics and its supplementation has been considered for the treatment of alcoholic liver injury, but some difficulties have been encoun-tered. Indeed, excess methionine was shown to have some adverse effects [113], including a decrease in hepatic adenosine triphosphate (ATP). Horowitz et al. [114] reported that the blood clearance of methionine after an oral load of this amino acid was slowed in patients with cirrhosis. Because about half of the methionine is metabolized by the liver, the previously mentioned observations suggest impaired hepatic metabolism of this amino acid in patients with alco-holic liver disease. For methionine to be utilized it has to be activated to S-adeno-sylmethionine (AdoMet) (Fig. 2). However, Duce et al. [115] found a decrease in AdoMet synthetase activity in cirrhotic livers, and AdoMet depletion ensues after chronic ethanol consumption [116]. Potentially, such AdoMet depletion may have a number of adverse effects. AdoMet is the principal methylating agent in various transmethylation reactions important for nucleic acid and protein synth-esis, as well as membrane fluidity and functions. It includes the transport of metabolites and the transmission of signals across membranes and maintenance of membranes. Thus, depletion of AdoMet may promote membrane injury docu-mented in alcohol-induced liver damage [117]. AdoMet is not only the methyl donor in almost all transmethylation reactions, but it also plays a key role in the synthesis of polyamines and, as already alluded to, it provides a source of cysteine for GSH production.

Orally administered AdoMet is a precursor for intracellular AdoMet, both as unchanged AdoMet and by the methionine it provides. Compared to methionine, the administration of AdoMet has the advantage of bypassing the deficit in Ado-Met synthesis (from methionine) referred to earlier (Fig. 2). The usefulness of AdoMet administration has been shown in various clinical studies [118,119]. It was also demonstrated in the baboon [116,120], with improvement of GSH depletion, and in the leakage, from the liver into the circulation of the enzymes, glutathione dehydrogenase (GDH) (Fig. 4) and aspartate aminotransferase (AST) (Fig. 5). Recently, in a multicenter placebo-controlled, randomized the double-blind clinical trial. Mato et al. [121] showed that AdoMet improves survi-val in patients with alcoholic liver cirrhosis.

3.2.2 Vitamin E deficiency

Bjøneboe et al. [122] reported a reduced hepatic α-tocopherol content after chronic ethanol feeding in rats receiving adequate amounts of vitamin E, as well as in the blood of alcoholics. Furthermore, hepatic lipid peroxidation was signifi-cantly increased after chronic ethanol feeding in rats receiving a low vitamin E diet [123], indicating that dietary vitamin E is an important determinant of hepa-

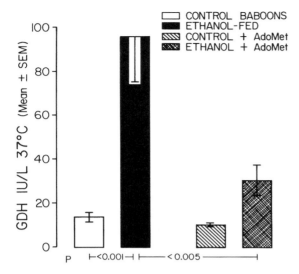

Fig. 4. Effect of S-adenosylmethionine (AdoMet) on the ethanol-induced increase in plasma glutamic dehydrogenase activity. The leakage of this mitochondrial enzyme into the blood stream was strikingly attenuated by AdoMet [116].

tic lipid peroxidation induced by chronic ethanol feeding. The lowest hepatic α-tocopherol was found in rats receiving a combination of low vitamin E and etha-

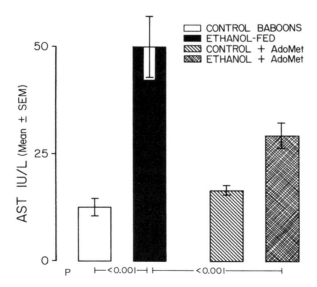

Fig. 5. Effect of S-adenosylmethionine (AdoMet) on the ethanol-induced increase of plasma AST activity. AdoMet corrected the ethanol-induced rise of AST [116].

nol: both low dietary vitamin E and ethanol feeding significantly reduced hepatic α-tocopherol content, the latter, in part, because of increased conversion of α-tocopherol to α-tocopherylquinone [123]. In patients with cirrhosis, diminished levels of hepatic vitamin E have been observed [77] (Fig. 6), as also shown by von Herbay et al. [124].

3.2.3 Phosphatidylcholine depletion

One of the key functions of phosphatidylethanolamine *N*-methyltransferase (PEMT) is to utilize AdoMet as a methyl donor in the methylation of phosphatidylethylanolamine to phosphatidylcholine (Fig. 2). However, it has been shown that chronic ethanol consumption is associated with a decrease of the activity in the enzymes, both in baboons [125] and in men [115]. The reduction in PEMT activity may have some secondary effects on liver phospholipids. Indeed, a decrease in PEMT activity after alcohol may be responsible, at least in part, for the associated decrease in phospholipids [120,125] which can be corrected by supplementation with a soybean extract, that is rich in polyunsaturated lecithin, namely polyenylphosphatidylcholine (PPC), about half of which consists of dilinoleoylphosphatidylcholine (DLPC) [120]. Thus, PEMT depression after alcohol may exacerbate the hepatic phospholipid depletion and the associated membrane abnormalities, thereby promoting hepatic injury, whereas PPC, by repleting hepa-

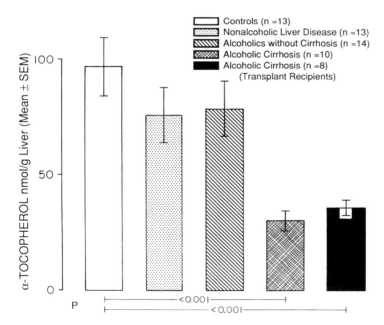

Fig. 6. Effects of various liver diseases on total hepatic tocopherol levels. The two cirrhotic groups had significantly lower α-tocopherol levels [77].

tic phospholipids and normalizing PEMT activity, may contribute to the protection against alcoholic cirrhosis provided by PPC supplementation [120,125] (Fig. 7).

PPC is especially suited to correct hepatic phospholipid depletion because phospholipids rich in polyunsaturated fatty acids (PUFA) have a high bioavailability. More than 50% of orally administered PPC is made biologically available for the organism either, to a low extent, by intact absorption or to a greater extent, by reacylation of absorbed lysophosphatidylcholine [126]. Pharmacokinetic studies in humans using tritiated hydrogen/^{14}C carbon radiolabeled (^{3}H/^{14}C) phosphatidylcholine showed the absorption to exceed 90% [127]. Similar observations were made in animals [128–130]. In addition to phosphatidylcholine repletion in the membranes, PPC may act more specifically as an antioxidant, despite the prevailing view that the polyunsaturated lipids favor peroxidation. It is generally believed that because of their multiple double bond configuration, polyunsaturated fats are much more susceptible, than saturated or monounsaturated ones, to free radical peroxidation [131]. Surprisingly, however, some reports suggest that the opposite may occur. Effects of high monounsaturated and polyunsaturated fat diets on plasma lipoproteins and lipid peroxidation were studied in type 2 diabetes mellitus [132]. All indices of plasma lipid peroxidation in the diabetic group and lipid peroxides in the controls were significantly lower on these than on the baseline diet. It was postulated that because both high monounsaturated and polyunsaturated fat diets increase hepatic metabolism of low-density lipoproteins and shorten their circulating half-life, they may be able to reduce lipid peroxidation, compared to high saturated fat diets;

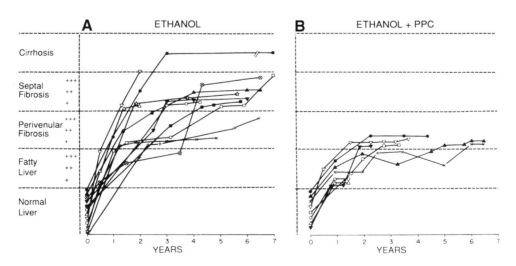

Fig. 7. Sequential development of alcoholic liver injury in baboons fed ethanol with an adequate diet (**A**), and prevention of septal fibrosis and cirrhosis by supplementation with polyunsaturated phosphatidylcholine (PPC) (**B**). Liver morphology in animals pair-fed control diets (with or without PPC) remained normal (not shown) [data from 120].

by this mechanism, polyunsaturated fat diets may offset any increased susceptibility of polyunsaturated-enriched low-density lipoproteins to peroxidation. Similarly, whereas the malondialdehyde concentration in plasma increased with increasing blood lipids, it was inversely proportional to linoleic acid in serum lipoprotein phospholipids, suggesting that oxidants and lipoprotein metabolism may be of greater importance for intravascular lipid peroxidation than the proportion of PUFA in the lipoprotein lipids. Furthermore, in newborn rats, it was demonstrated that a diet rich in PUFA confers protection against pulmonary oxygen toxicity [133,134]. Specifically, newborn rat offspring of dams fed diets high in PUFA had elevated concentrations of PUFA in their lung lipids and significantly improved survival in hyperoxia compared with offspring of dams fed regular rat chow; conversely, newborn offspring of dams fed low PUFA, high saturated fatty acid diets were most susceptible to pulmonary oxygen toxicity. In addition, when Intralipid, derived from soybean oil, containing a high percentage of n-6 family PUFA, and linolenic acid, a n-3 family PUFA, were given for 3 weeks before and then throughout pregnancy and lactation, 1- and 5-day-old offsprings of Intralipid diet-fed dams demonstrated significant increases in lung lipid, n-6 family PUFA plus elevated linolenic acid, compared to regular diet-fed offspring. Significantly improved hyperoxic survival rates were associated with these fatty acid changes. These findings supported the hypothesis that increasing lung PUFA content may provide enhanced O_2 free radical scavenging capacities [135].

In addition, evidence gathered in rodents and in nonhuman primates revealed striking antioxidant effects of PPC. It was found to prevent hepatic lipid peroxidation and attenuate associated injury induced by CCl_4 in rats [136]. Furthermore, PPC decreased oxidant stress and protected against alcohol-induced liver injury in the baboon [137]. Using gas chromatography/mass spectroscopy (GC/MS), hepatic F_2-isoprostanes (F_2IP), breakdown products of arachidonic acid peroxidation, and hydroxynonenal, were determined in liver needle biopsies. Whereas alcohol increased both, PPC administration resulted in a significant reduction, especially of hydroxynonenal (Fig. 8). The mechanism of the antioxidant effect has not been elucidated, but a radical "sink" hypothesis has been formulated (Fig. 9). Moreover, the alcohol-induced septal fibrosis and cirrhosis were fully prevented by PPC under these conditions. In addition, a 54% decrease in circulating free F_2-IP was also observed in the plasma of the animals given PPC with ethanol. Alcohol feeding also significantly decreased GSH, and the effect that was attenuated by either AdoMet [116] or PPC [120].

4   SUMMARY

1. The main pathway for the hepatic oxidation of ethanol to acetaldehyde proceeds via ADH, and is associated with the reduction of NAD to NADH, which produces striking redox changes with various associated metabolic disorders.

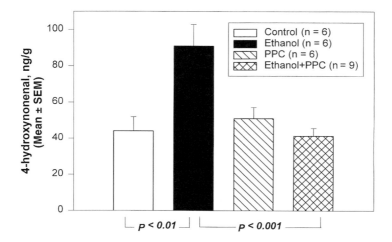

Fig. 8. Effect of ethanol and/or PPC on hepatic 4-hydroxynonenal in baboons. Whereas ethanol significantly increased hepatic 4-hydroxynonenal, PPC completely prevented this effect [137].

2. NADH also inhibits XD activity, resulting in a shift of purine oxidation from XD to the oxidase, thereby promoting the generation of oxygen-free radical species.

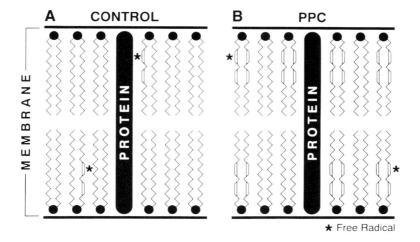

Fig. 9. Radical "sink" hypothesis for the antioxidant effect of polyenylphosphatidylcholine (PPC). Contrasting with the relative scarcity of polyunsaturated fatty acids in control membranes (**A**), after PPC (**B**), the membrane is enriched in polyunsaturated fatty acids and, therefore, for the same radical attack, it is much less likely for any given polyunsaturated fatty acid to be affected by the radical and to undergo severe peroxidation. As a consequence, less damage may ensue, and less peroxidation products may be released.

3. Contrary to the ADH pathway which is not inducible, ethanol can also be metabolized by an accessory pathway, namely MEOS, the induction of which involves a 4- to 10-fold increase of CYP2E1, its active enzyme.

4. This induction is associated with proliferation of the endoplasmic reticulum, both in experimental animals and in humans, and is accompanied by an increased oxidation of NADPH with resulting H_2O_2 generation.

5. The 2E1 induction also contributes to increased rates of superoxide radical production and lipid peroxidation which correlate with the amount of 2E1, there is also inhibition of hepatic microsomal lipid peroxidation by antibodies against 2E1.

6. Induction of the microsomal system results in enhanced acetaldehyde production which, in turn, impairs the defense systems against oxidative stress: it decreases GSH by various mechanisms, including binding to cysteine or by provoking GSH leakage out of the mitochondria and the cell. Hepatic GSH depletion after chronic alcohol consumption was shown both in experimental animals and in humans.

7. The ultimate precursor of cysteine (one of the three amino acids of GSH) is methionine. Methionine, however, must be first activated to AdoMet by an enzyme, the activity of which is depressed by alcoholic liver disease.

8. This block can be bypassed by AdoMet administration which restores hepatic AdoMet levels and attenuates parameters of ethanol-induced liver injury, such as the increase in circulating transaminases, mitochondrial lesions, and leakage of mitochondrial enzymes (e.g., glutamic dehydrogenase) into the bloodstream.

9. AdoMet also contributes to the methylation of phosphatidylethanolamine to phosphatidylcholine. The activity of the methyltransferase involved is strikingly depressed by alcohol consumption, but this can be corrected, and hepatic phosphatidylcholine levels restored, by the administration of a mixture of polyunsaturated phospholipids (polyenyl-phosphatidylcholine: PPC).

10. In addition, PPC provides protection against the alcohol-induced rise in hepatic F_2-IP and hydroxynonenal, products of lipid peroxidation. A similar effect was observed in rats given CCl_4.

11. At the same time as PPC prevented CCl_4 and alcohol-induced lipid peroxidation in rats and baboons, it also attenuated the associated liver injury, including fibrosis and cirrhosis.

5 PERSPECTIVE

Oxidative stress is an important cause of alcohol-induced liver injury. There are now therapeutic agents that can boost the body defenses against these toxic manifestations of alcohol excess by restoring the antioxidant status and repairing the phospholipid alterations in the membranes. Since the generation of radicals by the ethanol-inducible CYP2E1 is, in part, responsible for the stress, 2E1 inhibitors presently under investigation may eventually also provide useful tools for the prevention and treatment of the hepatotoxicity associated with heavy drinking.

6   ACKNOWLEDGMENTS

Original studies reviewed here were supported, in part, by NIH Grants AA05934, AA11160, AA11115 and AA07275 and by the Department of Veterans Affairs. Skillful typing of the manuscript by Ms Diana Perez is gratefully acknowledged.

7   ABBREVIATIONS

^{3}H/^{14}C:	tritiated hydrogen/^{14}C carbon radiolabeled
ADH:	alcohol dehydrogenase
AdoMet:	S-adenosylmethionine
ALDH:	aldehyde dehydrogenase
AST:	aspartate aminotransferase
ATP:	adenosine triphosphate
CCL_4:	carbon tetrachloride
CYP2E1:	cytochrome P4502E1
DLPC:	dilinoleoylphosphatidylcholine
DNA:	deoxyribonucleic acid
F_2 IP:	F_2-isoprostanes
GC/MS:	gas chromatography/mass spectroscopy
GDH:	glutamic dehydrogenase
GSH:	glutathione
H_2O_2:	hydrogen peroxide
IgA:	immunoglobulin A
IgG:	immunoglobulin G
MEOS:	microsomal ethanol-oxidizing system
NADH:	nicotinamide adenine dinucleotide-reduced form
NAD:	nicotinamide adenine dinucleotide
NADPH:	nicotinamide adenine dinucleotide phosphate-reduced form
NADP:	nicotinamide adenine dinucleotide phosphate
NDMA:	N-nitrosodimethylamine
O_2:	oxygen
PEMT:	phosphatidylethanolamine N-methyltransferase
PPC:	polyenylphosphatidylcholine
PUFA:	polyunsaturated fatty acids
XD:	xanthine dehydrogenase
XO:	xanthine oxidase

8   REFERENCES

1. Lieber CS. Cytochrome P-4502E1: Its physiological and pathological role. (In: Physiological Reviews) Am Phys Soc 1997;77:(2)517–544.
2. Domschke S, Domschke W, Lieber CS. Hepatic redox state: Attenuation of the acute effects of ethanol induced by chronic ethanol consumption. Life Sci 1974;15:1327–1334.
3. Greenway CV, Lautt WW. Acute and chronic ethanol on hepatic oxygen ethanol and lactate metabolism in cats. Am J Physiol 1990;258:411–418.
4. Lieber CS, Jones DP, Losowsky MS, Davidson CS. Interrelation of uric acid and ethanol metabolism in man. J Clin Invest 1962;41:1863–1870.
5. Kato S, Kawase T, Alderman J, Inatomi N, Lieber CS. Role of xanthine oxidase in ethanol-induced lipid peroxidation in rats. Gastroenterology 1990;98:203–210.
6. Lieber CS. Medical and Nutritional Complications of Alcoholism: Mechanisms and Management, New York, Plenum Press, 1992;579.
7. Lieber CS, Schmid R. The effect of ethanol on fatty acid metabolism: Stimulation of hepatic fatty acid synthesis in vitro. J Clin Invest 1961;40:394–399.
8. Israel Y, Kalant H, Orrego H, Khanna JM, Videla I, Phillips JM. Experimental alcohol-induced hepatic necrosis: Suppression by propylthiouracil. Proc Natl Acad Sci USA 1975;72:1137–1141.
9. Kessler BJ, Liebler JB, Bronfin GJ, Sass M. The hepatic blood flow and splanchnic oxygen consumption in alcohol fatty liver. J Clin Invest 1954;33:1338–1345.
10. Jauhonen P, Baraona E, Miyakawa H, Lieber CS. Mechanism for selective perivenular hepatotoxicity of ethanol. Alcohol Clin Exp Res 1982;6:350–357.
11. Sato N, Kamada T, Kawano S, Hayashin N, Kishida Y, Meren H, Yoshihara H, Abe H. Effect of acute and chronic ethanol consumption on hepatic tissue oxygen tension in rats. Pharmacol Biochem Behav, 1983;18:443–447.
12. Shaw S, Heller EA, Friedman HS, Baraona E, Lieber CS. Increased hepatic oxygenation following ethanol administration in baboon. Proc Soc Exp Biol Med 1977;156:509–13.
13. Stein SW, Lieber CS, Cherrick GR, Leevy CM, Ablemann WH. The effect of ethanol upon systemic hepatic blood flow in man. Am J Clin Nutr 1973;13:68–74.
14. Carmichael FJ, Saldivia V, Israel Y, McKaigney JP, Orrego H. Ethanol-induced increase in portal hepatic blood flow: interference by anesthetic agents. Hepatology 1987;97:89–94.
15. Lieber CS, Baraona E, Hernandez-Munoz R, Kubota S, Sato N, Kawano S, Matsumura T, Inatomi N. Impaired oxygen utilization: A new mechanism for the hepatotoxicity of ethanol in subhuman primates. J Clin Invest 1989;83:1682–1690.
16. Lieber CS, DeCarli LM. Ethanol oxidation by hepatic microsomes: Adaptive increase after ethanol feeding. Science 1968;162:917–918.
17. Lieber CS, DeCarli LM. Hepatic microsomal ethanol oxidizing system: In vitro characteristics and adaptive properties in vivo. J Biol Chem 1970a;245:2505–2512.
18. Teschke R, Hasumura Y, Joly JG, Ishii H, Lieber CS. Microsomal ethanol-oxidizing system (MEOS): Purification and properties of a rat liver system free of catalase and alcohol dehydrogenase. Biochem Biophys Res Commun 1972;49:1187–1193.
19. Teschke R, Hasumura Y, Lieber CS. Hepatic microsomal alcohol oxidizing system Solubilization, isolation and characterization. Arch Biochem Biophys 1974;163:404–415.
20. Ohnishi K, Lieber CS. Reconstitution of the microsomal ethanol-oxidizing system: qualitative and quantitative changes of cytochrome P-450 after chronic ethanol consumption. J Biol Chem 1977;252:7124–7131.
21. Miwa GT, Levin W, Thomas PE, Lu AYH. The direct oxidation of ethanol by catalase- and alcohol dehydrogenase-free reconstituted system containing cytochrome P-450. Arch Biochem Biophys 1978;187:464–475.
22. Koop DR, Morgan ET, Tarr GE, Coon MJ. Purification and characterization of a unique isozyme of cytochrome P-450 from liver microsomes of ethanol-treated rabbits. J Biol Chem

1982;257:8472–8480.

23. Morgan ET, Koop DR, Coon MJ. Catalytic activity of cytochrome P-450 isozyme 3a isolated from liver microsomes of ethanol-treated rabbits. J Biol Chem, 1982;257:13951–13957.

24. Morgan ET, Koop DR, Coon MJ. Comparison of six rabbit liver cytochrome P-450 isozymes in formation of a reactive metabolite of acetaminophen. Biochem Biophys Res Commun 1983; 112:8–13.

25. Ingelman-Sundberg M, Johansson I. Mechanisms of hydroxyl radical formation and ethanol oxidation by ethanol-inducible and other forms of rabbit liver microsomal cytochromes P-450, J Biol Chem, 1984;259:6447–6458.

26. Koop DR, Casazza JP. Identification of ethanol-inducible P-450 isozyme 3a as the acetone and acetol monooxygenase of rabbit microsomes. J Biol Chem 1985;260:13607–13612.

27. Yang CS, Tu YY, Koop DR, Coon MJ. Metabolism of nitrosamines by purified rabbit liver cytochrome P-450 isozymes. Cancer Res 1985;45:1140–1145.

28. Lasker JM, Raucy J, Kubota S, Bloswick BP, Black M, Lieber CS. Purification and characterization of human liver cytochrome P-450-ALC. Biochem Biophys Res Commun, 1987;148: 232–238.

29. Tsutsumi M, Lasker JM, Shimizu M, Rosman AS, Lieber CS. The intralobular distribution of ethanol-inducible P450IIE1 in rat and human liver. Hepatology 1989;10:437–446.

30. Shimizu M, Lasker JM, Tsutsumi M, Lieber CS. Immunohistochemical localization of ethanol-inducible P450IIE1 in the rat alimentary tract. Gastroenterology 1990;99:1044–1053.

31. Koivisto T, Mishin VM, Mak KM, Cohen PA, Lieber CS. Induction of cytochrome P-4502E1 by ethanol in rat Kupffer cells. Alcohol Clin Exp Res 1996;20:207–212.

32. Nordmann R, Ribière C, Rouach H. Implication of free radical mechanisms in ethanol-induced cellular injury. Free Radic Biol Med 1992;12:219–240.

33. Lieber CS, DeCarli LM. Reduced nicotinamide-adenine dinucleotide phosphate oxidase: Activity enhanced by ethanol consumption. Science 1970;170:78–80.

34. Dai Y, Rashba-Step J, Cederbaum AI. Stable expression of human cytochrome P4502E1 in HepG2 cells: characterization of catalytic activities and production of reactive oxygen intermediates. Biochemistry 1993;32:6928–6937.

35. Diluzio NR. Prevention of the acute ethanol-induced fatty liver by the simultaneous administration of antioxidants. Life Sci 1964;3:113–119.

36. Diluzio NR. The role of lipid peroxidation and antioxidants in ethanol-induced lipid alterations. Exp Molec Pathol 1968;8:394–402.

37. Ekstrom G, Ingelman-Sundberg M. Rat liver microsomal NADPH-supported oxidase activity and lipid peroxidation dependent on ethanol-inducible cytochrome P-450 (P-450IIE1). Biochem Pharmacol 1989;38:1313–1319.

38. Castillo T, Koop DR, Kamimura S, Triadafilopoulos G, Tsukamoto. Role of cytochrome P-450 2E1 in ethanol-, carbon tetrachloride- and iron-dependent microsomal lipid peroxidation. Hepatology 1992;16:992–996.

39. Albano E, Tomasi A, Goria-Gatti L, Poli G, Vannini B, Dianzani MU. Free radical metabolism of alcohols in rat liver microsomes. Free Rad Res Commun 1987;3:243.

40. Reinke L, Lai EK, DuBose CM, McCay PB, Janzen EG. Reactive free radical generation in vivo in heart and liver of ethanol-fed rats: Correlation with radical formation in vitro. Proc Natl Acad Sci USA. 1987;84:8223–8227.

41. Reinke LA, Kotake Y, McCay PB, Janzen EG. Spin trapping studies of hepatic free radicals formed following the acute administration of ethanol to rats: in vivo detection of L-hydroxyethyl radicals with PBN. Free Rad Biol Med 1991;11:31–39.

42. Cederbaum AI. Oxygen radical generation by microsomes: Role of iron and implications for alcohol metabolism and toxicity. Free Rad Biol Med 1989;7:559–567.

43. Albano E, Tomasi A, Goria-Gatti L, Persson JO, Terelius Y, Ingelman-Sundberg M, Dianzani MU. Role of ethanol-inducible cytochrome P-450 (P450IIE1) in catalyzing the free radical activation of aliphatic alcohols. Biochem Pharmacol 1991;411:1895–1902.

44. Clot P, Bellomo G, Tabone M, Aricò S, Albano E. Detection of antibodies against proteins modified by hydroxyethyl free radicals in patients with alcoholic cirrhosis. Gastroenterology 1995;108:201–207.
45. Hetu C, Dumont A, Joly JG. Effect of chronic ethanol administration on bromobenzene liver toxicity in the rat. Toxicol Appl Pharmacol, 1983;67:166–167.
46. Siegers CP, Heidbuchel K, Younes M. Influence of alcohol, dithiocard and (+)-catechin on the hepatotoxicity and metabolism of vinylidene chloride in rats. J Appl Toxicol 1983;3:90–95.
47. Tsutsumi R, Leo MA, Kim C, Tsutsumi M, Lasker JM, Lowe N, Lieber CS. Interaction of ethanol with enflurane metabolism and toxicity: Role of P450IIE1. Alcohol Clin Exp Res 1990;14: 174–179.
48. Takagi T, Ishii H, Takahashi H, Kato S, Okuno F, Ebihara Y, Yamauchi H, Nagata Y, Tashiro M, Tsuchiya M. Potentiation of halothane hepatotoxicity by chronic ethanol administration in rat: An animal model of halothane hepatitis. Pharmacol Biochem Behav, 1983;18(Suppl 1): 461–465.
49. Nakajima T, Okino T, Sato A. Kinetic studies on benzene metabolism in rat liver – possible presence of three forms of benzene metabolizing enzymes in the liver. Biochem Pharmacol 1987;36:2799–2804.
50. Beskid M, Bialck J, Dzieniszewski J, Sadowski J, Tlalka J. Effect of combined phenylbutazone and ethanol administration on rat liver. Exp Pathol 1980;18:487.
51. Sato C, Matsuda Y, Lieber CS. Increased hepatotoxicity of acetaminophen after chronic ethanol consumption in the rat. Gastroenterology 1981;80:140–148.
52. Lieber CS, Garro A, Leo MA, Mak KM, Worner TM. Alcohol and cancer. Hepatology 1986;6:1005–1019.
53. Garro AJ, Seitz HK, Lieber CS. Enhancement of dimethylnitrosamine metabolism and activation to a mutagen following chronic ethanol consumption. Cancer Res 1981;41:120–124.
54. Seitz HK, Garro AJ, Lieber CS. Enhanced pulmonary and intestinal activation of procarcinogens and mutagens after chronic ethanol consumption in the rat. Eur J Clin Invest 1981;11:33–38.
55. Seitz HK, Czygan P, Waldherr K, Veith S, Kommerell B. Ethanol and intestinal carcinogenesis in the rat. Alcohol 1985;2:491–494.
56. Farinati F, Zhou Z, Bellah J, Lieber CS, Garro AJ. Effect of chronic ethanol consumption on activation of nitrosopyrrolidine to a mutagen by rat upper alimentary tract, lung and hepatic tissue. Drug Metab Dispos 1985;13:210–214.
57. Garro AJ, Lieber CS. Alcohol and cancer. Annu Rev Pharmacol Toxicol 1990;30:219–249.
58. Leo MA, Lieber CS. Hepatic vitamin A depletion in alcoholic liver injury. N Engl J Med 1982;307:597–601.
59. Leo MA, Lieber CS. Hepatic fibrosis after long term administration of ethanol and moderate vitamin A supplementation in the rat. Hepatology 1983;2:1–11.
60. Sato M, Lieber CS. Hepatic vitamin A depletion after chronic ethanol consumption in baboons and rats. J Nutr 1981;111:2015–2030.
61. Leo MA, Lieber CS. New pathway for retinol metabolism in liver microsomes. J Biochem 1985;260:5228–5231.
62. Leo MA, Kim CI, Lieber CS. NAD$^+$-dependent retinol dehydrogenase in liver microsomes. Arch Biochem Biophys 1987;259:241–249.
63. Leo MA, Sato M, Lieber CS. Effect of hepatic vitamin A depletion on the liver in men and rats. Gastroenterology 1983;84:562–572.
64. Leo MA, Lowe N, Lieber CS. Interaction of drugs and retinol. Biochem Pharmacol 1986;35: 3949–3953.
65. Leo MA, Lieber CS. Hypervitaminosis A: A liver lover's lament. Hepatology 1988;8:412–417.
66. Leo MA, Arai M, Sato M, Lieber CS. Hepatotoxicity of vitamin A and ethanol in the rat. Gastroenterology, 1982;82:194–205.
67. Krinsky NI, Deneke SM. Interaction of oxygen and oxy-radicals with carotenoids. J Natl Cancer

Inst 1982;69:205–210.

68. Burton GW, Ingold KU. ß-carotene: An unusual type of lipid antioxidant. Science 1984; 224:569–573.

69. Krinsky NI. Antioxidant functions of carotenoids. Free Radic Biol Med, 1989;7:617–635.

70. Alam SQ, Alam BS. Lipid peroxide, α-tocopherol and retinoid levels in plasma and liver of rats fed diets containing ß-carotene and 13-cis-retinoic acid. J Nutr 1983;113:2608–2614.

71. Jenkins MY, Sheikh MN, Mitchell GV, Grundel E, Blakely SR, Carter CJ. Dietary carotenoids influenced biochemical but not morphological changes in adult male rats fed a choline-deficient diet. Nutr Cancer 1993;19:55–65.

72. Kunert KJ, Tappel AL. The effect of vitamin C on in vitro lipid peroxidation in guinea pigs as measured by pentane and ethane production. Lipids 1983;18:271–274.

73. Palozza P, Krinsky NI. The inhibition of radical-initiated peroxidation of microsomal lipids by both α-tocopherol and ß-carotene. Free Radic Bio Med 1991;11:407–414.

74. Kim-Jun H. Inhibitory effects of α- and ß-carotene on croton oil-induced or enzymatic lipid peroxidation and hydroperoxide production in mouse skin epidermis. Int J Biochem 1993;25: 911–915.

75. Mobarhan S, Bowen P, Andersen B, Evans M, Stacewicz-Sapuntzakis M, Sugerman S, Simms P, Lucchesi D, Friedman H. Effects of ß-carotene repletion of ß-carotene absorption, lipid peroxidation, and neutrophil superoxide formation in young men. Nutr Cancer 1990;14:195–206.

76. Leo MA, Kim C I, Lowe N, Lieber CS. Interaction of ethanol with β-carotene: Delayed blood clearance and enhanced hepatotoxicity, Hepatology 1992;15:883–891.

77. Leo MA, Rosman A, Lieber CS. Differential depletion of carotenoids and tocopherol in liver diseases. Hepatology 1993;17:977–986.

78. Ahmed S, Leo MA, Lieber CS. Interactions between alcohol and β-carotene in patients with alcoholic liver disease. Am J Clin Nutr 1994;60:430–436.

79. Forman MR, Beecher GR, Lanza E, Reichman ME, Graubard BI, Campbell MT, Yong LC, Judd JT, Taylor PR. Effect of alcohol consumption on plasma carotenoid concentrations in premenopausal women: a controlled dietary study. Am J Clin Nutr 1995;62:131–135.

80. α-Tocopherol, β-Carotene and Cancer Prevention Study Group. The effect of vitamin E and β-carotene on the incidence of lung cancer and other cancers in male smokers. N Engl J Med 1994;330:1029–1035.

81. Omenn GS, Goodman GE, Thornquist MD, Balmes J, Cullen MR, Glass A, Keogh JP, Meyskens FL, Jr., Barnhart S, Hammar S. Effects of a combination of β-carotene and vitamin A on lung cancer and cardiovascular disease. N Engl J Med 1996;334:1150–1155.

82. Albanes D, Heinonen, OP Taylor, PR, Virtamo J, Edwards BK, Rautalahti M, Hartman AM, Palmgren J, Freedman LS, Haapakoski J, Barrett MJ, Pietinen P, Malila N, Tala E, Liippo K, Salomaa ER, Tangrea JA, Teppo L, Askin FB, Taskinen E, Erozan Y, Greenwald P, Huttunen JK. α-Tocopherol and β-carotene supplements and lung cancer incidence in the α-Tocopherol, β-Carotene Cancer Prevention Study: Effects of base-line characteristics and study compliance. J Natl Cancer Inst 1996;88:1560–1571.

83. Leo MA, Lieber CS. Adverse effects of β-carotene. (Letter to the Editor). N Engl J Med 1994;331:612.

84. Leo MA, Aleynik S, Aleynik M, Lieber CS. β-carotene beadlets potentiate hepatototxicity of alcohol. Am J Clin Nutr 1997;66:1461–1469.

85. Keilin D, Hartree EF. Properties of catalase: Catalysis of coupled oxidation of alcohols, Biochem J, 1945;39:293–301.

86. Sies H, Chance B. The steady level of catalase compound I in isolated hemoglobin-free perfused rat liver. FEBS Lett 1970;11:172–176.

87. Oshino N, Chance B, Sies H, Bucher T. The role of H_2O_2 generation in perfused rat liver and the reaction of catalase compound I and hydrogen donors. Arch Biochem Biophys 1973;154: 117–131.

88. Handler JA, Thurman RG. Fatty acid-dependent ethanol metabolism. Biochem Biophys Res

Commun, 1985;133:44—51.

89. Williamson JR, Scholz R, Browning ET, Thurman RG, Fukami MH. Metabolic effects of ethanol in perfused rat liver. J Biol Chem 1969;25:5044—5054.

90. Handler JA, Thurman RG. Redox interactions between catalase and alcohol dehydrogenase pathways of ethanol metabolism in the perfused rat liver. J Biol Chem 1990;265:1510—1515.

91. Takagi T, Alderman J, Geller J, Lieber CS. Assessment of the role of non-ADH ethanol oxidation in vivo and in hepatocytes from deermice. Biochem Pharmacol 1986;35:3601—3606.

92. Kato S, Alderman J, Lieber CS. Respective roles of the microsomal ethanol oxidizing system (MEOS) and catalase in ethanol metabolism by deermice lacking alcohol dehydrogenase. Arch Biochem Biophys 1987;254:586—591.

93. Kato S, Alderman J, Lieber CS. Ethanol metabolism in alcohol dehydrogenase deficient deermice is mediated by the microsomal ethanol oxidizing system, not by catalase, Alcohol Alcoholism 1987;(Suppl 1):231—234.

94. Teschke R, Matsuzaki S, Ohnishi K, DeCarli LM, Lieber CS. Microsomal ethanol oxidizing system (MEOS): Current status of its characterization and its role. Alcohol Clin Exp Res 1977;1:7—15.

95. Thurman RG, Brentzel HJ. The role of alcohol dehydrogenase in microsomal ethanol oxidation and the adaptive increase in ethanol metabolism due to chronic treatment with ethanol. Alcohol Clin Exp Res 1977;1:33—38.

96. Kaikaus RM, Chan WK, Lysenko N, Ortiz P, Montellano D, Bass NM. Induction of liver fatty acid binding protein (l-FABP) and peroxisomal fatty acid ß-oxidation by peroxisome proliferators (PP) is dependent on cytochrome P-450 activity. Hepatology 1990;12:A248.

97. Hasumura Y, Teschke R, Lieber CS. Hepatic microsomal ethanol oxidizing system (MEOS): Dissociation from reduced nicotinamide adenine dinucleotide phosphate-oxidase and possible role of form 1 of cytochrome P-450. J Pharmacol Exp Ther, 1975;194:469—474.

98. Di Padova C, Worner TM, Julkunen RJK, Lieber CS. Effects of fasting and chronic alcohol consumption on the first pass metabolism of ethanol. Gastroenterology 1987;92:1169—1173.

99. Dicker E, Cederbaum AI. Increased oxygen radical-dependent inactivation of metabolic enzymes by liver microsomes after chronic ethanol consumption. FASEB J 1988;2:2901—2906.

100. Espina N, Lima V, Lieber CS, Garro AJ. In vitro and in vivo inhibitory effect of ethanol and acetaldehyde on O^6-methylguanine transferase. Carcinogenesis 1988;9:761—766.

101. Müller A, Sies H. Role of alcohol dehydrogenase activity and of acetaldehyde in ethanol-induced ethane and pentane production by isolated perfused rat liver. Biochem J 1982;206:153—156.

102. Müller A, Sies H. Inhibition of ethanol- and aldehyde-induced release of ethane from isolated perfused rat liver by pargyline and disulfiram. Pharmacol Biochem Behav, 1983;18:429—432.

103. Shaw S, Rubin KP, Lieber CS. Depressed hepatic glutathione and increased diene conjugates in alcoholic liver disease: evidence of lipid peroxidation. Dig Dis Sci 1983;28:585—589.

104. Morton S, Mitchell MC. Effects of chronic ethanol feeding on glutathione turnover in the rat. Biochem Pharmacol 1985;34:1559—1563.

105. Speisky H, MacDonald A, Giles G, Orrego H, Israel Y. Increased loss and decreased synthesis of hepatic glutathione after acute ethanol administration. Biochem J 1985;225:565.

106. Hirano T, Kaplowitz N, Tsukamoto H, Kamimura S, Fernandez-Checa JC. Hepatic mitochondrial glutathione depletion and progression of experimental alcoholic liver disease in rats. Hepatology 1992;6:1423—1427.

107. Lieber CS. Liver fibrosis: from pathogenesis to treatment. In: DF de Pretis (ed) Advances in Hepatobiliary and Pancreatic Diseases. Lancaster, UK: Kluwer Academic Press, 1995;62—81.

108. Shaw S, Lieber CS. Increased hepatic production of α-amino-n-butyric acid after chronic alcohol consumption in rats and baboons. Gastroenterology 1980;78:108—113.

109. Shaw S, Lieber CS. Plasma amino acid abnormalities in the alcoholic; respective role of alcohol, nutrition and liver injury. Gastroenterology 1978;74:677—682.

110. Shaw S, Jayatilleke E, Ross WA, Gordon ER, Lieber CS: Ethanol induced lipid peroxidation: Potentiation by long-term alcohol feeding and attenuation by methionine. J Lab Clin Med

1981;98:417—425.

111. Zhang H, Loney LA, Potter BJ. Effect of chronic alcohol feeding on hepatic iron status and ferritin uptake by rat hepatocytes. Alcohol Clin Exp Res 1993;17:394—400.

112. Valenzuela A, Fernandez V, Videla LA. Hepatic and biliary levels of flutathione andlipid peroxides following iron overload in the rat: Effect of simultaneous ethanol administration. Toxicol Appl Pharmacol, 1983;70:87—95.

113. Finkelstein JD, Martin JJ. Methionine metabolism in mammals. Adaptation to methionine excess. J Biol Chem 1986;261:1582—1587.

114. Horowitz JH, Rypins EB, Henderson JM, Heymsfield SB, Moffit SD, Bain RP, Chawla RK, Bleier JC, Rudman D. Evidence for impairment of transsulfuration pathway in cirrhosis. Gastroenterology 1981;81:668—675.

115. Duce AM, Ortiz P, Cabrero C, Mato JM. S-adenosyl-L-methionine synthetase and phospholipid methyltransferase are inhibited in human cirrhosis. Hepatology 1988;8:65—68.

116. Lieber CS, Casini A, DeCarli LM, Kim C, Lowe N, Sasaki R, Leo MA. S-adenosyl-L-methionine attenuates alcohol-induced liver injury in the baboon. Hepatology 1990;11:165—172.

117. Yamada S, Mak KM, Lieber CS. Chronic ethanol consumption alters rat liver plasma membranes and potentiates release of alkaline phosphatase. Gastroenterology 1985;88:1799—1806.

118. Vendemiale G, Altomare E, Trizzio T, Le Grazzie C, Di Padova C, Salerno T, Carrieri V, Albano O. Effects of oral S-adenosyl-L-methionine on hepatic glutathione in patients with liver disease. Scand J Gastroenterol 1989;24:407—415.

119. Lieber CS. Prevention and therapy with S-adenosyl-L-methionine and polyenylphosphatidylcholine. In: Arroyo V, Bosch J, Rodes J (eds) Treatments in Hepatology. Masson, SA: 1995; 299—311.

120. Lieber CS, Robins S, Li J, DeCarli LM, Mak KM, Fasulo JM, Leo MA. Phosphatidylcholine protects against fibrosis and cirrhosis in the baboon. Gastroenterology 1994;106:152—159.

121. Mato JM, Camara J, Fernandez de Paz J, Caballeria L, Caballero A, Buey-Garcia L, Beltran J, Benita V, Caballeria J, Sola R, Otero-Moreno R, Felix B, Duce-Martin A, Correa JA, Pares A, Barro E, Magaz-Garcia I, Puerta JL, Moreno J, Boissard G, Ortiz P, Rodes J. S-Adenosylmethionine in alcoholic liver cirrhosis: a randomized, placebo-controlled double blind, multicentre clinical trial. J Hepatology 1999;30:1081—1089.

122. Bjørneboe GEA, Bjørneboe A, Hagen BF, Morland J, Drevon CA. Reduced hepatic α-tocopherol content after long-term administration of ethanol to rats. Biochem Biophys Acta 1987; 918:236—241.

123. Kawase T, Kato S, Lieber CS. Lipid peroxidation and antioxidant defense systems in rat liver after chronic ethanol feeding. Hepatology 1989;10:815—821.

124. Von Herbay A, de Groot H, Hegi U, Stemmel W, Strohmeyer G, Sies H. Low vitamin E content in plasma of patients with alcoholic liver disease, hemochromatosis and Wilson's disease. J Hepatol 1994;20:41—46.

125. Lieber CS, Robins SJ, Leo MA. Hepatic phosphatidylethanolamine methyltransferase activity is decreased by ethanol and increased by phosphatidylcholine. Alcohol Clin Exp Res 1994;18: 592—595.

126. Fox JM. Polyene phosphatidylcholine: pharmacokinetics after oral administration — a review. In: Avogaro P, Macini M, Ricci G, Paoletti R (eds) Phospholipids and Atherosclerosis. New York: Raven Press, 1983;65—80.

127. Zierenberg O, Grundy SM. Intestinal absorption of polyenylphosphatidylcholine in man. J Lipid Res 1982;23:1136—1142.

128. Lekim D, Betzing H. The incorporation of essential phospholipids into the organs of intact and galactosamine intoxicated rats. Drug Res 1974;24:1217—1221.

129. Parthasarathy S, Subbaiah PV, Ganguly J. The mechanism of intestinal absorption of phosphatidylcholine in rats. Biochem J 1974;140:503—508.

130. Rodgers JB, O'Brien RJ, Balint JA. The absorption and subsequent utilization of lecithin by the rat jejunum. Am J Dig Dis 1975;20:208—211.

131. Halliwell B, Gutteridge JMC. Free radicals in biology and medicine, 2nd edn. Oxford: Clarendon Press, 1989;188—214.
132. Parfitt VJ, Desomeaux K, Bolton CH, Hartog M. Effects of high monounsaturated and polyunsaturated fat diets on plasma lipoproteins and lipid peroxidation in Type 2 diabetes mellitus. Diabetic Medicine 1994;11:85—91.
133. Sosenko IRS, Innis SM, Frank L. Polyunsaturated fatty acids and protection of newborn rats from oxygen toxicity. J Pediatr 1988;112:630—637.
134. Sosenko IRS, Innis SM, Frank L. Menhaden fish oil, n-3 polyunsaturated fatty acids and protection of newborn rats from oxygen toxicity. Pediatr Res 1989;25:399—404.
135. Sosenko IRS, Innis SM, Frank L. Intralipid increases lung polyunsaturated fatty acids and protects newborn rats from oxygen toxicity. Pediatr Res 1991;30:413—417.
136. Aleynik SI, Leo MA, Ma X, Aleynik MK, Lieber CS. Polyenylphosphatidylcholine prevents carbon tetrachloride induced lipid peroxidation while it attenuates liver injury and fibrosis. J Hepatology 1997;26:1—8.
137. Lieber CS, Leo MA, Aleynik SI, Aleynik MK, DeCarli LM. Polyenylphosphatidylcholine decreases alcohol-induced oxidative stress in the baboon. Clin Exp Res Alcohol 1997;21: 375—379.

©2000 Elsevier Science B.V. All rights reserved.
Handbook of Oxidants and Antioxidants in Exercise.
C.K. Sen, L. Packer and O. Hänninen, editors.

Part XI • Chapter 33

Cigarette smoking as an inducer of oxidative stress in relation to disease pathogenesis

Garry G. Duthie, John R. Arthur and Susan J. Duthie
Rowett Research Institute, Greenburn Road, Bucksburn, Aberdeen, AB21 9SB, Scotland, UK.
Tel.: +44-224-712-751.

1 INTRODUCTION
2 CHEMISTRY OF FREE RADICALS IN CIGARETTE SMOKE
3 OXIDANT STRESS AND SMOKING
   3.1   Lungs
   3.2   Blood
4 SMOKING AND ANTIOXIDANT NUTRIENTS
   4.1   Vitamin C
   4.2   Carotenoids
   4.3   Vitamin E
   4.4   Antioxidant enzymes
5 DIETARY ANTIOXIDANT INTAKES OF SMOKERS AND NONSMOKERS
6 SMOKING, ANTIOXIDANTS AND DISEASE
   6.1   Coronary heart disease
   6.2   Cancer
7 ANTIOXIDANT SUPPLEMENTATION OF SMOKERS
8 CONCLUSIONS
9 SUMMARY
10 ACKNOWLEGEMENTS
11 REFERENCES

1   INTRODUCTION

According to the latest report from the World Health Organisation [1] there are currently three million tobacco-related deaths worldwide each year. By the end of the 1990s, 30 million people will have been killed by smoking, more than half of them while in middle age. In the USA, smoking is implicated in one-sixth of all deaths each year and the American Lung Association estimates that medical treatment and lost production time ascribed to smoking-related disorders cost the US economy $97.2 billion/annum [2]. In the UK, smoking-attributable diseases account for 110,700 premature deaths annually and total annual in-patients costs to the National Health Service are estimated at £325 million [3]. The life expectancy of smokers is less than that of nonsmokers (Table 1) such that on average a 35 year old male smoker can expect to live seven years less than a nonsmoker. Moreover, exposure of nonsmokers to environmental tobacco smoke may also have damaging effects on health [3—10]. This premature mortality is due to habitual smoking increasing the risk of developing many diseases

Table 1. Life expectancy (additional number of years) at a given age.

Age	Male smokers	Male nonsmokers	Female smokers	Female nonsmokers
35	36.5	43.5	41.8	46.6
40	31.7	38.8	37.0	41.8
45	27.1	34.1	32.3	37.0
50	22.7	29.4	27.8	32.4
55	18.7	25.0	23.4	27.4
60	15.0	20.8	19.4	23.5
65	12.0	16.9	15.9	19.4
70	9.3	13.5	12.7	15.5
75	7.2	10.7	10.1	12.1

Data adapted from [3].

including coronary heart disease, lung cancer, stroke and emphysema (Table 2).

Many of the clinical conditions implicated with smoking are also associated with increased indices of free radical-mediated damage to proteins, lipids and DNA [11–15]. This suggests that smoking may exacerbate the initiation and propagation of oxidative stresses which are potential underlying processes in the pathogenesis of many diseases. However, it must be emphasised that the association of increased free radical activity with the occurrence of a disease does not indicate that the condition is caused by the radicals. Disruption and damage by radicals and subsequent further damage to cells which impairs or de-localises antioxidant defence systems against free radicals, will cause increased oxidant production. Moreover, many nonradical products such as alkaloids, nitrosamines

Table 2. Estimates of proportion of deaths from various clinical conditions that are attributable to smoking in the UK in 1988.

Disease	Attributal percentage		
	Men	Women	All
Coronary heart disease	24	11	18
Stroke	19	7	12
Aortic aneurism and atherosclerotic peripheral vascular disease	44	15	29
Chronic obstructive pulmonary disease	80	69	76
Lung cancer	86	69	81
Cancer of buccal cavity, oesaphagus, laryx	84	48	71
Cancer of bladder	45	29	40
Cancer of kidney	49	7	32
Cancer of the pancreas	22	30	26
Cancer of the cervix	–	29	29
Ulcer of stomach and duodenum	24	20	22

Data adapted from [3].

and hydrocarbons may also be of major importance in initiating smoking-related diseases [16].

Consequently, the aims of this chapter are to review how smoking challenges and perturbs the antioxidant defence system and to discuss whether increased antioxidant intakes can influence smoking-induced oxidative stress and disease morbidity.

2   CHEMISTRY OF FREE RADICALS IN CIGARETTE SMOKE

Cigarette smoke can be divided into two phases: particulate matter (tar) and gas phase smoke. Different free radicals are present in these fractions (Table 3). Tar contains more than 10^{17} stable long-lived radicals per gram. The gas phase smoke contains more than $\sim 10^{15}$ free radicals per puff [16,17]. These radicals can be divided into two distinct groups.

The first group consists mainly of long-lived quinone–semiquinone radicals that are associated with the particulate phase matrix and appear to be generated by oxidation of polycyclic aromatic hydrocarbons during the combustion process. When extracted into water the tar radical ($Q^\bullet$) can reduce oxygen to superoxide (O^-_2) and hydrogen peroxide (H_2O_2) and can also catalyse the conversion of H_2O_2 to the highly reactive hydroxyl radical ($OH^\bullet$) as follows:

$$O_2 + Q^\bullet \rightarrow O^-_2 + Q$$

$$O^-_2 + Q^\bullet + 2H^+ \rightarrow H_2O_2 + Q$$

$$H_2O_2 + Fe^{3+} \rightarrow OH^- + OH^\bullet + Fe^{2+}$$

Smokers deposit up to 20 mg of tar in their lungs per cigarette and aqueous extracts of the tar oxidise α-1-proteinase inhibitor and damage DNA in vitro presumably because of the production of $OH^\bullet$-type radicals. Moreover, tar consists

Table 3. Some oxidant species arising directly or indirectly from the combustion and inhalation of tobacco.

Oxidant species
Quinone/ semiquinone/ hydroquinone complexes
Carbon-centred free radicals
Oxygen-centered free radical
Hydrogen peroxide
Superoxide anion
Hydroxyl radical
Nitric oxide
Nitrogen dioxide

For recent review, see [23].

of an aerosol containing more than 5,000 organic compounds of a nonradical nature some of which may be tumor initiators, cocarcinogens, toxins and geno-toxins [16].

The second group are short-lived, reactive carbon- and oxygen-centered peroxy radicals, often detected by spin trapping methods [18−20]. Although the lifetime of these radicals is less than 1 s, they have an apparent lifetime of over 5 min because a steady state between production and destruction is attained as the smoke ages. This steady state of short-lived radicals may result from the slow oxidation of nitric oxide (NO) in cigarette smoke to the radical, nitrogen dioxide (NO_2) which reacts with smoke components such as aldehydes and olefins to continually produce peroxy radicals [21]. Moreover, NO and NO_2 may react with hydrogen peroxide to produce $OH^\bullet$:

$$NO + H_2O_2 \rightarrow HNO_2 + OH^\bullet$$

$$NO_2 + H_2O_2 \rightarrow HNO_3 + OH^\bullet$$

Potential sources of H_2O_2 in the above reactions include activated pulmonary macrophages and neutrophils; oxidant production by phagocytes may be stimulated by nicotine [22]. Cigarette smoke also contains Cu and Fe which can promote $OH^\bullet$ formation by Fenton-type reactions:

$$Fe^{2+} + H_2O_2 \rightarrow Fe^{3+} + OH^\bullet + OH^-$$

3   OXIDANT STRESS AND SMOKING

3.1 Lungs

Oxidants in cigarette smoke can damage the lungs through direct interactions with DNA, lipids and proteins [23]. Chemiluminescence and ESR studies have directly demonstrated the generation of O^-_2 in cigarette-smoke exposed aqueous solutions which then leads to the production of H_2O_2, $OH^\bullet$ and $^1O_2$ [24]. Thus, aqueous extracts of cigarette smoke cause DNA strand breaks probably through the continuous production of $OH^\bullet$. Moreover, $Q/QH_2/QH^\bullet$ complexes may cause nicking of DNA by preferentially binding to certain regions of the molecule [25]. Cigarette smoke also induces the oxidation of methyl linoleate and the free radicals in the gas phase induce the formation of lipid hydroperoxides thus contributing to the peroxidative destruction of the polyunsaturated fatty acid components of cell membranes [26]. Additionally, solutions of cigarette tar, whole cigarette smoke and gas-phase cigarette smoke all contain oxidants which can inactivate proteins such as α-1-proteinase inhibitor [25].

Another potential source of oxidants in the lungs of smokers are activated macrophages and neutrophils which can generate reactive oxygen species by activation of a membrane-bound NADPH-oxidase. Cigarette smoking is associated with increased numbers of neutrophils and macrophages in the airway lumen and alveoli [27,28] and these appear to be more activated than those in the lungs of nonsmokers [29—31]. Moreover, smokers may have increased activated pro-oxidant cytokines such as tumour necrosis factor α and interleukins 1 and 8 which could recruit and activate phagocytes in the lung epithelium [32].

Abnormalities in antioxidants concentrations in lungs of smokers also support the premise that smoking induces oxidative stress within the respiratory tract. The low concentrations of vitamin E in lung lavages from smokers [33] presumably result in part from a sustained exposure to the free radicals associated with tobacco combustion. In contrast, vitamin E concentrations in lung tissue of rats and guinea pigs increase following chronic exposure to tobacco smoke [34—36] suggesting an adaptive response to protect pulmonary tissues from oxidative damage. Moreover, alveolar macrophages of smokers have a higher total ascorbate content and an enhanced ability to accumulate ascorbate in vitro, which also suggests partial adaptation to oxidative stress [37]. Studies on animals indicate that adaptive increases in activities of antioxidant enzymes also occur in lung tissue, the exposure to cigarette smoke increasing the activities of glucose-6-phosphate dehydrogenase, glutathione reductase, glutathione peroxidase, catalase and superoxide dismutase [38,39]. Nutritional vitamin E status influences the cellular response to cigarette smoke as compensatory increases in lung antioxidants are more pronounced in vitamin E-deficient animals [39]. Acute cigarette smoking results in depleted glutathione concentrations in lungs, lavaged cells and lavaged fluids of rats, [38] although GSH was increased in rats chronically exposed to cigarette smoke [38,39]. Thus, acute exposure to cigarette smoke may cause a transient decrease in GSH and the lungs respond by increasing cysteine uptake to increase production of GSH. Such adaptive responses of the antioxidant defence system may partially explain why, despite the presence of oxidising species, increased formation of products of lipid peroxidation have not been clearly demonstrated in pulmonary tissue of smoke-exposed animal models [34].

3.2 Blood

One consequence of the production of free radicals in cigarette smoke is marked oxidising reactions in the blood. For example, exposure of plasma in vitro to gas phase cigarette smoke causes depletion in antioxidants such as vitamin C, vitamin E, urate, ubiquinol-10 and β-carotene, as well as increased products of free radical-mediated damage to lipids and proteins [40,41]. Moreover, as a result of this sustained oxidant load, many indices of oxidative damage to bio-molecules are elevated in the circulation of smokers in vivo. For example, plasma of smokers has a 2-fold higher concentration of F_2-isoprostanes than that of nonsmokers which is indicative of the enhanced peroxidation of arachidonic acid [42]. In addition, less specific indices of lipid peroxidation such as thiobarbituric acid reactive substances, conjugated dienes, fluorescent products and lipid peroxides are increased in plasma of smokers indicating that the inhalation of tobacco smoke induces a sustained oxidant stress which overwhelms the capacity of the antioxidant defence system [43—59] (Table 4). Moreover, smoking increases DNA damage in vivo as estimated by the enhanced detection of mutations in circulating T lymphocytes and 8-hydroxydeoxyguanosine in the urine and circulating leukocytes of smokers [55,56].

4   SMOKING AND ANTIOXIDANT NUTRIENTS

Abnormalities in concentrations of antioxidant nutrients and activities of antioxidant enzymes in plasma and red cells of smokers also supports the premise that smoking produces a systemic oxidative stress.

Table 4. Some studies indicating increased indices of oxidative stress in smokers.

Authors	Comments
Sakamoto [54]	Smokers have enhanced ethane expiration indicating higher peroxidation of n-3 fatty acids in vivo.
Duthie et al. [47,48]	Smokers have increased plasma concentrations of conjugated dienes and dehyroascorbate.
Hoshino et al. [52]	Increased pentane expiration by smokers indicates enhanced peroxidation of n-6 fatty acids in vivo.
Loft et al. [56]	Smoking increases oxidative DNA damage in vivo by approximately 50%, as indicated by increased urinary levels of the DNA repair product, 8-hydroxydeoxyguanosine.
Brown et al. [57]	Plasma lipid peroxides, thiobarbituric acid reactive substances and conjugated dienes elevated in smokers, suggesting increased lipid peroxidation.
Duthie et al. [55]	Increased DNA damage in smokers indicated by positive relationship between *hprt* mutant frequency of peripheral T lymphocytes and reported smoking intensity.
Morrow et al. [42]	Increased circulating levels of F_2 isoprostanes, a measure of lipid peroxidation, in smokers compared with nonsmokers.
Reilly et al. [58]	Increased levels of 8-epi-prostoglandinF_2-α, a stable product of lipid peroxidation, in urine of smokers.
Duthie et al. [129]	Increased oxidation of pyrimidines in DNA of lymphocytes of smokers.
Miller et al. [59]	Increased expired ethane and plasma thiobarbituric acid reactive substances in smokers compared with nonsmokers.

4.1 Vitamin C

Numerous studies indicate that plasma, serum and leukocyte vitamin C concentrations are approximately 20—40% less in smokers compared with nonsmokers [60—74]. The basis of the decrease in vitamin C could be biochemical or dietary. Some studies indicate that vitamin C intakes are similar in smokers and nonsmokers suggesting that altered dietary patterns do not completely explain the difference in ascorbate concentrations. Moreover, increased plasma concentrations of dehydroascorbate [47,48,75] suggest that smokers have an increased turnover of vitamin C possibly in response to a high and sustained oxidant load. This is supported by metabolic studies and dietary surveys which indicate that smokers have a nicotine-induced decrease in intestinal absorption efficiency, a decreased urinary excretion rate and a higher turnover of vitamin C [75—78] and the observation that after smoking cessation ascorbate levels increase [79].

4.2 Carotenoids

Plasma β-carotene concentrations of smokers are approximately 15—20% less than in nonsmokers [71,80—85]. Whether this is due to a reduced intake of β-carotene by smokers or to changes in metabolic turnover ascribed to oxidative stress is unclear. However, smoking is an independent factor in reducing plasma β-carotene following adjustment for dietary intakes [85]. Plasma concentrations of some other carotenoids such as α-carotene and β-cryptoxanthin are lower in smokers whereas concentrations of lycopene and phytofluene are similar to those of nonsmokers [86] (Table 5). The significant decrease in plasma concentrations of three of the six carotenoids in smoker's plasma may reflect dietary differences between smokers and never-smokers as intakes of fruit and fresh vegetables, which are rich sources of carotenoids, tend to be lower in smokers than in nonsmokers (see Section 5). Additionally, the greater alcohol consumption by smokers may also influence plasma carotenoid concentrations [86] The lack of a

Table 5. Example of the differences in plasma concentrations of dietary antioxidants between 50 smokers and 50 age-matched nonsmokers from the same Scottish population.

Parameter	Smokers	Nonsmokers	p values
α-Tocopherol (μg/ml)	11.38 ± 0.38	11.32 ± 0.33	0.574
γ-Tocopherol (μg/ml)	0.88 ± 0.04	0.85 ± 0.07	0.663
Vitamin C (μM)	25.6 ± 3.3	37.6 ± 2.4	**0.003**
α-Carotene (μg/ml)	0.042 ± 0.003	0.061 ± 0.004	**0.0006**
β-Carotene (μg/ml)	0.26 ± 0.02	0.32 ± 0.02	**0.026**
β-Cryptoxanthin (μg/ml)	0.042 ± 0.006	0.063 ± 0.007	**0.041**
Lycopene (μg/ml	0.27 ± 0.02	0.28 ± 0.02	0.879
Lutein/zeaxanthin (μg/ml)	0.24 ± 0.02	0.29 ± 0.02	0.052

Data adapted from Ross et al. [86] and compared using Students t test with p < 0.05 being taken as indicating statistical significance. Significant differences indicated by bold type.

significant difference between smokers and never-smokers in plasma concentrations of lycopene, lutein/zeaxanthin and phytofluene may, therefore, suggest that intakes of these carotenoids are unaffected by smoking or that they have limited metabolic and antioxidant function. This also indicates that it is unlikely that the differences in the other carotenoids are solely of dietary origin.

4.3 Vitamin E

Plasma concentrations of vitamin E are invariably reported to be similar in smokers and nonsmokers (Table 5) [45,57,87]. However, a recent study [88] indicates that smoking affects tocopherol uptake and possibly turnover as tocopherol concentrations in smokers were lower compared with nonsmokers following ingestion of similar oral doses of vitamin E. Moreover, there are indications that although plasma concentrations of vitamin E are similar between smokers and nonsmokers, red cell tocopherol concentrations of smokers are markedly decreased [89]. This difference reflects a lower binding activity for tocopherol by the erythrocytes of smokers, possibly due to a reduction in the number of vitamin E binding sites in the membrane and a lower affinity by these sites for tocopherol. Whether the decreased binding activity is due to enhanced smoking-induced oxidative damage to the binding protein is presently unclear but does suggest that smokers have an impaired vitamin E status.

4.4 Antioxidant enzymes

Smoking causes perturbations in the activities of blood antioxidant enzymes. For example, plasma ceruloplasmin activities are increased in smokers [48,90—92]; this change could reflect increased copper intake from the tar components of cigarettes or an acute phase stress response. Moreover, raised ceruloplasmin may provide antioxidant protection by preventing the oxidative inactivation of α1-proteinase inhibitor [90,91]. In the erythrocyte, catalase and superoxide dismutase activities are unchanged in smokers compared with nonsmokers, as are concentrations of metal cofactors such as copper and zinc [47—49,90,93,94]. However, a decrease in the activity of glucose-6-phosphate dehydrogenase in the erythrocytes of smokers [47—49] may reflect inhibition of the enzyme by extracellular or intracellular lipid hydroperoxides and contribute to the increased susceptibility of washed erythrocytes of smokers to hydrogen peroxide-induced peroxidation in vitro [47—49].

A decrease in glutathione peroxidase in smokers' erythrocytes has been inconsistently observed and may, therefore, reflect differences in selenium status rather than a direct response to a sustained oxidative stress [90,95—98]. Total body selenium may be depressed in smokers as indicated by a lower selenium content of toenail clippings [99].

5 DIETARY ANTIOXIDANT INTAKES OF SMOKERS AND NONSMOKERS

Part of the explanation for the observed decreases in concentrations of antioxidant nutrients in plasma of smokers may be ascribed to different dietary habits. This is difficult to establish for certain as the validity of measures of dietary intake in free living individuals rely on information given by the subjects themselves, which may not be accurate. A further complication is that daily variations in food intake mean that few dietary assessments measure true mean food or nutrient intake of individuals. Despite these caveats, it does appear that intakes of fruit and fresh vegetables, which are rich sources of vitamin C and carotenoids, tend to be lower in smokers than in nonsmokers [100–106] (Table 6). Moreover, recent analysis of the Multiple Risk Factor Intervention Trial data base [107] confirms that intakes of antioxidant nutrients are less in smokers than nonsmokers but that intakes increase once a smoker has managed to stop. Smoking may adversely affect the tastebuds and thus, alter the palatability and appeal of fruit and vegetables [108]. Consequently, the food choice by smokers may indirectly increase oxidant stress as a result of suboptimum intakes of antioxidant nutrients.

6 SMOKING, ANTIOXIDANTS AND DISEASE

Most data implicating tobacco use with increased incidence or susceptibility to disease come from epidemiological studies. Results have to be interpreted with caution as statistical associations between smoking and increased morbidity and mortality may not be causal but merely adventitious. Moreover, each type of study has particular advantages and disadvantages. For example descriptive eco-

Table 6. Summary of dietary studies suggesting lower fruit and vegetable intakes of smokers compared with nonsmokers.

Methodology	Reference	Comments
FFQ	100	Smokers less likely to eat vegetable and fruit.
7-day intake	101	Smokers ate less fresh fruit and carrots
FFQ	102	Smokers ate less fresh fruit
FFQ	103	Smokers had lower intakes of fruit
FFQ	104	Smokers ate less fresh fruit and raw vegetables
FFQ	105	Former smokers ate more fruit and vegetables than current smokers
FFQ	106	Smokers are less likely to eat fresh fruit and green vegetables

FFQ: food frequency questionnaire.

logical or correlational studies comparing disease rates within a population with average per capita consumption of tobacco are unable to link smoking to the occurrence of disease in the same person and also cannot exclude the possibility that a hidden, but associated, parameter is actually the causative factor. Cross-sectional retrospective and cohort studies often attempt to minimise confounding effects of other factors by multiple regression methods. However, Mead, for example, states; "Although each of the methods for multiple comparisons was developed for a particular, usually very limited situation, in practice these methods are used widely with no apparent thought to their appropriateness. For many experiments, and even for editors of journals, they have become automatic in the less desirable sense of being used as a substitute for thought" [109]. This suggests that results of epidemiological studies should be treated with caution particularly if good confirmatory mechanistic data are not available.

6.1 Coronary heart disease

Although cross-cultural studies do not reveal a strong, positive relationship between smoking levels and mortality from coronary heart disease (e.g., Fig. 1), longitudinal studies within a country support an association between smoking and disease incidence. One explanation for the poor cross-country association between smoking intensity and coronary heart disease may be due to cultural variation in antioxidant intakes which modify smoking-induced oxidative stress. In particular, there is now considerable evidence (for recent review see [111]) that the susceptibility of low-density lipoprotein (LDL) to oxidative modification

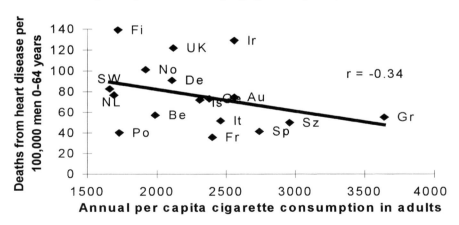

Fig. 1. The lack of a positive and strong cross-country relationship between standardised mortality rates for coronary heart disease calculated as an average from 1985–1987 and total adult cigarette consumption in adults over 15 years of age in Europe. Au, Austria; Be, Belgium; De, Denmark; Ge, Germany (former West); Fi, Finland; Fr, France; Gr, Greece; Ir, Ireland; Is, Israel; It, Italy; NL, Netherlands; No, Norway; Po, Portugal, Sp, Spain; Sw, Sweden; Sz, Switzerland; UK, United Kingdom. Adapted from [110].

to an atherogenic form is a key event in the development of atherosclerosis, and that such oxidation may be inhibited by increased antioxidant intakes [112]. This is corroborated by significant cross-cultural correlations [110] relating mortality from coronary heart disease and dietary intakes of antioxidant nutrients (Table 7). Moreover, coronary heart disease mortality is inversely related to a cumulative antioxidant index, defined as:

$$\frac{[\text{vitamin E}] \times [\text{vitamin C}] \times [\beta - \text{carotene}] \times [\text{selenium}]}{[\text{cholesterol}]}$$

where all concentrations are those in plasma [113]. Both plasma vitamin C and vitamin E concentrations are significantly correlated with mortality from coronary heart disease [114,115] particularly in populations with similar blood cholesterol concentrations [114]. One case-control study [116] suggests that low plasma concentrations of vitamins E and C and β-carotene are related to risk of angina in men.

6.2 Cancer

There are numerous early epidemiological studies linking smoking with the development of a range of cancers [117]. Mechanistically, free radicals in cigarette smoke may play a role in carcinogenesis which current theory suggests is a multi-stage process of genetic change affecting protooncogenes or tumour suppressor genes in a single cell or clone of cells. Reactive free radicals may abstract hydrogens from DNA causing strand breaks, base damage or adduct formation. Not all damage is repaired and persistent DNA lesions could result in permanent alterations in the genetic message when the cell replicates its DNA and divides. Smoking-related oxidative stress could, therefore, enhance mutagenesis and increase the probability of tumorigenesis.

In support of this, radicals in aqueous extracts of cigarette tar alter DNA bases

Table 7. Cross-country correlations between CHD mortality and intakes of antioxidants nutrients and antioxidant rich foods for 1985—1987.

Variable	Correlation coefficient (r)
Total vitamin E	−0.386
α-Tocopherol	−0.753
Vitamin C	−0.609
β-Carotene	−0.459
Vegetables	−0.653
Vegetable oils	−0.623
Wine	−0.798

Based on European countries, excluding Malta and Iceland. Significance levels for r with 15 degrees of freedom are: $p = 0.05$ when $r = 0.48$; $p = 0.01$ when $r = 0.61$; $p = 0.001$ when $r = 0.73$. Data adapted from [110].

and cause chromosomal abnormalities in the form of sister chromatid exchanges in human lymphocytes, and induce DNA single strand breaks in DNA from cultured lung cells [118,119]. Moreover, a number of studies have shown that smokers have a 50% increase in *hprt⁻* mutant frequency compared with nonsmoking individuals of a similar age [55,120]. This biomarker of genetic change is used in population studies to reflect long-term exposure to mutagenic influences. Such associations between mutant frequency and smoking are strengthened by findings of significant correlations between *hprt⁻* mutant frequency and the number of cigarettes smoked per day [55]. Damage is generally less in smokers with the greatest plasma vitamin C concentrations. As it is generally recognised that DNA damage, resulting in base change and mutation when replication occurs, is a very early event in carcinogenesis, it is feasible that enhanced vitamin C intake may have a protective role and account, in part, for both the difference in cancer rates in different countries [121] and the lack of consistency among studies relating *hprt⁻* mutant frequency in vivo and smoking [55].

7   ANTIOXIDANT SUPPLEMENTATION OF SMOKERS

The antioxidant status of smokers is compromised because of an inadequate dietary intake of antioxidant nutrients and the increased oxidant load incurred due to tobacco use. Consequently, several studies have assessed whether supplementation of smokers with antioxidants ameliorates enhanced biochemical and functional indices of oxidative stress. For example, increased pentane expiration by smokers can be reduced by supplementation with 800 mg vitamin E per day for 2 weeks [52,53] and the increased susceptibility of washed erythrocytes of smokers to hydrogen peroxide-induced peroxidation can be abolished by supplementing with 1,000 mg vitamin E per day for two weeks [45—47]. Lower doses of vitamin E may also be effective in reducing increased oxidative stress in smokers. Similarly, erythrocytes of male smokers from a Scottish population with a habitually low vitamin E intake were more susceptible to hydrogen-peroxide stimulated peroxidation than those from nonsmokers. Plasma concentrations of lipid peroxides, thiobarbituric acid reactive substances and conjugated dienes were also elevated in smokers compared with nonsmokers. These indices of oxidative stress were significantly decreased in the smokers following consumption of 280 mg dl-α tocopherol acetate per day for 10 weeks [122]. Supplementation of smokers for 10 days with 1000 mg vitamin E per day and 200 mg ʟ-Se-methionine reduced the enhanced respiratory burst reaction of neutrophilic granulocytes from the peripheral blood by 20—75% [123]. Similarly, short-term oral administration of vitamin C reduced oxidant release by blood phagocytes from cigarette smokers in a placebo-controlled, double blind crossover trial [124,125]. Supplementation of smokers with vitamin E and vitamin C in varying combinations, durations and doses decrease the enhanced susceptibility of LDL to oxidise to potentially atherogenic forms in vitro [126,127].

8   CONCLUSIONS

There is now a large body of biochemical, epidemiological and clinical data suggesting that diseases such as coronary heart disease and certain cancers may be preventable by improving in populations the dietary intake of antioxidant micronutrients. Establishing the optimum intakes of these nutrients is vitally important. In excess, antioxidants such as selenium and β-carotene could actually contribute to disease pathogenesis. In addition, there may be a distinction between the amount required by smokers and nonsmokers to reduce the risk of developing disease.

In most countries there is a large disparity between the officially recommended intakes and those amounts which may be actually required to maintain optimum health (Table 8). The large discrepancy between these various forms of dietary recommendations suggests that achieving a consensus of optimum intakes of antioxidant nutrients for smokers will be difficult. One of the first studies to attempt this [128] found that erythrocyte vitamin E concentrations of smokers increased in a dose-dependent manner during 20 weeks of supplementation with either 70, 140, 560 or 1,050 mg vitamin E per day. However, the lower dose was equally as effective as the higher doses in suppressing indices of lipid peroxidation, but consumption of over 1,000 mg/day demonstrated pro-oxidant activity.

It should be noted that such effects on indices of oxidative damage do not necessarily imply that increased intakes of antioxidants will prevent or promote the pathogenesis of major clinical conditions. As oxidative stress has been implicated both as a prime cause and a secondary consequence of many diseases, it is empirically desirable to ensure that dietary intakes of nutritional antioxidants of both smokers and nonsmokers are sufficient to keep oxidative damage to lipids, proteins and DNA to a minimum. Whether current recommended daily allowances for antioxidant vitamins are sufficient to achieve this and thus, maintain optimum health, is a matter of contention. However, it is likely that the antioxidant requirements for smokers are likely to be greater than for nonsmokers and sufficient antioxidant intake may require recourse to supplements. Notwithstanding, it should be emphasised that the most effective means for a smoker to reduce the induction of oxidative stress is to stop smoking.

Table 8. Various dietary recommendations for major antioxidant nutrients.

Nutrient	Probable nutritional requirement for public health	UK reference nutrient intake	US recommended daily allowance
Vitamin E (mg)	40—60	5—7	8—10
Vitamin C (mg)	150	40	60
β-Carotene (mg)	Not established	Not established	10—12

9   SUMMARY

1. The gas and tar phases of tobacco smoke contain a variety of long- and short-lived free radicals which directly and indirectly induce oxidative stress.
2. Lungs of smokers are deficient in vitamin E although in animal models chronic smoking is associated with adaptive increases in activities of antioxidant enzymes.
3. Concentrations of indices of free radical-mediated damage to lipids and DNA are elevated in smokers compared with nonsmokers suggesting that smoking overwhelms the protective capacity of the antioxidant defence system.
4. Plasma concentrations of antioxidants such as vitamin C and vitamin E are depressed in smokers in response to increased turnover and decreased dietary intakes.
5. Low-density lipoproteins of smokers are more susceptible to in vitro oxidative modification to a potentially atherogenic form.
6. Smokers may benefit from increased intakes of antioxidant nutrients, as supplementation with vitamins E and C decreases indices of oxidative stress.
7. It is unclear whether increased antioxidant intakes reduce the incidence of smoking-related diseases. The best way for a smoker to minimise the induction of oxidative stress is to stop smoking.

10   ACKNOWLEDGEMENTS

We are grateful for support from the Scottish Office Agriculture Environment and Fisheries Department (SOAEFD) and the Ministry of Agriculture Fisheries and Food (MAFF).

11   REFERENCES

1. World Health Organisation Report of the Director General. Geneva: WHO, 1997;162.
2. American Lung Association Fact Sheet — Smoking Policy in the Workplace. USA: ALA, 1997;3.
3. Health Education Authority: The Smoking Epidemic. UK: Martins of Berwick, 1992;A:81—98.
4. Steenland K. JAMA 1992;267:94—99.
5. Hole D, Gillis C, Chopra C. Br Med J 1990;299:423—427.
6. Humble C, Croft J, Gerber A et al. Am J Pub Health 1990;80:599—601.
7. Dobson A, Alexander H, Heller R et al. Med J Aust 1991;154:793—797.
8. Garland C, Barret-Connor E, Suarez L et al. Am J Epidemiol 1985;121:645—649.
9. Glantz S, Parmley W. Circulation 1991;83:1—12.
10. Smoking, Tobacco and Cancer Program. NIH publication, 1990;90-3107.
11. Duthie GG. Eur J Clin Nutr 1993;47:759—764.
12. Halliwell B. Am J Med 1991;91(Suppl 3C):14—22.
13. Halliwell B. Br J Exp Pathol 1989;70:737—757.
14. Ames BN. Science 1983;221:1256—1264.
15. Slater TF. Biochem J 1984;222:1—15.
16. Pryor WA, Stone K. Ann NY Acad Sci 1993;686:12—28.

17. Church DF, Pryor WA. Environ Health Perspect 1985;64:111—126.
18. Pryor WA. Science 1987;55(Suppl 8):18—23.
19. Pryor WA. In: Taylor J (ed) Pulmonary Emphysema and Proteolysis. New York: Academic Press, 1986;369—392.
20. Duthie GG, Wahle KJ. Biochem Soc Tranc 1990;18:1051—1054.
21. Cosgrove JP, Borish ET, Church DF, Pryor WA. Biochem Biophys Res Commun 1985;133: 780—786.
22. Nakayama T, Kodama M, Nagata C. Gann 1984;75:95—98.
23. Pryor WA. Environ Health Perspect 1997;105(Suppl 4):875—872.
24. Tsuchiya M, Suzuki YJ, Cross CE, Packer L. Ann NY Acad Sci 1993;686:39—52.
25. Pryor WA. Br J Cancer 1987;55(Suppl 8):19—23.
26. Niki E, Minamisawa S, Oikawa M, Komuro E. Ann NY Acad Sci 1993;686:29—38.
27. Wright JL, Hobson JE, Wiggs B et al. Lung 1988;166:277—286.
28. Van Antwerpen L, Theron AJ, Myer MS et al. Ann NY Acad Sci 1993;686:53—65.
29. Anderson R, Rabson AR, Sher R et al. Am J Clin Pathol 1974;61:879.
30. Hoidal JR, Fox RB, Lemarbe PA et al. Am Rev Respir Dis 1981;123:85—87.
31. Ludvig RW, Hoidal JR. Am Rev Respir Dis 1982;126:977—980.
32. Mio T, Romberger DJ, Thompson AB, Robbins RA, Heires A, Renard SI. Am J Respir Crit Care Med 1997;155:1770—1776.
33. Pacht ER, Kaseki H, Mohammed JR et al. J Clin Invest 1986;77:789—796.
34. Chow CK. Ann NY Acad Sci 1993;686:289—298.
35. Chow CK, Airriess GR, Changchit C. Ann NY Acad Sci 1989;570:425—427.
36. Airriess GR, Changchit C, Chen LC et al. Nutr Res 1988;8:653—661.
37. McGowen E, Parenti CM, Hoidal JR et al. J Lab Clin Med 1984;104:127—134.
38. York GK, Pierce TH, Schwartz LW et al. Arch Env Health 1976;29:286—290.
39. Chow CK, Chen LH, Thacker RR et al. Environ Res 1984;34:425—427.
40. Eiserich JJ, van der Vliet A, Handelman G, Halliwell B, Cross CE. Am J Clin Nutr 1996;995(2): 90S—1500S.
41. Handelman GJ, Packer L, Cross CE. Am J Clin Nutr 1995;63:559—565.
42. Morrow JD, Frei B, Longmire W, Gaziano M, Lynch SM, Shyr Y, Strauss W, Oates JA, Roberts LJ. N Eng J Med 1995;64:1198—1203.
43. Pre J, Le Floch A, Vassey R et al. Med Sci Res 1989;17:1029—1030.
44. Pre J, Le Floch A. Clin Chem 1990;36:1849—1850.
45. Duthie GG, Arthur JR, James WPT et al. Ann NY Acad Sci 1993;686:120—129.
46. Duthie GG, Shortt CT, Robertson JD et al. Nutr Res 1992;12:S61—S67.
47. Duthie GG, Arthur JR, James WPT et al. Ann NY Acad Sci 1989;570:435—438.
48. Duthie GG, Arthur JR, James WPT. Am J Clin Nutr 1990;570:435—438.
49. Duthie GG, Arthur JR. Fat Sci Technol 1990;92:456—458.
50. Duthie GG. Eur J Clin Nutr 1983;47:759—764.
51. Duthie GG, Morrice PC, Ventresca PG et al. Clin Chim Acta 1992;206:207—212.
52. Hoshina E, Shariff R, Van Gossum A et al. J Parenteral Enterl Nutr 1990;14:300—305.
53. Shariff R, Hoshino E, Allard J et al. Am J Clin Nutr 1988;47:758.
54. Sakamoto R. Jpn J Hyg 1985;40:835—840.
55. Duthie SJ, Ross M, Collins A. Mutat Res 1995;331:55—64.
56. Loft S, Virtisen K, Ewertz M, Tjønnland A, Overvad K, Poulsen HE. Carcinogenesis 1992;13: 2241—2247.
57. Brown KM, Morrice PC, Duthie GG. Am J Clin Nutr 1994;60:383—387.
58. Reilly M, Delanty N, Lawson JA, FitzGerald GG. Circulation 1996;94:19—25.
59. Miller ER, Appel LJ, Jiang L, Risby TH. Circulation 1997;96:1097—1101.
60. Brook M, Grimshaw JJ. Am J Clin Nutr 1968;21:1254—1258.
61. Calder JH, Curtis RC, Fore H. Lancet 1963;i:556.
62. Pelletier O. Am J Clin Nutr 1968;21:1259—1267.

63. Pelletier O. Am J Clin Nutr 1970;23:520—524.
64. Pelletier O. Ann NY Acad Sci 1975;258:156—168.
65. Elwood PC, Hughes RE, Hurley RJ. Lancet 1970;ii:1197.
66. Albanese AA, Wein EH, Mata LA. Nutr Rep Int 1975;12:271—279.
67. McLean HE, Dodds PM, Abernethy MH et al. NZ Med J 1976;83:226—229.
68. Murata A, Shiraishi I, Fukuzaki K et al. Int J Vit Nutr Res 1989;31:184—189.
69. Smith JL, Hodges RE. Ann NY Acad Sci 1987;498:144—152.
70. Bolton-Smith C. Ann NY Acad Sci 1993;686:347—360.
71. Chow CK, Thacker RR, Changit C et al. J Am Coll Nutr 1986;5:305—312.
72. Fehily AM, Philips KM, Yarnell JWG et al. Am J Clin Nutr 1984;40:827—833.
73. Keith RE, Mossholder SB. Nutr Res 1983;3:653—661.
74. Keith RE, Pelletier O. Can J Physiol Pharmacol 1973;51:879—884.
75. Lykkesfeldt J, Loft S, Nielsen JB, Poulsen HE. Am J Clin Nutr 1977;65:959—963.
76. Schectman G. Ann NY Acad Sci 1993;686:335—346.
77. Murata A. World Rev Nutr Diet 1991;64:31—57.
78. Kalner AB, Hartmann D, Hornig DH. Am J Clin Nutr 1984;34:1347—1355.
79. Lykkesfeldt J, Prieme H, Loft S, Poulsen HE. Br Med J 1996;313:91.
80. Gerster H. J Nutr Growth Cancer 1987;4:45—49.
81. Witter FR, Blake DA, Baumgardner R et al. Am J Obstet Gynecol 1982;144:857.
82. Davis C, Brittain E, Hunninghake D et al. Am J Epidemiol 1983;118:445.
83. Russel-Briefel R, Bates M, Kulner LH. Am J Epidemiol 1985;122:741—749.
84. Bolton-Smith C, Casey CE, Gey KF et al. Br J Nutr 1991;65:337—346.
85. Stryker WS, Kaplan LA, Stein EA et al. Am J Epidemiol 1988;127:283—296.
86. Ross M, Crosley KM, Brown KM, Duthie SJ, Arthur JR, Duthie GG. Eur J Clin Nutr 1995;49: 861—865.
87. McLaren DS, Loveridge N, Duthie GG et al. In: Garrow JS, James WPT (eds) Human Nutrition and Dietetics. London: Churchill Livingstone Press, 1993.
88. Munro LH, Burton G, Kelly FJ. Clin Sci 1997;92:87—93.
89. Bellizzi MC, Dutta-Roy AK, Duthie GG, James WPT. Free Radic Res Commun 1996;27: 105—112.
90. Strain JJ, Carville DGM, Barker ME et al. Biochem Soc Tranc 1989;17:498—498.
91. Gladstone M, Feldman JG, Levytska V et al. Am Rev Respir Dis 1987;24:783—787.
92. Bridges RB, Rehm SR. Basic Life Sci 1988;49:631—634.
93. Fischer PWF, L'Abbe MR, Giroux A. Nutr Res 1990;10:1081—1090.
94. Kuhnert BR, Kuhnert BR, Debanne S et al. Obstet Gynaecol 1987;71:67—70.
95. Kivela SL, Maenpaa P, Nissinen A et al. Int J Vit Nutr Res 1983;59:373—380.
96. Ellis NI, Lloyd B, Lloyd RS et al. J Clin Pathol 1984;37:200—206.
97. Lloyd RS, Lloyd B, Clayton BE. J Epidemiol Commun Health 1983;37:213—217.
98. Swanson CA, Longnecker MP, Veillon C. Am J Clin Nutr 1990;52:858—862.
99. Hunter DJ, Morris JS, Chute CG et al. Am J Epidemiol 1990;132:114—122.
100. Subar AF, Harlan LC, Mattson ME. Am J Pub Health 1990;80:1323—1329.
101. Margetts BM, Jackson AA. BMJ 1993;307:1381—1384.
102. Whichelow MJ, Golding JF, Treasure FP. Br J Addict 1988;83:295—304.
103. Herbert JR, Kabat GC. Eur J Clin Nutr 1990;51:784—789.
104. Le Marchard L, Ntilivamunda A, Kolonel LN et al. Asia Pas J Pub Health 1988;2:120—126.
105. Kato I, Tominaga S, Suzuki T. Int J Epidemiol 1989;18:345—354.
106. Thompson DH, Warburton DM. Psychol Health 1992;7:311—321.
107. Stamler JS, Rains-Clearman D, Lenz-Litzow K et al. Am J Clin Nutr 1997;65(Suppl): 374S—402S.
108. Morabia A, Wynder EL. Am J Clin Nutr 1990;52:933—937.
109. Mead R. The design of experiments. Statistical principles for practical applications. Cambridge University Press, 1988;617.

110. Bellizzi MC, Franklin MF, Duthie GG, James WPT. Eur J Clin Nutr 1994;48:822–831.
111. Steinberg D. J Biol Chem 1997;272:20963–20966.
112. Estebauer H, Gebicki J, Puhl H et al. Free Radic Biol Med 1992;13:341–390.
113. Gey KF. Bibl Nutr Diet 1986;37:53–91.
114. Gey KF. Int J Vit Nutr Res 1990;30:224–231.
115. Gey KF, Stanelin KB, Puska P et al. Ann NY Acad Sci 1987;498:110–123.
116. Riemersma RA, Wood DA, MacIntyre CCA et al. Lancet 1991;337:1–5.
117. Doll R, Peto R. J Natl Cancer Inst 1982;66:1192–1265.
118. Cross CE, Halliwell ET, Borisch WT et al. Ann Int Med 1987;107:526–545.
119. Wiley JC, Grafstrom CE, Moser Jr C et al. Cancer Res 1987;47:2045–2049.
120. Cole HJ, Green MHL, James L et al. Mutat Res 1988;204:493–507.
121. Diana JN. Ann NY Acad Sci 1993:686;1–11.
122. Brown KM, Morrice PC, Duthie GG. Int J Vit Nutr Res 1994;(In press).
123. Clausen J. Biol Trace Element Res 1991;31:281–291.
124. Theron AJ, Anderson R. Int J Vit Nutr Res 1988;58:218–224.
125. Harats D, Dabach Y, Hollander G et al. Atherosclerosis 1989;79:245–252.
126. Harats D, Ben-Naim M, Dabach Y et al. Atherosclerosis 1990;85:47–54.
127. Princen HMG, Van Poppel G, Vogelezang C et al. Arteriosclerosis Thrombosis 1992;12:554–562.
128. Brown KM, Morrice PC, Duthie GG. Am J Clin Nutr 1997;65:496–502.

©2000 Elsevier Science B.V. All rights reserved.
Handbook of Oxidants and Antioxidants in Exercise.
C.K. Sen, L. Packer and O. Hänninen, editors.

Part XI • Chapter 34

Regulation of inflammation and wound healing

John J. Maguire

Medical Scientist, Environmental Energy Technologies Division, Lawrence Berkeley National Laboratory, University of California, Berkeley, CA 94720, USA. Tel.: +1-510-642-1873. Fax: +1-510-642-8313. E-mail: jmaguire@socrates.berkeley.edu

1   INTRODUCTION
2   THE WOUND HEALING PROCESS
     2.1   Wound physiology
     2.2   Cell types in wound healing
     2.3   Cell activation, cytokines and cell adhesion
     2.4   Oxygen supply to wounds areas
3   THE INFLAMMATORY PROCESS
     3.1   The role of neutrophils and macrophages in wounds
     3.2   The respiratory burst
     3.3   Cytokines involved in oxidative stress, and healing
     3.4   Clinical implications
4   LINKS BETWEEN WOUND HEALING AND INFLAMMATION
     4.1   The balance of radical production and control by antioxidants
     4.2   The role of oxygen in wound healing and inflammatory resolution
     4.3   Wound healing and multiple cell signals
5   SUMMARY
6   PERSPECTIVES
7   ACKNOWLEDGMENTS
8   ABBREVIATIONS
9   REFERENCES

1   INTRODUCTION

Inflammation and wound healing involve a cellular "symphony" of signaling between cells, an alteration of a multitude of gene expressions and a massive mobilization of cellular resources that differs substantially from the quiescent state of cells. Wound healing is analogous to embryogenesis in that similar cellular processes of growth and (re)construction are occurring. Understanding wound healing is made far more complex when it occurs in pathological conditions where all of the cell's resources are not available. Well-known systemic pathologies and their effects on wound healing are well documented [1]. It is believed that there are numerous "subtle" pathologies that inhibit proper or adequate wound healing but these are not characterized as distinct pathological conditions. Medical practitioners frequently recognize differences in the healing of their patients that cannot be explained or treated.

Injuries in sports are a major cause of childhood morbidity and mortality [2]. The range of injuries include blunt trauma, head injuries, muscle, tendon and bone injuries [3—5]. Vascular injuries and neural injuries can also develop, for example, in cyclists [6,7]. The general descriptions of wound healing processes should be understood by clinicians and allied health professionals in order to facilitate optimal and rapid recovery from a sport-induced wound. While each sport has a profile of common injuries the range and extent of sport-induced wounding is extensive and should be of concern to athletes and trainers in order to optimize training and to minimize sports-related wounds and injuries.

In the past 15 years, there has been a vast increase in the understanding of cell biology, substantially because of newly developed laboratory tools. Some of these tools include the ability to clone virtually any gene from a eukaryotic cell, to quantitate messenger RNA in cells (which is a measure of the expression of genes) and to develop transgenic animals and "knock-out" animals that are missing specific genes. Using these tools (many of which were nonexistent at the beginning of this decade), scientists are now beginning to understand new cellular processes which are able to link cell responses from a wound or an inflammatory site to modified gene expression and control of cellular functions and ultimately the regrowth and healthy maintenance of the organism.

This explosion of new research is both exciting and daunting in that assimilation of this new knowledge in practical terms is frequently a challenge to anyone not active in the research area. It is in this light that this chapter will focus on two areas of intense research, inflammation and wound healing. This report will be limited to areas of research that are linked to inflammation and wound healing in the context of oxygen utilization and the production of oxidants. There are other more comprehensive reviews covering other related topics [8—15].

Leukocytes in physiological conditions, will produce copious quantities of oxidants and this includes superoxide ($O_2^{\cdot-}$), hydrogen peroxide, (H_2O_2), hypochlorous acid (HOCl), nitrogen monoxide (nitrous oxide or NO), and peroxynitrite ($OONO^-$), hydroxyl radical (OH·), chloramine and derivatives ($R\text{-}NH_2Cl$), thiyl radicals (R-S·) and a host of other secondary reactive radicals and oxidants. Collectively, these compounds are known as reactive oxygen species (ROS) [16—18]. There is a physiological role for ROS in the healing of a wound, notably in the killing of invading microorganisms. However, because of their reactivity and potential to cause unwanted oxidations, there is a fine balance between under- and overproduction of ROS. It is clear that in defined pathological conditions this balance is shifted. Some pathologies such as chronic granulomatous disease are the result of the underproduction of leukocyte radicals. Other diseases such as arthritis are the "result" of a hyperimmune response resulting in damage from the inflammation. In this chapter the focus will be on inflammatory responses that are essential for adequate wound healing and repair.

2   THE WOUND HEALING PROCESS

The source of a wound can be from trauma, excessive heat or cold, an inflammatory or infectious process or even from a metabolic or nutritional deficiency.

While wound origins certainly have a role in the host response, there are some basic tenets of wound repair that define the stages of repair. The first and foremost (local) response to a wound (not considering systemic events such as shock) is the control of blood loss through platelet aggregation and blood coagulation. Platelets are one of the first cell types to play an active role in wound repair. As the platelets develop blood clots to prevent blood and fluid loss from a wound, they also play a role in the activation of circulating leukocytes. Leukocytes are the first cells that actively proceed to the wound site by moving toward the wounded area. While the platelets are completing their task of preventing blood loss by forming blood clots in the wound area and stimulating vasoconstriction, simultaneously the circulating leukocytes begin their contribution to the repair process.

Following hemostasis, the wound site needs to be cleared of foreign material that may have entered the wound area. The host must begin a second stage of wound healing, which is to fend off assaults by microbial infections including bacteria, fungi, mycoplasma, and viruses. The wound site must be cleared of all of the clotted blood and related products and any foreign material rendered harmless and preferably removed. This process is accomplished mainly by neutrophils and macrophages which originate in the circulating blood. As these leukocytes clear the wound site, the next stage of repair can commence. The third stage is the regeneration stage. This involves angiogenesis (the formation of a new blood supply), and repair by fibroblasts, which are special cells that can generate and maintain the tissue fibers that hold us together. Certainly, wounds in different tissues result in different responses, by different cell types and with varying wound repair success. A broken bone heals somewhat differently than a lacerated arm but the core healing process in most tissues share many similarities. Brain tissue is an exception as it has specialized immune cells which act to circumvent the potentially lethal cellular infiltration that occurs in other part of the body [19,20]. The role of oxygen and oxidants are crucial to wound healing and studies can be undertaken in both animal and cell culture model systems to provide new insights into the clinical management of wounds and trauma. Figure 1 shows a schematic drawing of a wound and some of the cellular events that occur to facilitate wound healing.

This chapter will focus on the events that follow blood coagulation and cessation of blood loss. Of special interest will be the activation of leukocytes especially neutrophils. Neutrophils are also known as polymorphonuclear leukocytes or PMNs. Neutrophils are the first leukocytes to enter a wound area, and they precede the influx of circulating monocytes. Monocytes differentiate after leaving the circulation to become macrophages.

Neutrophils are known to be the "front line" of defense for a host. The area around a wound is usually noted for redness, increased temperature, and pain. The capillaries in the vicinity become filled with blood and the permeability of the capillary lining increases. Fluid accumulation in the wound area is notable. Neutrophils stick to the endothelial cells and then traverse between them, literally squeezing between adjacent endothelial cells which make up the capillary bed

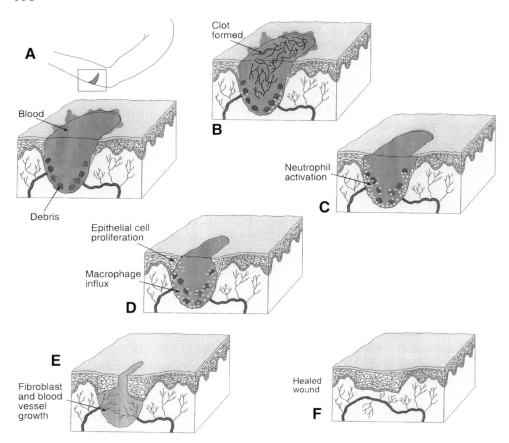

Fig. 1. **A:** *Stage:* Injury. *Cellular:* Physical disruption of cells at the wound site, contamination of the wound by debris and microorganisms. *Signals:* Activation of platelets, the primary immune response. **B:** *Stage:* Cessation of blood loss due to clotting. *Cellular:* Blood fills the wound site, forms a blood clot and there is a vasoconstriction of surrounding blood vessels to facilitate further blood loss. *Signal:* Signals are sent to the surrounding endothelium stating that there is an injury in a specific location. Neutrophils rapidly leave the circulation and traverse towards the injury site. **C:** *Stage:* Neutrophil activation. *Cellular:* Neutrophils move rapidly towards the wound site, initiate their cellular machinery to facilitate microbicidal activity and the removal of debris. *Signal:* Vasoconstriction is relaxed once the primary blood loss is controlled. As the neutrophils have completed their jobs circulating monocytes are recruited to the wound site these cells differentiate to become macrophages, and begin the next stage of the immune response. **D:** *Stage:* Macrophage infiltration. *Cellular:* Macrophages begin to outnumber neutrophils, fibroblasts are moving in towards the wound site and epithelial cells are growing rapidly to reseal the surface directly over the blood clot but below the drying scab. *Signal:* Fibroblasts are generating structural components required for the repair. Endothelium cells are initiating angiogenesis to allow new blood supply to the injured area. Epithelium and keratinocytes are generating a new surface in the outer skin. **E:** *Stage:* Fibroblast proliferation. *Cellular:* Fibroblasts begin to move into the wound area, epithelial cells cover the outer layers of the wound and angiogenesis causes growth of new blood vessels. *Signal:* Fibroblast growth factors, vascular tissue activity grows and epithelial cells grow over the surface. **F:** *Stage:* Completion of heat. *Cellular:* The area becomes oxygenated, leukocytes are no longer present, strength of the area increases as polymerization of collagen is completed. *Signals:* Cell-cell signaling is now the same as adjacent areas.

lining. Then they move to a location in the wound area. Each of these steps involves signals and messages to and from adjacent cells. The neutrophils cannot act alone but must communicate with the other cells that are involved in the mobilization of the repair of the host.

Neutrophils must know when, as well as where, to leave the circulating blood. The host must know how many neutrophils to "call" to a wound site. Too few could lead to a critical shortage of growth factors and cytokines, and implies that there will be a vulnerability to infection and too many may cause a shortage of cells at other wound sites or an overreactive immune response. The neutrophils must know when and in what capacity they are to activate their oxidative burst and the release of proteases, cytokines and oxidants. All of this requires a precise balance of cell to cell communication and activation of the neutrophils "arsenal" of antimicrobial resources.

2.1 Wound physiology

A basic function of living tissue is its ability to both replicate and to repair itself. The replication process (embryogenesis) occurs in a well-defined homeostatic environment. There is a predefined time (gestation time) that the organism has to replicate to an independently viable stage. While the healing of a wound often mirrors what is occurring in embryogenesis, the wound environment is constantly changing and it is often contaminated with foreign material, as well as infected by microorganisms. In wounding, there are frequently other stresses including such things as fluid loss, inadequate nutrition, and other factors that are involved in the physical surroundings of a wound.

In a wound, there is one unvarying feature that has been recognized for a considerable amount of time, specifically, the area around the wound becomes distinctly anaerobic. Since it is possible to make measurement of relatively small areas of wounds, it is possible to define the oxygen concentration in wounds [21]. The anaerobic area is incompatible to the proliferation of fibroblasts which must proceed to rebuild the structure of a wounded area. If the "anaerobic zone" is converted sooner to an aerobic area, the synthesis of collagen and the formation of new blood vessels occurs faster [22]. Studies with hyperbaric oxygen supplementation and wound healing demonstrate a strong positive correlation between enhanced oxygen tension in a wound and the resulting improved wound healing. There has been considerable discussion and research over many decades as to the advantages/disadvantages of the anaerobic "zone" of a wound [23,24].

Healing of chronic wounds is substantially dependent on the ambient oxygen concentrations in the wound areas. The availability of oxygen for the "final" healing of a chronic wound seems to be an oxygen- dependent function. There are several studies that have indicated that increasing the oxygen flow to a wound site enhances the rate of wound healing. Hyperbaric oxygen therapy can be helpful and is an important aid in the cure of human chronic wounds that are not healing [25].

Epithelial cells on the edge of a wound (but not in the actual wound itself) begin their proliferation almost immediately after the wound has occurred. In 4–6 h a notable proliferation of epithelial mitosis, glycogen accumulation and a migration of the appropriate cells towards the wound site follows. Migration of epithelial cells will occur throughout the dermis, as well as a stimulation of synthesis of new basement membrane which separates the dermis from the epidermis. When these cells encounter granulation tissue, they do not penetrate into this layer. Granulation tissue consists of a mix of macrophages, fibroblasts and endothelial cells. It is highly vascular and quite resistant to infection. Granulation tissue is fragile and is usually restricted to the nonepithelial tissues by an inhibitory process which is important to the resolution of repair but is not well understood. Granulation tissue contains active microbicidal neutrophils which are constantly replaced by macrophages. It can be regarded in some ways as a "space-filler" for a wound. Over a longer period of time, the granulation tissue resolves to fibrous scar tissue which holds the wound edges together. Granulation tissue is necessary for the healing of open wounds; in other cases, it is a detriment to good wound healing. In the event of a chronic irritation or infection, granulation tissue can persist for months or years [25,26].

Much of the wound healing "symphony" occurs in the extracellular environment. Debris, irritants and microbes are infrequently found within individual cells. Their removal in some cases involves phagocytosis which is the uptake of particles including bacteria by the cell. In other cases debris is removed by extrusion through fluid loss. In any case there is a compelling need to lay down a new matrix of connective tissue proteins and facilitate a remodeling of the tissue to replicate the original tissue as much as possible. Fibronectins are an important glycoprotein class that stimulate the adhesion of cells together, and facilitate the appropriate deposition of collagen to facilitate wound repair and closure. In addition to fibronectins, collagens, laminins and proteoglycans, mucopolysaccharides and glycoproteins are all active in the extracellular matrix and all have roles in the repair of a wound. The main source of strength of a healing wound is collagen [27–32].

2.2 Cell types in wound healing

As there are numerous stages of wound healing and each stage has different cells involved, the actual number of cells types in part depends on the location of the injury. The basic stages of wound healing are depicted in schematic form in Fig. 1. The blood that "leaks" to the wound area is the primary healing "inflammatory response" as the platelets in the blood are activated and form a clot. Clot formation is characterized by vasoconstriction and platelet aggregation and release of growth factors. The clotted blood contains mostly red cells but of course the full range of circulating white cells that are in circulating blood become part of the clot. After clot formation there is a mobilization of circulating neutrophils which come from the circulation, they are one of the two main cell types that kill microorganisms and remove debris by an arsenal of antimicrobial agents which includes phagocytosis, ROS and proteases [25]. During the early stages of the inflammatory infiltration, following clot formation and reduction of fluid loss there comes a stage of vasodilation in which there is a mobilization of several cells types. Fluid accumulates in the wound area along with leukocytes [25].

The next phase of the inflammatory response is the infiltration of circulating monocytes which differentiate to become macrophages [33]. These cells like their fast moving counterparts, the neutrophils, also produce ROS including potent and microbicidal oxidants. Macrophages have a host of additional facilities to remove debris and render potentially infectious microorganisms harmless and particularly to remove growth factors and other unwanted cell growth signals [33].

In regions peripheral to the wound, fibroblasts are activated to divide and to make collagen and other structural components that are required to repair the wound. Fibroblasts are not prepared to grow in or produce collagen in regions of very low oxygen tension or in infected areas. It is the task of the activated leukocytes (both neutrophils and macrophages) to facilitate the migration of new and dividing fibroblasts into the healing wound. In conjunction with fibroblast proliferation and migration into the healing area of the wound, new blood delivery must occur. This process is known as angiogenesis, the construction of new blood vessels [34]. Angiogenesis is an important function in both wound healing and tumorigenesis as cells will not grow well unless they have a good oxygen supply. The understanding of angiogenesis is of great medical importance as it represents an adaptation of wounds and tumors to get oxygen to their critical cells and facilitate growth. The cellular control mechanisms of angiogenesis are thus, of critical importance in several areas of medical research. The capillary beds are lined with endothelial cells which proliferate during angiogenesis. These sensitive cells form the barrier between a wound site and the circulating blood. They must be able to transmit messages to leukocytes to adhere to the endothelial wall and traverse between endothelial cells and subsequently migrate toward the wound [35]. Endothelial cells were important in the discovery of nitric oxide (NO) as a cell signal because they possess an NO sensitive receptor which causes vasodilation [36]. NO is both a cell signaling molecule in endothelial cells and neurons but it also plays a major role in microbicidal activity in leukocytes [37,38].

2.3 Cell activation, cytokines and cell adhesion

The activation of cells by cytokines and the need to stimulate cell adhesion represents a current frontier of research in the cellular basis of wound healing. Cell activation occurs by signaling, as do changes in cell adhesion. Some of the signals come from within a cell, however, there is a growing list of relatively small peptide messengers that are now recognized as important in the regulation of cellular differentiation and activation and these are called cytokines [13,15,39].

A definition of cell activation is important in the context of wound healing as such an activation differs from a "normal" physiologic replication or differentiation of a particular cell type or of apoptosis which involves a programmed cell death [40]. Activation of a cell involved in wound healing means that the cell is going to replicate and/or move to a new location prior to its "normal" replication time. In turn these activated cells will make more fibers, or material required to replicate the original wounded area and remove debris and microorganisms. "Activated cells" are going to move into an area where they would not have been if there were no wound. The process of activation involves intercellular messages. It is not known how many of these messages there are; however, small molecules such as NO, H_2O_2, and O_2^- are quite capable of traversing between cells and may well be intercellular messages [41]. Cytokines and their requisite receptors make up well-defined cellular communications that are essential for successful wound healing. Table 1 describes some of the known growth and signaling factors that have a role in wound healing. It is not known how many different cell types make each type of growth factor. This list is merely a brief summary of known cellular peptide messages. There is not much known about the interaction of these growth factors, notably which ones activate which cell types and what is

Table 1. Inflammation and related cell growth factors.

Growth factors	Sources	Targets	References
IGF Insulin-dependent growth factor	Plasma, fibroblasts, macrophages, kerationcytes	Mitogenic for most cell types	[185—187]
TGF-α Transforming growth factor	Macrophages, keratinocytes, fibroblasts and platelets	Keratinocytes and mitogenic	[188—190]
TNF Tumor necrosis factor	Macrophages, lymphocytes	Chemotactic and angiogenic	[80,191,192]
EGF Epidermal growth factor	Epithelial cells	Mitogenic	[193,194]
VEGF Vascular endothelial growth factor	Macrophages, keratinocytes	Stimulates angiogensis	[195,196]
IL Interleukins	Macrophages, fibroblasts, endothelial cells	Multiple targets	[197—200]
IF Interferons	Leukocytes, fibroblasts	Stimulates defence against viruses	[162—164]

the order of cell activation.

Receptors for a growth factor are also important in the functioning of a growth factor on a "remote cell". In the case of insulin-dependent growth factor (IGF), it has binding sites that are soluble in the serum. The expression and activation of growth factor receptors is equally as important in the functioning of growth factors as the expression and export of the growth factors themselves [42].

The adhesion systems of cells involved in wound healing represents a vast research effort that is reviewed in detail in many current reviews [8,12,15,32,43—55]. Stimulation of endothelial cells with cytokines tumor necrosis factor (TNF), inter-leukin-1 (IL-1), or bacterial-derived lipopolysaccharide (LPS), stimulate blood coagulation, white cell adhesion and migration through the endothelial cells [56—60] and leukocyte transendothelial migration [61,62]. Following stimulation, the endothelial cells will induce the expression of surface proteins that stimulate adhesion. These are called selectins, (the E and P selectin), intercellular adhesion molecule-1 (ICAM-1) and the vascular cell adhesion molecule-1 (VCAM-1) [63,64]. The expression of the stimulated adhesion molecules are transient events ranging from a few hours for the E-selectin [65,66], to VCAM-1 [67] and ICAM-1 . [60], which are stimulated for 12 h and can be found in chronic inflammatory sites after several days [68]. The adhesion molecules aid in direct cell to cell contact, as well as connecting the extracellular structural components to their cellular sources (principally fibroblasts). The adhesion molecules are required for movement of all the important cells into the healing environment.

2.4 Oxygen supply to wounds areas

An injury almost always results in a diminished oxygen supply to a wound area. Clinically, it is well-known that ischemic tissue will be more than likely become necrotic. An oxygen gradient can exist such that a region 1—2 mm away from ambient saturated oxygen (air) can be virtually anaerobic [69,70]. The evidence that an enhanced oxygen supply can improve wound healing is compelling [1,71—76]. Increasing the oxygen supply results in an aerobic metabolism for the cells, and aerobic metabolism is far more efficient for generation of ATP than anaerobic metabolism. In aerobic metabolism the NADPH-linked respiratory burst oxidase is also far more effective in generating superoxide. In fact recent studies in part from this author's laboratory have confirmed that NADPH oxidase from neutrophils has a high Km which results in a virtual shutdown of the respiratory burst in low, microaerobic conditions that are very prevalent in wound areas [77,78]. Finally, and certainly not the least in consideration, is that aerobic bacteria will consume oxygen and generate anaerobic areas if given the opportunity. There exists a balance between the growth rates of aerobic bacteria and their inhibition of growth by anaerobic conditions which are not conducive to rapid and effective wound healing especially as hypoxia diminishes leukocyte bactericidal activity.

The nitric oxide synthetase that is induced in macrophages [79], inducible NOS (iNOS) has been shown to have a low Km for oxygen compared to NADPH oxidase [80]. Recent studies have shown that superoxide (O_2^-) reacts in a diffusion limiting manner with nitric oxide (NO) to produce $ONOO^-$ which is a potent oxidant. It is important to recognize that in anaerobic conditions the ratio of NO/O_2^- will be higher than in aerobic conditions. As NO has been shown to be bactericidal in macrophages [38], the amount of oxygen and the corresponding activity of the NADPH oxygenase may well be very important for effective bactericidal activity and subsequent wound healing.

Measuring the oxygen tension in wound microenvironments is a difficult task. Physical measurement of the oxygen tension can be achieved by oxygen sensors, but the minimum volume of fluid needed to measured oxygen is on the order of a mm^3 [25]. From a cellular perspective this is a large oxygen probe. In vivo measurements of wound healing are hampered by the inability to observe directly the gradients of oxygen and other wound products that are known to exist. Understanding how, for example, a particular oxygen concentration may aid the stimulation of a new cell growth or expression of new gene products is difficult when cell localized oxygen tensions can only be estimated from known physical parameters including diffusion and consumption rates. There is no question that the concentration of oxygen in wound microenvironments is critical for the rapid and complete healing of a wound, and certainly oxygen is essential for the production of oxidants and ROS, which are becoming noted for an increasing role in cell signaling [81].

3   THE INFLAMMATORY PROCESS

Inflammation is a response involving many cell types and it initiates a response to an injury or an infection. In some cases the inflammatory response itself is the cause of pathological conditions, and this occurs when the inflammation response is inappropriate or inadequate to complete the task of repair and healing. Inflammation in an injury in which blood vessels are disrupted or broken represents the "typical" inflammatory response that would precede wound healing.

Leukocytes consist of the following categories of cells: the polymorphonuclear leukocytes includes neutrophils, eosinophils and basophils. By far the neutrophils are the most numerous of these cells in the blood. Eosinophils and basophils can increase during allergic reactions but usually the neutrophils are $>95\%$ of circulating the polymorphonuclear leukocytes [82]. Circulating monocytes represent a relatively small percentage of leukocytes (usually less than 10%). When these monocytes leave the circulation in response to signals indicating wounding or infection they differentiate to become macrophages. Their life cycle is complex and varied. The monocytes, like the neutrophils, have a broad arsenal of anti-microbial agents that are useful in the debridement and sterilization of infected areas [33].

Approximately 30% of circulating white cells are lymphocytes [25]. The lymphocytes are the key cells that develop and process antibody development. There are two major subdivisions of lymphocytes and these are the bone marrow-derived cells (B cells) and the thymus-derived lymphocytes (T cells). The understanding of the development of lymphocyte functioning has seen a rapid expansion in the last few years and describing these cells in wound healing has recently been reviewed [83—85].

The inflammatory response of clot formation, cessation of fluid loss and the initiation of neutrophil and macrophage infiltration into a wound site to initiate the repair process are the initial stages of wound healing. In Section 3.1, the role of neutrophils and macrophages in the wound healing process in terms of their ability to generate abundant free radicals and oxidants will be discussed.

3.1 The role of neutrophils and macrophages in wounds

The process of phagocytosis, using microscopic examination of tissue, was first noted by Metchnikoff about 100 years ago [86]. Investigators have been able to document the movement of neutrophils based on microscopic examination of tissue samples, but the understanding of the molecular events that signal and stimulate the activation of neutrophils is now a topic of intense current investigation.

Neutrophils contain a multilobed nucleus and granules that contain an assortment of enzymes such as myelperoxidase, lysozyme, collagenase, elastase, gelatinase and Cathepsin G [87]. Neutrophils are present in blood at a concentration of about $2,500-10,000/\mu l$ and they have a rather short life span in the range of $24-48$ h [88]. Certainly, when isolated from human blood, neutrophils undergo rapid degeneration such that their respiratory burst activation is rapidly diminished within a few hours of separation from the blood. The fate of healthy neutrophils is also somewhat elusive. Many of the neutrophils eventually are located in the gut in the absence of an acute injury [25]. The physiology and cell biology of the life cycle of neutrophils is at best poorly understood.

When neutrophils reach the site of an injury they have a finite time in which to aid in wound healing and then the cell degrades in a poorly understood process becoming among other fates, a major constituent of pus [25]. With the pus comes the removal of debris and microorganisms that impede the wound healing process. Probably the most studied and most intriguing aspect of neutrophil functioning at a wound site is its ability to phagocytose. In eukaryotes the cells that are able to phagocytose are know collectively as "professional phagocytes". Professional phagocytes are derived from bone marrow and includes neutrophils, macrophages and monocytes [89].

From an evolutionary perspective, the process of phagocytosis in higher organisms has likely derived from phagocytosis in more primitive unicellular cells such as amoebae. Amoebae phagocytose mainly for nutrition while the mammalian professional phagocytes are phagocytose in order to remove invading microorganisms. The mechanisms of the absorption of extracellular material in both cell types is, however, remarkably similar. Many mammalian cell types can pha-

gocytose and both endothelial and epithelial cells have been shown to phagocytose microorganisms. However, their efficiency at phagocytosis is far lower
than that of the professional phagocytes [89].

As neutrophils enter an environment where they may need to phagocytose an
invading microorganism they move through the endothelial capillary bed by
changing their cell membrane topology to develop pseudopodia which facilitate
the "squeezing" of the neutrophils between the endothelial cells [90,91]. The fluid
in a wound area contains many soluble antibodies which can bind to bacteria
and result in a coating of antibody on an invading microorganism. Some antibodies coat bacteria in a wound site and are called opsonins. Opsonins allow
for a more efficient recognition of the invading bacteria by the phagocytic cells
[92–94]. When bacteria and other microorganisms are taken up by neutrophils,
and the contents of the neutrophil granules fuse with the vacuole containing the
microorganism, then the granule contents are "poured" into the vacuole containing the microorganism. It is believed that the primary role of neutrophils is to
get to the wound site quickly and destroy bacteria rapidly [95].

Macrophages enter the wound environment later than the neutrophils, and
early studies on guinea pigs in which the neutrophils were depleted, demonstrated
that in the absence of a gross infection, macrophages supported adequate healing
[96,97]. In a healing wound, as the neutrophil numbers decline, there is a buildup
of macrophages. Histological examination of acute compared to chronic wound
sites reveals an inverse relationship of the number of neutrophils and macrophages at the respective wound sites. Studies in which the macrophages are
depleted show serious consequences for the animal as the wounds do not heal
well, even in the absence of infection. It is now known that macrophages secrete
numerous growth factors that stimulate adjacent cells to grow. This growth must
occur at the correct time! Failure to provide these signals results in dramatically
reduced wound healing [15,98–101].

Macrophages can originate from circulating monocytes or can be derived from
dividing resident tissue macrophages. Lung alveolar macrophages, for example,
are a combination of dividing and infiltrative cells. Similarly, liver Kupffer cells
are macrophages and are believed to be substantially derived from circulating
monocytes, but they can divide and proliferate within the liver [33]. However, in
an inflammatory condition, (and these can be pathological inflammatory conditions such as arthritis) the monocytes are recruited from the circulating blood
and differentiate into macrophages as they move from the blood to the site of
inflammation [33]. There is a notable differential migration of neutrophils and
macrophages. It is not surprising that there are chemotactic signals that are specific for the different types of professional phagocytes. For instance type I collagen can stimulate macrophages but not neutrophils [102]. Fibronectin is deposited by macrophages (as well as other cells), and it is believed to be a stimulating
protein for the formation of fibroblast orientation [103]. Fibronectin is an adhesive extracellular matrix protein and it plays important roles in embryogenesis,
as well as wound healing. The cellular effects of fibronectin are on the integrin

family of receptor/binding proteins on the surface of cells. The expression of integrins directs when and how the cells become attached. There is evidence that fibronectin may alter blood vessel formation, alveolar epithelial cell differentiation wound area growth and maturation [104,105].

Macrophages have other functions that are distinct from those of the neutrophil. As they come into a wound or inflammatory site, they are believed to be more likely involved in the breakdown of the extracellular degradation of connective tissue matrix than neutrophils. The macrophages can be stimulated to produce and secrete proteases [106,107]. Cathepsin S one class of proteases is present mainly in cells from a monocyte lineage including macrophages. Macrophage cathepsins have been noted to be involved in the destruction of basement membranes and extracellular matrix and cathepsin has recently been shown to degrade various extracellular matrix molecules [108].

Macrophages remove debris from a wound and are involved in the preparation of the wound area for angiogenesis. Angiogenesis occurs in the presence of and to a large extent is dependent upon macrophages. In addition to secreting macrophage-derived growth factors, macrophages must balance their activity between bactericidal and phagocytic activity, and the preparation of the area for new cell growth. There are at least 17 identified major cytokines and growth factors that are secreted by the macrophage. Growth of hematopoietic progenitor cells is coordinated by a number of both stimulatory and inhibitory cytokines [103].

3.2 The respiratory burst

The NADPH oxidase of leukocytes is an enzyme complex that is present in neutrophils, macrophages and certain other leukocytes [109]. It is a remarkable enzyme complex in that is reduces molecular oxygen (O_2) to superoxide ($O_2\cdot-$). The overall reaction is as follows:

$$2\, O_2\ +\ NADPH \rightarrow\ 2\, O_2^-\cdot\ +\ NADP^+\ +\ H^+$$

This reaction only occurs when the leukocyte is appropriately stimulated with a stimulant such as a phorbol ester, the LPS endotoxin from a gram negative bacteria, and certain peptide cell stimulants such as formyl-methione-leucine-phenylalanine (fMLP) [82]. The respiratory burst oxidase is not usually active in a circulating neutrophil or monocyte. In order to have activity, the enzyme requires activation, phosphorylation and protein assembly. This usually occurs when the cell has left the circulation and is at a site of injury or infection.

The respiratory burst oxidase has at least four components required for activation. Two of these components are membrane bound and two are soluble and located in the inactive state in the cytoplasm [110—113]. In addition, there are other peptides that are involved in the activation process. The regulatory enzymes protein kinase C (PKC) has a role [114], and dephosphorylases are important in maintaining the activity of the phosphorylated and activated enzyme.

In spite of over 20 years of research on this important enzyme complex, there is not much known about how it is maintained in an active state, how it functions *in vivo* in microaerobic environments that are encountered in wound sites, and whether the enzyme once activated can inactivate and reactivate at a later time. The mechanism of oxygen reduction is also quite elusive [109]. NADPH is the electron donor and molecular O_2 is the acceptor. The respiratory burst oxidase does contain a cytochrome b_{558} which is a likely candidate for electron transport and potentially a reduction site for oxygen. The binding site of NADPH is still elusive. The cytochrome b_{558} seems to complex between two of the membrane peptides and is present as two hemes per pair of membrane anchor peptides. Flavin adenine dinucleotide (FAD) is also present in this enzyme; however, the exact amount is also not clear [115,116]. There are some similarities to mitochondrial redox enzymes in that electrons reduce molecular O_2 in the mitochondria in two separate ways. One is the cytochrome oxidase, which is a highly efficient four electron reductant of water. This enzyme has never been shown to produce superoxide as a by-product. The NADH-ubiquinone reductase, as well as the succinate-ubiquinone reductase have both been shown to leak electrons and result in a small but certainly significant rate of formation of superoxide that is derived from mitochondrial electron transport [117]. Cells contain two distinct forms of superoxide dismutases (SOD), a copper-zinc and a manganese enzyme. SOD is believed to be present in order to trap superoxide from reacting with such substrates as reduced thiols on proteins, or with other hemes, flavins or quinones. The mitochondrial respiratory chain enzymes contain Fe-S clusters which are electron carriers and potentially reductants for oxygen [118,119]. The NADPH linked respiratory burst oxidase, however, it has no Fe-S clusters, and there are more similarities to cytochrome P-450, which is an enzyme family that is important in drug and toxin metabolism [120]. The evolution of the respiratory burst oxidase is not clear. It has likely evolved from more than one type of enzyme when one considers the transient nature of its activation and de-activation, via PKC. The rapid burst of oxygen reduction and the fact that it has at least four subunits that are mixed between membrane bound and cytosolic are special characteristics [109].

What is the function of the respiratory burst? The respiratory burst makes oxidants that are essential for microbicidal killing [109]. Exactly how leukocytes kill invading pathogens is not at all clear. The respiratory burst enzyme's main product is the precursor for a number of oxidants and radicals. Some of these are produced by enzymes such as SOD, which makes H_2O_2 and myeloperoxidase, which makes HOCl and other oxidants such as chloramines, which are produced by nonenzymatic reaction between HOCl and amines. There is compelling evidence that the respiratory burst is essential for microbicidal activity as there is a human disease called Chronic Granulomatous Disease in which the patients are very susceptible to infections, and their neutrophils do not have an adequate respiratory burst [109]. Does the respiratory burst generate molecules that are signals? There is a diverse literature that demonstrates that oxidants are very important in the modulation of cell differentiation and growth. As superoxide is formed and subsequently reacts forming H_2O_2 principally, and a secondary diverse range of oxidants and radicals, it is quite likely that signals derived from the respiratory burst enzyme cause modulation of function in other cells [41,121−125].

3.3 Cytokines and growth factors involved in oxidative stress, and healing

Growth factors and cytokines are involved in almost every step of every change in the differentiation and movement of cells during wound healing, it is apparent that what we know today is merely a small portion of what is a complex, redundant and reliable mechanism to regulate tissue regeneration. There are different mechanisms as to how growth factors operate. For example, transforming growth factor-α (TGF-α) is synthesized as a membrane-bound peptide that can act as a growth factor for an immediately adjacent cell (a juxtacrine) [126,127], or if the active portion of the peptide is cleaved by proteolysis then TGF-α becomes a potent soluble growth factor that can be active at remote sites and it becomes a paracrine and autocrine growth factor [128]. The synthesis and the release of the cytokine is one of the factors in establishing the activation and activity of these growth factors in wound healing and cell regeneration. However, each cytokine must have a receptor in order for it to be functional so there is a duality in understanding the role of growth factors in that both the factor and its receptor must be active and necessarily regulated in order for the growth factor to function. This does complicate the analysis of growth factor analysis in vivo. The transforming growth factor (TGF-β) signals cells through serine/threonine receptors. A number of these receptors have been recently identified and partially characterized. It is possible to use genetically altered truncated fragments of TGF-β or its receptor to block the signal from the cytokine [129]. Inactivation of the "type II" receptor reveals two receptor pathways for the diverse TGF-activities. There is a TGF-β that belongs to the epidermal growth factor (EGF) family [130]. Like other cytokines this peptide is also synthesized as a precursor that is transmembranous. The mature cytokine is released as a 50-amino acid peptide, and both the free and released forms have biological activity. This cytokine has a role in oncogenesis (as do many growth factors) and is associated with numerous tumor types including carcinomas, melanomas and hepatomas [128,131,132]. TGF-β is a potent inducer of angiogenesis and as such, has distinct and critical importance in wound healing and regeneration [133]. Recent studies have shown that activator protein-2 (AP-2) (a gene expression product involved in oxidative sensitivity of cells) regulates the TGF-β promoter may be involved in both tumorigenesis and growth [134].

Vascular endothelial growth factor (VEGF) is one of the more recently discovered growth factors, and it is a dimeric glycoprotein that is structurally similar to platelet-derived growth factor [135,136]. There are several isoforms of VEGF each of which has varying activity and presumably differing affinity to VEGF receptors [137]. VEGF is very specific for endothelial cell growth at least in vitro. As endothelial cells must proliferate to regenerate the capillary bed that is essential for reoxygenation VEGF is surely a critical cytokine for wound [135,136,138]. It has recently been shown that VEGF mRNA in keratinocytes is enhanced during wound healing and VEGF seems to act in a paracrine manner [139].

Tumor necrosis factor-α (TNF-α) is a macrophage-derived cytokine that has a multitude of signaling effects on different cell types. These effects include cell killing, induction of apoptosis (programmed cell death), DNA fragmentation (that indicates DNA damage), lipid peroxidation induction (indicating damage to membranes), and inhibition of mitochondrial electron transport (indicating a decrease in the oxidative ability of the cell to survive) [140]. It also induces activation of nuclear factor κ-B (NF-κB) [141]. NF-κB is a recognized cellular protein factor that is sensitive to oxidant stress. It activates a number of gene expression following its activation by oxidants [142,143].

Insulin-like growth factors Type I and II (IGF) are pleotropic polypeptides which have structural homologies to insulin. The IGF receptor binds IGF-I better than IGF-II or insulin. The receptor is a heterotetramer, consisting of subunits joined by disulfide. Insulin-like growth factors-I and -II differentially regulate endogenous acetylcholine released from the rat hippocampal formation [144]. Growth hormone stimulates peripheral tissue growth by involving the endocrine action of IGF-I from liver [145,146]. The IGF family of growth factors have a role in the wound healing process. The IGF-II circulates bound to an IGF receptor known as IGF-binding proteins. The IGF-II binds to the cation independent mannose-6-phosphate receptor. It reacts immunologically with the insulin, as well as the IGF-I receptor [147,148]. Conversely the IGF-I and insulin do not cross react with the IGF-II receptors [149]. The IGF-II receptor binds mannose-6-phosphate at different sites and there is no phosphorylation after binding that would suggest activation of a PKC. However, there is a redistribution of this receptor upon binding, and it involves an okadaic acid sensitive serine-threonine phosphatase [150].

When EGF binds to its receptor it can elicit a number of cell specific responses that result in differentiation and cell proliferation. The binding of EGF causes dimerization and phosphorylation of the receptor [151]. When epithelial cells are confluent (i.e., the cells are all in direct contact with one another), they are far more stable than if growing as independent "bundles" of cells. Single cells growing in culture initiate apoptosis and die. If cells are restricted in their ability to contact an adjacent cell they too initiate apoptosis [152]. The EGF-like growth factors, known as heparin-binding EGF-like growth factor (HB-EGF), increases in the kidney in vivo in response to acute renal tubular injury [153]. HB-EGF is synthesized as a membrane bound precursor and is believed to act as a juxtacrine, when it is in direct contact with an adjacent cell. In cultures, addition of EGF prevents apoptosis initiation and is good reason to suspect that EGF is modulating cell growth [154]. IL-1 has been long recognized as a cytokine that has a role in cell proliferation and wound healing. The expression of the IL-1 receptor is dependent on PKC. PKC and has a pivotal role in the activation of T cells. T cells are stimulated by the interaction of a specific antigen with T cell receptor-CD3 complex. This interaction activates the intracellular kinase cascade [155], one of which is mediated by PKC. Activated kinase cascade activates transcription factors which initiate transcription and expression of a variety of molecules including IL-2 and the high affinity IL-2 receptor chain (IL-2R). Due to IL-2 being a major T cell growth factor, the coordination of production IL-2 and IL-2 receptor is crucial for T cell proliferation and the immune response [156]. T cell stimulation with phorbal myristic acetate (PMA) alone is enough for IL-2R expression [157], and PKC is responsible for this effect [155]. Expression of IL-2R is transcriptionally regulated [158], and involves NF-κB activation [159]. NF-κB activation comprises of the phosphorylation and release of its inhibitory protein IκB [160]. The activated NF-κB translocates from the cytosol to the nucleus, where it binds to the (B consensus sequence of IL-2R gene promoter [159]. This binding is essential for NF-κB-regulated gene expression [114,161].

Interferons are a class of polypeptides that play a crucial role in the defense against viral and parasitic infections. They can stimulate the body's own immune system to acts against viral infections [162−164]. These cytokines can alter cell growth rates but have not yet proven to be useful in the treatment of cancers. There are several types of interferons which have a multitude of biological effects. The γ-interferon has been known for several years to stimulate the production of inducible nitric oxide synthase, iNOS in macrophages. β-Interferon is helpful in the treatment of multiple sclerosis and α-interferons have been partially successful in the treatment of chronic viral hepatitis B and C [165,166].

3.4 Clinical implications

Several well-characterized diseases inhibit wound healing directly due to "cellular" impairment. In diabetics there is a significantly increased problem in healing of surgical and traumatic wounds [25]. There are several possible causes for the wound healing problems associated with diabetes and these include the well-characterized degradation of capillary circulation in diabetics. The elevated serum glucose may result in an increased glycosylation of peripheral tissues, and the insulin deficiency or insulin resistance of the two types of diabetics are all factors that would likely disrupt normal wound healing. Diabetics have a propensity to develop infections from *Staphylococcus aureus, Escherichia coli* and *Candida* [167]. It is likely that a combination of diminished circulation, as well as the characteristic hyperglycemia are major contributing factors to diabetic wound healing retardation. Large vessel diseases such as atherosclerosis, due to sclerotic plaque buildup is exacerbated in diabetics. Whether this is due directly to the diabetes or its secondary effects of a tendency towards obesity and hypertension it is not immediately clear.

While diabetes is a very common disease there are many less common diseases that can provide insight into the mechanisms of leukocyte physiology by understanding what defects exist in the pathology. Chronic granulomatous disease [109] is a fairly well-characterized disorder in which the leukocytes of the patients cannot generate superoxides due to a defect in the respiratory burst enzyme. Such patients do not usually live very long as they are very susceptible to infections. It is possible to have neutropenia (a low neutrophils count), and have almost normal wound healing. Patients with chronic granulomatous disease who have a wound with no infection or debris, have no difference in healing compared to a healthy subject [25]. With antibiotic therapy often these patients can live for several years, however, few patients with severe chronic granulomatous disease live into adulthood. There are numerous sub types of chronic granulomatous disease. A recent study [168] demonstrates that there are possibilities to repair a genetic defect such as chronic granulomatous disease. In this recent study patients with a defective $p47^{phox}$ peptide, received intravenous infusions of autologous $CD34^{(+)}$ peripheral blood stem cells that had been transduced ex vivo with a recombinant retrovirus encoding normal $p47^{phox}$. These patients showed signs of development of neutrophils with a normal $p47^{phox}$. Corrected cells were detectable for as long as 6 months after infusion in some individuals although these cells represented a tiny fraction of total neutrophils.

As described in this brief survey of wounding and inflammation each of the steps involved in inflammation and wound repair involves a multitude of signals that must be transmitted to and from adjacent cells. There are many redundancies built into the inflammatory repair mechanism. Patients with a defective and impaired myeloperoxidase often don't have any major problems [169]. Primary inherited defects in neutrophil function: etiology and treatment [170,171]. Deficiency of myelperoxidase is not a lethal defect and this indicates that there are compensatory mechanisms for loss of a single enzyme even if myelperoxidase comprises a large portion of the protein in a leukocyte.

What we can learn from known pathologies? The known and characterized pathologies provide a clue that the balance of the inflammatory system can be disrupted without, necessarily, destroying the organism. Many subtle pathologies involved in wound healing are likely manifestations of defects in the inflammatory response. While some of these have now been identified, there is much to be learned about the pathophysiology of the immune system as it relates to wound healing.

4   LINKS BETWEEN WOUND HEALING AND INFLAMMATION

4.1 The balance of radical production and control by antioxidants

Leukocytes that generate copious quantities of reactive radicals that are important in the killing of bacteria, viruses and fungi have to have control systems for their own protection. Neutrophils contain considerably more ascorbate (vitamin C) than do other cells [172]. Ascorbate is an important reductive antioxidant that has been shown to reduce vitamin E radical directly [173]. The earliest wound healing research determined that ascorbate was essential for the prevention of scurvy. Subsequently the molecular role of ascorbate being involved in the formation of hydroxyproline from proline defined the role of ascorbate in the wound environment [174]. Vitamin E is strongly linked to the prevention of lipid peroxidation and it is believed to act as a chain breaking antioxidant which stops the progression of the nonenzymatic radical reactions of lipid peroxidation. Ascorbate is also believed to be important in the reduction of other radicals preventing radical damage to important cellular sites such as DNA, membranes and regulatory enzymes. Vitamin E is located in the membranes as it is very lipophilic. It can be recycled by enzyme linked reduction, such as in the mitochondrial respiratory chain where it is unlikely ascorbate in fact would remain oxidized [175].

When neutrophils have their respiratory burst stimulated by PMA they undergo a rapid respiratory burst. In an in vitro model system in which there is far more oxygen than in a "physiological" condition, there is no measurable decrease in the cell's ascorbate, vitamin E or glutathione [176]. This indicates that the neutrophils have a significantly enhanced cellular system to prevent their own oxidants from destroying the cell that made them. It is important to recognize that the production and protection of radicals in a cell such as a neutrophil is a balance. A diminution of one antioxidant such as ascorbic acid may not result in a measurable increase in oxidative damage as there are other antioxidant systems that can compensate for a decrease of one antioxidant. It is now common practice in the developed world to take vitamin supplements especially antioxidant vitamins such as vitamin C and E [177]. While the evidence that these vitamin supplements can actually result in any measurable health benefit is not very clear, there is a wealth of good scientific evidence that indicates that these two vitamins in particular are most influential in the prevention of cellular oxidative damage at all levels in the cell from the DNA to the cell membrane [178—183].

4.2 The role of oxygen in wound healing and inflammatory resolution

Oxygen in tissues is usually found in the range of 10—20% of ambient air saturated water (15—30 mmHg or 24—48 μM O_2). In the "center" of a wound the oxygen concentration can be decreased by an order of magnitude again [25]. When there is a stressful event for an organism such as a wound, the oxygen consumption will rise both locally and systemically. Accordingly the concentration of oxygen available for healing become a limiting and important aspect of a healing wound. In contrast, almost all cell cultures are performed in air saturated liquids that the cell would never be exposed to in a physiological condition.

It is becoming increasingly popular to utilize hyperbaric oxygen therapy clinically to stimulate wound healing. The logic is that increasing oxygen tension into an "anaerobic" wound environment can stimulate leukocyte antimicrobial activity in turn leading to wound resolution. A recent re-evaluation of several surgical cases has shown the effectiveness of hyperbaric oxygen and other procedures that can increase tissue oxygen tension and enhance clinical wound healing [71]. Sometimes a combination of rather simple, well-defined regimens can result in the resolution of wounds that might otherwise not heal well. For example, inexpensive techniques such as preoperative evaluation of nutrition, hyperglycemia, and steroid use can be controlled. Postsurgical considerations of maintenance of body warmth, adequate oxygen supply and the use of hyperbaric oxygen are all factors that aid wound resolution [25].

4.3 Wound healing and multiple cell signals

The complexities of wound healing and the interactions between intercellular messages and the eventual survival from an event such as a traumatic wound depend on a vast number of interacting events. A recent study [184] has begun to define a new way to evaluate leukocytes and their ability to encounter and respond to multiple chemoattractant signals in complex spatial and temporal patterns. As leukocytes are exposed to multiple chemoattractants (and potentially chemorepellants) they must process the signals that they receive so that they can move up a gradient of one type of attractant towards another. They must process signaling in a combinatorial manner in order not to be rendered immobile and unable to function properly. The "symphony" of cellular control of inflammation becomes more complex the more we have been able to understand it.

5   SUMMARY

The wound healing process is a complex cellular process that involves a number of cell types which must all interact harmoniously for the wound to resolve and heal. It differs in complexity from embryogenesis in that the wound is frequently infected or exposed to debris such as necrotic tissue that must be removed before the wound is completely healed. While the main cell types discussed in this chapter have been the neutrophils and macrophage, the interaction between platelets, fibroblasts, epithelial, endothelial cells, as well as specialized cells in selective tissues such as neural, bone, muscle are all tissues that are frequently damaged in injuries. Each cell type has specific requirements and limitations as to when and how it can replicate. Cytokines are a source of messages between cells and their production and subsequent interaction with "remote" cells can signal information about the wound environment that enables the wound peripheral cells to begin replicating and allow for the regrowth of the wounded area.

The necessity of having cells "stick" together is certainly critical in getting wound resolution. The expression and timing of the expression of adhesion molecules is a research area of considerable interest as it precedes tissue growth. The one item that is often overlooked in wound healing and in cell biology in general is the role of oxygen tension. At the very best most tissue concentrations of oxygen are far lower than might be found in a cell culture growing in ambient air. In wounds the oxygen supply substantially dictates the rate of neutrophil and macrophage production of O_2^- which precedes the production of numerous other oxidants. Oxygen is also required for generation NO·. NO· is certainly formed in human macrophages and has a role in the bactericidal arsenal of the immune system.

6   PERSPECTIVES

From a cellular and biochemical perspective the future for investigations into inflammation and wound repair are likely to unravel many new and currently ill-defined pathways of regulation. Understanding a concept such as how a cell can sense two separate chemoattractants, or how a cell can know when it must turn on a set of genes to reconstruct a wounded area in an area that is separated by microns from an environment that would destroy the cell, this represents an example of the balance that exists between the inflammatory "cleanup" cells and the reconstruction cells that follow into the wound site.

Clinically, as new pathways of cellular regulation and control are defined, there exist possibilities to understand the nature of pathological wound healing. As has been the case for centuries, observations made by clinicians about their patients can aid basic cellular sciences and clinicians can learn much by understanding the cellular events that result in wound healing. Keeping up with all the new information represents a major challenge. This brief review attempts to bridge this gap.

7   ACKNOWLEDGMENTS

The author is supported in part by a grant from The National Institutes of Health, Grant GM27345. I thank Prof Thomas K. Hunt and Dr John Feng for many helpful comments. The artwork of Fig. 1. was drawn by Fred Kim and Ronald Moy who have assisted in the manuscript preparation.

8   ABBREVIATIONS

AP:	activator protein
EGF:	epidermal growth factor
FAD:	flavin adenine dinucleotide
fMLP:	formyl-methione-leucine phenylalanine
HB-EGF:	heparin-binding EGF-like growth factor
IGF:	insulin-dependent growth factor
ICAM:	intercellular adhesion molecule
IL:	interleukin
IL-2R:	interleukin 2-receptor
iNOS:	inducible NOS
LPS:	lipopolysaccharide

NOS: nitric oxide synthase
PKC: protein kinase C
PMA: phorbal myristic acetate
ROS: reactive oxygen species
SOD: superoxide dismutase
TGF: transforming growth factor
TNF: tumor necrosis factor
VCAM: vascular cell adhesion molecule
VEGF: vascular endothelial growth factor

9   REFERENCES

1. Martin P. Science 1997;C 276:75–81.
2. Shafi S, Gilbert JC. Pediatr Clin N Am 1998;45:831–851.
3. Jones DC. Instr Course Lect 1998;47:419–427.
4. Fulcher SM, Kiefhaber TR, Stern PJ. Clin Sports Med 1998;17:433–448.
5. Perry J. Clin Sports Med 1983;2:247–270.
6. Abraham P, Chevalier JM, Leftheriotis G, Saumet JL Am J Sports Med 1997;25:581–584.
7. Maimaris C, Zadeh HG. Br J Sports Med 1990;24:245–246.
8. Shattil SJ, Ginsberg MH. J Clin Invest 1997;100:S91–S95.
9. Spotnitz WD, Falstrom JK, Rodeheaver GT. Surg Clin North Am 1997;77:651–669.
10. Brain SD. Immunopharmacology 1997;37:133–152.
11. Kerstein MD. Adv Wound Care 1997;10:30–36.
12. Menger MD, Vollmar B. Br J Surg 1996; 83:588–601.
13. Moulin V. Eur J Cell Biol 1995;68:1–7.
14. Polverini PJ. Exs 1997;79:11–28.
15. DiPietro LA. Shock 1995;4:233–240.
16. Jenner P, Olanow CW. Neurology 1996;47:S161–S170.
17. Halliwell B. Annu Rev Nutr 1996;16:33–50.
18. Packer L. J Sports Sci 1997;15:353–363.
19. Williams K, Ulvestad E, Antel J. Adv Neuroimmunol 1994;4:273–281.
20. Hartung HP, Jung S, Stoll G, Zielasek J, Schmidt B, Archelos JJ, Toyka KV. J Neuroimmunol 1992;40:197–210.
21. Jonsson K, Jensen JA, Goodson WHD, Scheuenstuhl H, West J, Hopf HW, Hunt TK. Ann Surg 1991;214:605–613.
22. Knighton DR, Hunt TK, Scheuenstuhl H, Halliday BJ, Werb Z, Banda MJ. Science 1983;221: 1283–1285.
23. Mader JT, Adams KR, Wallace WR, Calhoun JH. Infect Dis Clin N Am 1990;4:433–440.
24. Kuhne HH, Ullmann U. Kuhne FW. Infection 1985;13:52–56.
25. Hunt TK, Appleton-Century-Crofts, New York, 1980;303.
26. Egelberg J. J Periodontal Res 1987;22:233–242.
27. Clark RA. Am J Med Sci 1993;306:42–48.
28. Schwarzbauer JE. Bioessays 1991;13:527–533.
29. LeRoy EC, Trojanowska MI, Smith EA. Eur Cytokine Netw 1990;1:215–219.
30. Kittlick PD. Exp Pathol 1985;1(Suppl 10)1–174.
31. Mosher DF. Annu Rev Med 1984;35:561–575.
32. Grinnell F. J Cell Biochem 1984;26:107–116.
33. Lopez-Berestein GaK, J. Florida Boca Raton: CRC Press, Inc., 1993;239.
34. Polverini PJ. Crit Rev Oral Biol Med 1995;6:230–247.
35. Brown E. Sem Hematol 1997;34:319–326.

36. Ignarro LJ. Pharmacol Res 1989;6:651—659.
37. Haller H. Drugs 1997;53(Suppl 1):1—10.
38. Beckerman KP, Rogers HW, Corbett JA, Schreiber RD, McDaniel ML, Unanue ER. J Immunol 1993;150:888—895.
39. McFadden G, Kelvin D. Biochem Pharmacol 1997;54:1271—1280.
40. Duke RC, Ojcius DM, Young JD. Sci Am 1996;275:80—87.
41. Suzuki YJ, Forman HJ, Sevanian A, Free Radic Biol Med 1997;22:269—285.
42. Clemmons DR. Cytokine Growth Factor Rev 1997;8:45—62.
43. Albelda SM, Buck CA. FASEB J 1990;4:2868—2880.
44. Felding-Habermann B, Cheresh DA. Curr Opin Cell Biol 1993;5:864—868.
45. De Luca M, Pellegrini G, Zambruno G, Marchisio PC. J Dermatol 1994;21:821—828.
46. Jockusch BM, Bubeck P, Giehl K, Kroemker M, Moschner J, Rothkegel M, Rudiger M, Schluter K, Stanke G, Winkler J. Annu Rev Cell Dev Biol 1995;11:379—416.
47. Van Waes C. Head Neck 1995;17:140—147.
48. Shattil SJ. Thromb Haemostat 1995;74:149—155.
49. Vinatier D. Eur J Obstet Gynecol Reprod Biol 1995;59:71—81.
50. Etzioni A. Pediatr Res 1996;39:191—198.
51. Goligorsky MS, Noiri E, Peresleni T, Hu Y. Exp Nephrol 1996;4:314—321.
52. DiPietro LA. Exs 1997;79:295—314.
53. Mutsaers SE, Bishop JE, McGrouther G, Laurent GJ. Int J Biochem Cell Biol 1997;29:5—17.
54. Wilson AJ, Gibson PR. Clin Sci (Colch) 1997;93:97—108.
55. Schwartz SM. J Clin Invest 1997;100:S87—S89.
56. Bevilacqua MP, Schleef RR, Gimbrone MA Jr. Loskutoff DJ. J Clin Invest 1986;78:587—591.
57. Bevilacqua MP, Pober JS, Wheeler ME, Cotran RS, Gimbrone MA Jr. J Clin Invest 1985;76:2003—2011.
58. Gamble JR, Harlan JM, Klebanoff SJ, Vadas MA. Proc Natl Acad Sci USA 1985;82:8667—8671.
59. Klebanoff SJ, Vadas MA, Harlan JM, Sparks LH, Gamble JR, Agosti JM, Waltersdorph AM. J Immunol 1986;136:4220—4225.
60. Pober JS, Bevilacqua MP, Mendrick DL, Lapierre LA, Fiers W, Gimbrone MA Jr. J Immunol 1986;136:1680—1687.
61. Furie MB, McHugh DD. J Immunol 1989;143:3309—3317.
62. Moser R, Schleiffenbaum B, Groscurth P, Fehr J. J Clin Invest 1989;83:444—455.
63. Carlos TM, Harlan JM. Immunol Rev 1990;114:5—28.
64. Litwin M, Clark K, Noack L, Furze J, Berndt M, Albelda S, Vadas M, Gamble J. J Cell Biol 1997;139:219—228.
65. Bevilacqua MP, Stengelin S, Gimbrone MA Jr., Seed B. Science 1989;243:1160—1165.
66. Read MA, Whitley MZ, Williams AJ, Collins T. J Exp Med 1994;179:503—512.
67. Osborn L, Hession C, Tizard R, Vassallo C, Luhowskyj S, Chi-Rosso G, Lobb R. Cell 1989;59:1203—1211.
68. Koch AE, Kunkel SL, Burrows JC, Evanoff HL, Haines GK, Pope RM, Strieter RM. J Immunol 1991;147:2187—2195.
69. Niinikoski J, Hunt TK, Dunphy JE. Am J Surg 1972;123:247—252.
70. Silver IA. Adv Exp Med Biol 1973;37A:223—231.
71. Hunt TK, Hopf HW. Surg Clin North Am 1997;77:587—606.
72. Williams RL. J Am Pediatr Med Assoc 1997;87:279—292.
73. Davies KJ. Biochem Soc Symp 1995;61:1—31.
74. Roth RN, Weiss LD. Clin Dermatol 1994;12:141—156.
75. Cohen IK, Mast BA. J Trauma 1990;30:S149—S155.
76. Ninikoski J. Clin Plast Surg 1977;4:361—374.
77. Allen DB, Maguire JJ, Mahdavian M, Wicke C, Marcocci L, Scheuenstuhl H, Chang M, Le AX, Hopf HW, Hunt TK. Arch Surg 1997;132:991—996.

78. Gabig TG, Bearman SI, Babior BM. Blood 1979;53:1133—1139.

79. Marletta MA, Yoon PS, Iyengar R, Leaf CD, Wishnok JS. Biochemistry 1988;27:8706—8711.

80. Rengasamy A. Johns RA. J Pharmacol Exp Ther 1996;276:30—33.

81. Hopf HW, Hunt TK, West JM, Blomquist P, Goodson WH 3rd, Jensen JA, Jonsson K, Paty PB, Rabkin JM, Upton RA, von Smitten K, Whitney JD. Arch Surg 1997;132:997-1004; Discussion 1005.

82. Abramson JSaW, JG. Oxford: Oxford University Press, 1993;306.

83. Fulcher DA: Basten A. Immunol Cell Biol 1997;75,446—455.

84. Miller RA. Science 1996;273:70—74.

85. Rajewsky K. Nature 1996;381:751—758.

86. Shafrir E. Isr J Med Sci 1995;31:465.

87. Owen CA, Campbell EJ. Semin Cell Biol 1995;6:367—376.

88. Homburg CH, Roos D. Curr Opin Hematol 1996;3:94—99.

89. Brown EJ. Bioessays 1995;17:109—117.

90. Cassimeris L, Zigmond SH. Semin Cell Biol 1990;1:125—134.

91. Keller H, Niggli V, Zimmerman A. Adv Exp Med Biol 1991;297:23—37.

92. Klempner MS. Rev Infect Dis 1984;6(Suppl 1):S40—S44.

93. Brown EJ. J Leuk Biol 1986;39:579—591.

94. Ginsburg, I. Free Radic Res Commun 1989;8:11—26.

95. Levy O. Eur J Haematol 1996;56:263—277.

96. Hunninghake GW, Fauci AS. Immunology 1976;31:139—144.

97. Andersen L, Attstrom R, Fejerskov O. Scand J Dent Res 1978;86:237—247.

98. Leibovich SJ, Wiseman DM. Prog Clin Biol Res 1988;266:131—145.

99. Ganz T. New Horiz 1993;1:23—27.

100. Barbul A, Regan MC. Otolaryngol Clin North Am 1995;28:955—968.

101. Schaffer CJ, Nanney LB. Int Rev Cytol 1996;169:151—181.

102. Postlethwaite AE, Kang AH. J Exp Med 1976;143:1299—1307.

103. Clark RAF. The Molecular and Cellular Biology of Wound Repair. 2nd edn. New York and London: Plenum Press, 1998;611.

104. Roman J. Exp Lung Res 1997;23:147—159.

105. Hynes RO. Sci Am 1986;254:42—51.

106. Buck MR, Karustis DG, Day NA, Honn KV. Sloane BF. Biochem J 1992;282:273—278.

107. Maciewicz RA, Wotton SF, Etherington DJ, Duance VC. FEBS Lett 1990;269:189—193.

108. Petanceska S, Canoll P, Devi LA. J Biol Chem 1996;271:4403—4409.

109. Chanock SJ, el Benna J, Smith RM, Babior BM. J Biol Chem 1994;269:24519—24522.

110. Maly FE, Schuerer-Maly CC, Quilliam L, Cochrane CG, Newburger PE, Curnutte JT, Gifford M, Dinauer MC. J Exp Med 1993;178:2047—2053.

111. Chanock SJ, Faust LR, Barrett D, Bizal C, Maly FE, Newburger PE, Ruedi JM, Smith RM, Babior BM. Proc Natl Acad Sci USA 1992;89:10174—10177.

112. Zhen L, King AA, Xiao Y, Chanock SJ, Orkin SH, Dinauer MC. Proc Natl Acad Sci USA 1993;90:9832—9836.

113. Sekhsaria S, Gallin JI, Linton GF, Mallory RM, Mulligan RC, Malech HL. Proc Natl Acad Sci USA 1993;90:7446—7450.

114. Ogino T, Kobuchi H, Sen CK, Roy S, Packer L, Maguire JJ. J Biol Chem 1997;272:26247—26252.

115. Segal AW, Jones OT, Webster D, Allison AC. Lancet 1978;2:446—449.

116. Rotrosen D, Yeung CL, Katkin JP. J Biol Chem 1993;268:14256—14260.

117. Boveris A, Cadenas E, Stoppani AO. Biochem J 1976;156:435—444.

118. Turrens JF, Alexandre A, Lehninger AL. Arch Biochem Biophys 1985;237:408—414.

119. Gardner PR. Biosci Rep 1997;17:33—42.

120. Fujii H, Yonetani T, Miki T, Kakinuma K. J Biol Chem 1995;270:3193—3196.

121. Cerutti P, Larsson R, Krupitza G, Muehlematter D, Crawford D, Amstad P. Mutat Res 1989;

214:81—88.
122. Burdon RH, Gill V, Rice-Evans C. Free Radic Res Commun 1990;11:65—76.
123. Janssen YM, Van Houten B, Borm PJ, Mossman BT. Lab Invest 1993;69:261—274.
124. Zimniak L, Awasthi S, Srivastava SK, Zimniak P. Toxicol Appl Pharmacol 1997;143:221—229.
125. Amstad PA, Liu H, Ichimiya M, Berezesky IK, Trump BF. Carcinogenesis 1997;18:479—484.
126. Wong ST, Winchell LF, McCune BK, Earp HS, Teixido J, Massague J, Herman B, Lee DC. Cell 1989;56:495—506.
127. Brachmann R, Lindquist PB, Nagashima M, Kohr W, Lipari T, Napier M, Derynck R. Cell 1989;56:691—700.
128. Derynck R, Roberts AB, Winkler ME, Chen EY, Goeddel DV. Cell 1984;38:287—297.
129. Chen RH, Ebner R, Derynck R. Science 1993;260:1335—1338.
130. Marquardt H, Hunkapiller MW, Hood LE, Todaro GJ. Science 1984;223:1079—1082.
131. Derynck R, Goeddel DV, Ullrich A, Gutterman JU, Williams RD, Bringman TS, Berger WH. Cancer Res 1987;47:707—712.
132. Nister M, Libermann TA, Betsholtz C, Pettersson M, Claesson-Welsh L, Heldin CH, Schlessinger J, Westermark B. Cancer Res 1988;48:3910—3918.
133. Schreiber AB, Winkler ME, Derynck R. Science 1986;232:1250—1253.
134. Wang D, Shin TH, Kudlow JE. J Biol Chem 1997;272:14244—14250.
135. Keck PJ, Hauser SD, Krivi G, Sanzo K, Warren T, Feder J, Connolly DT. Science 1989;246:1309—1312.
136. Leung DW, Cachianes G, Kuang WJ, Goeddel DV, Ferrara N. Science 1989;246:1306—1309.
137. Houck KA, Ferrara N, Winer J, Cachianes G, Li B, Leung DW. Mol Endocrinol 1991;5:1806—1814.
138. Gospodarowicz D, Abraham JA, Schilling J. Proc Natl Acad Sci USA 1989;86:7311—7315.
139. de Vries C, Escobedo JA, Ueno H, Houck K, Ferrara N, Williams LT. Science 1992;255:989—991.
140. Lancaster JR Jr., Laster SM, Gooding LR. FEBS Lett 1989;248:169—174.
141. Duh EJ, Maury WJ, Folks TM, Fauci AS, Rabson AB. Proc Natl Acad Sci USA 1989;86:5974—5978.
142. Conner EM, Grisham MB. Nutrition 1996;12:274—277.
143. Sen CK, Packer L. FASEB J 1996;10:709—720.
144. Kar S, Seto D, Dore S, Hanisch U, Quirion R. Proc Natl Acad Sci USA 1997;94:14054—14059.
145. Daughaday WH. Perspect Biol Med 1989;32:194—211.
146. Isaksson OG, Jansson JO, Gause IA. Science 1982;216:1237—1239.
147. Morgan DO, Edman JC, Standring DN, Fried VA, Smith MC, Roth RA, Rutter WJ. Nature 1987;329:301—307.
148. Roth RA, Kiess W. Growth Regul 1994;4(Suppl 1):31—38.
149. Tally M, Enberg G, Li CH, Hall K. Biochem Biophys Res Commun 1987;147:1206—1212.
150. Braulke T, Mieskes G. J Biol Chem 1992;267:17347—17353.
151. van der Geer P, Hunter T, Lindberg RA. Annu Rev Cell Biol 1994;10:251—337.
152. Frisch SM, Francis H. J Cell Biol 1994;124:619—626.
153. Homma T, Sakai M, Cheng HF, Yasuda T, Coffey RJ Jr, Harris RC. J Clin Invest 1995;96:1018—1025.
154. Raff MC. Nature 1992;356:397—400.
155. Szamel M, Bartels F, Resch K. Eur J Immunol 1993;23:3072—3081.
156. Smith KA. Science 1988;240:1169—1176.
157. Shackelford DA, Trowbridge IS. J Biol Chem 1984;259:11706—11712.
158. Greene WC, Robb RJ, Depper JM, Leonard WJ, Drogula C, Svetlik PB, Wong-Staal F, Gallo RC, Waldmann TA. J Immunol 1984;133:1042—1047.
159. Bohnlein E, Ballard DW, Bogerd H, Peffer NJ, Lowenthal JW, Greene WC. J Biol Chem 1989;264:8475—8478.
160. Brown K, Gerstberger S, Carlson L, Franzoso G, Siebenlist U. Science 1995;267:1485—1488.

161. Jamieson C, McCaffrey PG, Rao A, Sen R. J Immunol 1991;147:416—420.
162. Billiau A. Mult Scler 1995;1(Suppl 1):S2—S4.
163. Williams CN. Can J Gastroenterol 1997;11:563—564.
164. Foster GR. Sem Liver Dis 1997;17:287—295.
165. Alberti A, Chemello L, Noventa F, Cavalletto L, De Salvo G. Hepatology 1997;26:137S—142S.
166. Schwartz CE, Coulthard-Morris L, Cole B, Vollmer T. Arch Neurol 1997;54:1475—1480.
167. Feigin RD, Shearer WT. J Pediatr 1975;87:677—694.
168. Malech HL et al. Proc Natl Acad Sci USA 1997;94:12133—12138.
169. Malech HL, Nauseef WM. Sem Hematol 1997;34:279—290.
170. Nauseef WM, Brigham S, Cogley M. J Biol Chem 1994;269:1212—1216.
171. Nauseef WM, Cogley M, McCormick S. J Biol Chem 1996;271:9546—9549.
172. Washko PW, Wang Y, Levine M. J Biol Chem 1993;268:15531—15535.
173. Packer JE, Slater TF, Willson RL. Nature 1979;278:737—738.
174. Hodges RE. World Health Organ Monogr 1976;Ser:120—125.
175. Maguire JJ, Kagan V, Ackrell BA, Serbinova E, Packer L. Arch Biochem Biophys 1992;292: 47—53.
176. Ogino T, Packer L, Maguire JJ. Free Radic Biol Med 1997;23:445—452.
177. Stahelin HB, Rosel F, Buess E, Brubacher G. J Natl Cancer Inst 1984;73:1463—1468.
178. Odeh RM, Cornish LA. Pharmacotherapy 1995;15:648—659.
179. Sardesai VM. Nutr Clin Pract 1995;10:19—25.
180. Jacob RA, Burri BJ. Am J Clin Nutr 1996;63:985S—990S.
181. Filiberti R, Giacosa A, Brignoli O. Eur J Cancer Prev 1997;1(Suppl 6):S37—S42.
182. Griendling KK, Alexander RW. Circulation 1997;96:3264—3265.
183. Ward JA. Drugs Aging 1998;12:169—175.
184. Foxman EF, Campbell JJ, Butcher EC. J Cell Biol 1997;139:1349—1360.
185. Mol JA, Selman PJ, Sprang EP, van Neck JW, Oosterlaken-Dijksterhuis MA. J Reprod Fertil Suppl 1997;51:339—344.
186. Marcus R. Horm Res 1997;48(Suppl 5):60—64.
187. Lee PD, Giudice LC, Conover CA, Powell DR. Proc Soc Exp Biol Med 1997;216:319—357.
188. Schmitt E, Rude E, Germann T. Chem Immunol 1997;68:70—85.
189. Heldin CH, Miyazono K, ten Dijke P. Nature 1997;390:465—471.
190. Letterio JJ, Roberts AB. Clin Immunol Immunopathol 1997;84:244—250.
191. Shanley TP, Warner RL, Ward PA. Mol Med Today 1995;1:40—45.
192. Gruss HJ, Dower SK. Cytokines Mol Ther 1995;1:75—105.
193. Mendelsohn J, Fan Z. J Natl Cancer Inst 1997;89:341—343.
194. Cho MI, Garant PR. Anat Rec 1996;245342—245360.
195. Carmeliet P: Collen D. Am J Physiol 1997;273,H2091—H2104.
196. Joukov V, Kaipainen A, Jeltsch M, Pajusola K, Olofsson B, Kumar V, Eriksson U, Alitalo K. J Cell Physiol 1997;173:211—215.
197. Rothwell N, Allan S, Toulmond S. J Clin Invest 1997;100:2648—2652.
198. Du X, Williams DA. Curr Opin Hematol 1995;2:182—188.
199. Fefer A, Robinson N, Benyunes MC, Bensinger WI, Press O, Thompson JA, Lindgren C. Cancer J Sci Am 1997;3 (Suppl 1):S48—S53.
200. Chougnet C, Shearer GM. Curr Opin Hematol 1996;3:216—222.

©2000 Elsevier Science B.V. All rights reserved.
Handbook of Oxidants and Antioxidants in Exercise.
C.K. Sen, L. Packer and O. Hänninen, editors.

Part XI • Chapter 35

Oxidative stress induced by the metabolism of medical and nonmedical drugs

Moreno Paolini[1] and Giorgio Cantelli-Forti[2]

[1]*Department of Pharmacology, Biochemical Toxicology Unit, The University of Bologna, Via Irnerio 48, 40126 Bologna, Italy. Tel.: +39-051-20917-83. Fax: +39-051-2488-62.*
[2]*Division of Environmental Toxicology and Community Health, University of Texas Medical Branch, Galveston, TX, USA.*

1   INTRODUCTION
2   DRUGS AND FREE RADICALS
3   DRUGS YIELDING FREE RADICAL METABOLITES
    3.1   Carbon tetrachloride
    3.2   Clozapine
    3.3   Aminopyrine
    3.4   Phenylbutazone
    3.5   Nitrofurantoin
    3.6   Doxorubicin
        3.6.1   Free radicals generation by redox-cycling
        3.6.2   Free radicals generation by drug iron complex
4   OXIDATIVE DAMAGE BY DRUGS DEPLETING GLUTATHIONE
5   INDUCERS OF CYTOCHROME P450 ISOZYMES
6   INDUCERS OF PEROXISOME PROLIFERATION
7   SUMMARY
8   PERSPECTIVES
9   ACKNOWLEDGEMENTS
10 ABBREVIATIONS
11 REFERENCES

1   INTRODUCTION

Reactive oxygen species (ROS) such as oxygen-derived free radicals, singlet oxygen, hydrogen peroxide, hypochlorite and peroxynitrite, are now known to be implicated in numerous pathologies, including the physical and mental decline associated with the aging process. However, it has been shown that certain ROS evidently form part of our immune system defenses against invading microorganisms and may also act as essentially intracellular second messengers for several cytokines and growth factors [1—3]. Indeed, oxy-radicals are able to mimic, in many ways, the actions of polypeptide factors. For example, calcium-ion mobilization from mitochondria and endoplasmic reticulum, and influx from the extracellular spaces are some of the earliest events occurring after ROS exposure [4]. The consecutive changes in the activities of phosphatases and kinases that transduce the initial signal to a family of transcription factors are only beginning to be explored [5,6]. These changes are a part of a highly complex network of activities that allows an immediate response to various forms of cellular stress.

In some instances, however, oxidative stress may result more directly in the alteration of the activity of trascription factors such as nuclear factor κ-B, tumor necrosis factor α, interleukin-1 and the oncoproteins Fos and Jun [7,8], followed by their enhanced synthesis and the transactivation of subfamilies of effector genes [9]. It is becoming increasingly recognised that activation of these gene expression circuits by oxy-radicals can contribute to various forms of cellular injury, including cancer [10] and the involvement of free radicals in many degenerative diseases. Nevertheless, with the exception of some conditions caused by environmental toxins and ionizing radiation, it is not currently known whether ROS generation is the causal factor of illnesses or the result of their progression.

Formation of ROS, like the superoxide anion $O_2^{·-}$ and its secondary radicals, is continuously induced by such factors as cellular respiration, oxidation during the metabolism of xenobiotics and arachidonic acid, and respiratory burst in phagocytic cells [11]. Under normal physiological conditions, about $1-3\%$ of the oxygen we breathe is used to make superoxide. Since human beings consume a lot of oxygen, it is possible to produce over 2 kg of superoxide in the body every year. Some examples of ROS generation during endogenous metabolism are shown in Table 1. The key role of constitutive levels of superoxide dismutase (SOD), catalase (CTS) and glutathione peroxidase (GPX) activities in protection against oxygen-mediated biological damage is extensively documented [12].

However, several unrelated phenomena that pose a risk to health, such as the metabolism of specific drugs, induction of the cytochrome P450 superfamily by drugs and environmental pollutants, inflammation and reoxygenation of ischemic tissues (Fig. 1), and alcoholism or tabagism can also lead to increased production of radicals. Tissues can often respond to mild oxidative stress by creating extra antioxidant defences, but severe increases of steady-state concentration of oxygen radicals can cause cell injury or even death by necrosis or apoptosis [13].

Here, we briefly summarize some of the scenarios where certain medical and nonmedical drugs can impose an oxidative stress either by the production of free radicals, (the toxin may itself be a free radical, be metabolized to a radical,

Table 1. Endogenous generation of ROS.

Enzyme or system	ROS produced
Mixed function oxidase	$O_2^{·-}$
Monoammine oxidase (brain)	H_2O_2
Xantine oxidase	$O_2^{·-}$
NADPH oxidase in neutrophils	$O_2^{·-}$
Nitric oxide synthase	$NO^·$
Superoxide dismutase	H_2O_2
Oxidative phosphorilation in mithocondria	$O_2^{·-}$
Fenton reaction (on surface of proteins)	$HO^·$

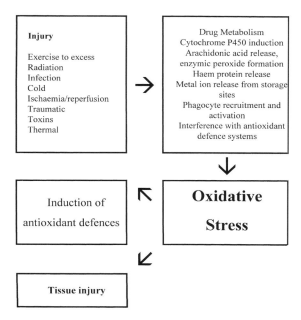

Fig. 1. ROS overproduction by tissue injury.

or generate oxygen free radicals), by depleting antioxidant defences, or also indirectly by the induction of cytochrome P450 isoenzymes and peroxisome proliferation.

2   DRUGS AS FREE RADICALS

Nitrogen dioxide ($NO_2^\cdot$) is a free radical contaminant member of an extended family of nitrogen oxides and oxy-acids interrelated by a number of reactions. Respiratory exposure to $NO_2^\cdot$, which is produced primarily by atmospheric oxidation of nitric oxide, produces a well-documented sequela of epithelial injury in both the conducting airways and the proximal alveoli. Since $NO_2^\cdot$ per se is eliminated by absorption, pulmonary-surface-lining-layer-derived products are probably critical to the genesis of $NO_2^\cdot$-induced lung disease. NO2$^\cdot$ exists in equilibrium with its dimer [14], N_2O_4:

$$2NO_2^\bullet \quad \rightleftharpoons \quad N_2O_4$$

which in aqueous solution forms nitrite and nitrate [15]:

$$N_2O_4 \xrightarrow{\text{water}} NO_2^- - \quad + \quad NO_3^-$$

Nitrogen dioxide is formed in the clean troposphere primarily through the rapid reaction of nitric oxide with ozone [16]:

$$NO^{\cdot} \; + \; O_3 \quad \rightarrow \quad NO_2^{\cdot} + O_3$$

and it is removed by photolysis:

$$NO_2^{\cdot} \; + \; h\nu \quad \rightarrow \quad NO \; + \; O(^3P)$$

leading to the generation of O_3.

$$O(^3P) \; + \; O_2 \quad \rightarrow \quad O_3$$

The net result is a photo-stationary state, where the relative concentrations are set by light intensity. $NO_2^{\cdot}$ can react with ozone [16]

$$NO_2^{\cdot} \; + \; O_3 \quad \rightarrow \quad NO_3^{\cdot} \; + \; O_2$$

and the nitrate radical so formed is also photolyzed [17].

$$NO_3^{\cdot} \; + \; h\nu \quad \rightarrow \quad NO \; + \; O_2 \text{ or}$$
$$NO_3^{\cdot} \; + \; h\nu \quad \rightarrow \quad NO_2^{\cdot} \; + \; O(^3P)$$

Further nitric oxide reactions yield:

$$NO_3^{\cdot} \; + \; NO^{\cdot} \quad \rightarrow \quad 2NO_2^{\cdot} \text{ or [16]}$$
$$NO_3^{\cdot} \; + \; NO_2^{\cdot} \quad \rightleftharpoons \quad N_2O_5$$

which is the major source of the highly reactive $NO_3^{\cdot}$ at night [18]. $NO_2^{\cdot}$ is also generated in the troposphere by the reaction of $NO^{\cdot}$ with the hydroperoxyl radical [17]:

$$NO^{\cdot} \; + \; HO_2^{\cdot} \quad \rightarrow \quad NO_2^{\cdot} \; + \; {}^{\cdot}OH$$

or with other peroxyl radicals, and finally by the reaction:

$$2NO^{\cdot} \; + \; O_2 \quad \rightarrow \quad 2NO_2^{\cdot}$$

which, however, is too slow to be an important source of $NO_2^{\cdot}$. In polluted atmosphere, the situation is far more complex, with the formation of many possible nitrogen-containing products [18].

Nitrogen dioxide can enter the body by inhalation and also can be generated in vivo [16—20] in many ways. Indeed, nitric oxide has been sound to constitute an intermediate key in a number of physiological processes, and this strongly supports the concept that $NO_2^{\cdot}$ might also be frequently reduced in biological systems. A fundamental reaction which may result in nitrogen dioxide generation in the body is:

$$NO^. + O_2^- \rightarrow {}^- OONO \text{ to give}$$
$$^- OONO \rightarrow NO_3^- \text{ or}$$

$$^- OONO \xrightarrow{H+} {}^. OH + NO_2$$

Nitric oxide also appears to react rapidly with organic peroxyl radicals:

$$NO^. + RO_2^. \rightarrow ROONO$$

forming peroxynitrites that have been proposed as intermediates in the nitrozation of organic hydroperoxides by N_2O_4. $NO_2^.$ might also be formed by the oxidation of nitrite in solution. For example, it has been suggested that the reaction of oxyhemoglobin with nitrite could yield $NO_2^.$ and hydrogen peroxide [21]:

$$HbO_2 + NO_2^- \rightarrow Hb^{+3} + NO_2^. + H_2O_2$$
$$NO_2^. + HbO_2 \rightarrow Hb^{3+} + NO_2^- + O_2$$

or, as occurs in gaseous phase, nitrogen dioxide might be formed in physiological systems through the reaction of NO with O_2.

$NO_2^.$ may undergo various different types of reactions [16]. These include hydrogen atom abstraction from C-H bonds [22,23] (e.g., n-alkanes, phenols), additions to unsaturated bonds [24,25] (dialkenes, alkenes, including polyunsaturated fatty acids), electron transfer reactions [25,26] (morpholine, ascorbate, α-tocopherol) and additions to many inorganic free radicals in atmospheric chemistry [27,28] and in liquid phase [29,30] (methanol, 2-propanol, benzene). These reactions, yielding oxygen- and carbon-centered radical formations, can lead to oxidative lesions (i.e., inflammation of the respiratory tract, lipid peroxidation) when the oxidant-antioxidant balance is altered [31]. It is well known, for example, that the interaction of nitrogen dioxide with plasma, can lead to depletion of antioxidants such as ascorbic acid, uric acid, protein thiol groups, α-tocopherol [32], thus damaging biological macromolecules [33–38].

3   DRUGS YIELDING FREE RADICAL METABOLITES

Free radicals are produced during the metabolism of many medical and non-medical drugs by enzymes such as cytochrome P450-dependent monooxygenases or peroxidases. In some cases, chemicals can redox cycle using reductases (e.g., cytochrome P450-reductase) by catalysing an electron reduction; some redox cycling drugs reduce molecular oxygen by one electron to generate superoxide which, in the presence of transition metals such as iron, can produce the very reactive hydroxyl radical (HO') by the well known iron-catalized Haber-Weiss reaction. Therefore, chemicals able to release iron from storage proteins can be very toxic, causing protein, lipid and nucleic acid oxidation.

A wide variety of chemical toxins, including some medical drugs, have been

Table 2. Free radicals by the metabolism of medical and nonmedical drugs.

Chemical	Radical metabolite	References
CCl_4	$\cdot CCl_3$	[39]
Daunomycin (daunorubicin)	$Q\cdot, O_2^{\cdot-}$	[40]
Adriamycin (doxorubicin)	$Q^{\cdot-}, O_2^{\cdot-}$	[40]
Mitoxantrone	$N\cdot$	[40]
Nitrofurantoin	$RNO_2^{\cdot-}, O_2^{\cdot-}$	[41]
Nitrofurazone	$RNO_2^{\cdot-}, O_2^{\cdot-}$	[41]
Metronidazole	$RNO_2^{\cdot-}, O_2^{\cdot-}$	[41]
Acetaminophen	$ArO\cdot$	[42]
6-Hydroxydopamine	$Q^{\cdot-}, O_2^{\cdot-}$	[42]
4-Hydroxyanisole	$Q^{\cdot-}, ArO\cdot$	[42]
Etoposide (VP-16)	$Q^{\cdot-}, \cdot OH$	[42]
Benzidine	$ArNH_2^{\cdot+}$	[42]
Aminopyrine	$RN(CH_3)_2^{\cdot+}$	[43]
Clorazil	$R^{\cdot-}$	[44]
Phenylhydrazine	$Ar\cdot, O_2^{\cdot-}$	[45]
3-Methylindole	$N\cdot$	[46]
Probucol	$ArO\cdot$	[46]
FeSO4	$\cdot OH$	[46]
Methimazole	$RS\cdot$	[46]
Chlopromazine	$CPZ^{\cdot+}$	[47,48]
Salicylanilides	$Ar\cdot$	[49]

found to metabolize to free radicals in biological systems (Table 2). In some cases, the free radical metabolite is responsible for the toxic effect of a given agent, while in others it may react further to give both radical and nonradical species. Below are some examples.

3.1 Carbon tetrachloride

One of the earliest free radical metabolites known to be implicated in the toxicity of a xenobiotic is the trichloromethyl radical ($\cdot CCl_3$). In 1961, Butler [39] proposed that this radical was responsible for the hepatotoxicity of carbon tetrachloride (CCl_4). It is generally accepted that the reductive dehalogenation product of CCl_4 results from metabolic activation by cytochrome P450-dependent monooxygenases. The immediate consequences of the metabolic activation of CCl_4 are the lipid peroxidation and covalent binding to proteins, but the subsequent events leading to centrolobular necrosis of the liver remain unclear. The mechanism probably involves reductive cleavage of the C-Cl bond [46,50,51], yielding the trichloromethyl radical:

$$CCl_4 \ + \ e^- \ \xrightarrow{\text{cytochromeP450}} \ \cdot CCl_3 \ + \ Cl^- \ \xrightarrow{O_2} \ Cl_3COO\cdot$$

A second carbon-centered radical derived from CCl_4 metabolism was discovered more recently by Connor et al. [52]. This is the carbon dioxide anion radical ($CO_2^{\cdot-}$), which was identified in the effluent perfusate of the isolated perfused liver following infusion of halocarbon. It was initially suggested that the formation of this second radical involved molecular oxygen [52]. In the proposed pathway, the trichloromethylperoxyl radical formed from the reaction of $\cdot CCl_3$ with O_2 was seen as a secondary product of the reductive CCl_4 metabolism. The decomposition of the trichloromethylperoxyl radical to $OC\cdot -Cl$ could be followed by hydrolysis to $CO_2^{\cdot-}$. The reaction sequence most likely responsible for $CO_2^{\cdot-}$ radical formation involves the trichloromethyl peroxyl radical ($CCl_3OO\cdot$), which is converted to the trichloromethoxy radical ($CCl_3O\cdot$) by a two-electron reduction followed by the promotion and elimination of a water molecule:

$$Cl_3COO\cdot \xrightarrow[-H_2O]{2e^- + 2H^+} Cl_3C\cdot O^- \xrightarrow{OH^-} ClC\cdot O + HOCl + Cl^-$$

The carbon dioxide anion radical $CO_2^{\cdot-}$ could be generated directly from hydrolysis of the chloro-carbonyl radical:

$$ClC\cdot O \xrightarrow[\substack{-HCl \\ -H^+}]{H_2O} CO_2^-$$

The carboin dioxide anion radical is known to reduce oxygen to superoxide:

$$CO_2^- \xrightarrow{O_2} CO_2 + O_2^-$$

forming also carbon dioxide, the final product of CCl_4 metabolism. However, recent investigations have cast doubt on this pathway and the most likely explanation foresees the cytosolic formation of $\cdot CO_2^-$ radical from water via an intermediate containing glutathione (GSH), which might play an important role in the overall process [53,54].

3.2 Clozapine

The use of clozapine, a unique antipsychotic drug, has been restricted due to a $1-2\%$ incidence of drug-induced agranulocytosis [55]. Hypersensitivity reactions in general appear to be linked to its metabolic activation by human myeloperoxidase (MEP) and horseradish peroxidase (HRP) in monocytes and neutrophils [56]. During phagocytosis, these cells are activated and release significant quantities of myeloperoxidase and hydrogen peroxide [57]. The peroxides are generally able to bioactivate aromatic amines via one-electron transfer reactions, leading to the formation of free radicals metabolites. MEP activity may thus, convert hydrogen peroxide and chloride ions to hypochlorous acid, which is a powerful oxidant catalyzing 2-electron oxidations [57]. The evidences currently available seem to indicate that clozapine is metabolized to a free radical by both HRP

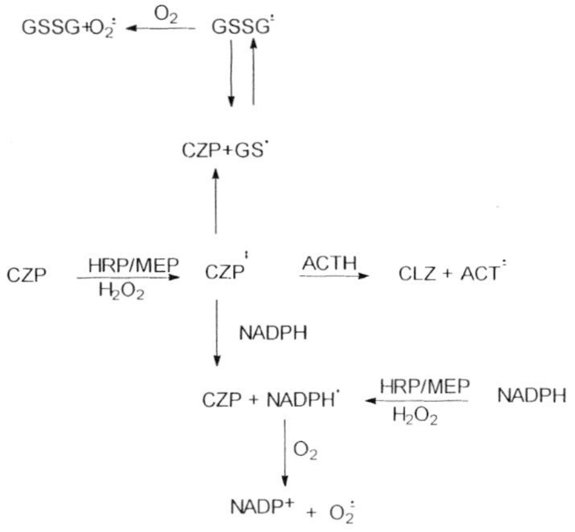

Fig. 2. Scheme for the clozapine (CZP)-metabolism by HRP/MEP system involving subsequent reactions with glutathione (GSH), NADPH or ascorbate (ACT). HRP: horseradish peroxidase; MEP: myeloperoxidase; ACTH: monodehydro-ascorbate.

and MEP systems. A clozapine cation radical would be a very electrophilic species, generated as reported in Fig. 2. The adduct formation could proceed through different mechanisms such as radical-radical coupling or addition of the nucleophilic glutathione anion to the clozapine radical cation, as depicted in Fig. 3. The resulting neutral radical adduct could then be oxidized by a second

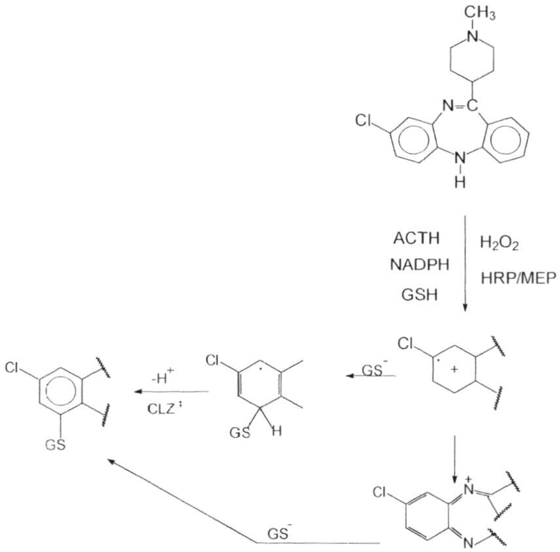

Fig. 3. Proposed clozapine (CZP) bioactivation. HRP: horseradish peroxidase; MEP: myeloperoxidase; ACTH: monodehydro-ascorbate.

clozapine cation radical or by another oxidant to produce the final stable adduct. Another possibility foresees a second-order radical disproportionation forming the two-electron oxidation product, di-imine [58].

Although glutathione conjugation is usually considered to be a detoxification process, conjugation with semiquinones or aminophenoxyl free radicals does not necessarily lead to less redox-active species [59—61]. The clozapine cation radical itself also behaves as a strong oxidant and, if thiyl radicals are formed in excessive amounts, oxidative stress may result, due to the depletion of the glutathione pool and the formation of the ROS that are probably responsible for clozapine-induced disorders. On the other hand, ascorbate at physiological concentration is able to reduce the clozapine cation free radical, thereby inhibiting not only oxidative stress but also protein and glutathione adduct formation [62—66]. The coadministration of clozapine with antioxidants such as ascorbic acid to patients should be beneficial in reducing the risk of agranulocytosis [57—67].

3.3 Aminopyrine

The clinical use of aminopyrine was sharply curtailed when it was found to be responsible for potentially fatal bonemarrow toxicity and agranulocytosis [68]. However, this substrate is still widely employed to assess either in vivo or in vitro the activity of the cytochrome P450-dependent monooxygenase system. It has been shown that the hypochlorous acid formed by the neutrophil myeloperoxidase system, is capable of producing free radical electrophilic metabolites as reported in the proposed scheme (Fig. 4), which are probably coresponsible for the drug toxicity [68].

3.4 Phenylbutazone

During the prostaglandin H synthase-(PHS)-catalyzed reduction of the hydroperoxy endoperoxide PGG_2, a number of xenobiotics including phenylbutazone are

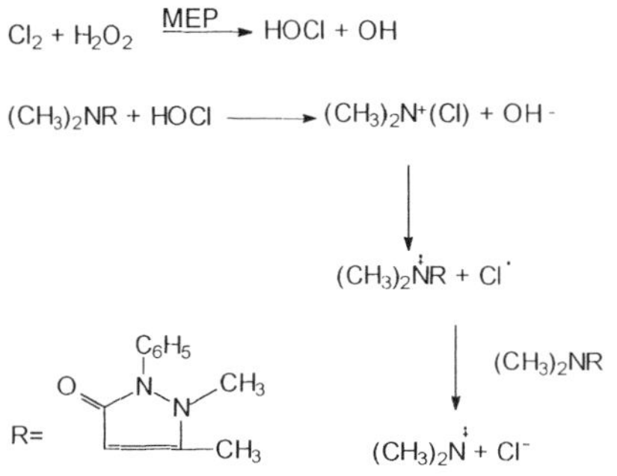

$$Cl_2 + H_2O_2 \xrightarrow{MEP} HOCl + OH$$

$$(CH_3)_2NR + HOCl \longrightarrow (CH_3)_2N^+(Cl) + OH^-$$

$$(CH_3)_2\overset{\cdot}{N}R + Cl^\cdot$$

$$(CH_3)_2NR$$

$$(CH_3)_2\overset{\cdot}{N} + Cl^-$$

R=

Fig. 4. Proposed scheme for the formation of aminopyrine (AMP) cation radical $AMP^{+\cdot}$ by the myeloperoxidase (MEP)-H_2O_2-Cl^- system. MEP: myeloperoxidase.

cooxidized by PHS-hydroperoxidase [69,70]. This nonsteroidal anti-inflammatory drug, firstly introduced in the 1950s to relieve the symptoms of rheumatoid arthritis, can produce serious side-effects [71]. The metabolic pathway of phenylbutazone to 4-hydroxyphenylbutazone occurs via the formation of a carbon-centered radical in the diketone moiety (position C-4). This radical can react with molecular oxygen to form a peroxyl radical [72]. The abstraction of a hydrogen atom results in the formation of 4-hydroperoxyphenylbutazone, which is thought to be reduced to 4-hydroxyphenylbutazone by PHS hydroperoxidase [72]. The proposed PHS-dependent metabolism is shown in Fig. 5.

A potential mechanism for the formation of 4-hydroxyphenylbutazone could involve the so-called "self-reaction", a chain termination reaction between two phenylbutazone peroxyl radicals forming a tetroxide [73]. The last intermediate rearranges to two alkoxy radicals and molecular oxygen in the triplet state [74], leading to production of 4-hydroxyphenylbutazone, after the abstraction of hydrogen atoms by the reactive alkoxy radical [75]. Therefore, it seems that the phenoxybutazone peroxyl radical can either abstract a hydrogen atom to yield 4-hydroxyperoxyphenylbutazone, or react with another peroxyl radical and eventually rearrange to 4-hydroxyphenylbutazone [76]. Considering the potency of phenylbutazone to inhibit PHS and prostacyclin synthase, the proposed inhibited species was the phenylbutazone peroxyl radical. Alternatively, if the peroxyl radicals self-react to form the tetroxide, the decomposition product of this intermediate, the alkoxy radical could be the inhibitor [76,77].

It was recently reported that, hem protein systems such as myoglobin- and hemoglobin-H_2O_2-dependent systems oxidize phenylbutazone into a free radical metabolite that is capable of initiating lipid peroxidation and inactivating α_1-anti-

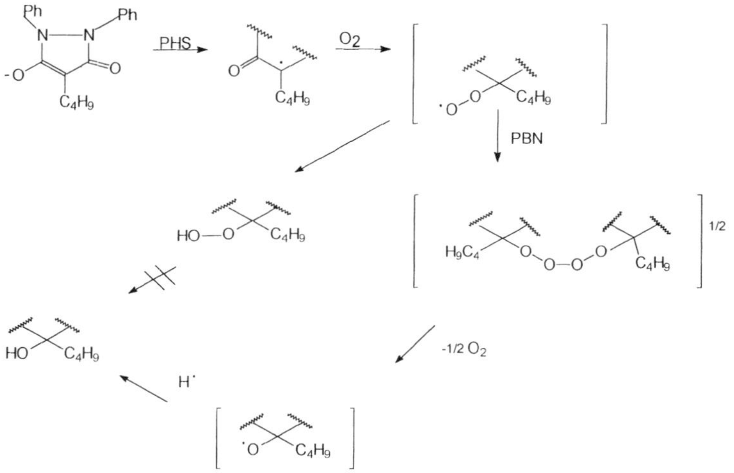

Fig. 5. Prostaglandine H syntase (PHS) hydroperoxidase-mediated metabolism of phenilbutazone (PNB).

proteinase [71]. This is particularly deleterious at the sites of chronic inflammation and tissue injury, where haem proteins can become available to catalyze
such reactions [77—79].

3.5 Nitrofurantoin

Nitrofurantoin (NTF) is widely used as an antibacterial agent known to be particularly effective in the treatment of acute urinary tract infections [80,81].
Although it does not seem to have carcinogenic properties [82], prolonged
administration of the drug has frequently been found to result in pulmonary
fibrosis [83]. NTF can be reduced by NADPH-cytochrome c-reductase and
xanthine oxidase [84]. In both enzymatic reactions, the drug is able to catalyze
or stimulate ethylene formation from methionine via the production of a strong
oxidant (cripto-HO$^{\cdot}$ radical) [85]. The production of this reactive species does
not need to involve $O_2^{\cdot-}$ directly, but the presence of high amounts of SOD in
the xanthine oxidation reaction resultes in a total inhibition of ethylene formation
[86]. It has been proposed that at or very close to the xanthine oxidase system,
the following reactions can take place:

$$NTF + e^- \rightarrow NTF^{\cdot-}$$
$$O_2 + e^- \rightarrow O_2^{\cdot-}$$
$$NTF^{\cdot-} + O_2 \leftrightarrow NTF + O_2^{\cdot-}$$
$$2O_2^{\cdot-} + 2H^+ \rightarrow H_2O_2 + O_2$$
$$NTF^{\cdot-} + H_2O_2 \rightarrow \underset{\text{crypto} - HO^{\cdot}}{(NTF^{\cdot-} - H_2O_2)}$$

Reactions occurring some distance away from xanthine oxidase may be:

$$NTF + O_2^{\cdot-} \leftrightarrow NTF^{\cdot-} + O_2$$
$$2O_2^{\cdot-} + 2H^+ \rightarrow H_2O_2 + O_2$$
$$NTF^{\cdot-} + H_2O_2 \rightarrow \underset{\text{crypto} - HO^{\cdot}}{(NTF^{\cdot-} - H_2O_2)}$$

depending on the capability of $O_2^{\cdot-}$ to diffuse away from the immediate vicinity
of the enzymatic system to the general reaction mileau, where the NTF/NTF$^{\cdot-}$
ratio would be greater than in proximity to the enzyme. The reaction between
superoxide and the drug is reversible, and near the enzyme the equilibrium would
be expected to favor the generation of $O_2^{\cdot-}$. Away from xanthine oxidase, the
equilibrium would be reversed and the NTF$^{\cdot-}$ radical increased. This radical
can subsequently react with H_2O_2, whether derived from the enzyme or $O_2^{\cdot-}$ dismutation, leading to the formation of crypto-HO$^{\cdot}$ radicals which can further oxidize the methionine to ethylene [86]. Additional evidence showed that even in
conditions of complete anaerobiosis, the reductase system was able to generate
the highly reactive crypto-HO$^{\cdot}$ radical from H_2O_2 and NTF$^{\cdot-}$ [87]. This radical,

together with ROS, may also play a central role in the mechanism of pulmonary toxicity of the compound [86,88—90].

3.6 Doxorubicin

The anthracycline antibiotic doxorubicin (DXC) exerts a powerful action against a wide range of human malignancies such as acute leukemia, non-Hodgkin lymphomas, breast cancer, Hodgkin's disease and sarcomas [91]. Apart from several side-effects that are common to many cancer chemotherapeutics, it is currently thought that free radical metabolites are critically involved in the cytotoxic mechanism of doxorubicin against tumor cells. It is known that suitable flavoproteins catalyze the formation of reduced semiquinone radicals by accepting electrons from NADPH or NADH and donating them to the drug. By reducing oxygen to superoxide the parental chemical is then regenerated. This "redoxcycling" reaction is potentially harmful to cells since a relatively small quantity of the drug is able to generate numerous superoxide radicals [92,93]. The formation of an oxidized semiquinone in a different ring of doxorubicin is known to occur in the presence of iron when no reducing system is available. The reaction of the semiquinone iron complex reacting with molecular oxygen yields a fully oxidized form of doxorubicin and oxygen radicals [94,95].

3.6.1 Free radicals generation by redox-cycling

The reductive redox-cycling of doxorubicin was first described in 1977 [96], using the NADPH cytochrome P450-reductase as a motor enzyme, and later NADH dehydrogenase and xanthine oxidase were also shown to catalyze the one-electron reduction of the drug [97,98]. For this reason, the metabolism can occur in mithocondria, endoplasmic reticulum, cytoplasm and nucleus. The nucleus-catalyzed redox-cycling of doxorubicin led to the knowledge of how site-specific activation of the drug after DNA binding lead to the formation of free radicals. Redox cycling, however, is rapid in the presence of oxygen and slow under hypoxic conditions.

The oxygen-dependent mechanism of doxorubicin metabolism involves the generation of hydroxyl radicals as DNA damaging species. The drug can be reduced by cellular flavoproteins to yield a 1-electron reduced semiquinone form. In the presence of oxygen, the semiquinone free radical is oxidized back to the parental quinone with the formation of superoxide radicals, as depicted in Fig. 6:

$$2O_2^- + 2H^+ \rightarrow H_2O_2 + O_2$$
$$O_2^- + Fe^{3+} \rightarrow O_2 + Fe_2^+$$
$$H_2O_2 + Fe_2^+ \rightarrow HO^\bullet + OH^- - + Fe$$

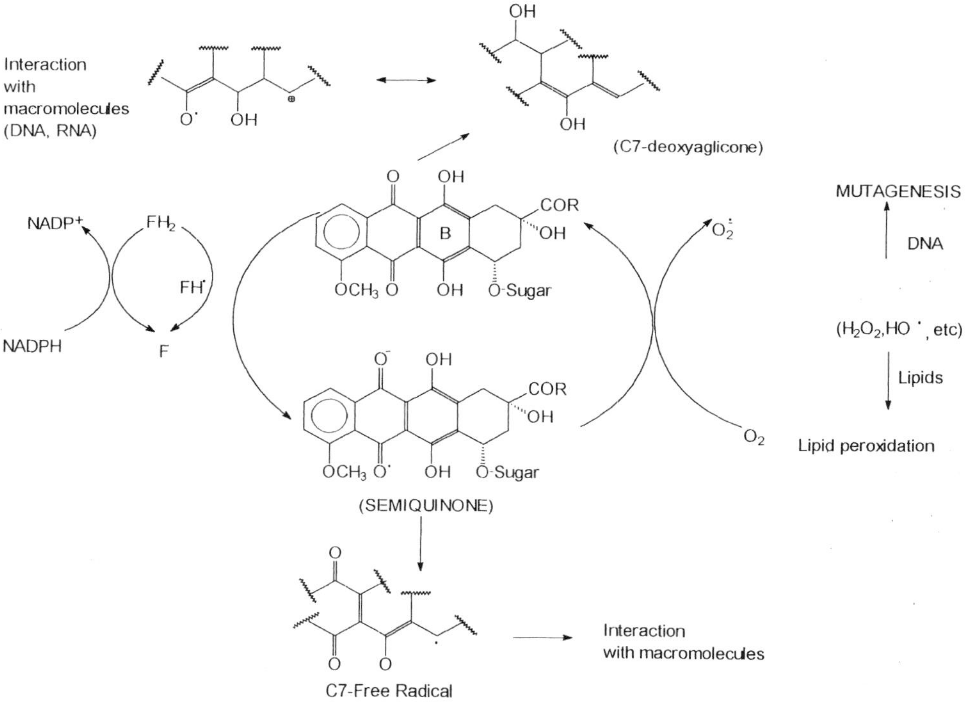

Fig. 6. Free radical generation by doxorubicin (DXC) metabolism.

These oxygen radicals are responsible for DNA damage, since the presence of SOD, CTS and iron chelator inhibit their cytotoxicity in several experimental models [99].

In the absence of molecular oxygen (Fig. 6), the unstable semiquinone loses its sugar moiety, yielding an intermediate C7 free radical which can bind covalently to cellular macromolecules or become again reduced forming a relatively stable product, the C7-deoxyaglicone [100,101]. A tautomer of C7-deoxyaglicone is the C7-quinone-methide, which is a strong DNA alkylating agent and is potentially toxic for tumor cells [102,103].

In the presence of submicromolar concentrations of iron and at low partial pressure of oxygen, the semiquinone of doxorubicin can react with H_2O_2 to cause the breakdown of deoxyribose [104]. The very low iron requirements for the reaction and the optimal oxygen tension required (approximatively 4 mmHg) may mimic the situation occurring in tumor cells [105]. Again, both in the presence or in the absence of oxygen, lipid peroxidation can be induced by the doxorubicin semiquinone radical, probably mediated by the HO species [106].

3.6.2 Free radicals generation by drug iron complex

Doxorubicin-iron complex can support free radical formation either by reducing system or by itself in the absence of reducing systems. The doxorubicin-iron III complex (DXC-Fe^{3+}), in the presence of a reducing system such as NADH cytochrome P450-reductase or of thiols like glutathione (GSH) and cysteine, may be reduced to DXC-Fe^{2+} (Fig. 7). The latter complex can react with oxygen or hydrogen peroxide leading to the generation of superoxide or hydroxyl radical while the complex is oxidized to yield DXC-Fe^{3+} again [95,107,108]. This GSH driven to HO$^{.}$ production is a typically cyclic process, which in the presence of sufficient amounts of GSH can proceed indefinitely, in a very similar manner to redox cycling [109]. Without the presence of a suitable reducing apparatus, DXC-Fe^{3+} can reduce its chelate irons by means of an intramolecular redox reaction either by oxidation on the C9 side chain or the hydrochinone moiety at ring B, producing a doxorubicin free radical chelated with Fe^{2+} [94,110,111]. This intramolecular reaction is probably catalyzed by DNA, which in the presence of oxygen yields superoxide radical and with H$_2$O$_2$ can also produce hydroxyl radical (Fig. 7) [112,113]. Oxidation of the side chain will ultimately lead to the gen-

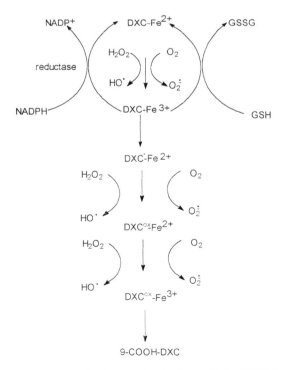

Fig. 7. Free radical generation by doxorubicin (DXC)-iron complex. GSH: glutathione.

eration of 9-dehydroxyacetyl-9-carboxyl doxorubicin (9-COOH-DXC) [111].

Contrary to intercalated doxorubicin, the drug-iron complex preserves its ability to catalyze oxygen radicals in the presence of double strand DNA [107]. Therefore, doxorubicin-iron complex-driver hydroxyl radical generation can proceed near DNA and has a high potential to induce DNA insults, especially in the light of its own probable ability to catalyze HO˙ production by this complex [112,113]. Free radical generation in cardiac cells is due to one-electron reduction of the drug occurring in several subcellular compartments, and seems to be responsible for the cardiotoxicity which is an important dose-limiting factor of its use in cancer treatment [106,114].

4   OXIDATIVE DAMAGE BY DRUGS DEPLETING GLUTATHIONE

Acetaminophen is an acetanilide widely used as an antipyretic and analgesic drug, which can cause hepatocellular necrosis in man and experimental animals [115,116]. Evidence from a variety of studies has indicated a model where the microsomal cytochrome P450-dependent system plays an important role in the oxidation of the drug to a chemically reactive and potentially toxic metabolite, highly reactive both as an electrophile and as reactive oxidant [117].

At low doses, the nonenzymatic conjugation of the reactive metabolite of acetaminophen with glutathione is believed to serve as a detoxification mechanism [117]. However, at high doses, intracellular glutathione levels are significantly depleted allowing the reactive metabolite to bind covalently to hepatic protein and to stimulate peroxidative events [118]. In other words, the cellular toxicity occurs only when glutathione stores fall below critical concentrations. In addition to the glutathione conjugate of acetoaminophen, other thioether metabolites have been identified (e.g., 3-mercapturic acid), and these are considered to represent biotransformation products of the glutathionyl precursor [119,120]. The 3-thioether structures of these conjugates support the contention that the reactive metabolite of acetaminophen is the quinone derivative, the *N*-acetyl-p-benzoquinone imine, which is prone to nucleophilic attack (e.g., by sulphydryl agents

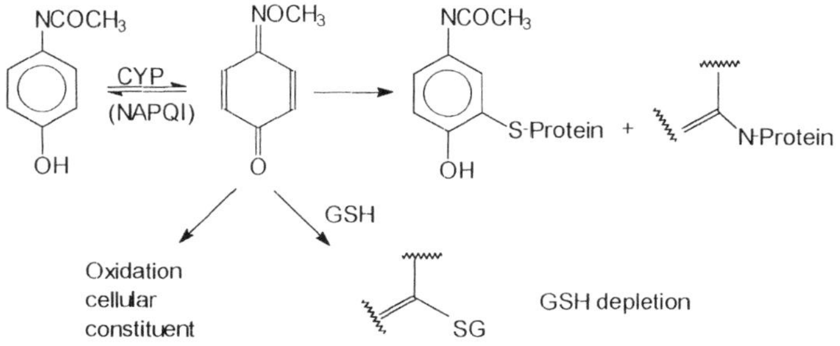

Fig. 8. Proposed pathway of acetaminophen metabolism. NAPQI: *N*-acetyl p-quinoneimine. GSH: glutathione.

such as glutathione) at the 3-position as shown in Fig. 8. The drug is initially metabolized by cytochrome P450 isoforms to give *N*-hydroxyacetaminophen which has been shown to be more toxic than the drug itself [121,122]. However, the formation of this intermediate has been questioned [123]. The metabolite is relatively instable at physiological pH and temperature and presumably undergoes water loss to form the *N*-acetyl-p-quinoneimine (NAPQI) [124]. This reactive metabolite can either react with GSH to form GSH-conjugates or can oxidize GSH to its disulfide GSSH with the concomitant production of acetaminophen. In cells with a functioning GSH-reductase, the rapid increase in GSSG is transient and is rapidly reduced back to GSH [118].

NAPQI may then undergo enzyme mediated conjugation or reduction by GSH. A number of investigations have shown that NAPQI is able to bind covalently to cellular macromolecules which, along with the concomitant GSH depletion, can have a pivotal role in acetaminophen cytotoxicity [125,126]. Because of these properties, NAPQI may stimulate lipid peroxidation, probably, with the aid of the released proinflammatory cytokines which are capable of mediating cytolytic effects by means of the induced overgeneration of ROS [123,127,128].

5   INDUCERS OF CYP ISOZYMES

The superfamily of cytochrome P450 genes encodes a variety of metal-isoenzymes with a wider but overlapping substrate specificity that catalyzes the metabolism of endo- and xenobiotics either into biologically inactive metabolites, or in some cases, into reactive ones. Reactions by these structurally different catalysts, involving the use of molecular oxygen and NADPH or NADH as a source of reducing power are considered to exhibit various types of activities such as monooxygenases, peroxidases, oxidases, reductases and desaturases.

The utilization of molecular oxygen for the combined oxidation of NADPH and target xenobiotics makes the cytochrome P450 superfamily of isoenzymes a potentially significant source of ROS. In protecting living organisms by facilitating the metabolism of various toxins, the cytochrome P450-dependent system potentially endangers an organism by causing activation of oxygen. During the monooxygenase catalytic cycle, this hemoprotein forms the pivot of the oxygen indispensable for its monooxygenase function:

$$RH + NADPH + H^+ \xrightarrow{\text{monooxygenase CYP}} ROH + NADP^+ + H_2$$

As observed by Gillette et al. [129] as long ago as 1957, the oxidation of NADPH also involves the generation of hydrogen peroxide:

$$NADPH + H^+ \xrightarrow{\text{oxidase CYP}} NADP^+ + H_2O_2$$

Although several possibilities have been hypothesized, the production of H_2O_2 either in the presence or in the absence of substrate, seems to originate via autoxidation of the oxy-cytochrome P450 complex:

$$Fe^{3+}O_2^- \longrightarrow Fe^{3+} + O_2^-$$

liberating O_2^-, which in turn spontaneously dismutates to give H_2O_2 [130]:

$$2H^+ + O_2^- + O_2^- \longrightarrow H_2O_2 + O_2$$

In the presence of transition metals hydrogen peroxide may be important for the microsomal generation of the very reactive hydroxyl radicals according to the Haber-Weiss reaction:

$$O_2^- + H_2O_2 \longrightarrow HO^. + O_2 + OH^-$$

Alternatively, hydrogen peroxide can also be reused by cytochrome P450 when operating in its peroxidase mode of activity, depicted as:

$$RH + H_2O_2 \xrightarrow{\text{peroxidase CYP}} ROH + H_2O$$

It should be noted that the overall significance of ROS generation by the cytochrome P450 apparatus would consider not only the toxicological consequences of the phenomenon, but also the role that O_2^-/HO$^.$ radicals may have in xenobiotic metabolism. Many chemicals such as adrenaline, benzoate, ethanol, aniline, safrole, dimethylsulphoxide and benzene are actually biotransformed by these active oxygen species that are derived from the cytochrome P450-system [130]. In some cases, the metabolic pathway involves the production of free radical metabolites (i.e., α-hydroxyethyl radical from ethanol or hydroxycyclohexadienyl radical and phenol from benzene) which can impose an oxidative stress [131].

The active oxygen production by the microsomal monooxygenase system is then increased by cytochrome P450 inducers, leading to a magnification of the processes described above [129,130]. It has recently been reported that the overproduction of O_2^- by cytochrome P450 overexpression, is not a prerogative of the induction of certain isozymes, as was initially discovered for cytochrome P450 2B1 and cytochrome P450 2E1 [130,132,133], but instead parallels the "unspecific" cytochrome P450 induction [134]. More generally, a strict correlation exists between the induction of each cytochrome P450 gene family and the O_2^- yield [134]. The importance of this phenomenon is underlined by the fact that an impressive number of chemical compounds, some of which are reported in Table 3, are to various extent capable of inducing cytochrome P450 enzymes. Many of these inducers are widely used medical drugs (Table 4).

Cytochrome P450 induction occurs by various mechanisms currently poorly understood in organisms that have diverged extensively during evolution. It is likely that the induction is advantageous from an evolutionary point of view, possibly as a mechanism by which terrestrial organisms confront potentially toxic

Table 3. Cytochrome P450 inducers.

Xenobiotics		References
1.	1,1,1,2-Tetrachloroethane	[135]
2.	1,1-Dichloroethylene	[136]
3.	1,2-Benzanthracene	[137]
4.	1,2-Dimethylhydrazine	[138]
5.	1,4-Bis[2-(3,5-chloropyridyloxy)]benzene	[139]
6.	1,4-Dioxane	[135]
7.	1,9-Cichlorotetrachloro-p-dibenzodioxin	[140]
8.	1-Aminoanthracene	[140]
9.	1-Aminomethyltetrachloro-p-dibenzodioxin	[140]
10.	1-Cyanotetrachlorodibenzodioxin	[140]
11.	1-Methylchrysene	[140]
12.	11-Aminoundecanoid	[135]
13.	16α-Cyanopregnenolone	[141]
14.	16α-Hydroxyestrone	[142]
15.	2,3,4,4′,5,5′-Hexachlorobiphenyl	[140]
16.	2,2′,4,4′,5,5′-Hexachlorobiphenyl	[140]
17.	2,2′,4,4′-Tetrachlorobiphenyl	[140]
18.	2,3-Terbutylhydroxyanisole	[143]
19.	2,3,3′,4,4′,5-Hexachlorobiphenyl	[140]
20.	2,3,3′,4,4′-Pentachlorobiphenyl	[140]
21.	2,3,4,4′,5,6-Hexachlorobiphenyl	[140]
22.	2,3,4,4′,5-Pentachlorobiphenyl	[140]
23.	2,3,4,4′-Tetrachlorobiphenyl	[140]
24.	2,3,4,5-Tetrachlorobiphenyl	[140]
25.	2,3,7,8-Tetrachloro-p-dibenzodioxin	[140]
26.	2,3,7,8-Tetrachlorodibenzofuran	[144]
27.	2,3,7,9-Tetrachloro-p-dibenzodioxin	[140]
28.	2,3,7-Trichloro-p-dibenzodioxin	[140]
29.	2,4,5-Trichlorophenol	[135]
30.	2,4,5-Trimethylaniline	[135]
31.	2,4,6-Trichlorophenol	[135]
32.	2,4-Dichlorophenoxyacetic acid	[139]
33.	2,4,5-Trichlorophenoxyacetic acid	[135]
34.	2,4-Dimethoxyaniline	[135]
35.	2,6 Bis(L-methylethyl)phenoxy]sulfonylcarbamic acid	[135]
36.	2,6 Bis(L-methylethyl)phenylester]carbamic acid	[145]
37.	2-Acetylaminfluorene	[140]
38.	2-Acetylfluorene	[140]
39.	2-Allylisopropylacetamide	[146]
40.	2-Aminoanthracene	[140]
41.	2-Aminobiphenyl	[140]
42.	2-Aminofluorene	[140]
43.	2-Chloro-p-phenylenediamine	[135]
44.	2-Chloroethanol	[136]
45.	2-Chloromethylpyridine	[136]
46.	2-Chloropromazine	[146]
47.	2-Hexanone	[147]

(Continued.)

Table 3. Continued.

Xenobiotics	References
48. 2-Methylcrysene	[140]
49. 3,3',4,4'-Tetrachlorobiphenyl	[144]
50. 3,3',4,4'-Tetrachloroazobenzene	[144]
51. 3,3',4,4'-Tetrachloroazoxybenzene	[144]
52. 3,3',4,4',5-Pentachlorobiphenyl	[140]
53. 3-Aminobiphenyl	[140]
54. 3-Methylchrysene	[140]
55. 3-Methylcholanthrene	[139]
56. 4,4'-Oxydianiline	[135]
57. 4-Aminobiphenyl	[140]
58. 4-Chloroacetylacetanilide	[136]
59. 4-Hydroxyestrone	[142]
60. 4-Methylchrysene	[140]
61. 5,5-Diphenylhydantoin	[144]
62. 5-Ethyl-5-phenylhydantoin	[148]
63. 5-Ethyl-5-phenyloxazolidinedione	[148]
64. 5-Methylchrysene	[140]
65. 6-Methylchrysene	[140]
66. 6-Aminochrysene	[140]
67. 6α-Methylprednisolone	[141]
68. 7-Br-Dichloro-p-dibenzodioxin	[141]
69. 7-CF$_3$-dichloro-p-dibenzodioxin	[140]
70. 7-Cl-dichloro-p-dibenzodioxin	[140]
71. 7-CN-dichloro-p-dibenzodioxin	[140]
72. 7-CO$_2$-methyldichloro-p-dibenzodioxin	[140]
73. 7-H-dichloro-p-dibenzodioxin	[140]
74. 7-1-Dichloro-p-dibenzodioxin	[140]
75. 7-Methyldichiloro-p-dibenzodioxin	[140]
76. 7-NH$_2$-dichloro-p-dibenzodioxin	[140]
77. 7-NO$_2$-dichloro-p-dibenzodioxin	[140]
78. 7-OH-dichloro-p-dibenzodioxin	[140]
79. 7-Phenyldichloro-p-dibenzodioxin	[140]
80. 8-Hydroxyquinoline	[135]
81. α-Hexachlorocyclohexane	[147]
82. α-Naphthylamine	[140]
83. Acetone	[139]
84. Acetylsalicylic acid	[139]
85. Acridine orange	[140]
86. Aflatoxin Bl	[135]
87. 5,5'-Diallylbarbituric acid	[139]
88. 3-(10,11-Dihydro-5H-dibenzo[a,d]cyclohepten-5-ylidene)–*N*,*N*-dimethyl-1-propanamine	[149]
89. 5-Ethyl-5-isopentylbarbituric acid	[139]
90. Anisole,2,3,5,6-tetrachloro-4-nitro	[136]
91. Anthracene	[140]
92. 2,3-Dimethyl-1-phenyl-3-pyrazolin-5-one	[150]
93. Aroclor 1254	[151]
94. Asbestos	[152]

(Continued.)

Table 3. Continued.

Xenobiotics	References
95. Ascorbic acid	[150]
96. β-Naphthoflavone	[139]
97. β-Naphthylamine	[140]
98. 5,5-Diethylbarbituric acid	[139]
99. 2-(4-Chlorophenyl)-α-methyl-5-benzoxazolacetic acid	[140]
100. Benzo[a]anthracene	[140]
101. Benzene	[139]
102. Benzo[a]chrysene	[140]
103. Benzo[a]pyrene	[140]
104. Benzo[b]chrysene	[140]
105. 1-([1,1′-Biphenyl]-4-ylphenylmethyl)-1H-imidazole	[153]
106. Bromobenzene	[139]
107. 5-sec-Butyl-5-ethylbarbituric acid	[139]
108. Butylated hydroxyanisole	[139]
109. Butylated hydroxytoluene	[135]
110. C.I. solvent yellow 14	[135]
111. Cannabidiol	[154]
112. 5H-dibenz[b,f]azepine-5-carboxamide	[150]
113. N-(aminocarbonyl)-2-bromo-2-ethyl-carbanamide	[155]
114. Chlordane	[146]
115. Chlorendic acid	[139]
116. Chlorometazole	[156]
117. 2-Chloro-N,N-dimethyl-10H-phenotiazine-10-propanamine	[139]
118. Chrysene	[140]
119. N-Cyano-N′-methyl-N″-[2-[[(5-methyl-1H-imidazol-4-yl)methyl]thio]ethyl] guanidine	[140]
120. 2-[4(2,2-Dichlorocyclopropyl)phenoxy]-2–methylpropanoic acid	[157]
121. 2-(4-Chlorophenoxy)-2-methylpropanoic acid	[153]
122. 5-(2-Chlorophenyl)-1,3-dihydro-7-nitro–2H-1,4-benzodiazepin-2-one	[139]
123. 1-[(2-Chlorophenyl)diphenylmethyl]-1H-imidazole	[147]
124. 5-(1-Cyclohexen-1-yl)-5-ethylbarbituric acid	[139]
125. Decabromodiphenyl oxide	[136]
126. Dehydroepiandrosterone	[139]
127. (11β,16α)-9-Fluoro-11,17,21trihydroxy-16–methylpregna-1,4-diene-3,20-dione	[158]
128. Diallyl sulfide	[147]
129. Dibenzo[a,h]antracene	[140]
130. Dichlorobenzene	[136]
131. Dichlorodiphenyltrichlorohetane	[140]
132. Dichlorvos	[136]
133. Dieldrin	[146]
134. Diphenylhydantoin	[150]
135. Disperse orange 11	[135]
136. 2-[α-(2-Dimethylaminoethoxy)-α-methylbenzyl]pyridine	[139]
137. Enldrin	[135]
138. Erythromycin	[139]
139. Ethanol	[139]
140. 1,2-Dichloroethylene	[139]

(Continued.)

Table 3. Continued.

Xenobiotics	References
141. Eucalyptol	[150]
142. Fluorine	[140]
143. *n*-Methyl-[4-(trifluoromethyl)phenoxy]-benzenepropanamine	[159]
144. 5-Methoxy-1-[4-(trifluoromethyl)-phenyl]-1-pentanone-o-(2aminoethyl)oxime	[160]
145. Geniconazole	[153]
146. 2-Ethyl-2-phenylglutarimide	[150]
147. 7-Chloro-2,4',6-trimethoxy-6'-methylspiro-[benzofuran-2(3H),1'-[2]cycloexene]-3,4'-dione	[150]
148. 5-(1-Cyclohepten-1-yl)-5-ethylbarbituric acid	[139]
149. 5-(1-Cyclohexen-1-yl)-1,5-dimethylbarbituric acid	[139]
150. α-Methyl-4-(2-methylpropyl)benzene acetic acid	[161]
151. 5-(3-Dimethylaminopropyl)-10,11-dihydro–5H-dibenzo[b,f]azepine	[149]
152. Indole-3-carbinol	[144]
153. Interferon	[162]
154. Interleukin-2	[163]
155. Imidazole	[144]
156. Isonicotinic acid hydrazide	[139]
157. Isopropanol	[144]
158. 5-(1-Propenyl)-1,3-benzodioxole	[139]
159. kepone	[135]
160. CI-1-actyl-4-[[2-(2,4-dichlorophenyl)-2–(1H-imidazol-1-ylmethyl)-1,3-dioxolan-2–yl]methoxy]phenyl]piperazine	[139]
161. Lansoprazole	[164]
162. Lindane	[150]
163. 4-(8-Chloro-5,6-dihydro-11H-benzo–[5,6]cyclohepta[1,2-b]pyridin-11-ylidene)--1-piperidinecarboxylic acid ethyl ester	[139]
164. Mandrax	[150]
165. (6α)-17-Hydroxy-6-methylpregn-4-ene-3,20-dione	[150]
166. 5-Ethyl-5-methyl-5-phenylbarbituric acid	[139]
167. 2-Methyl-2-propyl-1,3-propanediol dicarbamate	[150]
168. Methylpyrazole	[144]
169. Methyltrichlorometane	[139]
170. 2-Methyl-1,2-di-3-pyridyl-1-propanone	[165]
171. 1-[2,4-Dichloro-*β*-[(2,4-dichlorobenzyl)oxy]–phenethyl]imidazole	[139]
172. MK-0571	[139]
173. MK-7512	[144]
174. Monur	[136]
175. Musk ambrette	[143]
176. Musk xilene	[143]
177. *N*-esane	[139]
178. *N*-nitrosodimethylamine	[166]
179. *N*-phenyl-p-phenylenediamine	[135]
180. Nafenopin	[135]
181. Naphthalene	[140]
182. Nicotinic acid	[139]
183. *N,N*-diethylnicotinamide	[150]
184. Octachlorostyrene	[144]

(Continued.)

Table 3. Continued.

Xenobiotics	References
185. 5-Methoxy-2-[[(4-methoxy-3,5-dimethyl-2–pyridinil)methyl]sulfinyl]-1H. benzimidazole	[167]
186. 1,1-Dichloro-2,2-bis-(p-chlorophenyl)ethane	[135]
187. Pantoprazole	[168]
188. *trans*(-)-3-[1,3-Benzodioxol-5-yloxy)methyl]-4–(4-fluorophenyl)piperidine	[159]
189. Pentamethylbenzene	[144]
190. 5-Ethyl-5-(1-methylbutyl)barbituric acid	[139]
191. Perchloride ethylene	[139]
192. Perfluoroacetic acid	[169]
193. Perfluorobutyric acid	[169]
194. Perfluorodecanoic acid	[169]
195. Perfluorooctanoic acid	[169]
196. *N*-(4-ethoxyphenyl)acetamide	[170]
197. Phenantrene	[140]
198. 5-Ethyl-5-phenylbarbituric acid	[171]
199. Phenothiazine	[139]
200. 4-Butyl-1,2-diphenyl-3,5-pyrazolidinedione	[150]
201. 5,5-Diphenyl-2,4-imidazolinedione	[139]
202. Pentamethylbenzene	[144]
203. Propanol	[144]
204. 3-Hydroxypregn-5-en-20-one	[139]
205. Pyrazinecarboxamide	[172]
206. Pyrazole	[139]
207. Pyrene	[140]
208. Pyridine	[139]
209. RG-7512	[173]
210. Rifampicin	[175]
211. 5-(2-Propenyl)-1,3-benzodioxole	[140]
212. 5-Allyl-5-(1-methylbutyl)barbituric acid	[139]
213. SKF-525A	[174]
214. 7-(Acetylthio)-17-hydroxy-3-oxo-pregn-4-ene–21-carboxylic acid γ-lactone	[150]
215. 1,2-Diphenyl-4-[2-(phenylsulfinyl)ethyl]-3,5-pyrazolidinedione	[150]
216. 9-Amino-1,2,3,4-tetrahydroacridine	[175]
217. 5-Ethyl-5-(1-methylbutyl)-2-thiobarbituric acid	[139]
218. Toluidine	[140]
219. Toxaphene	[135]
220. *trans*-Retinoic acid	[176]
221. Tridiphane	[177]
222. Trichloroacetic acid	[139]
223. Trichloro ethylene	[144]
224. Oleandomycin triacetate ester	[139]
225. 5-[(3,4-Dimethoxyphenethyl)methylamino]-2–(3,4dimethoxyphyl)-2-isopropylvaleronitrile	[178]
226. 5-Ethyl-5-(1-methyl-1-buthenyl)barbituric acid	[139]
227. Vinyl chloride	[139]

Table 4. Cytochrome P450 inducers.

Medical drugs		References
1.	Acetylsalicylic acid	[139]
2.	Allobarbital	[139]
3.	Amitryptilyn	[149]
4.	Amobarbital	[139]
5.	Antipyrine	[150]
6.	Ascorbic acid	[150]
7.	Barbital	[139]
8.	Benoxaprofen	[140]
9.	Butobarbital	[139]
10.	Butabarbital	[139]
11.	Carbamazepine	[150]
12.	Carbromal	[136]
13.	Chlorimipramina	[150]
14.	Chlormetazole	[156]
15.	Chlorpromazine	[139]
16.	Cimetidine	[140]
17.	Ciprofibrate	[157]
18.	Clofibrate	[153]
19.	Clonazepam	[147]
20.	Clotrimazole	[147]
21.	Cyclobarbital	[139]
22.	Dehydroepiandrosterone	[139]
23.	Dexamethasone	[158]
24.	Doxylamine	[177]
25.	Eldrin	[135]
26.	Ethanol	[139]
27.	Erythromicin	[139]
28.	Fluoxetine	[159]
29.	Fluvoxamine	[160]
30.	Glutethimide	[150]
31.	Griseofulvin	[150]
32.	Heptabarbital	[139]
33.	Hexobarbital	[139]
34.	Ibuprofen	[161]
35.	Imidazole	[148]
36.	Imipramine	[149]
37.	Interferon	[162]
38.	Isoniazid	[139]
39.	Ketoconazole	[139]
40.	Lansoprazole	[164]
41.	Medroxyprogesterone	[150]
42.	Mephobarbital	[139]
43.	Meprobamate	[150]
44.	Miconazole	[139]
45.	Nikethamide	[150]
46.	Omeprazole	[167]
47.	Pantoprazole	[168]

(Continued.)

Table 4. Continued.

Medical drugs		References
48.	Paroxetina	[159]
49.	Pentobarbital	[139]
50.	Phenacetina	[170]
51.	Phenobarbital	[139]
52.	Phenothiazine	[139]
53.	Phenylbutazone	[150]
54.	Phenytoin	[139]
55.	Pregnenolone 16α-carbonitrile	[139]
56.	Pyrazinamide	[172]
57.	Rifampicin	[139]
58.	Secobarbital	[139]
59.	Spironolactone	[150]
60.	Sulfinpyrazone	[137]
61.	Tacrine	[175]
62.	Thiopental	[139]
63.	Troleandomycin	[139]
64.	Verapamil	[178]
65.	Vinbarbital	[139]

compounds in the diet and the environment [179]. From a more basic standpoint, however, along with the alteration of endogenous metabolism (where these catalysts are physiologically involved) coadministered drugs, and the metabolism of xenobiotics, cytochrome P450 induction determines a strong increase of O_2^- yield. This is particularly evident with drugs such as barbiturates (CYP2B1), ethanol (CYP2E1) and pregnenolone 16-α carbonitrile (cytochrome P450 3A) which are able to generate more severe oxidative stress [130–134]. This unremitting free radical production, imposed upon the cell by medical and nonmedical drugs, may perturb cellular defence mechanisms and thus, trigger cytotoxicity.

The induction phenomenon is even more complex since the overexpression of cytochrome P450 1A1, for example, which metabolizes polycyclic aromatic hydrocarbons, exibits a genetic polymorphism. Not surprisingly, in the presence of 100% oxygen, mice that are genetically unresponsive to cytochrome P450 induction survive significantly longer than responsive mice [180]. Again, the increase of certain cytochrome P450 isoforms such as cytochrome P450 1A1 and cytochrome P450 2B1 is associated to a pleiotropic response which involves the induction of metabolizing enzymes belonging to both phase-I and phase-II systems together with the induction of noncorrelated enzymes [134]. Under these conditions, the production of O_2^- from different cytochrome P450s can leads to a greater level of oxidative stress as compared to the one produced by the induction of single isoforms.

6 INDUCERS OF PEROXISOME PROLIFERATION

Peroxisomes are organelles widely distributed in most animal and plant cells with many vital cellular functions, such as the synthesis and the metabolism of complex biomolecules [180–185]. They contain over 40 enzymes (e.g., D-amino acid oxidase, α-hydroxyacid oxidase, polyamine oxydase and fatty acyl-CoA oxidase) including some that produce H_2O_2 (e.g., FAD-containing monooxygenases) and others that degrade H_2O_2 (e.g., CTS, GPX and SOD). A variety of structurally dissimilar xenobiotics including hypolipidemic drugs (such as clofibrate, ciprofibrate and nafenopin), phthalate ester plasticizers, trichloroethyl erbicides, and dietary factors and hormones have been reported to cause proliferation of peroxisomes [185–189]. The phenomenon of peroxisome proliferation has attracted considerable attention during the past decade due to the discovery that peroxisome proliferators have a role in the multistep process of carcinogenesis [188,189]. During an adaptive phase these compounds produce hepatomegaly and induction of peroxisomal and endoplasmic reticulum enzymes [190–194]. Chronic administration of proliferators results in the development of hepatocellular carcinomas by nonmutagenic mechanisms [194–196]. Peroxisome proliferators, which are also typical inducers of cytochrome P450 isoforms, in particular the one of the cytochrome P450 4A family, are included in Tables 3 and 4.

Under physiological conditions, peroxisomes are estimated to consume between 10 and 35% of the total oxygen utilized by liver, but since they are 10 times less abundant than mitochondria, individual peroxisomes must consume a significant amount of oxygen as compared to mitochondria [197,198]. The oxygen consumed is then converted into H_2O_2 and possibly to $O_2^{\cdot-}$, as suggested by the presence of $O_2^{\cdot-}$- and H_2O_2-producing and -degrading enzymes in peroxisomes [199–201]. Hydrogen peroxide is then degraded by catalases, but it is estimated that 2% of H_2O_2 may diffuse out into cytosol [202].

However, because of the fact that ciprofibrate-treated liver, for example, has a 25- to 30-fold increase in H_2O_2 producing oxidases, a high proportion of H_2O_2 is expected to escape from peroxisomes into cytoplasm [202]. This excessive release of H_2O_2 from peroxisomes due to a disproportionate induction of the H_2O_2-producing, FAD-containing oxidase may be a crucial factor in peroxisomal-proliferator-induced oxidative stress along with the simultaneous reduction in CTS activity in peroxisomes and an increased production of $O_2^{\cdot-}$, derived by the simultaneous cytochrome P450 induction [194]. This scenario is particularly important since it may lead to a situation of excessive H_2O_2 and $O_2^{\cdot-}$ escaping from organelles into the cytoplasm, which in turn could gain access to other intracellular compartments (e.g., nucleus), because of the parallel loss of cytosolic GPX and CuZn SOD activities [203], which could be responsible for the production of highly reactive $HO^{\cdot}$ derivatives and alteration in cellular proteins, enzymes and DNA [186–188]. Administration of clofibrate and other peroxisome proliferators also results in the induction of cell proliferation and in variable increases of a number of enzymes (pleiotropic response), and this provides support for the hypothesis that by generating active forms of oxygen the induction of the peroxisomal fatty acid β-oxidation system may play a key role in liver tumorigenesis [204].

7 SUMMARY

Although reactive oxygen species (ROS) have a prominent role in immune system defenses against invading microorganisms and in activating cytoplasmic signal transduction pathways that are related to differentiation, proliferation, cytoskeletal organization and cell death, they have been conventionally regarded as having pathological potential in a number of processes including aging, inflammation, cataract formation, arthritis, heart desease and cancer.

ROS are continuously produced in living cells as by-products of endogenous metabolism during metabolism of xenobiotics, and by radiation. However, because antioxidant defences are not completely efficient, increased ROS formation in the body (oxidative stress) is likely to induce damage.

One way of imposing oxidative stress is by the action of certain drugs, namely those that produce free radicals or deplete antioxidant defences. Thus, there is mounting interest in the possibility that the side-effects of several drugs involve increased oxidative damage.

8 PERSPECTIVES

A great deal of medical and nonmedical drugs are able to impose an oxidative stress and many pathologic states are known to involve the overgeneration of ROS. To date, however, it is not known to what extent these phenomena are due to ROS formation, or if their production is a result of the disease itself. In addition, the impressive amount of literature on this argument neither proves that ROS are involved in the induction of various illnesses, nor that drugs with anti-ROS activity are involved in their beneficial effects to these properties. However, there are models in which ROS generation is able to provoke illnesses, whose pathologic outcome can be attenuated by the use of anti-ROS drugs. Typical examples are the alloxan model of diabetes, the MTP-induced Parkinson's disease, experimental ischemia and inflammation.

ROS formations also form part of our immune system defenses and may be involved in some signaling processes. So, it would not be a medically sound approach to block their formation indiscriminately. Of course, our requirement for antioxidant vitamines evidences that ROS production must be carefully controlled, but abnormally high intakes of these vitamines appear to be of little benefit. Enzymes of antioxidant machinery have a fundamental role for the prevention of ROS-related diseases, but the overexpression of one or more of these catalysts may have a deleterious rather than a beneficial effect.

Considering that many people live in misery due to debilitating diseases such as polyarthritis, Parkinson's and Alzheimer's syndrome in which ROS generation is believed to play a leading role, appropriate site-specific anti-ROS drugs for the control of such diseases would be most welcome.

9 ACKNOWLEDGEMENTS

We thank Prof G.F. Pedulli of the Department of Organic Chemistry "A. Mangini" of the University of Bologna for critical comment and helpful advice. We also thank Drs L. Pozzetti, S. Trespidi, M.A. Antonelli for the assistance. The Authors are greatful to Drs B. Esposito, A. Camerino and Mr A. Caporali for their artwork.

This work was supported by the National Research Council of Italy (CNR) and MURST (Ministery of the University and of the Scientific and Technological Research) 40 and 60% grants.

10 ABBREVIATIONS

9-COOH-DXC: 9-dehydroxyacetyl-9-carboxyl doxorubicin
ACT: ascorbate
ACTH: monodehydro-ascorbate
AMP: aminopyrine
CTS: catalase
CYP: cytochrome P450
CZP: clozapine
DXC: doxorubicin
DXC-Fe^{3+}: doxorubicin-iron III complex
GPX: glutathione peroxidase
GSH: glutathione
HRT: horseradish peroxidase
MEP: myeloperoxidase
NAPQI: *N*-acetyl p-quinoneimine
NTF: nitrofurantoin
PHS: prostaglandin H synthase
PNB: phenylbutazone
ROS: reactive oxygen species
SOD: superoxide dismutase

11 REFERENCES

1. Bulkley GB. Lancet 1994;344:934—936.
2. Sundaresan M, Yu ZX, Ferrans VJ et al. Science 1995;270:296—299.
3. Irani K, Xia Y, Zweier JL et al. Science 1997;215:1649—1651.
4. Cerutti P, Trump C. Cancer Cells 1991;3:1—17.
5. Alessi C, Smythe C, Keise S. Oncogene 1993;8:2015—2020.
6. Larsson R, Cerutti P. J Biol Chem 1988;263:17452—17458.
7. Abate C, Patel L, Rauscher F, Curran T. Science 1990;249:1157—1161.

8. Schreck R, Rieber P, Baeuerle P. EMBO J 1991;10:2247—2258.
9. Kaina B, Stein B, Schönthal A, Rahmsdorf H. Life Sci 1990;63:632—654.
10. Cerutti PA. Lancet 1994;344:862—863.
11. Loft S, Vistien K, Ewertz M, Tionneland A. Carcinogenesis 1992;13:2241—2247.
12. Turrens JF. Xenobiotica 1990;21:1033—1040.
13. Sarafian TA, Bredesen DE. Free Radic Res Commun 1994;20:1—6.
14. Chao J, Wilhit RC, Zwolinsk BJ. Termochem Acta 1974;10:359—371.
15. England C, Corcoran WH. Ind Eng Chem Fundam 1974;13:373—381.
16. Atkinson R, Baulch DL, Cox RA et al. J Physiol Chem (Ref Data) 1992;21:1125—1444.
17. deMore Wb, Sander SP, Golden DM et al. YPL Publication. Jet Propulsion Laboratory, Posadene, California, 1992;92—120.
18. Huie RE. Toxicology 1994;89:193—216.
19. Huie RE, Padmaja S. Free Radic Res Commun 1993;18:195—197.
20. Pryor WA, Castle L, Church DF. J Am Chem Soc 1985;107:211—217.
21. Kosaka H, Himaizumi K, Tyuma I. Biochem Biopsys Acta 1981;702:237—241.
22. Titov AI. Tetrahedron Lett 1963;19:557—580.
23. Brunton G, Cruse HV, Riches KM, Whittle A. Tetrahedron Lett 1979;5:1093—1094.
24. Atkinson R, Aschman SM, Winer AM, Pitts JN. Int J Chem Kinet 1984;16:697—706.
25. Ohta T, Nagura H, Suzuki S. Int J Chem Kinet 1986;18:1—12.
26. Cooney RV, Ross PD, Bartolini GL, Ramseyen Y. Environ Sci Tecnol 1987;21:77—83.
27. Forni LG, Mora-Arellano VO, Packer JE, Willson RL. J Chem Soc Perkin Trans 1996;2:1—6.
28. Finlayson-Pitts BJ, Pitts JN. Atmospheric Chemistry. New York: Wiley-Interscience, 1986.
29. Padmaya S, and Huie RE. Biochem Biophys Res Commun 1993;195:539—544.
30. Elliot AJ, Simson AS. Can J Chem 1984;68:1831—1834.
31. Knispel R, Koch R, Siese M, Zetzsch C. Ber Bunsenger Phys Chem 1990;94:1375—1379.
32. O'Neill CA, Vander-Uliet A, Eiserich J. Pathol Biochem Soc Symp 1995;61:139—152.
33. Halliwell B, Huml ML, Louie S, Duval TL et al. FEBS Lett 1992;313:62—66.
34. Postlethwait EM, Langford SD, Jacobson LM, Bidani A. Free Radic Biol Med 1995;19:553—563.
35. Kikugawa K, Kato T, Okamoto Y. Free Radic Biol Med 1994;16:373—382.
36. Padmaja S, Huie RE. Biochem Biophys Res Commun 1993;195:539—544.
37. Bohm F, Tinkler JH, Truscot TG. Nature Med 1995;1:98—99.
38. Urban T, Hurbain I, Urban M et al. Ann Chir 1995;49:327—434.
39. Butler TC. J Pharmacol Exp Ther 1961;134:311—319.
40. Schreiber J, Mottley C, Sinha BK et al. J Am Chem Soc 1987;109:348—351.
41. Rao DNR; Harman L, Motten A, Schreiver J. Arch Biochem Biophys 1987;255:419—427.
42. Rao DNR, Fischer V, Mason RP. J Biol Chem 1990;265:844—847.
43. Griffin BW. FEBS Lett 1977;74:139—142.
44. Fischer V, Haar JA, Greiner R et al. Molec Pharmacol 1991;40:846—853.
45. Smith P, Maples KR. J Magn Res 1985;65:491—496.
46. Aust SD, Chignell CF, Bray TM et al. Toxicol Appl Pharmacol 1993;120:168—178.
47. Motten AG, Chignell CF. Magn Reson Chem 1985;23:834—841.
48. Motten AG, Buettner GR, Chignell CF. Photochem Photobiol 1985;42:9—15.
49. Chignell CF, Sik RH. Photochem Photobiol 1989;50:287—295.
50. Recknagel RO, Glende EA. Crit Rev Toxicol 1973;311—319.
51. McCay PB, Poyer JL. In: Martonosi A (ed) The Enzymes of Biological Membranes. New York: Plenum Press, 1976;239—256.
52. Connor HD, Thurman RG, Galizi MD, Mason RP. J Biol Chem 1986;261:4542—4548.
53. Lacagnin LB, Connor HD, Mason RP, Thurman RG. Molec Pharmacol 1988;33:351—357.
54. Connor Hd, Lacagnin LB, Knecht KT et al. Molec Pharmacol 1989;37:443—451.
55. Lieberman JA, Johns CA, Kane YM et al. J Clin Psychiatry 1988;49:271—277.
56. Vetrecht JP. Pharmacol Res 1988;6:265—273.

57. Babior BM. J Clin Invest 1984;73:599—601.
58. Fisher V, Haar JA, Greiner L et al. Biochem Pharmacol 1991;40:846—853.
59. Monks TJ, Lau SS, Highey RY, Gillette JR. Drug Metab Dispos 1985;13:553—559.
60. Eyer P Kiese M. Chem-Biol Interact 1976;14:165—178.
61. Takahashi N, Schreiber J, Fisher V, Mason KP. Arch Biochem Biophys 1987;252:41—48.
62. Washko P, Potrosen D, Levine M. J Biol Chem 1989;264:18996—19002.
63. Halliwell B, Foyer CH. Molec Pharmacol 1976;155:697—700.
64. Nishifimi M. Biochem Biophys Res Commun 1975;63:463—468.
65. Bando M, Obazawa H, Tanikawa T. J Free Radic Biol Med 1986;2:261—266.
66. Kataoka N, Shibata S, Immamura A et al. Chem Pharm Bull 1967;15:220—225.
67. Wainer D, Burton GW, Ingold KU et al. Biochem Biophys Acta 1987;924:408—419.
68. Kalyanaraman B, Sohnle PG. J Clin Invest 1985;75:1618—1622.
69. Mareniett L, Wlodawer P, Samuelsson B. J Biol Chem 1975;250:8510—8517.
70. Evans PJ, Cecchini R, Halliwell B. Biochem Pharmacol 1992;44:981—984.
71. Pagels WK, Sachs RJ, Marnett LJ et al. J Biol Chem 1983;258:6517—6523.
72. Ingold KU. Acc Chem Res 1969;2:1—9.
73. Howard YA, Ingold Ku. J Am Chem Soc 1968;90:1058—1059.
74. Font B, Torres JM. Qim Ind 1971;17:110—111.
75. Hughes MF, Mason RP, Eling TE. Molec Pharmacol 1988;34:186—193.
76. Reed GA, Griffin IO, Eling TE. Mol Pharmacol 1985;27:109—114.
77. Halliwell B, Hoult JRS, Blake DR. FASEB J 1988;2:2867—2873.
78. Kanner J, German JB, Kinsella JE. CRC Crit Rev Fod Sci Nutr 1987;25:317—364.
79. Odeh M. N Engl J Med 1991;324:1417—1420.
80. Boyd MR. CRC Crit Rev Toxicol 1980;103:23—40.
81. McCalla DR. In: Hahn FE (ed) Antibiotics, vol 4, part 1. Berlin: Springer, 1979;176.
82. Mason RP, Holtzman JL. Biochem Biophys Res Commun 1975;67:1267—1270.
83. Docampo R, Stoppani AOM. Arch Biochem Biophys 1979;197:317—321.
84. Wang CY, Behrens BC, Ichikawa M, Bryan GT. Toxicology 1974;23:3395—3399.
85. Sawada Y, Ohyama T, Yamazaki I. Biochem Biophys Acta 1972;268:305—308.
86. Yongman RJ, Osswald WF, Elstner EF. Biochem Pharmacol 1982;31:3723—3729.
87. Yongman RJ, Elstner EF. FEBS Lett 1981;129:265—269.
88. Buc-Calderon P, Roberfroid M. Life Sci 1990;46:207—215.
89. Martines PG, Winston GW, Metash-Ockey C et al. Toxicol Appl Pharmacol 1995;131:332—341.
90. Rao DNR, Jordan S, Mason RP. Biochem Pharmacol 1990;37:2907—2913.
91. Young RC, Ozols RF, Meyers CB. N Engl J Med 1981;305:139—153.
92. Dokoshow JR. Cancer Res 1983;43:460—472.
93. Suinger BA, Powis G. Arch Biochem Biophys 1981;209:119—126.
94. Gianni L, Zweyer JL, Levy A, Meyers CE. J Biol Chem 1985;260:6820—6824.
95. Zweyer JL. Biochem Biophys Acta 1985;839:209—213.
96. Goodman J, Hochstein P. Biochem Biophys Res Commun 1977;77:797—803.
97. Davies KYA, Doroshow JH, Chan T, Hochstein P. In: Greenwald RA, Cohen G (eds) Oxy Radicals and their Scavenger Systems: Cellular and Medical Aspects, vol 2. New York: Elsevier, 1990;313—316.
98. Doroshow JH. Cancer Res 1983;43:460—472.
99. Rowley DA, Halliwell B. Biochem Biophys Acta 1983;761:86—93.
100. Averbuch SD, Gaudiano GK, Koch TH, Bachur NR. Cancer Res 1985;45:6200—6240.
101. Moore HW. Science 1977;197:527—532.
102. Sinha BK, Chignell CF. Chem-Biol Interact 1979;28:301—308.
103. Sinha BK, Lewis-Gregory J. Biochem Pharmacol 1981;30:2626—2629.
104. Bates DA, Winterbourg CC. FEBS Lett 1982;145:137—142.
105. Winterbourg CC, Gutteridge JMC, Halliwell B. J Free Radic Biol Med 1985;1:43—49.
106. Keizer HG, Pinedo HM, Scuurhuis GJ, Hoenje H. Pharmacol Ther 1990;47:219—231.

107. Eliot H, Gianni L, Meyers C. Biochemistry 1984;23:928—936.
108. Meyers CE, Gianni L, Simone C et al. Biochemistry 1982;21:1707—1713.
109. Zweyer JL. Biochem Biophys Acta 1985;83:209—213.
110. Zweyer JL, Gianni L, Muindi J, Meyers CE. Biochem Biophys Acta 1986;884:324—336.
111. Gianni L, Vigano L, Lanzi et al. J Natl Cancer Inst 1988;80:1104—1111.
112. Muindi JRF, Sinha BK, Gianni L, Meyers CF. FEBS Lett 1984;172:226—230.
113. Muindi JRF, Sinha BK, Gianni L, Meyers CF. Molec Pharmacol 1985;27:356—365.
114. Green MD, Speyer JL, Muggia FM. Eur J Cancer Clin Oncol 1984;20:293—296.
115. Boyd EM, Bereczky GM. Br J Pharmacol 1996;26:606—614.
116. Boyer TD, Rouff SL. J Am Med Assoc 1971;218:440—441.
117. Jollow DJ et al. J Pharmacol Exp Ther 1973;187:195—202.
118. Albano E, Poli G, Chiarpotto et al. Chem Biol Interact 1983;47:249—263.
119. Nelson SD, Vaishnav Y, Kambara H, Baillie TA. Biomed Mass Spectrometry 1981;8:244—248.
120. Jollow DJ, Thorgeirsson SS, Potter WZ et al. Pharmacology 1974;12:251—256.
121. Gemborys MW, Gribble GW, Mudge GH. J Med Chem 1978;21:649—655.
122. Healey K, Calder IC, Yong AC et al. Xenobiotica 1978;8:40—44.
123. Holtzman JL. Drug Metab Rev 1995;27:277—297.
124. Miner DJ, Kissinger PT. Biochem Pharmacol 1979;28:3285—3290.
125. Streeter AJ, Dahlin DC, Nelson SD, Baillie TA. Chem Biol Interact 1984;48:349—366.
126. Devalia GL, Ogilvie RC, Mc Lean AM. Biochem Pharmacol 1982;31:3745—3749.
127. Sumoski W, Baquerizo H, Rabinovitch A. Diabetologia 1989;32:792—796.
128. Ruddle NH. Immun Today 1987;8:129—130.
129. Gillette JR, Brodie BB, Ladu BR. J Pharmacol Exp Ther 1957;119:532—540.
130. Persson YO, Terelius Y, Ingelman-Sundemberg M. Xenobiotica 1990;20:887—900.
131. Knecht KT, Bradford BU, Mason RP, Thruman RG. Molec Pharmacol 1990;38:26—30.
132. Bast A. Trends Pharmacol Sci 1996;7:266—270.
133. Ekstrom MG, Ingelman-Sundemberg M. Biochem Pharmacol 1989;38:1313—131.
134. Paolini M, Pozzetti L, Pedulli GF et al. J Invest Med Clin Res 1996;44:470—473.
135. Kitchin K, Brown J, Kulkarni AP. Mutat Res 1991;266:253—272.
136. Kitchin K, Brown J, Kulkarni AP. Teratogen Carcinogen Mutagen 1993;13;167—184.
137. Li SJ, Rodgers EH, Grant MH. Chem Biol Interact 1995;97:101—118.
138. Rosenberg DW, Mankowski DC. Carcinogenesis 1994;15:73—78.
139. Amdur OM, Doull J, Klaassen CD. Toxicology — the basic science of poison, 4th edn. New York: Pergamon Press, 1991.
140. David F, Lewis V. Drug Metab Rev 1997;29:589—650.
141. Douglas MH, Erin JG, Joyce LB et al. Molec Pharmacol 1981;21:753—760.
142. Martucci CP, Fishman J. Pharmacol Ther 1993;57:237—257.
143. Iwata N, Suzuki K, Minegishi K et al. Eur J Pharmacol 1993;248:243—250.
144. Okey AB. Pharmacol Ther 1990;45:241—298.
145. Robertson DG, Krause BR, Welty DF et al. Biochem Pharmacol 1995;49:799—808.
146. Whitlock JP, Denison MS. Induction of cytochrome P450 enzymes that metabolize xenobiotics. In: Ortiz di Montellano PR (ed) Cytochrome P450 — Structure, Mechanism and Biochemistry, 2nd edn. New York: Plenum Press, 1995;367—390.
147. Lubet RA, Dragnev KH, Chauhan DP et al. Biochem Pharmacol 1992;43:1067—1078.
148. Nims RW, Sinclair PR, Sinclair JF et al. Chem Res Toxicol 1993;6:188—196.
149. Hodgson AV, White TB, White JW, Strobel HW. Molec Cel Biochem 1993;120:171—179.
150. Gibson GG, Progress in Drug Metabolism, vol 11. London: Taylor and Francis, 1988.
151. Roelandt L, Dubois M, Todaro A et al. Ecotoxicol Environ Saf 1995;31:158—163.
152. Qamar R, Sikandar GK, Shahid A. Chem Biol Interact 1990;75:305—314.
153. Sabzevari, Hatcher M, O'Sullivan M et al. Xenobiotica 1990;25(4):395—403.
154. Bornheim LM, Everhart ET, Li J, Correia MA. Biochem Pharmacol 1994;48:161—171.
155. Ketter TA, Flockart DA, Post RM et al. J Clin Psycopharmacol 1995;15:387—398.

156. Hu Y, Mishin V, Johansson I et al. J Pharmacol Exp Ther 1994;296:1286—1291.
157. Leung LK, Glauert HP. Toxicol Lett 1996;85:143—149.
158. Sidhu JS, Omiecinski CJ. Pharmacogenetics 1995;5:24—36.
159. Shen WW. Int J Psychiat Med 1995;25:277—290.
160. Erling M, Lindstrom L, Bondesson U, Bertilsson. Ther Drug Monit 1994;16:368—374.
161. Rekka E, Ayalogu EO, Lewis DF et al. Arch Toxicol 1994;68:73—78.
162. Knickle LC, Spencer DF, Renton KW. Biochem Pharmacol 1992;44:604—608.
163. Kurokohchi K, Matsuo Y, Yoneyama H et al. Biochem Pharmacol 1993;45:582—584.
164. Steinijans VW, Huber R, Hartmann M et al. Int J Clin Pharmacol Ther 1994;32:385—399.
165. Wright MC, Paine AJ, Skett P, Auld R. J Steroid Biochem Mol Biol 1994;48:271—276.
166. Bhagwat SV, Boyd MR, Ravindranath V. Arch Biochem Biophys 1995;320:73—83.
167. McDonnell WM, Scheiman JM, Traber PG. Gastroenterology 1992;103:1509—1516.
168. Steinijans VW, Huber R, Hartmann M et al. Int Clin Pharmacol Ther 1996;36:243—262.
169. Permadi H, Lundgren B, Anderson K, Depierre J. Biochem Pharmacol 1992;44:1183—1191.
170. Nerurkar PV, Park SS, Thomas PE et al. Biochem Pharmacol 1993;46:933—943.
171. Burke MD, Thompson S, Weaver RJ et al. Biochem Pharmacol 1994;48:923—936.
172. Grange JM, Winstanley PA, Davies PD. Drug Saf 1994;11:242—251.
173. Gillum JG, Israel DS, Polk RE. Clin Pharmacokin 1993;25:450—482.
174. Griffith DA, Brown DE, Jezquel SG. Xenobiotica 1993;23:1085—1100.
175. Sinz MW, Woolf F. Biochem Pharmacol 1997;54:425—427.
176. Han IS, Choi JH. J Clin Endocrinol Metab 1996;81:2075—2096.
177. Hodgson E, Levi PE. Introduction to Biochemical Toxicology, 2nd edn. Norwalk-Connecticut: Appleton and Lange, 1994.
178. Fromm MF, Busse D, Kroemer HK, Eichelbaum M. Hepatology 1996;24:796—801.
179. Gonzales FJ, Nebert DW. Trends Genet 1990;6:182—186.
180. Gonder JC, Proctor RA, Will JA. Proc Natl Acad Sci USA 1985;82:6315—6319.
181. Hajra AK, Bishop JE. Ann NY Acad Sci 1982;386:170—182.
182. Lazarow PB, de Duve C. Proc Natl Acad Sci USA 1976;73:2043—2046.
183. Van de Bosch H, Schutgens RBH, Wanders RJA, Tager JM. Ann Rev Bichem 1992;61:157—197.
184. Singh I, Moser AE, Goldfisher SL et al. Proc Natl Acad Sci USA 1984;81:4203—4207.
185. Singh I. Peroxisome in biology and medicine: In: Malhotra SK (ed) Structural Biology, vol 3. Greenwich Ct: Jai Press, 1994;3:137—156.
186. Elliott BM, Dodd NJF, Elcombe CR. Carcinogenesis 1986;7:795—799.
187. Randernath E, Randernath K, Reddy R et al. Mutat Res 1991;64—76.
188. Kasai H, Okada Y, Nischimura S et al. Cancer Res 1989;49:2603—2605.
189. Singh I. Mammalian peroxisomes: antioxidant enzymes and oxidative stress. Oxygen Soc Meeting Proc 1994.
190. Vainio H, Linnainmaa K, Kahonen M et al. Biochem Pharmacol 1983;32:2775—2779.
191. Lazarow PB. J Biol Chem 1978;253:1522—1528.
192. Nemali MR, Usuda N, Reddy MK et al. Cancer Res 1998;48:5316—5324.
193. Reddy JK, Goel SK, Nemali MR et al. Proc Natl Acad Sci USA 1986;83:1747—1751.
194. Wu H, Masset-Brown J, Tweedie DJ et al. Cancer Res 1989;49:2337—2343.
195. Rao SM, Reddy JK. Environ Health Perspect 1991;93:205—209.
196. Rao SM, Reddy JK. Drug Metab Rev 1989;21:103—110.
197. De Duve C, Baudhuin PC. Physiol Rev 1966;46:323—357.
198. Leighton F, Poole B, Beaufay H et al. J Cell Biol 1968;37:482—513.
199. Keller G, Warner TG, Steiner KS et al. Proc Natl Acad Sci USA 1991;88:7381—7385.
200. Dhaunsi GS, Gulati S, Singh AK et al. J Biol Chem 1992;267:6870—6873.
201. Crapo JD, Oury T, Rabouille et al. Proc Natl Acad Sci USA 1992;89:10405—10409.
202. Poole B. J Theor Biol 1975;51:149—167.
203. Dhaunsi GS, Singh I, Orak JK et al. Carcinogenesis 1994;15:1923—1930.
204. Reddy JK, Usuda N, Rao MS. Arch Toxicol 1988;12:207—216.

©2000 Elsevier Science B.V. All rights reserved.
Handbook of Oxidants and Antioxidants in Exercise.
C.K. Sen, L. Packer and O. Hänninen, editors.

Part XI • Chapter 36

The paradoxical relationship of aerobic exercise and the oxidative theory of atherosclerosis

Robin Shern-Brewer[1], Nalini Santanam[1], Carla Wetzstein[1], Jill E. White-Welkley[2], Larry Price[2] and Sampath Parthasarathy[1]

Departments of
[1]Gynecology and Obstetrics,
[2]Physical Education,
Emory University Medical School, Atlanta, Georgia 30322, USA. Tel.: +01-404-727-8604. Fax: +01-404-727-8615. E-mail: spartha@emory.edu

1   INTRODUCTION
      1.1   Benefits of exercise
      1.2   Oxidative stress during exercise
      1.3   Oxidation theory of CAD
      1.4   Antioxidants and LDL oxidation
2   THE PARADOX
3   EXERCISE AND OXIDATION OF LDL
      3.1   Study 1
            3.1.1   Conclusion and limitations of study 1
      3.2   Study 2
4   COMPARISON OF STUDY 1 TO STUDY 2
      4.1 Definition of chronic exercise
5   IMPLICATIONS
6   SUMMARY
7   ACKNOWLEDGEMENTS
8   ABBREVIATIONS
9   REFERENCES

1   INTRODUCTION

The irony of the 20th century American health picture is that while many people strive for optimal health, the majority of Americans engage in very little physical activity as part of their daily life. Currently only about 24% of all adult Americans exercise regularly, a level that has remained basically unchanged since 1985 [1]. In 1990, the US Department of Health and Human Services published a report entitled Healthy People 2000: National Health Promotion and Disease Prevention Objectives [2]. The broad national goals proposed by this document are to increase the span of healthy life for all Americans, to reduce health disparities among Americans, and to secure access to preventive health services for all Americans. A major health promotion objective from this document is to increase the physical activity level of Americans. There is little doubt in the scientific community that regular aerobic exercise imparts important benefits. However, a degree of caution may be warranted with regard to specific health claims made by individuals or groups of people that are publicized largely via lay magazines, health clubs, health food stores, and/or health products concerning aerobic exercise, its benefits and its consequences. A case in point is the oxidative stress associated with aerobic exercise and the need for additional antioxidants. It is almost impossible to read through a medical journal, or even the newspaper, without encountering an article that deals with oxidative stress or antioxidant involvement in a disease process. It is imperative to develop a better understanding of the delicate balance between the pro-oxidant and antioxidant factors during aerobic exercise before nutrient supplementation recommendations can be made.

1.1 Benefits of exercise

Scientific research suggests that programmed, regular exercise have several important health benefits. In addition to enhancing physical fitness, exercise appears to reduce the risk of dying from heart disease, reduce the risks of developing diabetes and developing high blood pressure, help in the control of body weight, and promote psychological wellbeing [3—7]. Table 1 lists several potential benefits of exercise.

Table 1. Benefits of regular exercise and physical fitness.

Physical Benefits

1. Increased life expectancy	10. Increased protection against physiological effects of stress
2. Decreased risk of developing and dying from cardiovascular disease and stroke	11. Quicker recovery from illness and injury
3. Decreased risk of developing and dying from colon and rectal cancers	12. Increased resistance to fatigue
4. Decreased risk of adult-onset diabetes	13. Improved posture and body mechanics
5. Decreased risk of bone fractures from osteoporosis improved cardiac function	14. Strengthened tendons, bones, and muscles
6. Control of blood pressure levels	15. Increased lean body mass
7. Improved blood fat concentrations	16. Decreased body fat
8. Improved regulation of blood clotting	17. Decreased risk of injury
9. Improved ability to deliver oxygen to tissues	18. Reduced risk for low-back pain
	19. Improve joint health
	20. Improved performance in sport, work, and recreational activities

Mental Health Benefits

1. Tension relief and resistance to mental fatigue	5. Increased positive interaction with others
2. Reduced symptoms of stress	6. Improved appearance
3. Improved sleeping habits	7. Improved self-image
4. Increased energy level	8. Improved quality of life

Source: A report of the Surgeon General: physical activity and health. US Department of Health and Human Services, Centers for Disease Control and Prevention, 1996.

1.2 Oxidative stress during exercise

Conversely, strenuous exercise involves the consumption and utilization of oxygen, and cellular oxidative processes are enhanced. Free radicals are generated and if left unquenched can have deleterious effects on lipids, membranes, and other cellular macromolecules [8—10]. Damage can occur via oxidative reactions of polyunsaturated fatty acids in cellular membranes, nucleotides in DNA, and critical sulfhydryl bonds in proteins. Exercise has been shown to increase oxidative stress indices including lipid peroxidation, oxidative DNA damage, and intrinsic antioxidant defense systems as shown in Table 2. Antioxidants such as vitamin E and ascorbic acid are commonly thought to protect against oxidative damage by reacting with these free radicals [11]. As a result, they may be depleted in oxidative stress.

1.3 Oxidation theory of coronary artery disease (CAD)

It has been suggested that the oxidation of low density lipoprotein (LDL) is a key step in the pathogenesis of Coronary artery disease (CAD) [12—14]. Evidence for the in vivo occurrence of lipoprotein oxidation includes:
1) immuno cytochemical demonstration of epitopes formed during the oxidation of lipoproteins (malondialdehyde-MDA-lysine) in atherosclerotic lesions [15],
2) LDL extracted from lesions has physical and biological properties of oxidized LDL [16],
3) circulating antibodies against oxidized LDL are present in plasma of cardiac patients [17],
4) immune complexes between these autoantibodies and oxidized LDL are present in lesions [18], and
5) animal and human studies demonstrating the beneficial effects of antioxidants on the development of atherosclerotic lesions [19,20].
This oxidized LDL exhibits a number of potent pro-atherogenic properties, shown in Table 3.

1.4 Antioxidants and LDL oxidation

Lipophilic antioxidants, such as vitamin E, are carried in the lipoprotein and, it has been proposed that they may protect LDL against this oxidative modification [21—23]. When antioxidants are depleted from LDL, the LDL is more readily oxidized. Recent animal studies have shown that animals given antioxidants are protected against atherosclerosis despite very high levels of plasma cholesterol [24—26]. Human studies, although not as extensive as animal studies, are encouraging [27,28].

Table 2. Selected studies of exercise and oxidative indices.

Reference	Exercise	Sample	Assay
[78]	Running	Rat muscle	MDA—
[79]	Running	Rat muscle	MDA ↑
[80]	Running	Rat muscle	MDA ↑
[81]	Running	Rat muscle	MDA ↑
[82]	Running	Rat muscle	MDA ↑
[78]	Running	Rat liver	MDA ↑
[80]	Running	Rat liver	MDA ↑
[81]	Running	Rat liver	MDA ↑
[83]	Swimming	Rat heart	MDA ↑
[84]	Running	Rat urine	MDA ↑
[85]	Running	Mouse muscle	MDA —
[86]	Ergometer	Human plasma	MDA ↑
[86]	Ergometer	Human plasma	MDA —
[87]	Running	Human plasma	CD —
[88]	Ergometer	Human serum	MDA —
[89]	Running	Human serum	MDA ↑
[90]	Running	Human serum	MDA ↑
[91]	Running	Human serum	MDA ↑
[92]	Running	Human urine	MDA ↑
[93]	Walking	Human synovial fluid	MDA—
[80]	Running	Rat hind limb	EPR signals ↑
[94]	Electrically stimulated	Rat muscle	EPR signals ↑
[83]	Running	Rat heart	EPR signals ↑
[95]	Running	Human urine	8-Hydroxydeoxy Guanosine ↑
[87]	Running	Human plasma	GSH ↓ GSSG—
[96]	Running	Human plasma	GSSG ↑
		Rat plasma	GSSG ↑
[97]	Running	Rat heart	SOD activity ↑
[81]	Running	Rat liver	SOD activity ↑
[98]	Running	Rat liver	SOD activity ↑
[78]	Running	Rat liver	SOD activity ↑
[98]	Swimming	Rat skeletal muscle	SOD activity ↑
[99]	Running	Rat skeletal muscle	SOD activity ↑
[100]	Swimming	Rat skeletal muscle	GPX activity —
[99]	Running	Rat skeletal muscle	GPX activity ↓
[82]	Running	Rat skeletal muscle	GPX activity ↓
[101]	Running	Rat skeletal muscle	GPX activity ↑
[102]	Running	Rat heart	GPX activity ↑
[103]	Running	Rat platelet	GPX activity ↑
[83]	Running	Rat serum	Vitamin E ↓
[83]	Running	Rat heart	Vitamin E ↓
[104]	Running	Rat skeletal muscle	Vitamin E ↓
[105]	Running	Rat skeletal muscle	Vitamin E ↓
[106]	Running	Human plasma	Vitamin E ↑
[107]	Running	Rat plasma	Vitamin E ↓
[87]	Running	Human plasma	Vitamin E —

(Continued.)

Table 2. Continued.

Reference	Exercise	Sample	Assay
[108]	Running	Human expired air	Pentane ↑
[109]	Running	Rat expired air	Hydrocarbons ↑
[110]	Cycle ergometer	Human plasma	MPO protein ↑
[111]	Downhill Running	Human plasma	MPO protein ↑

↑: increase; ↓: decrease; —: no change; MDA: malondialdehyde; CD: conjugated diene; EPR: electron paramagnetic resonance spectroscopy; GSH: reduced glutathione; GSSH: oxidized glutathione; SOD: superoxide dismutase; GPX: glutathione peroxidase.

2   THE PARADOX

There is an apparent paradox between the beneficial effects of exercise on decreasing the risk for vascular disease and the potentially damaging consequences of exercise on vascular injury, i.e., promoting free radicals that may be generated in the course of physical exertion. The use of antioxidant supplements among exercisers to prevent free radical-induced injury appears to be widely promoted; yet our current understanding of the effect of exercise on oxidative processes provides little justification for their use. The oxidation of LDL is known to be involved in atherosclerosis. Current medical science considers sustained physical activity and exercise to be a deterrent to cardiovascular ailments. Yet, exercise represents a severe form of oxidative stress. Understanding this paradox will increase our understanding of when and how oxidation may have pro- and anti-atherogenic effects and how nutrition may be tailored to the oxidative demands of the exercising population.

Table 3. Atherogenic properties of oxidized LDL.

Reference	Atherogenic properties of oxidized low density lipoprotein.
[112—114]	Chemotactic for human monocytes, T-lymphocytes and smooth muscle cells
[113,115]	Inhibits macrophage chemotaxis
[116—118]	Avidly degraded by macrophages and generates foam cells
[119—122]	Inhibits endothelium-dependent relaxation of aorta
[123—125]	Cytotoxic to cells and causes endothelial injury
[126—128]	Modified LDL increases adhesive properties of endothelial cells; Ox-LDL induces VCAM-1 gene expression in endothelial cells
[129—131]	Causes DNA fragmentation and apoptosis of lymphoblastoid cells and smooth muscle cells
[132]	Stimulates collagen production
[133,134]	Enhances platelet aggregation
[135,136]	Is immunogenic and can elicit autoantibody formation

3   EXERCISE AND OXIDATION OF LDL

Few have investigated the potential differences in susceptibility of LDL to oxidative modifications isolated from chronic exercisers and sedentary subjects. In order to address this paradox, we performed two studies.

3.1 Study 1

In the first study, we compared the oxidizability of LDL from short-term "chronic" exercisers (aerobically active more than 6 h/week) with the LDL from sedentary subjects [29]. The exercisers and sedentary subjects were significantly different with regard to fitness and lipid profile parameters. The sedentary subjects had lower aerobic capacity, higher body fat composition and a more atherogenic profile than the exercisers. These findings are in agreement with many studies reporting the benefits of aerobic activity [3—7].

The lag time of isolated LDL subjected to in vitro 2.5 μM copper oxidation was significantly shortened in the exercisers as compared to the sedentary subjects (Fig. 1). This increased sensitivity was not due to the decreased presence of vitamin E since the amount of plasma and LDL vitamin E was not different between the two groups. Instead, these findings suggest that the LDL of exercisers contain increased amounts of preformed lipid peroxides, which could account for the increased susceptibility to oxidation. It is possible that plasma lipoproteins contain trace amounts of lipid peroxides [30—32]. Lipid peroxides could be formed by endogenous lipid peroxidation reactions and transferred to LDL. Sanchez-Quesada [33] reported an increase in minimally oxidized LDL following a prolonged exercise bout. The authors attributed this to acute oxidative stress concomitant with exercise.

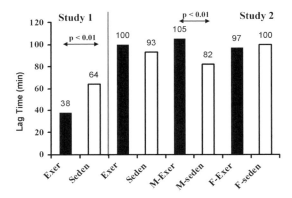

Fig. 1.

3.1.1 Conclusion and limitations of study 1

This study is the first to report the enhanced oxidizability of LDL from exercisers. If exercise has the potential to increase the susceptibility of LDL to undergo oxidative modification, the question should be asked: Is this phenomenon beneficial or is it hazardous? Exercise-induced oxidation of LDL might be beneficial if it occurred in the plasma. Exercise is known to increase the degranulation of neutrophils and subsequently increase the plasma levels of myeloperoxidase (MPO) [34—36]. Wieland et al. [37] and others [38—41] have reported that the oxidation of LDL by neutrophils and by MPO. Oxidized LDL is cleared rapidly from circulation by the liver as compared to native LDL [42,43]. In exercisers, the oxidation of LDL in the plasma may itself account for some of the lipid lowering effects of exercise and have a beneficial effect. Conversely, if this oxidation occurs in the artery wall, with subsequent foam cell formation, the supplementation of antioxidants might be warranted to help prevent this phenomenon.

Limitations of this study include the small sample size and the imbalance between the genders in the two groups. The exercise group was predominantly male and the sedentary group was predominantly female. This may suggest those females rather than sedentary subjects have a decreased susceptibility of their LDL to undergo oxidation. Other variables that could influence lag times such as fatty acid composition of the LDL [44—46], dietary intake of antioxidants [47—50] and dietary intake of fatty acids [44,47,51] were not measured.

3.2 Study 2

Study 2 was designed to investigate the impact of gender, body composition, diet, and LDL fatty acid composition on lag time in exercisers and sedentary control [29]. Both genders were represented in the two groups and the sample size was increased. The "chronic" exercisers (aerobically active more than 6 h/week) and sedentary subjects were significantly different with regard to fitness and lipid profile parameters. The sedentary subjects had a lower aerobic capacity, higher body fat composition and a more atherogenic profile than the exercisers.

The findings of study 2 suggest that "chronic" exercisers are undergoing an increased oxidative stress, indicated by a higher level of MPO protein in their plasma, as compared to the sedentary subjects. This was expected because exercise, like other oxidative stresses, has been shown to increase the demargination and degranulation of neutrophils with the subsequent release of MPO in plasma [35,36,52,53]. However, exercisers tended to have slightly longer lag times than the sedentary subjects using a 5-μM copper in vitro oxidation system, although this difference was not statistically significant (Fig. 1). This finding is in sharp contrast to the findings of study 1.

Although not statistically significant, mean LDL α-tocopherol levels were higher in the exercise group as compared to the sedentary group. This may help to explain the longer mean lag time of the exercise group since it has been demonstrated that lipid peroxidation starts only after LDL is depleted of antioxidants [54—57]. The mean polyunsaturated fatty acid (PUFA) composition of LDL was also higher in the exercisers. This suggests that their LDL should have an increased susceptibility to oxidation [44—45]. The additional availability of α-tocopherol may have outweighed the influence of the PUFAs.

Although not statistically significant, mean dietary intake of vitamin E, vitamin C and β-carotene were higher in the exercise group as compared to the sedentary group. This may also help to explain the longer mean lag time of the exercise group since all three antioxidants have been shown to prolong lag time of LDL in the copper oxidation system [58,59].

A review of the literature revealed no studies testing gender differences with regard to the susceptibility of LDL to undergo in vitro oxidation. Group by gender analysis in this study found that LDL isolated from sedentary males was significantly more susceptible to oxidation than LDL isolated from exercise males (Fig. 1). Both exercise and sedentary females had LDL with a similar susceptibility to oxidation as measured by lag time (Fig. 1). This held true when adjustments were made for age, body mass index (BMI), blood lipids, α-tocopherol levels, and MPO protein levels.

The longer lag time seen in these models of male exercisers may be explained by the increasing evidence that chronic exercise training upregulates antioxidant enzymes in skeletal muscle. Superoxide dismutase (SOD) activity has been shown to increase significantly after training [60—63]. Catalase (CAT) activity has been shown to increase [60,64], decrease [62,65], and remain the same [66] with training. With few exceptions, glutathione peroxidase (GPX) is reported to increase after training [62,65,67,68].

The similar lag times of women in these models, regardless of exercise status and concomitant oxidative stress, may be a reflection of the apparent cardiovascular protection they are afforded by virtue of their premenopausal status [69]. Premenopausal women (estradiol-rich) have a less atherogenic profile than their postmenopausal (estradiol-poor) counterparts [70,71]. Moreover, estradiol has been shown to scavenge free radicals and decrease the oxidation of LDL [72—74]. Another potential role for estradiol to influence LDL oxidation is its affect on nitric oxide (NO). Estradiol has been shown to induce the production of NO [75,76]. Shin et al. have demonstrated attenuation by NO on vascular smooth muscle cell activation thus, potentially inhibiting the entry of LDL into the intima. Chronic and acute exercise has been shown to increase nitrate in the plasma, which is a derivative of NO [77].

4   COMPARISON OF STUDY 1 TO STUDY 2

Study 1 found that exercisers had a greatly increased susceptibility to copper-induced oxidation compared to sedentary subjects. Study 2 found that male exercisers had a significantly decreased susceptibility to copper-induced oxidation compared to male sedentary subjects while females, regardless of exercise group, had a similar susceptibility. This remained the case when adjustments were made for fitness and blood lipid characteristics, as well as plasma and LDL α-tocopherol levels.

The findings of study 1 and study 2 are in direct opposition to each other. The lag time values of study 1 and study 2 cannot be directly compared because of the different copper oxidation systems used. Study 1 utilized a 2.5-μM copper system with 50 μg/ml of LDL while study 2 utilized a 5-μM copper system with 100 μg/ml of LDL. However, the general susceptibility to oxidation of the isolated LDL between groups can be contrasted between studies.

Both studies addressed the effect of "chronic" exercise on the susceptibility of LDL to oxidation. In study 1, the exercise group was predominantly male with a significantly shorter lag time as compared to the sedentary group, which was predominantly female. In study 2, the male exercisers had a significantly longer lag time as compared to the male sedentary subjects and a longer lag time, although not significant, to the females regardless of exercise group. This discrepancy might be explained by difference in the definition of "chronic" in the two studies.

4.1 Definition of chronic exercise

Study 1 used exercise subjects that had been recruited solely from undergraduate, beginning physical education classes at Emory University. These subjects reported greater than 6 h of aerobic activity each week, but the specific intensity of the exercise is unknown and most of the subjects had not exercised chronically over the preceding 6 months because of the summer break. Study 2 used exercise subjects that had been recruited from the Atlanta Track Club and the Emory University track team. These subjects also reported greater than 6 h of aerobic activity each week with many of them reporting 7 or more hours. Due to the competitive nature of clubs they were recruited from, it may be assumed that they were exercising at a higher intensity and greater frequency than were study 1 exercisers. These subjects, for the most part, reported that they had been in training for several years.

This difference of group exercise status, between the two studies may help to explain the difference in lag time findings. It is known that chronic exercise causes adaptations of the body's antioxidant enzyme systems [46,62,63,66,67]. This adaptation would likely decrease the susceptibility of an exerciser's LDL to undergo oxidation via a controlled and concomitant decrease in production of free radicals and ROS. It is not known how long it takes for these positive adaptations to occur. The findings of these two studies suggest that truly "chronic" exercise (aerobic intensity, over several months, perhaps years) decreases the susceptibility of a male exercisers LDL to undergo oxidation (as seen in study 2). Conversely, a regular aerobic stress of an overall shorter span of time creates a more oxidative environment in the body, increasing the susceptibility of LDL to undergo oxidation (as seen in study 1). The length of time it would take a human body to adapt and overcome the oxidative stress of aerobic exercise as measured by the oxidizability of LDL is not known.

5   IMPLICATIONS

Exercise is generally regarded as an oxidative stress to the body. The oxidative environment that may be present in the plasma of exercisers would likely increase the susceptibility of their LDL to undergo oxidation assuming the body's antioxidant systems are not performing at an optimal level. It is hypothesized that if LDL becomes oxidized in the artery wall, it becomes atherogenic. However, if it becomes oxidized in the plasma it may be rapidly cleared by the liver, thereby lowering blood cholesterol levels.

Given the generally accepted beneficial effects of aerobic exercise, the enhanced susceptibility to oxidation of LDL seen in study 1 exercisers (predominantly male) might suggest an ongoing oxidative clearance of LDL in exercisers from the plasma. If so, oxidation of LDL in the plasma may itself account for some of the lipid lowering effects of exercise and may actually be beneficial. The decreased susceptibility to oxidation of LDL seen in study 2 male exercisers might suggest an adaptation of their antioxidant enzyme systems, thereby decreasing the production of free radicals and ROS. It should be noted that study 1 male exercisers had higher mean blood lipid levels than study 2 male exercisers. This supports the hypothesis that short-term aerobic activity may cause oxidative modification of LDL in the plasma and clearance via the liver thus, lowering blood cholesterol. Long-term aerobic exercise may enhance the resistance of LDL to oxidation; thus, stabilizing already lowered blood lipid levels.

The presence of oxidized lipids in the plasma is often associated with disease states and there is no compelling reason to speculate that exercise-induced oxidation is different from other forms of oxidation. A corollary of this hypothesis would suggest that antioxidant supplements might raise plasma lipid levels in exercisers. Given the results of study 2, this seems unlikely. It may be prudent to assume that the oxidative stress induced by exercise is counteractive to its potential benefits, but the tissue exposed to recurrent oxidative stress generates defense strategies to minimize or negate the consequences of such stress.

Still, such systems may fail when compounded with other factors such as chronic inflammation, poor diet, inadequate antioxidants and genetic factors. Until the mechanism(s) that regulate the delicate balance between the pro-oxidant and antioxidant factors during chronic exercise are clearly understood, it may be judicious to ensure the adequate intake of dietary antioxidants for the sporadic exerciser, as well as the truly "chronic" exerciser.

Aerobic exercise does not appear to affect the oxidizability of LDL isolated from females regardless of their exercise status. Therefore, the many benefits of aerobic activity can be achieved without the potentially deleterious consequences of this oxidative stress.

6   SUMMARY

1. There is a paradox in the putative cardiovascular benefits derived from exercise and the oxidation theory of atherosclerosis.
2. We performed two studies to address this paradox. When low-density lipoprotein (LDL) from short-term/beginning exercisers was compared with LDL from sedentary subjects for its oxidizability, it was found that the former was more readily oxidized. Conversely, when LDL from well-trained exercisers was compared with LDL from sedentary subjects, there was no significant difference in lag time between the two groups.
3. However, a significant protection against oxidation could be demonstrated in LDL isolated from chronic male exercisers as compared to the LDL from sedentary male subjects.
4. These results suggest that initial exercise training is an oxidative stress and may warrant antioxidant protection. In contrast, chronic exercisers may be protected against oxidative stress by the induction of intrinsic antioxidant defense enzymes of the artery wall.

7   ACKNOWLEDGEMENTS

This work was supported by Grant #941120115 from the American Heart Association, Georgia Affiliate and generous funds from the Department of Gynecology and Obstetrics (Emory School of Medicine). Thanks go to Marquette Inc. for their generous loan of treadmills and financial support. R.S.B. thanks the Nutrition and Health Sciences Graduate Program of Emory University for its generous support.

8   ABBREVIATIONS

BMI:	body mass index
CAD:	coronary artery disease
CAT:	catalase
CD:	conjugated diene
EPR:	electron paramagnetic resonance spectroscopy
GPX:	glutathione peroxidase
GSH:	reduced glutathione
GSSH:	oxidized glutathione
HDL:	high density lipoprotein
LDL:	low density lipoprotein
MDA:	malondialdehyde
MPO:	myeloperoxidase
NO:	nitric oxide
PUFA:	polyunsaturated fatty acids
ROS:	reactive oxygen species
SOD:	superoxide dismutase

9   REFERENCES

1. Physical activity and cardiovascular health. National Institutes of Health Consensus Development Conference Statement, December 18—20, 1995. National Institute of Health, 1996. Online. Internet. Available at http://text.nlm.gov/nih/cdc/www/101.html
2. US Department of Health and Human Services 1990. Healthy People 2000: National Health Promotion and Disease Prevention Objectives. Washington, DC: US Government Printing Office. DHHS Pub (PHS) 91-50212.
3. Rejeski WJ, Brawley LR, Shumaker SA. Exer Sport Sci Rev 1996;24:71—108.
4. Paffenbarger R, Hyde RT, Wing AL, Steinmetz CH. JAMA 1984;252:491—495.
5. Haskell WL. Acta Med Scand 1986;711:25—37.
6. Gaisser GA, Rich RG. Med Sci Sports Exerc 1984;16:269—274.
7. Anderson AJ, Sobocinski KA, Freedman DS, Barboriak JJ, Rimm AA, Gruchow HW. Arteriosclerosis 1988;8:88—94.
8. Astrand PO, Rodahl K. Textbook of work physiology. New York: McGraw Hill, 1986.
9. Sjodin B, Westing YH, Apple FS. Sports Med 1990;10:236—254.
10. Alessio HM, Goldfarb AH. J Appl Phys 1988;64:1333—1336.
11. Ji LL. 1995. Exer Sports Sci Rev 1995;23:135—166.
12. Steinberg D, Parthasarathy S, Carew TE, Khoo JC, Witztum JL. N Eng J Med 1989;20: 915—924.
13. Parthasarathy S. Modified Lipoproteins in the Pathogenesis of Atherosclerosis. Austin, Texas: RG Landes Company, 1994;1—131.
14. Parhami F, Fang ZT, Fogelman AM, Andalibi A, Territo MC, Berliner JA. J Clin Invest 1993;92: 471—478.
15. Yla-herttuala S, Palinski W, Bulter SW, Picard S, Steinberg D, Witztum JL. Arterioscl Thromb 1994;14:32—40.
16. Aviram M. Atherosclerosis 1990;84:141—143.
17. Bergmark C, Wu R, de Faire U, Lefvret AK, Swedenborg J. Arteriosclerosis 1995; 15:441—445.
18. Khoo JC, Miller E, Pio F, Steinberg D, Witztum JL. Arterioscler Thromb 1992;12:1258—1266.
19. Steinbrecher UP. Can J Physiol Pharmacol 1995;75(3):228—233.
20. Hodis HN, Mack WJ, Labree L, Cashin-Hemphill L, Sevanian A, Johnson R, Azen SP. JAMA 1995;273:1849—1854.
21. Esterbauer H, Dieber-Rotheneder M, Striegl G, Waeg G. Am J Clin Nutr 1991;53:314S—321S.
22. Jialal I, Grundy SM. J Lipid Res 1992;33:899—906.
23. Princen HMG, van Poppel G, Vogelezang C, Buytenhek R, Kok FJ. Arterioscler Thromb 1992; 12:554—562.
24. Carew TE, Schwenke DC, Steinberg D. Proc Natl Acad Sci USA 1987;84:7725—7729.
25. Kita T, Nagano Y, Yokode M, Ishii K, Kume N, Ooshima A, Yoshida H, Kawai C. Proc Natl Acad Sci USA 1987;84:5928—5931.
26. Sparrow CP, Doebber TW, Olszewski J, Wu MS, Stevens KA, Chao Y. J Clin Invest 1992;89: 1885—1891.
27. Stephens NG, Parsons A, Schofield PM, Kelly F, Cheeseman K, Mitchinson MJ. Lancet 1996; 347:781—786
28. Azen SP, Qian D, Mack WJ, Sevanian A, Selzer RH, Liu CR, Liu CH, Hodis HN. Circulation 1996;94:2369—2372.
29. Shern-Brewer R, Santanam N, Wetzstein C, White-Welkley J, Parthasarathy S. Arterioscl Thromb Vasc Biol 1998;(In Press).
30. Itabe H, Takeshima E, Iwasaki H, Kimura J, Yoshida Y, Imanaka T, Tikano T. J Biol Chem 1994; 269:15274—15279.
31. Chang YH, Abdalla DS, Sevanian A. Free Radic Biol Med 1997;23:202—214.
32. Sevanian A, Bittolo-bon G, Cazzolato G, Hodis H, Hwang J, Zamburlini A, Maiorino M, Ursini F. J Lipid Res 1997;38:419—428.

33. Sanchez-Quesada JL, Ortega H, Payes-Romero A, Serrat-Serrat J, Gonzalez-Sastre F, Lasuncion MA, Ordonez-Llanos J. Atherosclerosis 1997;132:207—213.
34. Pyne DB. Sports Med 1994;17(4):245—258.
35. Hack V, Strobel G, Rau JP, Weicka W. Eur J Appl Physiol Occ Physiol 1992;65:520—524.
36. Nieman CC, Nehlsen-Cannarella SL. Endurance Sport 1992;487—504.
37. Wieland E, Parthasarathy S, Steinberg D. Proc Natl Acad Sci USA 1993;90:5929—5933.
38. Savenkova ML, Mueller DM, Heinecke JW. J Biol Chem 1994;269:20394—20400.
39. Daugherty A, Dunn JL, Rateri DL, Heinecke JW. J Clin Invest 1994;94:437—444.
40. Hazell LJ, Stocker R. Biochem J 1993;290:165—172.
41. Panasenko OM, Evgina SA, Aidyraliev RK, Sergienko VI, Vladimirov YA. 1994. Free Radic Biol Med 1994;16:143—148.
42. Steinbrecher UP, Witztum JL, Parthasarathy S, Steinberg D. Arteriosclerosis 1987;7:135—139.
43. Negelkerke JF, Barto KP, van Berkel TJ. J Biol Chem 1983;258:12221—12227.
44. Mata P, Alonso R, Lopez-Farre A, Ordovas JM, Lahoz C, Garces C, Caramelo C, Codoceo R, Blazques E, de Oya M. Arterioscl Thromb Vasc Biol 1996;16:1347—1355.
45. Thomas MJ, Thornburg T, Manning J, Hooper K, Rudel U. Biochem 1994;33:1828—1834.
46. Winklhofer-Roob BM, Ziouzenkova O, Puhl H, Ellemunter H, Greiner P, Muller G, van't Hof MA, Esterbauer H, Shmerling DH. Free Radic Biol Med 1995;19:725—733.
47. Reaven P, Grasse B, Barnett J. Arterio Thrombosis Vasc Biol 1996;16:1465—1472.
48. Abbey M, Noakes M, Nestel PJ. J Am Diet Assoc 1995;95:671—675.
49. Nyyssonen K, Porkkala E, Salonen R, Korpela H, Salonen JT. Eur J Clin Nutr 1994;48:633—642.
50. Meraji S, Ziouzenkova O, Resch U, Khoschsorur A, Tatzber F. Eur J Clin Nutr 1997;51:318—325.
51. Ziouzenkova O, Gieseg SP, Rames P, Esterbauer H. Lipids 1996;31(Suppl):S71—76.
52. McCarthy DA, Dale MM. Sports Med 1988;6:333—363.
53. Ndon JA, Snyder AC, Foster C, Wehrenberg WB. Int J Sports Med 1992;13:176—182.
54. Ferguson E, Singh RJ, Hogg N, Kalyanaraman B. Arch Biochem Biophys 1997;341:287—294.
55. Tribble DL, van den Berg JJ, Motchnik PA, Ames BN, Lewis BM, Chait A, Kraus RM. Proc Natl Acad Sci USA 1994;91:1183—1187.
56. Scheschonka A, Murphy ME, Sies H. Chem Biol Int 1990;74:233—252.
57. de Whalley CV, Rankin SM, Hoult JR, Jessup W, Leake DS. Biochem Pharm 1990;39:1743—1750.
58. Mosca l, Rubentire M, Mandel C, Rock C, Tarshis T, Tsai A, Pearson T. J Am Coll Cardiol 1997;30:392—399.
59. Abby M, Nestel PJ, Baghurst PA. Am J Clin Invest 1993;58:525—532.
60. Quintanilha AT. Biochem Soc Tranc 1984;12:403—404.
61. Higuchi M, Cartier LJ, Chen M, Holloszy JO. J Gerontol 1985;40:281—286.
62. Leeuwenburgh C, Fiebig R, Chandwaney R, Ji LL. Am J Physiol 1994;267:R439—455.
63. Powers SK, Criswell D, Lawler J. Am J Physiol 1994;266:R375—380.
64. Jenkins RR. Int J Sports Nutr 1993;3:356—375.
65. Laughlin MH, Simpson T, Sexton WL, Brown OR, Smith JK, Korthuis RJ. J Appl Physiol 1990;68:2337—2343.
66. Meydani M, Evans WJ. Free radicals, exercise, and aging. In: Yu BP (ed) Free Radical in Aging. Boca Raton, Florida: CRC Press, 183—204.
67. Ji LL, Stratman FW, Lardy HA. Arch Biochem Biophys 1988;263:137—149.
68. Lawler JM, Powers SK, Visser T, VanDijk H, Korthuis MJ, Ji LL. Am J Physiol 1993;265:R1344—1350.
69. Vaziri SM, Evans JC, Larson MG, Wilson PW. Arch Int Med 1993;153:2200—2206.
70. Bruckert E, Turpin G. Horm Ther 1995;43:100—103.
71. Manson JE. Am Heart J 1994;128:1337—1343.
72. Takanashi K, Watanabe K, Yoshizawa I. 1995. Biol Pharm Bull 1995;18:1120—1125.

73. McManus J, McEneny J, Young IS, Thompson W. Maturitas 1996;25:125—131.
74. Wilcox JG, Hwang J, Hodis HN, Sevanian A, Stanczyk FZ, Lobo RA. Fertil Steril 1997;67: 57—62.
75. Bobadilla RA, Henkel CC, Henkel EC, Escalante B, Hong E. Hypertension 1997;30:596—602.
76. Ma L, Robinson CP, Thadani U, Patterson E. J Cardiovasc Pharmacol 1997;30:130—135.
77. Jungersten L, Ambring A, Wall B, Wennmalm A. J Appl Physiol 1997;82:760—764.
78. Ji LL, Stratman FW, Lardy HA. Arch Biochem Biophys 1988;263:137—149.
79. Alessio HM, Goldfarb AH, Cutler RG. Am J Physiol 1988;255:C874—C877
80. Davies KJA, Quintanilha AT, Brooks GA, Packer L. Biochem Biophys Res Commun 1982;107: 1198—1205.
81. Alessio HM, Goldfarb AH. J Appl Phys 1988;64:1333—1336.
82. Ji LL, Fu R. J Appl Phys 1992;72:549—554.
83. Kumar CT, Reddy VK, Prasad M, Thyagaraju K, Reddanna P. Molec Cell Biochem 1992;111: 109—115.
84. Jenkins RR, Krause K, Schofield LS. Med Sci Sports Exerc 1993;25:213—217.
85. Salminen A, Vihko V. Exp Mol Pathol 1983;38:380—388.
86. Lovlin R, Cottle W, Pyke I, Kavanagh M, Belcastro N. Eur J Appl Physiol 1987;56:313—316.
87. Duthie GG, Robertson JD, Maughan RJ, Morrice PC. Arch Biochem Biophys 1990;282:78—83.
88. Viinikka L, Vuori J, Ylikorkala O. Med Sci Sports Exerc 1984;16:275—277.
89. Kanter MM, Nolte LA, Holloszy JO. J Appl Physiol 1993;74:965—969.
90. Kanter MM, Lesmes GR, Kaminsky LA, Ham-Saeger JH, Nequin ND. Eur J Appl Physiol 1988;57:60—63.
91. Maughan RJ, Donnelly AE, Gleeson M, Whiting PH, Walker KA, Clough PJ. Muscle Nerve 1989;12:332—336.
92. Meydani M, Evans WJ, Handelman G, Biddle L, Fielding RA, Meydani SN, Burrill J, Fiatarone MA, Blumberg JB, Cannon JG. Am J Physiol 1993;264:R992—998.
93. Merry P, Grootveld M, Lunec J, Blake D. Am J Clin Nutr 1991;53:362S.369S.
94. Jackson MJ, Edwards RHT, Symons MCR. Biochem Biophys Acta 1985;847:185—190.
95. Alessio HM, Cutler RG. 1990. Med Sci Sports Exerc 1990;22:751—754.
96. Sastre J, Asensi M, Gasco E, Pallardo FV, Ferrero JA, Furukawa T, Vina J. Am J Physiol 1992; 263:R992—995.
96. Ji LL. Med Sci Sports Exerc 1993;25:225—231.
98. Ji LL, Dillon D, Wu E. Am J Physiol 1990;258:R918—R923.
99. Lawlwer JM, Powers SK, Visser T, Van Dijk H, Korthuis MJ, Ji LL. Am J Physiol 1993;265: R1344—R1350.
100. Brady PS, Brady LJ, Ullrey DE. J Nutr 1979;109:1103—1109.
101. Ji LL, Fu RG, Mitchell EW. J Appl Physiol 1992;73:1854—1859.
102. Buczynski A, Kedziora J, Tkaczewski W, Wachowicz B. Int J Sports Med 1991;12:52—54.
103. Quintanilha AT. Biochem Soc Trans 1984;12:403—404.
104. Bowles DK, Torgan CE, Kehrer JP, Ivy JL, Starnes JW. Free Radic Res Commun 1991;14: 139—143.
105. Tiidus PM, Behrens WA, Madere R, Houston ME. Acta Physiol Scand 1993;147:2249—2250.
106. Pincemail J, Camus DCG, Pirnay F, Bouchez R, Massaux L, Goutier R. Eur J Appl Physiol 1988;57:189—191.
107. Lang JK, Gohil K, Packer L, Burk RF. J Appl Physiol 1987;63:2532—2535.
108. Dillard CJ, Litov RE, Savin RE, Dumelin EE, Tappel AL. J Appl Physiol Respir Env Exerc Physiol 1978;45:927—932.
109. Gee DL, Tappel AL. Life Sci 1981;28:2425—2429.
110. Pincemail J, Camus G, Roesgen A, Dreezen E, Bertrand Y, Lismonde M, Deby-Dupont G. 1990;61:319—322.
111. Camus G, Pincemail J, Ledent M, Juchmes-Ferir A, Lamy M, Deby-Dupont G, Deby C. Int J Sports Med 1992;13(6):443—446.

112. McMurray HG, Parthasarathy S, Fong LG, Steinberg D. J Clin Invest 1987;92:1004—1008.
113. Quinn MT, Parthasarathy S, Fong LG, Steinberg D. Proc Natl Acad Sci USA 1987;84: 2995—2998.
114. Weis JR, Pitas RE, Wilson BD, Rodgers GM. FASEB J 1991;5:2459—2465.
115. Harduin P, Tailleux A, Lestavel S, Clavey V, Fruchart JC, Fievet C. J Lipid Res 1995;36: 919—930.
116. Greenspan P, Ryu BH, Mao F, Gutman RL. Biochim Biophys Acta 1995;1257:257—264.
117. Zhang HF, Basra HJ, Steinbrecher UP. J Lipid Res 1990;31:1361—1369.
118 Ball RY, Bindman JP, Carpenter KL, Mitchinson MJ. Atherosclerosis 1986;60:173—181.
119. Mangin EL, Kugiyama K, Nguy JH, Kerns SA, Henry PD. Circ Res 1993;72:161—166.
120. Martin-Nizard F, Houssaini HS, Lestavel S, Duriez P, Fruchart JC. FEBS Lett 1991;293: 127—130.
121. Tanner FC, Noll G, Boulanger CM, Luscher TF. Circulation 1991;83:2012—2020.
122. Simon BC, Cunningham LD, Cohen RA. J Clin Invest 1990;86:75—79.
123. Holland JA, Ziegler LM, Meyer JM. J Cell Physiol 1996;166:144—151.
124. Boissonneault GA, Wang Y, Chung BH. Ann Nutr Metab 1995;39:1—8.
125. Nishio E, Arimura S, Watanabe Y. Biochem Biophys Res Commun 1996;223:413—418.
126. Frostegard J, Haegerstrand A, Gidlund M, Nilsson J. Atherosclerosis 1991;90:119—126.
127 Okada M, Sugita O, Miida T, Matsuto T, Inano K. Presse Medicale 1995;24:483:488.
128. Khan BV, Parthasarathy S, Alexander RW, Medford RM. J Clin Invest 1995;95:1262—1270.
129. Escargueil I, Negre Salvayre A, Pieraggi MT, Salvayre R. FEBS Lett 1992;305:155—159.
130. Escargueil-Blanc I, Salvayre R, Negre Salvayre A. FASEB J 1994;8:1075—1080.
131. Zwijesen RM, Japenga SC, Heijen AM, van den Bos RC, Koeman JH. Biochem Biophys Res Commun 1992;186:1410—1416.
132. Jimi S, Saku K, Uesugi N, Sakata N, Takebayashi S. Atherosclerosis 1995;116:15—26.
133. Weidtmann A, Scheithe R, Hrboticky N, Pietsch A, Lorenz R, Siess W. Arterioscler Thromb Vasc Biol 1995;15:1131—1138.
134. Schuff Werner P, Claus G, Armstrong VW, Kostering H, Seidel D. Atherosclerosis 1989;78: 109—112.
135. Parums DV, Brown DL, Mitchinson MJ. Arch Pathol Lab Med 1990;114:383—387.
136. Orekhov AN, Tertov VV, Kabakov AR, Adamova IY, Pokrovsky SN, Smirnov VN. Arterioscler Thromb 1991;11:316—326.

©2000 Elsevier Science B.V. All rights reserved.
Handbook of Oxidants and Antioxidants in Exercise.
C.K. Sen, L. Packer and O. Hänninen, editors.

Part XI • Chapter 37

Claudication, exercise and antioxidants

Paul V. Tisi and Clifford P. Shearman
Department of Vascular Surgery, E-level West Wing (Mail Point 67), Southampton General Hospital, Tremona Road, Southampton SO16 6YD, UK. Tel.: +44—1703—798801. Fax: +44—1703—798911.

1   INTRODUCTION
   1.1   Intermittent claudication: the scope of the problem
   1.2   Natural history of the disease
      1.2.1   Local disease
      1.2.2   Systemic disease
   1.3   Potential adverse effects of exercise on atherogenesis
2   THE EVIDENCE FOR EXERCISE-INDUCED OXIDATIVE DAMAGE IN CLAUDICATION
   2.1   Biochemistry of ischaemia-reperfusion injury
      2.1.1   Xanthine oxidase pathway
      2.1.2   Oxygen-derived free radicals and antioxidant mechanisms
      2.1.3   Role of vascular endothelium
      2.1.4   Neutrophil activation
   2.2   Animal experimental models of lower limb ischaemia-reperfusion
      2.2.1   Free radical formation
      2.2.2   Neutrophil activation
      2.2.3   Target organ damage
   2.3   Acute exercise in patients with intermittent claudication
      2.3.1   Changes in blood flow and oxygen metabolism
      2.3.2   Free radical formation and antioxidant consumption
      2.3.3   Neutrophil activation
      2.3.4   Effect on vascular endothelium
3   CHRONIC EXERCISE IN PATIENTS WITH INTERMITTENT CLAUDICATION
   3.1   Skeletal muscle adaptation
   3.2   Exercise training programmes for claudication
      3.2.1   Mode of benefit of exercise training
      3.2.2   Clinical trials of therapeutic exercise training
   3.3   Effect of training on the exercise-induced inflammatory response
4   SUMMARY
5   PERSPECTIVES
6   ABBREVIATIONS
7   REFERENCES

1   INTRODUCTION

Intermittent claudication is usually the earliest presenting symptom of peripheral arterial disease (PAD) of the lower limb. Claudication itself means "limping" and the typical description is of cramping calf pain following walking which resolves completely with rest. Claudication-type pain may also be a feature of other pathology, such as osteoarthritis or lumbar spinal stenosis, although this can usually be differentiated in the history and clinical examination. This chapter focuses on arterial (vasculogenic) claudication.

The term "intermittent claudication" was first used in 1831 by Bouley, a Parisian veterinary surgeon, who described recurrent lameness in the hind limb of a mare following walking which resolved completely on rest [1]. An autopsy revealed a "fusiform tumour" of the femoral artery containing fibrinous clot, which obstructed the lumen. He concluded that numerous "anastomoses" (i.e., collateral vessels) were sufficient to supply blood to the hind limb at rest, but that the blood supply was inadequate on exercise. Bouley termed this "spontaneous and intermittent claudication, determined by the interference with circulation". Charcot's classical case report of intermittent claudication in a human was presented to the Societe de Biologie of Paris in 1858 [2]. The man had been shot in the right flank during a military campaign in Africa in 1830. He now complained of weakness, paraesthesia and tightness of the lower limb after walking. The symptoms resolved rapidly with rest but recurred on repeated walking. Following death from gastrointestinal haemorrhage, an autopsy showed a traumatic right common iliac artery aneurysm that had eroded into the jejunum. The aneurysm was occluded by fibrinous clot and large collateral vessels reconstituted the femoral artery. Charcot suggested that these collaterals were adequate to supply the lower limb at rest, although were unable to increase blood flow on exercise. He suggested that resolution of the pain was due to a "chemical response which is accompanied by the presence of a certain quantity of oxygenated blood". In 1895, Goldflam presented a series of six patients with intermittent claudication, in whom three patients had absent foot pulses. He concluded that "intermittent claudication is not a disease but a clinical manifestation of arteriosclerosis" [3].

1.1 Intermittent claudication: the scope of the problem

Intermittent claudication is a common problem, but only comprises a subset of patients with PAD. The prevalence of asymptomatic PAD is 8—11.3% on population screening [4,5]. Only 10—50% of people with symptoms of claudication will ever consult their General Practitioner, and therefore, true prevalence rates are likely to be underestimated [6]. Prevalence rates depend on the age group, sex and diagnostic criteria used and range from 2.9% in the Speedwell Prospective Heart Disease Study [7] to 4.5% in the Edinburgh Artery Study [5]. An overall literature review suggests that claudication has a prevalence of > 5% in the over 50 age group.

The Framingham study has provided important information about the incidence of symptomatic claudication. A follow-up of 5,209 subjects over 26 years has shown a biannual incidence of 1.06% in 55- to 64-year-old men and 1.38% in 65- to 74-year-old men [8]. The Speedwell Prospective Heart Disease Study reported a similar incidence rate of 0.5% for men in their seventh decade [7].

1.2 Natural history of the disease

This section reviews the natural history of intermittent claudication, in terms of both local disease, (the lower limb), and the association between claudication and cardiovascular morbidity and mortality.

1.2.1 Local disease

From the patients point of view, the change in symptoms is the most important factor in considering the natural history of the disease. There is evidence that the atherosclerotic disease may progress locally despite an improvement in symptoms [9]. In 75% of patients, claudication symptoms will remain stable or improve [10,11]. The rate of progression to critical limb ischaemia is highest in the 1st year after diagnosis (7.5%) [12], but this risk is reduced if patients stop smoking [13]. The long-term major amputation rates for claudicants have been remarkably consistent (Table 1) and with the increasing trend towards more aggressive distal reconstruction for critical ischaemia, the amputation rate may be now as low as 1.7% [6,14].

1.2.2 Systemic disease

Claudicants have a high prevalence of coexisting cardiovascular disease. About one third of subjects have hypertension [15], while 34—58% of claudicants in hospital-based studies have either symptoms or ECG evidence of ischemic heart disease (IHD) [16—18]. The Edinburgh Artery Study revealed an even higher prevalence of IHD in 71% of claudicants [5]. The true prevalence of IHD is probably underestimated as invasive coronary angiography is only performed on symptomatic patients with failed medical treatment. Claudicants without other coexisting cardiovascular disease are at a high risk of developing atherosclerotic problems in these other sites. Dormandy and Murray [18] reported a 1.8% incidence of myocardial infarction and 1.4% incidence of stroke in 1,969 claudicants followed up over 1 year.

Claudicants have a significantly increased mortality compared to a control population, predominantly from cardiovascular disease. The reported mortality rates in major epidemiological studies are similar — 46.8% at 10 years in the Fra-

Table 1. Long-term amputation rates in patients with intermittent claudication.

No. of patients	Years follow-up	Amputation rate	Author
454	5	8.0%	Taylor and Calo (1962)
1476	5	7.0%	Bloor (1960)
104	2.5	5.8%	Imparato et al. (1975)
100	6	7.0%	McAllister (1976)
257	5	6.8%	Jelnes et al. (1978)

mingham Study [8], 38% at 17 years in the Whitehall Study [19], 47% at 10 years in the Speedwell Prospective Heart Disease Study [7] and 61.8% at 10 years reported by Criqui et al. [20]. More than three-quarters of these deaths were due to ischemic heart disease and cerebrovascular disease, corresponding to a relative risk of death of 3.8 compared to a control population [7]. The increased cardiovascular mortality in claudicants is in excess of that expected from subjects with previously diagnosed ischemic heart disease.

1.3 Potential adverse effects of exercise on atherogenesis

The poor long-term survival of this group of patients, despite a fairly benign prognosis for the claudicant limb, prompts the suggestion that the pathophysiological changes in claudication may have cumulative systemic effects that stimulate the progression of atherosclerosis. Evidence is accumulating that exercise to the onset of calf pain followed by rest in a claudicant may be considered as an ischaemia-reperfusion injury (I-RI). This is discussed further in the next section, but essentially this means that most of the tissue damage occurs on restoration of oxygenated blood flow. Repeated episodes of low-grade ischaemia-reperfusion as occurs in a claudicant may be an important factor in the natural history of atherosclerosis. Chronic inflammatory cells, such as macrophages and T-lymphocytes, have been demonstrated in atherosclerotic plaque, lending weight to the hypothesis that local release of cytokines may be important in plaque progression [21,22]. This potential exercise-induced injury obviously has important implications for the management of patients with this condition. The government in the UK and the US National Institutes of Health have actively promoted physical exercise to improve cardiovascular health in the general population [23,24]. The standard advice given to a claudicant is to "stop smoking and keep walking" [25] and it is usually suggested that walking is continued through the onset of ischemic pain in the hope of improving exercise tolerance. Are we wrongly advising patients on exercise in the face of evidence of exercise-induced vascular endothelial damage? The underlying mechanisms of atherogenesis are complex and not yet fully understood. Recent experimental work suggests that the common atherosclerotic risk factors such as diabetes, hypertension, smoking and hypercholesterolaemia lead to an increase in vascular permeability [26]. The vascular endothelium is therefore of vital importance in the pathogenesis of the disease. Current theories of atherogenesis suggest that the initial lesions, such as the fatty streak, represent a protective response to vascular endothelial damage. The subsequent excessive inflammatory proliferative response then becomes the pathological process, with a complex interaction between macrophages, T-lymphocytes, smooth muscle cells and endothelial cells [27]. The aetiological factor for vascular endothelial damage is likely to be multifactorial but oxidised low-density lipoprotein (OX-LDL) may be the critical factor [28]. Lipid peroxides, discussed in the following section, are involved in the oxidation of LDL and, by extrapolation, in the pathogenesis of atherosclerosis [29].

The aim of this chapter is, therefore, to review present evidence for exercise-induced oxidative damage both in animal experimental models of intermittent claudication and in clinical studies of patients with claudication. The effect of chronic exercise, including therapeutic exercise programmes will be explored in detail, with particular emphasis on skeletal muscle structural and metabolic adaptation, symptomatic improvement and potential adverse effects on vascular inflammation.

2 THE EVIDENCE FOR EXERCISE-INDUCED OXIDATIVE DAMAGE IN CLAUDICATION

2.1 Biochemistry of ischaemia-reperfusion injury

Physical exercise requires adenosine triphosphate (ATP) as an energy source, which is primarily produced during oxidative phosphorylation. In patients with intermittent claudication, ATP generation in skeletal muscle is limited by decreased blood flow as a result of atherosclerotic occlusive disease. Alternative sources of ATP are, therefore, required to sustain exercise. Hydrolysis of phosphocreatine and glycogenolysis to lactic acid both generate ATP with accumulation of hydrogen ions. Reperfusion with oxygenated blood, (i.e., rest in a patient with intermittent claudication), results in local and systemic effects which may cause more tissue damage than the original ischemic insult – ischaemia-reperfusion injury (I-RI) [30]. The metabolic changes of I-RI, e.g., acidosis, hyperkalemia, a decrease in tissue oxygen and glucose consumption and a rise in plasma lactate dehydrogenase and transaminases, are well known and have been termed the Legrain-Cormier [31] or myonephropathic-metabolic syndrome [32]. Recent work has shown that by controlling the rate of reperfusion, these adverse biochemical changes can be attenuated [33]. The above changes have usually been discussed in terms of acute limb ischaemia. The hypothesis in claudication is that lesser but repetitive ischaemia-reperfusion events may lead to similar changes.

2.1.1 Xanthine oxidase pathway

Experimental evidence suggests that endothelial xanthine oxidase (XO) is the major source of oxygen-derived free radicals (ODFR) which are important in the underlying mechanisms of reperfusion injury [34]. A clinical model of tourniquet-induced upper limb ischaemia showed an increase in XO on reperfusion with no change in xanthine dehydrogenase (XD), the reduced form of the enzyme complex. This was associated with an increase in plasma histamine (a catalyst of XO) and generation of superoxide (the product of XO) [35]. The concentration of XD (90% of the enzyme activity) is variable in different tissues, which may explain their susceptibility to I-RI [36].

As a consequence of inadequate oxidative phosphorylation, ATP is degraded to hypoxanthine via the purine metabolic pathway. Physiologically, hypoxanthine is converted to xanthine by xanthine dehydrogenase (XD) using oxidised nicotine adenine dinucleotide (NAD^+) as a co-factor. Hypoxia during tissue ischaemia disrupts cellular ionic gradients, and increases cytosolic calcium ion concentration [37]. This activates a protease attack on XD converting it to xanthine oxidase — the "D-O conversion" [36] (Fig. 1). In skeletal muscle ischaemia, endothelial cell hypoxanthine levels rise as no XD is available and the newly synthesised XO requires molecular oxygen as a substrate, which is not available. Reperfusion with oxygen allows XO to convert hypoxanthine to xanthine with generation of large amounts of superoxide [38].

2.1.2 Oxygen-derived free radicals and antioxidant mechanisms

ODFR are highly reactive molecules containing an unpaired electron in an atomic orbital [36]. They have a short half-life and low chemical specificity, resulting in widespread damage to cellular structures [39]. Physiologically, mitochondrial cytochrome p450 reduces molecular oxygen but the system leaks approximately 2% of the oxygen, which is converted to superoxide [34,37]. This is rapidly detoxified by intracellular superoxide dismutase (SOD), catalase and circulating antioxidants [40]. The principle sources of ODFR in reperfusion injury are XO (Fig. 1) and activated neutrophils [41]. The latter generate superoxide in a

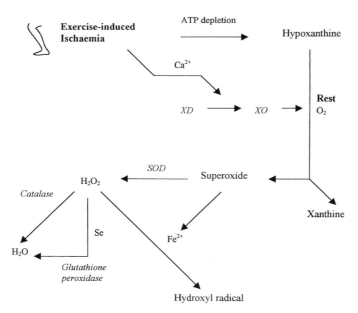

Fig. 1. Oxygen-derived free radical production in claudication. ATP: adenosine triphosphate, Ca^{2+}: calcium ions, Fe^{2+}: ferrous ions, O_2: oxygen, H_2O_2: hydrogen peroxide, Se: selenium, XD: xanthine dehyrogenase, XO: xanthine oxidase.

"respiratory burst" via oxidation of nicotine adenine dinucleotide phosphate (NADPH), which is catalysed by membrane-bound NADPH oxidase [42].

In vivo formation of superoxide is always accompanied by dismutation to hydrogen peroxide (H_2O_2), catalysed by intracellular superoxide dismutase (SOD). H_2O_2 increases intracellular calcium (Ca^{2+}) concentration resulting in oxidative damage to DNA. Physiological amounts of H_2O_2 in endothelial cells are detoxified by catalase and glutathione peroxidase, which requires selenium as a cofactor. Sublethal exposure of endothelial cells to H_2O_2 leads to an increase in vascular permeability and neutrophil adhesion [43].

Superoxide liberates ferrous ions (Fe^{2+}) from ferritin (containing Fe^{3+}) which catalyse the formation of the hydroxyl radical from H_2O_2 (the Fenton or Haber-Weiss reaction) [44,39]. The rate-limiting step in the reaction is the availability of H_2O_2. The hydroxyl radical is extremely reactive and attacks DNA causing free radical chain reactions and base mutations [45]. The hydroxyl radical was previously thought to directly damage vascular endothelium in small venules leading to an increase in permeability [46]. Current thought suggests that the hydroxyl radical attacks polyunsaturated fatty acid (PUFA) side-chains on endothelial cell membrane phospholipids forming a reactive carbon radical. Saturated fatty acids and monounsaturated fatty acids are less susceptible to oxidation. The carbon radical reacts with oxygen, forming the peroxyl radical which causes self-amplifying generation of lipid peroxides leading to widespread tissue damage [45]. Lipid peroxides are cytotoxic to endothelial cells and promote platelet aggregation by reducing endothelial prostacyclin and nitric oxide synthesis [47,48]. Copper ions (released from ceruloplasmin), the iron-based ferryl, as well as perferryl radicals and singlet oxygen may also be involved in lipid peroxidation. Lipid peroxides decompose to aldehydes such as 4-hydroxynonenal (toxic) and malondialdehyde (nontoxic). The latter is used as a marker of lipid peroxidation, although some authors disagree with this [49].

Free-radical scavengers limit the extent of ODFR tissue damage. Cytosolic and mitochondrial catalase reduce H_2O_2 to water and oxygen, acting in conjunction with SOD as a protective mechanism [50]. Cytosolic and mitochondrial selenium-dependent glutathione peroxidase keeps H_2O_2 concentration at $10^{-9}-10^{-7}$ M by oxidising reduced glutathione [39]. There are several naturally occurring antioxidants, e.g., vitamin E which are important in limiting ODFR-induced lipid peroxidation, particularly of low-density lipoprotein (see below). ODFR neutralise vitamin E but this can be regenerated by vitamin C or glutathione [51]. Ascorbic acid (vitamin C) is an electron donor and antioxidant, reacting with superoxide, H_2O_2 and hydroxyl radicals to form dehydroascorbic acid [39].

Recent work has shown that lipid peroxides are involved in oxidation of low-density lipoprotein (LDL). LDL is a complex of high molecular weight proteins, apolipoprotein B-100, phospholipids and antioxidants, predominantly vitamin E and to a lesser extent, β-carotene [28]. LDL is in constant flux between the circulation and the subendothelium and accumulates in certain sites, typical of the disease pattern of atherosclerosis [52]. Lipid peroxides attack PUFA side-chains in surface and core-lipids of subendothelial low-density lipoprotein forming minimally-modified LDL (MM-LDL) via a chain-reaction of lipid peroxidation. Oxidation mainly occurs within the intima of the vessel, as circulating antioxidants, e.g., vitamin E prevent intravascular oxidation of LDL [28,53]. MM-LDL is implicated in atherogenesis as it induces adhesion of monocytes to damaged endothelium and release of monocyte chemotactic protein-1 and macrophage-colony stimulating factor. This leads to loss of monocyte motility and conversion to macrophages [54,55]. MM-LDL inhibits macrophage chemotaxis, retaining cells within the subendothelial space. Some evidence also exists that T-cells release cytokines in response to MM-LDL. The intimal pool of MM-LDL may leak back into the circulation but is still recognised by the endothelial LDL receptor. Minimally oxidised LDL is thrombogenic, immunogenic (antibodies to MM-LDL and its epitopes have been demonstrated) and is cytotoxic to the vascular endothelium [56,53]. MM-LDL may also inhibit nitric oxide mediated vasodilatation. Subintimal MM-LDL may then be rapidly oxidised to highly oxidised LDL by reactive oxygen species from subendothelial macrophages. OX-LDL causes endothelial injury and recruits further monocytes and T-lymphocytes into the subendothelial space.

The lipid peroxide products in OX-LDL fragment into aldehydes and ketones (e.g., malondialdehyde and 4-hydroxynonenal) which covalently combine with lysine and other amino acid residues in apolipoprotein B-100. Epitopes on modified apo-B100 are recognised by "scavenger" receptors (acetyl-LDL receptors) on macrophages, which do not recognise native LDL [56,57]. Macrophages endocytose OX-LDL forming typical "foam cells" containing cholesteryl esters. Oxidised lipid may also induce macrophages to release cytokines, which initiate a hepatic acute-phase response [58] (Fig. 2). We have recently shown significantly higher resting levels of the acute-phase proteins fibrinogen, C-reactive protein and serum amyloid A protein in claudicants compared to control subjects [59] (Table 2). This warrants further investigation.

2.1.3 Role of vascular endothelium

The importance of the vascular endothelium was recognised by Brucke in 1857: "...in sound and living vessels the blood remains fluid, but it coagulates in dead ones" [60]. The vascular endothelium is a selectively permeable cell layer that has an active role in control of vascular permeability and tone, platelet aggregation and neutrophil adhesion. The endothelium produces mediators that are important in the pathophysiology of I-RI. Physiologically, a balance exists between protective and destructive mediators. Reperfusion shifts the balance towards the latter and endothelium then becomes the target organ of reperfusion injury.

The arachidonic acid pathway generates mediators that have significant effects on vascular endothelium. Superoxide increases endothelial cell calcium ion concentration, activating membrane-bound phospholipase A_2 which liberates arach-

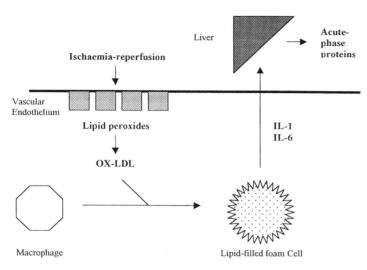

Fig. 2. The role of lipid peroxidation and oxidation of low-density lipoprotein (OX-LDL) in macrophage activation and hepatic acute-phase protein synthesis. IL-1: interleukin-1, IL-6: interleukin-6.

idonic acid [61]. Arachidonic acid is a PUFA (C20:4) derived from dietary γ-linoleic acid (C18:3) [47] and is the precursor for both pro-inflammatory, e.g., thromboxane A_2 (TXA_2) and leukotriene B_4 (LTB_4), and anti-inflammatory mediators, e.g., prostaglandin E_2 (PGE_2) and prostacyclin (PGI_2). These mediators act locally and systemically and are rapidly degraded. Dietary fish oils in the Eskimo diet provide eicosapentaenoic acid (EPA — C20:5) which competes with arachidonic acid for phospholipid binding sites [47]. Cyclooxygenase converts EPA to PGI_3 (with an equivalent antiplatelet effect to PGI_2) and TXA_3 (which is less active than TXA_2). The net effect is vasodilatation and antiplatelet activity [60]. This may explain the protective action of EPA in cardiovascular disease.

Leukotriene A_4 (LTA_4) is synthesised in endothelial cells by the action of lipooxygenase on arachidonic acid and is rapidly hydrolysed to LTB_4. There is controversy as to whether endothelial cells are the main source of LTB_4 in I-RI.

Table 2. Resting acute-phase protein levels in 67 claudicants and 15 control subjects. (CRP: C-reactive protein, SAA: serum amyloid A protein). Results are shown as the median (interquartile range) and levels are significantly higher in claudicants compared to control subjects (Mann-Whitney, p = 0.045 for fibrinogen, $p < 0.0001$ for CRP and p = 0.0009 for SAA). Data were obtained from Tisi et al. (1997).

	Controls (n = 15)	Claudicants (n = 67)
Fibrinogen (g/l)	3.5 (2.9—3.95)	3.7 (3.3—4.25)
CPR (mg/l)	2.1 (1.0—2.8)	4.7 (2.2—9.0)
SAA (mg/l)	30 (20—89)	72 (35—132)

Endothelial LTB_4 synthesis has been shown in cultured rabbit aortic endothelial cells [62]. Other authors, however, suggest that neutrophils are the main source of leukotrienes in reperfusion injury, as inhibition of endothelial xanthine oxidase by allopurinol does not affect leukotriene synthesis [63]. LTB_4 is chemotactic for neutrophils and monocytes [64] and upregulates neutrophil adhesion to the post-capillary venule by increasing surface expression of the CD11b/CD18 (Mac-1) adhesive glycoproteins [65]. Activated neutrophils also generate further leuko-trienes (LTC_4, LTD_4 and LTE_4) which mediate platelet aggregation and vasocon-striction [62].

Thromboxane A_2 has been implicated in the pathogenesis of coronary artery disease and Raynaud's syndrome, as well as peripheral arterial disease. TXA_2 may be synthesised by activated neutrophils, macrophages, endothelial cells and platelets [66]. Endothelial thromboxane is produced by the action of thrombox-ane synthetase on prostaglandin endoperoxides. TXA_2 has a half-life of 30–40 s in vitro [67] with a normal plasma level of < 3 pg/ml [68]. The stable metabolite TXB_2 has minimal biological activity. TXA_2 causes irreversible platelet aggrega-tion and degranulation [66], neutrophil chemotaxis, increased capillary perme-ability via disassembly of actin microfilaments and widening of interendothelial tight junctions [69], tissue necrosis, microcirculatory vasoconstriction and nega-tive inotropic effects on the heart [70]. Platelet aggregation is determined by the local balance of prostacyclin, as well as TXA_2, and the relative plasma levels of these two prostaglandin derivatives may be implicated in the development and clinical expression of atherosclerosis [47,61]. Neutrophil-derived TXA_2 is the main source in reperfusion injury. Goldstein et al. [67] showed that stimulation of neutrophils increased TXB_2 level while platelet depletion had no effect.

Prostacyclin is synthesised by vascular endothelium to help maintain a local nonthrombogenic surface [65]. Synthesis is induced by pulsatile pressure, throm-bin, bradykinin, 5-hydroxytryptamine, platelet-derived growth factor (PDGF) and interleukin-1 (IL-1) [50]. PGI_2 activity is greatest at the lumen and reduces throughout the vessel wall towards the adventitia. Its effects include vasodilata-tion, inhibition of platelet aggregation (via stimulation of adenylate cyclase), dis-aggregation of platelet clumps, inhibition of neutrophil aggregation and decreased neutrophil-endothelial adhesion [47]. In atherosclerosis there is a shift in the balance between protective PGI_2 and destructive TXA_2 [60]. This balance explains the therapeutic effect of low-dose aspirin in atherosclerotic disease. Aspirin irreversibly acetylates a serine residue on platelet cyclooxygenase inhibit-ing PGI_2 and TXA_2 synthesis, with little effect on thromboxane synthetase. Plate-lets cannot synthesise cyclooxygenase and therefore TXA_2 synthesis can only resume as new platelets enter the circulation (the platelet half-life is 8–11 days). Endothelial cells are able to continuously synthesise cyclooxygenase and therefore recover the ability to form PGI_2 [60]. The net result is cumulative inhibition of TXA_2 synthesis with preservation of PGI_2 synthesis [71].

ODFR stimulate phospholipase A_2 to synthesise platelet activating factor (PAF) from membrane phospholipids. PAF remains bound to vascular endothelium [72] and upregulates neutrophil-endothelial adhesion, promotes chemo-taxis and increases endothelin synthesis leading to an increase in microvascular permeability [37].

I-RI also results in synthesis of platelet-derived growth factor (PDGF) from activated vascular endothelium. Evidence for the importance of PDGF in the pathogenesis of atherosclerosis was reported by Cimminiello et al. [73] who found elevated levels in subjects with PAD compared to controls. Presumably PDGF encourages cell turnover to replace damaged vascular endothelium. What initially appears to be a protective mechanism may then become destructive as PDGF B-chain stimulates smooth muscle cells in the plaque to express the A-chain gene for PDGF [74].

Endothelin, an extremely potent vasoconstrictor described by Yanagisawa et al. [75], is important in the balance between protective and destructive endothelial products following I-RI. Endothelin-1 (ET-1) messenger RNA is synthesised by vascular endothelial cells in response to ischaemia-reperfusion, shear stress, thrombin, angiotensin-II, IL-1 and ODFR [60]. Endothelin synthesis is inhibited by increased nitric oxide levels [76]. The effects of endothelin are mediated by an increase in intracellular Ca^{2+}, activation of phospholipase C, phosphorylation of myosin light chains and smooth muscle contraction. This leads to profound arterio-venous vasoconstriction, as well as neutrophil-endothelial adhesion via the Mac-1 (CD11b/18) adhesive glycoproteins [50]. Endothelin also stimulates nitric oxide and prostacyclin production by the endothelium indicating that there is physiological attenuation of the constrictor effects of endothelin. Complement proteins also have a role in endothelial injury via the alternate pathway, with depletion of factor B and an increase in serum levels of C3a and C5a [49]. C3a and C5a are involved in neutrophil-endothelial adhesion, chemotaxis, neutrophil degranulation, increased microvascular permeability, stimulation of the arach-idonic acid pathway and vasodilatation [77].

Current evidence suggests that endothelial nitric oxide (NO) synthesis is important in the pathophysiology of I-RI. Endothelium-derived relaxing factor (EDRF) was isolated by Furchgott and Zawadzdki [78] and later shown to be identical to NO [79]. NO is synthesised from L-arginine by nitric oxide synthase (NOS) which exists in several isoforms, grouped into constitutive (cNOS) and inducible (iNOS) enzymes [80]. cNOS is continuously expressed in endothelial cells and platelets, in response to shear stress, catecholamines, bradykinin, his-tamine, thrombin and acetylcholine. The physiological effects of NO are mediated by guanylate cyclase resulting in vasodilatation and inhibition of both platelet aggregation and neutrophil adhesion [43]. Nitric oxide synthesis results in a basal vasodilatory tone, which is synergistic with prostacyclin [80]. NO is an unstable free radical and decomposes within a few seconds to nitrite and nitrate, catalysed by iron and haemoglobin. Experimental evidence suggests that in atherosclerosis there is failure of NO-mediated vasodilatation as both super-oxide and oxidised LDL are able to inactivate NO [81,37]. Superoxide inactivates NO by forming the peroxynitrite radical, which reduces the vasodilatory and antiplatelet protective effects. High concentrations of peroxynitrite are cytotoxic and may be involved in lipid peroxidation. Free radical scavengers have been shown to attenuate the reduction in NO-mediated relaxation following I-RI [81]. Recent experimental work has shown that activated neutrophils have an increased ability to inactivate NO in patients with intermittent claudication, compared to a control group [82]. The nitrate group of drugs, which are commonly used in the treatment of ischemic heart disease and hypertension, release NO directly to the luminal surface. This leads to vasodilatation and possible attenuation of these adverse effects.

iNOS is synthesised by neutrophils, macrophages, vascular endothelial and smooth muscle cells (i.e., the whole vascular wall) in response to inflammatory mediators such as TNF-α and IL-1. iNOS produces levels of NO $> 1,000$ times that of cNOS [81]. In the absence of L-arginine, iNOS generates large amounts of superoxide, which obviously has significant effects on vascular inflammation [37].

2.1.4 *Neutrophil activation*

Epidemiological evidence suggests that the neutrophil count appears to be an important cardiovascular risk factor, presumably a consequence of its important role in ischaemia-reperfusion. Friedman et al. [83] retrospectively reviewed records of 464 patients presenting with a myocardial infarction (MI) and found that a previously elevated leucocyte count (measured on health screening) predicted those patients who would subsequently present with a MI. Zalokar et al. [84] prospectively followed 7000 Parisians for an average of 6.5 years and found that smokers with a leucocyte count $> 9 \times 10^9$/l had 4 times the incidence of MI compared to smokers with a leucocyte count $< 6 \times 10^9$/l. The Multiple Risk Factor Intervention Trial concluded that white cell count was an independent predictive risk factor for incident cardiovascular disease and that lowering the leucocyte count by 1×10^9/l resulted in a 14% reduction in cardiovascular risk [85]. A white cell count decrease of 1×10^9/l was suggested to lower cardiovascular risk by 14%. Interestingly, Yemenite Jews are known to have a disproportionately low incidence of myocardial infarction, which may be a consequence of the widespread benign neutropenia seen in this ethnic group [86]. The Speedwell prospective heart disease study also demonstrated that an elevated leucocyte count predicted the development of intermittent claudication (mean 8.49×10^9/l in 84 future claudicants; mean 6.94×10^9/l in 2,010 controls) [7].

Activated neutrophils cause both local and remote tissue damage which is a major contributor to the morbidity and mortality of acute limb ischaemia, e.g., adult respiratory distress syndrome [87]. The changes in claudication may be more subtle, although having important long-term consequences. The mechanisms of neutrophil activation are undoubtedly complex. In the normal situation, 50–60% of neutrophils are sequestered in the pulmonary circulation although this pool is interchangeable with circulating neutrophils [87]. The precise mechanism of neutrophil activation is still not clear, although ODFR, PAF, complement, TXA_2 and LTB_4 have all been implicated [41,88,89]. Current theory suggests that a soluble "neutrophil activator", such as interleukin-8 (IL-8) generated during I-RI is responsible for activating systemic neutrophils. IL-8 (neutrophil activating peptide) is synthesised by monocytes and endothelial cells and is released into the systemic circulation [90]. IL-8 acts specifically on neutrophils promoting chemotaxis, upregulation of Mac-1 adhesive glycoprotein expression, extravascular accumulation and release of ODFR and proteases [91].

Activated neutrophils are less deformable than inactive cells as a result of increased cytoplasmic rigidity and pseudopodia. They are, therefore, less able to pass through the pulmonary capillary network [92]. This prolonged capillary transit time increases neutrophil adhesion to the endothelium of the precapillary sphincter and postcapillary venule. Plugging of the former by the large, stiff neutrophils after prolonged ischaemia may lead to the "low reflow" phenomenon on reperfusion, which exacerbates ischemic injury. The majority of neutrophils adhere to the postcapillary venule. High intracellular calcium levels results in degradation of Weibel-Palade bodies in endothelial cells and expression of P-selectin (previously known as GMP-140) which mediates early neutrophil adhesion [93]. Subsequent neutrophil adhesion is via a reversible calcium-dependent rolling of neutrophils on endothelial E-selectin (endothelial-leucocyte adhesion molecule (ELAM) [37]. Local production of inflammatory mediators, e.g., IL-1, IL-6, interferon-γ and tumour necrosis factor-α stimulates endothelial expression of intercellular adhesion molecule-1 (ICAM-1) and neutrophil expression of Mac-1 (CD11b/18) adhesive glycoproteins, via a phosphorylation-induced conformational change. This strong binding promotes neutrophil migration across the vascular endothelium and subsequent degranulation [94]. Monoclonal antibodies to Mac-1 or ICAM-1 have also been shown to reduce the extent of reperfusion injury [38]. Both ICAM and E-selectin require protein synthesis for maximal receptor expression and therefore are important late in the inflammatory response [87]. Activated neutrophils also aggregate forming microemboli which may explain the remote organ injury [65].

Neutrophil degranulation is an important event in the pathogenesis of I-RI. The mechanism of degranulation is via hydrolysis of cytosolic phosphatidyl inositol, increased intracellular Ca^{2+} and activation of protein kinase C [95]. Degranulation releases ODFR [96], proteolytic enzymes (e.g., elastase, collagenase and lactoferrin) and arachidonic acid products (e.g., TXA_2). Superoxide is a product of the neutrophil "respiratory burst" and rapidly dismutates to hydrogen peroxide (H_2O_2). Myeloperoxidase in neutrophil granules converts H_2O_2 into hypochlorous acid, which is a reactive oxygen species with a long half-life. Neutrophil elastase destroys the basement membrane of vascular endothelium, leading to an increase in endothelial permeability and adenosine diphosphate (ADP)-induced platelet aggregation. Neutrophil proteases may also influence the activity of coagulation factors, fibrinogen and complement. Eicosanoids are the third important product of neutrophil degranulation. Endothelial TXA_2 produced on reperfusion activates neutrophils which then produce TXA_2 forming a positive feedback mechanism.

The biochemical mechanisms of ischaemia-reperfusion in claudication are summarised in Fig. 3.

2.2 Animal experimental models of lower limb ischaemia-reperfusion

Several animal experimental models representing a claudicant limb have been designed to explore the biochemical mechanisms responsible for ischaemia-reperfusion injury. Other studies, discussed below, have used models of acute limb ischaemia followed by reperfusion to demonstrate their findings. This work can probably be extrapolated to the less severe situation of claudication. The adverse metabolic consequences of restoring blood flow to an acutely ischemic limb can be decreased by controlling the rate and the composition of the reperfusate (e.g., reperfusing with deoxygenated blood). This has been explored in several animal studies [33].

2.2.1 Free radical formation

The experimental evidence showing ODFR generation in animal models of claudication is limited. Punch et al. [97] studied the effect of ischaemia-reperfusion

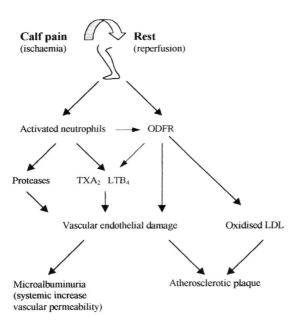

Fig. 3. An outline of the mechanisms of ischaemia-reperfusion injury in claudication. LDL: low-density lipoprotein, ODFR: oxygen-derived free radicals, TXA_2: thromboxane A_2, LTB_4: leukotriene B_4.

on xanthine oxidase formation and conjugated diene level (markers of lipid per-oxidation) in a rat model of acute hind limb ischaemia followed by reperfusion. Four-hour ischaemia followed by reperfusion led to an increase in XO, no change in XD and an increase in conjugated dienes, suggesting that the D-O conversion described by McCord [36] is responsible for ODFR generation. The increase in XO and conjugated diene was reduced by pretreatment with allopurinol, a xanthine oxidase inhibitor.

Homer-Vanniasinkam and Gough [48] reported the use of U74500A, an iron chelator which prevents lipid peroxidation, and found that it attenuated the adverse effects of I-RI in a rat model.

2.2.2 *Neutrophil activation*

Experimental work has attempted to determine the mechanisms of neutrophil activation. Patterson et al. [63] used an ex vivo chemotactic model in which human reperfusion plasma obtained during aortic aneurysm surgery was applied to a dermabrasion lesion on a rabbit. Human reperfusion plasma induced chemo-attraction of rabbit neutrophils with generation of ODFR, TXA_2 and LTB_4, and an increase in microvascular permeability. These changes were attenuated by neutropenia in the rabbit, confirming that a stable soluble factor was involved. Experimental work by Goldman et al. [98] using a rabbit hind limb ischaemia model showed that I-RI plasma induced neutrophil accumulation and micro-vascular injury when applied intratracheally to a different animal. Interestingly, when applied to a skin chamber of an animal with an ischemic hind limb, I-RI plasma prevented neutrophil diapedesis.

Neutrophil adhesion to endothelium is a prerequisite for neutrophil activation. Systemic mediators of neutrophil adhesion have been investigated by experimen-tal studies. Crinnion et al. [94], using a rat hind limb ischaemia model, demon-strated that pretreatment with a monoclonal antibody to Mac-1 prevented neutrophil recruitment, attenuated muscle necrosis and improved postischaemic muscle performance. Lehr et al. [99] used intravital fluorescent microscopy of skeletal muscle in the dorsal skin-fold chamber in a hamster to determine the role of leukotriene B_4 in mediating neutrophil adhesion. After 30 min reperfu-sion, LTB_4 accumulated in the tissue followed by neutrophil-endothelial adhe-sion. Adhesion was inhibited by MK886, an inhibitor of leukotriene synthesis.

Neutrophil degranulation is the main source of eicosanoids in I-RI. Crinnion et al. [100] reported a rat hind limb I-RI model in which the animals underwent 6 h ischaemia followed by reperfusion. At 10 min reperfusion, blood flow decreased — the "low reflow" phenomenon, which corresponded with peak TXA_2 synthesis. LTB_4 levels peaked at 120 min, while neutrophil elastase levels (degranulation) peaked at 240 min. Lelcuk et al. [69] demonstrated a rise in plas-ma and popliteal lymph TXB_2 following tourniquet-induced lower limb I-RI in dogs. Pretreatment with ketoconazole (an inhibitor of platelet thromboxane synthesis) had no effect on the increase in TXB_2 with reperfusion, suggesting that neutrophils were the main source of thromboxane. In a similar experimental model, neutrophil depletion using hydroxyurea or nitrogen mustard attenuated the increase in TXA_2 on reperfusion and reduced vascular permeability [101].

Thromboxanes generated by activated neutrophils also exert a positive feedback mechanism, promoting neutrophil accumulation in the lung. This has implications mainly for acute limb ischaemia, rather than claudication. Anner et al. [102] investigated the effect of 4 h ischaemia followed by reperfusion in a rat hind limb model of acute limb ischaemia. I-RI resulted in an elevation in TXB2 level, associated with neutrophil accumulation in the lungs at 4 h. Pretreatment with OKY-046 (a thromboxane synthetase inhibitor) prevented both the rise in thromboxane and the accumulation of neutrophils in the lung. Diethylcarbamazine (a lipooxygenase inhibitor) also resulted in a slight decrease in thromboxane and neutrophil accumulation. Further studies in other animal models have given similar results [103].

The end results of neutrophil activation is endothelial injury, resulting in reduced muscle blood flow and decreased muscle viability, (after acute ischaemia followed by reperfusion). In a well-described rat model of acute hind limb ischaemia, pretreatment with lipid-peroxidation inhibitors [48], thromboxane receptor antagonists, e.g., GR32191 [104], neutrophil depletion [105] and anti-Mac-1 monoclonal antibodies [94] results in increased tissue blood flow and improved muscle viability. None of these therapies reduce the extent of tissue oedema. Pretreatment with SC41930 (a leukotriene receptor antagonist) does reduce muscle oedema [48], suggesting that leukotrienes have important effects on vascular permeability, independent of activated neutrophils. Further confirmation of this was shown by Klausner et al. [101] who showed that pretreatment with diethylcarbamazine prevented an I-RI increase in popliteal lymphatic flow and the popliteal lymph to venous protein ratio.

2.2.3 Target organ damage

The target organ for oxygen-mediated vascular injury is vascular endothelium, both locally and systemically. This was well-demonstrated by Hickey et al. [106] who developed an in vivo model of claudication, in which rats were subjected to unilateral ligation of the common iliac artery and 2 weeks of intermittent hind limb stimulation. Control rats received either stimulation or ligation only. The ischaemia-reperfusion group had similar local endothelial cell swelling (extensor digitorum longus) to the ligation only group on electron microscopy, but had greater systemic endothelial cell swelling (diaphragm, left ventricular papillary muscle and spinotrapezius). Using the same animal model, Hickey et al. [107] showed that unilateral claudicant type ischaemia led to a bilateral increase in neutrophil-endothelial adhesion demonstrated by intravital fluorescence microscopy of the tibialis anterior postcapillary venule. This systemic effect from unilateral ischaemia was confirmed by an increase in urinary albumin excretion, suggesting a generalised increase in vascular permeability.

There is evidence that synthesis of endothelin-1 — responsible for endothelial injury — increases during reperfusion of ischemic tissue. Edwards et al. [108] reported a canine model of aortic cross clamping in which ischaemia led to an insignificant increase in ET-1, with a subsequent significant increase in ET-1 on reperfusion. Animal work has also confirmed the importance of complement proteins. Lindsay et al. [109] investigated the role of complement activation a feline model of I-RI. Four-hour limb ischaemia followed by reperfusion led to an increase in skeletal muscle permeability within 30 min of reperfusion and increased lung permeability within 4 h. This effect was blocked by SCR1, a soluble specific complement receptor antagonist.

Systemic vascular damage is difficult to assess both clinically and in animal experimental models. However, measurement of renal permeability to large molecules, e.g., urinary albumin appears to offer a straightforward method of determining underlying systemic changes [110]. Experimental work has shown that hamsters undergoing laparotomy and peritoneal contamination have an increase in microvascular permeability to fluorescein-labelled dextran in the cheek pouch, as well as increased urinary excretion of high molecular weight dextran, i.e., local injury has an effect on remote sites [111]. In the rat model described above, Hickey et al. [107] also found that unilateral claudicant type ischaemia led to an increase in urinary albumin excretion.

2.3 Acute exercise in patients with intermittent claudication

This section summarises the clinical evidence for biochemical changes induced by acute exercise in subjects with intermittent claudication.

2.3.1 Changes in blood flow and oxygen metabolism

It is well-established that following exercise to the onset of ischemic pain in claudicants, there is a delayed reactive hyperaemia corresponding to the severity of the ischaemia. This is likely to be a consequence of local acidosis within ischemic muscle leading to vasodilatation and its main purpose appears to be restoration of the oxygen debt established during exercise. The delay in hyperaemia is a result of inadequate blood flow through arterial stenoses or occlusions and may have diagnostic value in distinguishing between a mild claudicant with normal resting Doppler ankle pressures and subjects with no peripheral arterial disease. Transcutaneous oxygen tension ($TcPO_2$), measured in skin over the dorsum of the foot at rest and following exercise may enable differentiation between claudicants and control subjects [112]. The $TcPO_2$ recovery time may also reflect the severity of ischaemia. However, this method is a fairly crude estimation of the underlying physiological mechanisms. Depairon and Zicot [113] explored the association between blood flow and oxygen consumption in claudicants by using positron emission tomography of calf muscle and inhalation of $C^{15}O_2$ and $^{15}O_2$. At rest, there was no significant difference in muscle blood flow, oxygen consumption or oxygen extraction between normal and claudicant limbs. Ten min following exercise to the onset of calf pain, muscle blood flow and oxygen consumption were elevated in the ischemic limb, with parameters in the control limb returning to basal metabolic values. This lends support to the concept of a delayed hyperaemia, associated with recovery of the oxygen debt incurred during exercise. Kemp et al. [114] used ^{31}P magnetic resonance spectroscopy to measure ATP synthesis in claudicants and controls undergoing treadmill exercise. Recovery from exercise (spectra obtained over 13 min) was associated with a 42% decrease in maximal oxidative ATP synthesis compared to controls, prolonged acidosis and delayed recovery of phosphocreatine and ADP levels.

The above studies all suggest that acute exercise in claudicants has a marked effect on oxidative metabolism which continues for a significant period of time during reperfusion.

2.3.2 Free radical formation and antioxidant consumption

It is quite difficult to detect ODFR synthesis in claudicants, as they are highly reactive intermediates with short half-lives. Most studies have instead concentrated on measurement of lipid peroxides, which are the end-products of free radical induced oxidation. A number of assays have been developed to either measure total lipid peroxide concentration or specific end products. Stringer et al. [29] demonstrated elevated lipid peroxides in 50 claudicants compared to 75 control subjects. Levels were also increased in subjects with ischemic heart disease. Interestingly, there was no difference in lipid peroxide levels between subjects with claudication and critical ischaemia. In a case-control study, lipid peroxide levels at rest were found to be insignificantly higher in 10 claudicants compared to 10 matched controls [115]. However, following treadmill exercise, there was a significant increase in lipid peroxide generation at 1, 10 and 20 min in claudicants, with no corresponding change in controls. Hickman et al. [116] measured plasma malondialdehyde (a stable product of lipid peroxidation) and thrombomodulin (a marker of endothelial cell damage) in 15 claudicants and 15 controls before and 1 min after treadmill walking to maximum exercise tolerance. Both malondialdehyde and thrombomodulin increased following exercise in claudicants, with no significant change in controls.

A further method is to measure the activity of free radical scavenging systems, which scavenge newly formed ODFR, attenuating their harmful effects. Most studies, however, quote baseline levels only rather than changes with acute exercise. Significantly lower resting levels of red cell superoxide dismutase [117] and glutathione peroxidase, together with its co-factor selenium [118] have been demonstrated in claudicants compared to controls, suggesting that the free-radical scavenging systems are ineffective.

Perhaps a more appropriate measure of free radical activity is to assess the total antioxidant consumption, as this is independent of the various metabolic pathways of ODFR generation and degradation. Khaira et al. [119] used an enhanced

chemiluminescent assay to measure antioxidant capacity before and after treadmill exercise in 20 claudicants and 9 matched controls. The mean antioxidant
levels in claudicants and controls were similar at rest (mean 479, and 438 mmol/
l, respectively), while the claudicants showed a significant decrease 1 min following treadmill exercise (428 mmol/l), returning to baseline at 10 min. Control subjects showed an insignificant increase in antioxidant levels, probably reflecting a
protective mechanism against the adverse effects of exercise-induced disease.

2.3.3 Neutrophil activation

Clinical studies in claudicants have looked at several aspects of neutrophil activation. Absolute neutrophil count, although in itself not a measure of neutrophil
activation, obviously has important implications in terms of cardiovascular disease. Edwards et al. [118] found an increase in baseline neutrophil count in claudicants (5.6×10^6/l) compared to control subjects (2.8×10^6/l). The neutrophil
count increased immediately after exercise in claudicants only (7.1×10^6/l,
$p < 0.05$) with a return to baseline at 15 min. Activated neutrophils are larger
and have stiffer cytoplasm than their inactive counterparts, with a resultant
decrease in the ability to deform in order to pass through the microcirculation.
Neumann et al. [92] measured various neutrophil parameters in a group of claudicants exercising with repetitive toe stands. Exercise led to an immediate
increase in femoral venous neutrophil count (local circulation) compared to
femoral arterial blood (systemic circulation), an increase in the percentage of
activated neutrophils and a decrease in filtration of neutrophils through 8-μm
micropores. These changes were reflected in systemic venous blood after 10 min
of reperfusion. It has been shown that an increase in serum lysozyme (a product
of neutrophil degranulation) correlates with decreased filterability of neutrophils
in systemic venous blood following treadmill exercise in claudicants [120]. This
suggests that activated neutrophils are released locally into the circulation at the
site of injury and rapidly enter the systemic circulation, where many of the
adverse effects are mediated. The use of a sophisticated method of assessing
neutrophil activation (the cell transit analyser) has recently been reported in a
controlled study [121]. This technique measures neutrophil flow through 8-μm
pores, analysing 1,000 cells per sample. The study showed that claudicants had
an increase in the neutrophil transit time 5 min following exercise, with no significant change in controls. The decrease in median transit time correlated with
generation of plasma thromboxane, adding support to the idea that activated neutrophils are the main source of thromboxanes in I-RI.

Few studies have documented the effect of acute exercise on arachidonic acid
products in claudicants. Baseline plasma thromboxane levels are usually similar
in claudicants and control subjects. Following treadmill exercise to maximum
walking distance, claudicants show an increase in plasma thromboxane within
10 min of reperfusion which then peaks at between 15 and 60 min reperfusion
[118,121]. Control subjects show an insignificant rise in thromboxane level.

Wennmalm et al. [68] also found a significant increase in urinary excretion of thromboxane B_2 metabolites 20 min following maximal treadmill exercise in claudicants, suggesting that the plasma thromboxane level may peak earlier. Neutrophil degranulation also results in release of proteases. The Edinburgh Artery Study found an increase in basal neutrophil elastase level in patients with PAD [122]. This has been observed by other authors [123], although none have explored the effect of acute exercise on elastase levels.

2.3.4 Effect on vascular endothelium

Several clinical studies have measured biochemical mediators of the endothelial damage induced by I-RI. A significant increase in complement proteins C3a and C5a has been shown in 23 subjects with chronic lower limb ischaemia measured preoperatively [77]. The effect of acute exercise in a claudicant on complement has not been assessed.

Other studies have focussed on the assessment of vascular endothelial damage, as a measure of oxygen-mediated injury. There has been some interest in the use of von Willebrand factor (vWF) in the assessment of PAD. vWF is a specific product of damaged vascular endothelial cells and has a role in platelet aggregation and adhesion [124]. Elevated baseline vWF levels have been shown in subjects with positive cardiovascular risk factors such as diabetes, hypertension, smoking and hypercholesterolaemia [125]. A significant increase in vWF has also been shown in subjects with PAD compared to controls, presumably due to repetitive low-grade inflammatory events [123,126,128]. Treadmill exercise has been shown to lead to a further increase in vWF levels after 60 min rest (reperfusion) with no change in control subjects [118].

The systemic effects of repeated low-grade ischaemia-reperfusion events in claudicants are not fully known. Animal experimental work described above has shown that ischaemia-reperfusion in claudicant models leads to an increase in generalised vascular permeability, reflected by an increase in urinary albumin excretion. It has been suggested that an increase in permeability may be considered as an early disease marker of atherosclerosis, predating the development of atherosclerotic plaque [26]. This has been supported by evidence from the prospective Framingham Study which showed a 3-fold increase in cardiovascular mortality in subjects with proteinuria [128]. Urinary protein excretion may, therefore, reflect the degree of vascular endothelial damage and may have a role in determining progression of atherosclerosis and response to treatment [129,130]. Urinary albumin is normally excreted at a rate of < 25 µg/min [131]. The physiological mechanism for reabsorbing filtered protein in renal tubules is virtually saturated, and therefore a minor increase in glomerular permeability will be amplified by the renal concentrating mechanism leading to a significant increase in urinary albumin excretion — microalbuminuria [111]. Microalbuminuria is defined as a urinary albumin concentration which is not detectable by semiquantitative test strips [110]. This is equivalent to a urinary albumin level of 15–200 mg/l [132]. In most studies, microalbuminuria is expressed as the albumin-creatinine ratio (ACR) to allow for variation in urinary flow rate. The normal upper limit of the ACR is 0.95 [115], while an ACR > 3.0 confirms micro-albuminuria [110]. ACR levels between these two parameters must, by definition, reflect an increase in renovascular permeability. Microalbuminuria was originally described as a marker of early diabetic nephropathy and later shown to be associated with pancreatitis [133], the response to surgery [131], hypertension [134] and adult respiratory distress syndrome following aortic surgery [135].

Several studies have confirmed a clear association between microalbuminuria and patients with intermittent claudication. The baseline ACR cannot reliably distinguish between claudicants and control subjects [115,121], although other similar studies have shown a higher resting ACR in claudicants [136,137]. Perhaps an explanation for these differences may in the statistical tests used, as the ACR can vary by a factor of 10^3 between subjects, requiring nonparametric statistics for the analysis. Parametric tests may demonstrate a significant difference in the mean ACR between claudicants and controls, while the median values may not be significantly different. However, all of these reported studies have shown a significant increase in ACR in claudicants and not controls, following maximal treadmill exercise. For example, Hickey et al. [136] demonstrated a 153% increase in ACR in 23 claudicants after treadmill exercise (p < 0.001) with no significant change in 10 controls.

We have recently reported a further study in a larger group of patients, which confirms work from these previous studies [59]. Urinary ACR was measured at rest and at 60 min following maximal treadmill exercise in 67 claudicants and 15 age and sex-matched control subjects. Urinary albumin was measured with a double-antibody I^{125}-radioimmunoassay (Diagnostic Products Corporation, Caernavon, UK). Samples with urinary albumin levels > 60 mg/l were diluted and reassayed. These results were cross-checked with immunoturbidimetry, which is accurate to albumin concentrations of up to 250 mg/l. The data were not normally distributed, and therefore nonparametric statistics were used for the analysis. The most recent updated data is shown below.

The resting median (interquartile range) ACR in the claudicants was 1.36 mg/mmol (0.73—3.52) and in controls was 1.25 mg/mmol (0.72—1.96). There was no statistically significant difference in resting ACR between claudicants and controls (Mann-Whitney U test, z = −1.119, p = 0.23). In control subjects, the median percentage increase in ACR following treadmill exercise was 9.5% (IQR −18.8—72.7%). This increase was not statistically significant (Wilcoxon matched-pairs z = −1.1347, p = 0.18). In claudicants, the median percentage increase in ACR was 16.2% (IQR −12.2 to 53.6%). This increase is statistically significant (Wilcoxon matched-pairs z = −4.67, p < 0.0001). The data are shown in Fig. 4.

This exercise-induced increase in urinary albumin excretion has been shown to correlate with an increase in serum lipid peroxides [115], total antioxidant consumption [119], neutrophil activation and degranulation [120,121] and Doppler ankle pressure recovery time [136]. The change in ACR with exercise may have

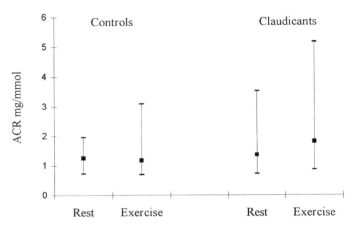

Fig. 4. Resting and postexercise albumin-creatinine ratio (ACR) in claudicants and control subjects. Results are shown as the median and interquartile range (mg/mmol).

use in assessing the effect of various treatment modalities. Tsang et al. [138] showed that treatment of claudicants with oxypentifylline, which has effects on neutrophil and platelet activation and microcirculatory blood flow, resulted in a reduction of the postexercise increase in ACR compared to placebo. Surgery also appears to have a significant effect on the ACR. Hickey et al. [120] demonstrated that bypass surgery had no effect on the resting ACR in 12 claudicants, but markedly reduced the postexercise increase in albumin excretion. These findings have been confirmed by other authors [137].

3 CHRONIC EXERCISE IN PATIENTS WITH INTERMITTENT CLAUDICATION

3.1 Skeletal muscle adaptation

Numerous authors have suggested that chronic exercise in claudicants leads to changes in skeletal muscle structure and metabolic function, with a resultant increase in exercise tolerance. The proposed mechanisms are thought to be similar to those seen in trained athletes.

Structurally, skeletal muscle consists of fast-twitch fibres (type II) which are required for phasic activity and are easily fatigued, and slow-twitch fibres (type I) which are more resistant to fatigue and are used for postural control. Type II fibres are subdivided into type IIa (fast oxidative) and type IIb (fast glycolytic). The fibre type in an individual muscle is usually related to the proportion of tonic and phasic activity required for normal function. It is tempting to postulate that chronic exercise in claudicants increases the percentage of type I fibres, improving exercise tolerance. Most methods of determining muscle fibre type are invasive, usually requiring biopsy of gastrocnemius muscle pre- and postexercise. A

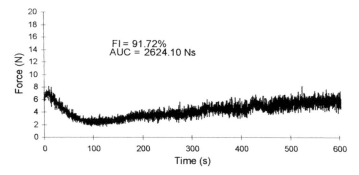

Fig. 5. Muscle performance in posterior compartment of a patient with intermittent claudication. The force of contraction (Newtons) is plotted against time. The fatigue index (FI) of 91.7% is the force of contraction at 10 min compared to the baseline value.

noninvasive method of assessing muscle performance has been described using isometric transcutaneous stimulation of anterior (tibialis anterior and extensor digitorum longus) and posterior (gastrocnemius-soleus) muscle groups in the leg and measuring the force of contraction against time, via a calibrated transducer linked to a computer [139,140]. The basis of this work is measurement of muscle fatigue, defined as the inability to sustain muscle function at a constant level of work over a fixed period of time. Skeletal muscle in claudicants, by definition, would be more susceptible to fatigue than muscle in control subjects and this can be shown clearly in the shape of the force-time curves (Figs. 5 and 6: results from our own work using the same technique). The force of contraction at rest is then compared to the force of contraction following muscle stimulation and a fatigue index (FI) derived: an FI of 100% would, therefore, indicate no change in muscle performance. Tsang showed a weak correlation between FI and tread-mill pain-free walking distance (PFWD), maximum walking distance (MWD)

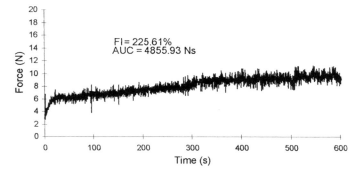

Fig. 6. Muscle performance in posterior compartment of a control subject with no peripheral arterial disease. The fatigue index (FI) of 225.61% is the force of contraction at 10 min compared to the baseline value.

and Doppler ankle pressure recovery time postexercise in a group of claudicants [139,140]. The advantage of this method is that is can be used repeatedly to assess the effect of treatment on muscle function. Tsang et al. [141] used this technique to assess the effect of chronic muscle stimulation on muscle performance. Both anterior and posterior muscle groups were stimulated at 8 Hz for 20 min, three times daily for a period of 4 weeks. This significantly reduced (normalised) the fatigue index and increased treadmill walking distances in comparison to a control group. This suggests an increase in type I muscle fibres, although further work is needed to clarify the relation between fatigue index and histological identification of fibre type.

Some authors have reported evidence that contradicts the hypothesis that chronic exercise increases type I fibres in skeletal muscle. Hiatt et al. [142] randomised 26 claudicants to 12 weeks of graded treadmill exercise training or control groups. Despite an increased exercise tolerance in the trained group, there were no changes in type I or type II muscle fibre distribution on gastrocnemius muscle biopsy. Interestingly, it was found that the percentage of denervated muscle fibres increased by > 100% from the baseline level in the trained group. This could perhaps explain the improvement in pain tolerance.

The metabolic changes within skeletal muscle cells in claudicants have been extensively studied over the past 40 years [143,144]. The response to exercise in claudicants is to increase mitochondrial oxidative capacity, with adaptation of enzymes of the citrate cycle, electron transport chain and fatty acid β-oxidation pathways [145] (Fig. 7). Despite this, mitochondrial function is impaired, with accumulation of intermediate products of oxidative metabolism, such as short-chain acylcarnitines in ischemic muscle and plasma [142]. These may be consid-

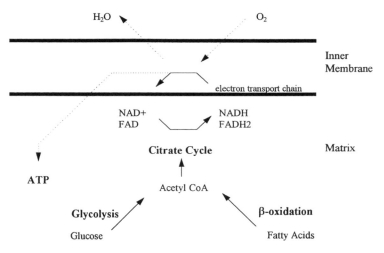

Fig. 7. Mitochondrial oxidative pathways indicating the potential sites for metabolic adaption with exercise training. (NAD: nicotinamide adenine dinucleotide, FAD: flavine adenine dinucleotide, ATP: adenosine triphosphate).

ered as biochemical markers of skeletal muscle function in claudication. Current theory is that exercise training improves mitochondrial oxidative capacity and normalises the metabolic pathways. Several historical studies have used repeated muscle biopsies to assess the effect of exercise training on mitochondrial function. Exercise training leads to an increase in succinate oxidase activity (citrate cycle), increased glycolysis, increased gluconeogenesis, decreased anaerobic glycolysis and lactate formation, as well as increased cytochrome oxidase [144—147]. Hiatt et al. [142] showed that 12 weeks treadmill exercise training decreased (normalised) plasma and muscle short-chain acylcarnitines, although having no effect on an already elevated citrate synthetase level. Metabolic adaptation, therefore, requires both physical activity and reduced blood flow.

An interesting mechanism for the metabolic adaptation to exercise was proposed by Capecchi et al. [148], who demonstrated an exercise-induced increase in plasma ATP and plasma adenosine in claudicants. It was suggested that exercise may lead to an adenosine-mediated metabolic adaptation, similar to the phenomenon of ischemic preconditioning in the heart, where repeated episodes of subacute ischaemia are protect the myocardium against an acute ischemic event and improve function after reperfusion [149]. The physiological effects of adenosine are ubiquitous, leading to inhibition of platelet aggregation and neutrophil activation, vasodilatation, increased microcirculatory blood flow and a relative resistance to ischaemia, mediated via A1 receptor activation.

3.2 Exercise training programmes for claudication

Exercise training programmes for claudication are widely reported in the literature and have conclusively shown an improvement in pain-free walking distance and maximum walking distances. Exercise is applicable to all patients with PAD, irrespective of age, sex, concurrent diabetes and the anatomical level of disease, although subjects with angina may achieve less benefit due to exercise-limiting chest pain [150]. Exercise training is also cost-effective in comparison to other treatment options. Recent work has suggested that for a 10% improvement in PFWD, twice-weekly exercise supervised for 2 h costs US$115 in comparison to US$3637 for percutaneous transluminal angioplasty [151]. Despite this evidence, exercise training is infrequently used as a therapeutic option in the UK, although perhaps is more widely available in the USA [152,153].

3.2.1 Mode of benefit of exercise training

Numerous mechanisms have been proposed to explain the improved exercise tolerance in claudicants subjected to exercise training, although many of these are speculative [154]. A review of the literature suggests the following are implicated:
Haemodynamic factors   — development of collaterals
                                     — increased lower limb blood flow
                                     — redistribution of blood flow distally

Structural factors	— muscle fibre adaptation
	— increased capillarization in skeletal muscle
Metabolic factors	— induction of muscle respiratory enzymes
	— increased size and number of mitochondria
	— increased oxygen delivery to the tissues
Haemorrheological factors	— reduction in plasma fibrinogen
	— reduction in plasma viscosity
	— activation of fibrinolysis
	— inhibition of platelet function
	— reduction in white cell count
Cardiovascular risk	— reduction in blood pressure
	— normalisation of serum lipids
	— weight loss
	— normalisation of glucose metabolism
	— stress reduction
	— regression of atherosclerosis

Improved walking technique [152]
Psychological factors [153,155]
Improvement in pain tolerance [150,154].
The effect of exercise training on skeletal muscle fibre adaptation and mitochondrial function is discussed in the previous section. Several of the above mechanisms are discussed below.

3.2.1.1 Haemodynamic effects. It has been suggested that exercise training increases the collateral circulation and therefore one would expect an associated increase in calf muscle blood flow [143,25]. The evidence for this increase is, however, conflicting. Few studies have conclusively shown an increase in lower limb blood flow following exercise training. An early study by Alpert et al. [156] used clearance of the radioisotope Xe^{133} to assess calf muscle blood flow in 19 claudicants subjected to exercise training. Six months training led to a significant increase in MWD which correlated with increased gastrocnemius blood flow at rest, during exercise and after exercise. Ericsson et al. [157] also demonstrated an increased resting and postexercise blood flow in claudicants following exercise training, using venous occlusion plethysmography. However, there is substantial published evidence that exercise training does not increase lower limb blood flow using both radio-isotope clearance and venous occlusion plethysmography techniques [144—147,158—161]. In view of this evidence, further mechanisms of action for the beneficial effects of exercise need to be explored.

3.2.1.2 Oxygen delivery to the tissues. Exercise training does not appear to increase tissue oxygen concentration. Mannarino et al. [160] found that basal $TcPO_2$ and $TcPO_2$ recovery time following treadmill exercise were unaffected by a 6-month exercise programme, despite increased walking distances. Several studies have confirmed that following exercise training there is increased oxygen consumption in the claudicant limb and a corresponding decrease in venous oxygen tension in the femoral vein [152,162].

3.2.1.3 Effect on serum lipids. Exercise training in normal subjects is known to have beneficial effects on lipoprotein metabolism. Kiens and Lithell [163] demonstrated that trained muscle has greater lipoprotein lipase activity, resulting in increased degradation of triglyceride-rich VLDL and increased synthesis of HDL_2-cholesterol. If similar mechanisms apply in claudicants, these changes may protect against the progression of atherosclerosis. Currently there is little data on the effect of exercise training on lipoprotein metabolism in claudicants.

3.2.1.4 Haemorrheological effects. The rheological properties of blood, particularly plasma viscosity, influence microcirculatory blood flow in ischemic muscle [150]. Epidemiological studies have shown that claudicants have an elevated blood viscosity [164] and therefore any treatment that reduces viscosity may have beneficial effects on the microcirculation. Ernst and Matrai [165] non-randomly assigned 42 claudicants to exercise training or observation. At baseline, no difference was found in haemorrheological parameters (blood viscosity, shear stress, plasma viscosity, haematocrit, blood cell filterability and red cell aggregation) between the two groups, although these were abnormal in comparison to normal subjects, confirming that claudicants have an haemorrheological deficit. Following exercise training, haemorrheological parameters returned towards normal levels, with no change in the observation group. Plasma fibrinogen level is an important component of blood viscosity. Binaghi et al. [161] showed that 3 months exercise training led to a slight reduction in plasma fibrinogen. Although not statistically significant, this change may have a beneficial effect on microcirculatory blood flow.

3.2.2 Clinical trials of therapeutic exercise training

The beneficial effects of exercise were first suggested by Erb in 1898 who reported an improvement in exercise tolerance in 12 claudicants treated with graded walking exercise [166]. Numerous clinical trials of exercise training have been reported, although few have been properly designed randomised controlled trials [144,146,152,158,159]. The problem with many of these studies is that the control group, having been informed about the potential benefits of the study prior to recruitment, may exercise more than anticipated and therefore may not represent a true control group. Gardner and Poehlman [167] recently performed a meta-analysis of 21 trials of exercise training and suggested an exercise programme should involve walking for at least 30 min to near maximum exercise tolerance, at least three times a week for a period of at least 6 months. The reported benefit from this was a 179% increase in PFWD (from a mean distance of 125.9—351.2 m) and a 122% increase in MWD (from a mean distance of 325.8—723.3 m). The greatest benefit from exercise is seen in those patients who have a supervised hospital-based exercise programme involving graded treadmill walking [152,153,168]. Supervised exercise training in the short-term leads to greater symptomatic improvement than percutaneous transluminal angioplasty [169]. Long-term results from this study found that maximum walking distance had deteriorated in the exercise group, with both distances in both groups not significantly different from baseline levels [170]. However, only 15 out of 26 patients randomised to exercise were reviewed at this time, with only five patients still complying with the exercise programme. Perhaps this underestimates the true benefit of exercise? Lundgren randomised 75 patients to exercise training, bypass surgery or exercise plus surgery [145,171]. Exercise alone was less effective than surgery in terms of walking distance, but the combined group showed the greatest improvement in exercise tolerance.

3.3 Effect of training on the exercise-induced inflammatory response

There is little data available on the effects of exercise training on the biochemical pathways of ischaemia-reperfusion outlined above. As previously discussed, surgical and pharmacological treatment of claudication attenuate the postexercise increase in urinary albumin excretion. The effect of exercise training on these parameters is not yet clear. The worst case scenario is that repeated episodes of exercise cause cumulative inflammation, which has adverse effects on cardiovascular morbidity and mortality. Current opinion suggests that this is not the case. Lower mortality rates in those treated by exercise have been shown in comparison to those treated surgically [166].

We have recently reported results from a randomised control of exercise training vs. 'observation' vs. angioplasty in 67 stable claudicants [59]. 22 patients were randomised to physiotherapist-supervised exercise and 17 patients randomised to observation. Experimental methods are mentioned above in section 2.34. Subjects were followed up at 3, 6 12 and 18 months following randomisation and resting and postexercise urinary albumin excretion determined. The latest data shows that claudicants in the observation group had a borderline increase in urinary ACR following treadmill exercise (median (interquartile range) 1.05 (0.69–1.57) mg/mmol at rest and 1.10 (0.65–1.97) mg/mmol postexercise, Wilcoxon matched pairs $p = 0.056$). The postexercise increase remained insignificant at 3, 6 and 12 months. Our concern was that the exercise group might show an increase in the postexercise ACR with repeated low-grade inflammatory events. Data for the exercise group are shown in Fig. 8. The significant increase in ACR following treadmill exercise was maintained at 3 months following commencement of exercise training, but from 6 months was attenuated with no significant difference between resting and postexercise values. Our concern regarding the adverse effects of exercise, therefore, appears to be unjustified. The trend at 18 months follow-up (although follow-up is incomplete at this time) suggests a long-term benefit from exercise.

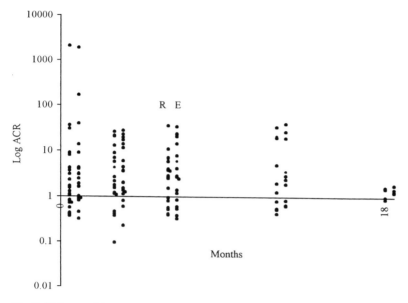

Fig. 8. Urinary albium-creatinine ratio (ACR) in claudicants following supervised exercise training. Data points (log ACR) for each subject at rest (R) and following exercise (E) are plotted against each time point (0, 3, 6, 12 and 18 months). At baseline, there was a significant increase in ACR postexercise (Wilcoxon matched pairs, p = 0.031). This was maintained at 3 months (p = 0.025). At 6 months (p = 0.463), 12 months (p = 0.386) and 18 months (p = 0.144) this rise was attenuated.

4   SUMMARY

1. Intermittent claudication is a common problem with a prevalence > 5% in the over 50 age group. The natural history of the disease suggests a benign prognosis for the limb. However, the 10-year mortality for this group of patients is 47—62%, which is significantly higher than an age-matched control population. Claudication may, therefore, be considered as a systemic disease.

2. Animal experimental models and clinical studies have demonstrated that exercise in a claudicant to the onset of calf pain results in oxygen radical generation, neutrophil activation and systemic vascular endothelial damage i.e., ischaemia-reperfusion injury. Does this matter in the long-term? The crucial question to answer is whether these repetitive low-grade inflammatory events are a transient phenomenon or whether they have significant effects on progression of atherosclerosis and subsequently on cardiovascular morbidity and mortality.

3. Therapeutic exercise training programmes are of proven benefit for patients with intermittent claudication in terms of improved walking ability. The mode of improvement is unclear but appears to be due to a skeletal muscle metabolic adaptation, a change in muscle fibre type, increased oxygen extraction in the ischemic limb, normalisation of serum lipids and reduction in plas-

ma viscosity. Exercise also has undoubted psychological benefit, as well as effects on general health and quality of life.

4. Current management of a patient with intermittent claudication involves advising on regular walking exercise through the onset of calf pain. Could the beneficial effects of exercise be outweighed by the adverse systemic changes resulting from an episode of acute exercise? Little evidence exists to confirm or refute this. Our own preliminary work suggests that long-term therapeutic exercise attenuates the changes seen with acute exercise and re-affirms the opinion that claudicants should be encouraged to exercise.

5   PERSPECTIVES

The inflammatory changes seen following treadmill exercise in a claudicant are unquestionable. Practically, many of these assays require complicated sample col-lection and specialist laboratory facilities and therefore could not be applied in the 'routine' clinical situation. If one were to identify a simple stable biochemical of disease reflecting cumulative inflammatory events, this would have potential use in the assessment of disease severity and in the evaluation of treatment such as exercise training programmes. Acute-phase proteins, such as serum amyloid A protein have potential use as markers of vascular inflammation, although further work is necessary to explore this. Although our early work suggests that exercise training may attenuate and not potentiate vascular inflammation, the study is not powerful enough to detect a change in cardiovascular morbidity or mortality with exercise. A prospective randomised multicentre trial comparing exercise training with "conservative" treatment may answer some of these ques-tions and would perhaps identify an association between change in inflammatory markers and cardiovascular disease. Another exciting prospect would be to modulate the vascular inflammatory response by dietary supplementation with antioxidants and/or fish oils, and determine whether the postexercise inflamma-tory changes can be reversed.

If we were to develop a clear understanding of the biochemical mechanisms involved in claudication and confirm that exercise is not harmful, then perhaps the majority of claudicants would be treated by a combination of exercise train-ing, low-dose aspirin and dietary antioxidant supplementation, reserving invasive treatment for those patients deteriorating to critical limb ischaemia.

6   ABBREVIATIONS

ACR:	albumin-creatinine ratio
ADP:	adenosine diphosphate
ATP:	adenosine triphosphate
Ca^{2+}:	calcium ions
CRP:	c-reactive protein
ELAM:	endothelial-leucocyte adhesion molecule

EPA: eicosapentaenoic acid
ET-1:   endothelin-1
HDL: high-density lipoprotein
H_2O_2:   hydrogen peroxide
ICAM-1:   intercellular adhesion molecule-1
IHD: ischemic heart disease
IL-:   interleukin
I-RI: ischaemia-reperfusion injury
LDL: low-density lipoprotein
LTB_4:   leukotriene B_4
MI: myocardial infarction
MM-LDL: minimally modified low-density lipoprotein
MWD: maximum walking distance
NAD^+:   nicotine-adenine dinucleotide
NO: nitric oxide
NOS: nitric oxide synthase
ODFR: oxygen-derived free radical
OX-LDL: oxidised low-density lipoprotein
PAD: peripheral arterial disease
PAF: platelet activating factor
PDGF: platelet-derived growth factor
PFWD: pain-free walking distance
PG: prostaglandin
PUFA: polyunsaturated fatty acids
SAA: serum amyloid A protein
Se: selenium
SOD: superoxide dismutase
$TcPO_2$:   transcutaneous partial pressure of oxygen
TXA_2:   thromboxane A_2
vWF: von Willebrand factor
VLDL: very low-density lipoprotein
XD: xanthine dehydrogenase
XO: xanthine oxidase

7   REFERENCES

1. Bouley jeune JF. Recueil de Medecine Veterinaire 1831;8:517—527.
2. Charcot JM. Comptes Rendres Seances Soc Biol Paris 1858;(2nd series)5:225—237.
3. Goldflam S. Dtsch Med Wschr 1895;21:587—590.
4. Criqui MH, Fronek A, Barrett-Connor E. Circulation 1985;71:510—515.
5. Fowkes FGR, Housley E, Cawood EHH et al. Int J Epidemiol 1991;20:384—392.
6. Dormandy JA. Hosp Update 1991;4:314—320.
7. Bainton D, Sweetnam P, Baker I, Elwood P. Br Heart J 1991;72:128—132.
8. Kannel WB, McGee DL. J Am Geriatr Soc 1985;3b:13—18.
9. Coran AG, Warren R. N Engl J Med 1966;274:643—647.

10. Bloor K. Ann Roy Coll Surg Eng 1961;28:36—42.
11. Imparato AM, Kim G, Davidson T, Crowley JG. Surgery 1975;78:795—799.
12. Jelnes R, Gaardsting O, Jensen K, Baekgard N. Br Med J 1978;293:1137—1140.
13. Nason P, Bergstrom R. Acta Med Scan 1987;221:253—260.
14. Dormandy JA, Mahir M, Ascady G, Balsano F, de Leeuw P. J Cardiovasc Surg 1989;30:50—57.
15. Coffman JD. N Engl J Med 1991;325:577—578.
16. Hughson WG, Mann JI, Woods HF, Walton I. Br Med J 1978;293:1377—1379.
17. Fowkes FGR. Eur J Vasc Surg 1988;2:283—291.
18. Dormandy JA, Murray GD. Eur J Vasc Surg 1991;5:131—133.
19. Davey Smith G, Shipley MJ, Rose G. Circulation 1990;82:1925—1931.
20. Criqui MH, Langer RD, Fronek A, Feigelson HS, Klauber MR. N Engl J Med 1992;326: 381—386.
21. Gown AM, Tsukada T, Ross R. Am J Pathol 1986;125:191—207.
22. Hansson GK, Holm J, Jonasson L. Am J Pathol 1989;135:169—175.
23. Secretary of State for Health. The Health of the Nation. A strategy for health in England. London: HMSO, 1992;46—47,62—64.
24. Powell KE, Pratt M. Br Med J 1996;313:126—127.
25. Housley E. Br Med J 1988;296:1483—1484.
26. Jellinek H, Detre Z. Path Res Pract 1986;181:693—712.
27. Ross R. Nature 1993;362:801—809.
28. Leake DS. Br Heart J 1993;69:476—478.
29. Stringer MD, Gorog PG, Freeman A, Kakkar VV. Br Med J 1989;298:281—284.
30. Parks DA, Granger DN. Am J Physiol 1986;250:G749—G753.
31. Larcan A, Mathieu P, Helmer J, Fieve G. J Cardiovasc Surg 1973;14:609—614.
32. Haimovici H. Surgery 1979;85:461—468.
33. Mitrev Z, Beyersdorf F, Hallmann R et al. Cardiovasc Surg 1994;2:737—748.
34. Zweier JL, Kuppusamy P, Lutty GA. Proc Natl Acad Sci USA 1988;85:4046—4050.
35. Friedl HP, Smith DJ, Till GO. Am J Pathol 1990;136:491—495.
36. McCord JM. N Engl J Med 1985;312:159—163.
37. Weight SC, Bell PRF, Nicholson ML. Br J Surg 1996;83:162—170.
38. Welbourn CRB, Goldman G, Paterson IS, Valeri CR, Shepro D, Hechtman HB. Br J Surg 1991; 78:651—655.
39. Sinclair AJ, Barnett AH, Lunec J. Br J Hosp Med 1990;43:344—341.
40. Bulkley GB. Surgery 1983;94:407—411.
41. Paterson IS, Klausner JM, Goldman G et al. Surgery 1989;106:224—229.
42. Tate RM, Repine JE. Am Rev Respir Dis 1983;128:552—559.
43. Halliwell B. Br Med J 1993;307:885—886.
44. McCord JM. Surgery 1983;94:412—414.
45. Halliwell B. Br J Exp Pathol 1989;70:737—757.
46. Parks DA, Bulkley GB, Granger DN. Surgery 1983;94:428—438.
47. Moncada S, Vane JR. N Engl J Med 1979;300:1142—1147.
48. Homer-Vanniasinkam S, Gough MJ. Br J Surg 1994;81:1500—1503.
49. Ward PA, Till GO, Hatherill JR, Annesley TM, Kunkel RG. J Clin Invest 1985;76:517—527.
50. Grace PA. Br J Surg 1994;81:637—647.
51. Defraigne JO, Detry O, Meurisse M, Lamy M, Limet R. Eur J Vasc Surg 1994;8:537—543.
52. Smith EB, Keen GA, Grant A, Stirk C. Arteriosclerosis 1990;10:263—275.
53. Witzum JL. Lancet 1994;344:793—795.
54. Quinn MT, Parthasarathy S, Fong LG, Steinberg D. Proc Natl Acad Sci USA 1987;84: 2995—2998.
55. Liao F, Andalibi A, Lusis AJ, Fogelman AM. Am J Cardiol 1995;75:65B—66B.
56. Witzum JL, Steinberg D. J Clin Invest 1991;88:1785—1792.
57. Steinberg D, Parthasarathy S, Carew TE, Khoo JC, Witzum JL. N Engl J Med 1989;320:

915—924.

58. Heinrich PC, Castell JV, Andus T. Biochem J 1990;265:621—636.
59. Tisi PV, Hulse M, Chulakadabba A, Gosling P, Shearman CP. Eur J Vasc Endovasc Surg 1997; 14:344—350.
60. Vane JR, Anggard EE, Botting RM. N Engl J Med 1990;323:27—36.
61. Hirsh PD, Campbell WB, Willerson JT. Am J Med 1981;71:1009—1025.
62. Nolan KD, Blair AK, Ramadan FM, Johnson G. J Vasc Surg 1990;12:298—304.
63. Paterson IS, Smith FCT, Tsang GMK, Hamer JD, Shearman CP. Ann Vasc Surg 1993;7:68—75.
64. Palmblad J, Malmsten C, Uden AM. Blood 1981;58(3):658—661.
65. Hickman P, McCollum PT, Belch JJF. Br J Surg 1994;81:790—798.
66. Ogletree ML. Fed Proc 1987;46:133—138.
67. Goldstein IM, Malmsten CL, Kindahl H. J Exp Med 1978;78:787—792.
68. Wennmalm A, Edlund A, Sevastik B, Fitzgerald A. Clin Physiol 1988;8:243—252.
69. Lelcuk S, Alexander F, Valeri R, Shepro D, Hechtman H. Ann Surg 1985;202:642—646.
70. Mathieson MA, Dunham BM, Huval WB, Lelcuk S, Stemp I, Valeri R. Surg Gynecol Obstet 1983;157:500—504.
71. FitzGerald GA, Oates JA, Hawiger J et al. J Clin Invest 1983;71:676—688.
72. Lewis MS, Whattley RE, Cain P, McIntyre JM, Prescott SM, Zimmerman GA. J Clin Invest 1988;82:2045—2055.
73. Cimminiello C, Arpaia G, Aloisio M et al. Angiology 1884;45:289—293.
74. Ross R. Lancet 1989;1:1179—1182.
75. Yanagisawa M, Kurihara H, Kimura S et al. Nature 1988;332:411—415.
76. Haynes WG, Webb DJ. Clin Sci 1993;84:485—500.
77. Bengtson A, Holmberg P, Heideman M. Br J Surg 1987;74:697—700.
78. Furchgott RF, Zawadzki JV. Nature 1980;288:373—376.
79. Palmer RM, Ferrige AG, Moncada S. Nature 1987;327:524—526.
80. Vallance P, Collier J. Br Med J 1994;309:453—457.
81. Davies MG, Fulton GJ, Hagen PO. Br J Surg 1995;82:1598—1610.
82. Akopov SE, Pogossian SS, Toromanian EN, Grigorian GG, Gabrielian ES. J Vasc Surg 1997;25: 704—712.
83. Friedman GD, Klatsky AL, Siegelaub AB. N Engl J Med 1974;290:1275—1278.
84. Zalokar JB, Richard JL, Claude JR. N Engl J Med 1981;304:465—488.
85. Grimm RH, Neaton JD, Ludwig W. JAMA 1985;254:1932—1937.
86. Shoenfeld Y, Pinkhas J. N Engl J Med 1981;304:1606.
87. Windsor ACJ, Mullen PG, Fowler AA, Sugerman HJ. Br J Surg 1993;80:10—17.
88. Klausner JM, Paterson IS, Mannick JA, Valeri CR, Shepro D, Hechtman HB. JAMA 1989;261: 1030—1035.
89. Klausner JM, Paterson IS, Kobzik L, Valeri CR, Shepro D, Hechtman HB. Surgery 1989;105: 192—199.
90. Donnelly SC, Strieter RM, Kunkel SL, Walz A. Lancet 1993;341:643—647.
91. Gross V, Andreesen R, Leser HG, Ceska M. Eur J Clin Invest 1992;22:200—203.
92. Neumann FJ, Waas W, Diehm C et al. Circulation 1990;82:922—929.
93. Homer-Vanniasinkam S, Crinnion JN, Gough MJ. Eur J Vasc Endovasc Surg 1997;14:195—203.
94. Crinnion JN, Homer-Vanniasinkam S, Parkin SM, Gough MJ. Br J Surg 1996;83:251—254.
95. Baggiolini M, Walz A, Kunkel SL. J Clin Invest 1989;84:1045—1049.
96. Granger DN. Am J Physiol 1988;255:H1269—H1275.
97. Punch J, Rees R, Cashmer B, Wilkins E, Smith DJ, Till GO. Surgery 1992;111:169—176.
98. Goldman G, Welbourn R, Klausner JM et al. Ann Surg 1990;211:196—200.
99. Lehr HA, Guhlmann A, Nolte D, Keppler D, Messmer K. J Clin Invest 1991;87:2036—2041.
100. Crinnion J, Homer-Vanniasinkam S, Parkin S, Gough M. Br J Surg 1993;80:S110.
101. Klausner JM, Paterson IS, Valeri R, Shepro D, Hechtman HD. Ann Surg 1988;208:755—760.
102. Anner H, Kaufman RP, Kobzik L, Valeri CR, Shepro D, Hechtman HB. Ann Surg 1988;

206:162—167.
103. Anner H, Kaufman RP, Kobzik L, Valeri CR, Shepro D, Hechtman HB. Ann Surg 1988;206: 642—648.
104. Homer-Vanniasinkam S, Crinnion JN, Gough MJ. Br J Surg 1994;81:974—976.
105. Crinnion J, Homer-Vanniasinkam S, Parkin S, Gough M. Br J Surg 1993b;80:S110—S111.
106. Hickey NC, Hudlicka O, Simms MH. Eur J Vasc Surg 1992;6:36—40.
107. Hickey NC, Hudlicka O, Gosling P, Shearman CP, Simms MH. Br J Surg 1993;80:181—184.
108. Edwards JD, Dovgan PS, Rowley JM, Agrawal DK, Thorpe PE, Adrian TE. Eur J Vasc Surg 1994;8:729—734.
109. Lindsay TF, Hill J, Ortiz F et al. Ann Surg 1992;216:677—683.
110. Winocour PH. Br Med J 1992;304:1196—1197.
111. Shearman CP, Gosling P, Simms MH. Br J Surg 1988;75:1273.
112. Caillard P, Mouren X, Pujade B, Blanchemaison P, Elbeze Y, Cloarec M. Angiology 1990;12: 469—478.
113. Depairon M, Zicot M. Angiology 1996;47:991—999.
114. Kemp GJ, Hands LJ, Ramaswami G et al. Clin Sci 1995;89:581—590.
115. Shearman CP, Gosling P, Gwynn BR, Simms MH. Eur J Vasc Surg 1988;2:401—404.
116. Hickman P, Harrison DK, Hill A et al. Adv Exp Med Biol 1994;36:P565—P570.
117. Hickman P, McClaren M, Hill H, McCollum PR, Belch JJ. Br J Surg 1994;81:616.
118. Edwards AT, Blann AD, Suarez-Mendez VJ. Br J Surg 1994;81:1738—1741.
119. Khaira HS, Maxwell SRJ, Shearman CP. Br J Surg 1995;82:1660—1662.
120. Hickey NC, Gosling P, Baar S, Shearman CP, Simms MH. Br J Surg 1990;77:1121—1124.
121. Khaira HS, Nash GB, Bahra PS, Sanghera K, Gosling P, Crow, AJ, Shearman CP. Eur J Vasc Endovasc Surg 1995;10:31—35.
122. Lowe GD, Fowkes FG, Dawes J, Donnan PT, Lennie SE, Housley E. Circulation 1993;87: 1915—1920.
123. Blann AD, Seigneur M, Adams RA, McCollum CN. Eur J Vasc Endovasc Surg 1996;12: 218—222.
124. Blann AD. J Rheumatol 1993;20:1469—1471.
125. Blann AD, McCollum CN. Eur J Vasc Surg 1994;8:10—15.
126. Blann AD, McCollum CN. Thromb Haemost 1994;72:151—154.
127. Blann AD, Dobrotova M, Kubisz P, McCollum CN. Thromb Haemost 1995;74:626—630.
128. Kannel WB, Stampfer MJ, Castelli WP, Verter J. Am Heart J 1984;108:1347—1352.
129. Gosling P, Shearman CP. Ann Clin Biochem 1988;25(Suppl):S150—S151.
130. Gosling P, Beevers DG, Goode GE, Hickey NC, Littler WA, Shearman CP. Lancet 1990;335: 349—350.
131. Gosling P, Shearman CP, Gwynn BR, Simms MH, Bainbridge ET. Br Med J 1988;296: 338—339.
132. Watts GF, Bennett JE, Rowe DJ et al. Clin Chem 1986;32:1544—1548.
133. Shearman CP, Gosling P, Walker KJ. J Clin Pathol 1989;42:1132—1135.
134. Gosling P, Beevers DG. Clin Sci 1989;76:39—42.
135. Smith FCT, Gosling P, Sanghera K, Green MA, Paterson IS, Shearman CP. Ann Vasc Surg 1994;8:1—5.
136. Hickey NC, Shearman CP, Gosling P, Simms MH. Eur J Vasc Surg 1990;4:603—606.
137. Matsushita M, Nishikimi N, Sakurai T, Yano T, Nimura Y. Eur J Vasc Endovasc Surg 1996;11: 421—424.
138. Tsang GM, Sanghera K, Gosling P, Smith FC, Paterson IS, Simms MH, Shearman CP. Eur J Vasc Endovasc Surg 1994;8:205—208.
139. Tsang GMK, Curry J, Smith FCT, Paterson IS, Hudlicka O, Shearman CP. Br J Surg 1992;79: 123.
140. Tsang GM. MD Thesis. University of Birmingham, 1995.
141. Tsang GM, Green MA, Crow AJ et al. Eur J Vasc Surg 1994;8:419—422.

142. Hiatt WR, Regensteiner JG,Wolfel EE, Carry MR, Brass EP. J Appl Physiol 1996;81:780—788.
143. Foley WT. Circulation 1957;15:689—700.
144. Holm J, Dahllof AG, Bjorntrop P, Schersten T. Scand J Lab Clin Invest 1973;31(Suppl 128): 201—205.
145. Lundgren F, Dahllof AG, Lundholm K, Schersten T, Volkmann R. Ann Surg 1989;209: 346—355.
146. Dahllof AG, Bjorntorp P, Holm J, Schersten T. Eur J Clin Invest 1974;4:9—15.
147. Sorlie D, Myhre K. Scand J Lab Clin Invest 1978;38:217—222.
148. Capecchi PL, Pasini FL, Cati G et al. Angiology 1997;48:469—480.
149. Ikonomidis JS,Weisel RD, Mickle DA. J Cardiac Surg 1994;9:526—531.
150. Radack K,Wyderski RJ. Ann Int Med 1990;113:135—146.
151. Rudofsky G, van Laak HH. J Cardiovasc Pharmacol 1994;23(Suppl 3):S22—S25.
152. Hiatt WR, Regensteiner J, Hargarten ME,Wolfen EE. Circulation 1990;81:602—609.
153. Regensteiner JG, Steiner JF, Hiatt WR. J Vasc Surg 1996;23:104—115.
154. Ernst E. Br J Hosp Med 1992;48:303—307.
155. Williams LR, Ekers MA, Collins PS, Lee JF. J Vasc Surg 1992;14:320—326.
156. Alpert JS, Larsen OA, Lassen NA. Circulation 1969;39:353—359.
157. Ericsson B, Haeger K, Lindell SE. Angiology 1970;21:188—192.
158. Larsen OA, Lassen NA. Lancet 1966;2:1093—1095.
159. Dahllof AG, Holm J. Scand J Rehab Med 1976;8:19—26.
160. Mannarino E, Pasqualini L, Menna M, Maragoni G, Orlandi U. Angiology 1989;40:5—10.
161. Binaghi F, Fronteddu PF, Carboni MR, Onnis A. Int Angiol 1990;9:251—255.
162. Zetterquist S. Scand J Clin Lab Invest 1970;25:101—111.
163. Kiens B, Lithell H. J Clin Invest 1989;83:558—564.
164. Dormandy JA, Hoare E, Colley J, Arrowsmith DE, Dormandy TL. Br Med J 1973;4:576—581.
165. Ernst EE, Matrai A. Circulation 1987;76:1110—1114.
166. Holm J. In: Bell PRF, Jamieson CW, Ruckley CV (eds) Surgical Management of Vascular Diseases. London: Saunders, 1992;111—118.
167. Gardner AW, Poehlman ET. JAMA 1995;274:975—980.
168. Regensteiner JG, Hargarten ME, Rutherford RB, Hiatt WR. Angiology 1993;44:1—10.
169. Creasy TS, McMillan PJ, Fletcher EWL, Collin J, Morris PJ. Eur J Vasc Surg 1990;4:135—140.
170. Perkins JMT, Collin J, Creasy TS, Fletcher EWL, Morris PJ. Eur J Vasc Endovasc Surg 1996;11: 409—413.
171. Lundgren F, Dahllof AG, Schersten T, Bylund Fellenius AC. Clin Sci 1989;77:485—493.

© 2000 Elsevier Science B.V. All rights reserved.
Handbook of Oxidants and Antioxidants in Exercise.
C.K. Sen, L. Packer and O. Hänninen, editors.

Part XI • Chapter 38

Exercise and oxidative stress in diabetes mellitus

David E. Laaksonen[1] and Chandan K. Sen[1,2]

[1] *Department of Physiology, University of Kuopia, 70211 Kuopio, Finland. Tel.: +358-17-163108. Fax: +358-17-163112. E-mail: david.laaksonen@uku.fi*

[2] *Lawrence Berkeley National Laboratory, University of California, One Cyclotron Road, Building 90, Room 3031, Berkeley, CA 94720-3200, USA. E-mail: cksen@socrates.berkely.edu*

1   INTRODUCTION
2   MECHANISMS FOR INCREASED OXIDATIVE STRESS IN DIABETES
     2.1   Advanced glycation endproducts
     2.2   Alterations in glutathione metabolism
            2.2.1   Glutathione homeostasis
                     2.2.1.1 Cell and animal studies
                     2.2.1.2 Human studies
            2.2.2   Glutathione-dependent enzymes
     2.3   Impairment of superoxide dismutase and catalase activity
            2.3.1   Cell and animal studies
            2.3.2   Human studies
     2.4   The polyol pathway
3   LIPID PEROXIDATION IN DIABETES MELLITUS
     3.1   Lipid peroxidation in experimental diabetes
     3.2   Lipid peroxidation in diabetic patients
     3.3   Lipid peroxidation and diabetic complications
     3.4   Insulin and lipid peroxidation
     3.5   Susceptibility of LDL cholesterol to oxidation
     3.6   Autoantibodies to oxidized cholesterol
4   EXERCISE, PHYSICAL FITNESS AND OXIDATIVE STRESS IN DIABETES MELLITUS
5   SUMMARY
6   PERSPECTIVES
7   ABBREVIATIONS
8   REFERENCES

1   INTRODUCTION

Diabetes mellitus (DM) is a major worldwide health problem predisposing to markedly increased cardiovascular mortality and serious morbidity and mortality related to development of nephropathy, neuropathy and retinopathy [1]. DM is characterized by derangements in carbohydrate and lipid metabolism, and is diagnosed by the presence of hyperglycemia. Diabetes has been traditionally divided mainly into type 1 and type 2 DM, with other less common forms [2]. Type 1 DM is marked by deficient or absent insulin secretion by the pancreas and tends to occur before middle age. Type 2 DM is characterized by insulin resistance coupled with an inability of the pancreas to sufficiently compensate by increasing insulin secretion, with onset generally in middle or old age. Type 1

DM is less common and tends to be more prevalent among more northern populations. The prevalence of type 2 DM among adults varies from less than 5% to over 40% depending on the population in question [1]. Due to increasing obesity, sedentariness and dietary habits in both developed and developing countries, the prevalence of type 2 DM is growing at an exponential rate [3,4].

Oxidative stress has been increasingly implicated in the accelerated atherosclerosis and microvascular complications of DM [5—8]. Oxidative stress can result in widespread lipid, protein and DNA damage [9], including oxidative modification of low-density lipoprotein (LDL) cholesterol, believed to be central in the pathogenesis of atherosclerois, and endothelial dysfunction [5,8,10,11].

Oxidative stress, assessed by mainly indices of lipid peroxidation has frequently, but not always, been shown to be elevated in diabetes [12—21], even in patients without complications [14,16—18,20,21]. Despite strong experimental evidence indicating a pathogenic role of oxidative stress in the development of atherosclerosis and microvascular complications in DM, controversy exists about whether the increased oxidative stress is merely associative rather than causal, or even whether oxidative stress is increased at all in DM. This is in part because measurements of oxidative stress are usually based on indirect and usually nonspecific measurement of products of reactive oxygen species (ROS) damage, and in part because most clinical studies in DM patients have been cross-sectional.

The mechanisms underlying the apparent increased oxidative stress in diabetes are not entirely clear. Accumulating evidence points to many, often interrelated mechanisms (Fig. 1) [5—8], increasing production of ROS such as superoxide [22—25] or hydrogen peroxide [26,27], or decreasing antioxidant defenses [21,28—30]. These mechanisms include glucose autoxidation [24,31] and the formation of advanced glycation products (AGE) [5,32], activation of the polyol pathway [6,7,33—36] and altered cell and glutathione redox status [33—36] and ascorbate metabolism [37], antioxidant enzyme inactivation [38—40], perturbations in nitric oxide and prostaglandin metabolism [8] and insulin resistance

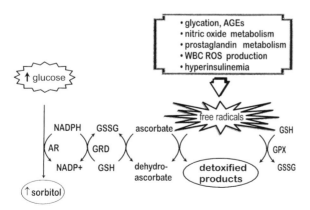

Fig. 1. Some hypothetical mechanisms for increased oxidative stress in diabetes mellitus.

[19,41,42]. No consensus has been reached as to the relative importance of these mechanisms.

Exercise has been widely recommended for DM patients [4]. The potential benefits and risks of exercise may be particularly important for diabetic patients, who at rest already show higher levels of oxidative stress. Many recent studies have shown that even moderate exercise may increase free radical production beyond the capacity of antioxidant defenses, resulting in oxidative stress [43−47]. Regular exercise can strengthen antioxidant defenses and may reduce resting and acute exercise-induced oxidative stress [45,47−49]. We [20] recently found increased oxidative stress, measured by plasma thiobarbituric acid reactive substances (TBARS) at rest and with exercise in young men with type 1 DM. Physical fitness as measured by maximal oxygen consumption (VO_2 $_{max}$), however, was strongly inversely correlated with plasma TBARS in the diabetic men only, suggesting a protective effect of fitness against oxidative stress. To our knowledge, only two articles have to date been published regarding acute exercise-induced oxidative stress in diabetes [20,50].

In this chapter we will first critically review the evidence for some of the mechanisms of increased oxidative stress in DM and the role of oxidative stress in the pathogenesis of diabetic macro- and microvascular disease. Due to the broadness of the topic, we will limit ourselves briefly to the role of AGEs and the polyol pathway, and discuss in greater detail glutathione and its related enzymes, catalase, superoxide dismutase (SOD) and lipid peroxidation in DM. We will then review our own work examining increased oxidative stress and its relationship to physical fitness in type 1 DM.

2   MECHANISMS FOR INCREASED OXIDATIVE STRESS IN DIABETES

2.1 Advanced glycation endproducts

Advanced glycation or glycosylation endproducts are the products of glycation and oxidation (glycoxidation), steps in the Maillard reaction. Glycation is the first step of the Maillard reaction, followed by reversible formation of Amadori products and Schiff bases. Subsequent reactions slowly give rise to AGEs and thereafter to cross-linking of collagen. AGEs increase with age, and at an accelerated rate in DM [51,52].

In vitro studies have suggested that glycation itself may result in production of superoxides [53,54]. Baker et al. [55], however, showed that the fructosamine assay proceeded faster under anaerobic conditions than aerobic conditions. Their data suggested that the Amadori compound itself directly reduced nitroblue tetrazolium, and that the inhibitory effect of catalase and SOD was likely because of oxygen regeneration in the assay mixture. Transformation of Amadori products into irreversible AGEs is oxidative. Oxidation has been hypothesized to result in the generation of superoxide, H_2O_2 and through transition metal catalysis, hydroxyl radicals [24]. In vitro studies have indeed shown that catalase and other antioxidants decrease cross-linking and AGE formation [32,56].

In addition to free radical formation during the generation of AGEs, AGEs have been shown to interact with receptors for AGEs (RAGE). Binding to RAGE in vitro has been shown to result in generation of TBARS and the induction of the transcription factor NF-κB, hemoxygenase (a marker of oxidative stress), vascular cell adhesion molecule-1 (VCAM-1), tissue factor, endothelin-1 and cytokines in endothelial cells [57−59]. In vitro studies have also shown mesangial growth factor release and extracellular matrix synthesis [60]. Diabetic red cells also have AGEs on their surfaces. These AGEs have been shown to bind to endothelial cell AGE receptors in vitro, with subsequent induction of NF-κB, platelet adhesion cell molecule-1 (PECAM-1) and TBARS [61,62].

Infusion of AGE-albumin at levels similar to those in diabetic patients in an animal model also resulted in induction of TBARS, VCAM-1, intercellular adhesion molecule-1 (ICAM-1) and heme oxygenase in vascular and other tissues [57,63]. Alteration in gene expression and induction of oxidative stress by AGEs was inhibited with antioxidants such as probucol or *N*-acetylcysteine [57]. Infusion of AGE-albumin into animals was also shown to increase basement membrane widening, extracellular matrix formation and growth factor mRNA levels, with consequent development of glomerulosclerosis and proteinuria [57,64]. In animal models the AGEs (N)epsilon-(carboxymethyl)lysine (CML) and pentosidine accumulated in the extracellular matrix and thickened capillary walls of early diabetic nephropathy and in nodular lesions and artery walls in advanced nephropathy lesions [65]. Immunostaining for malondialdehyde (MDA) has also shown collocalization of lipid peroxidation and AGEs in nodular glomerular lesions, suggesting that glycoxidation-induced lipid damage may be pathophysiologically relevant. Immunostaining has also shown collocalization of ICAM-1, VCAM-1 and AGEs with atheromatous lesions. Aminoguanidine, an AGE inhibitor, decreased AGE formation and the severity of nephropathy [64]. Infusion of AGE-albumin into nondiabetic rabbits for several weeks also produced marked endothelial dysfunction as measured by abnormal blood pressure responses to acetylcholine and nitroglycerine [66]. Coincubation of normal and diabetic LDL enhanced uptake of LDL into macrophages [67].

AGE content in skin, arterial wall and serum increases with age, and at an accelerated rate in DM [32,51,52,68]. Patients with end-stage renal disease had almost twice as much AGE in tissue as DM patients without renal disease, and serum AGE peptides were inversely related to creatinine clearance [68]. Phospholipids also react with glucose to form AGEs [69]. Both AGE-LDL and AGE-apolipoprotein B are increased in DM patients. Serum AGE-LDL levels have also been shown to be correlated with oxidized LDL levels, both of which were increased in DM patients. In type 1 DM skin collagen CML levels have been independently shown to increase progressively with development of early and proliferative retinopathy and micro- and macroalbuminuria, even when controlling for age and duration of DM [70,71]. Immunostaining of human atherosclerotic plaques revealed proliferated expression of AGE and AGE receptor anti-gen and mRNA [72,73]. Foam cells also contain high levels of CML [32].

Ortho-tyrosine and methionine sulfoxide, markers of protein oxidative damage, were formed concomitantly with CML and pentosidine during glycoxidation of collagen in vitro [74]. Ortho-tyrosine and methionine sulfoxide increased with age in human skin samples of collagen, these correlated with AGE levels in both DM and non-DM subjects. The age-adjusted levels of these oxidized amino acids in collagen was the same in diabetic and nondiabetic subjects, despite high-er AGE levels in the DM subjects. This suggests that in DM accumulation of AGEs and oxidative damage becomes uncoupled, and that diabetes per se does not cause an increase in oxidative stress. These results, although intriguing, may reflect only conditions in the extracellular matrix of skin, rather than conditions within the artery wall or in other tissues.

2.2 Alterations in glutathione metabolism

Tissue glutathione plays a central role in antioxidant defence [75,76]. Reduced glutathione detoxifies ROS such as hydrogen peroxide and lipid peroxides directly or in a glutathione peroxidase (GPX) catalyzed mechanism. Glutathione also regenerates the major aqueous and lipid phase antioxidants ascorbate and α-tocopherol. Glutathione reductase (GRD) catalyzes the NADPH-dependent reduction of oxidized glutathione, serving to maintain intracellular glutathione stores and a favorable redox status. Glutathione-S-transferase (GST) catalyzes the reaction between the -SH group and potential alkylating agents, rendering them more water soluble and suitable for transport out of the cell. GST can also use peroxides as a substrate [77].

2.2.1 Glutathione homeostasis

2.2.1.1 Cell and animal studies. In an in vitro study, insulin deficiency was found to decrease the activity of the rate limiting enzyme in glutathione synthesis, γ-glutamyl synthetase [78]. In an in vitro experiment, NADPH levels were decreased in human umbilical endothelial cells cultured in 33 mmol/l glucose [34,36]. Upon exposure to H_2O_2, glutathione disulfide (GSSG) release into the media decreased and intracellular GSSG increased, thus was likely to be due to decreased glutathione (GSH)-dependent H_2O_2 degradation and NADPH-dependent regeneration of GSH from GSSG. K562 cells grown in 27-mM glu-cose medium had decreased GSH levels, impaired γ-glutamyl transferase activity and impaired thiol transport [79].

Decreased [80−87] or normal [88] GSH levels, decreased [78] or increased [88] γ-glutamyl synthetase activity and an increased [89] or normal [88] GSSG/GSH ratio have been reported in hepatic tissue in streptozotocin (STZ)-induced dia-betic (insulin deficient) rats and in spontaneously obese diabetic mice, an animal model for type 2 DM diabetic rats. Decreased GSH content and GSH/GSSG ratio in the retina [90,91] and in the inner medulla of the kidney [33] in diabetic rats have also been found. Inner medulla glutathione synthetase and γ-glutamyl-cysteine synthetase activities were normal [33]. Ascorbic acid and vitamin E supplementation inhibited changes in retinal glutathione redox and antioxidant enzyme activity [90–92]. In contrast, Oster et al. [93] found no significant differences in GSH and GSSG in the liver of alloxan-induced diabetic rats. Rats with STZ-induced DM heve been reported to have increased renal total glutathione content, but normal liver and heart glutathione levels [94]. GSH content of endothelial cells in 10 rabbits with alloxan-induced DM decreased compared to 10 nondiabetic rabbits [95]. Alloxan-induced DM also decreased GSH levels and increased the GSSG/GSH ratio in rat red cells, with no effect on GSSG [96,97]. Nerve glutathione levels decreased in STZ-induced diabetic rats, with concomitant decreased neural blood flow and conduction velocity [98,99]. Administration of the thiol antioxidant α-lipoic acid alleviated these abnormalities in a dose-dependent manner [99]. On the other hand, normal GSSG and GSH levels have also been found in experiment diabetic rat nerves [100] and heart [86] tissue. Insulin restored hepatic [78,80–82], endothelial [95] and red cell [96] glutathione levels and γ-glutamyl synthetase activity [78]. Metformin has also restored hepatic and red cell glutathione homeostasis [86].

Most studies have found that GSH or total glutathione levels decrease in in vitro and animal models. GSSG levels or the GSSG/GSH ratio have also frequently been found to increase, although fewer studies have measured GSSG levels. Insulin and oral hypoglycemic agents have corrected these abnormalities.

2.2.1.2 Human studies. Diabetic patients have been shown to have decreased platelet GSH content, which was associated with increased thromboxane B2 production in response to arachidonic acid [101]. Murakami et al. [102] showed decreased GSH and increased GSSG levels in erythrocytes from type 2 DM patients. Platelet GSH content were 10-fold lower in type 1 DM patients with glycated Hb greater than 7%, but no further decrease was found when glycated Hb was greater than 11% [103]. Children with type 1 DM also had lower erythrocyte GSH than control subjects [104]. Hb_{A1c} was inversely correlated with red cell GSH content. Erythrocyte GSH levels decreased and GSSG levels increased in 18 type 2 DM patients compared to the 15 control subjects [35]. Blood GSH significantly decreased in 467 type 2 DM patients within 2 years of diagnosis and before development of complications [105]. Red cells from type 2 DM patients had decreased GSH levels, impaired γ-glutamyl transferase activity and impaired thiol transport [79]. Treatment was with an antidiabetic agent for 6 months corrected these changes. Erythrocyte GSH levels decreased and sorbitol levels increased in 29 type 2 DM patients [106]. Thornalley et al. [107] found an inverse correlation between erythrocyte GSH levels and the presence of DM complications in type 1 and 2 DM patients. Red cell GSH concentration was also related positively with duration of DM in type 1 DM and negatively with glycemic control in type 2 DM patients. Red cell GSH decreased in type 2 DM patients without complications and also in 105 patients with glucose intolerance and early hyperglycemia [42]. Twenty-six patients with type 2 DM who had poor glycemic control (mean Hb_{A1c} 11.2%) had decreased glutathione content [108]. Maintenance of euglycemia via intravenous glucose and insulin administration for 3 days decreased free MDA content and increased vitamin E levels, but did not have an affect on glutathione content.

In contrast, Costagliola et al. [109] found normal red blood cell GSH and GSSG levels in diabetic patients. No difference in red cell GSH levels were also found in elderly type 2 DM patients with and without retinopathy compared to nondiabetic control subjects [110]. Normal blood GSH levels were found in 43 patients with type 1 DM and in 107 patients with type 2 DM compared to 21 nondiabetic subjects [111]. Di Simplicio et al. [112] found normal GSH levels, increased GRD activity and decreased thiol transferase activity in platelets of 46 type 1 DM patients. Platelets from the DM patients also had a lower threshold for aggregation induced by arachidonic acid.

Glutathione infusion in 10 type 2 DM patients increased the plasma GSH:GSSG ratio, increased insulin secretion slightly and improved whole body glucose disposal, suggesting that the plasma GSH:GSSG ratio may play a major role in modulating glucose homeostasis in diabetic patients [113], since virtually all blood glutathione is intracellular, however, the mechanisms involved and physiological significance of these findings remain unclear.

Most studies have also found decreased blood or red cell glutathione levels in type 2 DM patients. Less firm conclusions can be drawn in type 1 DM patients. Further information is also needed about whether levels are decreased in patients without complications and whether patients with complications have even lower levels, although some studies do suggest this. The pathophysiological significance of decreased glutathione levels in DM remains to be shown.

2.2.2 Glutathione-dependent enzymes

In vitro glucose, glucose-6-phosphate and fructose all showed time-dependent inhibition of GRD, suggesting that glycation may play a role in GRD inactivation [39]. However, GRD activity has been reported to have an increasein the heart [82] and remain unchanged in the liver [89] in DM animal models. Conflictingly, GRD activity has been found to be decreased [114] and increased [115] in red blood cells in STZ-induced diabetic rats. GRD activities in endothelial cells of 10 alloxan-induced DM rabbits was unchanged compared to 10 nondiabetic rabbits [95].

Walter et al. [116] found no difference in whole blood GRD activity in 57 type 1 and type 2 DM patients compared to 28 nondiabetic control patients. Muruganandam et al. [103] also found normal red cell GRD enzyme kinetics in type 1 DM patients. On the other hand, blood GRD activity was lower in 11 children with type 1 DM compared to 49 healthy children [117].

Culturing of human endothelial cells in 20-mM glucose medium led to increased activity and mRNA expression of GPX [118]. Expression of mRNA for GPX also increased in the glomeruli of diabetic rats [119], and renal GPX activity showed an increased [82,119,120]. On the other hand, decreased GPX activity has been found in the liver [82,89,121], retina [90–92], soleus, gastrocnemius muscles and lymphoid tissue [122] in DM rats. On the other hand, GPX activity was found to be unchanged in the liver [123,124] and heart [124], but decreased in kidney [123], Asayama et al. [125,126] have shown increased GPX activity in heart, liver and kidney in STZ-induced DM rats. Aortic tissue Se-GPX activity has been found to be decreased [123] and unchanged [127] in DM rats. Alloxan-induced DM decreased GPX activity in endothelial cells of 10 DM rabbits compared to 10 nondiabetic rabbits [95]. Insulin treatment in diabetic animals restored GPX activity in the liver [82] and in endothelial cells [95]. Sukalski et al. [128] found decreased liver and increased kidney mitochondrial GPX activity. GPX activity in vascular tissue from the aorta and other major arteries in diabetic rats was normal [129], but in diabetic rats rendered euglycemic after pancreatic islet cell transplantation the catalase activity normalized. GPX activity increased in the pancreas and kidney, but not in liver or heart in STZ diabetic rats [120]. After 8 weeks of DM-induced by STZ, myocardial GPX activity was lower [130].

Erythrocyte GPX activity was also impaired in Asian diabetic patients [131]. On the other hand, Walter et al. [116] found no difference in whole blood GPX activity in 57 type 1 and type 2 DM patients compared to 28 nondiabetic control patients. GPX activity was normal in red cells of young type 1 DM patients [132] and in leukocytes of type 2 DM patients compared to age matched control subjects [133]. Red cell GPX activity was normal in 467 type 2 DM patients within 2 years of diagnosis and before development of complications [105]. In type 1 DM plasma selenium levels were normal, but red cell selenium content and GPX activity decreased [134].

In vitro studies have shown decreased liver GST activity in a hyperglycemic medium [135]. Hepatic [94,124] and heart [124] GST activity decreased in rat diabetes model, and insulin at doses sufficient to bring about euglycemia restored GST activity. Liver GST activity decreased in spontaneously obese diabetic mice [83]. Gupta et al. [96] also reported increased red cell GST activity in DM rats, which did not normalize with insulin treatment. Liver GST activity decreased in STZ DM rats, however, insulin partly normalized these changes. Normal red cell GST enzyme kinetics were found in type 1 DM patients [103]. GST activity has been reported to be decreased in the heart and the liver [124].

Changes in glutathione-dependent enzymes in experimental diabetic models have been contradictory. Most studies show tissue and time-dependent changes in enzyme activity. Even taking these factors into account, no consensus can be found among studies about the impact of DM on glutathione-dependent enzyme activity. Changes in glutathione dependent enzymes in diabetic patients are also inconsistent. Differences in results cannot be completely explained by study methodology.

2.3 Impairment of superoxide dismutase and catalase activity

SOD and catalase are also major antioxidant enzymes. SOD exists in three different isoforms. Cu,Zn-SOD is mostly in the cytosol and dismutates superoxide to hydrogen peroxide. Extracellular (EC)-SOD is found in the plasma and extracellular space. Mn-SOD is located in mitochondria. Catalase is a hydrogen peroxide decomposing enzyme mainly localized to peroxisomes or microperoxisomes. Decreased Cu,Zn-SOD activity coupled with the increased superoxide or H_2O_2 production that may occur in DM [23,24] could predispose to an increased oxidative stress, especially if not compensated with increased catalase or Se-GPX activity. Superoxide may react with other ROS such as nitric oxide to form highly toxic species such as peroxynitrite, in addition to direct toxic effects [8]. Alternatively, superoxide can be dismutated to much more reactive hydrogen peroxide, which through the Fenton reaction can then lead to highly toxic hydroxyl radical formation [24].

2.3.1 Cell and animal studies

Evidence for impairment of SOD or catalase activity is conflicting, especially in animal models of diabetes. In an in vitro study, human endothelial cells cultured in a 20-mM glucose medium increased mRNA and expression activity of Cu,Zn-SOD, Mn-SOD, catalase and GPX [118]. Elevated glucose [135] and hydrogen peroxide levels [136] have also been shown to inactivate catalase.

Loven et al. [80] reported decreased Cu,Zn-SOD activity in diabetic rat liver, kidney and erythrocytes. Oral glutathione or intramuscular insulin restored SOD activity in the liver and kidney but not in red cells. Increased catalase activity in cardiac tissue but decreased catalase and Cu,Zn-SOD activities in the liver and kidney were also found after 12 weeks of diabetes in rats, and corrected with insulin treatment [82]. In another study, catalase activity decreased in the liver, heart and blood but increased in the kidneys, Cu,Zn-SOD activity increased in the liver but not in the heart or kidneys [137]. Myocardial SOD activity decreased and catalase activity increased after 4 [138] and 8 [130] weeks of STZ-induced DM. Liver Mn-SOD increased in the liver but not in the kidney or heart in diabetic rats. Cu,Zn-SOD, on the other hand, decreased in the liver but not in the kidney or heart, and catalase activity also decreased in the liver and kidneys but increased in the heart [125,126]. These changes were similar in nondiabetic rats that were starved. Enzyme abnormailies corrected with respective insulin treatment and refeeding. Aorta catalase enzyme activity was accentuated without changes in SOD activity in a rabbit diabetes model [127]. In the liver and in endothelial cells prepared from 10 rabbits 17 days after induction of DM, catalase and Cu,Zn-SOD activities were depressed [95]. In 18 insulin treated animals, antioxidant enzyme activities were corrected. There was no effect on SOD activity after 8 to 12 weeks of DM enhanced large vessel catalase activity [129]. Pancreatic islet cell transplantation reversed catalase enzyme activity to normal levels.

Catalase and Cu,Zn-SOD activities steadily increased from 0 to 6 weeks after induction of DM in rat aorta [120]. On the other hand, vascular tissue from the aorta and other major arteries in diabetic rats were reported to have increased catalase but had normal levels of SOD activities [129]. Diabetic rats rendered euglycemic after pancreatic islet cell transplantation, catalase activity normalized. Cu,Zn-SOD, Mn-SOD and catalase showed variable changes in the heart, although by 6 weeks all enzymes had increased. Mn-SOD mRNA expression markedly decreased and that of Cu,Zn-SOD only slightly decreased in the aorta from STZ-induced DM rats [139]. Kaul et al. [130] reported decreased SOD, but increased catalase activities in rat myocardium 4 weeks after induction of DM. Probucol attenuated these changes. Liver mitochondria from DM rats 4 weeks after induction by STZ had lower levels of Mn-SOD [128]. SOD and catalase activities decreased in the liver of STZ DM rats. Kidney enzyme activities were also altered [121]. SOD and catalase activities decreased in the retina of DM rats [90,92,140]. Kaul et al. [138] reported slightly increased myocardial catalase activity but decreased SOD activity in rats 4 weeks after induction of DM. Probucol attenuated these changes. Kidney Cu,Zn-SOD and catalase mRNA levels were elevated in untreated and low dose insulin treated rats 17 days after indiction of DM with STZ [141]. With moderate dose insulin treatment catalase normalized, but Cu,Zn-SOD mRNA levels returned to normal only when insulin doses were sufficient to restore normoglycemia. Expression of mRNAs increased for Cu,Zn-SOD, but decreased for catalase in the glomeruli of diabetic rats [119]. Despite higher Cu,Zn-SOD mRNA expression, Cu,Zn-SOD activity decreased, whereas catalase activity correlated with catalase mRNA expression.

As in the case with glutathione-dependent enzymes, changes in SOD and catalase activity in experimental diabetic models have been contradictory. Most studies also show tissue- and time-dependent changes in enzyme activity. Even so, no consensus can be found among studies about the impact of DM on SOD or catalase activity in various tissues. Study design or assay methods do not completely explain differences in results.

2.3.2 Human studies

Superoxide levels as estimated indirectly by cytochrome c reduction were elevated in neutrophils from diabetic patients [22]. Decreased activity of cytoplasmic Cu,Zn-SOD and especially mitochondrial Mn-SOD in diabetic neutrophils was also found. Glycosylation of Cu,Zn-SOD has been shown to lead to enzyme inactivation both in vivo and in vitro [38], enzyme cleavage and release of Cu^{2+}, which in vitro resulted in transition metal catalyzed ROS formation [142]. Red cell Cu,Zn-SOD activity was similar between type 2 DM patients and normal subjects [116,131], irrespective of microvascular complications [116]. Erythrocyte Cu,Zn-SOD activity correlated inversely with indices of glycemic control in DM patients, however [143], red cell Cu,Zn/SOD activity has also been found to be decreased in DM patients [38,40]. Glycation may decrease cell-associated EC-SOD; however, this could predispose to oxidative damage. Jennings et al. [144] found decreased red cell Cu,Zn-SOD activity in 15 type 1 DM patients with retinopathy compared to type 1 DM patients without microvascular complications and nondiabetic control subjects. Yaquoob et al. [17] reported increased red cell SOD and serum MDA in patients with type 1 DM and normo- and microalbuminuria compared to healthy subjects. There was no difference, however, between DM patients with normo- or microalbuminuria.

In a study with 42 type 1 DM patients divided into groups based on the presence or absence of retinopathy, red cell Cu,Zn-SOD activity increased compared to healthy subjects [145]. No difference in SOD activity was found between patients with and without retinopathy. Red cell SOD levels in 22 patients with type 1 DM (10 had background retinopathy) were similar to reference levels in another study [146]. SOD activities were similar in 16 patients with micro- or macroalbuminuria compared to 69 normoalbuminuric patients in, young, type 1 DM patients [132]. Lipid peroxidation and antioxidant enzyme activity were also similar in the 39 smokers compared to nonsmokers. Red cell Cu,Zn-SOD and catalase activities decreased compared to 180 control subjects [105]. Plasma ascorbate and α-tocopherol levels also decreased. Leukocyte SOD activity was similar between 53 type 2 DM patients and 34 healthy control subjects, despite increased lipid peroxidation and decreased ascorbate levels [133]. In contrast to their earlier findings, Skrha et al. [147] found decreased red cell Cu,Zn-SOD activity in 47 type 1 and type 2 DM patients. An inverse relationship between tissue plasminogen activator and SOD was also noted. Red cell superoxide and catalase activities decreased in 105 subjects with impaired glucose tolerance (IGT) and early hyperglycemia and also in type 2 DM patients [42]. Red cell catalase and SOD activities were normal in 26 type 2 DM patients who had poor glycemic control [108].

EC-SOD can also be glycated, although glycation does not affect enzyme activity [148]. EC-SOD activity was found to be similar in 23 children with type 1 DM of varying duration compared to healthy children [149]. In contrast, Adachi et al. [148] found somewhat higher plasma EC-SOD levels in diabetic patients. Red cell glycosylated Cu,Zn-SOD levels were elevated in DM patients [38,40]. In another study, both diabetic and nondiabetic patients with peripheral vascular disease had elevated plasma EC-SOD activity [15].

The wide variability among studies does not allow conclusions to be drawn as to whether SOD isoform or catalase enzyme activities are abnormal in diabetic patients. Again, differences in methodology or study design do not completely explain the conflicting findings among studies.

2.4 The polyol pathway

Hyperglycemia induces the polyol pathway, resulting in induction of aldose reductase and production of sorbitol (Fig. 1) [7]. Importance of the polyol pathway may vary among tissues. Induction of oxidative stress may occur through many different mechanisms, including depletion of NADPH and consequent disturbance of glutathione and nitric oxide metabolism.

Activation of glucose oxidation by addition of 200 µM H_2O_2 was impaired in endothelial cells cultured in a 33-mM glucose medium, with concomitant NADPH depletion [34,36,150]. In GSH depleted cells, NADPH did not decrease, suggesting that consumption of NADPH by glutathione-dependent enzymes such as GRD in response to oxidative stress results in NADPH depletion in media with high glucose levels [151]. Addition of pyruvate decreased the NADH:NAD+ ratio as estimated by the pyruvate:lactate ratio, an enhanced glutathione-dependent degradation of H_2O_2 and decreased H_2O_2-induced endothelial cell damage. Thus, in endothelial cells induction of the polyol pathway by high glucose levels there is not only a depletion of NADPH and GSH but this also results in reductive stress by elevating the NADH/NAD+ ratio, predisposing to oxidative damage.

In homogenates of the inner medulla in diabetic rats the content of NADPH was about 32% lower than in the control rats, and the ratio of NADPH:NADP+ also decreased. GSH content and the GSH:GSSG ratio in diabetic rats also diminished [33].

Mean red cell GSH and NADPH levels and NADPH:NADP+ and GSH:GSSG ratios decreased in 18 type 2 diabetic patients compared to 16 non-diabetic control subjects [35,152]. One week of treatment with the aldose reductase inhibitor Tolrestat improved the NADPH and GSH levels in those patients whose NADPH levels were depressed (n = 8). Thus, in at least a subset of type 2 DM patients activation of the polyol pathway appears to deplete erythrocyte NADPH and GSH.

3   LIPID PEROXIDATION IN DIABETES MELLITUS

3.1 Lipid peroxidation in experimental diabetes

Culturing of human endothelial cells in 20-mM glucose medium led to increased TBARS and conjugated diene levels and enhanced production of platelet-derived growth factor [153]. Addition of SOD or glutathione prevented these changes. Elevated glucose concemtrations enhanced LDL oxidation as measured by TBARS formation, decreased electrophoretic mobility and decreased free lysine groups. Glucose mediated enhancement of LDL oxidation could be inhibited by SOD and buylated hydroxytoluene [154].

Red cells from rats with STZ-induced DM were more susceptible to lipid peroxidation as measured by MDA levels in response to H_2O_2 [115]. Lipid peroxide levels were elevated in the kidneys, unchanged in the heart and decreased in the liver of STZ-induced rats [155]. Induction of diabetes in rats resulted in accumulation of lipid peroxides in serum, liver [156], lymphoid tissue and soleus and gastrocnemius muscle [122]. Lipid peroxide content increased in the kidneys but decreased in the liver 2 weeks after induction of DM with STZ in rats [125,126]. Lipid peroxides were decreased [125] or unchanged [126] in the heart. Winkler and Moser [157] reported increased MDA levels; these correlated with glucose levels in STZ-induced DM rats. High-dose vitamin E supplementation decreased lipid peroxide levels to normal. Liver and kidney TBARS increased 1 week after induction of DM with STZ in rats [158]. Insulin reversed these changes. Plasma, red cell MDA and conjugated diene levels increased and ascorbate levels decreased in STZ diabetic rats [159,160]. Insulin treatment normalized these levels, although ascorbate homeostasis remained abnormal as indicated by increased dehydroascorbate levels. High-dose ascorbate supplementation without insulin restored ascorbate levels to normal and increased vitamin E levels. MDA and conjugated diene levels remained elevated, however, possibly because of increased iron availability. Serum TBARS increased in STZ-induced diabetic rats [161]. Vitamin E supplementation administered for 4 weeks decreased TBARS levels, although levels remained elevated compared to that of the normal rats. Induction of DM with STZ did not affect TBARS [85]. Insulin decreased lipid peroxidation and vitamin E-quinone levels to normal. Liver mitochondria from DM rats 4 weeks after induction by STZ were less susceptible to oxidative stress generated by an Fe^{3+}/ADP/xanthine/xanthine oxidase system as assessed by TBARS formation and sylfhydryl loss [128]. Kidney mitochondria were equally susceptible.

DM rats had higher levels of oxidized lipid in serum lipoproteins after being fed a diet containing high levels oxidized lipids [162]. Serum MDA antibodies and circulating immune complexes were similar in STZ-induced DM and control rats [163]. Liver mitochondria from DM rats were more resistant to Fe^{3+}/ADP-induced oxidation [128]. Kidney mitochondria from DM rats had similar susceptibility to oxidation and also had similar vitamin E contents. Oxidized lipid levels in DM rats on a fat-free diet were very low and did not differ from normal rat levels. Urinary MDA levels as measured by HPLC were markedly elevated in STZ-induced diabetic rats [164]. Heart ventricle TBARS increased in DM rats [165]. MDA content of the liver, serum and aorta were elevated in DM rats 4 weeks after induction of DM with STZ [166]. Brain MDA levels have been found to be elevated in alloxan-induced DM rats [167]. TBARS levels were higher in skeletal muscle but lower in lymphoid tissue in rats with STZ- induced DM [122]. Exhalation of ethane increased in response to acute hyperglycemia-induced by intravenus glucose administration and in response to chronic hyperglycemia in STZ-induced DM rats. Insulin attenuated ethane production in the DM rats [168], after injections of STZ in 4-, 7- and 8-fold increases in lipid peroxidation were found in the brain, liver and kidneys [169]. Pericyte and retinal capillary endothelial cell toxicity increased as LDL became glycated and later glycoxidized [170]. After the induction of DM with STZ for 10 weeks, rats had increased TBARS in the pancreas, heart and blood, but not in the liver or the kidneys [137]. Aorta, heart and blood TBARS were elevated at 2, 4 and 6 weeks after induction of the DM [120]. Kidney TBARS levels also rose 2 weeks after

DM [171]. Plasma TBARS were elevated in STZ-induced DM rats after 18 weeks [172], however, insulin treatment partly corrected the changes. Kaul et al. [130,138] reported markedly increased cardiac TBARS formation and impaired left ventricular function in rats 4 and 8 weeks after the induction of DM. Probucol attenuated these changes. N-acetylcysteine corrected the increased plasma lipid peroxide levels found in STZ-diabetic rats, in addition to correcting motor nerve conduction velocity Sagara et al. [173].

Studies have reported increased, decreased and unchanged levels of lipid peroxidation in various tissues of DM animal models. Although the tissue in question and the duration of DM seem to be important, no clear pattern can be found when comparing different studies. Again, these differences cannot be explained entirely based on differences in study design or assay method.

3.2 Lipid peroxidation in diabetic patients

Use of TBARS as an index of lipid peroxidation was pioneered by Yagi et al. [174], whose group also showed increased plasma TBARS levels in DM [12]. Diabetic red blood cells were shown to be more susceptible to lipid peroxidation as measured by TBARS in rats and humans [115,175]. Liposomes constructed from red cell membranes of DM patients were highly sensitive to superoxide-induced lipid peroxidation [176]. SOD and vitamin E inhibited lipid peroxidation. Walter et al. [116] found increased plasma peroxide concentrations in 57 type 1 and type 2 DM patients compared to 28 nondiabetic control patients. Higher plasma MDA levels were found in 67 middle aged diabetic patients (20 type 1, 47 type 2) than in 40 healthy subjects [177]. MDA levels showed a significant correlation with glycosylated Hb. LDL lipid peroxidation increased in 19 poorly controlled diabetic patients compared to age- and gender-matched subjects [178]. Serum lipid peroxides and plasma 11-dehydrothromboxane B2 (11-dehydro-TXB2), a stable metabolite of vasoactive thromboxane A2 released from platelets, were higher in 95 patients with normolipidemic type 2 DM than in control subjects [179]. A highly significant positive correlation existed between peroxide levels and 11-dehydro-TXB2 in the patients but not in the control subjects. Increased plasma MDA concentrations were found in poorly controlled type 2 diabetics when compared to well-controlled patients and to healthy normoglycemic subjects [180]. No difference was observed between the two latter groups. In diabetic patients a positive correlation was found between plasma MDA levels and HbA1 and plasma triglycerides. Furthermore, restoration of glycemic control in five poorly controlled patients lowered MDA levels to the normal range. Women with well-controlled type 1 DM had higher levels of lipid peroxidation during pregnancy than healthy women [181]. Serum levels of a conjugated diene isomer of linoleic acid was higher in DM patients with microalbuminuria than control subjects [14]. Increased basal and arachidonic acid stimulated MDA levels and enhanced platelet aggregation in response to ADP were found in 19 poorly controlled type 2 DM patients.

Plasma TBARS levels were higher in 117 type 1 and 2 DM patients than in 53 control subjects, independent of metabolic control [182]. There were no differences between type 1 and type 2 patients. Plasma MDA and lipid hydroperoxide levels were elevated in hospitalized ketotic type 1 DM patients [183]. One week after achieving glycemic control with insulin treatment, MDA levels approached reference values. Blood levels of the circulating form of ICAM-1 and MDA at baseline and 3 months after improved metabolic control were higher in 25 type 2 diabetic patients without signs of macroangiopathy than in 15 healthy subjects [184]. After improved metabolic control HbA$_{1c}$, circulating ICAM-1, and MDA significantly decreased. A significant correlation between circulating ICAM-1, HbA$_{1c}$, and MDA was found in diabetic patients. After 90 days of dietary and pharmacological treatment in 34 poorly controlled type 2 DM patients there was a decrease in plasma hydroperoxides, the susceptibility of LDL to in vitro oxidation, E-selectin levels and HbA$_{1c}$ [185]. E-selectin plasma concentration correlated with lag phase and lipid hydroperoxide values before and after 90 days of treatment. Plasma TBARS were elevated in women but not in men a study investigating lipid peroxidation in 56 young adult type 1 DM and 56 matched nondiabetic control subjects [186]. Basal and arachidonic acid stimulated MDA levels were 2.5-fold higher in 19 uncontrolled type 2 DM patients than in 26 normal subjects [187]. Platelet aggregation in response to ADP was also higher in the DM patients. Improvement of metabolic control in 11 of these patients decreased MDA levels and ADP induced platelet aggregation to normal levels. Plasma TBARS were elevated in women but not in men in a study investigating lipid peroxidation in 56 young adult type 1 DM and 56 matched nondiav=betic control subjects [188]. The peroxidative potential of whole plasma was studied in 13 control subjects and 23 diabetic patients divided into two groups on the basis of their metabolic control, defined as good (n = 12) or poor (n = 11) according to the fasting blood glucose, glycated hemoglobin and fructosamine levels. The lagtime for formation of plasma TBARS after Cu-dependent peroxidation were higher in 23 DM patients, especially those in poor metabolic control (n = 11) [189]. Baseline TBARS levels, however, were normal. Multivariate analysis showed a relation between the extent and duration of the diabetic pathology, and the decrease in the lag-time of oxidation. TBARS levels were elevated in 158 DM patients compared to control subjects [18]. TBARS levels were even higher in the 81 type 2 DM patients than in the 77 type 1 DM patients. TBARS levels were increased in 18 type 1 DM patients with no or mild retinopathy compared to previously established reference values [146]. Plasma lipid hydroperoxide levels were 2.5-fold higher in 22 type 2 DM patents than in control subjects, although plasma TBARS levels were similar [190]. The concentration of plasma esterified 8-epi-PGF2 α, considered to be a relatively specific index of lipid peroxidation, among type 2 DM patients was several-fold higher than in healthy individuals [191]. Baseline lipid hydroperoxide levels were similar in 75 subjects with normal glucose tolerance, IGT, and type 2 DM [192]. Oxidizability of plasma as measured by LPO formation in response to 2,2′-azobis-2-amidino-propane hydrochloride was greater in the DM group, however. There was no difference in lipid hydroperoxides between the normal glucose tolerance and impaired glucose tolerance groups. The initial plasma H_2O_2 and MDA levels in 15 patients with type 1 and 15 with type 2 diabetes before and after 2 weeks of intensive treatment were higher than in control subjects [26]. After 2 weeks of treatment, the values for both parameters were lower, although still higher than in the control group.

In a cross-sectional random urban sample of 595 elderly subjects in India, lipid peroxides were higher in patients with CAD and diabetes, and in those who smoked [193]. Plasma and urine TBARS were higher in 78 type 2 DM patients with and without microalbuminuria than in 28 healthy subjects [194]. There was no correlation between TBARS concentration and glycemic control. Plasma TBARS was higher in DM patients with hyperlipidemia than without [195]. Phosphatidylcholine hydroperoxide levels were higher in 50 DM patients without end-stage renal disease and in 33 uremic patients with DM nephropathy than in normal subjects [196]. Lipid peroxidation was increased and ascorbate levels were decreased in leukocytes from 53 type 2 DM patients compared to 34 age-matched control subjects [133]. Serum MDA levels were higher in 20 patients with newly diagnosed type 2 DM than in matched controls [197]. Lipid peroxide levels were higher in diabetic subjects in a study assessing lipid peroxide levels in 50 Mexican-American and 50 non-Hispanic whites [198]. Plasma TBARS levels were significantly increased in 467 type 2 DM patients already within the first two years of diagnosis compared to 180 control subjects, and increased with duration of disease and development of complications [105]. RBC-free and total MDA levels were elevated in 26 poorly controlled type 2 DM patients [108]. After 3 days of euglycemia maintained by constant insulin and glucose infusion, free MDA significantly decreased. Plasma TBARS were almost 30% higher in 42 normolipidemic type 2 DM patients, independent of lipid levels and glycemic control [199]. The vitamin E: lipid peroxide ratio was a major determinant of LDL susceptibility to oxidation. MDA levels were higher in DM patients compared to control subjects. Furthermore, LDL peroxidation was tightly correlated to the extent of LDL glycation. In men, TBARS was correlated with triglyceride levels and HbA1, but not in women. Dietary treatment decreased HbA_{1c} and MDA levels significantly. Lipid hydroperoxides and conjugated dienes were elevated in 72 patients with well-controlled type 1 DM and without complications, independent of metabolic control or diabetes duration [21]. Plasma TBARS but not oxysterols were higher in 14 normolipidemic DM patients than in control subjects [200]. Plasma lipid hydroperoxide levels were substantially higher in 41 type 2 diabetic patients compared to 87 control subjects [201]. Plasma lipid hydroperoxide levels were similar in diabetic patients with or without complications, as well as in smokers and nonsmokers. Plasma lipid peroxide levels, LPS-stimulated monocyte production of TNF-α and monocyte adhesion to endothelial cells were enhanced in eight poorly controlled type 2 DM patients on glyburide therapy compared to eight healthy subjects [202]. Gliclazide administration reversed these abnormalities.

On the other hand, no difference in serum conjugated diene levels between otherwise healthy diabetic patients and healthy control subjects were noted, although conjugated diene levels were increased in 26 diabetic patients with microangiopathy compared to 36 diabetic patients without microangiopathy and 36 control subjects [144]. TBARS levels in both poorly and well-controlled type 2 DM patients did not differ from the control subjects, whereas 2,3-dihydrobenzoate levels, a marker of hydroxyl radical formation, were elevated in DM patients [203]. Sinclaire et al. [110] reported no difference in plasma TBARS and conjugated diene levels between elderly DM patients with and without retinopathy and age matched control subjects, although ascorbate levels were markedly depleted. Conjugated diene and lipid peroxide levels were increased in patients with vascular disease, but levels were similar between diabetic and non-diabetic patients with vascular disease [15]. In 80 type 2 DM patients without cardiovascular or renal disease, MDA was elevated in those DM patients with microalbuminuria, but normoalbuminuric DM patients had similar MDA levels as matched healthy subjects [16]. Plasma TBARS levels were similar in 17- to 40-year-old type 1 DM patients as in control subjects, and were also similar in smokers [132]. Zoppini et al. [204] also found similar plasma TBARS levels in 56 type 1 DM patients as in 32 age and sex matched control subjects, but TBARS were higher in type 1 DM smokers.

Most published studies have found increased lipid peroxidation in both type 1 and type 2 DM patients. Conflicting results have also been found, however, and cannot be explained simply based on study design or methodology. Whether lipid peroxidation is increased in DM even before development of micro- and macrovascular disease is less clear. A causal role for lipid peroxidation in the development of diabetic macro- and microvascular complications is far from established.

3.3 Lipid peroxidation and diabetic complications

Jennings et al. [205] reported increased serum conjugated diene levels in 26 diabetic patients with microangiopathy compared to 36 diabetic patients without microangiopathy. Lipid peroxides were also significantly elevated in 15 type 1 patients with retinopathy compared to type 1 DM patients without microvascular complications [144]. In patients, both lipid peroxide levels and 11-dehydro-TXB2 increased according to the severity of their diabetic retinopathy [179]. Plasma TBARS levels correlated with albumin excretion in 64 type 1 and type 2 DM patients [206]. The degree of albumin excretion also correlated closely with indices of endothelial damage. Collagen stiffening as measured by metacarpopharyngeal joint angles correlated weakly with TBARS and serum lipid levels but not with duration of DM, blood glucose levels or HbA_{1c} in 205 elderly DM patients [207]. Type 2 patients with macrovascular disease had even higher TBARS levels than patients without macrovascular disease [182]. Twenty-one normotensive type 1 diabetic patients without microalbuminuria but with evidence of endothelial dysfunction (elevated plasma von Willebrand levels, soluble thrombomodulin content and angiotensin converting enzyme activity) had elevated levels of serum MDA compared to patients without evidence of endothelial dysfunction [208]. Microalbuminuric type 2 DM patients had higher MDA levels than normoalbuminuric patients and control subjects in a study of 80 patients free of cardiovascular disease, in good glycemic control and with a duration of DM of about ten years [16]. Type 1 and 2 DM patients in poor metabolic control or with angiopathy had higher levels of TBARS than those in good control or without angiopathy, independently of lipid levels [18]. In 78 type 2 DM patients, plasma but not urine TBARS concentrations were higher in patients with microalbuminuria than in those with normoalbuminuria [194]. Plasma phosphatidylcholine hydroperoxide levels of 33 DM patients undergoing hemodialysis were significantly higher than of DM patients without endstage renal disease [196]. In type 1 DM patients with microangiopathy, the oxidized LDL/normal LDL antibody ratio was paradoxically lower than in patients without complications, most likely due to oxidized LDL specific immune complexes found exclusively in antibody-negative patients [209].

In contrast, serum levels of a conjugated diene isomer of linoleic acid was higher in DM patients with microalbuminuria than control subjects, but levels were similar between DM patients with or without microalbuminuria [14]. No difference in plasma TBARS and conjugated diene levels was found reported between elderly DM patients with and without retinopathy, despite markedly depleted ascorbate levels [110]. Levels of serum MDA were similar between 33 type 1 DM patients with microalbuminuria and 49 patients without microalbuminuria [17]. TBARS levels were similar in 16 patients with micro- or macroalbuminuria compared to 69 normoalbuminuric patients in young type 1 DM patients [132]. Autoantibodies to copper-oxidized and MDA-modified LDL cholesterol were similar in 15 type 2 DM patients with no evidence of atherosclerosis and 17 type 2 DM patients previous myocardial infarction [210].

There seems to be no clear consensus as to whether patients who have developed diabetic complications have increased lipid peroxidation compared to patients without complications, although most studies have reported higher levels of lipid peroxidation in DM patients with complications than in patients without complications. Further studies are needed to clarify this issue and also whether such increased oxidative stress is pathologically important or merely a marker of micro- or macrovascular damage.

3.4 Insulin and lipid peroxidation

Insulin and IGF-1 increased monocyte superoxide production and LDL cholesterol oxidation [41]. A 5-h hyperinsulinemic euglycemic clamp had no effect on plasma TBARS; however, Niskanen et al. [19] showed for the first time that plasma TBARS were elevated in 22 patients with IGT in addition to 91 newly diagnosed type 2 DM patients, after 10 years follow-up fasting insulin and glucose levels were predictive of plasma TBARS levels in multiple regression analyses, suggesting a role for insulin resistance in inducing oxidative stress. Supporting these findings, lipid peroxidation was elevated in 105 subjects with IGT and early hyperglycemia and also in type 2 DM patients [42]. The susceptibility of LDL to copper-catalyzed oxidation was shortest in 22 familial hypertriglyceridemic patients while intermediate values were found in 24 type 1 DM, 16 type 2 DM and 14 abdominal obese patients compared to gluteal-femoral obese subjects and controls [185]. Thus, conditions commonly associated with insulin resistance were also characterized by increased LDL oxidizability. The different susceptibility to oxidation found in the different groups of patients was only partially explained by plasma triglyceride values.

On the other hand, baseline lipid hydroperoxide levels were similar in 75 subjects with normal glucose tolerance, IGT, and type 2 DM [192]. No difference was seen between normal glucose tolerance and IGT groups in oxidizability of plasma as measured by lipid hydroperoxide formation in response to 2,2'-azobis-2-amidino-propane hydrochloride, although oxidizability was greater in the DM group.

Although results to date on the role of insulin resistance as a mechanism for increased oxidative stress are intriguing, studies are surprisingly few. Given the attention focused on insulin resistance in the pathogenesis of DM and cardiovascular disease in general, future studies should also address the role of insulin resistance in oxidative stress.

3.5 Susceptibility of LDL cholesterol to oxidation

Incubation of LDL cholesterol with glucose at concentrations seen in the diabetic state increased susceptibility of LDL to oxidation as measured by TBARS and conjugated diene formation, electrophoretic mobility and degradation by macrophages [154]. Endothelial or smooth muscle cells cultured in glucose-enriched media resulted in a marked enhancement of the subsequent ability of cells to oxidize low-density lipoprotein, as assessed by the lipid peroxidation end product and conjugated diene content of the particle, its relative electrophoretic mobility and its degradation by macrophages [211].

LDL isolated from 10 normocholesterolemic and 10 hypercholesterolemic type 2 DM patients was much more susceptible to oxidation than LDL from normal subjects [212]. Susceptibility of LDL to oxidation was strongly correlated with degree of LDL glycosylation. LDL and RBC membranes in 11 normolipidemic type 1 and 18 type 2 DM patients were more susceptible to oxidation than in normal subjects [213]. The susceptibility of LDL to copper-catalyzed oxidation was shortest in 22 familial hypertriglyceridemic patients while intermediate values were found in 24 insulin-dependent, 16 non-insulin-dependent and 14 abdominal obese patients compared to gluteal-femoral obese subjects and controls [185]. The different susceptibility to oxidation found in the different groups of patients was only partially explained by plasma triglyceride values. Plasma TRAP (total peroxyl radical trapping potential) was lower and susceptibility of LDL to oxidation as measured by the lag phase of conjugated diene formation after initiation of LDL oxidation by the addition of copper was greater in poorly controlled type 1 diabetic subjects than in normal control subjects [29]. This could not be attributed to the presence of oxidation-susceptible, small, dense LDL particles in the diabetic subjects, whose lipoprotein particle distribution did not differ from the control subjects. LDL lipid peroxides and conjugated diene formation were higher in 10 type 2 diabetic patients than in control subjects [214,215]. LDL lipid peroxides and conjugated diene formation were related to LDL glycation, and decreased following diet [215]. The decrease in lipoprotein peroxidation was positively related to the percentage of linoleic acid in LDL. LDL from both type 1 (n = 20) and type 2 (n = 20) diabetic patients exhibited a shorter lag phase duration for conjugated diene formation, regardless of the presence of vascular complications [216]. LDL exhibited a shorter lagtime and a lower α-tocopherol/LDL ratio for 10 type 1 and 53 type 2 diabetic patients than for sex- and age-matched control subjects [217]. The lagtime was positively correlated to the LDL α-tocopherol/LDL and inversely correlated to HbA_{1c}. Recently diagnosed type 1 DM patients (n = 25) with poor glycemic control showed higher electronegative LDL, similar LDL subfraction phenotype and lower susceptibility to oxidation compared to 25 matched healthy control subjects [218]. After 3 months of intensive insulin therapy, HbA_{1c} and LDL electronegativity decreased, but no changes in LDL susceptibility to oxidation or LDL subfraction phenotype were observed. The vitamin E/lipid peroxide ratio and LDL susceptibility to oxidation were lower in 35 type 2 DM patients than in either hypertriglyceridemic or normolipidemic nondiabetic subjects [219].

In contrast, there was no difference between 20 type 1 diabetic patients in moderate glycemic control and nondiabetic subjects in the susceptibility of LDL cholesterol to either copper-dependent or non-transition-metal-dependent oxidation [220]. Furthermore, there was no difference between the groups for LDL vitamin E content, LDL fatty acid composition in cholesterol esters or triglycerides, but LDL glycation was elevated in the type 1 DM subjects. No significant difference in susceptibility to oxidation of LDL and VLDL could be detected in 30 diabetic patients compared to 30 healthy subjects [188]. There was no difference between 34 type 1 DM patients without clinical signs of vascular disease and 22 healthy control patients in the oxidizability of LDL and VLDL. There was no difference in the susceptibility to in vitro oxidation of LDL isolated from 15 type 1 DM patients in good glycemic control and with no evidence of macrovascular disease or proteinuria compared with control subjects [221]. The particle size, lipid composition, fatty acid content, antioxidant content, and glycation were similar for LDL isolated from both groups. LDL oxidizability was normal in 14 normolipidemic DM patients compared to healthy control subjects [200].

Most studies have found increased susceptibility of LDL cholesterol to oxidation in DM patients, although some well designed studies have had conflicting results. Studies carried out to date do not allow firm conclusions to be drawn about whether LDL is more susceptible to oxidation in DM patients without complications than in healthy subjects, or about what effect complications and glycemic control have on the susceptibility of LDL to oxidation.

3.6 Autoantibodies to oxidized cholesterol

Type 2 DM patients (n = 138) had an antibody ratio (calculated as the ratio of antibodies against modified vs. native LDL) significantly higher than control subjects (n = 80) for Cu^{2+}-oxidized LDL, MDA-modified LDL, and MDA-modified human serum albumin [222]. Autoantibodies to copper-oxidized LDL cholesterol were significantly higher in the 17 nondiabetic patients with previous myocardial infarction when compared to 18 nondiabetic patients without previous myocardial infarction, 15 type 2 DM patients with no evidence of atherosclerosis and 17 type 2 DM patients with previous myocardial infarction [210]. Autoantibodies to MDA-modified LDL were significantly higher in the nondiabetic subjects with heart disease and in both diabetic groups compared to nondiabetic subjects without coronary heart disease. Antiglycated LDL and antiglycoxidized LDL IgG was also higher in the type 2 DM patients. In 94 patients with type 1 DM the oxidized LDL/normal LDL antibody ratio was significantly higher than in control subjects [209].

In contrast, serum autoantibodies to oxidized LDL cholesterol did not differ between 91 newly diagnosed DM patients and 82 nondiabetic control subjects at baseline or after 10 years follow up [223]. Autoantibody titers also did not associate with development of cardiovascular morbidity, mortality or carotid media intima thickness. Antioxidized LDL antibodies and anti-MDA-modified LDL antibodies with similar levels in 16 type 1 DM patients free of macrovascular complications and 16 control subjects [224]. Both diabetic and normal individuals were found to have circulating immune complexes whose atherogenic potential appeared to be related to immune complex LDL levels and IgG and IgA antibodies. In 101 type 1 DM normo- and macroalbuminuric patients with a long duration of diabetes and 54 healthy subjects, antibodies against MDA-modified LDL did not differ among normoalbuminuric DM, albuminuric DM and control subjects [225].

No clear consensus has been found concerning the presence of increased oxidized LDL antibodies than for LDL cholesterol oxidizability or especially for indices of plasma or serum lipid peroxidation in DM patients. Although interesting results linking oxidized LDL antibodies to carotid atherosclerosis in the general population have been published [226], similar conclusions cannot be drawn from studies in diabetic patients. Whether this is an argument against increased oxidative stress or its role in the pathogenesis of atherosclerosis in DM or against the use of oxidized LDL autoantibodies as a marker of lipid peroxidation in DM remains unclear.

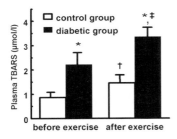

Fig. 2. Plasma TBARS levels were greater in the DM group than in the control group both at rest and after exercise. Reproduced with permission from Laaksonen et al. [20].

4   EXERCISE, PHYSICAL FITNESS AND OXIDATIVE STRESS IN DIABETES MELLITUS

Oxidative stress has been implicated in the accelerated atherosclerosis and micro-vascular complications of DM. Furthermore, physical exercise may acutely induce oxidative damage, although regular training appears to enhance antioxidant defenses, and in some animal studies, has decreased lipid peroxidation.

Exercise is a major therapeutic modality in the treatment of DM [4]. To maximize the benefits of exercise, it is important to understand the effect of acute and long-term physical exercise on oxidative stress and antioxidant defenses in diabetes.

With these goals in mind, we recruited 9 otherwise healthy type 1 DM and 13 control men aged 20–30 years [20,50]. They rode for 40 min on a bicycle ergometer at 60% of their $VO_{2\ max}$, after a 5-min warm-up. Blood samples were drawn at rest and immediately after exercise. We used as measures of oxidative stress plasma TBARS, and in response to exercise changes in GSSG levels and the GSSG/TGSH (total glutathione) ratio. For indices of antioxidant defenses, blood TGSH and GSSG levels and red cell GPX, GRD, GST, superoxide and

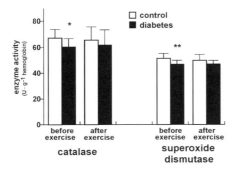

Fig. 3. Catalase and superoxide activities were less in the DM men than in the control men at rest. Reproduced with permission from M. Atalay et al. [50].

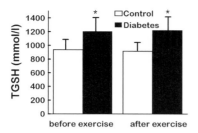

Fig. 4. Interestingly, TGSH was greater in the diabetic men at rest. Exercise did not affect overall TGSH levels. Reproduced by permission from Laaksonen et al. [20].

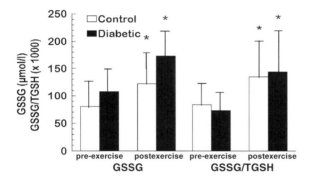

Fig. 5. In contrast, the GSSG and GSSG/TGSH ratio increased markedly in both DM and control men in response to exercise. The GSSG and GSSG/TGSH ratio did not differ between DM and control groups either at rest or after exercise. Reproduced with permission from Laaksonen et al. [20].

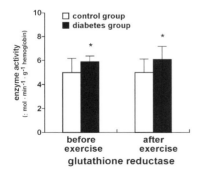

Fig. 6. Red cell GRD activity was greater in the DM men than in the control men at rest. Exercise affected only GPX activity in the control group, producing a small increase. Reproduced with permission from M. Atalay et al. [50].

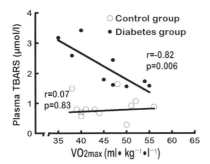

Fig. 7. Interestingly, plasma TBARS had a strong inverse correlation with VO$_2$ $_{max}$. There were no significant associations between glycemic control or lipid levels and plasma TBARS or antioxidant indices. Reproduced with permission from Laaksonen et al. [20].

catalase activities were measured. The results are summarized in Figs. 2–7.

We found increased plasma TBARS in the diabetic men both at rest and after exercise, showing for the first time increased exercise induced oxidative stress in DM. These results also support previous studies suggesting that type 1 DM patients have increased lipid peroxidation even in the absence of complications.

Decreased Cu,Zn-SOD activity coupled with increased superoxide production [22–25] could exacerbate oxidative stress, especially if not compensated with increased catalase or Se-GPX activity. Superoxide may react with other ROS such as nitric oxide to form highly toxic species such as peroxynitrite, in addition to direct toxic effects [8]. Alternatively, superoxide can be dismutated to the much more reactive hydrogen peroxide, which through the Fenton reaction can then lead to highly toxic hydroxyl radical formation [24]. Thus, decreased catalase activity could also contribute to the increased oxidative stress found in the type 1 DM subjects. Increased glucose [135] and hydrogen peroxide levels [136] have also been shown to inactivate catalase. As reviewed above, decreased red cell SOD and catalase activity have often but not always been found in DM patients.

Increased blood TGSH levels in the DM men could represent an adaptive response to increased oxidative stress, mediated possibly in part through increased red cell GRD activity. Most other studies have found either decreased or unchanged glutathione levels in DM patients. Relatively few studies have examined glutathione levels in type 1 patients. Frequently, patients have been older, have complications, or have been poorly described with respect to presence of diabetic complications or glycemic control. In the study by Di Simplicio et al. [112], however, type 1 DM patients without complications appeared to have increased platelet GSH.

The strongly negative association between plasma TBARS and VO$_2$ $_{max}$ suggests that good physical fitness may have a protective role against oxidative stress. The intriguing question, can lipid peroxidation be decreased through regular training in diabetes, is thus, raised. If so, this may have far reaching clinical implications should the role of oxidative stress in the development of diabetic micro- and macrovascular complications become firmly established.

5 SUMMARY

1. Many but not all studies show an increase in indices of lipid peroxidation and oxidative stress in DM. Whether lipid peroxidation is elevated in DM before development of complications or whether lipid peroxidation is greater in DM with complications than without is less clear. The causal role of oxidative stress in the development of diabetic micro- and macrovascular complications also remains to be shown, despite compelling evidence linking, e.g., AGEs, oxidative stress, cytokines and adhesion molecules to various pathological conditions in in vitro and animal models of diabetes.

2. Lack of specificity and sensitivity of various measures of oxidative stress is a major problem facing all investigators in free radical research. Furthermore, many studies have relied solely or mainly on TBARS as an index of lipid peroxidation. Although if proper precautions in preparation and measurement of samples are taken, TBARS remains a valid measure of lipid peroxidation, complementary measures should also be used. Additional indices of oxidative stress measuring protein or DNA oxidative damage have been virtually totally ignored and should also be employed.

3. Conflicting data also prevent drawing firm conclusions about impairments in antioxidant defenses in DM. Differences in assay, study design or study population do not seem to completely explain differences in results.

4. Most human studies have been limited to study of blood samples, which may not necessarily reflect conditions within the artery wall, where the major pathogenic processes of atherosclerosis are presumed to take place. Animal studies have been hampered by lack of a good experimental model of DM. With the exception of a few studies mimicking the DM state by injecting AGEs at levels similar to what is found in DM, most studies injected rats, mice or rabbits with STZ or alloxan, resulting in insulin deficient DM. Few studies have supplemented even subtherapeutic doses of insulin, however, resulting in very sick animals that suffer from extreme weight loss, diarrhea and impaired growth. It can be questioned whether such experimental models reflect the typical human type 1 diabetic condition. Animal models of type 2 DM have been less frequently employed.

5. The relative importance of various mechanisms leading to increased oxidative stress in DM is unclear. Furthermore, the role of various mechanisms leading to increased oxidative stress most likely differ between type 1 DM, characterized mainly by hyperglycemia due to insulin deficiency, and type 2 DM, generally linked to the insulin resistance syndrome, which includes abnormalities of lipid metabolism, obesity, and hypertension in addition to impaired glucose metabolism. Despite abundant research on the insulin resistance syndrome and the pathogenesis of DM and atherosclerosis, little research has been

done on the role insulin resistance may play in the pathogenesis of oxidative stress in type 2 DM.

6. Despite the importance of physical exercise for diabetic patients and the role of oxidative stress in acute and long term exercise, only two papers examining exercise-induced oxidative stress in DM have been published. We have recently completed a larger study in which 56 type 1 DM men aged 20—40 years were randomized into training and control groups. Blood samples were taken before and after a 12- to 16-week program consisting of 30- to 45-min running 4—5 times a week. The main measures of outcome will be the effect of training on decreasing indices of oxidative stress and increasing antioxidant defenses in blood and plasma. The training has been successfully carried out, and the samples are currently being analyzed. This study should provide additional information about the role of regular physical exercise in decreasing oxidative stress in DM, and will hopefully spur additional research into the role of exercise and oxidative stress in type 1 and 2 DM.

6   PERSPECTIVES

DM is associated with a markedly increased mortality from coronary heart disease, not explainable by traditional risk factors. Although data are not yet conclusive, oxidative stress has been increasingly implicated in the pathogenesis of diabetic micro- and macrovascular disease. Some evidence also supports a role for physical fitness in decreasing lipid peroxidation. If regular physical exercise can be shown to have a protective effect against oxidative stress in DM, this may have direct impact on the use of physical exercise as a therapeutic modality in diabetes.

7   ABBREVIATIONS

DM:	diabetes mellitus
LDL:	low-density lipoprotein
ROS:	reactive oxygen species
AGE:	advanced glycation products
TBARS:	thiobarbituric acid reactive substances
$VO_{2\ max}$:	maximal oxygen consumption
SOD:	superoxide dismutase
RAGE:	receptors for AGEs
VCAM-1:	vascular cell adhesion molecule-1
PECAM-1:	platelet adhesion cell molecule-1
ICAM-1:	intercellular adhesion molecule-1
CML:	(N)epsilon-(carboxymethyl)lysine
MDA:	malondialdehyde
GPX:	glutathione peroxidase
GRD:	glutathione disulfide reductase

GST: glutathione-S-transferase
GSSG: glutathione disulfide
GSH: reduced glutathione
STZ: streptozotocin
EC: extracellular
IGT: impaired glucose tolerance
MDA: malondialdehyde
TRAP: total peroxyl radical trapping potential
TGSH: total glutathione

8   REFERENCES

1. Zimmet PZ, McCarty DJ, de Courten MP. J Diab Comp 1997;11(2):60—68.
2. Expert committee on the diagnosis and classification of Diabetes Mellitus. Diabet Care 1997;20 (7):1183—1197.
3. Zimmet P, Lefebvre P. Diabetologia 1996;39(11):1247—1248.
4. American Diabetes Association. Clinical practice recommendations. Diabet Care 1998;21 (Suppl 1):S1—95.
5. Lyons TJ. Am J Cardiol 1993;71(6):26B—31B.
6. Cameron NE, Cotter MA, Hohman TC. Diabetologia 1996;39(2):172—182.
7. Cameron NE, Cotter MA. Diabet Med 1993;10(7):593—605.
8. Tesfamariam B. Free Radic Biol Med 1994;16(3):383—391.
9. Halliwell B. Lancet 1994;344(8924):721—724.
10. Haberland ME, Fong D, Cheng L. Science 1988;24(4862):215—218.
11. Witztum JL. Lancet 1994;344(8925):793—795.
12. Sato Y, Hotta N, Sakamoto N, Matsuoka S, Ohishi N, Yagi K. Biochem Med Metab Biol 1979; 1979(21):104—107.
13. Velazquez E, Winocour PH, Kesteven P, Alberti KG, Laker MF. Diabet Med 1991;8(8): 752—758.
14. Collier A, Rumley A, Rumley A et al. Diabetes 1992;41(8):909—913.
15. MacRury SM, Gordon D, Wilson R et al. Diabet Med 1993;10(4):331—335.
16. Neri S, Bruno CM, Raciti C, Dangelo G, Damico R, Cristaldi R. J Int Med 1994;236(5): 495—500.
17. Yaqoob M, McClelland P, Patrick AW, et al. Q J Med 1994;87(10):601—607.
18. Griesmacher A, Kindhauser M, Andert S et al. Am J Med 1995;98(5):469—475.
19. Niskanen LK, Salonen JT, Nyyssonen K, Uusitupa MI. Diabet Med 1995;12(9):802—808.
20. Laaksonen DE, Atalay M, Niskanen L, Uusitupa M, Hanninen O, Sen CK. Diabet Care 1996; 19(6):569—574.
21. Santini SA, Marra G, Giardina et al. Diabetes 1997;46(11):1853—1858.
22. Nath N, Chari SN, Rathi AB. Diabetes 1984;33(6):586—589.
23. Ceriello A, Giugliano D, Quatraro A, Dello—Russo P, Lefebvre PJ. Diabet Med 1991;8(6): 540—542.
24. Wolff SP, Jiang ZY, Hunt JV. Free Radic Biol Med 1991;10(5):339—352.
25. Dandona P, Thusu K, Cook et al. Lancet 1996;347(8999):444—445.
26. Wierusz-Wysocka B, Wysocki H, Byks H, Zozulinska D, Wykretowicz A, Kazmierczak M. Diabe Res Clin Care Pract 1995;27(3):193—197.
27. Ruiz Munoz LM, Vidal Vanaclocha F, Lampreabe I. Nephrol Dial Trans 1997;12(3):456—464.
28. Asayama K, Uchida N, Nakane et al. Free Radic Biol Med 1993;15(6):597—602.
29. Tsai EC, Hirsch IB, Brunzell JD, Chait A. Diabetes 1994;43(8):1010—1014.
30. Ceriello A, Bortolotti N, Falleti et al. Diabet Care 1997;20(2):194—197.

31. Hunt JV, Smith CC, Wolff SP. Diabetes 1990;39(11):1420—1424.
32. Schleicher ED, Wagner E, Nerlich AG. J Clin Invest 1997;99(3):457—468.
33. Grunewald RW, Weber, II, Kinne Saffran E, Kinne RK. Biochim Biophys Acta 1993;1225(1): 39—47.
34. Kashiwagi A, Asahina T, Ikebuchi et al. Diabetologia 1994;37(3):264—269.
35. De Mattia G, Laurenti O, Bravi C, Ghiselli A, Iuliano L, Balsano F. Metabolism 1994;43(8): 965—968.
36. Kashiwagi A, Asahina T, Nishio et al. Diabetes 1996;45(Suppl 3):S84—S86.
37. Sinclair AJ, Girling AJ, Gray L, Le-Guen C, Lunec J, Barnett AH. Diabetologia 1991;34(3): 171—175.
38. Arai K, Iizuka S, Tada Y, Oikawa K, Taniguchi N. Biochim Biophys Acta 1987;924(2):292—296.
39. Blakytny R, Harding JJ. Biochem J 1992;288(1):303—307.
40. Kawamura N, Ookawara T, Suzuki K, Konishi K, Mino M, Taniguchi N. J Clin Endocrinol Metab 1992;74(6):1352—1354.
41. Rifici VA, Schneider SH, Khachadurian AK. Atherosclerosis 1994;107(1):99—108.
42. Vijayalingam S, Parthiban A, Shanmugasundaram KR, Mohan V. Diabet Med 1996;13(8): 715—719.
43. Davies KJ, Quintanilha AT, Brooks GA, Packer L. Biochem Biophys Res Commun 1982;107(4): 1198—1205.
44. Alessio HM. Med Sci Sports Exerc 1993;25(2):218—224.
45. Sen CK, Packer L, Hanninen O (eds). Exercise and Oxygen Toxicity. Amsterdam: Elsevier, 1994;1—510
46. Ji LL. Exer Sport Sci Rev 1995;23:135—166.
47. Sen CK. J Appl Physiol 1995;79(3):675—686.
48. Kim JD, McCarter RJM, Yu BP. Aging Clin Exp Res 1996;8:123—129.
49. Kim JD, Yu BP, McCarter RJM, Lee SY, Herlihy JT. Free Radic Bio Med 1996;20(1):83—88.
50. Atalay M, Laaksonen DE, Niskanen L, Uusitupa M, Hanninen O, Sen CK. Acta Physiol Scand 1997;161(2):195—201.
51. Sell DR, Lapolla A, Odetti P, Fogarty J, Monnier VM. Diabetes 1992;41(10):1286—1292.
52. Dyer DG, Dunn JA, Thorpe S et al. J Clin Invest 1993;91(6):2463—2469.
53. Jones AF, Winkles JW, Thornalley PJ, Lunec J, Jennings PE, Barnett AH. Clin Chem 1987;33 (1):147—149.
54. Sakurai T, Tsuchiya S. FEBS Lett 1988;236(2):406—410.
55. Baker JR, Zyzak DV, Thorpe SR, Baynes JW. Clin Chem 1993;39(12):2460—2465.
56. Elgawish A, Glomb M, Friedlander M, Monnier VM. J Biol Chem 1996;271(22):12964—12971.
57. Yan SD, Schmidt AM, Anderson G et al. J Biol Chem 1994;269(13):9889—9897.
58. Schmidt AM, Hori O, Chen J et al. J Clin Invest 1995;96(3):1395—1403.
59. Zoukourian C, Wautier MP, Chappey et al. Int Angiol 1996;15(3):195—200.
60. Pugliese G, Pricci F, Romeo et al. Diabetes 1997;46(11):1881—1887.
61. Wautier JL, Wautier MP, Schmidt A et al. Proc Natl Acad Sci USA 1994;91(16):7742—7746.
62. Rattan V, Shen Y, Sultana C, Kumar D, Kalra VK. Am J Physiol 1997;273(2.1):E369—E375.
63. Vlassara H, Fuh H, Donnelly T, Cybulsky M. Molec Med 1995;1(4):447—456.
64. Vlassara H, Striker LJ, Teichberg S, Fuh H, Li YM, Steffes M. Proc Natl Acad Sci USA 1994;91 (24):11704—11708.
65. Horie K, Miyata T, Maeda et al. J Clin Invest 1997;100(12):2995—3004.
66. Vlassara H, Fuh H, Makita Z, Krungkrai S, Cerami A, Bucala R. Proc Natl Acad Sci USA 1992;89(24):12043—12047.
67. Dobrian A, Lazar V, Tirziu D, Simionescu M. Biochim Biophys Acta 1996;1317(1):5—14.
68. Makita Z, Radoff S, Rayfield E et al. N Engl J Med 1991;325(12):836—842.
69. Bucala R, Makita Z, Koschinsky T, Cerami A, Vlassara H. Proc Natl Acad Sci USA 1993;90 (14):6434—6438.
70. McCance DR, Dyer DG, Dunn J et al. J Clin Invest 1993;91(6):2470—2478.

71. Beisswenger PJ, Moore LL, Brinck-Johnsen T, Curphey TJ. J Clin Invest 1993;92(1):212—217.
72. Brett J, Schmidt AM, Yan S et al. Am J Pathol 1993;143(6):1699—1712.
73. Nakamura Y, Horii Y, Nishino T et al. Am J Pathol 1993;143(6):1649—1656.
74. Wells Knecht MC, Lyons TJ, McCance DR, Thorpe SR, Baynes JW. J Clin Invest 1997;100(4): 839—846.
75. Sen CK, Hanninen O. Physiological antioxidants. In: Sen CK, Packer L, Hanninen O (eds) Exercise and Oxygen Toxicity. Amsterdam: Elsevier, 1994:89—126.
76. Meister A. Meth Enzymol 1995;251:3—7.
77. Mannervik B, Danielson UH. CRC Crit Rev Biochem 1988;23(3):283—337.
78. Lu SC, Ge JL, Kuhlenkamp J, Kaplowitz N. J Clin Invest 1992;90(2):524—532.
79. Yoshida K, Hirokawa J, Tagami S, Kawakami Y, Urata Y, Kondo T. Diabetologia 1995;38(2): 201—210.
80. Loven D, Schedl H, Wilson et al. Diabetes 1986;35(5):503—507.
81. Grant MH, Duthie SJ. Biochem Pharmacol 1987;36(21):3647—3655.
82. Wohaieb SA, Godin DV. Diabetes 1987;36(9):1014—1018.
83. Barnett CR, Abbott RA, Bailey CJ, Flatt PR, Ioannides C. Biochem Pharmacol 1992;43(8): 1868—1871.
84. Thompson KH, Godin DV, Lee M. Biol Trace Elements Res 1992;35(3):213—224.
85. Thompson KH, McNeill JH. Res Commun Chem Pathol Pharmacol 1993;80(2):187—200.
86. Ewis SA, Abdel Rahman MS. J Appl Toxicol 1995;15(5):387—390.
87. Ewis SA, Abdel Rahman MS. J Appl Toxicol 1997;17(6):409—413.
88. McLennan SV, Heffernan S, Wright L et al. Diabetes 1991;40(3):344—348.
89. Saxena AK, Srivastava P, Kale RK, Baquer NZ. Biochem Pharmacol 1993;45(3):539—542.
90. Kern TS, Kowluru RA, Engerman RL. Invest Ophthalmol Vis Sci 1994;35(7):2962—2967.
91. Kowluru RA, Kern TS, Engerman RL, Armstrong D. Diabetes 1996;45(9):1233—1237.
92. Kowluru RA, Kern TS, Engerman RL. Free Radic Biol Med 1997;22(4):587—592.
93. Oster MH, Llobet JM, Domingo JL, German JB, Keen CL. Toxicology 1993;83(1—3): 115—130.
94. Mak DH, Ip SP, Li PC, Poon MK, Ko KM. Molec Cell Biochem 1996;162(2):153—158.
95. Tagami S, Kondo T, Yoshida K, Hirokawa J, Ohtsuka Y, Kawakami Y. Metabolism 1992;41(10): 1053—1058.
96. Gupta BL, Ansari MA, Singh JN, Baquer NZ. Biochem Int 1992;27(5):793—802.
97. Gupta BL, Ansari MA, Srivastava P, Baquer NZ. Biochem Molec Biol Int 1993;31(4):669—676.
98. Nickander KK, Schmelzer JD, Rohwer DA, Low PA. J Neurol Sci 1994;126(1):6—14.
99. Nagamatsu M, Nickander KK, Schmelzer JD et al. Diabet Care 1995;18(8):1160—1167.
100. Carroll PB, Thornton BM, Greene DA. Diabetes 1986;35(11):1282—1285.
101. Thomas G, Skrinska V, Lucas FV, Schumacher OP. Diabetes 1985;34(10):951—954.
102. Murakami K, Kondo T, Ohtsuka Y, Fujiwara Y, Shimada M, Kawakami Y. Metabolism 1989;38 (8):753—758.
103. Muruganandam A, Drouillard C, Thibert RJ, Cheung RM, Draisey TF, Mutus B. Thromb Res 1992;67(4):385—397.
104. Jain SK, McVie R. Metabolism 1994;43(3):306—309.
105. Sundaram RK, Bhaskar A, Vijayalingam S, Viswanathan M, Mohan R, Shanmugasundaram KR. Clin Sci Colch 1996;90(4):255—260.
106. Ciuchi E, Odetti P, Prando R. Diabetes Metab 1997;23(1):58—60.
107. Thornalley PJ, McLellan AC, Lo TW, Benn J, Sonksen PH. Clin Sci Colch 1996;91(5):575—582.
108. Peuchant E, Delmas Beauvieux MC, Couchouron A et al. Diabet Care 1997;20(2):202—207.
109. Costagliola C, Iuliano G, Menzione M, Nesti A, Simonelli F, Rinaldi E. Ophthalmic Res 1988; 20(5):308—316.
110. Sinclair AJ, Girling AJ, Gray L, Lunec J, Barnett AH. Gerontology 1992;38(5):268—274.
111. McLellan AC, Thornalley PJ, Benn J, Sonksen PH. Clin Sci Colch 1994;87(1):21—29.
112. Di Simplicio P, de Giorgio LA, Cardaioli E et al. Eur J Clin Invest 1995;25(9):665—669.

113. Paolisso G, Di Maro G, Pizza G et al. Am J Physiol 1992;263(3.1):E435—E440.
114. Reddi AS. Biochim Biophys Acta 1986;882(1):71—76.
115. Godin DV, Wohaieb SA, Garnett ME, Goumeniouk AD. Molec Cell Biochem 1988;84(2): 223—231.
116. Walter RM, Jr., Uriu Hare JY, Olin KL et al. Diabet Care 1991;14(11):1050—1056.
117. Stahlberg MR, Hietanen E. Scand J Clin Lab Invest 1991;51(2):125—130.
118. Ceriello A, dello Russo P, Amstad P, Cerutti P. Diabetes 1996;45(4):471—477.
119. Reddi AS, Bollineni JS. Biochem Biophys Res Commun 1997;235(3):598—601.
120. Kakkar R, Mantha SV, Kalra J, Prasad K. Clin Sci Colch 1996;91(4):441—448.
121. Srivastava P, Saxena AK, Kale RK, Baquer NZ. Res Commun Chem Pathol Pharmacol 1993; 80(3):283—293.
122. Pereira B, Rosa LF, Safi DA, Bechara EJ, Curi R. J Endocrinol 1994;142(1):161—165.
123. Dohi T, Kawamura K, Morita K, Okamoto H, Tsujimoto A. Horm Metab Res 1988;20(11): 671—675.
124. McDermott BM, Flatt PR, Strain JJ. Ann Nutr Metab 1994;38(5):263—269.
125. Asayama K, Hayashibe H, Dobashi K, Niitsu T, Miyao A, Kato K. Diabet Res 1989;12(2): 85—91.
126. Asayama K, Yokota S, Kato K. Diabet Res Clin Pract 1991;11(2):89—94.
127. Langenstroer P, Pieper GM. Am J Physiol 1992;263(1 Pt 2):H257—65.
128. Sukalski KA, Pinto KA, Berntson JL. Free Radic Biol Med 1993;14(1):57—65.
129. Pieper GM, Meier DA, Hager SR. Am J Physiol 1995;269(3.2):H845—H850.
130. Kaul N, Siveski Iliskovic N, Hill M, Khaper N, Seneviratne C, Singal PK. Molec Cell Biochem 1996;161:283—288.
131. Tho LL, Candlish JK. Biochem Med Metab Biol 1987;38(1):74—80.
132. Leonard MB, Lawton K, Watson ID, Patrick A, Walker A, MacFarlane I. Diabet Med 1995;12 (1):46—50.
133. Akkus I, Kalak S, Vural H et al. Clin Chim Acta 1996;244(2):221—227.
134. Osterode W, Holler C, Ulberth F. Diabet Med 1996;13(12):1044—1050.
135. Yadav P, Bhatnagar D, Sarkar S. Toxicol In Vitro 1994;8(3):471—476.
136. Ou P, Wolff SP. Biochem J 1994;303(3):935—939.
137. Kakkar R, Kalra J, Mantha SV, Prasad K. Molec Cell Biochem 1995;151(2):113—119.
138. Kaul N, Siveski Iliskovic N, Thomas TP, Hill M, Khaper N, Singal PK. Nutrition 1995;11(Suppl 5): 551—554.
139. Kamata K, Kobayashi T. Br J Pharmacol 1996;119(3):583—589.
140. Kowluru R, Kern TS, Engerman RL. Curr Eye Res 1994;13(12):891—896.
141. Sechi LA, Ceriello A, Griffin CA et al. Diabetologia 1997;40(1):23—29.
142. Kaneto H, Fujii J, Myint T et al. Biochem J 1996;320(Pt 3):855—863.
143. Tho LL, Candlish JK, Thai AC. Ann Clin Biochem 1988;25(Pt 4):426—431.
144. Jennings PE, McLaren M, Scott NA, Saniabadi AR, Belch JJ. Diabet Med 1991;8(9):860—865.
145. Skrha J, Hodinar A, Kvasnicka J et al. Clin Chim Acta 1994;229(1—2):5—14.
146. Faure P, Benhamou PY, Perard A, Halimi S, Roussel AM. Eur J Clin Nutr 1995;49(4):282—288.
147. Skrha J, Hodinar A, Kvasnicka J, Hilgertova J. Diabet Med 1996;13(9):800—805.
148. Adachi T, Yamada H, Yamada Y et al. Biochemical Journal 1996;313:(1):235—239.
149. Marklund SL, Hagglof B. Clin Chim Acta 1984;142(3):299—305.
150. Asahina T, Kashiwagi A, Nishio Y et al. Diabetes 1995;44(5):520—526.
151. Kashiwagi A, Nishio Y, Asahina T et al. Diabetes 1997;46(12):2088—2095.
152. Bravi MC, Pietrangeli P, Laurenti O et al. Metabolism 1997;46(10):1194—1198.
153. Curcio F, Pegoraro I, Dello Russo P, Falleti E, Perrella G, Ceriello A. Thromb Haemostat 1995; 74(3):969—973.
154. Kawamura M, Heinecke JW, Chait A. J Clin Invest 1994;94(2):771—778.
155. Dobashi K, Asayama K, Hayashibe H et al. Virchows Arch B Cell Pathol Incl Mol Pathol 1991; 60(1):67—72.

156. Pritchard KA, Jr., Patel ST, Karpen CW, Newman HA, Panganamala RV. Diabetes 1986;35(3): 278—281.
157. Winkler R, Moser M. Wien Klin Wochenschr 1992;104(14):409—413.
158. Rungby J, Flyvbjerg A, Andersen HB, Nyborg K. Acta Endocrinologica Copenh 1992;126(4): 378—380.
159. Young IS, Torney JJ, Trimble ER. Free Radic Biol Med 1992;13(1):41—46.
160. Young IS, Tate S, Lightbody JH, McMaster D, Trimble ER. Free Radic Biol Med 1995;18(5): 833—840.
161. Aoki Y, Yanagisawa Y, Oguchi H, Furuta S. Metabolism 1992;41(9):1025—1027.
162. Staprans I, Rapp JH, Pan XM, Feingold KR. J Clin Invest 1993;92(2):638—643.
163. Lung CC, Pinnas JL, Yahya MD, Meinke GC, Mooradian AD. Life Sci 1993;52(3):329—337.
164. Gallaher DD, Csallany AS, Shoeman DW, Olson JM. Lipids 1993;28(7):663—666.
165. Jain SK, Levine SN. Free Radic Biol Med 1995;18(2):337—341.
166. Chang KC, Chung SY, Chong WS et al. J Pharmacol Exp Ther 1993;266(2):992—1000.
167. Kumar JS, Menon VP. Metabolism 1993;42(11):1435—1439.
168. Habib MP, Dickerson FD, Mooradian AD. Metabolism 1994;43(11):1442—1445.
169. Mukherjee B, Mukherjee JR, Chatterjee M. Immunol Cell Biol 1994;72(2):109—114.
170. Lyons TJ, Li W, Wells Knecht MC, Jokl R. Diabetes 1994;43(9):1090—1095.
171. Kakkar R, Mantha SV, Radhi J, Prasad K, Kalra J. Life Sci 1997;60(9):667—679.
172. van Dam PS, Bravenboer B, van Asbeck BS, van Oirschot JF, Marx JJ, Gispen WH. Eur J Clin Invest 1996;26(12):1143—1149.
173. Sagara M, Satoh J, Wada R et al. Diabetologia 1996;39(3):263—269.
174. Yagi K. Biochem Med 1976;15(2):212—216.
175. Fujiwara Y, Kondo T, Murakami K, Kawakami Y. Klin Wochenschr 1989;67(6):336—341.
176. Urano S, Hoshi Hashizume M, Tochigi N, Matsuo M, Shiraki M, Ito H. Lipids 1991;26(1): 58—61.
177. Noberasco G, Odetti P, Boeri D, Maiello M, Adezati L. Biomed Pharmacother 1991;45(4—5): 193—196.
178. Watala C, Winocour PD. Eur J Clin Chem Clin Biochem 1992;30(9):513—519.
179. Katoh K. Diabet Res Clin Pract 1992;18(2):89—98.
180. Altomare E, Vendemiale G, Chicco D, Procacci V, Cirelli F. Diabet Metab 1992;18(4):264—271.
181. Carone D, Loverro G, Greco P, Capuano F, Selvaggi L. Eur J Obstet Gynecol Reprod Biol 1993; 51(2):103—109.
182. Gallou G, Ruelland A, Legras B, Maugendre D, Allannic H, Cloarec L. Clin Chim Acta 1993; 214(2):227—234.
183. Faure P, Corticelli P, Richard MJ et al. Clin Chem 1993;39(5):789—793.
184. Ceriello A, Falleti E, Bortolotti N et al. Met Clin Exp 1996;45(4):498—501.
185. Cominacini L, Garbin U, Pastorino AM, Fratta Pasini A, Campagnola M, De Santis A, Davioli A, Lo Cascio V. Diabetes Res 1994;26:173—184.
186. Evans RW, Orchard TJ. Metabolism 1994;43(9):1196—1200.
187. Srivastava S, Joshi CS, Sethi PP, Agrawal AK, Srivastava SK, Seth PK. Thromb Res 1994;76(5): 451—461.
188. Gugliucci A, Menini T, Stahl AJ. Biochem Mol Biol Int 1994;32(1):139—147.
189. Cestaro B, Gandini R, Viani P et al. Biochem Mol Biol Int 1994;32(5):983—994.
190. Nourooz-Zadeh J, Tajaddini-Sarmadi J, McCarthy S, Betteridge DJ, Wolff SP. Diabetes 1995;44 (9):1054—1058.
191. Gopaul NK, Anggard EE, Mallet AI, Betteridge DJ, Wolff SP, Nourooz Zadeh J. FEBS Lett 1995;368(2):225—229.
192. Haffner SM, Agil A, Mykkanen L, Stern MP, Jialal I. Diabetes Care 1995;18(5):646—653.
193. Singh S, Melkani GC, Rani C, Gaur SP, Agrawal V, Agrawal CG. Indian J Biochem Biophys 1997;34(6):512—517.
194. Ozben T, Nacitarhan S, Tuncer N. Int J Clin Lab Res 1995;25(3):162—164.

195. Nacitarhan S, Ozben T, Tuncer N. Free Radic Biol Med 1995;19(6):893—896.
196. Sanaka T, Takahashi C, Sanaka M et al. Clin Nephrol 1995;44(1):301—430.
197. Armstrong AM, Chestnutt JE, Gormley MJ, Young IS. Free Radic Biol Med 1996;21(5): 719—726.
198. Haffner SM, Miettinen H, Stern MP, Agil A, Jialal I. Metabolism 1996;45(7):876—881.
199. Freitas JP, Filipe PM, Rodrigo FG. Diabet Res Clin Pract 1997;36(2):71—75.
200. Mol MJ, de Rijke YB, Demacker PN, Stalenhoef AF. Atherosclerosis 1997;129(2):169—176.
201. Nourooz Zadeh J, Rahimi A, Tajaddini Sarmadi J et al. Diabetologia 1997;40(6):647—653.
202. Desfaits AC, Serri O, Renier G. Diabet Care 1998;21(4):487—493.
203. Ghiselli A, Laurenti O, De Mattia G, Maiani G, Ferro Luzzi A. Free Radic Biol Med 1992;13 (6):621—626.
204. Zoppini G, Targher G, Monauni T et al. Diabetes Care 1996;19(11):1233—1236.
205. Jennings PE, Jones AF, Florkowski CM, Lunec J, Barnett AH. Diabet Med 1987;4(5):452—456.
206. Knobl P, Schernthaner G, Schnack C et al. Diabetologia 1993;36(10):1045—1050.
207. Aoki Y, Yazaki K, Shirotori K et al. Diabetologia 1993;36(1):79—83.
208. Yaqoob M, Patrick AW, McClelland P et al. Clin Sci Colch 1993;85(5):557—562.
209. Festa A, Kopp HP, Schernthaner G, Menzel EJ. Diabetologia 1998;41(3):350—356.
210. Griffin ME, McInerney D, Fraser A et al. Diabet Med 1997;14(9):741—747.
211. Maziere C, Auclair M, Rose Robert F, Leflon P, Maziere JC. FEBS Lett 1995;363(3):277—279.
212. Bowie A, Owens D, Collins P, Johnson A, Tomkin GH. Atherosclerosis 1993;102(1):63—67.
213. Rabini RA, Fumelli P, Galassi R et al. Metabolism 1994;43(12):1470—1474.
214. Dimitriadis E, Griffin M, Owens D, Johnson A, Collins P, Tomkin GH. Diabetologia 1995;38 (11):1300—1306.
215. Dimitriadis E, Griffin M, Collins P, Johnson A, Owens D, Tomkin GH. Diabetologia 1996;39 (6):667—676.
216. Beaudeux JL, Guillausseau PJ, Peynet J et al. Clin Chim Acta 1995;239(2):131—141.
217. Leonhardt W, Hanefeld M, Muller G et al. Clin Chim Acta 1996;254(2):173—186.
218. Sanchez Quesada JL, Perez A, Caixas A et al. Diabetologia 1996;39(12):1469—1476.
219. Yoshida H, Ishikawa T, Nakamura H. Arterioscler Thromb Vasc Biol 1997;17(7):1438—1446.
220. O-Brien S, Mori TA, Puddey IB, Stanton KG. Diabetes Res Clin Pract 1995;30(3):195—203.
221. Jenkins AJ, Klein RL, Chassereau CN, Hermayer KL, Lopes Virella MF. Diabetes 1996;45(6): 762—767.
222. Bellomo G, Maggi E, Poli M, Agosta FG, Bollati P, Finardi G. Diabetes 1995;44(1):60—66.
223. Uusitupa MI, Niskanen L, Luoma J et al. Arterioscler Thromb Vasc Biol 1996;16(10): 1236—1242.
224. Mironova M, Virella G, Virella Lowell I, Lopes Virella MF. Clin Immunol Immunopathol 1997; 85(1):73—82.
225. Korpinen E, Groop PH, Akerblom HK, Vaarala O. Diabet Care 1997;20(7):1168—1171.
226. Salonen JT, Yla Herttuala S, Yamamoto R et al. Lancet 1992;339(8798):88.

©2000 Elsevier Science B.V. All rights reserved.
Handbook of Oxidants and Antioxidants in Exercise.
C.K. Sen, L. Packer and O. Hänninen, editors.

Part XI • Chapter 39

Exercise induces oxidative stress in healthy subjects and in chronic obstructive pulmonary disease patients

José Viña[1], Emilio Servera[2], Miguel Asensi[1], Juan Sastre[1], Federico V. Pallardó[1], Amparo Gimeno, Leo Heunks[4], P.N.R. Dekhuijzen[4] and José A. Ferrero[3]

[1]*Departamento de Fisiología, Facultad de Medicina, Universidad de Valencia, Av Blasco Ibanez 17, Valencia 46010, Spain. Tel.: +34-96386-4650. Fax: +34-96386-4642.*
Servicio de [2]Neumología; and [3]Cardiología, Hospital Clínico, Valencia, Spain.
[4]*Department of Pulmonary Diseases, University Hospital Nijmegen, Nijmegen, The Netherlands.*

1 INTRODUCTION
    1.1   Free radical generation in exercise
2 BLOOD GLUTATHIONE OXIDATION ASSOCIATED WITH EXERCISE: THE IMPORTANCE OF METHODOLOGY
3 EXERCISE GENERATES FREE RADICALS ONLY WHEN EXHAUSTIVE
4 GLUTATHIONE OXIDATION INDUCED BY EXERCISE IN CHRONIC OBSTRUCTIVE PULMONARY DISEASE (COPD) PATIENTS
    4.1   Lipid peroxidation in COPD patients who perform mild exercise
5 INDUCTION OF ANTIOXIDANT ENZYMES BY EXERCISE
6 TRAINING PROTECTS AGAINST FREE RADICAL DAMAGE CAUSED BY EXERCISE
7 SUMMARY
8 PERSPECTIVES
9 ACKNOWLEDGEMENTS
10 ABBREVIATIONS
11 REFERENCES

1   INTRODUCTION

1.1 Free radical generation in exercise

Physical exercise results in a number of benefits to health. Indeed, it increases high-density lipoprotein- cholesterol and lipoprotein lipase activity [1], attenuates diet-induced arteriosclerosis [2], increases bone density and can be considered as part of the treatment of diabetes mellitus. However, as stated in the old medical dictum, exhaustion prevents the beneficial effects of exercise.

Pioneer work carried out by Packer and his co-workers [3] using electron paramagnetic resonance showed that exercise generates free radicals and that vitamin E deficiency increases free radical formation by exercise. The finding that free radicals were involved in tissue damage caused by exercise [3,4] prompted a number of laboratories to test the possible protective effect of administration of antioxidants on free radical damage caused by exercise. Antioxidant vitamins proved effective [5,6,7]. Other antioxidants such as Coenzyme Q [8] were also useful. *N-*

acetyl cysteine was shown to inhibit muscle fatigue in humans [9]. The protective role of antioxidants has been extensively reviewed and thus, we will not do so in this chapter. The reader is referred to excellent reviews [10,11] for more detailed information on this matter.

2   BLOOD GLUTATHIONE OXIDATION: THE IMPORTANCE OF METHODOLOGY

Finding indexes of oxidative damage is of paramount importance in free radical research. Glutathione oxidation has been taken as an important index of free radical damage. Lang and his co-workers proposed that glutathione may serve as an index of aging [12]. We recently reported that oxidation of mitochondrial glutathione correlates with oxidative damage to mitochondrial DNA [13].

A major problem when measuring the glutathione status of cells [14] is that a small percentage of GSH oxidation may lead to large increases in GSSG concentration. In the 1970s we calculated that, if glutathione reductase is at equilibrium, the ratio GSH/GSSG in cells might be as high as 10^5 [15]. Even if the value of this ratio was only 100, a 2% oxidation of GSH would lead to an increase in GSSG of 100%. Thus, most methods used to determine GSSG are not effective to prevent glutathione oxidation and, are not useful to determine the extent of the oxidation of glutathione associated with exercise. A widely used HPLC method was reported by Reed and his co-workers [16].

Table 1 shows that, using Reed's method glutathione oxidation in many cell extracts is about 4%. Moreover, this percentage is much higher when measuring glutathione status in blood, in which glutathione oxidation can be as high as 25%. We have improved the method of sample treatment to decrease glutathione oxidation to about 0.3%. This was reported in [17] and we detailed this method to apply it to measuring glutathione oxidation in exercise [18]. Although a full explanation of our method of glutathione determination is outside the scope of this chapter, the reader is referred to our review [18] for more precise details.

Soon after the finding that free radicals are involved in exercise-induced oxidative damage, changes in the glutathione status of plasma, liver and muscle following exhaustive exercise in experimental animals were reported [19,20]. Furthermore, blood glutathione oxidation during human exercise was observed [21].

3   EXERCISE GENERATES FREE RADICALS ONLY WHEN IT IS EXHAUSTIVE

We used our method to determine glutathione redox ratio in exercise in rats and humans which confirmed that exercise causes glutathione oxidation in both humans and in rats [22]. Glutathione oxidation could be prevented by oral administration of the antioxidant vitamins C and E. When exercise was performed at submaximal intensities, glutathione oxidation did not occur. In fact we found that glutathione oxidation is related to an increase in the blood lac-

Table 1. Glutathione oxidation in biological samples.

A. Using iodoacetic acid as thiol trapping agent (Reed's method).

	GSSG level		% Oxidation
	−GSH	+GSH	
Blood (μM)	221 ± 46 [6]	475 ± 99 [6][a]	24 ± 6 [6]
Liver (nmols/g)	316 ± 54 [3]	468 ± 50 [3][a]	2.9 ± 0.3 [3]
Kidney (nmols/g)	90 ± 38 [3]	329 ± 17 [3][a]	4.1 ± 0.4 [3]

B. Using NEM as thiol trapping agent (our method).

	GSSG level		% Oxidation
	−GSH	+GSH	
Blood (μM)	19.3 ± 6.2 [5]	20.8 ± 4.9 [5]	0.13 ± 0.28 [5]
Liver (nmols/g)	19 ± 11 [4]	30 ± 22 [4]	0.22 ± 0.34 [4]
Kidney (nmols/g)	26 ± 17 [4]	55 ± 40 [4]	0.59 ± 0.49 [4]

We measured GSSG levels following Reed's method (**A**) or by using our method (**B**). Values are means ± standard deviation with the number of experiments in parentheses. The percentage of GSH oxidation was calculated as follows: % of oxidation = $(A - B - C) \times 2 \times 100 \times D^{-1}$; where A = GSSG levels in blood or tissue samples treated with PCA containing exogenous GSH, B = GSSG levels in blood or tissue samples, C = GSSG levels in PCA containing exogenous GSH. A, B and C are expressed as nmol/ml for blood and in nmol/g for tissues. D = final concentration of the exogenous GSH added (expressed in nmol/ml for blood and in nmol/g for tissues). A factor of 2 is used to convert GSSG to GSH equivalents. A significant difference in GSSG level between with and without addition of exogenous GSH is shown as [a]$p < 0.05$.

tate/pyruvate ratio [22]. Figure 1 shows this linear relationship. This suggested that only exhaustive exercise causes oxidative damage to cells. Indeed, when lactate levels were low, oxidation of glutathione did not occur. The fact that an increase in oxidation of glutathione was correlated with an increase in the reduction of the lactate/pyruvate ratio led us to think that the cause of oxidative damage associated with exercise might not be an increase in electron leakage in the respiratory chain. Conversely, pioneer work by Chance and co-workers [23] showed that free radical formation by mitochondria which were actively phosphorylating ADP (as is the case in exercise), produce considerably fewer peroxides than those in resting cells.

The fact that glutathione oxidation was related to increases in lactate levels, led us to think that exercise-induced free radical formation could be related to exhaustion and not to an increased oxygen utilization. This could be tested in chronic obstructive pulmonary disease (COPD) patients who become exhausted when they perform exercise that is of low intensity but that is exhaustive for them. We thus decided to test the effect of exercise on glutathione status in COPD patients.

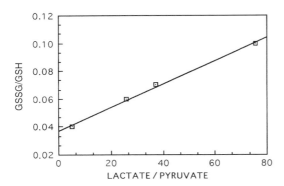

Fig. 1. Linear relationship between GSSG/GSH and lactate/pyruvate ratios in blood from humans subjected to physical exercise. Human blood was obtained from subjects before, immediately after, and 30 or 60 min after physical exercise to exhaustion on a treadmill using Bruce's protocol.

4   GLUTATHIONE OXIDATION INDUCED BY EXERCISE IN COPD PATIENTS

COPD patients become exhausted when they perform exercise of low intensity. Thus, they lend themselves as an excellent model to test the effect of exhaustion in persons who do not perform high-intensity exercise. Furthermore, COPD patients may become exhausted daily in their life when they perform light exercise necessary to carry out their ordinary activities. In this respect they are different from healthy persons who become exhausted only when they voluntarily perform heavy exercise, whereas COPD patients become exhausted when they perform their everyday activities.

There is no statistically significant difference between resting blood GSH and GSSG levels in healthy subjects and in COPD patients. Indeed we reported in [22] that blood GSH and GSSG levels in resting healthy subjects were 800 ± 300 μmol/l (n = 19) and 29 ± 10 μmol/l (n = 15), respectively. We have also found that in COPD patients, resting GSH and GSSG levels are 776 ± 62 μmol/l (n = 5) and 31.7 ± 7 μmol/l (n = 5), respectively (see Table 2).

Table 2 shows that submaximal exercise causes glutathione oxidation in COPD patients. This was evidenced by an increase in GSSG and a slight decrease in GSH levels in blood. The fact that changes in GSH after exercise are not statistically significant is due to the high interindividual variability found in blood GSH values, a fact extensively discussed by Mills et al. [24]. The patients performed exercise (approximately 40 W for up to 6 min), i.e., the kind of exercise a person is expected to perform in usual day-to-day activity. Thus, blood glutathione is oxidized in these patients many times a day as they perform light exercise, which is, nevertheless, hard for them, in the course of their ordinary life [25].

Table 2. Effect of physical exercise on glutathione status and lactate levels in arterial blood.

	Control		Oxygen therapy	
	Rest	Post-exercise	Rest	Post-exercise
GSH (µM)	776 ± 62	598 ± 103^a	788 ± 198	808 ± 227
GSSG (µM)	31 ± 7	50 ± 12^b	28 ± 6	36 ± 6^b
Lactate (mM)	1.27 ± 0.23	3.20 ± 0.47^b	1.25 ± 0.53	2.70 ± 0.27^b

Results are means ± standard deviation for five COPD patients. Statistical analyses were performed by Student's t test for paired samples and is expressed as follows: $^a p < 0.05$; $^b p < 0.01$ between rest and exercise.

4.1 Lipid peroxidation in COPD patients who perform mild exercise

As stated before, glutathione oxidation is considered a good index of oxidative stress. However, after we found that mild exercise causes oxidation of glutathione in COPD patients, we decided to test whether exercise causes an increase in lipid peroxidation, made evident by an increase in malondialdehyde levels in plasma. Malondialdehyde was determined using an HPLC method that is useful in measuring it specifically. The widely used thiobarbituric acid reactive substance (TBARS) is inadequate because of its lack of specificity.

Figure 2 shows that blood levels of malondialdehyde are significantly higher in COPD patients after a bout of low-intensity exercise that is, however, exhaustive for them. In contrast with the oxidation of glutathione, which occurred immedi-

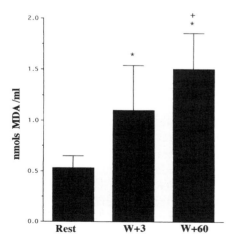

Fig. 2. Effect of physical exercise on serum malondialdehyde levels in COPD patients. W+3: 3 min after maximal workload; W+60: 60 min after maximal workload. Statistical difference between rest and exercise groups is shown as * ($p < 0.05$). Statistical difference between W+3 and W+60 is shown as + ($p < 0.005$).

ately after exercise, the increase in malondialdehyde occurred 1 h after the completion of the bout of exercise. This lag period may be required for lipid peroxidation to occur after the initial oxidative stress has taken place.

5   ENZYME INDUCTION BY EXERCISE

The fact that exhaustive exercise causes an increase in free radical formation suggested that antioxidant enzymes might be induced by exercise. Indeed, Ji et al. [26] and also Sen et al. [27] studied the effect of training on antioxidant enzymes. Exhaustive exercise resulted in an increase in glutathione peroxidase, glutathione reductase, superoxide dismutase and catalase activities. Ji and Fu [28], studying the effect of physical exercise on the glutathione system, hypothesized that both exhaustive exercise and hydroperoxide can cause severe oxidative stress to the body by a similar mechanism.

The original work by Davies et al. [3] suggested that muscle mitochondriogenesis associated with exercise might be caused by repeated free radical formation. Indeed, cells react against free radical formation associated with exercise by inducing the synthesis of enzymes which tend to detoxify such radicals. This may be very important in determining the possible protective effects of training against damage associated with exercise as discussed in the following section.

6   TRAINING PROTECTS AGAINST FREE RADICAL DAMAGE
CAUSED BY EXERCISE

The majority of persons who practice strenuous exercise do so after training. Thus, an important question was whether training protects against oxidative damage caused by exercise. Shortly after the observation of the free radical formation by exercise, Salminen and Vihko [29] found that endurance training protected against muscle lipid peroxidation in vitro. They also reported that muscle catalase activity and the concentration of vitamin E in red muscle fibers is significantly higher after training than in controls. No changes were reported in total sulfhydryl contents.

In spite of much effort devoted to studying the effect of training on enzyme activities, especially on antioxidant enzymes (see previous section), little work has been dedicated to testing the protective effect of training on metabolites that might be an index on oxidative stress. To our knowledge this question had been tested only on malondialdehyde, measured as TBARS [28]. This method of malondialdehyde determination might be flawed by technical errors, as already mentioned above. Thus, we determined the effect of training on changes of glutathione redox status in human blood. For this purpose we used volunteers from the Spanish army. These young recruits were not previously trained. They performed exercise graded to exhaustion, and venous blood was collected before and after exercise. This was followed by 2 months of aerobic training in the army and then the exercise test was repeated.

In untrained sedentary male volunteers, exhaustive physical exercise caused an oxidation of blood glutathione. Indeed we found a significant decrease in GSH (from 841 to 664 μM) and an increase in GSSG (from 45 to 83 μM). However, when the same subjects performed exercise to exhaustion after a period of training, blood glutathione oxidation was lower than in untrained subjects. As expected, blood lactate and pyruvate levels rose both in controls (untrained) and in trained subjects.

By using an adequate method to determine blood GSSG [17,18], we were able to observe that there is a linear relationship between lactate/pyruvate and GSSG/GSH ratios [22]. We have measured the effect of training on the "slope" of the line that relates the oxidation of glutathione and the lactate/pyruvate ratio (see Fig. 3). This Figure shows that at a given level of effort (indicated by the lactate/pyruvate ratio) the oxidative stress caused by exercise is higher in untrained than in trained subjects. We have calculated this from the data shown in Fig. 3 and have found that the slope for untrained subjects was 5.8 and that for the same subjects after training it was 1.4. These values show that for the same increase in lactate/pyruvate due to exercise, the oxidation of the glutathione redox pair is 4-fold greater (5.5 vs. 1.4) in untrained than trained subjects. Thus, although training did not entirely protect against exercise-induced glutathione oxidation (the line for "trained" in Fig. 3 would then be horizontal), it indeed confers significant protection against oxidative stress (evident by the oxidation of glutathione) caused by exhaustive physical exercise.

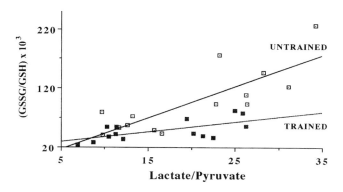

Fig. 3. Relationship between blood glutathione oxidation and lactate/pyruvate in untrained volunteers under four experimental conditions, i.e., rest and postexercise in untrained subjects (empty squares), and rest and postexercise in the same subjects after a period of 2 months of training (filled squares). The slopes of the lines were 5.31 for untrained, and 1.65 for trained volunteers. The standard errors of the slopes were 1.11 and 0.57 for untrained and trained volunteers, respectively.

7 SUMMARY

1. Blood glutathione oxidation serves as an index of oxidative stress associated with exercise, both in humans and in experimental animals.
2. Oxidative stress occurs only when exercise is exhaustive.
3. Chronic obstructive pulmonary disease patients who perform light exercise that is, nevertheless, exhaustive for them also show signs of oxidative stress.
4. The occurrence of oxidative stress does not depend on the absolute intensity of exercise but on the degree of exhaustion.
5. Training partially, but not completely, prevents exercise-induced oxidative stress.
6. Antioxidant administration prevents some of the undesirable effects of exhaustive exercise.

8 PERSPECTIVES

Oxidative stress occurs during exhaustive physical exercise. The possible causes of this oxidative stress, however, remain elusive. Future directions of research involve testing the possible role of the mitochondrial machinery in the generation of reactive oxygen species and also the involvement of extramitochondrial enzymes that can produce ROS under conditions of exhaustive physical exercise. According to our findings, antioxidants can ameliorate recovery after a bout of exhaustive physical exercise and can even, in the long-term, protect muscle and joint injuries associated with overtraining. The above-reviewed data clearly show that much remains to be done to elucidate the role of ROS during exhaustive physical exercise in both healthy and COPD patients. Certain lines of available information are at least starting points which suggest working hypotheses for further research.

9 ACKNOWLEDGEMENTS

This work was supported by grants FIS 98/1462 to JV, GV-3277/95 to MA and FIS 96/1207 to FVP.

10 ABBREVIATIONS

COPD: chronic obstructive pulmonary disease
GSH: reduced glutathione
GSSG: oxidized glutathione
HPLC: high-performance liquid chromatography
TBARS: thiobarbituric acid reactive substance

11 REFERENCES

1. Kantor MA, Culliane EM, Sady SP, Herbert PN, Thomson PD. Exercise acutely increases high-density lipoprotein-cholesterol and lipoprotein lipase activity in trained and untrained men. Metabolism 1987;36:188—192.
2. Hasler CM, Rothenbacher H, Mela DJ, Kris-Etherton PM. Exercise attenuates diet-induced arteriosclerosis in the adult rat. J Nutr 1987;117:986—993.
3. Davies KJA, Quintanilha AT, Brooks GA, Packer L. Free radicals and tissue damage produced by exercise. Biochem Biophys Res Commun 1982;107:1198—1205.
4. Zerba E, Komorovsky TE, Faulkner JA. Free radical injury to skeletal muscles of young, adult and old mice. Am J Physiol 1990;258:C429—C435.
5. Packer L. Protective role of vitamin E in biological systems. Am J Clin Nutr 1991;53: S1050—S1055.
6. Bendich A. Exercise and free radicals — effects of antioxidant vitamins. Adv Nutr Top Sport 1991;32:59—78.
7. Meydani M, Evans WJ, Handelman G, Biddle L, Fielding RA, Meydani SN, Burill J, Fiatarone MA, Blumberg JB, Cannon JG. Protective effect of vitamin E on exercise-induced oxidative damage in young and older adults. Am J Physiol 1993;264:R992—R998.
8. Shimomura Y, Suzuki M, Sugiyama S, Hanaki Y, Ozawa Y. Protective effect of coenzyme Q10 on exercise-induced muscular injury. Biochem Biophys Res Commun 1991;176:349—355.
9. Reid MB, Stokic DS, Koch SM, Khawli FA, Leis AA. *N*-acetylcysteine inhibits muscle fatigue in humans. J Clin Invest 1994;94:2468—2474.
10. Ji LL. Oxidative stress during exercise: implication of antioxidant nutrients. Free Radic Biol Med 1995;18:1079—1086.
11. Witt EH, Reznick A, Viguie CA, Starke- Reed P, Packer L. Exercise, oxidative damage and effects of antioxidant manipulation. J Nutr 1992;122:766—773.
12. Lang C, Narshkin S, Schenider DL, Mills BJ. Low glutathione levels in healthy aging adults. J Lab Clin Med 1992;120:720—725.
13. Garcia de la Asuncion J, Millan A, Pla R, Bruseghini L, Esteras A, Pallardo FV, Sastre J, Viña J. Mitochondrial glutathione oxidation correlates with age-associated oxidative damage to mito-chondrial DNA. FASEB J 1996;10:333—338.
14. Kosower NS, Kosower EM. The glutathione status of cells. Int Rev Cytol 1978;54:109—160.
15. Viña J, Hems R, Krebs HA. Maintenance of glutathione content in isolated hepatocytes. Bio-chem J 1978;170:627—630.
16. Reed DJ, Babson JR, Beatty PW, Brodie AE, Ellis WW, Potter DW. High-performance liquid chromatography analysis of nanomole levels of glutathione, glutathione disulfide, and related thiols and disulfides. Anal Biochem 1980;106:55—62.
17. Asensi M, Sastre J, Pallardó FV, García de la Asunción J, Estrela JM, Viña J. A high-performance liquid chromatography method for measurement of oxidized glutathione in bio-logical samples. Anal Biochem 1994;21:323—328.
18. Viña J, Juan Sastre J, Miguel Asensi M, Packer L. Assay of blood glutathione oxidation during physical exercise. Meth Enzymol 1995;251:237—243.
19. Lew H, Pyke S, Quintanilha A. Changes in the glutathione status of plasma, liver and muscle following exhaustive exercise in rats. FEBS Lett 1985;185:262—266.
20. Pyke S, Lew H, Quintanilha A. Severe depletion in liver glutathione during physical exercise. Biochem Biophys Res Commun 1986;139:926—931.
21. Gohil K, Viguie C, Stanley WC, Brooks G, Packer L. Blood glutathione oxidation during human exercise. J Appl Physiol 1988;64:115—119.
22. Sastre J, Asensi M, Gascó E, Ferrero JA, Furukawa T, Viña J. Exhaustive physical exercise causes and oxidation of glutathione status in blood. Prevention by antioxidant administration. Am J Physiol 1992;263:R992—R995.
23. Chance B, Sies H, Boveris A. Hydroperoxide metabolism in mammalian organs. Physiol Rev

1979;59:527–604.

24. Mills BJ, Ritchie JP, Lang CA. Glutathione variability in normal human blood. Anal Biochem 1994;222:95–101.

25. Viña J, Servera E, Asensi M, Sastre J, Pallardó F, Ferrero JA, García de la Asunción J, Antón V, Marín J. Exercise causes blood glutathione oxidation in chronic obstructive pulmonary disease. Prevention by oxygen therapy. J Appl Physiol 1996;81(5):2199–2202.

26. Ji LL, Stratman FW, Lardy HA. Antioxidant enzyme systems in rat liver and skeletal muscle. Influences of selenium deficiency, chronic training and acute exercise. Arch Biochem Biophys 1988;263:150–160.

27. Sen CK, Atalay M, Hanninen O. Exercise-induced oxidative stress: Glutathione supplementation and deficiency. J Appl Physiol 1994;77:2177–2187.

28. Ji LL, Fu R. Responses of glutathione system and antioxidant enzymes to exhaustive exercise and hydroperoxide. J Appl Physiol 1992;72:549–554.

29. Salminen A, Vihko V. Endurance training reduces the susceptibility of mouse skeletal muscle to lipid peroxidation in vitro. Acta Physiol Scand 1983;117:109–113.

©2000 Elsevier Science B.V. All rights reserved.
Handbook of Oxidants and Antioxidants in Exercise.
C.K. Sen, L. Packer and O. Hänninen, editors.

Part XI • Chapter 40

Hypoxia, oxidative stress and exercise in rheumatoid arthritis

S. Jawed[1], S.E. Edmonds[2], V. Gilston[1] and D.R. Blake[3]

[1] *ARC Clinical Research Fellow, The Bone and Joint Research Unit, The London Hospital Medical College, 25—29 Ashfield Street, London E1 2AD, UK. Tel.: +44 171-377-7000. Fax: +44 171-377-7763. E-mail: sjawed@mds.qmw.ac.uk*
[2] *Department of Rheumatology, Stoke Mandeville Hospital, Ayelsbury, Bucks HP21 8AL, UK*
[3] *Department of Rheumatology, Royal National Hospital for Rheumatic Diseases, Upper Borough Walls, Bath, BA1 1RL, UK*

1 INTRODUCTION
   1.1 What is rheumatoid arthritis?
   1.2 The role of T cells and macrophages in rheumatoid arthritis
   1.3 Joint physiology in health and disease
   1.4 Synovial metabolism, hypoxia and immune function
2 HYPOXIA, OXIDATIVE STRESS AND CELL SIGNALING
   2.1 Activation of AP-1
   2.2 Activation of NFκB
   2.3 Hypoxia-inducible factor-1
3 THE ROLE OF XANTHINE OXIDOREDUCTASE IN RHEUMATOID ARTHRITIS
   3.1 Conversion of XD to XO
   3.2 Localisation of XO
   3.3 Measurement of XO in human plasma
   3.4 XO and nitric oxide generation
4 THE GENERATION OF REACTIVE OXYGEN SPECIES BY SYNOVIUM
   4.1 ROS-induced damage to proteins
   4.2 ROS-induced damage to other biomolecules
5 MICROBLEEDING, IRON AND SYNOVITIS
6 OXIDATIVE INDUCTION OF BONE RESORPTION
   6.1 Oxidative damage to nerves
   6.2 Understanding the typus robustus patient
7 THE COMPLEX INFLUENCES OF REST AND EXERCISE ON THE CLINICAL OUTCOME OF RHEUMATOID ARTHRITIS
   7.1 Rest
   7.2 Exercise
   7.3 Speculation as to the mechanism of exercise-induced suppression of synovitis
8 SUMMARY
9 PERSPECTIVES
10 REFERENCES

1 INTRODUCTION

Many of the disorders of joints that fall under the broad label of "arthritis" have an inflammatory basis. In this review we deal primarily with the disease rheumatoid arthritis (RA), one of the more common, destructive and eventually disabling of the inflammatory polyarthritides.

It is perhaps unnecessary to state that the inflammatory reaction is not designed to cause disease but to prevent or limit it. The multiple, complex and iterating cascades that make up an inflammatory reaction are designed to prevent or inhibit infection and minimise tissue damage. In order to focus the inflammatory response to a certain site, a degree of tissue damage will ensue as a consequence of the otherwise salutatory inflammatory reaction, but the primary purpose of the process is containment and destruction of pathogens with full return of function. Reactive oxygen intermediates (ROI) play a critical role in all aspects of the inflammatory process, from initiation to resolution. What then goes wrong in RA that allows the inflammatory reaction to persist into a chronic phase for the rest of the patients' life? In this review we provide evidence that the complex biochemical influences of hypoxia and oxidative stress that are induced by joint movement, provide an answer to this question.

1.1 What is rheumatoid arthritis?

As a defined causative factor is lacking, no exact definition of RA exists, but clinically the disease presents as a systemic disorder with manifestations in multiple organs. An inflammatory synovitis affecting mobile diarthrodial joints dominates the clinical picture and the pattern of joint involvement usually forms the basis for a clinical diagnosis.

The basic pathology within the joint centres on the synovial membrane and there are several key features which are illustrated in Fig. 1. The lining layer, normally two cells thick, is much thickened, with increased numbers of macrophage and fibroblast cells, both expressing "activation markers". The deeper layers are infiltrated with bone marrow-derived cells, with perivascular accumulations and follicles. These are rich in CD_4^+ (T_4) cells — helper T cells. Some CD_8 (T_8) or cytolytic T cells are also present — found in between perivascular accumulations along with abundant plasma cells and a few B cells. Macrophages are found in the follicles. Plasma cells and B cells are involved in the production of rheumatoid factors (see below). Between synovial tissue, cartilage and bone, is the site for early bone erosion and the tissue filling this area and covering the bone surface is referred to as pannus and is vascularised.

Synovial fluid volumes are increased in RA, often markedly so, and the cellularity is also increased. Despite a paucity of polymorphonuclear cells within the synovial membrane, this cell type predominates within the synovial fluid. In a typical synovial fluid during an acute flare of synovitis, approximately 10^6/ml polymorphs are present.

The disease has been found in all populations that have been examined although prevalence figures vary between 0.2 and 5.3% [1]. The age distribution of the populations studied explains some, though not all, of the differences in prevalence as the disease is 6 times more common in the sixth decade than the second. Women are affected 2.5 times more commonly than men, suggesting an

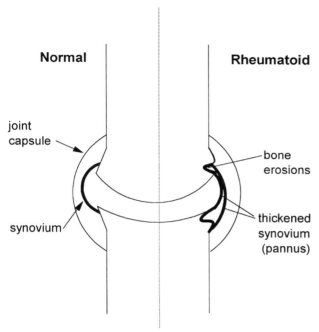

Fig. 1. The main pathological features of rheumatoid synovitis. The inflamed synovium (pannus) gradually causes erosive damage of bone and cartilage.

hormonal influence and indeed the disease often remits during pregnancy only to return postpartum.

A symmetrical synovitis of the small joints of the hands and feet with sparing of the distal interphalangeal joints is the single most characteristic clinical feature of RA [2]). The dominant side is often, though not always, most severely affected [3] and heavy manual workers often develop marked destructive changes in bone in a relatively painless joint. This form of disease is referred to as typus robustus arthritis [4] and is described in more detail below. The converse of heavy exercise is of course, immobility, which has a complex influence on synovitis. Immobility, used as a therapy and created by external splinting suppresses synovitis [5], whilst in a hemiparetic patient, the paretic side of the body is usually much less affected [6]. The disease is most varied both with regard to severity and the rate of progress but once joint damage has started, remission of synovitis is rare until the joint fuses — then synovitis settles.

Although RA is primarily a disease confined to mobile joints, extra-articular manifestations can be found in many organs and occasionally antedate the synovitis. A full description of such complications is out with the scope of this article and is well reviewed elsewhere [7]. However, we wish to draw attention to one common extra-articular manifestation of the disease, namely, rheumatoid nodules. These are found in about one third of patients and consist of firm subcutaneous swellings that occur on the extensor surface of the forearms and other regularly pressurized areas of the skin. They are invariably present in patients with typus robustus arthritis and are associated with the presence of antibodies directed at self IgG — otherwise known as "rheumatoid factor".

Rheumatoid factors are antibodies directed against antigenic determinants on the Fc fragment of IgG. In RA the antibody is polyclonal, reacting with a range of determinants on both the CH_2 and CH_3 domains, including sites expressed by aggregated or denatured IgG. As discussed in detail below, exercise-induced oxidative modification of IgG appears to be one mechanism by which the antigenicity of IgG may be altered and the production of rheumatoid factors generated.

1.2 The role of T cells and macrophages in rheumatoid arthritis

The role of the T cell in RA is been the subject of much controversy. The various hypothesis range from those that suggest T cells initiate and perpetuate RA to those which suggest that the T cell is only of transient importance in the initial phase of the disease. There is evidence to support both these theories including studies which show anti-T cell therapy [8] to be ineffective and studies showing efficacy of cyclosporin (a T cell inhibitor) in some RA patients [9]. We have also seen the emergence of HIV infection which results in a depleted numbers of T helper cells in infected individuals and there have been case reports of disease remission in patients with RA who have contracted HIV infection and there are also case reports of patients with HIV presenting with an RA-like inflammatory arthropathy for the first time [10].

Recent advances in T cell research have shown there to be subsets of T helper cells present in autoimmunity [11]. These have been divided into Th1 and Th2 subsets, each have different roles in immunity and produce a different cytokine profile (Fig. 2). Th1 cells primarily produce interferon-γ and interleukin 2 where as Th2 cells produce interleukin 4 which may have an inhibitory effect on Th1 activity [12]. In RA there appears to be a shift towards a Th1 cell cytokine response [13] and the ratio in Th1/Th2 cells in RA may have important implications in designing future anti-T cell therapies.

In contrast to T cells and their products, macrophages are easily found in RA synovium. Macrophage-derived cytokines are easily found in synovial tissue and fluid. These include IL-1, IL-6, IL-10, GM-CSF and TNFα amongst others [14]. This response is similar to that observed in hypoxic conditions and there exists the possibility that RA, once initiated, is then a 'fibroblast-macrophage' driven process largely independent of T cells.

1.3 Joint physiology in health and disease

The synovial fluid volume of the normal human knee joint is up to 4 ml, spread evenly throughout the joint and having a thickness of approximately 26 μm [15].

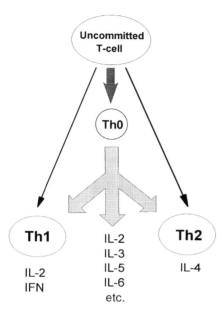

Fig. 2. In rheumatoid arthritis (RA) the T cells divide into two subsets (Th1 and Th2) each with a distinct cytokine profile. In RA there may be a shift towards a Th1 cytokine response (interferon-γ and interleukin-2).

The synovial intra-articular pressure (IAP) in the knees of normal humans, cats, rabbits and dogs is subatmospheric (between −2 and −10 mmHg) [16,17] whether or not the joint is weight-bearing and irrespective of whether it is mobile or not: this is of considerable physiological importance.

Bone ends are covered by cartilage which lies within the synovial cavity. Cartilage is avascular and is subjected to compressive forces that would lead to repeated episodes of vasoconstriction if it were a vascular tissue. Intermittent vasoconstriction responses may result in bursts of oxidants from endothelial reductases (e.g., xanthine oxido-reductase) which act as part of our bactericidal defense mechanism in traumatic situations, where vasoconstriction (hypoxia) and vasodilation (reperfusion) are early features of such injury. These oxidants would damage the cartilage cell (the chondrocyte) and the cartilage matrix, which is composed of collagen and proteoglycans bound to hyaluronan, a glycosaminoglycan. Cartilage is metabolically active and requires constant nutrition; this is achieved via the synovial microvessels and synovial fluid.

In the normal joint the synovial membrane is only a few cells thick, but incorporated into it is a dense vascular plexus. The important vascular parameters which govern the efficacy of the oxygen delivery system are: capillary density; capillary spatial distribution and blood flow. Morphometry of tissue sections of normal synovium has supplied data on the first two of these features [18,19] which are much altered in disease. The synovium is considerably more vascular than the structures supporting the joint such as the capsule, ligaments and tendons. The first description of the vasculature within the joint was by Hunter in 1743 who described the circulus articuli vasculosus — the vascular plexus of the joint. At the margins of the articular cartilage the synovium forms villi and folds into which the plexus sends arcades of capillaries. These capillaries are much more densely distributed in the superficial layers of the synovium (approximately 240 capillaries per mm^2) than in the deeper layers. The negative IAP effectively means that the joint space or cavity is only a potential space and the synovium and its multiple blood vessels are maintained in close physical proximity to the cartilage edges. The maintenance of the negative cavity pressure on exercise or weight-bearing ensures that these vessels remain patent and the cartilage nourished irrespective of the amount of exercise taken as illustrated in Fig. 3.

   In inflammatory RA the situation is much altered. Assuming that the data on capillary density and depth, which were determined in normal joints, represent the optimal situation, there is a significant reduction in vascularity in the functionally important superficial region of the synovium. The capillary density in RA is reduced to about one third of the normal value and the mean intercapillary distance increases, reflecting not only an increase in spatial distribution of the vasculature, but also the thickened synovial lining. The vasculature is also buried more deeply with the average capillary distance from the joint cavity increased, probably in response to the intra-articular hypoxia [20]. In addition to these changes, multilamination of the basement membrane surrounding the blood vessels also occurs, creating a further barrier to nutrient exchange. Vascular changes are accompanied by changes to both synovial fluid volume and viscosity, which

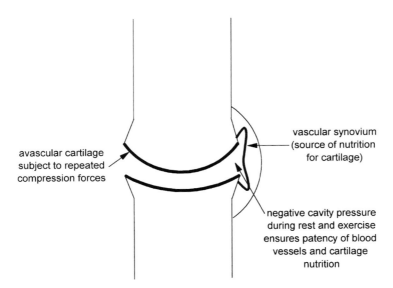

Fig. 3. The physiology of the normal synovial joint.

are in part associated with changes in synovial IAP.

Synovial fluid, feeding the avascular cartilage, is an ultrafiltrate of plasma to which components secreted by the synovial cells are added. The most important of these is hyaluronate. Hyaluronate is a linear repeating disaccharide, β-D-glucuronyl-β-D-N-acetylglucosamine of molecular mass in excess of 10^7 Da. Hyaluronate forms the central axis of the proteoglycan aggregates necessary for the functional integrity of articular cartilage and within the synovial fluid, along with "lubricin", is responsible for the remarkable viscoelastic properties of synovial fluid. In RA, the synovial macrophages secrete increased amounts of hyaluronan. However, the synovial fluid has a decreased viscosity compared to normal. This reduction in viscosity is a consequence of a decrease in molecular weight which may be explained in two ways: either by defective synthesis with premature termination of the nascent polysaccharide chain, or by fragmentation of the intact chain after secretion into the synovial cavity. Pulse chase experiments support the view that the presence of short chain molecules of hyaluronan in arthritis synovial fluid is due to degradation after synthesis rather than defective synthesis [21]. As outlined below, oxidative fragmentation seems the most likely explanation for the presence of low MW fragments of hyaluronan and such fragments have interesting biological properties that may perpetuate synovitis. In addition, hyaluronan plays an important role in normal tissue homeostasis and interacts with matrix hyaluronan-binding proteins (hyaluronan receptors) to influence cell behaviour [22] suggesting further implications for its fragmentation.

Associated with the increased synovial fluid volume is a marked change in the synovial intra-articular pressure (IAP) profile and responses. In 1875, Ranke [23] observed that in an acute haemarthrosis the IAP can rise as high as 200 mmHg and thereby diminishes effective synovial blood flow. More recently, Jayson and Dixon [24] observed that patients with RA had significantly higher resting IAP pressures than normal control subjects with a simulated effusion of an equal volume of isotonic saline. The effusion pressure/volume curves obtained rose smoothly in both groups, although the rheumatoid IAP pressures were invariably higher, probably as a result of a decreased compliance of the joint wall due to synovial membrane swelling and fibrosis of the capsule. Merry et al. [25] performed a detailed comparative study of the IAP's in joints with acute traumatic and chronic inflammatory effusions before and after exercise. In patients with chronic knee effusions due to RA the mean (SD) IAP during exercise was 222.5 (158.6) mmHg. In patients with acute traumatic effusions of greater than one day but less than 3 days duration the results were barely above atmospheric — 2.0 (2.8) mmHg — and the mean IAP during exercise was very modest at 13.7 (8.6) mmHg. Clearly the rise postexercise in the chronic inflammatory group is well in excess of the estimated capillary perfusion pressure of the synovial membrane in disease (35—60 mmHg), whilst this is not the case in those with traumatic effusions. In a further study [26] we measured exercise-related IAP in four different groups of patients with knee effusions. These included patients with acute traumatic effusions (ATE), those with an acute synovitis on the background of a chronic inflammatory arthropathy (RA and psoriatic arthritis) and those with a chronic low grade inflammatory arthropathy (osteoarthritis) and those with an acute intermittent inflammatory arthropathy (pyrophosphate arthropathy, amyloidosis and Behcet's disease). The results showed a significant rise in exercise-related IAP in all groups except the ATE (Fig. 4). Interestingly the volume of synovial fluid aspirated in the non-ATE groups correlated significantly with the magnitude of the IAP change (Fig. 5). We can, therefore, conclude that the IAP rise during exercise is a feature of all patients with an inflammatory-based effusion irrespective of the duration of the effusion. This is not the case in patients with an ATE. Also, in inflammatory synovitis the rise in intra-articular pressure with isometric quadriceps contraction relates to effusion volume. The most likely explanation for this is that the inflammatory process prevents reflex muscle inhibition (RMI), a locally protective mechanism that minimises the potential for intermittent ischaemia/oxidative injury. The rise in IAP in RA is not restricted to the large lower limb joints and has also been demonstrated in smaller upper limb peripheral joints using similar methodology [27].

In order to assess whether such pressure changes induced by exercise were associated with changes in synovial capillary blood flow, a laser Doppler flow meter with a specially designed 16 gauge sideview optical probe was used to directly measure the synovial blood flow. In normal knees, the mean baseline capillary flow rates ranged from 10–22 perfusion units and during exercise

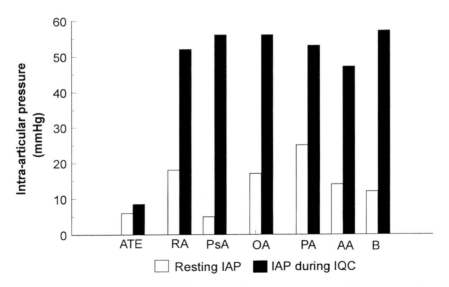

Fig. 4. Intra-articular pressure (IAP) at rest and during isometric quadriceps contraction (IQC) in patients with acute traumatic effusions (ATE), rheumatoid arthritis (RA), psoriatic arthritis (PsA), osteoarthritis (OA), pyrophosphate arthropathy (PA), Behcet's syndrome (B) and amyloid arthropathy (AA).

Synovial fluid volume (ml)

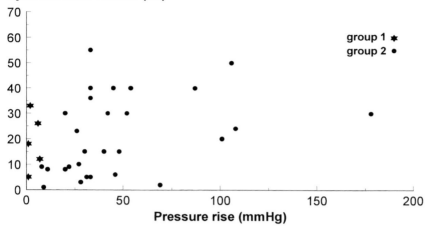

Fig. 5. The relationship between intra-articular pressure rise and volume of synovial fluid aspirated in groups 1, (patients with acute traumatic knee effusions), and 2, (patients with knee effusions secondary to rheumatoid arthritis, psoriatic arthritis, osteoarthritis, pyrophosphate arthropathy, Behcet's syndrome and amyloid arthropathy). There is a significant positive correlation in group 2 (r = 0.45, p < 0.05) but not in group 1 (r = 0.21, p = 0.74).

(quadriceps setting) there was no significant change. In inflamed knees, however, the situation was very different. Mean basal capillary flow rates ranged widely between 33 and 372 perfusion units, but during exercise fell sharply to means of 4–47 units. After exercise, flow returned to basal or suprabasal levels within 10–15 s although in some recordings, reperfusion was delayed for up to one min after cessation of exercise. James et al. [28] confirmed these findings and demonstrated that in rheumatoid patients with knee effusions increases in IAP in the range encountered during normal daily activity will compromise blood flow. This is associated with an increase in the concentration of synovial fluid lactate, an elevated pCO_2 and a decrease in pH. In rabbits, IAP's as low as 19 mmHg cause synovial capillaries to assume a more flattened elliptical profile [29]. During the course of these studies, we have confirmed the observation, reported by others, that if one adds "normal saline" to a healthy knee in order to simulate an effusion, for a short while (5 min) the volunteer can generate a raised IAP but fails to sustain it due to RMI. This would explain why patients with traumatic effusions of greater than one days duration do not generate raised pressures and suggests that RMI is a defense mechanism. It is not understood why this is overcome in patients with chronic inflammatory synovitis. However, as discussed below, oxidative injury damages sensory nerves and it is reasonable to speculate that receptors may be damaged in a similar fashion.

The rise in IAP and constriction of synovial blood flow is associated with a fall in the synovial O_2 tension. Measurement of synovial fluid pO_2 has been performed after 2 min isometric quadriceps contraction. The initial O_2 tension, measured after a period of rest, was approximately 60 mmHg; immediately after the short exercise programme, the pO_2 fell to 40 mmHg, rebounding to suprabasal levels after 5 min [30]. Short-term exercise clearly affects blood flow and reduces the pO_2 rapidly. Synovial metabolism is disturbed for other reasons and we now discuss how these may influence the inflammatory responses, both innate and acquired.

1.4 Synovial metabolism, hypoxia and immune function

The oxygen consumption of the rheumatoid synovial membrane per gram of excised tissue is approximately 20 times that of normal [31,32] and the activity of the glycolytic (Embden-Meyerhof) pathway is markedly increased in the rheumatoid compared to normal synovium. The raised metabolic rate of the rheumatoid synovium concomitantly raises the demand for ATP. The intracellular production of this molecule can be achieved by either the aerobic or anaerobic oxidation of glucose via the tricarboxylic acid (Kreb's) cycle or the glycolytic pathway, respectively. The oxygen-dependent Kreb's cycle is a much more efficient producer of ATP than the anaerobic system and is generally favoured in normoxic tissues. The fact that the rheumatoid synovium favours the anaerobic glycolytic pathway suggests its hypoxic nature. In support of this, synovial intimal cells in RA contain significantly more glyceraldehyde-3-phosphate and lactate dehydrogenase activity than those of normal tissue [33]. These are the major enzymes of the glycolytic pathway. This increase in their activity is most easily explained by a response to tissue hypoxia rather than by elevated metabolic activity, as mitochondrial oxidation is not similarly enhanced [34].

Synovial fluid oxygen tension is more easily quantifiable than synovial tissue ischaemia. The oxygen tension within the inflamed joint cavity is generally much lower than in traumatic effusions [35] and as demonstrated above will rise with rest and fall with exercise. Even the aggressive angiogenesis seen in RA does not improve oxygenation. The distribution of the new vasculature is not conducive to complete perfusion of the joint through to the joint space as demonstrated in Fig. 6 [20]. As expected, joints with the lowest pO_2 also exhibit the largest increases in pCO_2 and lactate: the same joints also show evidence of microvascular obliteration in the synovial membrane. The end-product of the anaerobic oxidation of glucose is lactate and the ratio of lactate to glucose should, therefore, give an indication of the oxygen status in the synovium. This is indeed the case: it has been shown that lowered glucose and raised lactate correlate well with falls in pH [36]. More recently, our own studies utilising proton nuclear magnetic resonance spectroscopy confirm the peculiar anaerobic environment in the inflamed joint. Comparison of paired samples of synovial fluid and sera shows that the concentration of lactate and the ketone bodies, 3-D-hydroxybutarate and acetoacetate, are all much higher in the synovial fluid than the serum and levels increase after exercise [37].

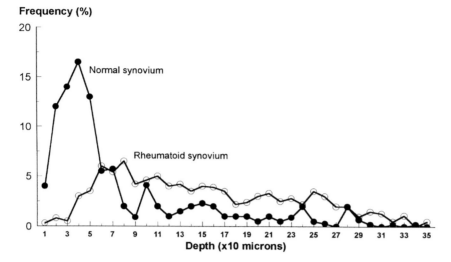

Fig. 6. Microvessel distribution at defined depths from the surface of rheumatoid and normal control synovium.

The hypoxic conditions prevailing in the inflamed joint lead to an increase in fatty acid oxidation. However, the unavailability of NAD^+ results in an inability of the citric acid cycle to oxidise fully acetylcoenzyme A. This process leads to a build up of unoxidisable metabolites — ketone bodies — recently demonstrated by NMR spectroscopy. Such products may have profound effects on immune function.

A major feature of RA is the laboratory demonstration of a significant immune response of undetermined specificity. As discussed, this usually includes production of polyclonal rheumatoid factors and the accumulation of plasmacytes and CD_4 T cells within the synovial membrane. However, cytokine production in the joint is more characteristic of activated macrophages and fibroblasts rather than of T cells, suggesting that T cells are rendered hyporesponsive after they arrive in the synovium.

Many workers have shown unresponsiveness in synovial T cells or inhibitory effects of synovial fluid on T cell activity [38]. Such samples also inhibit responses of synovial mononuclear cells to PHA as measured by production of IL-2. Several mechanisms appear to be involved, although products of polyamine oxidation which include hydrogen peroxide and aldehydes inhibit IL-2 production [39]. Aldehydes identified within rheumatoid synovial fluid include 4-hydroxy-trans-2-nonenal at a concentration of approximately 0.5 μM [40] — this has potent cytotoxic [41,42] and pro-inflammatory properties [43].

Normal immune responses involve an interaction between antigen presenting cells (APC) and CD_4 positive T cells. Ligation of the T cell receptor by peptide antigens bound to MHC class II molecules at the surface of the APC induces T cell activation, but can also result in specific nonresponsiveness, or anergy, if costimulatory signals provided by the APC are defective. At the chemical level, reversible covalent events take place during APC:T cell conjugation between reactive ligands on the APC and T cell surface. These take the form of transient carbonyl-amino condensation or Schiff base formation between constitutive carbonyl and amine functions which are expressed reciprocally on the APC and T cell [44,45]. The reactions probably depend on conventional interactions between adhesion molecules (such as LFA1:ICAM 1 and 2; CD_2:LFA3; B7:CD_{28}) bringing reactive ligands into sufficiently close proximity. Small molecules that participate in carbonyl-amino condensation reactions have marked effects on T cell activation in vitro; inhibition of T cell responses may occur depending on the species and concentration of Schiff-base forming aldehydes [46]. Because Schiff base formation is essential in specific T cell activation and is susceptible to modification by exogenous Schiff base forming compounds, it seems likely that low molecular weight species, generated by anaerobic metabolism and augmented by exercise cycles, explain T cell hyporesponsiveness in rheumatoid disease. As discussed, although T cells appear activated, for instance, 50% express HLA class II, cytokine production is aberrant. For instance, despite early reports using unsatisfactory assays, of raised IL-2 in synovial fluid, more recent studies suggest this is not the case. Brennan has shown that although IL-2 mRNA is present in synovial T cells, there is no detectable secreted protein [47]. IL-4 and IFNγ are two other cytokines produced almost exclusively by T lymphocytes and found in small quantities in the RA joint [13]. IL-4 inhibits the production by monocytes of pro-inflammatory cytokines such as IL-1, TNFγ and IL-6. The presence of only certain T cell cytokines may in part be explained by the existence of different subsets of T cells with different levels of activation in different disease processes, as discussed earlier. We hypothesise that the hypoxic-induced anergy of T cells caused by the production of low MW aldehydes leads to an abnormal control by T cells of macrophages with excessive production of pro-inflammatory cytokines. Rather than directing therapies to inhibiting such individual cytokines, we believe an alternative strategy would be to reverse the hypoxic and oxidative insult that appears to drive the system.

2   HYPOXIA, OXIDATIVE STRESS AND CELL SIGNALLING

A key feature of inflammatory diseases such as rheumatoid arthritis is the increased expression of certain genes which encode inflammatory cytokines and proteinases involved in tissue destruction, such as collagenases, gelatinases and stromelysins. In turn, an important characteristic of gene expression is the control of gene transcription by specific proteins, transcription factors, which bind to short DNA sequence elements located adjacent to the promoter or in enhancer regions of genes. Once bound to DNA, transcription factors interact with each other and with the proteins of the transcriptional apparatus itself (e.g., RNA polymerase) to regulate gene expression. Recently, there has been considerable interest in the idea that transcription factors may be useful targets for novel thera-peutic strategies in the treatment of human diseases, including inflammatory dis-eases [48].

The two transcription factors, activator protein-1 (AP-1) and nuclear factor kB (NFkB), can both be regulated by intracellular ROI [49,50]. They have been implicated in the transcriptional regulation of a wide range of genes involved in cellular inflammatory responses and tissue destruction. Inappropriate activation, such as the overexpression of pro-inflammatory genes, may be involved in the progression of inflammatory diseases, such as rheumatoid arthritis.

2.1 Activation of AP-1

AP-1 is a protein dimer composed of the proto-oncogene products, Fos and Jun. mRNA levels for c-fos and c-jun are strongly induced in response to hydrogen peroxide and other oxidative stresses such as ultraviolet light and ionising radia-tion, in both fibroblasts and T-cells [51]. In contrast, AP-1 binding activity is only weakly induced by hydrogen peroxide [52]. The AP-1 site, also referred to as the tetradeconyl phorbol acetate responsive element (TRE) is found in various genes, including those encoding human collagenase, stromelysin, transforming growth factors (TGFs) a and b, IL-2 and tissue inhibitor of metalloproteinases-1 (TIMP-1) [53].

AP-1 binding has been shown to be modulated by the reduction-oxidation of a single conserved cysteine residue in the DNA recognition site of the two sub-units. Since the reduced state of the conserved cysteines is critical for DNA bind-ing, it has been suggested [52] that redox modification of this domain, may con-tribute to the mechanism of transcriptional activity.

Furthermore, a nuclear protein has been identified that was able to reduce the Fos and Jun heterodimer thus, stimulating DNA binding in vitro [54]. This ubiquitous nuclear protein, known as redox-factor-1 (Ref-1), is a bifunctional protein which also possesses apurinic/apyrimidinic endonuclease DNA repair activity [55]. However, both the redox and DNA repair activities of Ref-1 can be distinguished biochemically, which suggests that a link may exist between tran-scription factor regulation, oxidative signaling and DNA repair processes.

Abate and colleagues [54] showed that the oxidation of Ref-1 significantly diminished its ability to stimulate the DNA binding activity of AP-1. However, upon the addition of thioredoxin, an enzyme that catalyses the reduction of cysteine residues, the stimulatory activity of Ref-1 was restored and AP-1 binding resumed. Thioredoxin alone was unable to enhance AP-1/DNA binding, suggest-ing that it increases the reducing efficiency of Ref-1, rather than acting directly on the Fos and Jun subunits of AP-1 [55].

The same group has now shown that both Ref-1 and AP-1 can be activated in the response of HT29 colon cancer cells to hypoxia [56]. Elevation of the Ref-1 gene steady state mRNA levels occurs as an early event following induction of hypoxia and persists when cells are restored to a normally oxygenated environment. This is supportive of the data recently published by Rupec and Baeuerle, who showed the activation of AP-1 in hypoxic conditions [57]. AP-1 activation during hypoxia appeared to rely on the activation of so called "primary transcription factors", such as the serum responsive factor (SRF), which is also activated by antioxidants [52]. These newly synthesised "primary transcription factors" are then able to up regulate c-fos and c-jun gene transcription and, therefore, AP-1 activation. Earlier we mentioned how c-fos and c-jun could be upregulated by oxidative stress [51], yet AP-1 binding to DNA is only weakly induced by hydrogen peroxide [52]. Thus, it appears that both antioxidant and pro-oxidant conditions increase the expression of the genes encoding the components of AP-1, but AP-1/DNA binding occurs preferentially during hypoxia. Meyer et al. [52] showed that the induction of c-fos and c-jun mRNAs by both hydrogen peroxide and the antioxidant PDTC, occurred with very similar kinetics, suggesting that antioxidant and oxidant conditions in the cell may funnel into the same pathway. On the other hand, AP-1 may exist in a latent form which is only fully activated when cells regain a "normoxic" or hypoxic state. Figure 7 illustrates the mechanisms involved in the upregulation of AP-1.

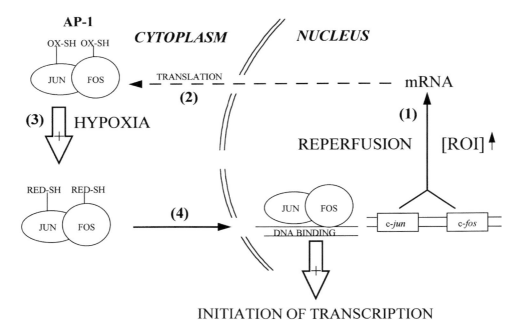

Fig. 7. The activation of AP-1. (1) Reperfusion increases levels of ROI which can upregulate the genes c-jun and c-fos. (2) The protein products of these genes Jun and Fos then combine to form the heterodimer AP-1. (3) Under hypoxic conditions AP-1 is activated by the reduction of critical sulphydryl groups. (4) The activated form of AP-1 can then bind DNA and initiate transcription.

2.2 Activation of NFκB

The target genes for NFκB comprise a growing list of genes intrinsically linked to a coordinated inflammatory response. These include genes encoding tumour necrosis factor (TNF-a), interleukin-1, interleukin-6, interleukin-8, the interleukin-2 receptor b chain, inducible nitric oxide synthase (iNOS), MHC class I antigens, E-selectin, vascular cell adhesion molecule-1, serum amyloid A precursor, c-Myc [49] and the H-chain of ferritin [59]. The DNA binding, nuclear form of NFkB is a protein heterodimer made up of one Rel-A (p65) subunit and one p50 subunit. In nonstimulated cells, NFkB exists in an inactive, cytosolic form bound to its inhibitor, IkB. Activators of NFkB (such as TNF-a, IL-1, phorbol esters, viruses, lipopolysaccharide, calcium ionophores, cycloheximide and ionising radiation) induce the dissociation of IkB from the NFkB-IkB complex and positively charged nuclear location sequences (NLS) in Rel-A and p50 are unmasked. NFkB is then translocated to the nucleus, where it controls gene expression. The events of NFkB activation are summarised in Fig. 8. The importance of ROI in the expression of the genes coding for these proteins was highlighted by Baeuerle and colleagues [60]. They showed that NFkB activity was induced by hydrogen peroxide in an human T cell line. This effect was blocked by the antioxidant N-acetylcysteine. Other more recently reported activators include oxidised LDL [61] and nitric oxide [62] although the latter effect is disputed [63].

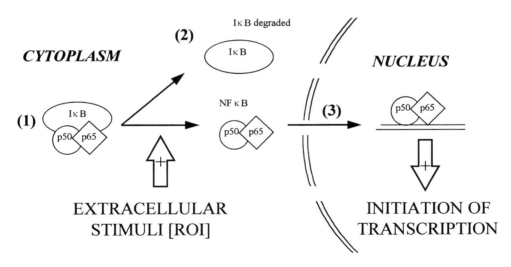

Fig. 8. The activation of NFκB. (1) Within the cell NFκB exists in an inactive form bound to its inhibitory subunit, IκB. (2) When the cell is challenged by extracellular stimuli (e.g., ROI) IκB is released and proteolytically degraded. (3) The release of IκB "unmasks" the nuclear location sequence of NFκB enabling it to move into the nucleus and initiate transcription.

IkB dissociation from NFkB involves its phosphorylation-controlled proteolytic degradation (64,65,66] whilst ROI appear to control this IkB phosphorylation. This explains why NFkB activation is blocked by a host of antioxidants. The precise mechanism by which ROI control the phosphorylation of IkB is unclear [64]. ROI might either activate an IkB kinase or suppress a phosphatase activity. Experiments using specific inhibitors of different protease classes indicated that the intracellular proteinase activity responsible for the degradation of the phosphorylated form of IkB was the 26S proteosome [49,64,66].

2.3 Hypoxia-inducible factor-1

Hypoxia-inducible factor-1 (HIF-1) is a heterodimeric basic helix-loop-helix DNA-binding protein tightly regulated by cellular oxygen tension. HIF-1 regulates hypoxia inducible genes such as erythropoietin (EPO), vascular endothelial growth factor (VEGF) and inducible nitric oxide synthase. Hypoxia response elements (HRE) from these genes contain a HIF-1 binding site, as well as additional DNA sequences [67].

Studies of solid tumour growth and angiogenesis suggest that HIF-1 activation occurs in hypoxic regions of tumours and this may have a significant influence on gene expression [68]. HIF-1 has also been implicated in the activation of VEGF gene transcription in hypoxic Hep3B cells [69]. These results suggest that the HIF-1/HRE system of gene regulation may provide a common pathway for hypoxic cells to respond to their environment and may in the future provide a target for therapeutic intervention. It may also play a key role in synovitis as both VEGF and EPO are elevated in RA, however, its exact role in the pathophysiology of RA is yet to be determined.

3   THE RHEUMATOID SYNOVIUM AND XANTHINE OXIDOREDUCTASE

Xanthine oxidoreductase (XOR) is a 300,000 MW homodimer [70], each monomer containing a molybdenum (Mo) atom, two nonhaem iron-sulphur (Fe/S) groups and one flavine adenine nucleotide (FAD) molecule, all of which have the capacity to accept and donate substrate-derived electrons [71,72]. XOR is best recognised for its role in the terminal oxidation of the purines hypoxanthine and xanthine to uric acid. Mammalian XOR exists in two forms, a dehydrogenase (XD) and an oxidase form (XO), both participate in the purine degradation pathway oxidising hypoxanthine to xanthine, and xanthine to uric acid. These reactions are illustrated in Fig. 9.

Both isoforms have the capacity to accept and donate substrate-derived electrons. However, the electron acceptor specificity is different for the two forms. In the XD catalysed reaction, NAD^+ is utilized as the sole electron acceptor whereas XO utilizes molecular oxygen and its univalent reduction leads to the formation of the superoxide radicals. XD is the predominant form of the enzyme

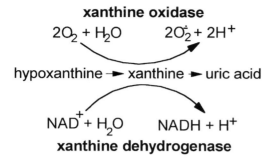

Fig. 9. Purine degradation by xanthine oxidase (XO) and dehydrogenase. XO is capable of generating superoxide in the process.

in vivo. It can be converted to XO through reversible sulphydryl oxidation or by irreversible proteolytic modification.

It is generally accepted that the Mo centre is the site at which xanthine and all other substrates (except NADH) donate electrons to the enzyme [73]. The oxidation of NADH by both XO and XD occurs at the FAD centre with the production of NAD. Studies on enzyme which has had the flavin removed suggests that it is the FAD that interacts with the oxygen in the course of reoxidation [74]. As the enzyme is capable of accepting six electrons (two at each site: Mo, FAD and Fe/S) the reduction and reoxidation of the enzyme involve its sequential reaction with either xanthine or oxygen, respectively. Electrons enter and leave the enzyme at physically separate locations indicating that electron transfer within the enzyme must be an integral part of catalysis. Electron transfer between the three redox centres of XOR is illustrated in Fig. 10.

3.1 Conversion of XD to XO

The enzyme may be converted from the D form to an O form by means of the oxidation of critical thiol groups, or a proteolytic cleavage, possibly near such a thiol group by a calcium ion-dependent protease [75]. The rise in intracellular Ca^{2+} induced by hypoxia, therefore, augments oxidative damage if oxygen returns to the system. This we have demonstrated takes place in an exercised joint, where multiple cycles of hypoxia and reperfusion are occurring in rapid succession; in a system sensitised to hypoxia due to a cellular infiltrate outstripping the vascular supply. Oxidative damage may also augment a calcium influx which then, by activating a calcium or calmodulin sensitive phospholipase A_2, will generate lysophospholipids and arachidonic acid and feed the generation of pro-inflammatory prostaglandin products, again contributing to the perpetuation of inflammation.

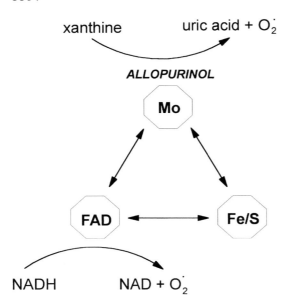

Fig. 10. The three redox centers of xanthine oxidase (XO). XO is capable of utilising xanthine and NADH as substrates to generate superoxide. Allopurinol inhibits the oxidation of xanthine by binding to the Mo center.

3.2 Localisation of XO

Given the potential importance of xanthine oxidoreductase in sustaining multiple pro-inflammatory cascades we sought its presence within the synovium by two techniques. Utilising a carbon 14 radioassay which detects the conversion of ^{14}C xanthine to ^{14}C uric acid, we found that normal synovium contained relatively small amounts of activity (up to 5.0 μU/g tissue), whilst in rheumatoid synovial tissue, levels were very scattered but generally higher (up to 305 μU/g tissue). The activity of both was independent of NAD^+ indicating that conversion to the O form is possible [76].

An antibody to bovine xanthine oxidase was subsequently used to localise the enzyme by immunohistochemistry. The antigen was found to be localised to capillary endothelium in all the specimens of both normal and rheumatoid synovium. In larger vessels, the endothelial staining was less intense [77]. This capillary endothelial location is in accordance with a previous sequence of immunohistochemical studies on a variety of human tissues including heart, gut and liver [78].

3.3 Measurement of XO in human plasma

Although the evidence for the presence of XO in the rheumatoid joint is substantial, attempts to demonstrate its presence in the plasma of RA patients have largely been unsuccessful. Several methods have previously been described to measure XO in biological tissues and fluids. The pterin-based fluorometric assay [79] and the uric acid radioimmunoassay [80] have probably been the most successful and widely used. However, these have failed to detect XO activity in human plasma. Kojima et al. [81] have previously published an assay to measure XO activity in human plasma using high performance liquid chromatography (HPLC) and electrochemical detection. Interestingly, they found no relationship between plasma XO levels and plasma uric acid levels in their results which, therefore, questions the validity of the uric acid-based assays in human plasma. Miesel and Zuber [82] reported a xanthine-based chemiluminescence (CL) assay for measuring XO activity in human plasma. They reported XO levels up to 50-fold higher in inflammatory conditions than in normal controls. However, the activity in their assay was not allopurinol inhibitable and correlation's with disease activity were not made. We were not able to reproduce these results in our own studies. Although some plasma samples do produce luminescence when xanthine and lucigenin are added if this is not allopurinol inhibitable then the activity is unlikely to be due to XO.

Recent studies by Harrison et al. [83] have changed the way we investigate XO. Their work demonstrated that human XO has a different substrate specificity to the much researched bovine enzyme. The human form is far more effective at generating superoxide from NADH than xanthine (up to 20-fold). This discovery largely explains the difficulties in measuring XO activity in humans. The clear evidence that hXO has far greater NADH oxidase activity than xanthine oxidase activity suggests that NADH should be the substrate used in assays which attempt to measure hXO activity. In our own study [84] we measured the plasma NADH oxidase activity in normal controls and in patients with RA using an NADH-based CL assay and correlated the results in the RA patients with their erythrocyte sedimentation rate (ESR) and C-reactive protein (CRP). The results demonstrated the presence of significantly increased NADH oxidase activity in RA plasma when compared to controls (Fig. 11). In the RA patients this activity sig-

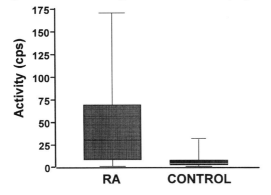

Fig. 11. Plasma from rheumatoid arthritis (RA) patients shows significantly ($p < 0.001$) higher levels of NADH oxidase activity (in counts per second, cps) than normal controls when measured by lucigenin-enhanced chemiluminescence.

nificantly correlated with biochemical markers of disease activity (ESR and CRP). We then used an immunoprecipitation technique to show that xanthine oxidase constitutes most of the NADH oxidase activity in RA. Figure 12 demonstrates the removal of activity from 3 RA patients using antihuman XO antibody coated Sepharose beads. The remainder of the observed activity may be due other circulating NADH oxidases.

These findings support the hypothesis that human XO shows a specificity for NADH as its superoxide generating substrate rather than xanthine. This activity is not allopurinol inhibitable as its inhibits XO by binding tightly to the Mo center of the enzyme. The redox reaction with xanthine occurs at this centre but the reaction with NADH occurs at the FAD centre and is, therefore, unaffected by allopurinol.

From these results the question arises; What is the purpose of circulating hXO which has NADH oxidase activity? We know that RA is characterised by a profound hypoxic metabolism and that tissue NADH levels rise under hypoxic conditions. These facts would lead us to hypothesise that a circulating NADH oxidase would serve a useful bactericidal function in acute traumatic ischaemic injury where it would locate its substrate. In RA its effect would be to potentate damage and specific hXO inhibitors acting at the FAD redox centre may have a therapeutic role in active RA in the future. This hypothesis can be further modified by the work of Freeman et al. [85]. They suggest that circulating intravascular XO found in hypercholesterolemic rabbits may bind to endothelial cell glycosaminoglycans thereby concentrating cell surface XO which in areas of high sub-

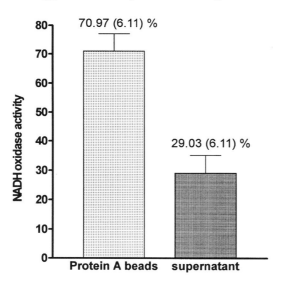

Fig. 12. Immunoprecipitation of NADH oxidase activity from plasma (from rheumatoid arthritis patients) using protein A beads coated with rabbit antihuman xanthine oxidase antibody. Approximately 70% of the total NADH oxidase activity is attributable to xanthine oxidase.

strate would generate superoxide and impair nitric oxide-dependent vasorelaxation. In RA the circulating XO could potentially bind to synovial membrane endothelial cells or the abundant glycosaminoglycans in articular cartilage thereby causing tissue damage directly.

3.4 XO and nitric oxide generation

Sergeev et al. [86] have shown that XO related to pH has the ability to convert nitrate (NO_3^-) to nitrite (NO_2^-). As described above human XO can generate superoxide from NADH but in ischaemic conditions NADH or xanthine can donate electrons which can reduce NO_3^- to NO_2^-· in our studies we have found that XO converts NO_3^- into NO_2^- using the Mo centre of the enzyme when oxygen is restricted [87]. This activity is detectable at physiological pH but is increases with decreasing pH. Activity is blockable by oxypurinol irrespective of electron donor.

XO also has NO_2^- reducing activity when exposed to a limited oxygen supply. This activity can utilise either xanthine or NADH as electron donors, and it appears that either the Mo or the FAD centre can receive the electrons which may be passed to NO_2^- at the Fe/S centre (Fig. 13). One product of this reaction is nitric oxide (NO) as detected by an isolated probe and an ozone chemiluminescence system [87,88]. These findings have potentially important consequences. In hypoxic conditions XO may convert dietary NO_3^- to NO_2^- and then go on to form NO. The effect of NO in inflammation and its possible interaction with ROI to form peroxynitrite suggests that XO may play an important role in diseases where hypoxic episodes are a factor.

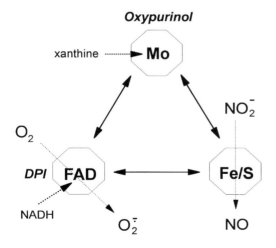

Fig. 13. Proposed mechanism for nitrite reductase activity of xanthine oxidase. Since this activity is not inhibitable by either oxypurinol or diphenyleneiodonium (DPI), we propose that it occurs at the Fe/S centre although the electrons required can be accepted at the other redox centres.

4 THE GENERATION OF REACTIVE OXYGEN SPECIES BY SYNOVIUM

It is possible to detect the generation of reactive oxygen species (ROS) in biological tissue in spite of their short half-lives, by adding nonradicals such as nitrones or nitroso compounds which act as spin traps, forming stable radical adducts with a characteristic electron spin resonance (ESR) spectrum. ESR spectroscopy is an unequivocal method of detecting free radicals and exploits the magnetic properties of the unpaired electron(s) in free radical species. In our studies we have utilised the spin-trap DBNBS: 3,5, dibromo-4-nitrosobenzenesulphate. The 3-line ESR spectrum of this species has been characterized [89]. Pulse radiolysis studies have shown that though DBNBS reacts rapidly with $O_2^{\bullet-}$, the product formed is very unstable. However, DBNBS can be used to detect oxidising species which are capable of forming the cation $DBNBS^+$ by one electron oxidation. This characteristic 3-line spectrum has been characterised in the horseradish peroxidase catalysed oxidation of DBNBS by hydrogen peroxide. Synovial membrane tissue from a patient with seropositive nodular RA was subjected to an episode of hypoxia (30 min under nitrogen) followed by normoxia (up to 40 min under 95% air and 5% carbon dioxide) in the presence of DBNBS. We observed an ESR signal characteristic of the stable adduct of DBNBS in the bathing medium of the synovium incubated in air/CO_2. Levels were increased if the synovium was subjected to an hypoxic/normoxic cycle. The inclusion of either the xanthine oxidase inhibitor allopurinol (2×10^{-6} mol/l) or the enzyme superoxide dismutase (SOD; 600 U/ml) in the bathing medium suppressed the production of the DBNBS adduct. These data are interpreted as confirming that reperfusion cycles result in the production of ROS by the rheumatoid synovium and that the "O" or ROS producing form of xanthine oxidase contributes to their production [48].

Given the endothelial cell location of xanthine oxidase, we now turn our attention to how such ROS may damage biomolecules and influence cells pertinent to joint pathology.

4.1 ROS-induced damage to proteins

4.1.1 Immunoglobulin G

As outlined above in the clinical description of rheumatoid synovitis, nodular RA — a feature of "typus robustus" arthritis — is invariably associated with an autoantibody directed against abnormal determinants on the heavy chain fragment of IgG. The most commonly measured rheumatoid factor is an IgG directed against IgM, although IgG directed against IgA and IgG are also described. Circulating immune complexes of rheumatoid factors and their antigens have been thought to be a contributing factor to the systemic vasculitis that may accompany RA. It has been assumed that the reactive epitopes arise from localised denaturation and/or chemical modification of amino acid side chains. In conjunction with Prof J. Lunec, we proposed that oxidative damage to IgG might be responsible for such changes.

When human IgG was exposed to ROS generating systems ex vivo, characteristic autofluorescent monomeric and polymeric IgG was formed [90]. The fluorescent complexes, when generated in vitro could stimulate the release of $O_2^{\bullet-}$ from neutrophils and in the presence of excess unaltered IgG further fluorescent damage to IgG occurred. Measurement and isolation of fluorescent monomeric and polymeric IgG by HPLC from fresh rheumatoid sera and synovial fluid indicated that identical complexes are present in vivo [90]. Oxidatively modified IgG acquired increased reactivity with both IgM and IgA rheumatoid factors in a modified ELISA assay [91]. In patients successfully treated for active RA with the "disease-modifying" drug D-penicillamine, IgG fluorescence fell in parallel with indices of inflammation such as the ESR and CRP [84], illustrated in Fig. 14.

When oxidatively modified IgG was added to an existing model of inflammation, it exacerbated the acute phase and prolonged the chronic phase [92]. In addition, the proportion of IgG, which on resolution showed the characteristic fluorescence, increased. This study clearly demonstrated how the presence of free radical altered IgG might convert an otherwise self-limiting inflammatory event into a persistent process if the stimulus to oxidative injury continued. We therefore asked the simple question — would exercise, with its capacity to induce a temporary ischaemic insult and thereby activate xanthine oxidase to generate ROS, increase the amount of pro-inflammatory IgG?

We examined 19 patients in all and they were randomly divided into an exercise and a control group. The exercise programme was similar to that utilised for

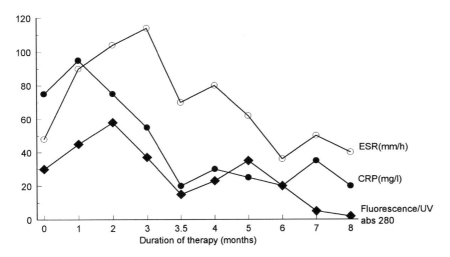

Fig. 14. The effect of long-term penicillamine therapy on the relationship between changes in ESR, CRP, fluorescent IgG antigen and IgM rheumatoid antibody in rheumatoid sera. Adapted from Lunec et al. [84].

pressure and synovial blood flow studies and synovial fluid was aspirated pre and post the exercise regime. Samples were batch assayed for both total and fluorescent IgG (*IgG) by gel permeation HPLC separation and subsequent quantitation with ultraviolet and fluorescence detectors. Fluorescence was expressed as a ratio of the UV absorbance to the IgG peak. The chromatogram contains a peak attributable to albumin and this is measured to control for any dilutional effects and cytochrome C included as an internal molecular mass standard. In the exercise group there was a significant rise in *IgG/UV IgG from baseline; the effect was greatest immediately after the exercise period. The albumin concentration was unaltered. Our results indicate that when a joint is exercised, proteins are oxidised [93]. The consequences of this are potentially profound, as illustrated from our studies of α-1-proteinase inhibitor.

4.1.2 α-1-antitrypsin

α-1-antitrypsin (AAT) is the major protease inhibitor of human serum, limiting tissue damage by the leukocyte protease, elastase — an enzyme implicated in the destruction of cartilage [94]. AAT forms a stable 1:1 complex with elastase, in which form the protease is inactive. Elastase has a very broad substrate specificity acting upon elastin, fibrinogen, proteoglycans, structural collagen, complement, and immununoglobulins. Congenital AAT deficiency is associated with pulmonary emphysema [95] and some groups have suggested that severe rheumatoid arthritis is also associated with an abnormal AAT phenotype [96,97].

Cigarette smoking is associated with pulmonary emphysema in normal individuals, as well as those deficient in AAT. In these patients, though absolute levels of AAT are normal, elastase inhibitory activity is depressed [98]. There is strong evidence to suggest that this is due to the oxidation of a critical reactive methionine residue (Met 358) to methionine sulphoxide [99]. Likewise, a large proportion of AAT is also inactivated in the rheumatoid joint cavity [100,101]. This has been found even when synovial fluid samples have been analyzed immediately after aspiration [102]. Again, methionine sulphoxide has been detected in AAT isolated from rheumatoid synovial fluid [103]. Because free elastase activity is not normally detectable in rheumatoid synovial fluid, it has been suggested that elastase is not important in joint destruction. This assumption neglects the effect of the microenvironment of the cartilage surface. In contrast to the "bulk phase" synovial fluid, cartilage interferes with the interaction between AAT and elastase [104], probably because of the relative inability of α-1-antitrypsin to diffuse into the cartilage by virtue of its charge and molecular weight.

Using free radicals produced in a Fenton system (H_2O_2/copper ions), Dean et al. [105] have shown that human neutrophil elastase is just as susceptible to inactivation as AAT. However, the oxidant species which is most likely to be important in inactivating AAT in vivo is hypochlorous acid, a product of the neutrophil myeloperoxidase-H_2O_2-Cl$^\bullet$ system [106]. Furthermore, the equal inactivation of elastase and its inhibitor was demonstrated using a high dose of H_2O_2 (5 mM)

– a possible differential effect at lower doses was not tested.

It has recently been suggested that a contribution to AAT inactivation might be made by a metalloproteinase with collagenase activity released from neutrophils [107,108], although the activation of the metalloproteinase is itself dependent on myeloperoxidase-catalyzed hypochlorous acid (HOCl) generation [94]. Additionally, the connective tissue metalloproteinases, endothelial cell collagenase and stromalysin are capable of catalyzing the proteolytic inactivation of AAT. These enzymes cleave at the exposed loop of AAT which contains the reactive centre. Fragments of AAT of molecular weight consistent with such cleavage have been identified by Western blotting in rheumatoid synovial fluids [109]. Although the precise role of oxygen radicals in the activation of these metalloproteinases in vivo is as yet unclear, the above observations suggest that hypoxia-reperfusion cycle driven production of oxygen radicals may have resulted in their local activation thereby having the indirect consequence of AAT inactivation by proteolysis.

To test this hypothesis, we recently studied the elastase inhibitory activity of sequential synovial fluid samples taken from patients over a 30 min period following standardized exercise of the sampled joints [102]. A significant decrease in the specific elastase-inhibition activity of synovial AAT was seen in the samples taken from exercised patients but not in those taken from resting controls. Western blotting of the samples showed that the inactivation of AAT was not accompanied by increased AAT cleavage. Exercise-induced AAT inactivation in the inflamed joint, therefore, is not due to proteolysis but rather to direct ROS-mediated oxidative damage.

4.2 ROS-induced damage to other biomolecules

4.2.1 Lipids

One site of ROS attack is the cell membrane. This is composed of polyunsaturated fatty acids and a ROS attack on the membrane results in the process of lipid peroxidation (rancidification). Polyunsaturated fatty acids have methylene-interrupted unconjugated double bonds. ROS attack at this point will abstract the "vulnerable" hydrogen atom causing rearrangement of the double bond and the formation of a conjugated diene radical species [110]. Diene conjugates can be measured by their characteristic ultraviolet (UV) absorbance at 233 nm. Further peroxidation will yield conjugated diene hydroperoxides and cytotoxic aldehydes which can be detected by their reaction with thiobarbituric acid (TBA) to form a chromophobe [111]. In vivo, lipid peroxides can be produced both enzymically (eg. by the arachidonic acid cascade) and nonenzymically by lipid peroxidation. Muus et al. [112] measured TBA reactivity (TBARS) in synovial fluids of RA patients and found correlation with clinical severity of the disease. However, they could not differentiate between TBA reactivity generated from prostaglandin metabolism and radical-induced peroxidation. At about the same time Lunec and Dormandy [113] developed a simple assay which simultaneously measured

Schiff base fluorescence and diene conjugation in chloroform-methanol extracts of synovial fluids from RA. These assays did not suffer from interference by prostaglandins, and products of lipid peroxidation were identified. Lunec et al. [114] reported that conjugated dienes were detectable in synovial fluid from patients with inflammatory and noninflammatory effusions but those with inflammatory effusions had higher levels. Sera from patients with RA had significantly higher levels of conjugated dienes than normal controls with the levels declining after treatment. These levels correlated with inflammatory disease activity. The serum TBARS probably originated from the liver. In addition, the amount of TBARS in the synovial fluid was found to correlate with bleomycin-detectable iron salts (iron that is capable of catalysing the formation of $OH\cdot$), indicating the important catalytic effect of iron on free radical reactions. The lipid peroxidation products measured in sera were always higher than in corresponding synovial fluids, strongly suggesting that some of the synovial fluid lipid peroxidation products originated from sera. However, the correlation between bleomycin-detectable iron salts supports the intra-articular generation of lipid peroxides.

4.2.2 Oxidation of lipoproteins and the role of vitamin E

As we know that lipid peroxidation is occurring within the rheumatoid synovium, we speculated that lipoprotein may be similarly oxidised. Low density lipoprotein (LDL) is, however, protected by the presence of several antioxidants of which the most important is α-tocopherol (Vitamin E) — there being about 7 molecules of vitamin E to each LDL particle. We therefore ascertained the α-tocopherol status of synovial fluid in comparison to paired serum and found them to be significantly lower [115]. Lower concentrations of cholesterol, triacylglycerol and LDL were also observed in patients' synovial fluid compared with serum. However, multiple regression analysis indicated that there remained a significant depletion of α-tocopherol which was largely independent of these covariables.

We then proceeded to assess whether oxidatively modified LDL was present in rheumatoid synovium [116]. A polyclonal antiserum raised in rabbits against o-LDL was used to perform an immunohistochemical study of rheumatoid patients. Collections of positively stained macrophages, arranged in a linear fashion and with the morphological characteristics of foam cells were identified around blood vessels within the intimal connective tissue. In addition, scattered, positively stained foam cells were present in association with deposits of fibrin. These staining patterns were absent from control synovial membranes. As o-LDL is a specific chemoattractant for circulating human monocytes and oxidation of LDL at or near endothelial cells results in monocyte binding [117], it is reasonable to propose that the oxidative modification of LDL sustains inflammatory synovitis.

4.2.3 Glycosaminoglycans

In rheumatoid arthritis and other inflammatory arthritides as discussed above, synovial hyaluronic acid is fragmented and depolymerized with a corresponding reduction in synovial fluid viscosity and an increase in the synovial concentration of dialysable hyaluronate saccharide fragments and saccharide monomers. As normal and inflammatory synovial fluids contain no measurable hyaluronidase activity, it has been suggested that oxygen-derived free radicals may be involved in this process. Broadly, the evidence for this derives from two approaches, viz: (a) the demonstration of potential free-radical generating systems within the joint and (b) the demonstration of hyaluronate degradation by such systems in vitro as evidenced by decreased viscometric parameters and apparent hyaluronate molecular weight measured by gel filtration and analytical ultrafiltration [118]. Phillips et al. [119] obtained evidence that the fragmentation of hyaluronic acid proceeds by the direct oxidative cleavage of the glycosidic bonds. McNeil et al. [120] found that the smallest degradation products of hyaluronic acid obtained by exposure to oxygen free radicals generated by several systems in vitro had molecular weights of around 10^4 and that re-exposure to the radical generating systems failed to degrade these products further. They interpreted their data to suggest that hyaluronate depolymerization by hydroxyl radicals may at least in part proceed by an ordered chain reaction with a rapid reduction from high to low molecular weight material.

Using high resolution proton Hahn spin-echo nuclear magnetic resonance spectroscopy, we have recently characterized several intermediates and end products of free-radical attack on hyaluronic acid in vitro and demonstrated their elevation in the synovial fluids and sera of rheumatoid patients over those of normal controls [121]. The results demonstrated an increase in a single resonance at 2.044 ppm after γ irradiation. This was attributed to the N-acetyl methyl protons of a mobile low molecular weight oligosaccharide derived from the OH$^\bullet$ radical-mediated fragmentation of hyaluronate rather than from damaged N-acetylated glycoproteins whose broader signals slightly downfield appeared unchanged. While this may represent the limit fragment seen in the McNeil experiments, we believe the line-width of this proton resonance indicates that it arises from a much smaller oligosaccharide with a molecular weight of the order of 10^3.

Subsequent SEFT-NMR analyses of a series of synovial fluid samples taken from patients with a variety of inflammatory joint diseases demonstrated this resonance peak in only a minority of cases. In this series, however, no account of the exercise status of the patients at the time of joint aspiration was taken. Serial joint aspirations from similar patients following the exercise protocol described above were then analyzed. These spectra revealed an increase in the postexercise 2.044 ppm resonances over pre-exercise baseline reaching its maximum value at 4 min and declining to pre-exercise baseline values by 8 min. We interpret these data to imply that, in the inflamed knee, hyaluronate-derived oligosaccharide fragments generated by hypoxia-reperfusion cycle-induced free radical oxidation are either rapidly cleared from the synovial fluid and/or are further degraded by nonradical mechanisms, such as phagocyte-derived terminal glycosidase activity, within the synovial fluid [122].

5   MICROBLEEDING, IRON AND SYNOVITIS

The generation of the hydroxyl radical, the most toxic of the potential reactive oxygen species, is dependent upon the presence of transition metals, particularly ferric and cupric ions. Firstly, the superoxide anion radical reduces iron to its ferrous state and then ferrous iron reacts with hydrogen peroxide to produce the hydroxyl radical (the Fenton Reaction):

$$Fe^{3+} + O_2^{\bullet-} \rightarrow O_2 + Fe^{2+}$$
$$Fe^{2+} + H_2O_2 \rightarrow OH^- + OH^{\bullet} + Fe^{3+}$$

The hydroxyl radical is highly unstable, reacting within one to five molecular diameters of its site of formation, with a rate constant almost diffusion controlled [123,124]. Because of the toxicity of the hydroxyl radical, iron is compartmentalised intracellularly, thereby limiting its formation. The protein apoferritin subserves this purpose. Extracellularly, iron is for the most part, bound to transferrin or lactoferrin and intravascularly in haemoglobin. These proteins not only protect against the toxicity of iron, but allow for the delivery of oxygen to tissues and the controlled release of iron for a multitude of critical enzymatic processes. How may this system break down and promote an inflammatory synovitis?

Iron microbleeding and joint inflammation were first associated by Hochstatter in his description in 1674 of the arthritis associated with excessive bleeding [125] — effectively a description of the synovitis associated with haemophilia. Haemophilic arthropathy is characterised by a florid and proliferative synovitis and associated with erosive bone damage and cartilage destruction [126]. Bleeding into an otherwise normal joint is clearly associated with damage. In patients with an abnormal joint, for instance, rheumatoid synovitis, iron also plays a role in perpetuating inflammatory damage. Intermittent intra-articular haemorrhage is a feature of inflammatory synovitis [127], and the iron released is taken up by synovial cells and stored intracellularly within the protein apoferritin as ferritin. In early rheumatoid synovitis, the amount of synovial membrane ferritin has been significantly associated with the activity of the disease at the time of biopsy. The amount of Perls' (ferric) iron is associated with the persistence of disease [128]. We have performed a very detailed ultrastructural study of a variety of synovitides, and found iron deposits occurring as siderosomes in the B (or fibroblast-like) cells of rheumatoid synovia, and postulated that the iron is probably initially incorporated into ferritin within macrophages which synthesise apoferritin where, as levels increase, it causes oxidative damage to the cells, liberating the iron which is then taken up by fibroblast-like cells in the more stable form of haemosiderin [129].

The cytokine-driven uptake of iron by the reticulo-endothelial (RE) system leads to "the anaemia of chronic disease". As the synovium functions as an extension of the RE system, iron can be redirected to it via this mechanism, as well as by traumatic microbleeding. The anaemia was previously thought worthy of correction and attempts were made to overcome the so called "RE block" in iron release by intravenously infusing iron dextran. A variety of groups found this to promote synovitis [130,131]. The clinical features are worthy of note: the synovitis is very common, and the sensitive technique of infrared thermographic imaging indicated that the majority of the patients had some degree of worsening of synovitis. Only previously inflamed joints were worsened and the worsening was maximal in joints that were mobile and exercised. Conversely, patients rested in bed for three days after the synovitis had significantly less problems than ambulant patients, whose exacerbations were most noticeable in the lower limb joints. The flare occurred 24 to 48 h after the infusion, when serum and synovial fluid transferrin became saturated with iron, leading to the production of iron not bound to protein and capable of causing oxidative injury [132]. Concomitant with the presence of such iron there was extensive evidence of oxidative damage to lipids and the concentration of oxidised ascorbic acid increased in both serum and synovial fluid, whilst red cell glutathione levels fell. Similar effects can be seen in animal models of inflammation. Intravenous (iv) iron dextran or intramuscular (im) iron sorbitol given to rats with adjuvant arthritis, at the onset of clinical joint symptoms, led to a significant flare in joint inflammation. This was associated with the presence of Perls' positive ferric iron in the synovial membrane and extensive bone erosion and focal osteoporosis [133]. Using a hydrogen peroxide initiated model of rat knee joint inflammation, where glucose oxidase was used to generate hydrogen peroxide in vivo [134,135] we have demonstrated that iv but not im iron dextran exacerbates this model of joint inflammation [136]. This, and the non pro-inflammatory effects of iv iron dextran on another joint inflammatory model where reactive oxygen species are not a predominant feature, led us to conclude that iron exacerbates joint inflammation by its interaction with reactive oxygen species, leading to extensive oxidative damage within the joint.

Oral iron has also induced a flare of rheumatoid synovitis [137]. This effect is not common, but again is predominantly associated with a flare in mobile joints that are already inflamed. Oral iron does not of course saturate the iron binding capacity and the mechanism of the reaction remains unclear.

Iron overload, as in idiopathic haemochromatosis [138], or in transfusional secondary haemochromatosis [139], clearly promotes synovitis. Is iron deficiency or removal of iron associated with less disease? This is, of course, not necessarily the other side of the same coin. There is no clear clinical evidence that iron deficiency is associated with less severe rheumatoid disease, though in animal models, nutritional iron deficiency of modest degrees will suppress joint inflammation found in adjuvant disease [140]. One striking observation was the apparent joint selectivity of the anti-inflammatory effects of iron deficiency on a widespread inflammatory condition. Other indices of adjuvant disease, such as increased levels of serum acute phase reactants, characteristic pathological changes in inguinal lymph nodes and granuloma formation at the site of the adjuvant injection, were not different from those of control animals. The moderate level of iron deficiency induced did not affect the acute inflammatory response to a range of irritants and was not sufficient to suppress immune function. Both the hypersensitivity reaction of oxazolone and lymphocyte incorporation of ^{3}H-thymidine were normal, the observation, therefore, supporting the view that iron had a selective and possibly "nonimmune influence on joint-mediated inflammation". Iron chelation with desferrioxamine also decreased the incidence and severity of joint inflammation associated with adjuvant disease in rats, but did not alter the local primary response or the systemic sequelae [141]. Within the joint, both soft tissue swelling and bone erosion were suppressed. Such effects of desferrioxamine on the inflammatory response are not, however, joint specific, similar doses suppressing the response in a wide variety of animal model systems [142–144].

We have attempted to suppress rheumatoid synovitis in man with iron chelation therapy using desferrioxamine. The approach cannot be recommended as desferrioxamine induced both cerebral and ocular toxicity [145]. In a pilot study, seven patients with rheumatoid disease were treated with desferrioxamine. Two of these patients who also received the anti-emetic prochlorperazine for nausea lost consciousness for 48 to 72 h, and then fully recovered. It is suggested that the nausea was induced by the effect of iron chelators on the iron-dependent enzyme ribonucleotide reductase in the gut. Electroencephalographic studies showed abnormalities associated with the metabolic disturbance. Analysis of cerebral spinal fluid showed a decrease in loosely bound catalytic iron, and an increase in loosely bound (catalytic) copper, total iron and products of lipid peroxidation, with values approaching normal as symptoms resolved. This patient showed pyramidal features and developed an optic neuropathy and pigmentary retinopathy subsequently. Two other patients, not receiving concomitant prochlorperazine, developed retinal problems which later improved. Our ongoing investigations suggest a mechanism dependent on the ability of desferrioxamine to mobilise copper, to which it has an appreciable affinity (10^{14} for Cu^{2+}, 10^{32} for Fe^{3+}) [146]. An animal-based model for studying desferrioxamine-induced retinopathy was established in the albino rat [147,148]. The model measured the electro-retinogram b wave amplitude. Ocular damage was exacerbated by increased levels of white light and oxygen. Studies in the model intriguingly showed that darkness, and in particular red light, protected the eye against desferrioxamine toxicity.

6   OXIDATIVE INDUCTION OF BONE RESORPTION

Rheumatoid arthritis is characterised by articular erosions of bone and as discussed are most marked in the "typus robustus" subset of rheumatoid patients. Erosions, a form of bone resorption along the surfaces of subchondral compact bone, are the most destructive radiographic feature of the disease. Erosions are usually preceded by synovial inflammatory swelling and focal osteopaenia: they start at the margins of the joint where the cartilage ends and the capsule inserts – an area that is very richly vascularised and innervated in health.

Various agents, including parathyroid hormone (PTH), 1,25-dihydroxyvitamin D_3, cytokines, prostaglandins and growth factors enhance bone resorption. These substances interact with "modulator" osteoblasts (cells which induce bone formation), not with "effector" osteoclasts – the cells responsible for bone resorption. In response to stimulation, osteoblasts induce osteoclastic bone resorption by secreting into the medium a soluble "osteoclast resorption stimulatory activity"; this is referred to by the acronym ORSA. Excessive osteoclastic activity causes bone destruction in a variety of diseases including osteoporosis, Paget's bone disease, tumour-induced osteolysis, as well as RA. However, it is not clear how many of these states are ORSA driven.

In a simple study design we have found that nanomolar concentrations of H_2O_2 produce a stimulation of osteoclastic bone resorption and enhance cell motility in the absence of a response to PTH and 1,25-dihydroxyvitamin D_3 and independent of a pH change [149]. More recently we have demonstrated that the osteoblast is capable of generating H_2O_2 and have preliminary data that the osteoblast contains the enzyme xanthine oxidase (T Sahinoglu; personal communication). This raises the possibility that xanthine oxidase inhibitors, such as allopurinol, (Wellcome) or amflutazole (Eli Lilly) may have a part to play in inhibiting bone resorption.

The most common of the bone resorptive states is of course osteoporosis, a condition that primarily affects postmenopausal women. Intriguingly, xanthine oxidase is under hormonal control and although levels are higher in males, activity appears to be significantly altered by changes in sex hormone levels [150]. To our knowledge, no attempt has been made to examine the influences of hormonal fluxes on the rate of conversion of the D form of xanthine oxidase to the radical-generating O form. Clearly a hormonal influence on xanthine oxidase activity may be relevant to the female propensity for RA, its remission during pregnancy and its worsening immediately postpartum and would warrant more detailed study.

6.1 Oxidative damage to nerves

Pain is probably the commonest symptom of the rheumatoid patient and a major therapeutic target of the pharmaceutical industry. It is unfortunately very difficult to describe and to quantify. Although a mobile rheumatoid joint is painful, particularly on initiation of movement, if a patient with RA is perfectly rested, with all joints supported and all surrounding muscles and ligaments are relaxed, their joints are no longer painful. This implies that the pain in rheumatoid disease does not come from the inflamed synovial membrane which should be uninfluenced by such a procedure. In order to ascertain why pain was absent in a completely rested synovium we reanalysed the distribution of nociceptive (pain responsive) nerves in the synovium utilising antisera directed to neural cytoskel-

etal proteins and neuroactive peptides [151]. The entire innervation of the synovium was assessed with the marker protein gene product 9.5 (PGP 9.5), a major
protein component of neuronal cytoplasm and the most sensitive marker of
innervation. Sensory fibres were identified using antisera to substance P (SP)
and calcitonin gene-related peptide (CGRP). SP and CGRP are considered to
be good markers of sensory nerves with CGRP being present in approximately
half of all primary sensory neurones. An antisera to the C-flanking peptide of
neuropeptide Y (NPY) was utilised to distinguish sympathetic nerves (where
excessive tone may contribute to synovial hypoxia).

In normal synovium, PGP 9.5 active nerves were numerous, in particular, the
vasculature was densely innervated. Free fibres were less numerous but present
in all synovia examined and in many cases extended to the intimal layer. Neuropeptide immunostaining was predominantly found in perivascular networks and
NPY staining exclusively located around blood vessels. In contrast to normal
synovium, rheumatoid synovium showed an absence of staining in superficial
synovium for PGP 9.5, substance P, CGRP and NPY. In deeper tissues staining
was present but weaker. The lack of staining for specific neuropeptides is most
easily explained by their release, but this would not explain the lack of staining
to PGP 9.5, which indicates that the nerves were destroyed. We speculated that
inflammatory responses damaged such nerves directly and have recently tested
this hypothesis in model systems.

To investigate how inflammation may initiate nerve depletion, three animal
model systems were established. The first involved the induction of a mild synovitis by latex spheres injected intra-articularly. This model induces a foreign body
type mild synovitis with the recruitment of macrophages and few, if any lymphocytes. In the second model, hydrogen peroxide-induced inflammation was created by the intra-articular injection of glucose oxidase. This model causes acute
tissue damage from the hydrogen peroxide which gives rise to a rapid polymorphonuclear leucocyte response. The third model was more chronic. Animals
were sensitised to an antigen — methylated bovine serum albumin in Freunds'
adjuvant — and subsequently challenged by injection into the joint of the antigen
alone. Nerve fibres were assessed as described above. In the synovitis induced
by latex spheres no nerve depletion was seen. In contrast, both in the antigen
and hydrogen peroxide-induced model of arthritis, nerve depletion was extensive:
both sensory and sympathetic nerve fibres were affected equally. The depletion
was seen only in areas with an inflammatory cell infiltrate, indicating that a
mixed lymphocyte and macrophage population of cells may be necessary for
this effect [152].

6.3 Understanding the typus robustus patient

As we have already discussed, "robustus" type RA is most commonly seen in men
and is said to represent "a special reaction to the disease of a strong body supported by a tough mind", but is in no other way a separate entity from RA — it

is part of the spectrum of the disease [153]. Understanding the far points of a spectrum disorder can clearly assist in understanding the process as a whole.

Pain thresholds in these patients are normal away from the joints, as in all RA patients, but "show a distinctive tendency to be raised at the finger joints" [4]. This implies a genuine decrease in sensory input. In addition, such patients have substantial numbers of rheumatoid nodules, high titres of rheumatoid factor and show marked destructive bone and cartilage changes in joints that have been heavily exercised. The process of hypoxic reperfusion injury will explain all these features. Continuing heavy exercise, will, as described, induce a sustained oxidative insult. The oxidative modification of synovial plasma cell produced IgG will account for the "autoimmune" generation of rheumatoid factors and the oxidative stimulation of osteoclasts the extensive bone destruction. The inactivation of α_1-antitrypsin will account for the increase in elastase and the destruction of cartilage, whilst the relatively anaesthetic nature of the joint is easiest explained by the oxidative destruction of fine nociceptor nerves.

The X-ray illustrated in Fig. 15 is of the hands of a jazz drummer who has long standing RA, compared with those of a patient with only moderate disease. Quite remarkably, the patient was able to maintain his profession and did not experience pain on joint movement. The extensive destruction of the small bones of the carpus and metacarpophalangeal joints is evident. Arrows indicate those joints relatively little used whilst drumming; these show less bony damage.

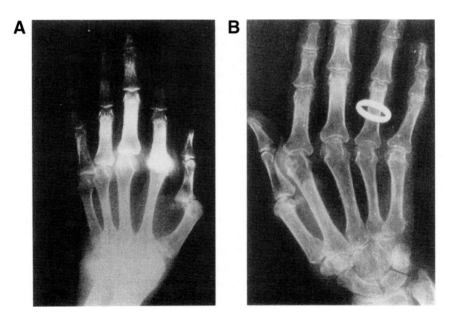

Fig. 15. Comparative radiographs of the hands of a patient with "typus robustus" arthritis (A) and a patient with moderate rheumatoid arthritis (B).

7 THE COMPLEX INFLUENCES OF REST AND EXERCISE ON THE CLINICAL OUTCOME OF RHEUMATOID SYNOVITIS

7.1 Rest

Rest in bed has been a traditional therapeutic maneuver since the time of Hippocrates in all branches of medicine. With the development of specific and directed therapies for most diseases its use has declined, but in rheumatological practice remains a major therapeutic strategy for treating rheumatoid synovitis. Does it work, how does it work and what are the dangers?

To deal first with the dangers: immobilisation of a limb may lead to ankylosis — fusion of the joint. A joint with synovitis that fuses will lose its inflammation, but at the cost of ceasing to be a functional joint. On occasion, isolated joint fusing (arthrodesis) is used clinically, but for the most part, joint ankylosis is to be avoided. Very few studies have specifically examined the mechanism of ankylosis despite its clinical importance. Michelsson and Hunneyball, in developing a model with some features of osteoarthritis [154], provided some intriguing insights.

One normal knee of each of 33 rabbits was immobilised by means of a plastic splint with the knee in extension, for up to 5 weeks. The splint was then removed and the animals allowed to move freely for up to 8 weeks. The animals were sacrificed at various times from 4 days after immobilisation through to the end of remobilisation at 13 weeks to examine the synovial reaction.

At the first assessment point, 4 days, the synovium contained a marked mononuclear cell infiltrate with synovial lining cell proliferation. The proliferation decreased towards the end of the remobilisation period but reappeared in a more severe form during remobilisation when severe macroscopic lesions of the cartilage and bone occurred. Bone changes were both erosive, a feature of RA, but osteophytes were also evident, a feature of osteoarthritis. Pannus tissue overlaid cartilage, proteoglycan was depleted and areas of cartilage adjacent to the pannus were acellular — as described above, these are features of rheumatoid synovitis. By day 11, synovial vascular changes were reported, with an increase in the vascularity which increased further on remobilisation.

Clearly, a marked synovial reaction occurs as a consequence of immobilising a normal joint and includes many of the pathological features we associate with rheumatoid disease. Such studies have not been performed in man, but it is reasonable to presume similar changes; we must conclude that a mobile joint inhibits the development of synovitis and that the synovium has a marked tendency to an inflammatory response. Given that an infiltrate occurs as a consequence of the expression of select adhesion molecules within the vasculature, we would speculate that the synovium has a propensity to express adhesion molecules most readily and that some event associated with movement inhibits this reaction.

Despite these unexpected "inflammatory" findings in the normal rabbit synovium, there is no evidence that inflammatory synovitis worsens as a consequence of immobilisation, indeed, all available data suggests the opposite — that immobility suppresses synovitis. We analyse the limited number of trials that have studied this question.

John Hunter (1835) was one of the first to make a clinical observation on the subject. He reported that "nothing can promote the contraction of a joint so much as motion before the disease is removed". In 1936, Kindersley reported that he had immobilised inflamed joints for two weeks and notes a reduction in joint inflammation [155] but few controlled studies of immobilisation by splinting have been performed.

In a study of 18 hospitalised rheumatoid patients with active synovitis of both knees, the latter were immobilised in casts for 4 weeks. On one side after day 4, the joint was passively mobilised briefly each day. Pain and swelling were suppressed on both sides and a full range of movement regained rapidly in the continuously immobilised knees [156]. Intermittent splinting of severely affected upper extremity joints and hands of seven patients with chronic synovitis was reported to result in sustained improvement in comparison with the nonsplinted side [157]. The authors reported an interesting incidental finding — "a well immobilised joint never flared, even when moderate flares were occurring in other joints of the body" and they concluded that "it is interesting to speculate that the local trauma of joint motion might predispose to local joint disease activity in rheumatoid arthritis". Such a finding is very similar to our observation that a splinted joint does not flare following intravenous iron dextran (vide supra).

A controlled trial of the effect of complete immobilisation of all four limbs was performed, compared with patients hospitalised and rested in bed with splints and daily mobilisation exercises. In this study of two well-rested groups, both groups improved in terms of disease activity, a composite assessment of synovitis assessed clinically and systemic disturbance determined by change in weight and two laboratory tests reflecting disease activity, the ESR and haemoglobin. However, there was no change in the amount of rheumatoid factor detected. The most active patients, with the highest ESR's showed the greatest propensity for improvement [5].

A subsequent study, however, comparing bed rest in hospital coupled with graded resisted exercises for up to 1 h a day, with similar exercises but much less bed rest, failed to show either the same degree of improvement to that reported in the "immobilisation" study or any difference between the groups [158]. A very similar result was found by Alexander et al. who studied 36 patients before and after 1 week's bed rest. The improvement that was seen was marginal and of little clinical relevance and a considerable number of patients actually worsened [159]. Generally, those that improved had the worst disease and those that worsened the least severe.

In conclusion, rigid immobilisation of a joint appears to lead to a fairly rapid resolution of synovitis and a clinically meaningful response that is reasonably well sustained. Hospitalised bed rest, however, whether movement is simply "allowed" or whether exercise is deliberately encouraged, has little effect.

7.2 Exercise

Exercise has varied effects on rheumatoid arthritis. Rheumatoid patients have demonstrated a very low level of physical performance ability when measured by aerobic capacity [160–162] and regular conditioning exercise improved aerobic capacity, speed of walking, depression, anxiety and physical activity after a 12-week programme [163] and this is to be anticipated. More surprising, in view of the disease suppressing effects of immobilisation, is that moderate exercise appears to have a similar effect. This we examine in more detail.

One of the most impressive studies performed examining the influence of physical training on the rheumatoid process was based at the Karolinska Hospital, Sweden [164,165]. The study was impressive not because patient numbers were large, but because the duration of the study was prolonged — up to 8 years. Twenty-three patients with RA were given physical training for 4–5 years. The training programme consisted of different types and intensities of exercise designed to be acceptable to the individual patient. All the patients predominantly exercised the lower limbs, starting training on a bicycle ergometer which was used at home. Group training exercise was performed under the direction of a physiotherapist for one h every two weeks and all patients were encouraged to train regularly for 30 min a day. Patients experiencing more symptoms post-training periods were taught to reduce the loading on the joint concerned. A control group, not randomly selected, was treated in a similar fashion except for the training programme. The results were encouraging over a 4-year period. The control group suffered more rapid progression of bone destruction than the trained group, required more time off work and spent more time as hospital inpatients. A pain index was reduced in the trained group although laboratory indices of inflammation (haemoglobin, ESR and rheumatoid factor titre) showed no such change.

A Danish study reported 6 years later gave somewhat different results. Using the minimisation method, 18 patients were allocated into two groups and entered into a controlled crossover study. Training was performed twice weekly with aerobic conditioning and strengthening exercises, progressing to strenuous exercise over an 8 week period. After training,, the patients, all of whom had moderately active synovitis at the commencement of the study, had significantly fewer swollen joints than before and the haemoglobin increased significantly after the training period although the ESR and the number of sore joints remained the same [166].

A further short-term exercise study has been reported from Michigan [167]. Twenty women with RA performed one of three low intensity aerobic exercise protocols with a nontraining group serving as controls. Exercises were performed in a group setting, consisting of bicycle ergometry exercises performed 3 times a week for 12 weeks. The three exercise protocols differed in the initial length of total exercise time, the rate of progression and the final total duration of activity achieved after 6 weeks (15, 25 and 35 min). Exercise intensity was measured by heart rate and was maintained in all groups at 70% of the maximal heart rate measured during the baseline exercise tolerance test. The load on the bicycle ergometer was applied at a resistance which achieved and maintained 70% of the maximal heart rate at 50 rpm. All exercised groups significantly improved their "joint count" (an assessment of both pain and swelling) and their aerobic capacity, whilst the control group showed no such improvement.

7.3 Speculation as to the mechanism of exercise-induced suppression of synovitis

Both gold and D-penicillamine are partially effective treatments of rheumatoid synovitis, working slowly over a period of months, in contrast to nonsteroidal anti-inflammatory drugs (NSAIDs) which show efficacy over hours or days. The precise mechanism of action of either drug is not known and it is clear that they affect multiple pathways. Nevertheless, Matsubara et al. reported that the antiproliferative effects of D-penicillamine on endothelial cells were Cu^{2+}-dependent and inhibited by catalase, implying that they are mediated by ROS derived from hydrogen peroxide [168]. We have observed that gold, also cytotoxic to endothelial cells results in a shift in the ratio of the xanthine dehydrogenase/oxidase system, favouring the production of ROS [169]. This led us to hypothesise that both drugs and exercise exert their effects via a common pathway — by impairing microvascular function they cause involution of the inflamed synovium, thereby achieving a polyarticular synovectomy.

To test this hypothesis we made use of the observation that von Willebrand factor (vWF), a 220 kDa glycoprotein produced by endothelial cells, was present in plasma and released by a calcium-dependent mechanism following a variety of stimuli including oxidant stress [170,171]. Several studies have shown increased levels of vWF in the presence of vasculitis, however, levels of vWF are not increased in uncomplicated rheumatoid synovitis. We hypothesised that vWF might be an in vivo marker of hypoxic reperfusion injury during joint exercise; to test this, 12 rheumatoid patients with active synovitis of the knee were admitted to hospital and rested supine for 45 min before plasma sampling. All patients and controls performed a standard exercise of walking for 15 min at their own pace. There were no differences between mean basal levels of vWF in patients and controls. Controls showed no significant change in levels of vWF after exercise; however, in patients with RA, levels of vWF increased significantly as illustrated in the figure, with approximately an 80% increase occurring in the rheumatoid group. The peak levels of vWF all occurred in the first 20 min after exercise, although in half the subjects, the peak level of vWF was immediately after exercise [148]. Clearly, exercising rheumatoid patients will drop the O_2 tension, and this appears to lead to a rise in intracellular calcium and the release of vWF. Repetitive strenuous exercise should amplify the process, and by further exacerbating synovial hypoxia lead to synovial involution — a polyarticular synovectomy.

8   SUMMARY

1. The synovial cavity has a negative pressure in health. When the joint is exercised, vascular patency is maintained, allowing for nutrition of the avascular cartilage.
2. In rheumatoid synovitis, the situation is altered:
   a. the cavity pressure is raised
   b. on exercise this pressure exceeds the capillary perfusion pressure.
3. This leads to the production of multiple episodes of "hypoxic-reperfusion injury" generating reactive oxygen species (ROS).
4. Circulating xanthine oxidase is increased in rheumatoid arthritis. It is potentially capable of generating both ROS and nitric oxide depending on its physiological environment.
5. ROS may be involved in the upregulation of the transcription factors AP-1 and NFκB.
6. ROS oxidise:
   a. IgG, inducing rheumatoid factor production
   b. α_1-antitrypsin, increasing both elastase and TNF activity, inducing cartilage destruction
   c. hyaluronan, leading to hyaluronan fragmentation products which may alter immune function
   d. lipids, generating aldehydes which are toxic and may alter T cell/macrophage interactions
   e. lipoproteins, leading to the production of monocyte chemotactic peptides.
7. ROS also:
   a. stimulate osteoclasts to destroy bone, creating bone erosions
   b. damage fine "pain" nerves, creating the clinical picture of "typus robustus" synovitis
8. Immobilisation suppresses synovitis by reversing such processes, although bed rest has a
   minimal effect.
9. Exercise may have a similar effect by killing the synovial lining — an auto-synovectomy.

9   PERSPECTIVES

An understanding of the complex influences of hypoxia and oxidative insult in synovitis may lead to a more rational and targeted therapeutic approach. However, the complex and iterating nature of the cascading systems suggest that no single antioxidant therapy will be of outright benefit. Polypharmacy, with multiple antioxidants is clearly a difficult therapeutic and commercial approach. Bio-reductive drugs that are cytotoxic to hypoxic tissues [172], may be a more rational and feasible way forward by creating a polyarticular synovectomy, not dissimilar to the proposed mechanism of exercise-induced suppression of synovitis.

10 REFERENCES

1. Spector TD. In: Hochberg MC (ed) Epidemiology of Rheumatic Diseases. Philadelphia: Saunders, 1990;513—537.
2. Wollheim FA. In: Maddison PJ, Isenberg DA, Woo P, Glass DN (eds) Oxford Textbook of Rheumatology vol 2. Oxford Medical Publications, 1993;639—661.
3. Owsianik WDJ. Ann Rheum Dis 1980;39:508—510.
4. De Haas WHD, De Boer W, Griffioen F, Oosten-Elst P. Ann Rheum Dis 1974;33:81—85.
5. Partridge REH, Duthie JJR. Ann Rheum Dis 1963;22:91—99.
6. Thompson M, Bywaters EGL. Ann Rheum Dis 1961;21:370—377.
7. Maddison PJ, Isenberg DA, Woo P, Glass DN (eds) Oxford Textbook of Rheumatology vol 1. Oxford Medical Publications, 1993;section 1.3.
8. Van der Lubbe, Dijkmans BAC, Markusse HM et al. Arthritis Rheum 1995;38:1097—1106.
9. Pasero G, Priolo F, Marubini E et al. Arthritis Rheum 1997;40:791—792.
10. Ornstein MH, Kerr LD, Spiera H. Arthritis Rheum 1995;38:1701—1706.
11. De Carli M, D'Elios MM, Zancuoghi G et al. Autoimmunity 1994;18:301—308.
12. Van Roon JA, van Roy JL, Duits A et al. Ann Rheum Dis 1995;54:836—840.
13. Dolhain RJ, van der Heiden AN, ter Haar NT et al. Arthritis Rheum 1996;39:1961—1969.
14. Firestein GS. Mech Therap 1995;47:37—51.
15. Levick JR Blood flow and mass transport in synovial joints. In: Renkin EM, Michel CC (eds) Handbook of Physiology II, Cardiovascular IV, The Microcirculation. American Physiology Society, Bethesda 1984.
16. Reeves B. Nature 1966;212:1046.
17. Levick JR. J Physiol 1979;289:69—82.
18. Stevens CR, Revell PA, Blake DR, Levick JR. Br J Rheumatol 1989;28(suppl 2):62.
19. Wilkinson LS, Edwards JCW. J Anat 1989;167:129—136.
20. Stevens CR, Williams RB, Farrell AJ, Blake DR. Ann Rheum Dis 1991;50:124—132.
21. Henderson EB, Grootveld M, Farrell A, Blake DR et al. Ann Rheum Dis 1991;50:196—200.
22. Knudson CB, Knudson W. FASEB J 1993;7:1233—1241.
23. Ranke HR. Zent Bl Chir 1875;39:609—613.
24. Jason MIV, Dixon A St J. Ann Rheum Dis 1970;29:261—265.
25. Merry P, Williams R, Cox N, Blake DR et al. Ann Rheum Dis 1991;50:917—920.
26. Jawed S, Gaffney K, Blake DR. Ann Rheum Dis 1997;56:686—689.
27. Gaffney K, Williams RB, Jolliffe VA, Blake DR. Ann Rheum Dis 1995;54:611—612.
28. James MJ, Cleland LG, Rofe AM, Leslie AL. J Rheum 1990; 17: 521—527.
29. Levick JR. J Rheumatol 1990;17:579—582.
30. Unsworth J, Outhwaite J, Blake DR et al. Ann Clin Biochem 1988;25:8—11.
31. Page-Thomas DP, Dingle JTM. Br J Exp Pathol 1955;36:195.
32. Dingle JTM, Page-Thomas DP. Br J Exp Pathol 1956;37:318—336.
33. Henderson B, Bitensky L, Chayen J. Ann Rheum Dis 1979;38:63—67.
34. Henderson B, Bitensky L, Chayen J. Ann Rheum Dis 1978;37:548—551.
35. Lund-Olsen K. Arthritis Rheum 1970;3:766—769.
36. Falchuk KH, Goetzel EJ, Kulka JP. Am J Med 1970;49:222—231.
37. Naughton D, Whelan M, Blake DR, Grootveld M. FEBS Lett 1993;317:135—138.
38. Millenburg AM, van Laar JM, de Kuiper P et al. Clin Exp Immunol;82:499—503.
39. Hovdenen J, Hovdenen AB, Egeland T et al. Scand J Rheumatol 1990;19:398—406.
40. Selley ML, Bourne DJ, Bartlett MR et al. Ann Rheum Dis 1992;51:481—484.
41. Hauptlorenz S, Esterbauer H, Moll W et al. Biochem Pharmacol 1985;34:3803—3809.
42. Kaneko T, Kaji K, Matsuo M. Chem-Biol Interact 1988;67:295—304.
43. Benedetti A, Ferrali M, Casini AF et al. Biochem Pharmacol 1980;29:121—124.
44. Rhodes J. J Immunol 1989;143:1482—1489.
45. Gao XM, Rhodes J. J Immunol 1990;144:2883—2890.

46. Rhodes J, Zheng B, Lifely MR. Immunology 1992;75:623—631.
47. Brennan FM, Field M, Chu CQ et al. Br J Rheumatol 1991;30:76—80.
48. McKay IA, Winyard PG, Leigh IM, Bustin SA. Br J Dermatol 1994;131:591—597.
49. Baeuerle PA, Henkel T. Annu Rev Immunol 1994;12:141—179.
50. Blake DR, Winyard PG, Marok R. NY Acad Sci 1994;723:308—317.
51. Amstad PA, Krupitza G, Cerutti PA. Cancer Res 1992;52:3952—3960.
52. Meyer MR, Schreck R, Baeuerle PA. EMBO J 1993;12:2005—2015.
53. Karin M. In: Cohen P and Foulkes JG (eds) Molecular Aspects of Cellular Regulation, vol 6. The Hormonal Control of Gene Transcription. Amsterdam: Elsevier, 1991;235—253.
54. Abate C, Patel L, Rauscher FJ, Curran T. Science 1990;249:1157—1161.
55. Xanthoudakis S, Miao G, Wang F, Yu ching E, Pan, Curran T. EMBO J 1992;11:3323—3335.
56. Yao KS, Xanthoudakis S, Curran T, O'Dwyer PJ. Molec Cell Biol 1994;14:5997—6003.
57. Rupec RA, Baeuerle PA. Eur J Biochem 1995;234:632—640.
58. Hayashi T, Ueno Y, Okamato T. J Biol Chem 1993;268:11380—11388.
59. Kwak EL, Larochelles DA, Beaumont C et al. J Biol Chem 1995;270:15285—15293.
60. Schreck R, Rieber P, Baeuerle PA. EMBO J 1991;10:2247—2258.
61. Liao F, Andalibi A, deBeer FC et al. J Clin Invest 1993;91:2572—2579.
62. Lander HM, Sehajpal P, Levine DM, Novogrodsky A. J Immunol 1993;150:1509—1516.
63. Schreck R, Albermann K, Baeuerle PA. Free Radic Res Commun 1992;17:221—237.
64. Tasinato A, Boscoboinik D, Bartoli GM et al. Proc Natl Acad Sci USA 1995;92:12190—12194.
65. Drury PL, Rudge SR, Perrett D. Br J Rheumatol 1984;23:100—106.
66. Traenckner EB-M, Wilk S, Baeuerle PA. EMBO J 1994;13:5433—5441.
67. Semenza GL, Agani F, Booth G et al. Kidney Int 1997;51:553—555.
68. Maxwell PH, Dachs GU, Gleadle JM et al. Proc Natl Acad Sci USA 1997;94:8104—8109.
69. Forsythe JA, Jiang BH, Iver NV et al. Molec Cell Biol 1996;16:4604—4613.
70. Waud WR, Brady FO, Wiley RD, Rajagopalan KV. Arch Biochem Biophys 1975;169:695—701.
71. Komai H, Massey V, Palmer G. J Biol Chem 1969;244:1692—700.
72. Rajagopalan KV, Johnson JL. J Biol Chem 1992;267(15):10199—10202.
73. Bray RC. The enzymes, vol 12, 3rd edn. NY Academic Press, 1975;229—419.
74. Della Corte E, Stirpe F. Biochem J 1972;126:739—745.
75. Allen RE, Outhwaite JM, Morris CJ, Blake DR. Ann Rheum Dis 1987;46:843—845.
76. Stevens CR, Benboubetra M, Harrison R, Blake DR et al. Ann Rheum Dis 1991;50:760—762.
77. Jarach E-D, Bruder G, Heid HW. Acta Physiol Scand 1986;548:39—46.
78. Beckmann JS, Parks DA, Pearson JD et al. Free Radic Biol Med 1989;6:607—615.
79. Decker DE, Levinson DE. Arthritis Rheum 1982;25:326—332.
80. Kojima T, Nishina T, Yamanaka H. Rinsho Byori 1992;40:1096—1100.
81. Miesel R, Zuber M. Inflammation 1993;17:551—561.
82. Sanders SA, Eisenthal R, Harrison R. Eur J Biochem 1997;245:541—548.
83. Jawed S, Stevens CR, Harrison R, Blake DR. Biochem Soc Tranc 1997;25:531S.
84. Sergeev NS, Ananiadi LI, L'vov NP, Kretovich WL. J Appl Biochem 1985;7:86—92.
85. White CR, Darley-Usmar V, Berrington WR. Proct Natl Acad Sci USA 1996;93:8745—8749.
86. Millar TM, Stevens CR, Blake DR. Biochem Soc Tranc 1997;25:528S.
87. Zhang Z, Naughton DP, Blake DR et al. Biochem Soc Tranc 1997;25:524S.
88. Nazhat NB, Yang G, Allen RE, Blake DR et al. Biochem Biophys Res Commun 1990;166(2): 807—812.
89. Lunec J, Blake DR, Brailsford S, Bacon PA. J Clin Invest 1985;76:2084—2090.
90. Lunec J, Wakefield A, Brailsford S, Blake DR. In: Rice-Evans C (ed) Free radicals, cell damage and disease. London: Richelieu Press, 1986;241—263.
91. Hewitt SD, Lunec J, Morris CJ, Blake DR. Ann Rheum Dis 1987;46:866—874.
92. Blake DR, Merry P, Unsworth J et al. Lancet 1989;i:289—293.
93. Carrell RW and Travis J. Trends Biochem Sci 1985;10:20—24.
94. Carrell RJ. Clin Invest 1986;78:1427—1431.

95. Cox DW and Huber O. Clin Genetics 1988;17:153—160.
96. Sanders PA, Thomson W, Browne DA et al. Ann Rheum Dis 1986;45:450—453.
97. Carrell R. Nature 1984;312:14.
98. Carp H, Miller F, Hoidal JR, Janoff A. Proc Natl Acad Sci USA 1982;79:2041—2045.
99. Schtacher G, Maayan R, Feinstein G. Biochem Biophys Acta 1973;303:138—147.
100. Lewis DA, Parrott DP, Bird J et al. IRSC Med Sci 1984;12:304—305.
101. Chidwick K, Winyard P G, Zhang Z, Blake DR et al. Ann Rheum Dis 1991;50:915—916.
102. Wong PS, Travis J. Biochem Biophys Res Commun 1980;96:1449—1454.
103. Burkhardt H, Kasten M, Rauls S, Rehkopf E. Rheumatol Int 1987;7:133—138.
104. Dean RT, Nick HP, Schnebli HP. Biochem Biophys Res Commun 1989;159:821—827.
105. Weiss SJ, Regiani S. J Clin Invest 1984;73:1297—1303.
106. Desrochers PE, Weiss SJ. J Clin Invest 1988;81:1646—1650.
107. Vissers MCM, George PM, Bathurst IC et al. J Clin Invest 1988;82:706—711.
108. Zhang Z, Winyard PG, Chidwick K, Blake DR et al. Biochem Soc Tranc 1990;18:898—899.
109. Aust SD, Svingen BA. In Pryor WA (ed) Free radicals in biology, vol 5. NY Academic Press, 1982;1—28.
110. Satoh K. Clin Chim Acta 1978;90:37—43.
111. Muus P, Bonta IL, den Oudsten SA. Prostaglandins Med 1979;2:63—65.
112. Lunec J, Dormandy TL. Clin Sci (Colch) 1979;56:53—59.
113. Lunec J, Halloran SP, White AG, Dormandy TL. J Rheumatol 1981;8:233—245.
114. Fairburn K, Grootveld M, Ward RJ, Blake DR et al. Clin Sci 1992;83:657—664.
115. Winyard PG, Tatzber F, Esterbauer H, Blake DR et al. Ann Rheum Dis 1993;52:677—680.
116. Brown MS, Goldstein JL. Ann Rev Biochem 1983;52:223—261.
117. Greenwald RA, Moy WW. Arthritis Rheum 1980;23:255—463.
118. Phillips GO, Filby WG, Moore JS, Davies JV. Carbohydr Res 1971;16:79—111.
119. McNeil JD, Weibkin OW, Betts W, Cleland LG. Ann Rheum Dis 1985;44:780—789.
120. Grootveld MC, Henderson EB, Farrell A, Blake DR et al. Biochem J 1991;273:459—467.
121. Grootveld MC, Henderson EB, Farrell A, Blake DR. Br J Rheumatol 1990;29(Suppl 1):97.
122. Lunec J, Blake DR. In: Ching Quang Chow (ed) Critical reviews in chemistry. Cellular antioxidant defense mechanisms, vol 3. 1988;143—159.
123. Lunec J, Blake DR. In: Cohen RD, Alberti KGMM, Lewis B, Denman AM (eds) The metabolic and molecular basis of acquired disease. Bailliere Tindall Ltd, 1990.
124. Bullock W, Fildes P. In: A treasury of human inheritance, vol 1. London: Dulau and co., 1912;Section XIVa:169—354.
125. Morris CJ, Wainwright AC, Steven MM, Blake DR. Virchows Arch B Pathol Anat 1984;404:75—85.
126. Bennet RM, Williams ED, Lewis SM, Holt PJL. Arthritis Rheum 1973;16:298—304.
127. Blake DR, Gallagher P, Potter A et al. Arthritis Rheum 1984;27:495—501.
128. Withdrawn.
129. Morris CJ, Blake DR, Wainwright AC, Steven MM. Ann Rheum Dis 1986;45:21—26.
130. Blake DR, Lunec J, Ahern M et al. Ann Rheum Dis 1985;44:183—188.
131. Winyard PG, Blake DR, Chirico S et al. Lancet 1987;1:69—72.
132. Rowley D, Gutteridge JMC, Blake DR, Halliwell B. Clin Sci 1984;66:691—695.
133. Dabbagh AJ, Blake DR, Morris CJ. Ann Rheum Dis 1992;51:516—521.
134. Dabbagh AJ, Morris CJ, Sahinoglu T, Blake DR. Eur J Exp Path(In press).
135. Dabbagh AJ, Trenam CW, Morris CJ, Blake DR. Ann Rheum Dis 1992;52:67—73.
136. Blake DR, Bacon PA. Lancet 1982;1:623.
137. Schumacher HR. Arthritis Rheum 1964;7:41—50.
138. Sella EJ, Goodman AH. J Bone Joint Surg 1973;55(A):1077—1081.
139. Andrews FJ, Morris CJ, Blake DR. Ann Rheum Dis 1987;46:859—865.
140. Andrews FJ, Morris CJ, Kondratowicz G, Blake DR. Ann Rheum Dis 1987;46:327—333.
141. Blake DR, Hall N, Bacon P et al. Ann Rheum Dis 1983;42:89—93.

142. Yoshino S, Blake DR, Bacon PA. J Pharmacy Pharmacol 1984;36:543—545.

143. Sedgewick AD, Blake DR, Winwood P et al. Eur J Rheumatol Inflam 1984;7:87—94.

144. Blake DR, Winyard PG, Lunec J, Hider R et al. Q J Med 1985;56:344—355.

145. Pall HS, Brailsford S, Williams AC, Lunec J, Blake DR. J Neurol Neurosurg Psychiat 1990;53: 803.

146. Good PA, Blake DR, Claxson A, Morris CJ. In: Rice-Evans C (ed) Free radicals, disease states and antiradical interventions. Richelieu Press, 1989;167—182.

147. Good PA, Claxson A, Morris CJ, Blake DR. Ophthalmologica 1990;201:32—36.

148. Bax BE, Towhidul Alam ASM, Blake DR, Zaidi M et al. Biochem Biophys Res Commun 1992; 183:1153—1158.

149. Stevens CR, Abbot SE, Harley SL, Blake DR et al. J Bone Min Res 1993;8(1):S124.

150. Mapp PI, Kidd BL, Blake DR, Polak JM et al. Neuroscience 1990;37:143—153.

151. Mapp PI, Walsh DA, Garrett NE, Blake DR et al. Ann Rheum Dis(In press).

152. Dequeker J. Ann Rheum Dis 1992;51:561—562.

153. Michelsson JE, Hunneyball IM. Scand J Rheumatol 1984;13:273—281.

154. Kindersley CE. Proc R Soc Med 1936;29:237.

155. Harris R, Copp EP. Ann Rheum Dis 1962;21:353—359.

156. Gault SJ, Spyker RPT. Arthritis Rheum 1969;12:34—44.

157. Mills JA, Pinals RS, Ropes MW et al. N Engl J Med 1971;284:453—458.

158. Alexander GJM, Hortas C, Bacon PA. Br J Rheum 1983;22:134—140.

159. Beals C, Lampman R, Figley B et al. Clin Res 1980;28:752A.

160. Beals C, Lampman R, Figley B et al. Clin Res 1981;29:780A.

161. Ekblom B, Lovgren O, Alderin M et al. Scand J Rheumatol 1975;4:80—86.

162. Minor MA, Hewett JE, Webel RR et al. Arthritis Rheum 1989;32:1396—1405.

163. Nordemar R, Ekblom B, Zachrisson L, Lundqvist K. Scand J Rheumatol 1981;10:17—23.

164. Nordemar R. Scand J Rheumatol 1981;10:25—30.

165. Lyngberg K, Danneskiold-Samsøe B, Halskov O. Clin Exp Rheumatol 1988;6:253—260.

166. Harkcom TM, Lampman RM, Figley Banwell B, Castor CW. Arthritis Rheum 1985;28:32—39.

167. Matsubara T, Saura R, Hirohata K, Ziff M. J Clin Invest 1989;83:158—167.

168. Sahinoglu T, Grootveld M, Stevens CR, Blake DR et al. Agents Actions 1991;325:71—75.

169. Hamilton KK, Sims PJ. J Clin Invest 1987;79:600—608.

170. Patel KD, Zimmerman GA, Prescott SM et al. J Cell Biol 1991;112:749—759.

171. Farrell AJ, Williams RB, Stevens CR, Blake DR et al. Ann Rheum Dis 1992;51:1117—1122.

172. Adams GE, Stratford IJ. In: Peckham MJ (ed) Oxford Textbook of Oncology. Oxford University Press, 1993;785—795.

Index of authors

Aiken, J.M. 831
Alessio, H.M. 115
Ames, B.N. 755
Aratri, E. 403
Arthur, J.R. 977
Asensi, M. 1137
Asmus, K-D. 3
Azzi, A. 403

Beard, J. 129
Beckman, K.B. 755
Blake, D.R. 1147
Blumberg, J.B. 177
Bonifai, M. 3
Boscoboinik, D. 403

Cannon, J.G. 177
Cantelli-Forti, G. 1021
Chance, B. 485
Chung, S.S. 831
Clarkson, P.M. 323

Darley-Usmar, V. 69
Das, D.K. 655
Decker, E.A. 323
Dekhuijzen, P.N.R. 1137
Duthie, G.G. 977
Duthie, S.J. 977

Edmonds, S.E. 1147

Ferrero, J.A. 1137
Fujii, J. 243

Gerber, M. 927
Gilston, V.D.R. 1147
Gimeno, A. 1137
Goldfarb, A.H. 297

Hamaoka, T. 485
Han, D. 433
Hartmann, A. 195
Hellsten, Y. 153

Heunks, L. 1137
Husain, K. 713

Jackson, M.J. 57
Jawed, S. 1147
Jenkins, R.R. 129
Ji, L.L. 689
Jo, H. 69

Katsumura, T. 485
Kizaki, T. 243
Kondo, H. 631

Laaksonen, D.E. 1105
Leeuwenburgh, C. 881
Lieber, C.S. 951
Lopez, M.E. 831
Loukianoff, S. 433

Maguire, J.J. 995
Maulik, N. 655
McCarter, R.J.M. 797
McCully, K.K. 485
McLaughlin, L. 433
Meacher, D.M. 513
Menzel, D.B. 513
Moellering, D. 69

Niess, A.M. 195

Oh-ishi, S. 243
Ohno, H. 243
Ookawara, T. 243
Özer, N.K. 403

Pallardó, F.V. 1137
Paolini, M. 1021
Parthasarathy, S. 1053
Patel, R.P. 69
Pollack, M. 881
Powers, S.K. 221
Price, L. 1053

Radák, Z. 243
Reid, M.B. 599
Reznick, A.Z. 89
Ricciarelli, R. 403

Santanam, N. 1053
Sastre, J. 1137
Sen, C.K. 221, 297, 375, 1105
Servera, E. 1137
Shearman, C.P. 1069
Shelton, J.E. 69
Shern-Brewer, R. 1053
Shimomitsu, T. 485
Simon-Schnass, I.M. 555
Somani, S.M. 713
Suzuki, K. 243

Taniguchi, N. 243
Tirosh, O. 89
Tisi, P.V. 1069
Traber, M.G. 359

Viña, J. 1137

Weber, S. 579
Weindruch, R. 831
Wetzstein, C. 1053
White, C.R. 69
White-Welkley, J.E. 1053

Zainal, T.A. 831

Subject index

abstraction reaction, 24
acetaldehyde, 951, 958–960
  toxicity, **958**
acetylcholinesterase, 723, 725
acetylcysteine, 44, 303, **313**, 380, 390, 392,
  393, 414, 561, 609, 611, 784, 906
acid, 33
aconitase, **442**, 763, 773, 787, 901
acrolein, 111
actin, 410, 607
action potential, 607
activation energy, 9
activator protein-1, 278, 383, **385**, 413, 414,
  1159
acute
  exercise, **247**–249, 261, 266, 268, 722, 727
  heart infarction *see* heart infarction
  kidney failure, 147
  leukemia, **286**
  phase protein, 1098
  phase response, **177**–190
adaptation, **79**
addition reaction, 33, 34
adenine nucleotide, **156**
adenosine, 348, 745
  agonist, 745
  antagonist, 745
adenosine-5′-diphosphate, 156, 157, 490
adenosine-5′-monophosphate, 156–159
adenosine-5′-triphosphate, 77, 156, 488, 490,
  503, 504, 841, 1073
s-adenosylmethionine, 959
adhesion molecule, 1158
adiposity *see* obesity
ADP *see* adenosine-5′-diphosphate
Adriamycin *see* doxorubicin
adult respiratory distress syndrome, **287**
advanced glycation end product, 771, 772,
  1107
aerobic
  exercise, 60, 61, 118, **119**, 812, **1053**–1068
  metabolism, 607, 620, 833, 841, 1003
  performance, **143**

age, **188**, **769**, **775**, **777**, 816, 844
aging, **103**, 108, 109, 188, 274, **503**, **674**,
  706, 755–830, 834, 854, **881**–926
agranulocytosis, 1027, 1029
Ah gene battery, **386**
Ah receptor, 386, 387
Ah receptor nuclear translocator protein, 387
AIDS, 394
air
  pollutant, **535**
  pollution, **513**–554, 582, 583
airway
  inflammation, 518, 521, 522, 529, **530**,
    531–533, **537**, **539**, 584
  reactivity, **533**, 534, **536**
  resistance, 526, 527, 530, 537
alanine aminotransferase, 262
albumin-creatinine ratio, 1089, 1096
albuminuria, 1085, 1088, 1121, 1122
alcohol *see* ethanol
  dehydrogenase, 952
  liver cirrhosis, 961, 964
aldehyde, 33, 96, **101**, 102, 111, 116, **466**,
  542, 546, 716, 763, 1157
aliphatic amino acid, **97**
alkoxyl radical, **35**
allantoin, 163
allopurinol, 73, 75, 79, 165, 666, 678, 680,
  954, 1177
Alzheimer disease, **107**, **728**, 772, 895, **911**
amflutazole, 1177
amino acid, 472–474, 619
  oxidation, **97**, **100**, 898–900
aminophenazone, **1029**
aminopyrine *see* aminophenazone
α-amino radical, 24
AMP *see* adenosine-5′-monophosphate
amyloid A protein, 1094
amyloid-β-peptide, 729, 772
amyotrophic lateral sclerosis, 269, **270**, 736,
  738, 896
anaerobic
  area, 999, 1003

exercise, **119**
threshold, 560, 561
anemia, 134, 138, 140, **142**, 143, 1175
angina pectoris, 662, **663**
angiogenesis, 997, 1001, 1007
angioplasty, **677**
angiotensin II, 382
anoxia, 146
anserine, 346, 347
antagonistic pleiotropy, 767, 768
anthocyanin derivative, 340
antibody, **469**
antigen presenting cell, 1157
antimycin A, 761
antioxidant, 5, 64, 75, 80, 115–123, **180**, **184**,
        187, 188, **221**–**239**, **297**–**317**,
        323–352, 384, **446**, 458, 474, 518,
        547, **555**–574, **584**, 586, **589**, 666,
        696, 704, 716, 717, 722, **727**, 741,
        764, 775, 779, 783, 787, 858, **881**–
        950, 981, **982**, **985**, **988**, 1012,
        1055, 1060, 1062, **1069**–1104,
        1173, **1184**
    activity, 342, 344–347, **361**, 377, 378, 422,
        807, 858–861
    deficiency, **306**
    enzyme, **546**, 674, 675, **696**, 707, 721, **743**,
        858–861, 905, 911, 984, 1060,
        1061, 1142
    index, 987
    interaction, **316**
    reserve, 681
    supplementation, **307**, 865, 905, **988**, 1086
antithrombin III, 566, 568
α-1-antitrypsin, **1170**
AP-1 *see* activator protein-1
apoptosis, **204**, 415, **667**, **788**, 932, 934
apoferritin, 1174
apotransferrin, 134
arachidonic acid, 1076
arginine, 72, 100
arteriosclerosis *see* atherosclerosis
arthritis, 887
arthrodesis, 1180
artifact, 436
asbestos, 940, 942
ascorbic acid, 5, 8, 13, 29, 40, 110, 122, 131,
        184–186, 189, **229**, **302**, **311**, 315,
        316, **334**, 349, 350, 361, 377, 434,
        447, 452, 453, **455**–458, 518, 520,
        522, 547, 556, 557, 560, 570, 573,

584–586, 666, 698, 705, 714, 742,
        866, 890, 893, 906, 909, 930, 936,
        939, 943, 944, 983, 988, 1013,
        1029
    deficiency, 705
ascorbyl radical, 13, 438, 439, 585, 714
aspartate aminotransferase, 262
asthma, 521, 526, 533–538, 584
atherogenesis, 909, 1055, 1057, 1072, 1076
atheroma, 71, 72
atherosclerosis, **71**, **72**, **106**, **405**, 406, 408,
        412, 413, 415, 423, **661**, 698, 888,
        892, 895, 900, 908–910, 987,
        1011, **1053**–1068, 1071, 1072,
        1079, 1088, 1125
athlete, 210, 247, **501**, 502, 529, 533, 538,
        556, 560
ATP *see* adenosine-5'-triphosphate

barbituric acid derivative, 1044
basic fibroblast growth factor, 183, 407
Becker dystrophy, 490
benzene, 33
benzoic acid, 341
bilirubin, **231**
binding protein, 136
bioaccumulation, **770**
bioavailability, **323**, 336, 341, 342, 348
biomarker, 434
biomolecule, **459**
biradical, 6
bioreductive agent, 1184
bleeding, **1174**
ß-blocker, 182, 691, 694
blood, 981
    brain barrier, 562, 726
    clotting, 566–569, 997, 1000
        disorder, 566–569
    donation, 139
    flow, 1085, 1094
    rheology, 565–569, 571, 1095
    toxicity, 540
    transfusion, **140**
    viscosity, 565, 566
BMK1 *see* mitogen activated protein kinase
bone resorption, **1176**, 1177
bovine serum albumin, 764
brain, 107
    cortex, 562
    edema, 562, 569, 714
    hemorrhage, 740

ischemia, 740
breast cancer, 936, 937
bromine, 6, 39
bronchitis, 521
buthionine sulfoximine, 697
butylated hydroxyanisole, 337, 338
tert-butylated hydroxyquinone, 337
butylated hydroxytoluene, 337, 338, 453, 906
tert-butylperoxyl, 32

CA 125 antigen, 286
caffeic acid, 338, 350
calcineurin, 418
calcitonin gene related peptide, 1178
calcitriol, 1177
calcium
    accumulation, **64**
    antagonist, 390, 392, 745
    ATPase, 607, 618, 715
    cell level, **389**–392, 638, 643
    homeostasis, 62, 64, 615
    release channel, 607, 617
    restriction, **266**
caloric restriction, **797**–830**,** 856, 866, 882,
        900–903, 906
cancer, **107**, 139, 209, 210, 890, **927**–950,
        987
    epidemiology, 209–212, 934, 943
    growth, **933**
    intervention studies, 938
    mortality, 936, 940
    prevention, 347, 349, 932, 938–945
    risk, 934, 942, 943
canthaxanthin, 332
capillary density, 1152
captopril, 656, 678, 679
carbon monoxide, 39
carbon tetrachloride, 7, 27, 34, 38, **1026**
carbon-halogen bond cleavage, 39
carbonyl group, 99, 100, 104–110, **472**, 587
carbonyl iron, **139**
carcinogenesis, 107, 196, 198, 209, 338, 808,
        819, **928**, **931**, 955–7, 1045
cardiomyopathy, **657**, 698, 820
cardioplegia, 678–680
cardiotoxicity, 706, 1035
cardiovascular disease, **124**, 138, 698, 708,
        908, 1071, 1080
carmustine, 395, 726
carnitine, 247
carnosic acid, 338

carnosine, 345–347, 349
carnosol, 338, 341
α-carotene, 330, 332, 334, 935, 983
β-carotene, 186, 314–316, 329–331, **332**–
        334, 349, 350, 547, 556, 557, 570,
        573, 720, 742, 783, 866, 930, 933–
        936, 938–944, 957
γ-carotene, 330
carotenoid, 186, **230**, **300**, **330**–334, 556,
        557, 570, 929, 933, 935, 944, 957,
        983, 985
carvedilol, 413
catalase, 165, 180, **225**, **236**, 267, **444**, 445,
        546, 584, 585, 587, 637, 648, 660,
        666, 678, 693, 696, 720, 860, 889,
        952, 958, 1113
cataract, **274**, 890
catechin, 338, 340
    derivative, 339–341, 350
catecholamine, **63**, 253, **694**
cathepsin, 1007
cell
    activation, 1001
    adhesion, 1001
    cycle, 931, 932
    damage, 65, 663
    differentiation, **410**
    growth, 420
    pH, **145**, 488
    proliferation, **383**, **408**, 411, 412, **419**–421,
        931
    protection, 824, 826
cellular defense, 800, 858
cellular mechanism, **615**
2-center-3-electron bond, 44
central nervous system, **713**–751
central nervous system disease, **727**, 745
cereal, 325, 326, 331, 335
cerebrovascular injury, 737, **740**
ceruloplasmin, 180, 337, 663, 984
Chapman reaction, 583
chelating agent, **140**, 743
chemical
    agent, 824
    mixture, 535
    structure, **360**
chemiluminescence, 440, 442, 464, 1165
chemokinesis, 408
chemotaxis, 408
chloramine, 1008
chlorination, 96

chlorine, 39
chlorofluorocarbon, 583
chlorogenic acid, 338
chloromethylperoxyl radical, 29
3-chlorotyrosine, 96, 97, 106, 899
cholesterol, 805, 908, 1062
cholinesterase, 262
chromanoxyl radical, 40
chromosome, 196
chromosome-21, 270
chromosome alteration, 204
chronic
    exercise, **248**, **253**, **263**, 267, 1058, 1061,
        1090
    granulomatous disease, 1008, 1012
    lung disease, 533
    obstructive lung disease, **1137**–1146
chylomicron, 332, 333, 363
cigarette smoking *see* smoking
cinnamate derivative, 340
circulus articuli vasculosus, 1152
cisplatin, 394, 395, 726, 742, 743
citrate synthase, 501, 841
claudication, **1069**–1104
    prevalence, 1070
clozapine, **1027**
coagulopathy *see* blood clotting disorder
coenzyme
    Q *see* ubiquinone-10
    Q9, 781
    Q10, **311**, 743, 781
collagen, 106, 587, 588, 1000, 1001
collagenase, 588, 589
colon cancer, 937, 939, 941
comet assay, 199
complement activation, 181, 182, 1085
concentration-response, 527
congestive heart failure *see* heart failure
conjugated diene, **465**
conjugated linoleic acid, **344**
cooking, 335
copper, 130, 146, 335, 337, 640, 984, 1060
copper zinc superoxide dismutase, 245, 253–
        269, **270**–279, 546, 635, 636, 649,
        650, 701, 1113–1115, 1128
coronary artery disease, 422, 1055
C-reactive protein, 1165
creatine, 78
    kinase, 188, 262, 674
cross-termination, 43
crotonaldehyde, 111

β-cryptoxanthin, 330, 332, 334, 935, 983
cyclic guanosine monophosphate, 610
cycline, 931, 932
cyclooxygenase, 530, 531, 539, 540
    inhibitor, 530, 531
cyclopiazonic acid, 392
cysteamine, 43, 44
cysteine, 35, 43, 44, 101, 556
cytochemistry, 637
cytochrome, 494
    c oxidase, 505, 760, 849–852
    p450, 762, 954–956, 1036
    p450 isoenzyme, **1036**
cytogenetics, **204**
cytokine, 177–180, **183**, 262, 408, 410, 541,
        740, 981, 1001, 1002, 1009, 1072,
        1150
cytoplasm, 638
cytotoxicity, 1044

daidzein, 338, 340–342
daidzin, 340
dauer larva, 782
deamination, 98
decarboxylation, 23, 97
defense mechanism, **80**, 833
deferoxamine, 60, 137, 139, 140, 641, 642,
        646, 666, 678, 680, 771, 1176
degradation, 33, 36
dehydration, 555, 571, **572**
dehydroascorbic acid, 334, 336, 377, 378,
        447, 456–458, 698
denervation, **648**
Deprenyl *see* selegiline
dermatoheliosis, 588
dermis, 580, 581
Desferal *see* deferoxamine
desmin, 411
detoxification, **222**
dexamethasone, 279, 540
diabetes mellitus, **105**, **124**, **272**, **659**, 964,
        1011, **1105**–1136
diabetic
    cardiomyopathy, 659, 660
    microangiopathy, 1121, 1122
    nephropathy, 659, 1108
    retinopathy, **274**, 1121, 1122
diamide, 394
3,5-dibromo-4-nitrosobenzenesulfate, 1168
dicarbonyl, 412
dichlorofluorescein, **444**, 700

3,5-dichlorotyrosine, 96
diet, 132, 298, **305**–308, **323**, 368, 662, **783**, **985**
  restriction, **781**, 799, 902
  supplementation, 298, 299, 303–305, **307**–316, **349**, **368**, **555**, 570, **602**, 696
dietary
  fat, 331
  fiber, 331
  source, **325**, 330, 334, 339
differential path length factor, 500
diffusion controlled process, 6, 9
dihydrolipoic acid, 110, 348, 393, 700, 743
2,3-dihydroxybenzoic acid, 441, 643, 664
dihydroxyphenylalanine, 95
dimercaptopropanol, 666
5,5-dimethyl-1-pyrroline-N-oxide, 437, 439, 440
dimethyl sulfoxide, 73, 609, 611, 743
2,4-dinitrophenylhydrazine, 472, 473
dipeptide oxidation, **99**
disease, **138**, **268**, **281**, 502, **503**, **881**–926, **977**–994, 1150
  model, **123**
  prevention, 808, 809, 814, 817, 823
displacement reaction, 24
disulfide reduction, 43, 44
5,5′-dithiobis-(2-nitrobenzoic acid), 449
dithiothreitol, 387, 609
dityrosine, 94, 106, 856, 857, 898–900, 902
diurnal cycle, 519
DNA, **196**, **587**
  binding, 385–388, 414
  damage, 141, **195**–213, 587, 855, 988
  fragmentation, **204**, 667
  mutation, 886
  oxidation, 107, 110, 437, **460**, 855
  repair, 196, 197, 203
  strand breakage, 107, 137, 198, 206, 980
docosahexaenoic acid, 187
dosimetry, **524**–526, 549
Down syndrome, 270, 736, **739**
doxorubicin, 394, 395, 706, **1032**
  iron complex, 1034
drug
  interaction, **725**
  metabolism, 541, **705**, **1021**–1052
  metabolite, **1025**, 1035
  radical, **1023**, **1025**
DTNB *see* 5,5′-dithiobis-(2-nitrobenzoic acid)

Duchenne muscular dystrophy, 108, 490, **650**

eccentric exercise, 163, 169, 170, 182, 184, **188**
EGb 761 *see* Ginkgo biloba extract
EGTA-AM, 390, 391
eicosanoid, 566, 1081, 1083
eicosapentaenoic acid, 187, 1077
elastase, 187, 1088, 1170
electrochemical detection, **451**–456, 461
electron paramagnetic resonance *see* electron spin resonance
electron spin resonance, **14**, **21**, 274, **438**–441, 600, 601, 700, 1168
electron transport, 29, 42, 43, 620, 690, 760, 778, 846, 849, 884, 903, 904
elimination reaction, 42
ELISA *see* enzyme linked immunosorbent assay
Ellman reagent *see* 5,5′-dithiobis-(2-nitrobenzoic acid)
embryogenesis, 995, 999
emoxipine, 667
endonuclease, 202
endoperoxide radical, 31
endothelin, 1079
endothelin-1, 1085
endothelium, **72**
  cell, **71**, **279**
  damage, 1072, 1084, 1088, 1121
endurance, 81, 815, 865
  running, 65, 200, 203, 253–260, 265, 266, 306, 816–819
energy metabolism, **486**, **487**, **558**
environmental manipulation, **781**
environmental temperature, 555, 571, 572
enzymatic method, **461**, **465**
enzyme
  activation, 64
  assay, **245**, **246**
  distribution, **155**
  expression, **277**
  fragmentation, **273**
  function, **154**
  inactivation, **273**
  induction, **277**, **279**, 956, **1036**, **1142**
enzyme linked immunosorbent assay, 244, 246
enzyme structure, **154**
epicatechin, 340–342
  gallate, 340, 341

epidemiology, **209**–211
epidermal growth factor, 1010
epidermis, 580, 581
epigallocatechin, 329, 340–342
    gallate, 340, 341
epilepsy, 740, 741
epinephrine, 122, 123, 694
epithelium cell permeability, 533, **537**
epoxide, 31
ergogenic acid, 603
erythema, 587, 588
erythorbic acid, 334, 336
erythrocyte
    aggregation, 565, 566
    filterability, 563–565
    sedimentation rate, 1165
erythropoiesis, 565
erythropoietin, 1162
esophagus
    cancer, 940
    dysplasia, 939
estradiol, 1060
ethane, 775
ethanol, 726–728, **951**–976, 1044
    metabolism, **952**
ethyl radical, 17
etoposide, 395
excitation-contraction coupling, **616**
exercise, **58**, 59, **69**–88, 109, **115**–322, 496,
    526, 529, 532, **557**, **689**–754, 788,
    797–830, 863, 904, 1054, 1055,
    1058, **1069**–1188
    performance, **528**, 602
    training, **79**, **221**, **232**, 697, 714, 722, **723**,
        725, 728, 1093–1096
exhaustion, 248–252, 265, **1138**
extensor digitorum longus muscle, 648, 649
extracellular superoxide dismutase, 245, 246,
        261, 263, 264, 266, 269, 1113,
        1115

F2-isoprostane, **470**, 965, 981
familial amyotrophic lateral sclerosis *see*
            amyotrophic lateral sclerosis
fatty acid binding protein, 666
fatty acid metabolism, 958
fatty liver, 953
fenozan, 666
Fenton reaction, **140**, 604, 764, 1170, 1174
Fenton reagent, 141
Fenton-Haber-Weiss process, 36

ferrireductase, 134
ferritin, 133, **134**, 137, **138**, 142, 146, 764,
        1174
fibrinogen, 1095
fibroblast, 1001
fibronectin, 532, 1000, 1006
fish oil, 187, 309, 1077
flavonoid, 186, 329, 338, 941
flavonol derivative, 340
flaxseed oil, 910
flow cytometry, 437, 444, 447, **451**
fluid balance, 572
fluorescent
    probe, 440
    product, **469**
fluorometric
    detection, 453
    assay, 1165
food, 326, 331, 339, 342, 345, **349**, 941
    restriction, 799
    storage, 335
forced expiratory volume, 525, 526, 529, 530,
        532, 534, 536, 539
formaldehyde, 583
free radical, 3–54, **59**, 63, **65**, 140, **206–208**,
        435, 437, 541, 555, 558, 563, 570,
        585, 600, **655**–688, **690**, **757**, **766**,
        807, 811, 843, 844, 846, **881**–926,
        928, 933, 959–962, 965, 978, **979**,
        981, 987, 1012, 1021–**1023**, **1025**,
        1057, 1082, 1086, 1108, 1137,
        1138–**1142**
    scavenger, 162, 570, 663, **743**
    molecule interaction, 9
Freund adjuvant, 1178
frost bite, 569
fruit, 326, 331, 334, 335, 941, 985

GA-binding protein, **388**
gallic acid, 338
gallocatechin, 340
gas chromatography, 436, 437, 441, 460, **461**,
        463–**465**, 467–**469**, 470, 473, 474,
        542
gastrointestinal bleeding, 146
gene, 196
    damage, 930
    deletion, 849–852
    expression, 65, **413**, **423**
    induction, 677
genetic information, **196**

genetics, 103
genistein, 340–342
genistin, 340
genotoxicity, 200, 928
genotype, 211
Ginkgo biloba extract, 341, 671 912
glucocorticoid hypothesis, 811
glucose, 161, 714
glucose-6-phosphate dehydrogenase, 674,
    772, 773
glutamate synthetase, 775
glutamine synthase, 715, 764
γ-glutamylcysteine synthetase, 699
γ-glutamyltransferase, 246
γ-glutamyltranspeptidase, 699
glutaredoxin, **226**
glutathione, 8, 35, 79, 110, **227**, **236**, **302**,
    306, 307, **312**, 338, 345, 348, 349,
    376, 377–**379**, 434, 436, 443,
    447–452, 472, 518, 539, 546, 547,
    556, 584–586, 602, 611, 632–634,
    650, 660, **699**, 702, 703, 720, 723–
    725, **742**, 861, 890, 891, 959,
    1035, 1056, 1109–1112, 1116,
    1140, 1143, 1178
  deficiency, 306, 307, 705
  -dependent enzyme, 1111
  disulfide, 303, 436, **447**–451, 561, 584,
    585, 632, 699, 723–725, 1056,
    1109–1111, 1138, 1140, 1143
    reductase, **446**–450, 1111
  homeostasis, 1109
  metabolism, 1035, 1109
  oxidation, **1138**, **1140**
  peroxidase, 80, **224**, **235**, 267, 302, 436,
    445, **446**, 546, 562, 584, 585, 636,
    649, 650, 658, 696–698, 723–725,
    861, 889, 1056, 1112
  reductase, 546, 584, 585, 632, 650, 660,
    696, 721, 1111
  s transferase, 302, 451, 546, 637, 696, 1112
s-glutathionylcaftaric acid, 340
glycation *see* glycosylation
glycitein, 340
glycitin, 340
glycolysis, 836, 840
glycoprotein, 1000
glycosaminoglycan, **75**, **1173**
glycosylation, 105, 106, 271, **272**–**274**, 771,
    811, 1115, 1124
gold, 1183

granulation tissue, 1000
granulocyte, 201, 567, 568
granulocyte macrophage colony stimulating
    factor, 539
grape juice, 340
growth factor, 408, 932, 1001, 1003, 1006,
    1009
  receptor, 1003
growth hormone, 109
GSH *see* glutathione
gynecologic cancer, **286**, 938

H7, 279
Haber-Weiss reaction, **141**
Hahn spin-echo, 1173
halogenated acetic acid, 38
halogenated organic compound, 33
halogenated oxyl radical, 38
health benefit, 1054
healthy subject, **118**, 281
heart
  arrhythmia, 662, **671**
  attack *see* heart infarction
  damage, **703**
  failure, 502, 505, **656**
  hypertrophy, **659**
  infarction, 138, 165, **281**, 282, 284, 662,
    908
  ischemia, 662, **663**–**665**, 678, 776, 784, *see*
    also ischemic heart disease
  metabolism, **690**
  mitochondrion, 691, 703, 706
  performance, **655**–687
  protection, **655**–687
  surgery, 677, **678**
  transplantation, **680**
  ventricle fibrillation, 672, 673
heat shock protein, 65
heat shock protein-70, 206
helicobacter pylori, 937
hematocrit, 566
hematoma *see* primary hematoma
heme oxygenase 1, 206
hemochromatosis, 137, 139, 1175
hemoglobin, 142, 143, **146**, 494, 495, 498–
    500
hemolysis, 146, 247
hemolytic anemia *see* anemia
hemophilia, 1174
hemophilic arthropathy, 1174
hemosiderin, **135**, 1174

heparan sulfate, 75
heparin, 75, 76, 418
heparin binding epidermal growth factor,
    412
high altitude, **555**–577
high density lipoprotein, 328, 363
high energy electron, 12
high performance liquid chromatography,
    436, 437, 441, 447, 448, **450**, 451,
    453, 454, **456**, 460, **461**–**463**, 465,
    467, **468**, **469**, 470, 473, 474
hippuric acid, 341
histamine, 168, 170
histidine, 100, 556
    dipeptide, **346**
HIV *see* human immunodeficiency virus
    infection, 1150
homovanillic acid, 341
hormesis, 824
horseradish peroxidase assay, **445**
human immunodeficiency virus, 393, 394
Huntington disease, 107, 737, **740**
hyaluronic acid, 1153, 1173
hyaluronan binding protein, 1153
hydrated electron, 13
hydrogen, 16
    abstraction, 91, 92
    peroxide, 32, 43, 60, 382, 390, 391, 395,
        437, **443**–**445**, 446, 603, 604, 609,
        637, 643, 691, 760, 884, 885, 1075
1,2-hydrogen shift, 37
hydroperoxide, 31, 36
hydrophobicity, 108
hydroquinone, 41
hydroxycinnamic acid derivative, 338
8-hydroxy-2′-deoxyguanosine, 202, 203
8-hydroxy-7,8-dihydro-2′-deoxyguanosine,
    198
hydroxyl adduct, 24
α-hydroxyl peroxyl radical, 30
α-hydroxyl radical, 25
ß-hydroxyl radical, 26
hydroxyl radical, 4, 10, 13, **22**, 33, 34, 60, 90–
    93, 95, 98, 108, 141, 180, 437–
    439, **441**, 531, 585, 590, 604, 640,
    643, 664, 693, 715, 757, 759, 883,
    895, 898, 911, 1025, 1075
hydroxylation, 91, 92, 93, 95, 441
4-hydroxyalkenal, 117, 542, 716
4-hydroxynonenal, 101, 462, 466, 468, 469,
    542–544, 546, 773, 965

hyperbaric oxygen, 714, 717–719, 999, 1013
hypercholesterolemia, 72, 661, 1166
hyperemia, 1085
hyperglycemia, 1115
hyperoxia, 718, 719, 776, 783
hypertension, **407**, 659
hyperthyroidism, 690
hypochlorous acid, **99**, 106, **446**, 882, 1029
hypodermis, 580
hypothermia, 571
hypoxanthine, 62, 78, 79–80, 153, 154, 157–
    167, 170, 348, 638, 693
    phosphoribosyl transferase, 161, 162, 988
hypoxia, **267**, **557**, 558, 571, 572, 783, **1147**,
    1156, **1158**
    inducible factor-1, **1162**
    responsive element, 1162

ibuprofen, 530, 531, 696
immobilization, **109**, **632**
immune
    complex, 1168
    function, **1156**
    response, 185–**187**, 190
immunoglobulin G, **1168**
immunosuppression, 186, 187
immunosuppressive agent, 418
IMP *see* inosine monophosphate
in vitro study, **539**
in vivo study, **540**
indapamine, 666
indometacin, 530
indoor air pollution, 524
infection, 178, 209
inflammation, 108, **168**, 188, 190, **208**, **537**,
    539, 588, 928, **995**–1020, 1096
inflammatory cell, 533
inorganic particle, 519
inorganic phosphate, 488–491
inosine, 157
    monophosphate, 157–161
inspiratory resistive loading, 601
insulin, 1105, 1109–1114, 1117, 1122
insulin-like growth factor I, 415, 1010
insulin-like growth factor II, 1010
insulin resistance, 1123, 1130
γ-interferon, 170
interferon, 168, 1011
interleukin-1, 170, 178, 179, 262, 276, 285,
    286, 410, 541, 568, 1011
interleukin-1ß, 279

interleukin-2, 380, 1011
interleukin-6, 178, 179, 531, 532
interleukin-8, 539
intermittent claudication, **1069**–1104
intestine absorption, **362**
intraarticular pressure, 1151, 1153, 1154
iodometric method, **465**
ionizing radiation, 99, 101
IRFI 16, 667
iron, **129**–152, 180, 334, 337, 589, **641**–643,
      764, 771, 911, 1025, **1174**, 1175
  absorption, 132–134
  ascorbate, 145
  blood level, 133, **146**
  containing protein, **65**
  cycle, **133**
  deficiency, 142, **143**
  dextran, 1175, 1181
  homeostasis, 136
  loading, **139**
  mobilization, **143**
  movement, **640**
  overload, **137**, 1175
  pool, 136, 142
  related disease, **138**
  sorbitol, 1175
  storage, **134**
  -sulfur protein, **388**
  transport, **131**, **134**
  uptake, **135**
ischemia, 1073, 1074, 1079, 1081
ischemic heart disease, **662**, 698, **986**, 1071,
    see also heart ischemia
ischemic preconditioning, **665**
isoenzyme, 245
isoflavone derivative, 339–342
isoflavonoid, 341
isomer, **332**
isoprenaline, 694
isopropanol radical, 34

joint
  physiology, 1150
  immobilization, 1180, 1181
  splinting, 1181

ketone, 33
knee effusion, 1153
knockout mouse, **269**
Krebs cycle, 1156
kynurenine, 90

lactate dehydrogenase, 561, 840
lactic acid, 79, 560, 1139
lactosylceramide, 383
laser flash radiolysis, 11
lazaroid, 743
leukemia *see* acute leukemia
leukocyte, **179**, **184**, 201, 567, 888, 996, 997,
    1004, 1007, 1012, 1080
leukocytosis, 182, 263
leukotriene
  A4, 1077
  B4, 540
  C4, 539
  D4, 539
  E4, 539
life
  expectancy, 798, 825, 978
  prolongation, **902**
  span, **788**, 797, 798, 802, 815–822, 824,
    902–907
lifestyle, 811, 945
limb amputation, 1071
limb ischemia, 1071, 1073–1085
lipid, **586**, **1171**
  hydroperoxide, 437, 463, **464**, 465, 586,
    717, 1119
  oxidation, 79, 342, 346, 348, 423
  peroxidation, 92, 101, 109, **115**–128, 137,
    144, 145, 166, 188, 244, 419, 435–
    437, 452, 454, 459, **462**, 463, 466,
    470, 475, 531, 541–547, 562, 570–
    572, 586, 591, 602, 632, 641, 661,
    698, 715, **717**–719, 722, 723, 807,
    854, 863, 894, 955, 959, 964, 981,
    1013, 1075, 1076, 1083, 1106,
    1115, **1116**–1126, 1141
  peroxide, 116, 1058, 1075, 1076, 1086,
    1116, 1119, 1121, 1124
  radical, 116, 585
lipoate radical, 44
lipofuscin, 770, 771, 778, 782, 855
α-lipoic acid *see* thioctic acid
lipopolysaccharide, 277, 279
lipoprotein, 328, 332, 333, 366, 405, 412
  a, 412
  lipase, 328, 366
  metabolism, 1095
  oxidation, 1055, 1057, **1058**, 1061, 1072,
    1076, 1122–1125, **1172**
lipoxygenase, 540
liver, 363, 364

cancer, 939, 1045
injury, 953, 955, 961, 963
secretion, **363**
steatosis, 953
longevity, 798, 800–802, 807, 809, 810, 814–817, 821, 825, 826, 903, 904
low density
lipoprotein, 71, 92, 106, 363, 405, 661, 895, 909, 986, 1055, **1058**, 1075, 1108, 1120, 1122, 1172
lipoprotein cholesterol, 1122, 1123
autoantibody, 1125
low molecular weight iron, 134, **136**
lucigenin, 442
luminol, 442, **446**
lung, 980
absorption, 514–516, 525, 526
cancer, 935–937, 940, 942
damage, 980
deposit, 516, 521
edema, 569
fibrosis, 532
function, **527**–532, **534**–536
injury, 519–521, 533
surfactant, 514, 515
transplantation, **680**
lutein, 330, 332–334, 984
LY333531, 422
lycopene, 330, 332, 333, 935, 936, 984
lymphocyte, 201
lysine residue, 273

macrophage, 64, 170, 183, 284, 531, 909, 980, 1001, 1005, 1150
inflammatory protein-2, 540
macula degeneration, 570
magnetic resonance spectroscopy, 486, **487**, 489, 490, **501**–503
Maillard reaction, 273, 811, 1107
malnutrition, 555, **572**
malondialdehyde, 117, 462, **466**–469, 562, 591, 656, 661, 691, 707, 716, 725, 729, 854, 938, 965, 1056, 1086, 1118, 1119
manganese, 130
superoxide dismutase, 244–**269**, **276**–289, 546, 635, 636, 649, 691, 1113, 1114
mannitol, 743
margarine, 325, 326
mass spectrometry, 436, 437, 441, 460–**465**,

467, **469**, 470, 473, 474, 542
mast cell, 170
maximal oxygen uptake, 529
maximum life span potential, 759, 762, 766, **778**–781, **783**, 787
mechanical stress, 121
melanin, 494, 581
melanoma, 588
MELAS syndrome, 848
melatonin, 911, 913
membrane
damage, 558, 562, 646
fluidity, 562, 566
integrity, 558, 566
menadione, 900
mercaptan derivative, 375
2-mercaptoethanol, 35, 906
messenger RNA, 264, 265
metabolic acidosis, 559
metabolic rate, 806, 807, 809, 810, 820–822, 824, 903
metabolism, **362**, **367**, 800, 804, 813, **1156**
metal binding agent, **129**
metal chelate, 131
metal ligand, 131
metal-catalyzed oxidation, 90, 98, 100
metallothionein, 141, 180
metastasis, 933
meteorology, 523
methionine, 23, 29, 101, 961
sulfoxide, 1109, 1170
methoxatin *see* pyrroloquinoline quinone
methyl radical, 16
microalbuminura *see* albuminuria
microcirculation, 566, 569, 1011, 1090, 1094, 1095
microsomal ethanol-oxidizing system, 954
mineral, 342
minimal erythemal dose, 582
mitochondrial
biogenesis, 601
disease, 502, 505
DNA, 197, 198, 769, 774, 846–849, 886
dysfunction, **620**
encephalomyopathy, 848
mutation aging theory, 886
myopathy, 848
respiration, 841, 884
mitochondrion, 59, 680, 690, **691**, 703, 706, 760, 767, **769**, 778, 780, 781, 883, 885, 1092

mitogen activated protein kinase, **382**, 383, **417**

mitomycin C, 395

mitosis, 1000

mobilferrin, 133

modeling, **524**

mongolian gerbil, **139**, 772

monobromobimane, 451

monochlorobimane, 451

monoclonal antibody, 246, 286

morphine, 726

mortality, 211, 798, 815, 822, 825, 977, 978, 987, 1071, 1130

motor control, 606, **621**

motor unit, 838, 842

mountain sickness, 568

mountaineer, 560, 563, 573

mucopolysaccharide, 1000

multiple system atrophy, 736, **739**

muscle, **156**
  atrophy, 145, **631**–653, 812, 834, 842, 852
  blood flow, 621
  contraction, 58–60, **606**, **608**, 813, 839, 843
  damage, 58, 59, 64, 65, **166**, 167, 182, 189, 195, 208, 813, 843, 846
  denervation, 834, 838, 842
  deoxygenation, 496
  disease, **647**, 848, 849
  endurance, 839
  exercise, **496**, 839, 863
  fatigue, **599**–630, 1091
  fiber, 834, 836, 1090
  force, 608, 610
  function, 839, 1093
  injury *see* muscle damage
  integrity, **145**
  ischemia, 61, 166, **496**
  mass, 805, 813, 832, 834, 835, 845, 864, 867
  metabolism, **485**, 813, 840, 1092
  mitochondrion, 607, 833, 846
  oxygenation, **496**
  regeneration, 844, 845
  reinnervation, 842
  strength, 839, 863, 865
  twitch, 264, 609

mutagenicity, 588, 956, 987

mutation, 196, 738, 777

myeloperoxidase, 93, 95, 96, 208, 267, 887, 1012, 1059

myocardial
  adaptation, **665**
  infarction *see* heart infarction
  stunning, **670**

myofilament, 607, 615, **619**, 623

myoglobin, 65, **146**, 494, 495, 498, 669

myoglobinuria, 147

myoinositol hexaphosphate *see* phytic acid

myosin, 410, 607, 619
  adenosine triphosphatase, 836

N′-formylkynurenine, 90–92

N-ethylmaleimide, 450

N-tert-butyl-α-phenylnitrone, 743, 784, 907

NADH oxidase, 1165, 1166

NAD(P)H oxidase, **63**, 695, 1008

NADH dehydrogenase, 760

naringein, 341

naringin, 341

near infrared spectroscopy, 486, **493**, 494, 498, **501**, **502**, **504**

nedocromil, 539

neointima formation, 415

nephropathy, 819

nerve damage, **1177**

nerve fiber C, 530

neurodegenerative disease, **107**, 198, 895, **910**

neurologic disease, **107**

neuromuscular junction, 842

neurotoxicity, **717**

neutral endopeptidase, 530

neutrophil, 154, 168, 170, 179, 182, 183, 189, 208, 284, 531, 532, **695**, 997–999, 1005, 1013
  activation, 980, 1080, 1083, 1087
  degranulation, 1081, 1083

neutrophilia, 182, 532

NF-kappa B *see* nuclear factor kappa B

NF-Y *see* nuclear factor-Y

nicotine, 980

nifedipine, 390

nitrate, 1167

nitration, 93–96, 857, 895

nitric acid, 535

nitric oxide, 69, 70, **71**–73, **80**, 81, 90, 93, 95, 96, 378, 437, 605, **610**, **613**, 618, **643**, **668**, 745 761, 762, **786**, 857, 882, 894, 898, 900, 909, 980, 1023, 1060, 1079, 1080, **1167**
  derivative, **605**, 606

synthase, 605, 643, 644, 857, 885, 1080, 1162
  inhibitor, 745
nitrite, 95, 1167
nitrofurantoin, **1031**
nitrogen, 16
  dioxide, 95, **513**–554, 1023–1025
  radical, 45
nitrones, 18
3-nitrotyrosine, 93–95, 97, 857, 858, 894–896, 899, 900
nitrous acid, 583
nitroxyl radical, 18
nitrylchloride, 97
nociceptive nerve, 1177
nonheme iron, 132
nonsteroidal anti-inflammatory agent, 1183
noradrenalin, 571
nuclear factor kappa B, 265, 385, **389**–392, 413, 414, 772, 1159, **1161**
nuclear factor-Y, **387**
nuclear magnetic resonance spectroscopy, 1173
nucleoside, **203**
nucleotide, **347**, 349
  degradation, **156**
nutrient, **298**, **314**, 325, **329**, **704**, 941, 944, **982**, 989
  absorption, 326, 330, 336, 341, 343, 345, 346, 348, 362
  interaction, **329**, **337**, **342**
  storage, 328, 333, 336, 341, 346
  transport, 327, 333, 336, 341, 346, 362
nutrition, **131**, **142**, **188**, 298, 305, 321, 573, **602**, 704
nutritional deficiency *see* malnutrition

obesity, 809
ONO-3144, 666
optic neuropathy, 1176
ornithine carbamoyltransferase, 263
osteoarthitis, 1180
osteopenia, 1176
osteoporosis, 1177
outdoor air pollution, **538**
ovary cancer, **286**
ovary carcinoma antigen *see* CA 125 antigen
ovary epithelium carcinoma, 286
oxidant, **70**, **75**, **78**, 412, 416, **579**, **603**, **755**, **759**, **762**, **777**, **787**, **788**, **883**, 888, 937, 996, 1008

oxidant stress *see* oxidative stress
oxidant/antioxidant balance, 896, 937, 943, 945, 1025
oxidation, 43, 63, 71, 97, **771**, **774**, 896, **900**, 933, 1062, 1076, 1123
oxidative
  adaptation, 681
  burst, 179
  damage, 763, **765**, **766**, **769**, **778**, 807, 833, 845–848, 852, 856, 866, 867, 882, 894, **896**, 902, **1035**, 1055, **1073**, 1138, 1139
  metabolism, 59, **486**, **490**–493, 1092
  stress, 64, 65, 69, 70, **77**, 103, 122, 143, 145, 195, 239, 268, **433**–484, **513**–578, **586**, **590**, 602, **631**–654, **676**, **689**–754, 811, 819, 822, **831**–995, 1009, **1021**–1052, 1054, 1055, 1062, **1105**–1188
oxidized
  amino acid, **473**
  biomolecule, **459**
  DNA base, **202**, **203**
  low density lipoprotein, 1055, 1057, **1058**, 1061, 1072, 1076, 1122–1125
  nucleoside, **203**
oxidopamine, 726
8-oxo-7,8-dihydroguanine, 587
8-oxodeoxyguanosine, 460–**462**, 763, 774, 779
8-oxoguanine, 460, 461, 763, 779
oxygen, 6, 34, **98**, **446**, **713**, 716
  consumption, 499, 646, 690, 800, 865, 1085, 1095
  metabolism, 1085
  radical, 3, **21**, 45, 72, 73, 116, 166, 167, **179**, 208, 437, 663, 702, 703, 759–763, 768, 769, 846, 1022, 1032, 1035, 1073, 1074, 1078, 1083, 1086
  sufficiency, 486
  supply, 1003, 1013
  tension, **782**, 999, 1004, 1014, 1155
  toxicity, 714–**717**, 744, 965
oxyl radical, 4, 26, 34, 37, 38
oxypurinol, 73, 75, 165, 166, 1167
ozone, 100, 101, 208, **513**–554, 579, 580, **582**, **590**, 593
  hole, 583

pannus, 1148, 1149

paracetamol, 956, 1035
parathion, 726
parathyroid hormone, 1177
cis-parinaric acid, **470**
Parkinson disease, 107, **729**, 732–736, 762,
    896, 911, **912**
pathology, 799, **808**
Pax-8 *see* transcription factor
PEBP2/CBF *see* transcription factor
penicillamine, 43, 44, 1169, 1183
pentane, 562, 775
pentosidine, 771, 772, 778
peptide bond, **97**
peripheral vascular disease, 502, 504
peroxide, 36
peroxisome, **693**
   proliferator, **1045**
peroxy radical, 97
peroxyacetyl nitrate, 536
peroxyl radical, 4, **27**, 30–34, 43, 536, 541,
    590, 980
peroxynitrite, **73**, 93–95, 106, 437, 613, 619,
    761, 894, 895, 1080
phagocyte, **64**, 887
phagocytosis, 64, 887, 1005
pharmacokinetics, **365**
phenobarbital, 541
phenol, 33
phenolic acid derivative, 341
phenolic compound, **337**–342
phenothiazine, 28
phenotype, **410**, 411
phenoxyl radical, 8, 39
phenylalanine, 95, **441**
phenylbutazone, 1029
phenyl-tert-butylnitrone, 437, 439
phorbol ester, 382, 415
phorbol myristate acetate, **277**–279
phosphatase, 416, **417**
phosphatidylcholine, 963
phosphatidylinositol 3-kinase, 380
phosphocreatine, 77, 488–492, 501–503
phospholipid, 959, 963–965
photoaging, **588**
photocarcinogensis, 582
photochemical smog, 522
photolysis, 583
photooxidative damage, **586**
photoreaction, 586
photosensitizing agent, 586
physical

activity, **142**, **782**, 799–801, 811–816, 823,
    1054, 1182
   exercise *see* exercise
   fitness, **1126**
   inactivity, 812, 823, 1059
   performance, 558, 560
physiological parameter, 804, 813
physostigmine, 726
phytate, 131, 345
phytic acid, **349**, 667
phytofluene, 984
pigeon, 780
PKC *see* protein kinase C
plant, 570, 941
plant compound, **337**–339, 342
plant oil, 325, 326
platelet activating factor, 1079
platelet derived growth factor, 183, 382, 408,
    409, 411, 419, 1079
polyamine, 345, **347**, 349
polyaromatic hydrocarbon, 519
polyclonal antibody, 246
polycythemia, 565
   vera, 143
polyol pathway, 1115
polyphenol, 131
polyunsaturated fatty acid, **187**, 359, 542,
    543, 938, 965
   radical, 34
pomace, 340
precancer, 939
primary bilairy cirrhosis, **285**
primary hepatoma, **285**
probucol, 72, 661, 909
procarbazine, 726
product analysis, **19**
proline, 100
propyl gallate, 337
prostacyclin, 696, 1078
prostaglandin, 63, 530, 531
   E2, 530–532, 539
prostanoid metabolism, **63**
prostate cancer, 936, 940
protease, 62, **418**, 777, 1081
protein, 342, 587
   bcl 2, 934
   C, 566, 568
   carbonyl, **472**, 772, 773, 776, 777, 779–
     782, 784, 856, 895–897, 908
   cleavage, **98**
   cross-linking, 587

damage, **101**, 646, 896
degradation, **108**, **896**–898
denaturation, 108
disulfide, **471**
DNA interaction, **384**
expression, 423, 424
gene product-9.5, 1178
inactivation, **108**
kinase C, **382**, 409, **415**, **420**
   inhibitor, 745
oxidation, **89**–111, 435, **470**, 471, **544**,
      602, 764, 773, 855, **893**
phosphorylation, **379**–384
repair, **896**
sulfhydryl, 856
thiol, **471**
tyrosine kinase, **379**
tyrosine phosphatase, **381**
proteoglycan, 1000
proteolysis *see* protein degradation
protooncogene expression, **418**
pulmonary hypertension, 561
pulse radiolysis, 11
purine, **157**, 161
   degradation, **77**
   metabolism, **156**, 954
   salvage, **161**
putrescine, 347
pyridostigmine, 726
pyrrolidine dithiocarbamate, 414
pyrroloquinoline quinone, 339, **342**

quercetin, 329, 338–341
quercetin derivative, 339
quinoid, 40
quinone, 40, 41, 60, 726, 979

radiation, 824
radioimmunoassay, 1165
radiolysis, 98
ragged red fiber disease, 848
rate constant, **21**
rate of living hypothesis, 759, 762, 780, 807,
      809, 810
reaction kinetics, **8**
reactive nitrogen species, **383**, 857, 858, 896
reactive oxygen species, 71, 90, 104, 178–
      181, 197, 221, **222**, **403**–432, 434,
      437, 459, 460, 474, 475, 559, **603**,
      606, 608, 611, 614, 689, 691, 692,
      700, 708, 714, 715, **727**, 780, 846,

      848, 852, 853, 896, 901, 932, 955,
      996, 1021, 1022, 1046, 1106,
      1119, 1148, **1168**, 1171
reactivity selectivity principle, 26
receptor, 772, 900, 901
recommended dietary allowance, **305**, 368
redox, 301, **375**, **392**, 412, 413, **471**, **606**, 614
   cycle, 378, 379, 1032
   factor-1, 1159
   potential, 43, 44
   state, 953
reduced glutathione, 379
reducing agent, 137
reduction, 36, 43, 44
   potential, **19**–21, 28
reflux muscle inhibition, 1154
rehabilitation, **501**
reperfusion injury, 162, **163**–165, 171, 172,
      659, **663**, **667**, 678, 776, 784,
      1073–1085, 1183
resonance structure, 8
respiratory burst, 887, 1007
rest, **1180**
restenosis, **406**, 415
retina hemorrhage, 569
retinoid, 955
retinol, 329, 330, 334, 349, 350, 938–940, 957
retinopathy, **1176**
reversible oxygen addition, **33**
rhabdomyolysis, 147
rheumatoid
   arthritis, 108, 139, 163, **1147**–1188
   factor, 1150, 1168, 1169, 1179
   nodule, 1149
   synovitis, **1162**, **1180**
riboflavin, 573
ribose-5-phosphate, 161
risk assessment, **555**
roentgen radiation, 776
rosemary, 338, 341
Russell mechanism, 32
rutin, 340, 341

salicylic acid, 437, **441**, 643
Salvia Miltiorrhiza Bunge, 910
sarcolemma, 607, **617**
sarcomere, 843
sarcopenia, **831**–880
sarcoplasmic reticulum, 607–**617**
satellite cell, 844
scavenger receptor, 406, 415

Schiff base, 102, 105, 1158

β-scission, 37–39

season, 519, 523

sedentary *see* physical inactivity

selectin, 1003, 1081

selegiline, 905, 914

selenium, **305**, 306, 314, 573, 930, 937, 940, 984

   deficiency, 697

selenocysteine, 305

selenomethionine, 305

semidehydroascorbate radical, 698, 699

semiquinone radical, 60, **41**, 700, 979, 1032

serum responsive factor, 1160

sesamin, 329

sesamol, 350

sex difference, 138, 816, 1061

signal transduction, **375**, **787**

single oxygen, 32

sister chromatid exchange, 204

skeletal muscle, **232**, **603**, **632**, **834**, 1090

skin

   aging, 582

   anatomy, **580**

   barrier pertubation, 592

   cancer, 579, 587, **588**

   excretion, 367

   inflammation, 570

   pathophysiology, **579–596**

   physiology, **580**

smoking, **110**, 334, 336, 956, **977–994**, 1170

sodium selenite, 394

SOK-1 see mitogen activated protein kinase

soleus muscle, 632, 648, 649

somatic mutation, 767, **768**, 777

soybean, 338, 340, 341

species difference, **778**, 810

spectrophotometry, 447–**449**, **457**

spermidine, 345, 347

spermine, 345, 347

spin trapping, **18**, 435, 437–440, 442, 980

sports, **142**

steady state, **490**

stomach cancer, 936, 940

stratum corneum, 581, 591

streptozotocin, 274, 275

stress, 824

stroke, 908

substance P, 530, 1178

succinate dehydrogenase, 561, 760, 850–852

sulfhydryl group, 559, 561

sulfide, 29

sulfonyl

   free radical, 35

   peroxyl radical, 35

sulfoxide, 29

sulfur centered free radical, 35, **43**, 45

sulfur dioxide, 535

sulfuranyl radical, 23

sulfuric acid, 535, 536

sunburn, **587**

superoxide, **42**, 69, **71**, **74**, 131, 437, 439, **441**, **442**, 884, 885, 928, 1003, 1008, 1074, 1075, 1114, 1128

   anion, 4, 15, 244, 438–440, 603, 604, 635, **638**, 643

   dismutase, 73, 75, 79, 80, 93, 103, 163, 165, 180, 224, **232**, **243**–296, 562, 584, 585, 611, 632, 635, 636, 659, 666, 678, 702, 720, 859, 883, 888, 889, 1056, 1113

   deficiency, 269

   probe, **442**

   radical, 4, 60, 62, **439**, **441**, 691, 715, 852

swimming, 254–260, 264, 266, 701

synovial

   fluid, 1153, 1155

   joint, 1152, **1168**

   membrane, 1148

synovitis, 1148, 1149, **1174**, 1175, **1183**, 1184

T cell leukemia, 394

T helper cell, 1150

T lymphocyte, 530, 1150

t-tubule, 607

tar radical, 979

target organ damage, 1084

taurine, 556

TBARS *see* thiobarbituric acid reactive substances

tea, 339–342, 352

temperature difference, **571**

tepoxalin, 392

tetroxide, 31, 32

thalassemia, 138, 140

thapsigargin, 390–392

thearubigens, 340

thermolysin, 96

thiobarbituric acid assay, 436, 466, 467

thiobarbituric acid reactive substances, 117, 121, 122, 268, 564, 565, 570, 632,

633, 643, 645, 650, 755, 854,
1107, 1117–1122, 1128, 1141,
1171
thioctic acid, **229**, **303**, **314**, 348, 390, 392,
393, 556, 743, 784
thiol compound, 43, **348**, 361, **375**–401
thiolate, 43, 44
S-thiolation, **472**
thioperoxyl radical, 35
thioredoxin, **226**, **376**, **377**, 385, 387, **393**–
395, 1159
  peroxidase, 377, 395
  reductase, 378
thiyl radical, 4, 8, 34, 35, 43–45, 361
thrombocyte, 997
  aggregation inhibition, 422
thrombomodulin, 568, 1086
thromboxane, 1084, 1087
  A2, 1078
  B2, 531, 539, 540
thymidine glycol, 779
thymine glycol, 779
time resolved optical spectroscopy, **10**, 12
tissue
  delivery, **366**
  injury, **163**
  ischemia, 154, 163–168, 171, 172
  reperfusion, 154, 163–166, 168, 283
TNF *see* tumor necrosis factor
α-tocopherol, 5, 7, 8, 40, 109, 110, 122, 144,
184–189, 207, **228**, **237**, **298**, 306,
307, 314–316, **324**, 333, 334, 337,
342, 344, 349, 350, **359**–374,
403–432, 434, 447, **452**, 453, 459,
518, 522, 530, 540, 541, 543, 545–
557, 560–570, 572–574, 584, 585,
586, 589, 590, 645, 647, 649, 650,
658, 666, 691, 741, 783, 863, 865,
892, 893, 906, 909, 930, 936, 938–
944, 981, 984, 988, 1013, 1056,
1172
  acetate, 589
  binding protein, **364**
  blood level, **365**
  deficiency, 328, 344, 347, 348, 361, 602,
698, 704, 741, 961, 981
  recycling, 361
  sorbate, 589
  transfer protein, 328, 363, **364**, 386
β-tocopherol, 324, 325, 327, 359
δ-tocopherol, 324, 325, 327, 360

γ-tocopherol, 324, 325, 327–329, 360, 584,
585
α-tocopheroxyl radical, 337, 361, 438, 439,
452
α-tocotrienol, 324, 325, 327, 360
β-tocotrienol, 325, 360
δ-tocotrienol, 325, 327, 360
γ-tocotrienol, 327, 360
TPA *see* phorbol myristate acetate
trace element, 573
training, **184**, **501**, **1142**
transcription factor, 65, 1160
transferrin, 132, **134**, 764
  receptor, 134
transforming growth factor, 1009
transforming growth factor-ß, 183, 409
transition metal, 130, 640
transport protein, 328, 329, 333
trauma, 178, 189, 1153
trichloromethyl radical, 27
trichloromethylperoxyl radical, 7, 9
1,2,3-trioxolane, 541, 542
triplet state, 6
trolox, 40, 458, 666
α-tropomyosin, 423, 424
troponin, 619
troposphere, 583
tryptophan oxidation, **90**
TTF-1 *see* transcription factor
tumor necrosis factor, 170, 178, 179, 276,
277–279, 285, 286
tumor necrosis factor-α, 382, 410, 539, 541,
1010
tungsten, 165, 166
typus robustus arthritis, 1149, **1178**
ortho-tyrosine, 531, 902, 1109
tyrosine
  chlorination, **96**
  kinase, **381**, **416**, 417
  nitration, **93**
  oxidation, **93**
  phosphorylation, 380, **382**, 417, 418
tyrosyl radical, 106, 856, 898

ubiquinol, 361, 447, 452, **454**, 455, 760
ubiquinone, **231**, **301**, **343**, 447, **454**, 455,
586, 700, 714, 760, 778, 783
ubiquinone-9, 454
ubiquinone-10, 60, 231, 343, 454, 584, 585,
743
ubisemiquinone, 760

ultraviolet
  detection, 453, 454, 456, 465
  radiation, 555, **569**, 579, 580, **582**, 585,
      586, 588, 593
unpaired electron, 6
unsaturated fatty acid, 519
uracil, 24
urate *see* uric acid
urban area, **537**
uric acid, 78–80, 110, 154, 158–160, **162**,
      163, **230**, 348, **455**, 456, 547, 556,
      584, 638, 693, 700, 1162
urinalysis, 462
urinary excretion, **203**
uterine cervix carcinoma, 937
utilization pool, **136**

valvular heart disease, **657**
vascular
  control, **621**
  endothelial growth factor, 415, 1009, 1162
  endothelium, 422, 1076, 1088
  injury, **70**, **74**, 1084, 1085
  permeability, 1083, 1084, 1088
  smooth muscle cell, **403**–430
  wall elasticity, 566
vasorelaxation, **72**
vegetable, 325, 326, 330, 331, 334, 335, 941,
      985
very low density lipoprotein, 327, 328, 333,
      363
vimentin, 411
vinylperoxyl radical, 27
2-vinylpyridine, 450

vitamin, **184**, **698**, **741**
vitamin A *see* retinol
vitamin C *see* ascorbic acid
vitamin E *see* α-tocopherol
vitamin K, 329
volatile hydrocarbon, **469**
voltage sensor, 617
von Willebrand factor, 1088, 1183
vulnerability, 825

walking, 1095
Werner syndrome, **275**, 773, 895
wine, 339, 340, 342, 352
wound healing, **995**–1020
wound healing cell, 1000
wound physiology, 999
wound repair *see* wound healing

xanthine, 78, 154, 159, 348, 638
  dehydrogenase, 61, 153, **154**–156, 159,
      160, 162, **163**–171, 954, **1163**
  oxidase, **61**, 69, 73, **74**, **153**–156, 159, 160,
      162–171, 246, 638, 659, **693**, 694,
      953, 1073, **1163**–1167
  oxidoreductase, **1162**
xenobiotic
  agent, 955
  metabolism, 956, **1021**–1052
xeroderma pigmentosa, 587

zeaxanthin, 332–334, 984
zinc, 130, 334, 573
  deficiency, 260
zinc-finger protein, **388**